CLINICAL TRIALS IN CARDIOVASCULAR DISEASE

CLINICAL TRIALS IN CARDIOVASCULAR DISEASE

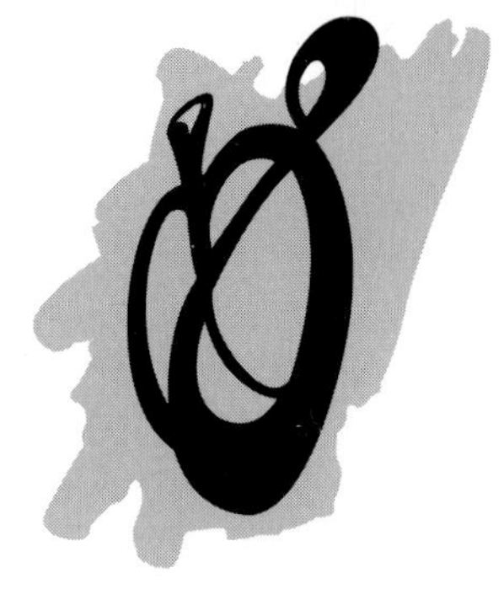

A Companion to Braunwald's Heart Disease

Charles H. Hennekens, M.D., Dr.P.H.
Eugene Braunwald Professor of Medicine
Harvard Medical School

Chief, Division of Preventive Medicine
Brigham and Women's Hospital
Boston, Massachusetts

Section Editors

Julie E. Buring, Sc.D.
Professor of Ambulatory Care and Prevention
Harvard Medical School

Deputy Director
Division of Preventive Medicine
Brigham and Women's Hospital
Boston, Massachusetts

JoAnn E. Manson, M.D., Dr.P.H.
Associate Professor of Medicine
Harvard Medical School

Co-Director of Women's Health and Director of Endocrinology
Division of Preventive Medicine
Brigham and Women's Hospital
Boston, Massachusetts

Paul M. Ridker, M.D., M.P.H.
Associate Professor of Medicine
Harvard Medical School

Director of Cardiovascular Disease Research
Division of Preventive Medicine
Brigham and Women's Hospital
Boston, Massachusetts

W.B. SAUNDERS COMPANY
A *Harcourt Health Sciences Company*
Philadelphia London New York St. Louis Sydney Toronto

W.B. SAUNDERS COMPANY
A Harcourt Health Sciences Company

The Curtis Center
Independence Square West
Philadelphia, Pennsylvania 19106

Library of Congress Cataloging-in-Publication Data

Clinical trials in cardiovascular disease: a companion to Braunwald's heart disease / [edited by] Charles H. Hennekens.—1st ed.

p. cm.

ISBN 0–7216–6867–4

1. Cardiovascular agents—Testing. 2. Clinical trials. 3. Heart—Diseases—Treatment. I. Hennekens, Charles H. II. Braunwald, Eugene, Heart disease. [DNLM: 1. Heart Diseases. 2. Clinical Trials. WG 200 C6417 1999]

RM345.C58 1999

616.1′06—dc21

DNLM/DLC 98–48479

CLINICAL TRIALS IN CARDIOVASCULAR DISEASE: A Companion to Braunwald's Heart Disease

ISBN 0–7216–6867–4

Printed in the United States of America.

Last digit is the print number: 9 8 7 6 5 4 3

Contributors

Robert Allan, Ph.D.
Clinical Assistant Professor of Psychology, Departments of Medicine and Psychiatry, Cornell University Medical College; Professional Associate, The New York Hospital, New York, New York
Psychosocial Factors

Keaven M. Anderson, PhD
Director of Biostatistics, Centocor, Inc., Malvern, Pennsylvania
Platelet Glycoprotein IIb/IIIa Receptor Inhibitors

Elliott M. Antman, M.D.
Associate Professor of Medicine, Harvard Medical School; Director, Samuel A. Levine Cardiac Unit, Brigham and Women's Hospital, Boston, Massachusetts
Direct Thrombin Inhibitors

Colin Baigent, B.M., B.Ch., M.A., M.Sc.
Medical Research Council Scientist, Clinical Trial Service Unit and Epidemiological Studies Unit, University of Oxford, Oxford, United Kingdom
Large-Scale Randomized Trials; Aspirin and Heparin; Thrombolytic Therapy

Malcolm R. Bell, M.B.B.S., F.R.A.C.P.
Associate Professor of Medicine, Mayo Medical School; Consultant, Internal Medicine and Cardiovascular Diseases, Mayo Clinic and Mayo Foundation, Rochester, Minnesota
Angioplasty and Bypass Surgery

Catherine S. Berkey, D.Sc., M.A.
Lecturer in Medicine and in Biostatistics, Harvard Medical School and School of Public Health, Boston, Massachusetts
Meta-Analysis of Randomized Trials

John A. Bittl, M.D.
Interventional Cardiologist, Ocala Heart Institute and Munroe Regional Medical Center, Ocala, Florida
Direct Thrombin Inhibitors

B. Greg Brown, M.D., Ph.D.
Professor of Medicine, University of Washington School of Medicine; Attending Cardiologist and Director, Coronary Atherosclerosis Research Laboratory, Cardiology Division, University of Washington Medical Center, Seattle, Washington
Lipid-Lowering Therapy

Julie E. Buring, Sc.D.
Professor of Ambulatory Care and Prevention, Harvard Medical School; Deputy Director, Division of Preventive Medicine, Brigham and Women's Hospital, Boston, Massachusetts
Contributions of Basic Research, Observational Studies, and Randomized Trials; Aspirin

William P. Castelli, M.D.
Adjunct Associate Professor of Medicine, Boston University School of Medicine, Boston; Medical Director, Framingham Cardiovascular Institute, Framingham, Massachusetts
Cholesterol Reduction

Claudia U. Chae, M.D., M.P.H.
Instructor, Harvard Medical School; Associate Physician, Division of Preventive Medicine, Brigham and Women's Hospital and Clinical Assistant in Medicine, Cardiology Division, Massachusetts General Hospital, Boston, Massachusetts
Beta Blockers; Postmenopausal Hormone Replacement Therapy

David Chiriboga, M.D.
Director, Claudio Benati Hospital, Zumbahua, Cotopaxi, Ecuador
Prevention Strategies: From the Office to the Community

Graham A. Colditz, M.D., Dr.P.H.
Associate Professor of Medicine, Harvard Medical School; Boston, Massachusetts
Meta-Analysis of Randomized Trials

Barry S. Coller, M.D.
Murray M. Rosenberg Professor and Chairman, Samuel Bronfman Department of Medicine, Mount Sinai School of Medicine; Director and Chief of Medicine, Mount Sinai Hospital, New York, New York
Platelet Glycoprotein IIb/IIIa Receptor Inhibitors

Rory Collins, M.B., B.S., M.A., M.Sc.
British Heart Foundation Professor of Medicine and Epidemiology, Clinical Trial Service Unit and Epidemiological Studies Unit, University of Oxford, Oxford, United Kingdom
Large-Scale Randomized Trials; Aspirin and Heparin; Thrombolytic Therapy

Jeffrey A. Cutler, B.A., M.D., M.P.H.
Director, Clinical Applications and Prevention Program, Division of Epidemiology and Clinical Applications, National Heart, Lung, and Blood Institute, National Institutes of Health, Bethesda, Maryland
Comparative Features of Primordial, Primary, and Secondary Prevention Trials

David L. DeMets, Ph.D.
Professor of Statistics and Biostatistics, Department of Biostatistics and Medical Informatics, University of Wisconsin, Madison, Wisconsin
Principles of Data and Safety Monitoring Boards in Randomized Trials

Marcus D. Flather, M.B.B.S., M.R.C.P.
Honorary Senior Lecturer, Imperial College of Science Technology and Medicine; Director, Clinical Trials and Evaluation Unit, Royal Brompton Hospital, London, United Kingdom
Angiotensin-Converting Enzyme Inhibitors

Barry A. Franklin, Ph.D.
Professor of Physiology, Wayne State University School of Medicine, Detroit; Program Director, Cardiac Rehabilitation and Exercise Laboratories, William Beaumont Hospital, Royal Oak, Michigan
Exercise

Laurence S. Freedman, M.A., Dip.Stats.
Professor of Statistics, Department of Mathematics, Statistics, and Computer Science, Bar Ilan University, Ramat Gan; Head Statistician, Department of Clinical Epidemiology, Chaim Sheba Medical Center, Tel Hashomer, Israel
Methodology of Randomized Trials

Lawrence M. Friedman, M.D.
Director, Division of Epidemiology and Clinical Applications, National Heart, Lung, and Blood Institute, Bethesda, Maryland
Comparative Features of Primordial, Primary, and Secondary Prevention Trials

Peter L. Friedman, M.D., Ph.D.
Associate Professor of Medicine, Harvard Medical School; Co-Director, Cardiac Arrhythmia Service and Clinical Electrophysiology Laboratory, Cardiovascular Division, Brigham and Women's Hospital, Boston, Massachusetts
Antiarrhythmic Drug Therapy

J. Michael Gaziano, M.D., M.P.H.
Assistant Professor of Medicine, Harvard Medical School, Boston; Director, Massachusetts Veterans Epidemiology Research and Information Center, and Director, Cardiac Rehabilitation and Prevention, Brockton/West Roxbury, Veterans Affairs Medical Center, West Roxbury, Massachusetts
Cholesterol Reduction; Antioxidant Vitamins

Bernard J. Gersh, M.B., Ch.B., D.Phil, F.R.C.P.
W. Proctor Harvey Teaching Professor of Cardiology and Chief, Division of Cardiology, Georgetown University Medical Center, Washington, D.C.
Angioplasty and Bypass Surgery

C. Michael Gibson, MS., M.D.
Assistant Professor of Medicine, Harvard Medical School, Boston; Chief of Cardiology, Brockton/West Roxbury Veterans Affairs Medical Center, West Roxbury, Massachusetts
Primary Angioplasty, Rescue Angioplasty, and New Devices

Jacqueline A. Hart, M.D.
Instructor in Medicine, Harvard Medical School; Associate in Medicine, Beth Israel Deaconess Medical Center, Boston, Massachusetts
Multiple Risk Factor Intervention Trials

Jiang He, M.D., Ph.D.
Assistant Professor of Biostatistics and Epidemiology, Tulane University School of Public Health and Tropical Medicine, New Orleans, Louisiana
Blood Pressure Reduction

Charles H. Hennekens, M.D., Dr.P.H.
Eugene Braunwald Professor of Medicine, Harvard Medical School; Chief, Division of Preventive Medicine, Brigham and Women's Hospital, Boston, Massachusetts
Contributions of Basic Research, Observational Studies, and Randomized Trials; Beta Blockers; Aspirin

Elaine M. Hylek, M.D., M.P.H.
Instructor of Medicine, Harvard Medical School; Assistant Physician in Medicine, Massachusetts General Hospital, Boston, Massachusetts
Anticoagulation and Antiplatelet Drug Therapy in Atrial Fibrillation

David M. Kerins, M.D.
Assistant Professor of Medicine, Vanderbilt University; Staff Physician, Vanderbilt University Medical Center and Nashville Veterans Affairs Medical Center, Nashville, Tennessee
Antithrombotic and Anticoagulant Therapy

Ari D. Levinson, B.Sc.(Med), M.B.Ch.B., F.R.C.P.(C)
Clinical Fellow in Cardiology, McMaster University and Hamilton Health Sciences Corporation, General Division, Hamilton, Ontario, Canada
Nitrates

JoAnn E. Manson, M.D., Dr.P.H.
Associate Professor of Medicine, Harvard Medical School; Co-Director of Women's Health and Director of Endocrinology, Division of Preventive Medicine, Brigham and Women's Hospital, Boston, Massachusetts
Postmenopausal Hormone Replacement Therapy; Antioxidant Vitamins

Peter A. McCullough, M.D., M.P.H.
Director, Cardiovascular Informatics and Associate Director, Center for Clinical Effectiveness, Henry Ford Health System, Detroit, Michigan
Exercise

Frederick Mosteller, Ph.D.
Professor of Mathematical Statistics, Emeritus, Department of Statistics, Harvard University, Cambridge, Massachusetts
Meta-Analysis of Randomized Trials

Ira S. Ockene, M.D.
Professor of Medicine, University of Massachusetts Medical School; Associate Director, Division of Cardiovascular Medicine, and Director, Preventive Cardiology Program, University of Massachusetts Medical Center, Worcester, Massachusetts
Prevention Strategies: From the Office to the Community

Dean Ornish, M.D.
Clinical Professor of Medicine, University of California, San Francisco, School of Medicine; Attending Physician, California Pacific Medical Center, San Francisco, California
Multiple Risk Factor Intervention Trials

Richard C. Pasternak, M.D.
Associate Professor, Harvard Medical School; Director, Preventive Cardiology and Cardiac Rehabilitation, Massachusetts General Hospital, Boston, Massachusetts
Smoking Cessation

Richard Peto, F.R.S.
Professor of Medical Statistics and Epidemiology, University of Oxford; Co-Director, Clinical Trial Service Unit, Radcliffe Infirmary, Oxford, United Kingdom
Large-Scale Randomized Trials

Marc A. Pfeffer, M.D., Ph.D.
Professor of Medicine, Harvard Medical School; Staff Physician, Cardiovascular Division, Brigham and Women's Hospital, Boston, Massachusetts
Angiotensin-Converting Enzyme Inhibitors

Hanne Berg Ravn, M.D., Ph.D.
Assistant Professor, Institute of Clinical and Experimental Research, Aarhus University Hospital, Aarhus N, Denmark
Magnesium

Sharon C. Reimold
Assistant Professor of Medicine, Harvard Medical School; Associate Physician, Cardiovascular Division, Brigham and Women's Hospital, Boston, Massachusetts
Antiarrhythmic Drug Therapy in Supraventricular Tachycardia

Paul M. Ridker, M.D., M.P.H.
Associate Professor of Medicine, Harvard Medical School; Director of Cardiovascular Disease Research, Division of Preventive Medicine, Brigham and Women's Hospital, Boston, Massachusetts
Antithrombotic and Anticoagulant Therapy

Nancy A. Rigotti, M.D.
Assistant Professor of Medicine, Harvard Medical School; Director, Tobacco Research and Treatment Center, Massachusetts General Hospital, Boston, Massachusetts
Smoking Cessation

Frank M. Sacks, M.D.
Associate Professor in Nutrition, Harvard School of Public Health, and Associate Professor of Medicine, Harvard Medical School; Staff Physician, Brigham and Women's Hospital, Boston, Massachusetts
Dietary Factors

Stephen Scheidt, M.D.
Professor of Clinical Medicine, Cornell University Medical College; Staff Physician, The New York Hospital, New York, New York
Psychosocial Factors

Norman Sharpe, M.D.
Professor and Head, Department of Medicine, University of Auckland School of Medicine; Cardiologist and Chief of Medicine, Auckland Hospital, Auckland, New Zealand
Congestive Heart Failure

Denise G. Simons-Morton, M.D., Ph.D.
Leader, Prevention Scientific Research Group, Division of Epidemiology and Clinical Applications, National Heart, Lung, and Blood Institute, Bethesda, Maryland
Comparative Features of Primordial, Primary, and Secondary Prevention Trials

Daniel E. Singer, M.D.
Associate Professor of Medicine, Harvard Medical School, and Associate Professor of Epidemiology, Harvard School of Public Health; Director, Clinical Epidemiology Unit, General Medicine Division, Massachusetts General Hospital, Boston, Massachusetts
Anticoagulation and Antiplatelet Drug Therapy in Atrial Fibrillation

Marcia L. Stefanick, Ph.D.
Associate Professor of Medicine (Research) and Associate Professor of Gynecology and Obstetrics, Stanford University School of Medicine, Stanford, California
Exercise and Weight Loss

William G. Stevenson, M.D.
Associate Professor of Medicine, Harvard Medical School; Co-Director, Cardiac Arrhythmia Service and Clinical Electrophysiology Laboratory, Brigham and Women's Hospital, Boston, Massachusetts
Antiarrhythmic Drug Therapy

Gerald C. Timmis, M.D.
Medical Director, Cardiovascular Research, Division of Cardiology, William Beaumont Hospital, Royal Oak, Michigan
Exercise

James L. Velianou, M.D., F.R.C.P.(C)
Clinical Fellow in Cardiology, McMaster University School of Medicine and General Division of the Hamilton Health Sciences Corporation, Hamilton, Ontario, Canada
Nitrates

David Waters, M.D.
Professor of Medicine, University of Connecticut School of Medicine; Director of Cardiology, Hartford Hospital, Hartford, and the University of Connecticut Health Center, Farmington, Connecticut
Calcium Channel Blockers

Harlan F. Weisman, M.D.
Vice President of Clinical Research, Centocor, Inc., Malvern, Pennsylvania
Platelet Glycoprotein IIb/IIIa Receptor Inhibitors

Paul K. Whelton, M.D., M.Sc.
Professor of Biostatistics and Epidemiology, and Dean, Tulane University School of Public Health and Tropical Medicine New Orleans, Louisiana
Blood Pressure Reduction

Kent L. Woods, M.D., S.M., F.R.C.P.
Professor of Therapeutics, University of Leicester, Leicester, United Kingdom
Magnesium

Salim Yusuf, F.R.C.P., D.Phil.
Professor of Medicine and Director, Division of Cardiology, McMaster University School of Medicine; Staff Physician, Hamilton General Hospital, Hamilton, Ontario, Canada
Nitrates

Xue-Qiao Zhao, M.D.
Research Assistant Professor of Medicine, University of Washington School of Medicine; Research Cardiologist and Associate Director, Coronary Atherosclerosis Research Laboratory, Cardiology Division, University of Washington Medical Center, Seattle, Washington
Lipid-Lowering Therapy

Foreword

Since the development of antibiotics in the middle of this century, no area in medicine has moved forward as rapidly as has cardiology. This has resulted from notable advances in cardiovascular biology and pathophysiology, as well as from the development of several classes of important new cardiovascular drugs and of a variety of effective new procedures and devices. The clinical impact of these new therapeutic modalities requires rigorous assessment in clinical trials, which have become *the* principal method of judging the efficacy and safety of interventions. Clinical trials serve as the critical interface between initial studies that have offered "proof of concept" of a therapeutic or preventive modality and its widespread clinical application. Clinical trials are also required for the registration of new drugs and devices. It is no exaggeration to say that the randomized clinical trial now provides the key to rational, evidence-based cardiac care and prevention of cardiovascular disease.

I am especially delighted that Drs. Hennekens, Buring, Manson, and Ridker, from the Preventive Medicine and Cardiovascular Divisions of Harvard Medical School's Department of Medicine and the Brigham and Women's Hospital, have produced this splendid text—*Clinical Trials in Cardiovascular Disease: A Companion to Braunwald's Heart Disease.* The first section provides the understanding required to design, conduct, and interpret trials. The second section consists of a systematic review of the key cardiovascular treatment trials, and the third section details the growing number of trials designed to prevent or at least delay the development of cardiovascular disease.

This important book thus provides an up-to-date review and analysis of this very important segment of cardiology. It should be of great interest not only to clinical trialists and trainees in this field but to all physicians responsible for the care of patients with cardiovascular disease. I am proud that *Clinical Trials in Cardiovascular Disease* is the newest Companion to *Heart Disease: A Textbook of Cardiovascular Medicine.*

EUGENE BRAUNWALD, M.D.
Boston, Massachusetts

Preface

Cardiovascular disease (CVD) is the leading cause of death in the United States, as well as in most developed countries. In the United States, CVD is responsible for nearly 1 million annual fatalities, or two of every five deaths. CVD also carries a tremendous economic burden, with U.S. direct health care costs and indirect costs due to lost productivity from CVD in 1999 estimated at $286.5 billion.[1]

Since the late 1960s, the United States and several Western European countries have experienced a decline in CVD mortality, with reductions in the United States of about 2% each year. This markedly favorable trend has been attributed to advances in both prevention[2] and treatment[3] of CVD. However, despite more than two decades of sustained decline in mortality rates, CVD remains the leading cause of death in the United States. With regard to coronary heart disease (CHD), which accounts for the largest share of CVD deaths, age-specific rates are lower for women than for men. Further, CHD becomes the leading killer of U.S. men by 45 years of age and women by 65 years of age. Nonetheless, heart disease remains responsible for one of every three deaths among both sexes.

There are also troubling trends in CVD rates in both developed and developing countries. With respect to developed countries, U.S. age-adjusted stroke rates have risen slightly in the 1990s, while the slope of the age-adjusted rate of CHD may be increasing or leveling following several decades of decline.[4] In addition, trends among U.S. adolescents toward greater obesity,[5] increased smoking prevalence,[6] and decreases in physical activity levels,[7] if not reversed, will have far-reaching consequences for future morbidity and mortality from CVD.

In developing countries, between the years 1990 and 2020, the proportion of worldwide deaths due to CVD is projected to increase from 28.9% to 36.3%.[8] Moreover, CVD will increase from fourth to first in number of years of life lost, and from fifth to first as a cause of premature death and disability. In developing countries, the projected increases in CVD are related principally to two trends: (1) the eradication of malnutrition and infectious diseases as primary causes of death, which is allowing for an aging of the population; and (2) marked increases in rates of cigarette smoking.[9]

Thus, the continuing enormous burden of CVD in developed countries, alarming trends in cardiovascular risk profiles of young people, as well as the emerging increases in CVD in developing countries, all underscore the crucial need to redouble both treatment and prevention efforts.[10]

With respect to clinical trials, for most therapeutic and preventive interventions, they have been neither necessary nor desirable. For example, in malignant hypertension the benefits of pharmacologic treatment were so large and obvious in uncontrolled clinical observations that randomized trials would in fact have been unethical. Even with respect to cigarette smoking and CVD, a totality of evidence that included basic research, clinical investigation, observational epidemiology, case-control, and cohort studies was clearly sufficient for the U.S. Surgeon General to declare smoking a cause of CHD. However, with respect to most treatment and prevention strategies, increasingly the most plausible effects are small to moderate (i.e., 10% to 40%), such as drug treatment of mild-to-moderate hypertension[11] or aspirin in the primary prevention of CVD.[12] Such interventions are clearly worthwhile, especially for such a common and serious disease as CVD. Indeed, such interventions might avoid 10,000 or more premature deaths for therapies and 100,000 or more for prevention strategies. Nonetheless, they are difficult to detect reliably, because the amount of uncontrolled and, indeed, uncontrollable confounding inherent in case-control or cohort studies is about as large as the most plausible effects being sought.[13] For these reasons, clinical trials are the most reliable design strategy capable of evaluating definitively the many new promising hypotheses in the treatment and prevention of cardiovascular disease.

With each new advance in cardiovascular medicine, randomized clinical trials generally—and those of large sample size in particular—have become even more crucial to achieving further gains. Advances in the treatment of acute myocardial infarction (MI), for example, have led to substantial decreases in short-term mortality following hospitalization for acute MI, from approximately 20% in 1970 to 10% in 1990.[14, 15] As a consequence, although a 20% mortality benefit in 1970 would have yielded an absolute reduction of 4 percentage points, from 20% to 16%, a new treatment today that confers a comparable 20% benefit would yield an absolute mortality reduction only half as great (a 2-percentage-point decrease, from 10% to 8%). Thus, the reliable detection of such a benefit on acute MI today requires clinical trials of even larger sample sizes to rule out the statistical possibility that the play of chance accounts for any observed treatment effect. Moreover, therapeutic trials increasingly are not comparing a promising treatment to no treatment, but are evaluating whether a new agent confers greater benefit than an already established treatment. For promising interventions in primary prevention, clinical trials of large size are also crucial, since study populations in such trials are, by definition, at lower baseline risk of disease and will accrue outcomes at a much slower rate than a population with prior disease. Nevertheless, effective primary prevention measures may have an even larger public health impact than treatments for those with a CVD history, since they can be implemented broadly among a much larger proportion of the population.

No area of medicine has likely been the focus of more large, randomized clinical trials than CVD. Efforts to compile listings of completed and ongoing trials in CVD have easily identified hundreds of investigations.[16–18] In the crowded alphabet soup of trial acronyms, more than a few selections have wound up serving multiple trial masters, with the popular choices ranging from the predictably wellness oriented (e.g., CARE, three separate trials listed) to the (coronary) patently incongruous (e.g., BIGMAC, two separate trials listed).[17] Keeping up with this vast and rapidly expanding literature is a daunting task for increasingly busy academic researchers and clinical practitioners, committed to applying the most scientifically sound, current knowledge to the care of their patients.

This book, therefore, is intended to serve as a resource on clinical trials in CVD for those in research and in clinical practice. In the ensuing chapters, leading authorities in more than two dozen areas of CVD treatment and prevention research provide clear distillations of current knowledge from clinical trials. While they are large in number, clinical trials in cardiovascular disease are certainly not all equal in quality or in their ability to provide definitive evidence that can reliably guide clinical practice. Critically reviewing the results of studies requires an understanding of the basic principles of clinical trials. Section I provides an overview of these issues, with chapters ranging from reviews of the contributions of different types of evidence to discussions of various aspects of trial methodology, the role of data monitoring boards, and the principles of meta-analysis. Sections II and III then provide substantive, critical assessments of clinical trials in the treatment and prevention of CVD. Section II focuses on treatment trials, with the first half devoted to interventions for acute ischemia and the second half devoted to interventions for long-term secondary prevention. Section III focuses on prevention trials among those without prior CVD, an area that will assume increasing importance in the face of constraints on health care resources in developed countries and the severely limited medical care available in developing countries now confronting the CVD pandemic.

CHARLES H. HENNEKENS
JULIE E. BURING
JOANN E. MANSON
PAUL M. RIDKER

REFERENCES

1. American Heart Association. 1999 Heart and Stroke Statistical Update. Dallas, American Heart Association, 1998.
2. Goldman L, Cook EF. The decline in ischemic heart disease mortality rates: An analysis of the comparative effects of medical interventions and changes in lifestyle. Ann Intern Med 1984; 101:825–836.
3. Hunink MGM, Goldman L, Tosteson ANA, et al. The recent decline in mortality from coronary heart disease, 1980–1990. JAMA 1997; 277:535–542.
4. National Heart, Lung, and Blood Institute. Fact Book, Fiscal Year 1996. Bethesda, MD, U.S. Department of Health and Human Services, National Institutes of Health, 1997.
5. Troiano RP, Flegal KM, Kuczmarski RJ, et al. Overweight prevalence and trends for children and adolescents. Arch Pediatr Adolesc Med 1995; 149:1084–1091.
6. Johnson LD, Bachman JG, O'Malley PM. Cigarette smoking continues to rise among American teen-agers in 1996. Ann Arbor, Michigan, University of Michigan News and Information Services, December 19, 1996.
7. U.S. Department of Health and Human Services. Physical Activity and Health: A Report of the Surgeon General. Atlanta, U.S. Department of Health and Human Services, Centers for Disease Control and Prevention, National Center for Chronic Disease Prevention and Health Promotion, 1996.
8. Murray CJL, Lopez AD. The global burden of disease: A comprehensive assessment of mortality and disability from diseases, injuries, and risk factors in 1990 and projected to 2020. Cambridge, MA, Harvard University Press, 1996.
9. Murray CJL, Lopez AD. The global burden of disease: Summary. Cambridge, MA, Harvard University Press, 1996.
10. Hennekens CH. Increasing burden of cardiovascular disease: Current knowledge and future directions for research on risk factors. Circulation 1998; 97:1095–1102.
11. Hebert PR, Fiebach NH, Eberlein KA, et al: The community-based randomized trials of pharmacologic treatment of mild-to-moderate hypertension. Am J Epidemiol 1988; 127:581–590.
12. Hennekens CH, Buring JE, Sandercock P, et al. Aspirin and other antiplatelet agents in the secondary and primary prevention of cardiovascular disease. Circulation 1989; 80:749–756.
13. Hennekens CH, Buring JE. Observational evidence. Ann NY Acad Sci 1993; 703:18–24.
14. McGovern PG, Folsom AR, Sprafka JM, et al. Trends in survival of hospitalized myocardial infarction patients between 1970 and 1985. The Minnesota Heart Survey. Circulation 1992; 85:172–179.
15. McGovern PG, Pankow JS, Shahar E, et al, for the Minnesota Heart Survey Investigators. Recent trends in acute coronary heart disease—mortality, morbidity, medical care, and risk factors. N Engl J Med 1996; 334:884–890.
16. Astra AB. What's What: A guide to Acronyms for Cardiovascular Trials. Göteborg, Sweden, Astra Hässle AB, 1996.
17. Cheng TO. Acronyms of clinical trials in cardiology—1996. J Am Coll Cardiol 1996; 27:1293–1305.
18. Parmley WW. TOTAL ABC CHAOS. J Am Coll Cardiol 1996; 27:1292.

Acknowledgments

Collaboration and teamwork are critical elements in clinical trials in cardiovascular diseases. So, too, were they critical elements in preparing this companion text to Braunwald's *Heart Disease.* The vast majority of chapter authors accepted our initial invitation and provided outstanding, comprehensive summaries of the current state of knowledge on clinical trials in their areas of expertise. Our medical editor, Michael Jonas, performed yeoman's work. His expert editing and organizational skills were crucial. Finally, we would like to thank our families for their unfailing support and forbearance.

CHARLES H. HENNEKENS
JULIE E. BURING
JOANN E. MANSON
PAUL M. RIDKER

Contents

SECTION I
METHODOLOGY 1

1 Contributions of Basic Research, Observational Studies, and Randomized Trials 3
- Julie E. Buring
- Charles H. Hennekens

2 Methodology of Randomized Trials 9
- Laurence S. Freedman

3 Comparative Features of Primordial, Primary, and Secondary Prevention Trials 17
- Lawrence M. Friedman
- Denise G. Simons-Morton
- Jeffrey A. Cutler

4 Large-Scale Randomized Trials 24
- Colin Baigent
- Rory Collins
- Richard Peto

5 Principles of Data and Safety Monitoring Boards in Randomized Trials 31
- David L. DeMets

6 Meta-Analysis of Randomized Trials 43
- Graham A. Colditz
- Catherine S. Berkey
- Frederick Mosteller

SECTION II
TREATMENT TRIALS 53

PART I
Interventions for Acute Ischemia 55

7 Aspirin and Heparin 55
- Colin Baigent
- Rory Collins

8 Thrombolytic Therapy 65
- Colin U. Baigent
- Rory Collins

9 Beta Blockers 76
- Claudia U. Chae
- Charles H. Hennekens

10 Angiotensin-Converting Enzyme Inhibitors 95
- Marcus D. Flather
- Marc A. Pfeffer

11 Calcium Channel Blockers 106
- David Waters

12 Magnesium 119
- Kent L. Woods
- Hanne Berg Ravn

13 Nitrates 131
- Ari D. Levinson
- James L. Velianou
- Salim Yusuf

14 Direct Thrombin Inhibitors 145
- Elliott M. Antman
- John A. Bittl

15 Platelet Glycoprotein IIb/IIIa Receptor Inhibitors 166
- Keaven M. Anderson
- Harlan F. Weisman
- Barry S. Coller

16 Primary Angioplasty, Rescue Angioplasty, and New Devices 185
- C. Michael Gibson

PART II
Interventions for Secondary Prevention 199

17 Lipid-Lowering Therapy 199
- B. Greg Brown
- Xue-Qiao Zhao

18 Antiarrhythmic Drug Therapy 217
- William G. Stevenson
- Peter L. Friedman

19 Antiarrhythmic Drug Therapy in Supraventricular Tachycardia 231
- Sharon C. Reimold

20 Antithrombotic and Anticoagulant Therapy 245
- David M. Kerins
- Paul M. Ridker

21 Anticoagulant and Antiplatelet Drug Therapy in Atrial Fibrillation 257
- Daniel E. Singer
- Elaine M. Hylek

22 Angioplasty and Bypass Surgery 267
- Malcolm R. Bell
- Bernard J. Gersh

23 Exercise 278
- Barry A. Franklin
- Peter A. McCullough
- Gerald C. Timmis

24 Congestive Heart Failure 296
- Norman Sharpe

25 Psychosocial Factors 315
- Robert Allan
- Stephen Scheidt

SECTION **III**
PREVENTION TRIALS 325

26 Cholesterol Reduction 327
- J. Michael Gaziano
- William P. Castelli

27 Blood Pressure Reduction 341
- Paul K. Whelton
- Jiang He

28 Smoking Cessation 361
- Nancy A. Rigotti
- Richard C. Pasternak

29 Exercise and Weight Loss 375
- Marcia L. Stefanick

30 Aspirin 392
- Julie E. Buring
- Charles H. Hennekens

31 Postmenopausal Hormone Replacement Therapy 399
- Claudia U. Chae
- JoAnn E. Manson

32 Antioxidant Vitamins 415
- J. Michael Gaziano
- JoAnn E. Manson

33 Dietary Factors 423
- Frank M. Sacks

34 Multiple Risk Factor Intervention Trials 432
- Dean Ornish
- Jacqueline A. Hart

35 Prevention Strategies: From the Office to the Community 447
- Ira S. Ockene
- David Chiriboga

Index 461

Section Editor
▶ **Julie E. Buring**

SECTION

I METHODOLOGY

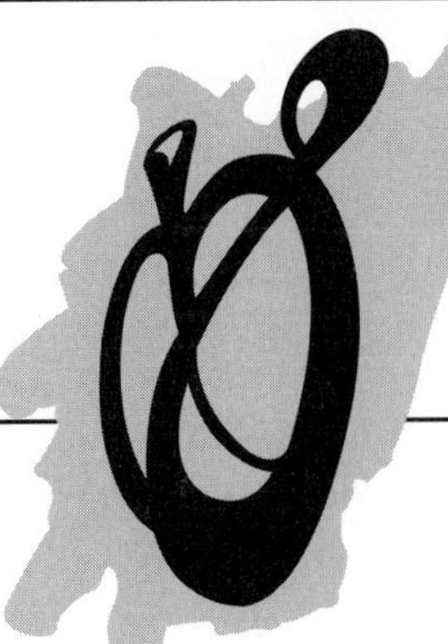

1 Contributions of Basic Research, Observational Studies, and Randomized Trials

▶ **Julie E. Buring**
▶ **Charles H. Hennekens**

In cardiovascular disease, as in all areas of medicine, advances in our knowledge proceed on several fronts, optimally, simultaneously. Basic researchers provide biologic mechanisms to answer the crucial question of why an agent or intervention reduces the risk of premature death. Clinicians are providing enormous benefits to affected patients through advances in diagnosis and treatment, and they formulate hypotheses from their clinical experiences in case reports and case series. Clinical investigators address the relevance of basic research findings to affected patients and healthy people. Epidemiologists and statisticians, optimally collaborating with researchers in other disciplines, formulate hypotheses from descriptive studies and test these in analytic studies, both observational case-control and cohort as well as, where necessary, randomized trials. This answers the equally crucial and complementary question of whether an agent or intervention reduces premature morbidity or mortality. Thus, each discipline and, indeed, every strategy within a discipline provides importantly relevant and complementary information to a totality of evidence upon which rational clinical decisions for individuals and policy decisions for the health of the general public can be safely based.[1, 2] It is crucial to consider the totality of evidence for any question because each research discipline has its unique strengths and limitations.

BASIC RESEARCH

Basic laboratory and animal research has the unique strength of precision, in that it can achieve virtually complete control of exposures, environment, and even genetics. Because of this, basic research can provide the scientific underpinnings for all applied research in humans, with unique and crucial information concerning disease mechanisms. However, basic research also has the disadvantage of potential lack of relevance to free-living humans owing to such differences as species specificity, dose, and routes of administration of exposures. Thus, the results from basic research may differ so greatly from those that apply to free-living humans as to render them of questionable direct relevance. The inability to predict the applicability of findings from a particular species of animals to humans was underscored by John Cairns, who wrote:

> Who could have guessed that *Homo sapiens* would share with the humble guinea pig the unenviable distinction of being incapable of synthesizing ascorbic acid, or share with armadillos a susceptibility to the bacterium that causes leprosy, or that intestinal cancer usually occurs in the large intestine of humans and the small intestine of sheep?[3]

Because of such issues, the results from animal research may be limited in their ability to provide a reliable quantitative estimate of human disease risk. However, the precision possible in such research provides unique and crucial information of great value in setting priorities for studies in free-living humans to test their relevance.[4]

Although basic research may add to our biologic understanding of why an exposure causes or prevents disease, only epidemiology allows the quantification of the magnitude of the exposure-disease relationship in humans and offers the possibility of altering risk through intervention. Indeed, epidemiologic research has often provided information that has formed the basis for public health decisions long before the basic mechanism of a particular disease was understood. In striving to identify factors that cause or prevent disease, laboratory testing and theoretic speculation about possible mechanisms are important, but no more so than direct, straightforward observation of what actually happens in human populations. If epidemiologic studies are well designed and conducted, and if the data are properly analyzed and interpreted, they can provide strong and reliable evidence on which to base clinical care of individual patients and, ultimately, policy decisions affecting the health of the general public.

EPIDEMIOLOGIC STUDIES

Epidemiology, because it is based directly on observations of free-living humans, has the unique advantage of relevance. However, for this reason, epidemiologic studies have the potential disadvantage of imprecision. Indeed, in contrast with basic research, epidemiology is crude and inexact, since observations in free-living humans can never take place under the controlled conditions possible to achieve in the laboratory. Nonetheless, epidemiology contributes essential information to a totality of evidence, which then can support a judgment of a cause-effect relationship.

Making such a judgment involves several steps, the first being to establish whether there is a valid statistical association. To conclude that an association is valid, alternative explanations for the finding must be ruled out, including the potential roles of chance, bias, and confounding. If a valid statistical association is present, the question then becomes, is it one of cause and effect? To render this judgment, the totality of evidence from all sources must be considered, with particular attention to the strength of the association, the consistency of the evidence from different studies, and the existence of a plausible biologic mechanism to explain the findings.

The basic design strategies used in epidemiologic research can be broadly categorized according to whether such investigations focus on describing the distributions of disease or on elucidating its determinants (Table 1–1). Descriptive epidemiology is concerned with the distributions of disease, including consideration of what populations or subgroups do or do not develop a disease, in what geographic locations it is most or least common, and how the frequency or occurrence varies over time. Information on each of these characteristics can provide clues leading to the formulation of an epidemiologic hypothesis that is consistent with existing knowledge of disease occurrence. Analytic epidemiology focuses on the determinants of a disease by testing the hypotheses formulated from descriptive studies, with the ultimate goal of judging whether a particular exposure causes or prevents disease.

TABLE 1–1 • Design Strategies in Epidemiologic Research

Descriptive
Case reports and case series
Correlational (ecologic) studies
Cross-sectional surveys

Analytic
Observational
  Case-control studies
  Cohort studies
Randomized clinical trials

There are a number of specific analytic study design options that can be employed. These can be divided into two broad design strategies: observational and interventional (i.e., randomized clinical trials). The major difference between the two approaches lies in the role played by the investigator. In observational studies, the investigator simply observes the natural course of events, noting who is exposed and nonexposed and who has and has not developed the outcome of interest. In randomized clinical trials, the investigators themselves allocate the exposure and then follow the subjects for the subsequent development of disease.

OBSERVATIONAL EPIDEMIOLOGIC STUDIES

There are two basic types of observational analytic investigations: case-control and cohort. In a case-control study, a case group, or series of patients who have a disease of interest, and a control group, or comparison series of people without the disease, are selected for investigation, and the proportions with the exposure of interest in each group are compared. In contrast, in a cohort study, subjects are classified on the basis of the presence or absence of exposure to a particular factor and then followed for a specified period to determine the development of disease in each exposure group.

Case-control and cohort studies are often criticized because of the potential for bias and confounding that is inherent in the fact that the design is observational. Since the use of a particular drug or treatment, or the adoption of a certain lifestyle is self-selected, people who use that drug, for example, may be systematically different from those who do not in ways that will affect the outcome of interest. Moreover, since the outcome of interest has already occurred at the time exposure is assessed, case-control studies have the potential for bias in the selection of subjects into the study and in their recall of prior events. In a cohort study, the often long latent period between exposure and disease can lead to bias owing to losses to follow-up. However, despite these inherent limitations, many exposure-disease relationships have been well established from observational evidence.[5]

There are two chief strengths of observational evidence. The first relates to the evaluation of exposures that require long duration, the second to detection of moderate- to large-sized effects, which can be roughly translated to mean those effects with relative risks greater than 1.5. With respect to the evaluation of exposures that require long duration, one example of the strength of observational studies is the evaluation of the relationship between blood pressure and risk of myocardial infarction (MI). Basic research had suggested mechanisms for a benefit of blood pressure lowering on risks of stroke and MI, and observational studies had consistently demonstrated a statistically significant 40% to 45% increased risk of stroke and a 25% to 30% increase in risk of MI associated with a 6 mm Hg difference in diastolic blood pressure.[6] In contrast, although individual randomized trials of pharmacologic therapy of mild-to-moderate hypertension indicated that blood pressure lowering by 6 mm Hg resulted in a comparable 40% decrease in risk of stroke, there was a far smaller and less certain benefit on MI than that suggested by the observational evidence. The apparent inconsistency remained even after the availability of results from 14 individual randomized trials of drug therapy in 37,000 subjects. This led some researchers to conclude that treatment of hypertension did not benefit risk of subsequent MI. However, a comprehensive overview, or meta-analysis, of the trials demonstrated that a decrease of 6 mm Hg in diastolic blood pressure significantly reduced stroke by 42% and MI by a smaller, but statistically significant, 14%.[7] A subsequent meta-analysis, which included three additional trials, demonstrated the reduction in risk of MI to be 16%.[8] The 14% to 16% reduction in risk of MI seen in the randomized trials over 3 to 5 years of treatment was about half the 28% reduction one would predict from the results of observational studies of blood pressure lowering over decades. This discrepancy may well have been due to chance but also could have been due to the fact that stroke risk immediately decreases following lowering of blood pressure levels, whereas MI risk may be affected by prolonged effects of hypertension on more chronic processes of atherogenesis and thus would require far longer than the usual 3 to 5 years of treatment in trials to observe the full impact. Thus, basic research and observational studies with long durations of exposure have been crucial components of the totality of evidence concerning the relationship of blood pressure lowering with risk of MI.

The second strength of observational studies lies in evaluating associations where the relative risk is moderate to large—relative risks above 1.5. In this regard, observational evidence has provided both the necessary and sufficient information on which to judge a cause-effect relationship for a large number of important questions of clinical importance and public health significance. Chief among these has been the health effects of cigarette smoking. Starting in 1950 with case-control studies by Doll and Hill in the United Kingdom[9] and Wynder and Graham in the United States,[10] observational epidemiologic studies established a clear association between smoking and lung cancer, with risks among long-term smokers about 20 times greater than those of nonsmokers. Based on their observational evidence, Doll and Hill judged smoking to be a cause of lung cancer years before there was any clear understanding of the actual mechanism of alterations in DNA by initiators or promoters of cancer. In 1964 the U.S. Surgeon General also judged smoking to be a definite cause of this disease, still years before the biologic mechanism was clearly understood.[11] Thus, although basic research is crucial to identify mechanisms to explain causal or preventive factors, direct answers to the questions of whether particular exposures are associated with risks of disease may derive from straightforward observation of what actually happens in free-living human populations.

With regard to smoking and coronary heart disease (CHD), the finding that current cigarette smokers have about an 80% increased risk has been consistently demonstrated over the last 30 years by different investigators in a large number of case-control and cohort studies involving millions of person-years of observation.[12] It is interesting that smoking was not judged to be a cause of CHD until far later than the judgment that it caused lung cancer. Part of this related to the lack of a clear biologic mechanism. However, another reason related directly to a limitation in interpreting the findings from any observational study, namely, that as the relative risk gets smaller, there is increasing concern that some factor other than the exposure being studied may explain all or at least part of the findings. For example, cigarette smokers may share other characteristics or lifestyle practices that independently affect their risk of CHD. Information can be collected on any potential confounding variables known to the investigator and then used in the data analysis to adjust for any impact of these factors. However, there can be no adjustment for the effects of unmeasured or unmeasurable confounding variables.

When a large effect is seen, such as with smoking and lung cancer, the amount of uncontrolled confounding may affect the magnitude of the relative risk estimate, making it, for example as high as 22 or as low as 18, rather than the observed value of 20. However, it is unlikely that complete control of confounding would materially change the conclusion that there is a strong positive association between smoking and lung cancer. Even in the case of current smoking and CHD, while uncontrolled confounding may mean that the true relative risk is as small as 1.6 or as large as 2.0, instead of the 1.8 most consistently seen in observational studies, that range of uncertainty does not materially affect the conclusion that current cigarette smoking increases the risk of CHD. On the other hand, when the most plausible magnitude of benefit or harm is only 20% to 40%—as is the case with most promising interventions today—a small amount of uncontrolled confounding in an observational study could mean the difference between a relative risk of 0.8, indicating a 20% decreased risk, 1.0, indicating no effect, or 1.2, indicating a 20% increased risk. In such circumstances, randomized trials represent the most reliable research design strategy.

RANDOMIZED CLINICAL TRIALS

Randomized clinical trials, also referred to as experimental studies or intervention studies, may be viewed as a type of cohort study, because participants are identified on the basis of their exposure status and followed to determine whether they develop the disease. The distinguishing feature of the intervention design is that the exposure status of each participant is assigned by the investigator.

Intervention studies are often considered as providing the most reliable evidence from epidemiologic research because of the unique strength of randomization as the means of allocating exposure status in a trial. When participants are allocated to a particular exposure group at random, such a strategy achieves, on average, control of all other factors that may affect disease risk. While such variables, if they are known to the investigators, could be controlled in the design and/or analysis of observational studies, the unique feature of randomization is that it also, on average, controls the effects of risk factors that are unrecognized or unmeasurable. It is this ability to control both known and unknown confounders that makes the randomized trial such a powerful epidemiologic strategy, especially for studying small-to-moderate effects. Of course, ethical concerns preclude the allocation of exposures that are known to be hazardous. Such exposures can properly be assessed in intervention studies only by attempts to eliminate them, as in the Multiple Risk Factor Intervention Trial,[13] which was designed to evaluate the effects of smoking cessation, blood pressure reduction, and cholesterol lowering on decreasing risk of CHD. There are also particular concerns of costs and feasibility for intervention studies. Nevertheless, when well designed and conducted, randomized clinical trials can indeed provide the most direct epidemiologic evidence on which to judge whether an exposure causes or prevents a disease.

If the treatments are allocated at random in a sample of sufficiently large size, intervention studies have the potential to provide a degree of assurance about the validity of a result that is simply not possible with any observational design option. It is rare that the introduction of a new treatment or procedure is accompanied by benefits as striking and as unequivocal as those that followed the introduction of the antibiotic penicillin, namely, an immediate reduction in death rates from pneumococcal pneumonia from about 95% to 15%. A randomized trial of the efficacy of penicillin seemed neither necessary nor, for ethical reasons, desirable, in part because the mortality reduction was so large and immediate that it seemed clearly due to the drug itself. Most often, however, the effects of therapeutic or preventive measures are small to moderate, on the order of 20% to 40% differences in disease outcomes. Such effects can be extremely important from a clinical or public health standpoint, especially when the outcome of interest is mortality from common diseases. Although important, small-to-moderate differences are difficult to establish reliably from observational studies, since the magnitude of the observed effect of the treatment may be about the same as the amount of uncontrolled confounding. In these circumstances, the conduct of a randomized trial will yield the strongest and most direct epidemiologic evidence on which to base a judgment of whether an observed association is one of cause and effect.

A recent example that illustrates the contributions of the various types of research strategies to the totality of evidence relates to the possible role of antioxidant vitamins in the prevention of cardiovascular disease. Basic research has provided evidence of plausible mechanisms for antioxidant vitamins in the prevention of cardiovascular disease as well as cancer. For cardiovascular disease, antioxidant vitamins can inhibit the oxidation and/or uptake of low-density lipoprotein cholesterol, the particularly atherogenic form of cholesterol. In addition to descriptive studies, a large number of analytic observational studies have examined the antioxidant hypothesis. Several large-scale prospective cohort studies have found decreased cardiovascular disease risks on the order of 20% to 40% among subjects with higher intake of antioxidant vitamins, either through diet or supplements.[14]

However, as in any observational study, it may be, for example, that those with greater intake of antioxidant vitamins share other dietary or nondietary lifestyle practices that account for all or some of the observed association with antioxidant vitamins. While adjustments can be made for known confounding variables for which data are collected, observational studies are unable to control for the potential effects of confounding variables not collected or known to the investigators, and when searching for the proposed modest-sized effects, the amount of uncontrolled confounding may be as large as the most likely effect.

For all these reasons, randomized trials of sufficient

sample size and duration of treatment and follow-up were necessary to detect reliably any small-to-moderate treatment effects. If the trials were large enough, the randomization process would, on average, evenly distribute among treatment groups known as well as unknown confounding variables. In addition, extremely large trials were necessary to avoid the possible uninformative null result of no benefit when in fact a modest-sized benefit truly exists.

Four large-scale randomized trials of β-carotene supplementation have been completed.[15–18] Overall, their results for CHD have not supported the promising evidence that accumulated from basic research, descriptive studies, and analytic observational investigations. The results certainly do not preclude the possibility that some benefit may yet emerge for antioxidants. Indeed, there are several ongoing trials evaluating antioxidants in both primary and secondary prevention of cardiovascular disease, and the evidence remains particularly promising for vitamin E. However, with respect to β-carotene supplementation, the data presently available from completed trials indicate no overall benefits on cardiovascular disease among well-nourished populations. These data suggest that the findings from observational studies of possible benefits may, indeed, have reflected some influence of other confounding variables associated with β-carotene intake that explain all or some of the decreased risks of cardiovascular disease among those with high intake levels. The findings also raise the possibility that the antiatherogenic mechanisms for β-carotene described in basic research may not have direct relevance to the effects of supplementation with this antioxidant on human disease risk.

SUMMARY

The evaluation of an epidemiologic hypothesis involves the consideration of the totality of evidence, including basic research, observational epidemiologic studies, and randomized clinical trials. Each of these strategies provides unique and complementary information to the totality of evidence on which rational clinical decisions for individuals and policy decisions for the health of the general public can be safely based.

For many if not most hypotheses, randomized trials are neither necessary nor desirable. For detecting small-to-moderate effects, however, they represent the most reliable research design strategy. Randomized trials certainly can be more difficult to design and conduct than observational epidemiologic studies, owing to their unique problems of ethics, feasibility, and costs. However, randomized trials that are sufficiently large, as well as carefully designed, conducted, and analyzed, can provide the strongest and most direct epidemiologic evidence on which to make a judgment about the existence of a cause-effect relationship.

REFERENCES

1. Hennekens CH, Buring JE. Epidemiology in Medicine. Boston, Little, Brown, 1987.
2. Hennekens CH. The increasing burden of cardiovascular disease: Current knowledge and future directions for research on risk factors. Circulation 1998; 97:1095–1102.
3. Cairns J. The treatment of diseases and the war against cancer. Sci Am 1985; 253:51–59.
4. Doll R, Peto R. The Causes of Cancer. New York, Oxford University Press, 1981.
5. Hennekens CH, Buring JE. Observational evidence. *In* Warren KS, Mosteller F (eds). Doing More Good than Harm: The Evaluation of Health Care Interventions. Ann N Y Acad Sci 1993; 703:18–24.
6. MacMahon S, Peto R, Cutler J, et al. Blood pressure, stroke, and coronary heart disease: I. Prolonged differences in blood pressure: Prospective observational studies corrected for the regression dilution bias. Lancet 1990; 335:765–774.
7. Collins R, Peto R, MacMahon S, et al. Blood pressure, stroke, and coronary heart disease: II. Short-term reductions in blood pressure: Overview of randomized drug trials in their epidemiologic context. Lancet 1990; 335:827–838.
8. Hebert PR, Moser M, Mayer J, et al. Recent evidence on drug therapy of mild to moderate hypertension and decreased risk of coronary heart disease. Arch Intern Med 1993; 153:578–581.
9. Doll R, Hill AB. Smoking and carcinoma of the lung: Preliminary report. BMJ 1950; 2:739–748.
10. Wynder EL, Graham EA. Tobacco smoking as a possible etiologic factor in bronchiogenic carcinoma: A study of 684 proved cases. JAMA 1950; 143:329–336.
11. U.S. Department of Health, Education, and Welfare. Smoking and Health: Report of the Advisory Committee to the Surgeon General of the Public Health Service. PHS Publication No. 1103. Bethesda, U.S. Department of Health, Education, and Welfare; Public Health Service; Centers for Disease Control, 1964.
12. Hennekens CH, Buring J, Mayrent SL. Smoking and aging in coronary heart disease. *In* Bosse R, Rose C (eds). Smoking and Aging. Lexington, MA, DC Heath, 1984, pp 95–115.
13. Multiple Risk Factor Intervention Trial Research Group. Multiple Risk Factor Intervention Trial: Risk factor changes and morbidity results. JAMA 1982; 248:1465–1477.
14. Hennekens CH, Gaziano JM, Manson JE, Buring JE. Antioxidant vitamin–cardiovascular disease hypothesis is still promising, but still unproven: The need for randomized trials. Am J Clin Nutr 1995; 62:1337S–1380S.
15. Blot WJ, Li JY, Taylor PR, et al. Nutrition intervention trials in Linxian, China: Supplementation with specific vitamin/mineral combinations, cancer incidence, and disease-specific mortality in the general population. J Natl Cancer Inst 1993; 85:1483–1492.
16. Alpha-Tocopherol, Beta Carotene Cancer Prevention Study Group. The effect of vitamin E and beta carotene on the incidence of lung cancer and other cancers in male smokers. N Engl J Med 1994; 330:1029–1035.
17. Omenn GS, Goodman GE, Thornquist MD, et al. Effects of a combination of beta carotene and vitamin A on lung cancer and cardiovascular disease. N Engl J Med 1996; 334:1150–1155.
18. Hennekens CH, Buring JE, Manson JE, et al. Lack of effect of long-term supplementation with beta carotene on the incidence of malignant neoplasms and cardiovascular disease. N Engl J Med 1996; 334:1145–1149.

2 Methodology of Randomized Trials*

▶ Laurence S. Freedman

Randomized clinical trials are the most reliable method available for comparing alternative preventive or therapeutic interventions. Since the conduct and publication of the earliest randomized trials in the 1940s, clinicians have increasingly accepted this method as the gold standard for evaluating new treatments. This trend has been more rapid in some specialties, such as cardiovascular disease and oncology, than in others, but the trend is evident in nearly all areas of medicine. In the last 15 years, a number of excellent textbooks have been published, describing comprehensively the methodology of randomized trials.[1–3] In this chapter, I discuss some selected topics that seem pertinent to cardiovascular disease trials. The reader is referred to the just-mentioned texts for more details.

Most of the issues surrounding the methodology of clinical trials revolve around three principles: *achieving unbiasedness, achieving adequate precision,* and subject to these two principles, *increasing efficiency* (Table 2–1).

The main aim of any clinical trial should be to provide an estimate of the effect of a (usually new) treatment on clinical outcome compared with that achieved by another (usually standard) treatment. By *unbiasedness,* I mean the ability of the trial, through proper design, conduct, and analysis, invariably to obtain the correct estimate of the treatment effect, given as large a number of participating subjects as desired. Many study designs, mostly nonrandomized, lead to bias and fail to satisfy the unbiasedness criterion. Furthermore, even when randomization is used, certain other design features or types of statistical analysis give biased results.

Unbiasedness is a theoretical concept (although nonetheless important for this). In practice, the number of participating subjects is always limited. Limited sample sizes introduce another type of error into the estimation of the treatment effect that is distinct from bias and is referred to as *random error.* When the random error is large, we cannot estimate the treatment effect accurately, that is, with good *precision.* The larger the sample size, however, the more we reduce the random error, and the better is the precision of our estimate.

Important as they are, randomized clinical trials often require a large investment of money and time. Furthermore, many of these trials are financed by public money. It is therefore important for investigators continually to search for ways of reducing the costs of randomized clinical trials. There are many ways to design trials so that they provide unbiased estimates of treatment effects with good precision. Two different designs that achieve unbiasedness and the same level of precision may have different costs. In particular, since the costs often depend heavily on the number of participating subjects, interest often focuses on how to achieve the same precision with fewer participants. The ratio of the reciprocals of the number of participants required by the two designs to achieve the same precision is known as their *relative efficiency.* Clearly we should be interested in finding new designs with large efficiency relative to the standard design.

Table 2–1 shows how the six topics discussed in this chapter relate to these basic principles.

THE NEED FOR RANDOMIZATION

Until recently it was unusual to conduct a formal medical experiment. However, lack of controlled experiments sometimes led to conflicting claims and

TABLE 2–1 • Three Principles in Clinical Trials Methodology

Principles	Concept	Topics
Unbiasedness	Getting the correct estimate of treatment effect "with unlimited sample size"	Randomization Intention-to-treat analysis
Precision	Getting an accurate estimate of the treatment effect	Sample size Length of follow-up
Efficiency	Reducing costs subject to unbiasedness and good precision	Reducing noncompliance Factorial designs

*All the material in this chapter is in the public domain, with the exception of any borrowed figures or tables.

even to adoption of treatments that later were demonstrated to be harmful, such as gastric freezing for duodenal ulcer.[4] A basic element of the controlled experiment is the use of a control group of patients who receive the standard therapy with which the new treatment is to be compared. The control group may be formed by a number of different methods, not necessarily involving randomization. Controls may be chosen from patients who refuse the new treatment or from patients who are not offered the new treatment for a variety of reasons. It is now quite widely accepted that patients who are offered and refuse a new treatment are likely to be characteristically different from those who accept, and in a manner that will affect their overall prognosis. Such prognostic differences naturally lead to bias in the comparison of the treatment and control groups.

More controversial is the value of using "historical controls," that is, patients who were treated with the standard therapy before the new treatment became available. However, several problems arise when using this method. First, the eligibility criteria for the study of the new treatment may cause a different disease profile of patients from that in the historical control group. Friedman and associates[1] observe that an annual total mortality rate of 6% was anticipated in the control group of the Coronary Drug Project[5] based on rates from previous myocardial infarction (MI) patients. In fact, an annual mortality rate of approximately 4% was observed in the trial in the control and in the treatment groups. If historical controls had been used, then the conclusion would have been that the new treatments were effective.

Gehan and Freireich[6] advocate the use of historical controls, particularly when these are participants in previous studies using similar criteria for eligibility and evaluation. However, even in these circumstances, time changes in the nature of the patients referred for treatment, in diagnostic criteria, or in supportive care can introduce hidden bias into the comparison. Byar and colleagues[7] report that, in the Veterans Administration Cooperative Urological Research Group trial of treatments for prostate cancer, patients admitted in the last half of the trial and randomized to estrogen had significantly better survival than the controls who entered in the first half of the trial. There was no survival difference, however, when the same patients allocated estrogen were compared with their concurrent control subjects.

Gehan and Freireich[6] advocate controlling for hidden biases by adjusting for differences in known prognostic factors between the treatment and control groups using a multivariate regression model. However, only if one has knowledge of all relevant prognostic factors can one be sure that this method will work. In reality, known prognostic factors for most chronic diseases account for only a small fraction (<15%) of the observed variation among patients of their clinical outcomes.[8] Thus, there is little hope of controlling for all hidden biases by this device. When the treatment difference is large, these biases may not be sufficient to mask the underlying difference, and a randomized design may not be necessary. However, for moderate and small treatment differences the biases using historical controls are likely to distort the comparison and lead to erroneous results.

More recently, there has been much interest in using medical databases to evaluate the comparative effects of treatments.[9] This approach suffers from many of the problems of historical controls and more besides. Perhaps the most serious problem is that database information is rarely sufficient to describe *why* a patient receives a particular treatment. Very often, the choice of treatment is heavily confounded with the current health of the patient, including the extent of the disease, concurrent illnesses, and general fitness.[10] As a result, comparison often leads to apparent advantages for less invasive procedures, even after adjustment for known prognostic factors. Byar[11] describes the analysis of data from a thyroid cancer register that appeared to show that surgery followed by x-ray therapy was harmful compared with surgery alone. However, because it was unknown whether x-ray treatment was given selectively to those with an incomplete resection of the tumor, the result was uninterpretable.

Allocating the treatment to a patient by randomization avoids confounding of the treatment choice with the patient's state of health or with other characteristics that can affect prognosis. This property represents the principal advantage that randomization carries over other methods of forming a control group and is the reason why the randomized, controlled trial is regarded as the gold standard of evaluation designs. However, the act of randomization does not by itself guarantee a trial to be free from hidden bias. For example, one sometimes prepares in advance a list of the treatments to be allocated in sequence as patients enter the trial. If the clinician in charge of entering patients into the trial has seen the list and remembers the next treatment to be allocated, then he or she has the possibility of encouraging or discouraging the next patient to enter, depending on the clinician's subjective opinion about the suitability of the treatment for that patient. Such selection can introduce bias and nullifies the advantage of randomization. It is therefore important that the randomized allocation remains unknown before the decision of the patient to enter the trial is made.

Other ways in which bias can be introduced, even though randomized treatment allocation is used, are in the conduct of the outcome assessment and in the statistical analysis. Often, to avoid biased assessment, the trial is designed to be double blind, that is, the control group receives an inert medication in place of the active medication received by the treatment group, and neither patients nor clinicians are informed whether they have been given the active or inert treatment (see Chapter 6 in Reference 2 for more details).

Another commonly encountered problem related to bias—the statistical analysis of the data—is discussed in the next section.

INTENTION-TO-TREAT ANALYSIS

The treatment protocol that is to be followed in a clinical trial comprises a number of details. For example, even in the simple case of use of aspirin for patients who have had an MI, the protocol would specify the dose and frequency of administration, the delay between the MI attack and starting the medication, and the duration of continuing the medication. Commonly, some patients do not receive the randomized treatment according to protocol. Treatment protocol deviations may involve minor changes in the dose or schedule, or they may involve gross departures, the most extreme being the failure to receive any of the medication. Similarly, those allocated to the control group may not receive the standard treatment and may even receive the therapy offered to the treatment group.

A question arises at the time of statistical analysis regarding the handling of the data from patients who have deviated from the treatment protocol. On first consideration it seems natural to compare the outcomes of patients who have received the new treatment approximately according to protocol with those who have received the standard treatment approximately according to protocol. In this analysis, a patient allocated to the treatment group but receiving only standard therapy would be moved to the control group and vice versa. However, this analysis strategy, which is sometimes called *analysis by treatment received*, frequently introduces bias into the comparison.

The Coronary Drug Project Research Group[5] reported results of a comparison of clofibrate with placebo given for up to 5 years to men with a previous MI. The investigators presented mortality rates according to whether subjects were more than 80% compliant with taking the allocated clofibrate capsules or not. The 5-year mortality rate among the good compliers with clofibrate was 15.0%. Analysis by treatment received requires that this rate is compared with the total control group, since any noncompliance with a placebo should have no medical effect. The mortality rate in the total control group was 19.4%, and the difference between the two rates is statistically significant ($P < 0.01$). Thus, from this analysis of compliers with the active drug one would conclude that clofibrate reduced the mortality rate in males following MI.

As pointed out in the same article, there was a strikingly lower mortality rate among good compliers with clofibrate (15.0%) than among poor compliers with clofibrate (24.6%). This seems to support the conclusion that clofibrate reduces mortality. However, when the control group was considered, it was found that those who complied well with placebo had a 15.1% mortality rate, nearly identical to that of the good compliers with clofibrate, whereas those who complied poorly with placebo had a mortality rate of 28.2%, quite similar to the poor compliers with clofibrate. It is clear that the higher mortality rate in the placebo poor compliers compared with the placebo good compliers could not be caused by their failure to take placebo but must result from innate differences in the health and characteristics of poor versus good compliers. Consequently, it becomes clear that analysis by treatment received can cause serious biases in treatment comparisons.

An alternative strategy that avoids the bias introduced from using analysis by treatment received is to retain all patients in the group to which they are randomized, regardless of the treatment they received. This strategy has come to be known as *intention-to-treat analysis,* since when a patient is first randomized to a treatment group, the clinician intends to administer that treatment according to the protocol. Applying intention to treat analysis to the Coronary Drug Project example, the mortality in the total clofibrate group was 18.2% compared with 19.4% in the total control group, a difference that is not significant ($P > 0.25$). Thus in this example, when an unbiased analysis strategy is employed, the apparent treatment difference, seen when using analysis by treatment received, disappears.

When there is considerable noncompliance in a clinical trial, some argue that intention to treat analysis itself gives a biased (under)estimate of the real treatment difference. The truth of this statement depends on one's understanding of the term *real treatment difference.* If one means that the real difference is the difference that would occur under conditions of perfect compliance with the treatment protocol, then the assertion is correct: an intention-to-treat analysis would underestimate this difference. However, the intention-to-treat analysis does provide an unbiased estimate of the treatment difference that would occur under the same compliance conditions as occurred in the trial. If the noncompliance that occurred in the trial were due to adverse side effects of the treatment or to the unpleasant nature of the treatment administration, then one might anticipate the same levels of noncompliance in general practice. In this instance the treatment effect under these same levels of noncompliance would be the most relevant effect to estimate.

Sometimes noncompliance is avoidable or at least can be reduced by modifications of the trial design. This topic is addressed later when I discuss questions of efficiency.

SAMPLE SIZE AND STATISTICAL POWER

The precision with which we can estimate the treatment effect is directly related to the ability of the trial to detect reliably a real treatment difference as statistically significant. Trials with poor precision may be able to detect a large treatment effect but will have low probability of detecting moderate or small effects. The probability of detecting a given treatment difference is known as the *statistical power* of the trial.

Increasing the sample size improves the precision of the estimate of the treatment effect and increases statistical power. Suppose that we were designing a trial to prevent early deaths (events) following a first acute MI. Suppose we have evidence that with current standard therapy the 5-week event rate will be approximately 12%. We expect that the new treatment will reduce this rate to 9%. Assuming that we will use a two-sided 5% significance level, Figure 2–1 shows how sample size affects the statistical power. Clearly, small trials with fewer than 1000 patients have little chance of detecting the postulated reduction in event rate. To achieve a probability of at least 9 in 10 (power of 90%) of detecting the effect, we would need approximately 4500 patients or more in our trial.

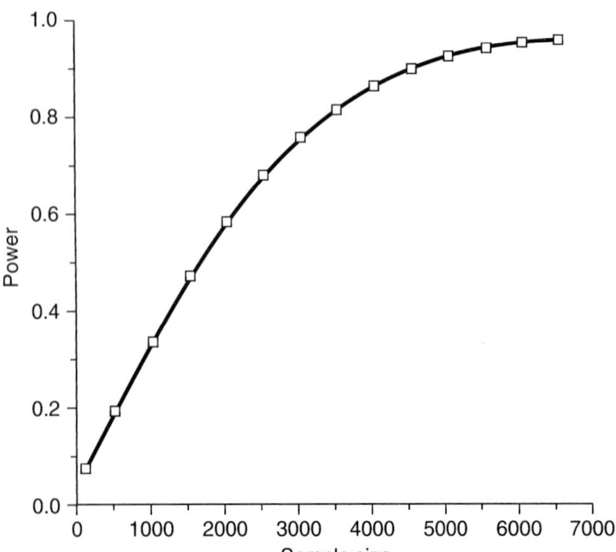

Figure 2–1 Effect of sample size on statistical power for detecting a reduction in event rate from 12% to 9% as statistically significant at the 5% level.

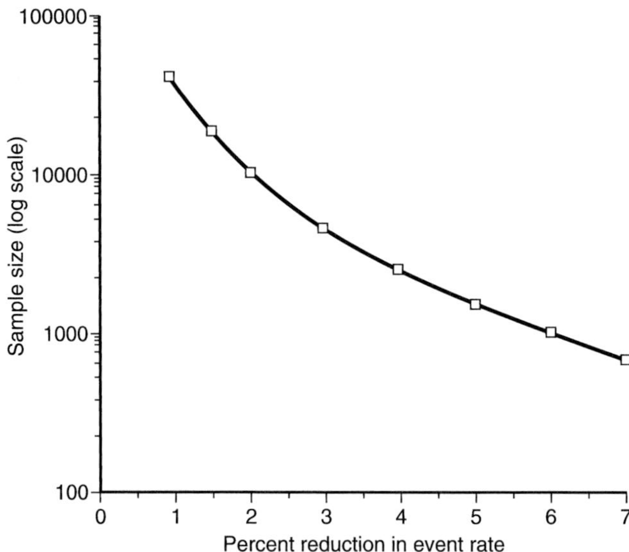

Figure 2–2 Sample size required for 90% power of detecting a given percent reduction in event rate as statistically significant (e.g., 3% means that the event rate is reduced from 12% to 9%).

The sample size requirements in a trial are extraordinarily sensitive to the magnitude of the treatment effect that one aims to detect. In the earlier example, if we were unwilling to miss detecting a smaller reduction, say from 12% to 10%, and wished to have 90% power for that effect, then our sample size would need to be increased from 4500 to 10,300. Figure 2–2 shows in more detail the relationship between sample size requirements and the magnitude of treatment differences. The sample size axis has been drawn on a logarithmic scale to accommodate the wide range of sizes. The rapid rise of sample size with decreasing treatment effect is readily appreciated.

Limited resources preclude us from designing all our trials with sample sizes that are large enough to be sure of detecting small effects. Nevertheless, for important questions involving common diseases carrying a risk of mortality, such an aim is only reasonable given the public health benefits that could result from even small improvements in therapy. The example par excellence of large trials conducted to detect small but worthwhile effects is the series of International Studies of Infarct Survival (ISIS) trials of treatment for MI. For example, the data from ISIS-2[12] showed 791 vascular deaths (9.2%) in the first 5 weeks among 8592 patients allocated streptokinase infusion compared with 1029 vascular deaths (12.0%) among 8595 patients allocated placebo infusion. The difference of 2.8% is highly significant ($P < 0.00001$). Moreover, the 90% confidence interval for this difference is 2.0% to 3.6%, indicating a remarkably precise estimate of the vascular mortality reduction. Armed with such precise information, clinicians are far better equipped to form rational policies for managing the treatment of the many patients who suffer an MI.

For trials that do not have these large sizes, it is possible that we will often get a nonsignificant result even when a useful benefit really exists. To protect ourselves from premature discarding of such useful therapies, caution is required in our interpretation of nonsignificant results. Freiman and coworkers[13] have commented on this problem. They collected 71 published reports of randomized clinical trials that reported negative (i.e., nonsignificant) results. Eighty percent of these results were not precise enough to exclude (using 90% confidence limits) the possibility of a 25% absolute reduction in the event rate. The authors concluded that "many of the therapies discarded as ineffective after 'negative' trials may still have a clinically meaningful benefit."

The antidote to this problem, aside from increasing the size of trials, is to adopt caution in the interpretation of "nonsignificant" results. In the face of nonsignificance it is best to focus on the confidence interval for the estimate of treatment effect. Treatment benefits that lie within this interval are quite consistent with the trial results. If the interval includes benefits that are clinically useful, then the nonsignificant result has not excluded a clinical benefit from the new treatment.

It is also prudent to reserve judgment concerning large, statistically significant treatment differences reported from small trials. In areas of medicine that have not seen dramatic improvements for many years, the emergence of a new treatment that is much superior to the standard is not a likely occurrence. For a small trial to demonstrate a statistically significant difference, the observed treatment difference must necessarily be large and is likely to overestimate the true difference. Thus, although it may be true that the new treatment does have *some* added benefit, the small trial is likely to have seriously exaggerated the magnitude of this benefit.

Other factors in addition to sample size can strongly influence the statistical power of a trial. One of these—the duration of trial follow-up—is the topic of the next section.

LENGTH OF FOLLOW-UP

In the hypothetical example used in the previous section to illustrate the choice of sample size at the design stage of a trial, I postulated a control group 5-week event rate of 12% compared with an anticipated treatment group rate of 9%, a 25% proportional reduction. For this trial at least 4500 patients are needed to attain good statistical power.

Suppose instead that we wished to design the trial based on a longer-term follow-up of patients, say 2 years. Previous data suggest that the control group event rate after 2 years will be about 20%. If the proportional reduction in events were maintained at 25%, then we would expect the 2-year event rate of the controls to be about 15%. The number of patients needed to achieve a 90% power for detecting this effect is approximately 2500, compared with the 4500 calculated for the 5-week follow-up design.

A useful rule of thumb related to this example is that the number of *events* rather than the number of patients is what really determines power. Thus, the 5-week design is expected to lead to 4500 × (12% + 9%)/2 or about 470 observed events, and the 2-year design is expected to yield 2500 × (20% + 15%)/2 or about 440 events, demonstrating the approximately equal power of the two designs.

However, this rule of thumb is only valid under circumstances where the same level of benefit from the treatment is expected to extend throughout the period of follow-up. In fact, several large trials of treatment following acute MI demonstrate that reductions in event rates are often limited to the early recovery period following MI. In ISIS-2[12] the vascular mortality rate over the first 5 weeks was 12.0% in the control group and 9.5% in the aspirin group, a proportional reduction of 21%. In the course of the next 99 weeks (up to the end of the second year) the vascular mortality rate among the surviving patients was 9.1% in the control group and 9.7% in the aspirin group, indicating no further reduction in vascular mortality. Similarly, in the same trial streptokinase reduced 5-week vascular mortality proportionally by 23%, but there was no observed reduction in vascular mortality among the survivors over the following 2 years.

Returning to the hypothetical example, if, anticipating a 25% proportional reduction in events throughout the period, we had planned the trial with 2500 patients followed for 2 years, but the reduction occurred only in the first 5 weeks with no effect thereafter, then the power of the trial would drop from the projected 90% to below 50%. Thus, making optimistic assumptions about the duration of the treatment effect can lead to a seriously underpowered trial design. Generally speaking, prevention trials require longer analysis follow-up periods, whereas for treatment trials a shorter planned analysis period appears wise, as demonstrated by the examples just provided. A good understanding of the biology of the disease and the biologic mechanism of the intervention is the best guide to decisions regarding the appropriate follow-up period for the planned analysis of a trial.

REDUCING NONCOMPLIANCE

In a previous section, I discussed patients' noncompliance with the therapy allocated by randomization, its impact on the statistical analysis of a trial, and the merits of intention-to-treat analysis versus analysis by treatment received. Noncompliance also affects the design of a trial. Its main effect is to reduce the treatment difference that is observed in the trial, and as shown in Figure 2–2, this in turn necessitates an increase in the sample size to maintain good statistical power.

Returning again to the hypothetical trial in acute MI, suppose that the new treatment carried an acute side effect that made it intolerable to 20% of patients and that these would have to terminate treatment almost immediately and cross over to receive the standard therapy. Assume also that those suffering the side effect carry the same prognosis as other patients. Using intention-to-treat analysis, the anticipated event rate in the treatment group will be increased from 9% under perfect compliance to $0.8 \times 9\% + 0.2 \times 12\% = 9.4\%$. This decreases the absolute reduction in event rate from 3% to 2.6% and necessitates an increase in sample size from 4500 to 6000 to maintain 90% power (see Fig. 2–2). Thus, seemingly minor levels of noncompliance can necessitate substantial increases in the sample size and therefore the cost of the trial.

Noncompliance is a particularly important issue in prevention trials for several reasons. First, the participants are healthy volunteers who are likely to be less well motivated than patients in complying carefully with a prescribed treatment. Second, prevention interventions tend to involve longer-term medication than therapeutic interventions. Third, some prevention strategies require lifestyle changes, such as dietary modification and smoking cessation, that are difficult for people to achieve and maintain. Fourth, people in the control group may "drift" closer toward adopting the intervention of the treatment group as a result of population trends. All of these phenomena were met in the Multiple Risk Factor Intervention Trial (MRFIT),[14] which involved dietary intervention, smoking cessation, and blood pressure reduction. This trial has since served as an object lesson in the practical importance of noncompliance.

Considerable thought and effort are needed in first assessing the level of noncompliance that is likely, and then finding ways of reducing this level, if at all possible. If the noncompliance level is not assessed properly before the trial begins, then there is a danger that it will be underestimated and the trial will consequently be seriously underpowered. If no effort is put into reducing the noncompliance level, then the trial may be designed to be larger and more expensive than it need be.

An excellent example of coping with noncompliance was provided by the investigators of the Physicians' Health Study. This trial of aspirin and β-carotene for preventing cardiovascular disease and cancer, respectively, is being conducted in approximately 22,000 volunteer U.S. male physicians. The investigators arranged an 18-week run-in period during which potential participants were asked to take daily capsules similar to those used in the main trial.[15] Compliance at the end of the run-in period was assessed by questionnaires. Approximately 11,000 of the 33,000 volunteers decided not to participate in the main study, took less than than two thirds of the capsules, or became ineligible during the run-in period and were not admitted to the trial. The investigators calculated that exclusion of these potentially noncompliant participants actually increased the power of the trial and reduced considerably the cost of the trial.

Another cost-efficient measure taken in the design of the Physicians' Health Study is discussed in the following section.

FACTORIAL DESIGNS

With the considerable amount of resources and money that are invested in large long-term clinical trials, it is worth carefully considering whether the trial can be designed to answer more than one primary question about the therapy or prevention of disease. Factorial designs allow the effects of two or more interventions to be assessed in the same trial.

The simplest version is the 2 × 2 factorial design, which allows two separate treatments to be assessed. Suppose the new treatments are A and B and the control treatment is C. The design requires that at randomization one fourth of the patients are allocated treatment C, one fourth treatment A, one fourth treatment B, and one fourth a combination of treatments A and B (A + B). In this way one may estimate the effect of treatment A and of treatment B from the same trial. Moreover, if the effects of the treatments are *additive,* then the effects of treatment A and treatment B can both be estimated with the same precision as in a two-group trial of the same size. In other words, the 2 × 2 factorial design provides as much information about these treatments as would two separate equally sized trials, at approximately half the cost.

The reasoning underlying this surprising cost saving lies in the notion of additivity of effects. *Additivity* means that when considering the effect of treatment A, the difference between treatment A and treatment C is the same as the difference between treatment A + B and treatment B. Thus, when estimating the effect of treatment A, we can employ information from all the patients participating in the trial. Treatment group A is compared with treatment group C to obtain one estimate of A's effect, while treatment group A + B is compared with treatment group B to obtain another independent estimate, and the two estimates are statistically combined. The effect of treatment B is estimated in an analogous manner, using comparisons of treatment groups B with C and treatment groups A + B with A.

This design has been used in a number of large trials recently. For example, ISIS-2 involved randomization to 1 month of daily aspirin (A), a 1-hour intravenous infusion of streptokinase (B), both of these (A + B), or neither (C). Table 2–2 shows the 5-week vascular mortality rates in the four groups, calculated from the information provided in Figure 2 of the ISIS-2 Collaborative Group's report.[12] The treatment differences shown in the margins demonstrate that the additivity assumption is well supported in this trial, with the addition of streptokinase effecting an estimated 2.8% to 2.9% absolute decrease in vascular mortality in the presence or absence of aspirin treatment, and the addition of aspirin effecting an estimated 2.4% to 2.5% absolute reduction in vascular mortality whether or not streptokinase is given.

Another example of the use of a 2 × 2 factorial design is provided by the Physicians' Health Study, which was designed to study simultaneously the effects of aspirin on cardiovascular disease and β-carotene on cancer. In this case the factorial design takes on a new twist in that the two interventions studied target different diseases. The additivity assumption is again quite reasonable, since it would be unlikely (although not impossible) that a treatment targeting one disease would interact with another treatment's action on a different disease, and because the metabolic pathways and the hypothesized mechanisms of action of these agents are quite distinct.

The reason to be vigilant with respect to the additivity assumption is that the 2 × 2 design could be compromised if the effect of the combination of the treatments were *subadditive*.[16] Returning for the last time to the hypothetical example, suppose the effect of new treatment A in the absence of B is to reduce the event rate from 12% down to 9%, and that when B is given the event rate is 9% with or without treatment A. The combination effect is subadditive because A + B is no more effective than A alone or B alone. In our analysis of this 2 × 2 trial we would combine an estimated reduction of about 3% (A vs. C) with an estimated zero reduction (A + B vs. B). The estimated overall reduction would then be approximately 1.5%, the average of the two estimates. In other words, introduction of the second treatment B into the design would reduce the magnitude of the treatment effect and consequently seriously reduce the power of the trial.

TABLE 2–2 • Estimated 5-Week Vascular Mortality Rates in the 2 × 2 Factorially Designed ISIS-2 Trial, Showing Support for the Additivity Assumption

	Aspirin	No Aspirin	Difference
Streptokinase	8.1% (A + B)	10.5% (B)	−2.4% (A + B vs. B)
No streptokinase	10.9% (A)	13.4% (C)	−2.5% (A vs. C)
Difference	−2.8% (A + B vs. A)	−2.9% (B vs. C)	

Data from information in Figure 2 of Reference 12: ISIS.

Conservative investigators have opposed the use of 2 × 2 factorial designs on the grounds that one cannot exclude the possibility of subadditivity. A more balanced view is that these designs should be avoided if the nature and postulated mechanisms of action of the treatments are similar or are likely to interact but should otherwise be encouraged. The experience with several such large trials in cardiovascular disease and in cancer prevention has so far been positive, with little or no evidence that negative interactions have compromised the results.

CONCLUSION

The foundation principles of evaluation of clinical interventions rests on avoidance of biased comparisons, achieving adequate precision, and finding efficiencies in design. As new funding for health care research becomes increasingly difficult to obtain, the pressure on large long-term studies will increase. Some of the most important questions regarding the prevention and treatment of common diseases, including cardiovascular disease, can only be reliably answered by such studies. Alternatives, such as historical control studies and database analyses, have been carefully considered. So far, for small-to-moderate treatment effects, these alternatives have been found to fall far short of the scientific standards that should be applied to evaluate one of our closest concerns, the maintenance of our own health.

REFERENCES

1. Friedman LM, Furberg CD, DeMets DL. Fundamentals of Clinical Trials, 2nd Ed. Boston, John Wright, 1996.
2. Pocock SJ. Clinical Trials: A Practical Approach. Chichester, UK, John Wiley & Sons, 1983.
3. Meinert CL. Clinical Trials: Design, Conduct, and Analysis. Oxford, Oxford University Press, 1986.
4. Ruffin JM, Grizzle JE, Hightower NC, et al. A cooperative double-blind evaluation of gastric "freezing" in the treatment of duodenal ulcer. N Engl J Med 1969; 281:16–19.
5. Coronary Drug Research Group. Influence of adherence to treatment and response of cholesterol on mortality in the coronary drug project. N Engl J Med, 1980; 303:1038–1041.
6. Gehan EA, Freireich EJ. Nonrandomized controls in cancer clinical trials. N Engl J Med 1974; 290:198–203.
7. Byar DP, Simon RM, Friedewald WT, et al. Randomized clinical trials: Perspectives on some recent ideas. N Engl J Med 1976; 295:74–80.
8. Korn EL, Simon RM. Measures of explained variation for survival data. Stat Med 1990; 9:487–503.

9. Hui SL, McDonald C, Katz B. Methods of using large databases in health care research: Problems and promises. Stat Med 1991; 10:505–674.
10. Miettinen OS. The need for randomization in the study of intended effects. Stat Med 1983; 2:267–271.
11. Byar DP. Why data bases should not replace randomized clinical trials. Biometrics 1980; 36:337–342.
12. ISIS-2 Collaborative Group. Randomized trial of intravenous streptokinase, oral aspirin, both, or neither among 17,187 cases of suspected acute myocardial infarction: ISIS-2. Lancet 1988; 2:349–360.
13. Freiman JL, Chalmers TC, Smith H, et al. The importance of beta, the type II error, and sample size in the design and interpretation of the randomized control trial: Survey of 71 "negative" trials. N Engl J Med 1978; 299:690–694.
14. Neaton JD, Broste S, Cohen L, et al. The multiple risk factor intervention trial (MRFIT): VII. A comparison of risk factor changes between the study groups. Prev Med 1981; 10:519–543.
15. Lang JM, Buring JE, Rosner B, et al. Estimating the effect of the run-in on the power of the Physicians' Health Study. Stat Med, 1991; 10:1585–1594.
16. Brittain E, Wittes J. Factorial designs in clinical trials: The effects of noncompliance and subadditivity. Stat Med 1989; 8:161–172.

3 Comparative Features of Primordial, Primary, and Secondary Prevention Trials*

▶ Lawrence M. Friedman
▶ Denise G. Simons-Morton
▶ Jeffrey A. Cutler

The basic features of a good clinical trial apply whether the study population is healthy, at high risk of a disease or condition, or already stricken with the condition. These basic features include specification of the question being addressed, the intervention to be tested, and the primary outcome, as well as a properly justified sample size, randomization, unbiased measurement, and an intention-to-treat analysis. The differences in design and conduct of trials of primordial, primary, or secondary prevention are mostly matters of degree, rather than of kind.

Primary prevention is the prevention of the onset of disease. The primary prevention of risk factors is referred to as *primordial prevention.*[1] In the case of cardiovascular disease, primordial prevention would mean intervening to prevent the development of recognized risk factors such as hypertension, elevated serum cholesterol level, or cigarette smoking. An example of a primordial prevention trial is the Child and Adolescent Trial for Cardiovascular Health (CATCH), a study of school-based interventions to lower fat in the diet, increase physical activity, and prevent smoking to reduce the likelihood of children developing risk factors in the future.[2]

Primary prevention also can be conducted in people at high risk for disease due to existing risk factors, with the aim of reducing the risk factors to decrease the probability of developing disease. Examples of primary prevention trials in high-risk populations are trials of blood pressure lowering in hypertensive people such as the Hypertension Detection and Follow-up Program (HDFP)[3, 4] and the Systolic Hypertension in the Elderly Program (SHEP)[5]; trials of lipid lowering in those with elevated blood cholesterol levels such as the Lipid Research Clinics—Coronary Primary Prevention Trial (LRC-CPPT)[6, 7]; trials of smoking cessation in smokers[8, 9]; and trials of reduction of several risk factors such as the Multiple Risk Factor Intervention Trial (MRFIT).[10, 11] Sometimes primordial prevention and primary prevention are combined in population-wide intervention strategies. Studies of community interventions to encourage lower-fat diets for reducing blood cholesterol, to foster smoking cessation and prevention, and to encourage physical activity are aimed at reducing the population distribution of risk factors associated with cardiovascular disease. The Minnesota Heart Health Program (mhHP),[12, 13] the Stanford Five-Community Study,[14, 15] and the Pawtucket Heart Health Program[16, 17] are examples.

In secondary prevention, the disease or condition is already present. Secondary prevention trials include those that test strategies for early detection and treatment of subclinical disease, such as trials of screening mammography. Secondary prevention also includes interventions to forestall, delay, or reduce in intensity sequelae of disease, including mortality. Trials of interventions in patients with clinical coronary heart disease (CHD) or with acute myocardial infarction (MI) are secondary prevention studies. Examples include trials testing the effects on mortality of drug treatment of elevated cholesterol levels in men with previous MI, such as the Coronary Drug Project (CDP)[18, 19] and the Scandinavian Simvastatin Survival Study (4S),[20, 21] trials testing the effects of beta blockers in reducing mortality after acute MI,[22] trials of thrombolysis during acute MI,[23–25] and trials of angiotensin-converting enzyme inhibitors in people with heart failure.[26]

STUDY DESIGN

The design of any clinical trial, as of any scientific study, starts with the primary, or main, question to

*All the material in this chapter is in the public domain, with the exception of any borrowed figures or tables.

be answered. This main question drives whether the study will be one of primordial, primary, or secondary prevention. The conceptual framework for conducting prevention trials posits that the natural history of disease goes from no or low risk, to elevated risk because of the presence of risk factors, to detectable disease, to disease sequelae (which may include mortality). Primordial, primary, and secondary prevention trials are asking research questions at different places in this continuum. An example of how one topic can be addressed by any of the three types of studies is high blood cholesterol and heart disease. Trials to lower blood cholesterol level or prevent its increase in people who do not yet have hypercholesterolemia[2] are primordial prevention trials; trials testing approaches to lowering blood cholesterol level in people with hypercholesterolemia to prevent heart disease[7] are primary prevention trials in high-risk participants; and trials testing whether cholesterol level lowering in patients with CHD will prevent a subsequent MI or mortality[21] are secondary prevention trials.

The study design traditionally used in clinical trials is that people are selected from the population at risk for developing the risk factor or disease in question and are randomly assigned (randomized) to either one or several intervention groups and a control group. Randomization of large numbers results in groups that tend to be comparable in factors that are known to be associated with the outcome of interest (e.g., age) as well as factors that are unknown and yet may be associated with the outcome of interest. Thus, the randomization process allows the inference that differences in outcomes are the result of the intervention being administered rather than of any other initial factors that may differ between the groups (i.e., potential confounders). The randomized, controlled trial is the preferred design for all types of intervention studies.

Generally, individual subjects are randomized into intervention and control groups. In some situations, however, entire groups, rather than individuals, may be randomized. These groups may be schools,[2] worksites,[27] medical practices,[28] or entire communities.[29, 30] Group randomization (also called *cluster* or *unit randomization*) often is used in primordial or primary prevention trials, because such larger units are particularly relevant for interventions that are aimed at preventing or reducing risk factors. Advantages of randomizing groups are that (1) mass intervention techniques can be implemented, (2) the inherent social interaction within the group may reinforce adherence to the intervention, and (3) multilevel interventions can be tested (e.g., individual instruction for healthful eating plus cafeteria changes in food offerings). In group randomization, the primary sample size is considered the number of groups randomized, not the number of individuals in each group, although the latter does contribute to the study power.[31] The main disadvantage of group randomization is that if the group sizes are very large, as with communities, it may be difficult to find or afford enough communities to have adequate power and comparable intervention and control groups. Some studies have successfully recruited and randomized groups, such as schools, for a true randomized, controlled trial; for example CATCH recruited and randomized 96 schools.[2] When fewer groups are being studied, matching of groups may be used and randomization carried out within each matched pair.[32] An example of a study randomizing within matched community pairs was the Community Intervention Trial (COMMIT) study of smoking cessation.[29, 30] Communities may be matched on the basis of size, location, or demographic characteristics of the population. If enough groups are included, this approach has the advantage of being a true randomized design and increases the likelihood that the intervention and control communities will be comparable on potential confounding factors.

Sometimes, rather than conducting a randomized, controlled trial an investigator may undertake an intervention study with no control or comparison group. An effort is made to intervene in a participant or a community to see if changes occur, and the comparison is before and after intervention. An example is the Gothenborg study of community education to reduce delay in seeking care for acute MI symptoms (a secondary prevention question), which examined delay before and after the intervention.[33] It is unclear from a preintervention-to-postintervention design, however, whether changes are the result of the intervention or of other factors. Other studies have been conducted where a comparison group is chosen by some method other than randomization, often called a *quasi-experimental design*. An example is a school study for lowering fat in children's diets (a primordial prevention question) with two intervention and two comparison schools where assignment was made by the investigator.[34] Although substantially better than not having any control, the quasi-experimental design suffers from some of the same problems as nonrandomized studies of individuals, in that various important characteristics may not be balanced between intervention and control groups. Whether they are used for primordial, primary, or secondary prevention studies, preintervention-to-postintervention and quasi-experimental designs do not eliminate selection bias, secular changes, or confounding due to uncontrolled variables. Such studies, however, can be used to determine the feasibility of an intervention for primordial or primary prevention or to determine the side effects or dose of treatment for secondary prevention. A randomized, controlled trial could be conducted subsequently to provide a more definitive determination of the effect of intervention on outcome.

OUTCOMES

The outcomes to be measured in any trial are directly linked to the research question being posed. Outcomes in trials of primordial or primary prevention often are the amount of change in a lifestyle behavior, a risk factor, or an intermediate or surrogate measure of disease. A surrogate measure may be a noninvasive assessment of subclinical disease, for example, assessment of atherosclerosis by carotid ultrasonography or some other measure of the disease process that would be a surrogate for a clinical outcome. Although changes in behaviors, risk factors, or disease measures are most commonly operationalized as average levels at the end of intervention (usually the least demanding choice for sample size), the rate of crossing a threshold value may better fit the idea of prevention and may also conform to clinical or pathophysiologic concepts, for example, hypertension or a critical arterial stenosis. The notion of slowing a disease process may be best satisfied by a measure of rate of change, although if change is not linear, such a rate may be difficult to define from multiple measurement during follow-up. Unless the trial is very large and long, the measurement of a clinical outcome (e.g., disease morbidity or mortality) in a primordial prevention trial usually is not feasible, because an insufficient number of clinical events will occur over the duration of the trial.

A trial of a primary prevention in a high-risk population or of secondary prevention may use surrogate disease endpoints but will more often have as its primary question whether a major clinical event, such as an acute MI or death, will be reduced by the intervention to be tested. Thus, the outcomes for primary prevention and secondary prevention trials are often disease incidence or recurrence, acute events (such as MI), or mortality.

All clinical trials have, in addition to the primary outcome, one or more secondary outcomes. These secondary outcomes will be similar in character to the primary outcomes for all types of trials but are usually not used to determine sample size or power. Quality of life as an outcome is useful in all kinds of trials, and all trials also examine, to a greater or lesser extent, adverse effects of the interventions being tested. Adverse effects are perhaps less likely when the intervention is a change in lifestyle, but impairment of quality of life with such interventions may be considered an important adverse effect to detect.

For primordial prevention trials, one is less tolerant of adverse effects of an intervention than one would be for secondary prevention, or even primary prevention high-risk trials. Caution is needed to ensure that healthy people are not harmed in an effort to prevent a possible future disease or condition. Lifestyle change is generally believed to be relatively harmless, except perhaps for some decrease in quality of life, and therefore is readily accepted as a possible primordial or primary prevention intervention. There are theoretical exceptions, such as risk of musculoskeletal injury from an exercise program or risk of delayed growth and development from a dietary intervention. In contrast, drug treatment for any type of prevention carries risks. Even drugs such as aspirin may not be worth testing for primordial prevention in those at low risk of developing heart disease in the short or medium term. One of the reasons for the controversy over the trial of tamoxifen in women at high risk of developing breast cancer is the expectation that tamoxifen will increase the risk of endometrial cancer and thromboembolic events. These risks might be acceptable in women with diagnosed breast cancer but may raise ethical questions about studying tamoxifen in women who, although at high risk of developing breast cancer, do not yet have it.[35] This debate is relevant to cardiovascular disease as well, because tamoxifen has been reported to reduce low-density lipoprotein cholesterol levels and ischemic heart disease.[36, 37]

SETTINGS AND POPULATIONS

The settings and participant enrollment strategies may be quite different for primordial, primary, or secondary prevention trials. Primordial prevention trials are generally conducted in community settings such as schools or worksites. Primary prevention trials can be conducted in medical facilities, for example, smoking cessation in pregnant women,[38, 39] but also have been conducted in communities or in community settings. Medical settings such as inpatient facilities, whether general medical or surgical units, or special units, such as emergency departments, operating rooms, or coronary care units, would almost always be used for identifying participants for and conducting secondary prevention trials. Primary or secondary prevention trials also could be implemented in outpatient facilities or physicians' offices. In the era of managed care with its controls on use of specialized services, such settings are becoming increasingly important.

Mass recruitment approaches should be helpful in both primordial and secondary prevention trials but may be less so for primary prevention trials in high-risk populations. For primordial prevention trials, mass mailings and mass media may be used effectively to encourage large numbers of potentially eligible participants to contact the study investigator. For secondary prevention trials, most people will know if they have had an MI or been otherwise diagnosed with heart disease. However, for primary prevention trials in high-risk participants, most of the respondents to mass media or mailings may be incorrect or unknowledgeable about their risk factor status, such as blood pressure or cholesterol levels, diabetes, or even family history. One exception is cigarette smoking as a risk factor. Nevertheless, even in primary prevention trials mass recruitment is effective at inducing large numbers of people to present themselves for in-person or telephone screening.

In clinical settings, potential participants are identified by record or chart review, by examining lists of patients who have undergone special procedures (surgical or diagnostic), or by referrals from physicians and other health care providers. Trials of high-risk participants could also identify people through community risk factor screening activities such as at health fairs, worksites, apartment complexes, churches, or other areas where large numbers of people live, work, or congregate.

All three types of prevention trials require specific eligibility criteria for including participants in the study. Criteria are usually specified by defining both inclusion and exclusion criteria. In all cases, the eligibility criteria must create a study population that is relevant to the primary research question in terms of age, gender, and other characteristics. Eligibility criteria for primordial prevention trials are usually much broader than for primary and secondary prevention trials. For example, a primordial prevention trial may target all children in a school, so that the only eligibility is childhood age and that the child attends a particular school. In contrast, a primary prevention trial would require knowledge of an individual's risk factor status and so would require, for example, blood cholesterol or blood pressure levels that indicate a high-risk condition; the specific cutpoints for cholesterol and blood pressure and the method of measurement would need to be specified. A primary prevention trial also would exclude someone with diagnosed disease, for example, CHD, because it is not possible to prevent a condition that already exists. A secondary prevention trial, by definition, requires that the clinical disease be present, so eligibility must contain the criteria by which one determines presence of disease. For example, self-reported prior MI may be sufficient, or confirmed acute cardiac ischemia by electrocardiographic tracing may be required.

The size of the study and the complexity of the eligibility criteria are not so much a function of whether the trial is primordial, primary, or secondary prevention, as they are a function of the primary question and the intervention being tested. For example, a primary prevention trial can be extremely large, with a simple intervention (e.g., aspirin), and broad eligibility criteria (e.g., no clinical evidence of heart disease, no indications for or contraindications to aspirin). On the other hand, it can be small, with a complicated intervention (e.g., a specially prepared diet given in a metabolic unit) and narrow eligibility criteria (e.g., a willingness to eat a specially prepared diet and no other food for some weeks). Similarly, a secondary prevention trial may be extremely large, with a simple intervention (aspirin), and broad eligibility criteria (physician's impression that the patient is suffering an acute MI). Alternately, a secondary prevention trial can be small, with an intervention requiring special training and experience (e.g., ablation of arrhythmia focus) and highly specific eligibility criteria (specified rhythm disturbance, resistance to pharmacologic therapy).

DURATION, EFFICACY, AND EFFECTIVENESS

The duration of a trial, and therefore the problem of maintaining participant involvement and adherence to the protocol, is not dependent on whether it is for primordial, primary, or secondary prevention. Depending on the nature of the question and intervention, primordial, primary, and secondary prevention trials all may be either short or long. If the outcome of interest is a clinical event, the primary prevention trial will be much larger and longer than the secondary prevention trial to accrue enough events for sufficient statistical power. In such a situation, the primary prevention trial may have more of a problem with competing risk. For example, in a primary prevention trial for cardiovascular disease a greater proportion of the overall events may be noncardiovascular than in a secondary prevention trial in patients with acute MI. This competing risk may affect the ascertainment of the primary outcomes of interest.

A distinction between studies of efficacy and effectiveness is sometimes made. An efficacy trial is one where a well-controlled intervention is assessed under optimal circumstances with high compliance to ask how beneficial (or harmful) is the regimen (or diet or behavior) itself. An effectiveness trial is conducted in more generalizable circumstances and assumes that a certain proportion of the participants will not adhere to the regimen, either by failing to take the intervention as prescribed, or, if in the control group, starting to take the intervention. Thus, an effectiveness trial more truly reflects a "real life" situation. Only reasonably short studies can be done as efficacy trials because of the problem with long-term compliance with interventions in longer studies.

Primordial, primary, or secondary prevention interventions can be tested either for efficacy or for effectiveness. For example, the Dietary Approaches to Stop

Hypertension (DASH) study tested the efficacy of two dietary patterns compared with a reference diet in reducing elevated blood pressure.[40] All the food was provided to the participants, so the actual dietary intake has a high compliance for the patterns being tested. If the same dietary patterns were to be tested for effectiveness, dietary education would be delivered in a more typical situation, and the effect of the diet would be a function of both the diet itself and the compliance with the diet. If the outcome is a clinical event, efficacy assessment is more feasible in a secondary prevention trial than a primary prevention trial. Since the high compliance necessary for an efficacy assessment may be reasonable only over the short term, participants with relatively high event rates are required, which usually are persons with existing disease.

STUDY MANAGEMENT AND MONITORING

As with study design, study management and monitoring depend more on the nature of the intervention and outcome than on whether the study is one of primordial, primary, or secondary prevention. If the intervention is easy to perform and the outcome is simple to assess, quality monitoring and assurance is not as extensive, regardless of the population being studied. When the intervention is more complex, however, quality assurance of intervention delivery is important, no matter what size or type of study. For example, a small primordial prevention trial of exercise, with the outcome being long-term change in physical function, may require the same degree of quality assurance as a small secondary prevention trial of coronary artery stents for long-term vessel patency. Not only are the procedures of comparable complexity, so may also be the forms and assessment of adverse effects. Monitoring of adherence to the intervention and the protocol, on the part of the participants, is also more similar than different, as long as the study sizes are similar and interventions are of similar complexity. A large, multicenter, primary prevention trial of aspirin with cardiovascular mortality as the outcome requires the same adherence assessment as a large, multicenter, secondary prevention trial of angiotensin-converting enzyme inhibitors with either total mortality or cardiovascular mortality as the outcome.

One possible difference in monitoring is that in primordial or primary prevention trials, the intervention may be more available to the control group, because it consists of either lifestyle change or use of a drug that is readily obtained, such as aspirin. Furthermore, compliance with lifestyle changes on the part of the intervention group may not be high. Therefore, primary prevention trials may be more likely to have crossovers, that is, intervention participants not receiving the intervention and control participants receiving the intervention. In secondary prevention trials of physician-prescribed interventions, clinical decisions can also lead to large crossover rates, such as in medical treatment versus coronary artery bypass graft surgery.[41]

Crossover rates do need to be carefully monitored, because if they are large, they can reduce the observed effect size and therefore the likelihood of detecting a significant effect.

As noted earlier, data monitoring may be considerably different in primordial, primary, and secondary prevention trials. In primordial prevention trials, one is less likely to accept serious or even bothersome adverse effects as the possible price of benefit. Not only does the likelihood of adverse events affect the choice of intervention, it means that if adverse trends emerge in the accumulating data, one is more apt to stop the study before its planned end. One might be willing to continue longer a study of high-risk patients, but not as long as a secondary prevention trial. Even in secondary prevention trials, there may be gradations, depending on the severity of the condition being studied. For example, one would be willing to accept a fair amount of adverse events in the hope of improving duration or quality of life if testing an intervention in people with advanced heart failure, as opposed to a trial in patients with stable CHD.

These monitoring concepts are often built into the formal stopping guidelines of a trial. In primordial and primary prevention trials, the statistical boundaries for deciding if benefit or harm has been demonstrated may be asymmetric. That is, it would require more evidence to declare an intervention beneficial than harmful, with respect to the primary outcome. Even secondary prevention trials may employ asymmetric monitoring boundaries, but if the condition being studied is serious, one may be willing to continue the trial even in the face of a strong adverse trend in the data, in the hope that the trend may change with the accumulation of additional data.

ANALYSIS AND INTERPRETATION

For analysis and interpretation of results of the typical trial, where individuals are the unit of randomization, there are no important differences between primordial, primary, and secondary prevention studies. In all cases, the magnitude of effect one wishes to detect should be identified before the study begins based on the main research question of the study, and the magnitude of effect should be relevant either clinically or to public health.

As noted earlier, some trials, generally but not exclusively in primordial or primary prevention, employ group allocation. The analysis of such studies should take design effects into consideration, that is, the level of correlation between individuals within each unit randomized. The CATCH study, for example, used a two-stage analysis that took into account both the individual and school-level variance.[2] Trials sometimes use outcomes that yield more than one measure per randomized participant. An example is assessment of coronary artery lesion progression or regression. It may be important to assess more than one area of narrowing or a global evaluation of all coronary arteries. Because the lesions in an individual are not independent, it is inappropriate simply to count the total number of progressions or regressions, for example. Statistical techniques allow one to take into account in the analysis the degree of dependence among the lesions.[42] This is a similar analysis issue for group allocation, as mentioned earlier, where correlations among individuals in each unit are likely to be present.

SUMMARY

Most of the design, management, and analysis features are common to all trials, whether they are primordial, primary, or secondary prevention types. Differences are more often a matter of degree than of kind. In all trials, the major issues are driven by the primary question posed. The study design best employed in all three types is the randomized, controlled trial. Even in primordial or primary prevention trials of whole communities, a randomized design is preferred. In all trials, eligibility criteria must be explicit. Primordial prevention trials often require recruitment methods that reach out to whole communities to recruit individuals or recruit entire communities for more broad-based interventions. Primary and secondary prevention trials, on the other hand, often recruit patients in clinical settings. All three types of trials could vary in duration and complexity of the intervention being tested. Primordial and primary prevention trials address questions of low-risk interventions and their effects on precursors or early manifestations of disease. Data monitoring for safety varies depending on the risk for adverse effects of the intervention being tested. Analysis methods are similar in that all randomized participants or groups should be analyzed according to the group (intervention or control) to which they are assigned.

REFERENCES

1. Expert Committee, Prevention in Childhood and Youth of Adult Cardiovascular Diseases. Time for Action: Report of a WHO Expert Committee, Technical Report Series No. 792. Geneva, World Health Organization, 1990.
2. Luepker RV, Perry CL, McKinlay SM, et al. Outcomes of a field trial to improve children's dietary patterns and physical activity: The Child and Adolescent Trial for Cardiovascular Health—CATCH Collaborative Group. JAMA 1996; 275:768–776.
3. Hypertension Detection and Follow-up Program Cooperative Group. Five-year findings of the hypertension detection and follow-up program: I. Reduction in mortality of persons with high blood pressure, including mild hypertension. JAMA 1979; 242:2562–2571.
4. Anonymous. Effect of stepped-care treatment on the incidence of myocardial infarction and angina pectoris: Five-year findings of the Hypertension Detection and Follow-Up Program. Hypertension 1984; 6(2 Pt 2):I198–I206.
5. SHEP Cooperative Research Group: Prevention of stroke by antihypertensive drug treatment in older persons with isolated systolic hypertension: Final results of the Systolic Hypertension in the Elderly Program (SHEP). JAMA 1991; 265:3255–3264.
6. Lipid Research Clinics Coronary Primary Prevention Trial. The Lipid Research Clinics Coronary Primary Prevention Trial results: I. Reduction in incidence of coronary heart disease. JAMA 1984; 251:351–364.
7. Lipid Research Clinics Coronary Primary Prevention Trial. The Lipid Research Clinics Coronary Primary Prevention Trial results: II. The relationship of reduction in incidence of coronary heart disease to cholesterol lowering. JAMA 1984; 251:365–374.
8. Rose G, Hamilton PJ, Colwell L, et al. A randomised, controlled trial of antismoking advice: Ten-year results. J Epidemiol Community Health 1982; 36:102–108.
9. Rose G, Colwell L. Randomised, controlled trial of antismoking advice: Final (20-year) results. J Epidemiol Community Health 1992; 46:75–77.
10. Multiple Risk Factor Intervention Trial Research Group. Multiple risk factor intervention trial: Risk factor changes and mortality results. JAMA 1982; 248:1465–1477.
11. Multiple Risk Factor Intervention Trial Research Group. Mortality after 16 years for participants randomized to the Multiple Risk Factor Intervention Trial. Circulation 1996; 94:946–951.
12. Jacobs DR, Luepker RV, Mittelmark MB, et al. Community-wide prevention strategies: Evaluation design of the Minnesota Heart Health Program. J Chronic Dis 1986; 39:775–788.
13. Luepker RV, Murray DM, Jacobs DR, et al. Community education for cardiovascular disease prevention: Risk factor changes in the Minnesota Heart Health Program. Am J Public Health 1994; 84:1383–1393.
14. Farquhar JW, Fortmann SP, Maccoby N, et al. The Stanford Five-City Project: Design and methods. Am J Epidemiol 1985; 122:323–334.
15. Farquhar JW, Fortmann SP, Flora JA, et al: Effects of community-wide education on cardiovascular disease risk factors: The Stanford Five-City Project. JAMA 1990; 264:359–365.
16. Carleton RA, Lasater TM, Assaf A, et al. The Pawtucket Heart Health Program: I. An experiment in population-based disease prevention. RI Med J 1987; 70:533–538.
17. Carleton RA, Lasater TM, Assaf A, et al. The Pawtucket Heart Health Program: Community changes in cardiovascular risk factors and projected disease risk. Am J Public Health 1995; 85:777–785.
18. Canner PL, Klimt CR. The coronary drug project: Experimental design features. Control Clin Trials 1983; 4:313–332.
19. Canner PL, Berge KG, Wenger NK, et al. Fifteen-year mortality in coronary drug project patients: Long-term benefit with niacin. J Am Coll Cardiol 1986; 8:1245–1255.
20. The Scandinavian Simvastatin Survival Study Group. Design and baseline results of the Scandinavian simvastatin survival study of patients with stable angina and/or previous myocardial infarction. Am J Cardiol 1993; 71:393–400.
21. The Scandinavian Simvastatin Survival Study Group. Randomised trial of cholesterol lowering in 4444 patients with coronary heart disease: the Scandinavian simvastatin survival study (4S). Lancet 1994; 344:1383–1389.
22. Yusuf S, Peto R, Lewis J, et al. Beta blockade during and after myocardial infarction: An overview of the randomized trials. Prog Cardiovasc Dis 1985; 27:335–371.

23. Yusuf S, Collins R, Peto R, et al. Intravenous and intracoronary fibrinolytic therapy in acute myocardial infarction: Overview of results on mortality, reinfarction, and side effects from 33 randomized controlled trials. Eur Heart J 1985; 6:556–585.
24. Gruppo Italiano per lo Studio della Streptochinasi nell'Infarto Miocardico. Effectiveness of intravenous thrombolytic treatment in acute myocardial infarction: Gruppo Italiano per lo Studio della Streptochinasi nell'Infarto Miocardico (GISSI). Lancet 1986; 1:397–402.
25. ISIS-2 (Second International Study of Infarct Survival Collaborative Group). Randomized trial of intravenous streptokinase, oral aspirin, both, or neither among 17,187 cases of suspected acute myocardial infarction: ISIS-2. J Am Coll Cardiol 1988; 12(6 Suppl A):3A–13A.
26. Garg R, Yusuf S. Overview of randomized trials of angiotensin-converting enzyme inhibitors on mortality and morbidity in patients with heart failure: Collaborative group on ACE inhibitor trials. JAMA 1995; 273:1450–1456.
27. Glasgow RE, Terborg JR, Hollis JF, et al. Take heart: Results from the initial phase of a work-site wellness program. Am J Public Health 1995; 85:209–216.
28. Ammerman A, Caggiula A, Elmer PJ, et al. Putting medical practice guidelines into practice: The cholesterol model. Am J Prev Med 1994; 10:209–216.
29. The COMMIT Research Group. Community Intervention Trial for smoking cessation (COMMIT): II. Changes in adult cigarette smoking prevalence. Am J Public Health 1995; 85:193–200.
30. The COMMIT Research Group. Community Intervention Trial for smoking cessation (COMMIT): I. Cohort results from a four-year community intervention. Am J Public Health 1995; 85:183–192.
31. Hsieh FY. Sample size formulae for intervention studies with the cluster as unit of randomization. Stat Med 1988; 7:1195–1201.
32. Martin DC, Diehr P, Perrin EB, et al. The effect of matching on the power of randomized community intervention studies. Stat Med 1993; 12:329–338.
33. Blohm M, Herlitz J, Hartford M, et al. Consequences of a media campaign focusing on delay in acute myocardial infarction. Am J Cardiol 1992; 69:411–413.
34. Simons-Morton BG, Parcel GS, Baranowski T, et al. Promoting physical activity and a healthful diet among children: Results of a school-based intervention study. Am J Public Health 1991; 81:986–991.
35. Bush TL, Helzlsouer KJ. Tamoxifen for the primary prevention of breast cancer: A review and critique of the concept and trial. Epidemiol Rev 1993; 15:233–243.
36. Bagdade JD, Wolter J, Subbaiah PV, et al. Effects of tamoxifen treatment on plasma lipids and lipoprotein lipid composition. J Clin Endocrinol Metab 1990; 70:1132–1135.
37. McDonald CC, Alexander FE, Whyte BW, et al. Cardiac and vascular morbidity in women receiving adjuvant tamoxifen for breast cancer in a randomized trial: The Scottish Cancer Trials Breast Group. BMJ 1995; 311:977–980.
38. Ershoff DH, Mullen PD, Quinn VP. A randomized trial of a serialized self-help smoking cessation program for pregnant women in an HMO. Am J Public Health 1989; 79:182–187.
39. Mayer JP, Hawkins B, Todd R. A randomized evaluation of smoking cessation interventions for pregnant women at a WIC clinic. Am J Public Health 1990; 80:76–78.
40. Appel LJ, Moore TJ, Obarzanek E, et al. A clinical trial of the effects of dietary patterns on blood pressure. N Engl J Med 1997; 336:1117–1124.
41. Yusuf S, Zucker D, Peduzzi P, et al. Effect of coronary artery bypass graft surgery on survival: Overview of 10-year results from randomised trials by the Coronary Artery Bypass Graft Surgery Trialists Collaboration. Lancet 1994; 344:563–570.
42. Kelsey SF. Strategies for statistical analysis of angiographic data: Individual lesions versus individual patients. *In* Glagov S, Newman WP, Schaffer SA (eds). Pathobiology of the Human Atherosclerotic Plaque. New York, Springer-Verlag, 1990, pp 525–533.

4 Large-Scale Randomized Trials

▶ Colin Baigent
▶ Rory Collins
▶ Richard Peto

NEED TO ASSESS *MODERATE* DIFFERENCES IN OUTCOME

If a widely practicable treatment can achieve just a moderate reduction in a common cause of premature death or of serious disability, reliable recognition of this could prevent much suffering. Consider, for example, aspirin, which is cheap, practicable, and widely available and provides just a moderate degree of protection against recurrence in people with a previous history of myocardial infarction (MI) or occlusive stroke[1] (with a moderate but definite additional benefit if treatment starts as soon as the diagnosis is made[2–4]). Worldwide, there are more than 10 million deaths each year from MI or stroke,[5] plus a comparable number of nonfatal (but often seriously disabling) episodes, and appropriately widespread use of aspirin for the treatment and secondary prevention of vascular disease could well avoid more than 100,000 premature deaths annually. This is obviously important, but it is the type of moderate benefit that may be reliably demonstrable only by large-scale randomized evidence.

Similarly, congestive heart failure is an important cause of mortality and of progressive disability, with much suffering and with the substantial costs of recurrent hospitalization. Converting-enzyme inhibitors produce moderate (but, in large trials, definite) reductions in the risk of death and in the rates of hospitalization for worsening heart failure,[6] and the addition of digoxin further reduces the need for recurrent hospitalization.[7] Hence, the appropriately widespread use of these two treatments would make a significant additional contribution to the management of cardiovascular disease worldwide, but again the benefits for individuals are only moderate, and hence have been long disputed.

Conversely, if a widely used treatment has no material effect on fatal or seriously disabling outcomes (or if an easy, inexpensive treatment is about as good as a more complex one), then reliable demonstration of this could avoid a lot of trouble, toxicity, and expense in future medical practice. Thus, clinical research into the avoidance of major outcomes needs to be able to distinguish reliably between a moderate benefit, a moderate hazard, and a negligible difference in such outcomes. Research of this type is particularly important because moderate benefits may quite commonly await discovery. By contrast, large differences in major outcomes are rarely encountered—indeed, when unusually large treatment effects are claimed, they often turn out to have been substantially inflated by the play of chance or by various biases.[8] Clinical research strategies should, therefore, not be distorted by unrealistic hopes.

The need to be able to recognize moderate differences in the major outcomes that are of most relevance to patients (e.g., dead/alive; disabled/not disabled) leads, in many instances, to the need for large-scale randomized evidence and for appropriate analysis of it once it has been generated. The reasons are obvious[8–11]: nonrandomized methods cannot generally guarantee the avoidance of moderate biases; small-scale studies cannot guarantee the avoidance of moderate distortion by the play of chance; and even when large-scale randomized evidence is available, either in one or two mega-trials or in a large "meta-analysis" (see later) of many smaller trials, serious distortions can be introduced by inappropriate analysis of it—especially if this involves unduly data-dependent emphasis on particular parts of the evidence (e.g., on particular trials or on particular subgroups of the patients).

HOW LARGE A REDUCTION IN THE RISK OF A MAJOR OUTCOME WOULD BE PLAUSIBLE?

Enthusiasm for the biologic foundations of a particular therapeutic approach often leads to exaggerated hopes for the effects of treatment on major clinical outcomes. These hopes may be based on dramatic laboratory measures of efficacy or on the types of surrogate outcomes that are commonly studied before drugs go into Phase III or IV studies: for example, a drug may virtually completely inhibit an important enzyme, prevent experimental ischemia progressing to infarction, or practically abolish experimental thrombosis. But, only rarely do these large effects on surrogate endpoints translate into large effects on major clinical outcomes, and many of the important recent improvements in outcome in the major cardiovascular diseases have been only moderate in size. Proportional reductions of only about 10% or 20% in major outcomes are, therefore, the most that should generally be anticipated when planning Phase III or IV trials in cardiovascular disease. Studies of the effects of treatments on major outcomes should often start with the premise that any risk reductions are unlikely to be large, but that even a moderate risk reduction would be worthwhile. Thus, although it may be appropriate to design a trial to see whether 12% mortality can be reduced to 10% mortality (a reduction of one sixth in the risk of death), it might well be unwise to design a trial to see whether 12% can be reduced to 6% mortality. For, proportional reductions of 50% in the major outcomes of interest* are often implausible.

TABLE 4–1 • Requirements for Reliable Assessment of *Moderate* Treatment Effects[8]

Negligible Biases: Guaranteed Avoidance of *Moderate* Biases

Proper *randomization* (nonrandomized methods cannot guarantee the avoidance of moderate biases)
Analysis by *allocated* treatments (i.e., an "intention-to-treat" analysis)
Chief emphasis on *overall* results (with no unduly data-derived subgroup analyses)
Systematic *meta-analysis* of all the relevant randomized trials (with no unduly data-dependent emphasis on the results from particular studies)

Small Random Errors: Guaranteed Avoidance of *Moderate* Random Errors

Large numbers (with minimal data collection because detailed statistical analyses of masses of data on prognostic features generally add little to the effective size of a trial)
Systematic *meta-analysis* of all the relevant randomized trials

FUNDAMENTAL REQUIREMENT FOR RELIABLE ASSESSMENT OF MODERATE TREATMENT EFFECTS

Any clinical study whose main objective is to assess moderate treatment effects must ensure that any biases and any random errors that are inherent in its design are *both* substantially smaller than the effect that is to be measured. This requirement limits the range of study designs that can be informative (Table 4–1).[8]

Negligible Biases

If moderate differences are to be assessed, the study design must guarantee the exclusion of moderate biases, and this generally requires appropriate analysis of properly randomized evidence. For, if the allocation of treatment is not properly randomized, characteristics of the disease (or of the patient) that affect the prognosis may also affect the choice of treatment. For example, patients with acute MI whose physicians choose to use thrombolytic therapy may differ systematically from those whose physicians choose not to. Such pre-existing differences could well bias a nonrandomized study of thrombolysis. It may well be difficult or impossible to avoid such biases or to adjust fully for their effects. Therefore, even if nonrandomized comparisons happen to get the right answer, nobody will really know that they have done so, unless the difference in outcome is extraordinarily large (or the outcome is one that could not plausibly be associated with those aspects of the disease that might influence the choice of treatment). Thus, because nonrandomized study designs cannot generally be guaranteed to exclude moderate biases, they are of little practical value if the primary aim is to assess moderate treatment effects (whether beneficial or adverse) on major outcomes.[12]

Even when studies have been properly randomized and well conducted, moderate biases can still be introduced by inappropriate analysis or interpretation. One well-recognized circumstance is when patients are excluded after randomization, particularly when the prognosis of the excluded patients in one treatment group differs from that in the other (such as might occur, for example, if noncompliers were excluded after randomization). If there is, in reality, virtually no difference in outcome between two treatments, then the least-biased assessment of the treatment effect is that which compares all those allocated to one treatment versus all those allocated to the other (i.e., an "intention-to-treat" analysis), irrespective of what treatment they actually received.[9] Thus, whether analyzing just one trial or undertaking a meta-analysis of many smaller randomized trials, it is generally best to avoid postrandomization withdrawals in the main analysis.

*For rare side effects, however, there may be large proportional differences between one treatment and another, or between treatment and control. For example, some nonsteroidal anti-inflammatory drugs may substantially increase the risk of gastrointestinal bleeding. Rare side effects with extreme relative risks can often be recognized reliably by careful clinical observation or by other nonrandomized methods, and such relative risks are sometimes best quantified in case-control or cohort studies that are designed and analyzed appropriately.

In the current medical literature (and at many medical conferences) a particularly important source of bias is unduly data-dependent emphasis on particular trials or on particular subgroups of patients. Such emphasis is often entirely inadvertent, arising from a perfectly reasonable desire to understand the randomized trial results in terms of exactly who to treat, exactly which treatments to prefer, or disease mechanisms. But, whatever its origins, unduly selective emphasis on particular parts of the evidence can often lead to seriously misleading conclusions. This is because reliable identification of categories of patients for whom treatment is particularly effective (or ineffective) requires surprisingly large quantities of data. Even if the real sizes of the effects of treatment do vary substantially among subgroups of patients, subgroup analyses are so statistically insensitive that they may well fail to demonstrate these differences. On the other hand, if the real proportional risk reductions are about the same for everybody, subgroup analyses can vary so widely just by the play of chance that the results in selected subgroups may be exaggerated. Consequently, even when highly significant "interactions" are found, they may be a poor guide to the sizes (or even the directions) of any genuine differences in the proportional improvements in particular outcomes among specific categories of patients, as the more extreme such results may still owe more to the play of chance than to reality. This is particularly the case when such interactions have emerged after an overzealous examination of multiple subgroups. Despite these difficulties such subgroup analyses still get widely reported, and widely believed, in ways that may lead to the inappropriate management of hundreds of thousands of patients.

An example of the potential for subgroup analyses to mislead is provided by the large Italian Gruppo Italiano per lo Studio della Streptochinasi nell'Infarto Miocardico (GISSI)-1 Trial comparing streptokinase versus control after acute MI. The overall results favored streptokinase, but in retrospective subgroup analyses streptokinase appeared to be beneficial only among patients without prior MI. Fortunately, the GISSI investigators were circumspect about this "finding,"[13] and their caution turned out to have been wise, since a subsequent overview of all the large fibrinolytic trials showed that the benefits were similar irrespective of a history of MI.[14] Many thousands of patients with a previous history of MI might well have been denied fibrinolytic therapy, however, if the apparent pattern of the results in the GISSI-1 subgroups had been believed.

A converse example is provided by the early results on the use of aspirin to prevent the recurrence of occlusive cerebrovascular disease, where inappropriate emphasis on the results in one sex only led to a situation where, for almost 20 years, the U.S. Food and Drug Administration approved the use of aspirin in transient cerebral ischemia only for men; more recent evidence shows this to have been mistaken.[1] In general it is preferable to emphasize the overall results of trials and to regard the results of subgroup analyses with healthy skepticism. (For further discussion of this key issue, see Reference 8, or see the analyses of the Second International Study of Infarct Survival [ISIS-2][2] that, if interpreted incautiously, would have indicated that aspirin works only for patients with acute MI who were not born under the astrologic star signs of Libra or Gemini!)

Such examples also reinforce the importance of considering *all* the randomized evidence relating to the effects of a given treatment on major outcomes, preferably within a thorough meta-analysis. Appropriate meta-analyses help to avoid unduly data-dependent emphasis on especially striking results within particular trials and, hence, to provide a better guide to the true effects of treatments. Occasionally, when detailed information on individual patients is available within a really large meta-analysis that includes several thousand major outcomes, such as death[14] or cancer recurrence,[15] it may be feasible to identify particular groups of patients in whom the benefits or hazards of treatment really are especially great. (Where it has been possible to establish cooperation between trialists before any of the trial results are known, having just a few prespecified subgroup hypotheses can provide some protection against unduly data-dependent emphasis on particular results in a large meta-analysis.[16]) More commonly, however, even a meta-analysis of all the trials in the world is too small for reliable subgroup analyses. Indeed, in many meta-analyses the total number of randomized patients is too small for even the main analyses to be statistically reliable, let alone the analyses of subgroups (see later).

Small Random Errors

Although avoidance of moderate biases chiefly requires careful attention both to the randomization process and to the analysis and interpretation of the available trial evidence, the avoidance of moderate random errors chiefly requires large numbers of events. Since major outcomes such as death may affect only a small proportion of those randomized, very large numbers of patients often need to be studied before the results can be guaranteed to be statistically (and hence medically) convincing. To observe thousands of deaths, tens of thousands of patients may need to have been randomized, and such large-scale evidence is difficult to organize. For many therapeutic questions, the scale of randomized evidence that is necessary for the assessment of major outcomes may well not yet be available even through a meta-analysis of all of the completed randomized trials in the world. In that instance, the key need is to find some practicable way of generating new trials that provide really large-scale evidence.

Randomized trials of the treatment of vascular disease have become larger in recent years, but still the numbers randomized rarely exceed a few thousand patients. Even though such trials may seem "large" to those who do the hard work, they may still not be large enough. Consider, for example, a widely practicable treatment among patients with acute MI that reduces inhospital mortality from 10% to 8%. If just 1 million out of the 10 million such cases that occur annually were to be treated, this would prevent about 20,000 deaths a year, which would be a substantial achievement. However, such benefits would be surprisingly easy to miss: if, for example, just 2000 patients were to be randomized, 1000 to active treatment and 1000 to control, then about 80 deaths would be expected in the active group and 100 in the control group. Even if exactly this result was to be seen, it would not be conventionally significant ($2P > 0.1$)—and, by chance alone, the results from such a trial might well be about 90 versus 90 deaths instead of about 80 versus 100, misleadingly suggesting the treatment to be completely useless. After randomizing 2000 patients, therefore, the real effects of this particular treatment might remain unclear.[8] Instead, what is needed in this case is to randomize 20,000 patients: this would allow the clear demonstration of a 20% reduction with about 800 treated and 1000 control deaths ($2P < 0.0001$); and somewhat smaller benefits, which might still be worthwhile, could also be detected.

RANDOMIZED TRIALS CAN BE LARGE IF THEY ARE KEPT SIMPLE

If trials of the effects of treatments on major outcomes are to become substantially larger, then as many as possible of the main barriers to rapid recruitment need to be removed. One of the most effective ways to guarantee the recruitment of small numbers of patients is to burden busy clinicians with obtaining large amounts of information. The information that really needs to be recorded at entry can often be surprisingly brief and should concentrate on those few clinical details that are of paramount importance (including at most only a few major prognostic factors and only a few variables that are believed likely to influence substantially the benefits or hazards of treatment). Similarly, the information recorded at follow-up need not be extensive and can be limited largely to those major outcomes that such studies have been designed to assess and to approximate measures of compliance. (Other outcomes that are of interest but do not need to be studied on such a large scale may best be assessed in separate smaller studies or in subsets of these large studies when this is practicable.) Likewise, complicated eligibility criteria, inappropriately detailed consent procedures,[17] and unnecessarily extensive auditing of data all can deter physicians from entering large numbers of patients into studies. Furthermore, if trials are complex, they are likely to involve a high cost per patient, which again tends to limit their size.

Complexity is rarely a virtue in trials designed to assess major outcomes, whereas extreme simplicity can sometimes lead to the rapid randomization of large numbers of patients and to results that may lead to appropriate worldwide changes in practice within short periods.[2, 19] Thus, in clinical trial design, less information per patient may mean much better science.

THE "UNCERTAINTY PRINCIPLE": ETHICALITY, HETEROGENEITY, AND MAXIMAL SAMPLE SIZE

For ethical reasons, randomization is appropriate only if both the physician and, to the extent that they are part of the process of determining which treatments to use, the patient feel substantially uncertain as to which trial treatment is best. The "uncertainty principle" maximizes the potential for recruitment within this ethical constraint (see Box).

The "Uncertainty Principle"

- A patient can be entered in a randomized trial if, and only if, the responsible physician is substantially uncertain as to which of the trial treatments would be most appropriate for that particular patient.
- A patient should not be entered if the responsible physician, or the patient, is for any medical or nonmedical reasons reasonably certain that one of the treatments that might be allocated would be inappropriate for that particular patient (either in comparison with no treatment or in comparison with some other treatment that could be offered to the patient in or outside the trial).[18]

If many hospitals are collaborating in a trial, wholehearted use of the uncertainty principle encourages clinically appropriate heterogeneity in the resulting trial population, and this, in large trials, may add substantially to the practical value of the results. Among the early trials of fibrinolytic therapy, for example, most of the studies had restrictive trial entry criteria that precluded the randomization of elderly patients, so those trials contributed nothing of direct relevance to the important clinical question of whether treatment was useful among older patients. Other trials that did not impose an upper age limit, however, did include some elderly patients, and were therefore able to show that age alone is not a contraindication to fibrinolytic therapy.[14] Similarly, exclusion from the earlier fibrinolytic trials of patients presenting more than a few hours after the onset of the symptoms of MI delayed the emergence of clear evidence that such treatment is beneficial for most of the patients presenting up to at least 12 hours from symptom onset.[14] Thus, homogeneity of those randomized may be a serious defect in clinical trial design, whereas heterogeneity may be a scientific strength; after all, trials do need to be relevant to a heterogeneous collection of future patients.

The uncertainty principle not only ensures ethicality and clinically useful heterogeneity but also is easily understood and remembered by busy collaborating clinicians, which in turn helps the randomization of large numbers of patients. There is scope, therefore, for many more trials to adopt this as the fundamental principle that determines who is eligible.

CAN ALTERNATIVE STUDY DESIGNS SUBSTITUTE FOR LARGE-SCALE RANDOMIZED EVIDENCE?

As the resources will never be available to design large, simple trials to address all the questions of clinical interest, it is reasonable to ask whether there are circumstances when it might be possible to circumvent the need for large trials, either by using routinely collected observational data (sometimes referred to as *outcomes research*) or perhaps by analyzing previously published randomized trials (within meta-analyses).

Outcomes Research

Outcomes research means various things to various people but, as commonly used, the term refers to the use of routinely collected nonrandomized data to compare the effects of various treatments. Even within a carefully designed observational study, where specific arrangements to minimize sources of bias and confounding are planned and monitored, the guaranteed avoidance of biases that would correspond to a moderate increase or decrease in risk may well not be feasible.[12] The effects of uncontrolled, and often uncontrollable, biases or confounding may be at least as big as the sort of moderate effect that is to be assessed (as is the case for the so-called indication bias that occurs when there is selective use of particular treatments in particular patients considered to have specific indications). It follows, therefore, that routinely collected data from outcomes research projects are unlikely to be able to assess reliably any moderate effects on outcome and should generally not be considered as providing credible evidence if attempts are made to use them for this purpose.[20] This is particularly important when nonrandomized studies suggest that certain treatments have surprisingly large effects, because such findings are often refuted when those treatments are assessed in large randomized trials.[21] For example, the claims of hazards with digoxin in heart failure,[22] based on nonrandomized evidence, have not been confirmed by the very large randomized Digitalis Investigation Group (DIG) Trial.[7] Many of the nonrandomized studies currently supposed to indicate hazards of calcium antagonists similarly may be found by future large-scale randomized trials to have been misleading.[12]

Biases and Random Errors in Small-Scale Meta-Analyses

Since meta-analyses are appearing in medical journals with increasing frequency, it is important that those responsible for the delivery of health care and the planning of future research are able to judge the reliability of such reviews and, in particular, the extent to which confounding, biases, or random errors could lead to mistaken conclusions. (In randomized trials, "confounding" exists when a comparison of some particular treatment in one group versus a control group involves the routine coadministration in one group, but not the other, of some cointervention that might affect the outcome.) To avoid any possibility of confounding and to avoid any flexibility in the question of which trials to include, those who perform or interpret meta-analyses should generally adopt the rule that they will include only unconfounded properly randomized trials. The main problems that then remain are those of biases and random errors.

Two types of bias could affect the reliability of a meta-analysis: those that occur within individual trials and those that relate to the selection of trials. For example, it is clear that inadequate concealment of the likely treatment allocation does quite often result in exaggerated estimates of treatment effect[23] and that the inappropriate postrandomization exclusion of particular patients is common.[24] Such defects have unpredictable consequences for particular trials, however, and no generalizations about the likely size, or even direction, of the resultant biases are possible.

A further problem involves the process of identifying all relevant trials (or, occasionally, the failure to include all such trials once they have been identified). Unfortunately, the subset of trials that are eventually published (and, hence, are conveniently available) is often a biased sample of the trials that have been done, since trials may well be more likely to be submitted for publication if their results are strikingly positive than they are if they are negative or null.[25–28] Such "publication bias" can, along with other sources of bias, produce surprisingly impressive-looking evidence of effectiveness for treatments that are actually useless.[29] The particular circumstances in which publication bias has contributed to producing misleading estimates of treatment are difficult to identify, and it is still more difficult to generalize about the exact size of any such bias when it does occur.

The problem of incomplete ascertainment is likely to be particularly acute within small meta-analyses that contain no more than a few hundred major outcomes and consist chiefly of small published trials. This is because results from trials with only a limited number of endpoints are subject to large random errors, and such trials are therefore particularly likely to generate implausibly large effect estimates. If publication bias then results in unduly selective emphasis on the more promising of these small trial results, the resulting summary odds ratios might well be unreliable.[30, 31] Hence, unless the particular circumstances of a small-scale meta-analysis suggest that publication bias is unlikely, it may be best to treat such results as no more than "hypothesis-generating." On the other hand, a thoroughly conducted meta-analysis that in aggregate contains sufficient numbers of major outcomes to constitute "large-scale" randomized evidence[1, 14, 15] is unlikely to be materially affected by publication bias. In addition, provided there are no serious uncontrolled biases (see earlier) within the individual component trials, it is likely to be fairly trustworthy, at least in its overall conclusions, although even then inappropriate subgroup analyses may generate wrong answers.

SUMMARY

Many medical interventions produce only moderate effects on major outcomes such as death or serious disability. But, even a moderate effect of treatment, if demonstrated clearly enough for that treatment to be adopted widely, may well prevent substantial numbers of premature deaths. Moreover, if more than one moderately effective treatment for the particular condition can be identified, then the combination of two or three individually moderate improvements in outcome may collectively result in substantial health gains. There is often no reliable alternative to large-scale randomized evidence for the reliable identification of moderate effects on major outcomes. For most of the important clinical questions in which the existing trials do not provide such evidence, the only medically and financially practical way to obtain it is to plan, design, and conduct some large, simple randomized trials.

The success of this approach is well illustrated by the progress that has already been made in the management of acute MI during recent years: international collaborations have yielded large-scale randomized evidence of the value of fibrinolytic therapy,[2, 13, 32] aspirin,[1, 2, 32] converting enzyme inhibitors[30, 33, 34] and, less reliably, beta blockers[35] (and of the lack of value of some other treatments, such as magnesium[30]). Likewise, the first really large-scale trials in acute ischemic stroke have recently shown small but real benefits from aspirin, and an unexpected lack of clinical benefit from either 5000 IU or 12,500 IU twice daily of subcutaneous heparin.[3, 4] Finally, large-scale randomized evidence on the long-term management of MI, stroke, and heart failure patients has now established the value of the prolonged use of various treatments (such as beta blockers, aspirin, diuretics, converting enzyme inhibitors, and digoxin), all of which were previously disputed.

In some instances, sufficient information is already available from large-scale randomized trials or, better still, from meta-analyses of those trials to allow the balance of risk and benefit of particular treatments to be defined for particular patients. However, many important questions still have not been answered reliably, and there remains a need for many more large, "streamlined" mega-trials to help resolve some of the outstanding clinical uncertainties in the management of cardiovascular disease.

REFERENCES

1. Antiplatelet Trialists' Collaboration. Collaborative overview of randomised trials of antiplatelet therapy: I. Prevention of death, myocardial infarction, and stroke by prolonged antiplatelet therapy in various categories of patients. BMJ 1994; 308:81–106.
2. ISIS-2 (Second International Study of Infarct Survival) Collaborative Group. Randomised trial of intravenous streptokinase, oral aspirin, both, or neither among 17,187 cases of suspected acute myocardial infarction: ISIS-2. Lancet 1988; 2:349–360.
3. Chinese Acute Stroke Trial Collaborative Group. CAST: A randomised, placebo-controlled trial of early aspirin use in 20,000 patients with acute ischaemic stroke. Lancet 1997; 349:1641–1649.
4. International Stroke Trial Collaborative Group. IST: A randomised trial of aspirin, subcutaneous heparin, both or neither among 19,435 patients with acute ischaemic stroke. Lancet 1997; 349:1569–1581.
5. Murray CJL, Lopez AD (eds). The Global Burden of Disease. Boston, Harvard University Press, 1996, pp 465–468.
6. The SOLVD Investigators. Effect of enalapril on survival in

patients with reduced left ventricular ejection fractions and congestive heart failure. N Engl J Med 1991; 325:293–302.
7. The Digitalis Investigation Group. The effect of digoxin on mortality and morbidity in patients with heart failure. N Engl J Med 1997; 336:525–533.
8. Collins R, Peto R, Gray R, Parish S. Large-scale randomized evidence: Trials and overviews. *In* Weatherall D, Ledingham JGG, Warrell DA (eds). Oxford Textbook of Medicine, Vol 1. Oxford, Oxford University Press, 1996, pp 21–32.
9. Peto R, Pike MC, Armitage P, et al. Design and analysis of randomized clinical trials requiring prolonged observation of each patient: I. Introduction and design. Br J Cancer 1976; 34:585–612.
10. Peto R, Pike MC, Armitage P, et al. Design and analysis of randomized clinical trials requiring prolonged observation of each patient: II. Analysis and examples. Br J Cancer 1977; 35:1–39.
11. Yusuf S, Collins R, Peto R. Why do we need some large simple randomized trials? Stat Med 1984; 3:409–420.
12. Ad Hoc Sub Committee of the Liaison Committee of the World Health Organization and the International Society of Hypertension. Effects of calcium antagonists on the risks of coronary heart disease, cancer, and bleeding. J Hypertens 1997; 15:105–115.
13. GISSI (Gruppo Italiano per lo Studio della Streptochinasi nell'Infarto Miocardico). Effectiveness of intravenous thrombolytic treatment in acute myocardial infarction. Lancet 1986; 1:397–402.
14. Fibrinolytic Therapy Trialists' Collaborative Group. Indications for fibrinolytic therapy in suspected acute myocardial infarction: Collaborative overview of early mortality and major morbidity results from all randomised trials of more than 1000 patients. Lancet 1994; 343:311–322.
15. Early Breast Cancer Trialists' Collaborative Group. Systemic treatment of early breast cancer by hormonal, cytotoxic, or immune therapy: 133 randomised trials involving 31,000 recurrences and 24,000 deaths among 75,000 women. Lancet 1992; 339:1–15 (Part I); 71–85 (Part II).
16. Cholesterol Treatment Trialists' (CTT) Collaboration. Protocol for a prospective collaborative overview of all current and planned randomized trials of cholesterol treatment regimens. Am J Cardiol 1995; 75:1130–1134.
17. Doyal L. Journals should not publish research to which patients have not given fully informed consent with three exceptions. BMJ 1997; 314:1107–1111.
18. Collins R, Doll R, Peto R. Ethics of clinical trials. *In* Williams CJ (ed). Introducing New Treatments for Cancer: Practical, Ethical and Legal Problems. New York, John Wiley & Sons, 1992, pp 49–65.
19. Collins R, Julian D. British Heart Foundation surveys (1987 and 1989) of United Kingdom treatment policies for acute myocardial infarction. Br Heart J 1991; 66:250–255.
20. Sheldon TA. Please bypass the PORT: Observational studies of effectiveness run a poor second to randomised controlled trials. BMJ 1994; 309:142–143.
21. Peto R. Clinical trial methodology. Biomedicine Special Issue 1978; 28:24–36.
22. Yusuf S, Wittes J, Bailey K, Furberg C. Digitalis—a new controversy regarding an old drug: The pitfalls of inappropriate methods. Circulation 1986; 73:13–18.
23. Schulz KF, Chalmers I, Hayes RJ, Altman DG. Empirical evidence of bias: Dimensions of methodologic quality associated with estimates of treatment effects in controlled trials. JAMA 1995; 273:408–412.
24. Schulz KF, Grimes DA, Altman DG, Hayes RJ. Blinding and exclusions after allocation in randomised controlled trials: Survey of published parallel group trials in obstetrics and gynaecology. BMJ 1996; 312:742–744.
25. Dickersin K, Chan S, Chalmers TC, et al. Publication bias and clinical trials. Control Clin Trials 1987; 8:343–353.
26. Easterbrook PJ, Berlin JA, Gopelan R, Matthews DR. Publication bias in clinical research. Lancet 1991; 337:867–872.
27. Dickersin K, Min Y-I, Meinert CL. Factors influencing publication of research results: Follow-up of applications submitted to two institutional review boards. JAMA 1992; 267:374–378.
28. Dickersin K, Min Y-I. Publication bias: The problem that won't go away. Ann NY Acad Sci 1993; 703:135–146.
29. Counsell CE, Clarke MJ, Slattery J, Sandercock PAG. The miracle of DICE therapy for acute stroke: Fact or fictional product of subgroup analysis? BMJ 1994; 309:1677–1681.
30. ISIS-4 (Fourth International Study of Infarct Survival) Collaborative Group. ISIS-4: A randomised factorial trial assessing early oral captopril, oral mononitrate, and intravenous magnesium sulphate in 58,050 patients with suspected acute myocardial infarction. Lancet 1995; 345:669–685.
31. Davey Smith G, Egger M. Misleading meta-analysis. BMJ 1995; 310:742–754.
32. Collins R, Peto R, Baigent C, Sleight P. Aspirin, heparin, and fibrinolytic therapy in suspected acute myocardial infarction. N Engl J Med 1997; 336:847–860.
33. Gruppo Italiano per lo Studio della Sopravvivenza nell'Infarto Miocardico. GISSI-3: Effects of lisinopril and transdermal glyceryl trinitrate singly and together on 6-week mortality and ventricular function after myocardial infarction. Lancet 1994; 343:1115–1122.
34. Chinese Cardiac Study Collaborative Group. Oral captopril versus placebo among 13,634 patients with suspected acute myocardial infarction: Interim report from the Chinese Cardiac Study (CCS-1). Lancet 1995; 345:686–687.
35. ISIS-1 (First International Study of Infarct Survival) Collaborative Group. Randomised trial of intravenous atenolol among 16,027 cases of suspected acute myocardial infarction: ISIS-1. Lancet 1986; 2:57–66.

5 Principles of Data and Safety Monitoring Boards in Randomized Trials

▶ David L. DeMets

During the past three decades, clinical trials have evolved to become a major research methodology for clinical medicine. Many statistical principles have been applied to the design, conduct, and analysis of clinical trials, and these statistical methodologies continue to evolve as we apply clinical trials to an increasing array of research settings.[1–3] As the methodology for clinical trials began to develop, the National Institutes of Health (NIH) commissioned a task force to establish the administrative structure and process for conducting multicenter Phase III clinical trials that are designed to establish the cost:benefit ratio of new therapies and interventions. This task force issued a report, known as the *Greenberg Report*,[4] in 1967. In addition to the trial chair, the executive committee or steering committee, and a statistical or coordinating center, the Greenberg Report established the need for an independent Policy Advisory Board. This is illustrated in Figure 5–1. Although the functions of this board were not specified in detail, this unit came to be known in most trials of the National Heart, Lung, and Blood Institute (NHLBI) at the NIH as the *Data and Safety Monitoring Board* (DSMB) or the *Data Monitoring Committee* (DMC).[5] In the current clinical trial structure, the DSMB is a critical component of the administrative structure in the comparative Phase III trial.[6–21] The DSMB is an independent group of experts who provide informed advice on the progress of a trial to the principal investigator or trial chair and the sponsor of the trial. One possible outcome of a trial is early termination due to convincing evidence of benefit, harm, or equivalence of the treatments. The focus of this chapter is the special role and responsibilities of the DSMB in monitoring a clinical trial. In particular, issues to be discussed include the rationale for data monitoring, the complexity of the decision process for early termination, the need for DSMB expertise, the constitution of a DSMB, as well as the format and content of DSMB meetings. There is no single or simple prescription for the role of a DSMB, but principles have emerged over the past three decades that seem useful. Examples from several cardiovascular trials are used to illustrate the issues that can arise in monitoring trials.

RATIONALE FOR DATA MONITORING

Clinical trials are designed to evaluate the usefulness of a newly emerging or an existing device, procedure, or therapeutic treatment, or a disease prevention strategy. The goal may be to establish the most effective dose or identify side effects and toxicity. Patients who participate in these clinical trials trust that a trial will not continue if clear evidence of unacceptable adverse events or toxicity is observed. Furthermore, patients also trust that a trial will not continue if convincing evidence of treatment benefit emerges and the risk:benefit ratio is favorable. In addition, during their conduct equivalence trials may reach their goal and patients would want to receive the treatment that is less invasive or costly or has fewer side effects. If a design flaw is identified early in the conduct, modifications should be made when possible to preserve the integrity of the trial and maximize its potential for success. Finally, trials that have little or no chance of achieving their stated goals, either primary or secondary, should be identified and considered for termination since further patient participation may be wasted effort. Thus, whether stated directly or implied in the informed consent, patients put their trust in the clinical trial process to consider these issues while the trial is ongoing. Trials are both a patient and scientific investment. For these ethical and scientific reasons, data monitoring is an essential part of the clinical trial process.

Clinical trials are often classified into one of four categories. *Phase I trials* attempt to identify the maximum tolerated dose of a drug or biologic, or the conditions for using a device. *Phase II trials* are designed to screen for possible biologic effectiveness and identify side effects or toxicity rates. *Phase III trials* are the comparative trials, designed to test the

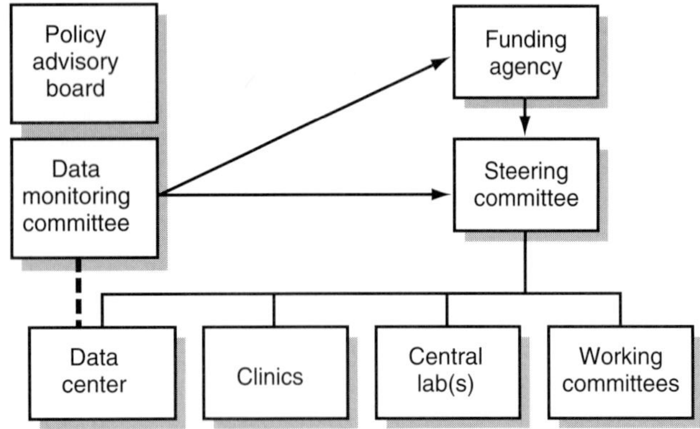

Figure 5–1 National Heart, Lung, and Blood Institute (NHLBI) clinical trial model[5] based on Greenberg's Heart Special Project Review.

effectiveness of a therapy and estimate the cost:benefit ratio. *Phase IV trials* typically are long-term follow-up studies to scrutinize approved or accepted therapies for potential harm not observed in the Phase III trial. By their design, Phases I and II trials have a required data-monitoring process because each step in their designs is based on the results of previous steps. That is, in Phase I trials dose is not escalated until results of the current dose are known. In Phase II trials, if no positive results are observed in the first 12 or 24 patients, additional patients are not entered. Phase I and II trials typically do not have independent DSMBs perform the monitoring process but rely on the investigators involved in the trial.

Phase III trials are larger, take longer to complete, and are more costly than Phase I or II trials because their goal is to provide a definitive answer to the treatment effectiveness question. Not all Phase III trials need to be monitored. However, if the primary or secondary outcomes involve mortality or irreversible morbidity or if safety issues could be a concern, then careful monitoring is critical and mandatory.[8] Balancing potential benefit with potential risks is exactly where the role of the DSMB is most important, and often that evaluation is complex and involves several factors.

MONITORING: A COMPLEX PROCESS

A clinical trial has several components, all of which must be functioning for success to be achieved. In the interim review of these components, if results suggest that a trial may need to be modified or terminated early, then several factors need to be taken into consideration before that decision is made.[21–25]

Early in the trial, administrative issues such as the validity of design assumptions, recruitment success, and patient compliance must be considered. Modifications to the design may be required, including changing entry criteria to improve recruitment, increasing sample size to compensate for lower-than-anticipated event rates or increased variability, or dose adjustment to improve compliance. The purpose of these types of administrative analyses is to keep the design as close to the original goals as possible. If done early, such modifications have more of a chance to correct any identified problems.

Fleming[24] has noted that for a DSMB to carry out its responsibilities, it must have relevant high-quality data that are reasonably current. The Thrombolysis in Myocardial Infarction (TIMI) II trial[26] was designed to evaluate the use of a tissue plasminogen activator (t-PA), a thrombolytic agent, in percutaneous transluminal coronary angioplasty procedures. TIMI-I had established that t-PA was more effective in rapidly resolving blood clots. However, in the process of scaling up the manufacturing of the t-PA, a change in the methodology increased the potency of the agent. Thus, in the very early stages of TIMI-II, bleeding complications became a serious issue. Recruitment was suspended and the matter investigated. Ultimately a dose adjustment was made to account for the change in potency, and TIMI-II was completed successfully. However, it was critical that the data flow was rapid so that timely decisions could be made before more bleeding complications had occurred. In the Diabetes Control and Complications Trial (DCCT),[27, 28] a central laboratory with an excellent research record was unable to keep up with the volume and turn around required by the protocol on critical parameters for glucose control. Careful administrative monitoring quickly discovered this problem and another laboratory was found with the necessary capability. Had this not been discovered early, patient safety could have been compromised.

Later in a trial, decisions are often related to early termination due to emerging evidence of benefit or harm. Previous experience suggests that this is a particularly complex decision process.[8, 10, 21–23] Comparability between the experimental and the control group needs to be examined carefully. Assessment of the primary, secondary, and side effect measurements must be unbiased or results are not interpretable. Lack of treatment effect may be the result of poor patient compliance to the protocol. Differential compliance rates may suggest bias. Another consideration is whether the results are internally consistent across other outcome measures and across risk groups or subgroups. Although magnitude of effect, either beneficial or harmful, may differ quantitatively, qualitative consistency is reassuring in terminating a trial early. External consistency with other trials or observational trials must be weighed as well. Finally, the therapeutic index or risk:benefit ratio must be carefully considered. Benefit might be significant but the toxicity is substantial, and these must be balanced before a trial can be terminated and recommendations made. Early benefits that appear to wane with follow-up may not be considered important.

Most trials measure numerous outcomes, and some outcomes may be measured repeatedly. Data monitoring requires repeatedly testing these outcome measures, but this process also increases the chances of a false-positive result.[29, 30] For example, if the normal P value of 0.05 is used on each of five interim analyses, the true false-positive error is not 5% but almost 15%. Methods have been developed to guard against this, but they are limited mostly to one or two primary outcome measures. A common method, referred to as the *group sequential procedure*,[31–36] increases the level of evidence required at each interim analysis before statistical significance can be achieved. By being more conservative at each analysis, the overall trial false-positive error rate can be maintained at conventional levels (e.g., 0.05). There are several proposed group sequential methods, each producing different statistical criteria or interim boundaries for being conservative, although each can achieve the same overall false-positive error rate.[31–37] Another approach, referred to as *conditional power* or *stochastic curtailment*,[38, 39] computes the probability at interim analysis of reaching a statistically significant result, for either benefit or harm, if the trial continued to its scheduled end. If this probability is very low, the trial may be hopeless and not worth continuing. If this probability is extremely high, the results may already be so overwhelming that continuation is not necessary. This method is most often used in the circumstance of an observed negative or harmful trend, computing the probability of recovering from this negative deficit to ever achieving a positive and statistically significant benefit. If this probability is very low, considering a variety of reasonable postulated treatment effects, then the trial is unlikely to demonstrate benefit and may in fact show harm. Finally, the impact of any decision to terminate early on the practice of medicine and public health policy must be taken into account. Early termination that does not have an impact wastes the investment of patients, investigators, and sponsors. These factors are summarized in Table 5–1.

Given the number of factors that must be considered and weighed carefully, no single person would likely have all the required expertise in clinical medicine, epidemiology, biostatistics, clinical trials, and medical ethics. Furthermore, it is not likely that any single person would want the responsibility for such a complex decision process. For that reason, major Phase III trials are monitored through an independent committee, referred to here as the *DSMB*.[5, 8, 21–23]

TABLE 5–1 • Early Termination Considerations

Baseline comparability	External consistency
Unbiased evaluation	Benefit/risk
Compliance	Length of follow-up
Internal consistency	Public impact
Other outcomes	Repeated testing
Subgroups	Multiple comparisons

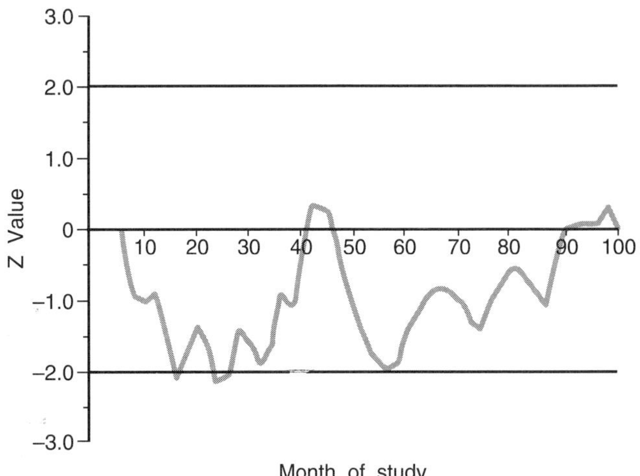

Figure 5–2 Interim analyses in the Coronary Drug Project if performed almost continuously. The horizontal lines at Z values of +2.0 and −2.0 represent the nominal 0.05 significance levels. The graph shows the interim standardized test statistic comparing event rates in the placebo group and the clofibrate group. A positive Z value indicates placebo is better and a negative that clofibrate is better.

To illustrate the complexity of the decision making, several cardiovascular trials with early termination are briefly described. Each presents different issues that a DSMB must be prepared for as a possibility. The Coronary Drug Project (CDP) compared several cholesterol-lowering drugs in men who had recently experienced a myocardial infarction (MI).[40] One of the drugs was clofibrate. As the interim data emerged and were reviewed by the DSMB, the standardized test statistic or Z value comparing mortality curves approached the nominal 0.05 boundaries on four occasions in favor of clofibrate, but these trends did not sustain themselves (Fig. 5–2). The horizontal boundaries correspond to using a 0.05 significance level or critical values of ± 2.0 for the test statistic at each analysis. The final comparisons produced nearly identical mortality curves.[22] This phenomenon is a consequence of repeatedly testing accumulating data, and the process leads to an increase in the false-positive error rate.[30] The CDP DSMB was well aware of this danger and did not respond prematurely in terminating this treatment arm and claiming a treatment benefit.

Another trial was terminated early for treatment benefit. The Beta-Blocker Heart Attack Trial (BHAT) compared propranolol with placebo in a multicenter, randomized, double-blind trial.[41] A positive trend emerged early and continued to increase, eventually meeting statistical criteria used to control the false-positive error rate (Table 5–2). While determining that a statistical boundary was crossed may not require much discussion, the monitoring process was still not simple for the BHAT DSMB.[42] Even though propranolol appeared to be effective in the short follow-up period of 2 or 3 years, the question of how long a postinfarct patient should remain on propranolol had not been resolved. Issues listed in Table 5–1 had to be evaluated. In addition, other trials of beta blockers, such as the Norwegian Timolol trial,[43] were becoming available suggesting that a placebo control may no longer be ethical when combined with the BHAT results. The BHAT DSMB had to consider what further information would be learned if the trial went to its planned termination date; it was determined that not enough information would be gathered to answer definitively the long-term question. Thus, after considerable discussion, the BHAT DSMB recommended early termination for treatment benefit over the period observed.

In contrast to early termination for benefit, the Cardiac Arrhythmia Suppression Trial (CAST) was terminated very rapidly for unexpected but convincing evidence of treatment harm.[44] Cardiac arrhythmias are associated with sudden cardiac death, and drugs such as encainide and flecainide were known to be effective in suppressing arrhythmias. Drugs of this type were becoming widely used because of this effect. CAST was designed to evaluate the effectiveness of suppressing arrhythmias with these drugs on total mortality. The expectation was a reduction, but how large the effect was not known. With only 10% to 15% of the expected deaths observed, the statistical comparison indicated a large effect but in the negative direction, contrary to expectation (Table 5–3). In addition, although the statistical criteria used to protect against false-positive errors were very conservative at this early stage of the trial, the test statistic for the mortality comparison had already been exceeded.[45] Given this dramatic result, which was contrary to conventional wisdom and expectation, the DSMB had to move quickly but carefully. A mistake in not terminating early would cause more deaths, but a mistake in jumping to a decision prematurely about treatment harm would cause confusion in a widely used treatment of a high-risk population. After weighing carefully all the evidence, including treatment group comparability, compliance, and outcome ascertainment, the DSMB concluded that CAST needed to be terminated and the results disseminated immediately.[46] However, these results caught the cardiology community by surprise, and patients on encainide and flecainide had to be dealt with rapidly.

The most agonizing complex decision is the slowly emerging negative or harmful trend. This occurred in two trials in congestive heart failure (CHF), the Prospective Randomized Milrinone Survival Evaluation (PROMISE) trial[47] and the Prospective Randomized Flosequinan Longevity Evaluation (PROFILE)[48] trial. PROMISE was a randomized, double-blind, placebo-controlled trial testing the effect of a drug, milrinone, on total mortality for severe Class III and Class IV CHF. Milrinone had already been shown to be effective in exercise testing. The DSMB observed early on a negative trend, but one not as overwhelming as the CAST negative trend. As the trend continued to become more negative, the ethical question arose whether this trial should prove harm or just that a positive benefit was not likely. In this setting, a neutral or equivalent result on mortality might mean that milrinone could still be used for its effect on exercise functioning. The DSMB determined that PROMISE should distinguish between a neutral result and a harmful effect. When the negative trend continued and passed the statistical criteria for significance, PROMISE was terminated early and the investigators concluded that milrinone had in fact a harmful effect on mortality. Later, another trial in CHF, PROFILE, had a similar experience.[48] PROFILE was very similar in design to PROMISE, but it evaluated another drug, flosequinan, for a mortality effect. While the trial was just getting started, this drug was approved by the Food and Drug Administration (FDA) for use because

TABLE 5–2 • Interim Analyses for the BHAT

Planned Analysis	Calendar Time (mo)	Total Observed Deaths (*d*)	Logrank Z	Critical Boundary Value*
1	11	56	1.68	5.88
2	16	77	2.24	5.04
3	21	126	2.37	3.79
4	28	177	2.30	3.19
5	34	247	2.34	2.64
6	40	318	2.82	2.30*
7	48	—	—	—

*If the logrank statistic (*Z*) exceeds the critical boundary value in absolute value, the mortality comparison is significant at the 0.05 level, adjusting for repeated testing.

TABLE 5–3 • CAST Interim Results for Encainide and Flecainide

Time	Placebo†	Active†	Total†	Logrank	Lower Critical Boundary*
09/01/88	7 (576)	22 (571)	29 (1147)	−2.82	−3.18
03/30/89	9 (725)	33 (730)	42 (1455)	−3.22	−3.04*

*If the logrank statistic is below the lower critical boundary, the mortality comparison is significant at the 0.05 level.
†Number of deaths; sample size is shown in parentheses.

of its positive effect on exercise tolerance. However, just as in PROMISE, the PROFILE DSMB began to observe a negative trend. In this instance, however, the drug had just been approved for use. Again, the DSMB had to weigh the impact of terminating a trial for not showing a beneficial effect, or waiting to distinguish between a neutral effect and a harmful effect. Since flosequinan had just been approved by the FDA, the DSMB concluded that PROFILE must distinguish between a neutral and a harmful result. Unfortunately, flosequinan, like milrinone, proved to have a statistically significant harmful effect on mortality.

In contrast with PROMISE and PROFILE, the Cooperative North Scandinavian Enalapril Survival Study (CONSENSUS) II trial terminated early with a negative trend that did not reach statistical significance.[49] CONSENSUS II was evaluating enalapril in the treatment of MI patients. The primary outcome in this randomized, double-blind, placebo-controlled trial was 6-month total mortality. The sample size calculation assumed a one-sided 0.05 significance level for treatment benefit. During the trial, conditional probabilities were to be calculated for accepting or rejecting the hypothesis of no treatment benefit. If this probability was very high (e.g., 90%), then the trial might be considered for early termination. In this case, a negative trend in 6-month mortality emerged, favoring placebo over enalapril (9.9% vs. 11.1%). This trend did not reach levels of statistical significance proving that treatment was harmful. However, the DSMB made a recommendation to terminate early on the basis that the trial was highly unlikely to show a positive benefit unless the current negative effect was reversed dramatically for the rest of the patient follow-up, a reversal that would be extremely implausible.[15, 50] This decision resulted in considerable discussion between investigators and the DSMB, but the recommendation was accepted by the investigators. In this instance, the issue for the CONSENSUS II investigators was whether termination was appropriate while not showing either benefit or harm. These types of agonizing negative trends require considerable judgment, expertise, and experience.

Another type of difficult and complex decision is whether to terminate a trial where no apparent trends on the primary endpoint are emerging but other factors seem compelling for early stopping. The Physicians' Health Study (PHS) is an excellent example. The PHS was a trial of unique design where more than 22,000 individual health physicians were randomized in a factorial design to receive beta carotene, aspirin, both, or neither.[51] The aspirin component was designed to test the effect on reducing total cardiovascular mortality, with total mortality and nonfatal MIs as secondary outcomes. After 5 years of the scheduled 7 years of follow-up, the aspirin component was terminated by the PHS DSMB[52] (results are shown in Table 5–4). Several factors played a role in their decision. The first issue was that the primary event rate of cardiovascular mortality in the placebo group was extremely low, less than 50% of that used in the design. This caused the power to detect the effect of aspirin on cardiovascular mortality to be extremely low. The total mortality rate was also extremely low. From this perspective, the PHS had little or no chance of success for the primary goal unless the trial was

TABLE 5–4 • Physicians' Health Study: Five-Year Results

	Aspirin	Placebo	RR	*P*
Total mortality	217	227	0.96	0.64
Cardiovascular	81	83	0.96	0.87
Myocardial infarction	10	28	0.31	0.004
Nonfatal myocardial infarction	129	213	0.59	<0.00001
Total stroke	119	98	1.22	0.15
Ischemic	91	82	1.11	0.50
Hemorrhagic	23	12	2.14	0.06

RR, relative risk.

extended for 10 or more years of follow-up. However, the effect of aspirin on the secondary outcome of fatal and nonfatal MI, most of which were nonfatal, was overwhelmingly positive (44% reduction; $P < 0.00001$). This result had been becoming increasingly positive as the trial progressed, ultimately exceeding the conservative statistical criteria used to control the false-positive error rate. However, the decision had an added complexity. A possible adverse risk of hemorrhagic stroke was observed in the aspirin group (23 vs. 12; $P = 0.06$). Although the number of hemorrhagic strokes was small, and the rate much smaller than the nonfatal infarctions, the consequences of this event were nonetheless worrisome. As a further complexity, aspirin was already approved as a secondary prevention for cardiovascular mortality in an MI population, and PHS physicians who just had an MI began taking aspirin. This further decreased the likelihood of detecting any aspirin effect on mortality. The DSMB decided the following:

- The aspirin effect on nonfatal MI was important for public health
- The total mortality effect would not be detected
- The stroke adverse-event rate was small and already an expected risk for both primary and secondary use
- Not much more would be learned in the next 2 years of scheduled follow-up to further resolve the stroke issue
- Physician crossover to aspirin was becoming increasingly nontrivial

These were among the major factors that led to the early termination of the aspirin component.

CONSTITUTION OF A DSMB

As already indicated, the DSMB is an independent group of people not directly involved with the conduct of the trial and has no special vested interest in the outcome.[4, 5, 8, 21, 23] The DSMB usually provides recommendations to the principal investigators of the trial, through its chair or executive committee, and to the sponsor (see Fig. 5–1). This reporting role should be clearly stated before the start of the trial. In some instances, the DSMB reports only to the study executive committee and not directly to the sponsor, whereas in other cases it may report to both. Either structure is feasible but must be understood at the initiation of the study. The DSMB is usually given the authority to make recommendations and not final decisions, being primarily an advisory body to either sponsor, investigators, or both.

The authority to appoint the DSMB must also be identified in the protocol. Either the sponsor or the investigators may make the appointments. Since DSMB decisions ultimately impact on both sponsor and investigators, both parties should ideally agree to the appointments, regardless of who makes the invitation to individuals. Thus, it is recommended that this process be done jointly. As described by Armstrong and Furberg,[23] whatever reporting relationship is agreed to, the independence of the DSMB from both sponsor and investigator is in the best interest of the trial and the participants.

Given the complexity of most clinical trials and the decisions that must be made, the DSMB collectively must have expertise in the disciplines related to the disease, treatment, and populations being studied. This often requires both clinicians and laboratory scientists. In addition, the DSMB must have expertise in clinical trials, biostatistics, epidemiology, data management, and research ethics. NIH-sponsored trials traditionally appoint to the DSMB someone with medical ethics or sociology training to particularly reflect patients' point of view in the monitoring process. This is not as common in industry-sponsored trials. To cover this wide range of expertise, between three and seven people are likely to be needed. Often a DSMB of five members is adequate and is an ideal committee size for complex discussions. The chair of the DSMB should be someone either familiar with the specific scientific question being addressed or experienced in monitoring clinical trials, and ideally should be expert in both areas.

The DSMB should be kept independent of investigators entering or caring for patients in the trial.[11] Otherwise, the ethical dilemmas arise for the investigator as trends emerge or fail to emerge. Investigators should remain in equipoise about the benefits of the treatment until the trial is terminated.[53] Oncology trials as a routine used to share interim results with investigators. This practice, however, led to many trials not being completed presumably owing to investigators drawing inferences from nonsignificant trends.[54] Thus, although the investigators have a great deal of relevant expertise, they should not be eligible for the DSMB.

Although the DSMB technically reports to either the investigators through their study chair or executive committee and to the sponsor, DSMB members must feel primarily responsible to the participants in the trial. During the conduct of the trial, they bear the major burden of monitoring patient safety, especially in double-blind trials. The next level of responsibility is to the investigators and to the integrity of the trial since investigators have turned over many of their concerns to the DSMB. Any DSMB will recognize the important role of the sponsor, whether it is federal or private, and will attempt to reflect those interests following those of the patient and investigator. Finally, the DSMB does not routinely interact with regulatory agencies such as the FDA, but regulatory requirements must also be recognized in DSMB deliberations and decisions.[55, 56] However, although all of these four constituencies must be considered, their priority must be in the order described, starting with the participants in the trial.

Since the DSMB has the responsibility for monitoring the interim results of the trial and making recommendations about conduct, benefit, and safety to the investigators and sponsor, the DSMB members need to be independent of the trial.[5, 8, 11, 21, 23] That is, the DSMB members should not be entering patients into the trial or into any competing trials. Furthermore, they must be free of any real conflicts of interest, especially those that might appear to be financial. Conflict of interest in itself may not be bad unless it would influence decision making. Most scientists have some intellectual conflict just by being an expert in the field. However, undisclosed financial conflicts can be problematic. In addition to consulting and travel, another especially sensitive conflict is having financial investments in the company whose product is being tested by the trial. The members of the DSMB cannot have any financial investment in the sponsor. This policy has been described for one recent cardiovascular trial.[57] A good policy is for DSMB members to annually report their activities outside their own institution in terms of travel, speaking engagements, and honoraria for consulting as well as any financial investments in the sponsor. These activities should be reviewed annually by the DSMB chair, the study chair, and the sponsor as appropriate. If the appearance of a conflict exists and cannot be resolved, the best action may be for that board member to either refrain from further activity on that issue or not continue on the DSMB.

In addition, representatives from the sponsor and the regulatory agency should not be members of the DSMB since they obviously are not independent.[5, 8, 11, 21, 23] Sponsor representatives have either a programmatic interest or a financial interest and thus cannot be totally independent. Furthermore, the DSMB is advisory either directly or indirectly to the sponsor, so it is inconsistent for a DSMB member to be independently advising his or her own institution. Similarly, representatives of regulatory agencies such as the FDA should also not be members of a DSMB. If the trial results are to be reviewed by the regulatory agency, it would be extremely awkward for the agency to fairly critique those results if they essentially participated in the trial decision making. This would be especially true if the trial was terminated early. The roles of the regulatory agency and the DSMB are quite different. The DSMB primarily focuses on the conduct of a specific trial or set of trials. The regulatory agency must make judgments based on a much larger set of evidence, some of which may not even be fully known in scientific circles. Both sponsors and regulatory representatives may have a limited participation in DSMB meetings, according to guidelines on who should attend, described later. As Walters described it, the independence of the DSMB is not an end in itself but an essential means to achieving knowledge and maximum objectivity about new interventions, and the DSMB respects the patients making those contributions.[11] This is maximized by sponsors and regulators not being DSMB members.

In addition to being free of conflict of interest, DSMB members must be able to maintain absolute confidentiality. Interim data may reflect transient trends that, if shared, could be not only misleading but damaging to the trial, even precluding continuation. As already described, oncology trials demonstrated that routine presentation of interim data often precluded further recruitment as trends emerged.[54] Investigators may willingly turn over the monitoring responsibility to the DSMB, but it is only natural that they remain interested in how the trial is going and curious as to interim results. Thus, comments or inferences made by DSMB members in the presence of an investigator, sponsor, or regulator may be interpreted, correctly or incorrectly, and thus it is paramount that DSMB members are absolutely silent on DSMB matters outside their meetings. Even acknowledging that a DSMB member is going to a DSMB meeting can be informative to an interested party.

STATISTICAL ANALYSIS CENTER

To fulfill its monitoring responsibilities, the DSMB is heavily dependent on the statistical analysis or coordinating center.[4, 5] This center must have statistical, data management, and clinical trials expertise. The center is often responsible for the statistical aspects of the protocol design and preparing the data collection instruments. At the conclusion of the trial, this center is involved in the preparation of final analyses and the trial publication. During the trial, it collects, enters, and edits the data in a timely manner and prepares interim reports for the DSMB. The DSMB may also request additional analyses from the statistical center as issues arise during its deliberations. Thus, the smooth working relationship between the DSMB and the statistical center is essential.[24]

DSMB MEETINGS

DSMB meetings should be held often enough so that patient safety can be protected, but not so often that there is only a small increment in information from one meeting to the next. One guide is that the DSMB should meet at least once, and perhaps twice, per year. Another variation is a once-per-year meeting with an in-between conference call meeting to at least review safety. From the statistical point of view, one guideline is to meet with every 20% increment in information (e.g., deaths or primary events). However, if events are slow in accruing, the once- to twice-per-year guideline should override because safety issues should not go on too long before review.

Attendance at DSMB meetings needs to be clearly understood at the beginning of the trial. Communication between the DSMB, investigators, and sponsor about some aspects of the trial progress and conduct is essential. Yet information on treatment comparisons for benefit or safety should not be shared among all parties. The NIH special report recommended that investigators not be aware of interim results since that knowledge may influence their decisions as to which patients to recruit or on the evaluation of treated patients, either influence biasing the trial and seriously damaging its scientific goal. In some special cases, such as Multiple Risk Factor Intervention Trial (MRFIT)[58] or BHAT,[41] the chair of the trial was intentionally selected to represent the investigators while not entering or caring for patients in the trial. In those instances, the study chair has attended the DSMB meetings. For most NIH trials and some industry-sponsored trials (e.g., PROMISE and Prospective Randomized Amlodipine Survival Evaluation [PRAISE]), representatives of the sponsor have attended the entire DSMB meetings. However, the question of who should attend DSMB meetings has generated discussion for cardiovascular and noncardiovascular trials.[11] A general format has evolved that appears to meet the needs of all parties, using an open-session, closed-session, and executive-session process.[59]

During the open session, representatives from the investigators (usually the chair or co-chair), from the sponsor, and from the FDA may attend. During this session, information is shared on the conduct of the trial, including recruitment, compliance, data quality, and general operational issues. Exchange of this information may identify logistical problems or scientific issues that, if resolved early, may strengthen the trial and enhance the likelihood of a meaningful answer.

Following this interchange, the major portion of the DSMB meeting should be conducted in strict confidence. Generally, only DSMB members plus representatives from the statistical center who present the interim analyses should be present. Traditionally, NIH-sponsored trials have an NIH representative at this closed session. Some industry-sponsored trials' representatives have been at the closed session (PROMISE, PRAISE), whereas others have not (GUSTO[60]). If sponsors do attend, they must not under any circumstances interfere with the business and responsibility of the DSMB. Furthermore, information learned at the closed session should not be shared with their colleagues within the sponsor. This requires a strong commitment and understanding by the sponsor with their designated trial representative. Walters[11] argues that neither sponsors nor regulators should attend the closed session, except when the sponsor is a federal agency such as the NIH. NIH project offices should be mostly representing the general public and the scientific community and not commercial interests. Even in this instance, however, NIH officials should have at most only a minor role in the DSMB deliberations. Otherwise, the DSMB soon loses the independence on which it is based.

An executive session at the end of each meeting, and during if necessary, is recommended where only DSMB members attend so that candid and frank comments can be made that may have been inhibited by the presence of any sponsor or statistical center representative at the closed session.

DSMB REPORTS

Since the monitoring is a complex process and many factors must be considered, the data report presented to the DSMB must be both thorough and focused. Detailed analyses as to patient recruitment, baseline risk factors, treatment group comparability, compliance to therapy, primary and secondary outcomes, subgroup comparisons, and measures of safety and adverse events must be included. Graphical presentations whenever possible, with tables as backup, are recommended to make the most efficient use of the DSMB meeting. A standard format from meeting to meeting is also useful and should be developed early in the trial. As the trial progresses, new issues will inevitably arise so that a standard format will allow for new analyses to be included in a meaningful and efficient manner. Given the amount of data typically collected in a clinical trial, data reports can easily become voluminous and overwhelm a DSMB. DSMB reports with dozens or even hundreds of tables soon become uninformative. Graphs and executive type summaries with detailed tables in an appendix often serve the DSMB needs most effectively.

For an interim data report to be useful to the DSMB, the data base itself must be relatively up to date.[24] A DSMB should be reluctant to make any decision, especially early termination decisions, based on data that are several months behind. Good standard practice should allow for a data base to be delayed no more than 3 months. For mortality trials, information should be only a few days old if appropriate communication channels are developed. However, the need for current data for the interim analysis and the DSMB meeting may not be appreciated by investigators and sponsors, so this critical aspect must not be taken for granted. The Nocturnal Oxygen Therapy

(NOT) trial evaluated continual verses nocturnal use of oxygen supplementation in patients with advanced chronic obstructive lung disease. Nott reported[61, 62] that a differential, perhaps biased, delay in reporting results from one or two centers almost led that DSMB to make a decision for early termination. However, an inquiry of all the clinical centers revealed a delay that modified the interim results. A premature early termination would have altered the inferences about the effectiveness of continual oxygen therapy. For trials such as CAST, reliable and updated interim results proved to be critical in the DSMB's ability to make rapid and correct decisions.

In presenting data to the DSMB, one issue is whether or not the DSMB should be blinded to treatment groups where possible.[10] Two approaches are being used successfully: One traditional approach is to label all tables by treatment identification, or by codes (e.g., A vs. B) with codes known to the DSMB. Another is to label tables by these codes, which are consistent across all tables, except perhaps for those that may unblind the DSMB. This approach keeps the DSMB blind until a point is reached in the trial where a decision point may be approaching. The DSMB may want to discuss how knowledge of treatment assignment would affect their decision. Since decisions about early termination may not be symmetric, knowledge of whether an emerging, possibly convincing, trend is suggesting benefit or harm might make a difference in the decision. Thus, before any decision is made, the DSMB would unblind itself. The CAST DSMB used this latter approach. This latter approach allows any member of the DSMB to request that the code be broken at any time. Since the DSMB must keep strict confidence about the treatment comparisons, the tradeoff between these two approaches is mainly for the benefit of the DSMB, and the latter approach may require more reflection on how knowledge of the treatment code would change their decision. One approach that should not be considered is to have a data report that changes treatment code from table to table or between categories of tables for the purpose of ensuring that the DSMB is blind. For the DSMB to carry out its responsibility, it must assess the total risk-benefit profile, which can be done only with all tables presented consistently. Ultimately, however, the welfare of the patients is paramount and the traditional approach where the DSMB knows the treatment code from the beginning is quite satisfactory and recommended.

Since each clinical trial has large data bases that must be summarized and interpreted, most DSMB reports are somewhat lengthy, even where graphic presentations are used extensively. In addition, issues can be complex and may take several reviews of the report to grasp subtleties in the data. For that reason, statistical reports should be sent to the DSMB a few days prior to the meeting or conference call. Express mail is an efficient and secure method to distribute these confidential reports. DSMB reports should be carefully accounted for and collected by the statistical center following the meeting. This provides a little more assurance that these highly confidential data reports do not get left in a nonsecure place. This prior distribution of DSMB reports, however, places even more pressure on the data flow and data management process. Each delay forces the report to be more out of date and less useful to the DSMB.

EXTERNAL INFORMATION

During the conduct of a trial, additional information may become available that is relevant. This may be the discovery of new basic science or the results of other trials, perhaps in similar populations with a similar treatment. In some instances, it may even be the same population and the same treatment. The issue becomes how much the DSMB should take this into account in the monitoring of their trial. During the BHAT study, which tested a beta-blocker drug in a postinfarct population, results of two other trials showing a treatment benefit became available, one using the drug timolol (Norwegian Timolol Trial[43]) and another trial using metoprolol.[63] Although the BHAT results had passed their own statistical criteria for termination for benefit, the discussion to terminate was not straightforward since it was not known how long the beta-blocker therapy should be given. However, the results of the other two trials certainly gave the DSMB confidence about the 2-year results of BHAT. Given all the available information, both internal and external, the DSMB recommended that BHAT be terminated almost a year early.

Another cardiovascular trial testing arrhythmia-suppressing drugs, CAST, was terminated early owing to an observed harmful effect. Conventional wisdom and practice in cardiology were to use this new class of drugs (encainide and flecainide), which was known to be highly effective in suppressing arrhythmias, and arrhythmias were known to be associated with sudden death and cardiovascular death. Quite early in the trial, the statistical evidence was strikingly showing a harmful effect of encainide and flecainide. In this instance, most of the external information favored these drugs' effectiveness, yet the DSMB had to rely heavily on the internal consistency of the CAST data to make their ultimate judgment.

Although external information should be used informally, such information should not be combined formally with the ongoing trial in a meta-analysis. A recent NIH-sponsored workshop discussed the concept of a formal sequential meta-analysis of all ongoing relevant trials. However, such an approach was not judged to be feasible[64] in most circumstances. Each trial should attempt to come to its own conclusions and use the external information as secondary support.

DOCUMENTATION OF THE DSMB

Since the DSMB plays such a central role in the conduct of Phase III trials with mortality or irreversible morbidity outcomes, the activities of the DSMB need to be documented carefully for scientific as well as regulatory reasons. Before the initiation of a trial, the DSMB should develop a brief guideline on its operational procedures, including any statistical guidelines for early termination. The DSMB statistical reports for each meeting provide a summary of the analyses conducted. In addition, minutes of those DSMB meetings should be kept and filed along with the reports. Any correspondence between the DSMB and either the sponsor or the investigators should also be retained.

COMMUNICATION OF THE DSMB

In the event a decision is made to recommend a protocol modification or early termination, the DSMB must be prepared to communicate those recommendations quickly to the study chair and the sponsor as agreed on. The rationale for the recommendation must be clearly laid out along with the data analyses that led to the recommendation. This communication may require a special meeting between the full DSMB and the study executive committee where the details of the DSMB report are gone over. However, there is usually not much time to prepare for such meetings, so the communication between the two chairs is the most efficient. If the sponsor was not present for the closed session of the DSMB meeting, then the sponsor must be fully briefed as soon as possible as well. In instances where an investigational new drug is being tested, communication between the DSMB and the FDA may also be requested. Since the final authority to modify a protocol or terminate the trial rests with the investigators and the sponsor, they must be given sufficient information to implement the recommendations as soon as possible.

CAST results were conveyed rapidly to both the FDA and investigators because of the harmful effects of the drugs being evaluated.[44–46] However, once the information was released, it became a challenge to rapidly get the detailed results through the peer review and into the scientific community. A special short presentation in a leading medical journal was arranged and a more detailed manuscript followed as rapidly as possible through regular peer review. Press coverage, however, caused the public and especially all the many patients on the drugs tested to get in touch with their physicians before many of those physicians were even aware of the general CAST results, much less the detailed results. The PHS aspirin results appeared in the medical literature a few weeks following the DSMB recommendation for termination.[51] Generally, such rapid communication requires some anticipation by the DSMB that early termination might be possible and early drafts of manuscripts are prepared that can be modified at the time of the final decision. This was the case for both CAST and BHAT. In the PRAISE trial,[65] the chair of the DSMB and the director of the statistical center attended a briefing of the FDA by the sponsor to reflect their thoughts and deliberations.

Although the DSMB has typically no formal role in further dissemination of the trial results, many executive committees seek the advice and counsel of the DSMB in the preparation of the final manuscript. For example, the PRAISE chair met with the DSMB to get their advice on the conclusions of the trial, taking advantage of the extensive knowledge of the data base and analyses. This interchange is especially prudent if the trial was terminated early based on the recommendations of the DSMB, and the essential features of their rationale need to be included. BHAT and CAST study chairs met with their DSMBs as well in preparation for dissemination of those results. In one NIH-sponsored trial,[66] some DSMB members were so displeased with the conclusions of the paper that they[67, 68] took the unusual step of publishing their opinion that differed with the trial authors.

Hasty presentation of results shortly after termination can lead to mistaken conclusions or misunderstandings. Thus, as the DSMB senses that the trial may be terminated early, they should guide the statistical center and the chair of the trial in early preparation or at least rapid release of the information. In addition, the DSMB can provide the authors a first-pass peer review with their detailed knowledge of the trial and yet be somewhat independent. Through this interchange, the trial publication and communication of results are likely to be improved, which is to everyone's benefit.

SUMMARY

The concept of a DSMB has existed since the mid 1960s with the planning of the CDP. Since then, numerous DSMBs have existed for a wide variety of clinical trials across different diseases and sponsors. The success of the DSMB concept during this period has been outstanding. Confidentiality has been maintained. Trials have been terminated early for safety reasons or evidence of benefit or lack of feasibility.

Although useful statistical guidelines exist for interpreting interim analyses, they are still limited, and the judgment and experience of the DSMB are essential to the clinical trial process.

REFERENCES

1. Friedman L, Furberg C, DeMets DL. Fundamentals of Clinical Trials, 3rd ed. St. Louis, Mosby-Yearbook, 1996.
2. Meinert CL. Clinical Trials: Design, Conduct, and Analysis, New York, Oxford University Press, 1986.
3. Pocock SJ. Clinical Trials: A Practical Approach. New York, John Wiley & Sons, 1983.
4. Heart Special Project Committee. Organization, Review, and Administration of Cooperative Studies (Greenberg Report): A Report from the Heart Special Project Committee to the National Advisory Council, May 1967. Control Clin Trials 1988; 9:137–148.
5. Friedman L. The NHLBI model: A 25-year history. Stat Med 1993; 12:425–432.
6. Ellenberg SS, Geller NL, Simon R, Yusuf S (eds). Proceedings of Practical Issues in Data Monitoring of Clinical Trials. Bethesda, MD, January, 27–28, 1992. Stat Med 1993; 12:415–616.
7. Fleming TR. Evaluating therapeutic interventions: Some issues and experience. Stat Sci 1992; 7:428–456.
8. Fleming TR, DeMets DL. Monitoring of clinical trials: Issues and experiences. Control Clin Trials 1993; 14:183–297.
9. Hawkins BS. Data monitoring committees for multicenter clinical trials sponsored by the National Institutes of Health: I. Roles and membership of data monitoring committees for trials sponsored by the National Eye Institute. Control Clin Trials 1991; 12:424–437.
10. Task Force of the Working Group on Arrhythmias of the European Society of Cardiology. The early termination of clinical trials: Causes, consequences, and control. Circulation 1994; 89:2892–2907.
11. Walters L. Data monitoring committees: The moral case for maximum feasible independence. Stat Med 1993; 12:575–580.
12. O'Neill RT. Some FDA perspectives on data monitoring in clinical trials in drug development. Stat Med 1993; 12:601–608.
13. Peto R, Pike MC, Armitage P, et al. Design and analysis of randomized clinical trials requiring prolonged observations of each patient: I. Introduction and design. Br J Cancer 1976; 34:585–612.
14. Rockhold FW, Enas GG. Data monitoring and interim analyses in the pharmaceutical industry: Ethical and logistical considerations. Stat Med 1993; 12:471–480.
15. Williams GW, Davis RL, Getson AJ, et al. Monitoring of clinical trials and interim analyses from a drug sponsor's point of view. Stat Med 1993; 12:481–492.
16. Buyse M. Interim analyses, stopping roles, and data monitoring in clinical trials in Europe. Stat Med 1993; 12:509–520.
17. Wittes J. Behind closed doors: The data monitoring board in randomized clinical trials. Stat Med 1993; 12:419–424.
18. DeMets DL, Ellenberg SS, Fleming TR, et al. Data and safety monitoring board and acquired immune deficiency syndrome (AIDS) clinical trials. Control Clin Trials 1995; 16:408–421.
19. Liberati A. Conclusions: I. The relationship between clinical trials and clinical practice: The risks of underestimating its complexity. Stat Med 1994; 13:1485–1492.
20. O'Neill RT. Conclusions: II. The relationship between clinical trials and clinical practice: The risks of underestimating its complexity. Stat Med 1994; 13:1493–1500.
21. DeMets DL. Data monitoring and sequential analysis—an academic perspective. J AIDS 1990; 3(Suppl 2):s124–s133.
22. Coronary Drug Project Research Group. Practical aspects of decision making in clinical trials: The Coronary Drug Project as a case study. Control Clin Trials 1981; 2:363–376.
23. Armstrong PW, Furberg CD. Clinical trial data and safety monitoring boards: The search for a constitution. Circulation 1995; 91:901–904.
24. Fleming TR. Data monitoring committees and capturing relevant information of high quality. Stat Med 1993; 12:565–570.
25. Pocock SJ. Statistical and ethical issues in monitoring clinical trials. Stat Med 1993; 12:1459–1469.
26. The TIMI Study Group. Comparison of invasive and conservative strategies after treatment with intravenous tissue plasminogen activator in acute myocardial infarction. N Engl J Med 1989; 320:618–627.
27. Diabetes Control and Complications Trial Research Group. Diabetes Control and Complications Trial (DCCT): Design and methodologic considerations for the feasibility phase. Diabetes 1986; 35:530–545.
28. Diabetes Control and Complications Trial Research Group. The effect of intensive treatment of diabetes on the development and progression of long-term complications in insulin-dependent diabetes mellitus. N Engl J Med 1993; 329:977–986.
29. Armitage P. Interim analysis in clinical trials. Stat Med 1991; 10:925–937.
30. McPherson K. Statistics: The problem of examining accumulating data more than once. N Engl J Med 1974; 290:501–502.
31. Pocock SJ. Group sequential methods in the design and analysis of clinical trials. Biometrika 1977; 64:191–199.
32. Pocock SJ. Interim analyses for randomized clinical trials: The group sequential approach. Biometrics 1982; 38:153–162.
33. O'Brien PC, Fleming TR. A multiple testing procedure for clinical trials. Biometrics 1979; 35:549–556.
34. Lan KKG, DeMets DL. Discrete sequential boundaries for clinical trials. Biometrika 1983; 70:659–663.
35. DeMets DL, Lan KKG. Interim analyses: The alpha spending function approach. Stat Med 1994; 13:1341–1352.
36. DeMets DL, Lan KKG. The alpha spending function approach to interim data analyses. *In* Thall P (ed). Recent Advances in Clinical Trial Design and Analysis. Amsterdam, Kluwer Academic, 1995, pp 1–27.
37. DeMets DL, Ware JH. Asymmetric group sequential boundaries for monitoring clinical trials. Biometrika 1982; 69:661–663.
38. Lan KKG, Simon R, Halperin M. Stochastically curtailed tests in long-term clinical trials. Communicat Stat Sequent Analys 1982; 1:207–219.
39. Lan KKG, Wittes J. The *B* value: A tool for monitoring data. Biometrics 1988; 44:579–585.
40. Coronary Drug Project Research Group. The Coronary Drug Project: Design, methods, and baseline results. Circulation 1973; 47(Suppl 1):II–179.
41. Beta-Blocker Heart Attack Trial Research Group. A randomized trial of propranolol in patients with acute myocardial infarction: I. Mortality results. JAMA 1982; 247:1707–1714.
42. DeMets DL, Hardy R, Friedman LM, Lan KKG. Statistical aspects of early termination in the Beta-Blocker Heart Attack Trial. Control Clin Trials 1984; 5:362–372.
43. Norwegian Multicenter Study Group. Timolol-induced reduction in mortality and reinfarction in patients surviving acute myocardial infarction. N Engl J Med 1981; 304:801.
44. Cardiac Arrhythmia Suppression Trial (CAST) Investigators. Preliminary report: Effect of encainide and flecainide on mortality in a randomized trial of arrhythmia suppression after myocardial infarction. N Engl J Med 1989; 321:406–412.
45. Pawitan Y, Hallstrom A. Statistical interim monitoring of the Cardiac Arrhythmia Suppression Trial. Stat Med 1990; 9:1081–1090.
46. Friedman LM, Bristow JD, Hallstrom A, et al. Data monitoring in the Cardiac Arrhythmia Suppression Trial. Online J Curr Clin Trials 1993; Jul 31:Doc no 79.
47. Packer M, Carver JR, Rodeheffer RJ, DeMets DL, et al, for the PROMISE Study Research Group. Effect of oral milrinone on mortality in severe chronic heart failure. N Engl J Med 1991; 325:1468–1475.
48. Packer M, Rouleau J, Swedberg K, et al, and the PROFILE Investigators. Effect of flosequinan on survival in chronic heart failure: Preliminary results of the PROFILE study. Circulation 1993; 88(Suppl I):1–301.
49. Swedberg K, Held P, Kjekhus J, et al. Effects of early administration of enalapril on mortality in patients with acute myocardial infarction—results of the Cooperative North Scandinavian Enalapril Survival Study II (Consensus II). N Engl J Med 1992; 327:678–684.

50. Furberg C, Campbell R, Pitt B. Letter to the editor (on Consensus II). N Engl J Med 1993; 328:967–968.
51. Steering Committee for the Physicians' Health Study Research Group. Preliminary Report: Findings from the Aspirin Component of the Ongoing Physicians' Health Study. N Engl J Med 1988; 318:262–264.
52. Cairns J, Cohen L, Colton T, et al. Issues in the early termination of the aspirin component of the Physicians' Health Study: Data Monitoring Board of the Physicians' Health Study. Ann Epidemiol 1991; 1:395–405.
53. Freedman B. Equipoise and the ethics of clinical research. N Engl J Med 1987; 317:141–145.
54. Green S, Fleming T, O'Fallon J. Policies for monitoring and interim reporting of results. J Clin Oncol 1987; 5:1477–1484.
55. FDA Guideline. Guideline for the Format and Content of the Clinical and Statistical Sections of an Application. Bethesda, MD, Center for Drug Evaluation and Research, Food and Drug Administration, Department of Health and Human Services, July, 1988.
56. PMA Ad Hoc Committee on Interim Analysis. Interim analysis in the pharmaceutical industry. Control Clin Trials 1993; 14:160–173.
57. Healy B, Campeau L, Gray R, et al, and the Investigators of the Post Coronary Artery Bypass Graft (CABG) Surgery Trial. Conflict-of-interest guidelines for a multicenter clinical trial of treatment after coronary artery bypass graft surgery. N Engl J Med 1989; 320:949–951.
58. Multiple Risk Factor Intervention Trial Research Group. Multiple Risk Factor Intervention Trial: Risk factor changes and mortality results. JAMA 1982; 248:1465–1477.
59. DeMets DL, Fleming TR, Whitley RJ, et al. The Data and Safety Board and acquired immune deficiency syndrome (AIDS) clinical trials. Control Clin Trials 1995; 16:408–421.
60. GUSTO Investigators. An international randomized trial comparing four thrombolytic strategies for acute myocardial infarction. N Engl J Med 1993; 329:673–682.
61. Nocturnal Oxygen Therapy Group. Continuous or nocturnal oxygen therapy in hypoxemic chronic obstructive lung disease. Ann Intern Med 1980; 93:391–398.
62. DeMets DL, Williams GW, Brown BW Jr, and the NOTT Research Group. A case report of data monitoring experience: The Nocturnal Oxygen Therapy Trial. Control Clin Trials 1982; 3:113–124.
63. Hjalmarson A, Elmfeldt D, Herlitz J, et al. Effect on mortality of metoprolol in acute myocardial infarction: A double-blind randomized trial. Lancet 2:823, 1981.
64. Pocock SJ. The role of external evidence in data monitoring of a clinical trial. Stat Med 1996; 15:1285–1293; discussion 1295–1297.
65. Packer M, O'Connor C, Ghali J, and the Prospective Randomized Amlodipine Survival Evaluation (PRAISE) Study Group. Effect of Amlodipine on Morbidity and Mortality in Severe Chronic Heart Failure. Presented at the American College of Cardiology Meetings, March 18, 1995, New Orleans.
66. Berson EL, Rosner B, Sandberg MA, et al. A randomized trial of vitamin A and vitamin E supplementation for retinitis pigmentosa. Arch Ophthalmol 1993; 111:761–772.
67. Marmor MF. A randomized trial of vitamin A and vitamin E supplementation for retinitis pigmentosa [comments]. Arch Ophthalmol 1993; 111:1460–1461.
68. Norton EWD. A randomized trial of vitamin A and vitamin E supplementation for retinitis pigmentosa [comments]. Arch Ophthalmol 1993; 111:1460.

6 Meta-Analysis of Randomized Trials

▶ Graham A. Colditz
▶ Catherine S. Berkey
▶ Frederick Mosteller

RESEARCH SYNTHESIS

Research synthesis offers an effective approach for dealing with the growing volume of the medical research database by offering a formalized, usually quantitative, method for the review of published data. A research synthesis ordinarily addresses a single clinical issue—typically the efficacy of a therapeutic intervention—or the risk associated with a treatment, a condition, or other factors, possibly environmental or behavioral. The synthesis of research findings has long been a central part of a research review that identifies areas of agreement in a field of clinical medicine as well as areas that have discrepancies or require further research. The large number of scientific publications concerning any single topic makes it nearly impossible for the clinician to keep abreast of the results of studies that bear on clinical practice. Further, the practicing clinician does not have the time required (or the specialized skills) to do all the work involved in synthesis of the published results. So people with the specialized skills need to carry out syntheses, and clinicians need to be able to interpret the subsequent reports.

For example, when searching the databases of the National Library of Medicine, one notes a large number of meta-analyses bearing on cardiovascular problems. The use of the term *meta-analysis* by the National Library of Medicine makes it easy for the reader to search and identify published reports of meta-analyses. In 1996 alone, there were at least 25 references to meta-analysis identified bearing on coronary disease. These included risk factors predicting disease, cholesterol lowering, psychosocial issues as predictors of disease and in treatment, apolipoprotein E, diet and activity, antihypertensive therapy, nifedipine, and interventional cardiology. As an example of the role of meta-analysis in the synthesis of a field of study, we might review the results from the quantitative assessment of plasma homocysteine as a risk factor for vascular disease.[1] This meta-analysis identified and combined data from 27 studies relating homocysteine to arteriosclerotic vascular disease and from an additional 11 studies of folic acid effects on homocysteine. After combining the data the authors concluded that the variable of elevations in homocysteine is an independent risk factor for arteriosclerotic vascular disease; they also concluded that the risk of disease increases by 60% for each 5 μmol/L increase in homocysteine. Using different assumptions regarding the benefit of reduction in homocysteine through folate supplementation, the authors estimated that 13,500 to 50,000 cases of coronary disease could be prevented annually.[1]

Formalizing the methods of research synthesis, including the requirement of a protocol, is important to limit the biases that may be introduced through more traditional reviews that rest on authoritative pronouncements. Among the many examples that illustrate the potential bias in such reviews is a study that examined the citation of trials of cholesterol-lowering drugs. Trials with positive results were cited more frequently than those that failed to show benefit of therapy, thereby distorting the reported benefit of therapy (see Reference 2). Where appropriate, a research synthesis may use quantitative methods to combine and summarize the results of several studies. Such a quantitative summary should include a measure of location (mean effect) and its uncertainty (variability), including the variability among studies as well as within studies.

Through the Potsdam Consultation, which included scientists from nine countries, guidelines have been published for the systematic review of randomized, controlled trials.[3] We review these guidelines in this chapter, focusing on the reading and interpretation of a meta-analysis rather than on its actual conduct.

We note that not all meta-analyses are based on randomized trials in which steps are deliberately taken to equate the treated and control groups being compared (e.g., making them similar with regard to age or tobacco use). Instead, many meta-analyses encompass observational studies, which may compare groups that have not been or cannot be equated. This lack of control over the treatment or exposure of interest, or other known or unknown confounders, makes conclusions riskier in observational studies. Despite these limitations, numerous meta-analyses of observational data have informed consensus opinion on topics such as the causes and prevention of cardiovascular disease. For example, Berlin and Colditz have summarized the observational evidence that physical activity is protective against coronary heart disease,[4] and Law and colleagues have combined data from cohort studies, international comparisons, and randomized trials to quantify the reduction in ischemic heart disease associated with lowering of serum cholesterol levels.[5]

Several comprehensive texts have addressed the many statistical issues relevant to combining study results[6–8] and the use of meta-analysis for exploration of new issues beyond those addressed in the primary studies[9] and, more generally, summarize the many issues in research synthesis.[10–12] The U.S. Preventive Services Task Force has offered an extended collection of examples in which a consistent set of criteria has been applied to an evaluation of the strength of evidence supporting the efficacy of preventive services.[13] That work summarizes results from both randomized trials and observational studies that bear on preventive services. Perhaps Light and Pillemer give the broadest overview of this field for the general reader who wishes to understand and interpret meta-analysis.[11]

The Oxford database attempted to meta-analyze all clinical trials dealing with obstetrics.[14] A somewhat larger group headed by the same team, now called the *Cochrane Collaboration,* has set out to do for all medicine what the Oxford document, "Effective Care in Pregnancy and Childbirth" (ECPC),[14] has done for obstetrics. Because of this movement, we may hope for many additional medical meta-analyses in the future. The investigators who developed the Oxford database of perinatal trials, which encompasses an entire field of medicine and public health, have summarized the methodologic issues encountered in the process.[15]

We do not attempt to cover all the material in those texts but refer the reader interested in conducting a meta-analysis to these works. Here we focus on issues arising when one reads and interprets a meta-analysis.

Quantitative methods have been used in research synthesis for much of the twentieth century. Olkin gave a brief history of methods for combining results from individual studies.[16] He traced methods that have been used to combine results of studies on a variety of subjects, from the effectiveness of inoculation on enteric fever[17] to topics in agricultural[18, 19] and the social sciences. Smith and Glass first used the term *meta-analysis* in the 1970s when combining results from studies evaluating the effectiveness of psychotherapy.[20] Despite early applications of meta-analysis by Beecher in analgesic research,[21] and Gilbert and colleagues in summarizing outcomes of surgical research,[22] it was not until the 1980s that the methods were widely applied in the health sciences.[23, 24] Among the fields in medicine adopting meta-analysis, cardiovascular disease has been a leading area of application. Early efforts to combine results applied to aspirin in the prevention of recurrent myocardial infarction (MI) and death after hospitalization for acute MI. More recently, meta-analyses have addressed a broad range of topics on the etiology, treatment, and prevention of cardiovascular diseases.

Benefits of Meta-Analysis

The purpose of meta-analysis has been described in numerous writings and spans a broad range of applications. Sacks and colleagues[25] and Ingelfinger and associates[26] have described the following benefits of meta-analysis:

1. Increase in statistical power for comparing primary endpoints and for comparing subgroups
2. Resolution of uncertainty when reports disagree
3. Improvement in estimates of the size of effect
4. Answers to new questions not posed at the start of individual trials
5. Improvements in the quality of primary research
6. Contribution to medical technology assessment
7. Production of more objective summaries of the literature than unaided intellectual interpretation can supply

An example of the benefits of meta-analysis comes from the Antiplatelet Trialists' Collaboration, which combined results from 145 randomized trials of antiplatelet therapy among high-risk patients and low-risk populations.[27] In addition to demonstrating the benefits of aspirin therapy in patients with acute MI, this collaborative analysis showed that the magnitude of benefit is comparable in younger and older patients (<65 versus ≥ 65 years of age) and in men and women. Within the individual studies combined in this meta-analysis, analyses of these subgroups had insufficient power to be definitive. Further, the analysis of other subgroups showed that antiplatelet therapy benefits a wide range of high-risk patients, including those with stable angina, those undergoing vascular procedures, and those with peripheral vascular disease.

MODELS USED IN META-ANALYSIS

Two models are widely used in quantitative data synthesis, and controversy continues over which approach is better. Homogeneity of the outcomes of results of the studies is the key issue. When the outcomes of studies are about as alike as sampling variation would predict, the mean or a simple weighted mean of the study outcomes may summarize them well. However, if the results of different studies vary substantially, too much to be explained by within-study sampling error, the extent of this variability among studies also needs to be evaluated and taken into account.

The *fixed-effects model* is based on the homogeneity assumption, that is, the assumption that the group of study results all estimate the same true result and that the observed variation is due to within-study sampling error. Under this model, we do not consider that the true values may differ from one situation to another. The weakness of this assumption is that, in practical research applications, we cannot know whether it is true, and we are sure that it is not. Many investigators use statistical tests of homogeneity to see whether the assumption is correct and to evaluate the test at the $P = 0.05$ level. Because we cannot believe that the among-study variance of the results can ever be zero and because the tests for homogeneity have low power, we should not uncritically accept the assumption of homogeneity. That is, the purpose of the test is not to determine whether heterogeneity exists at all but to get an idea of *how much* heterogeneity exists. We prefer to act as if there is heterogeneity among the study results when the chi-square goodness-of-fit test statistic is greater than the number of studies minus 1, which is the mean value when there is no heterogeneity.

Some authors suggest that, when the test for heterogeneity yields a significant result, we should not combine the results since the combined value is not interpretable as the single true value. However, if the purpose of a meta-analysis is to study a broad issue (e.g., the evaluation of a treatment that may be administered in different ways to many different kinds of patients), then we can expect true values to vary from study to study, and both an estimate of this variability and the mean of these true values are important.[28]

In this second situation, when variation among study results is too large to be explained solely by within-study sampling error, we employ the *random-effects model.* We suppose that there is a universe of study situations and that each situation has its own true value (treatment effect). Over the universe of different study situations, there is a grand mean effect as well as variance among the studies. Thus, the variance of the result from a given study includes two components: the within-study variance and the among-study variance. The assumption that a random sample of studies has been drawn from this universe is rarely met in practice. When we treat the data as if we had a random-effects model, we are making an inference to the universe of populations that is generated by the scientific process.

If we use the fixed-effects model and assume no variance among the true treatment effects of the studies, then—to the degree that the assumption is false—we will report better precision in estimates of treatment effect than we are justified in using. On the other hand, when we apply the random-effects model to study results that are homogeneous, it reverts to the fixed-effects model. Consequently, the random-effects model gives back the fixed-effects model when the situation deserves it. Therefore it is reasonable to use the random-effects model as the starting point for a combined analysis,[8] not because we believe in the random-effects model, but because its analysis is satisfactory for either situation.

Use of Quantitative Methods in Meta-Analysis: An Illustration

In 1982 Stampfer and colleagues identified eight randomized trials of intravenous streptokinase therapy in acute MI and combined their published results.[29] The data from the eight trials are summarized in Table 6–1. (The authors noted that four additional trials were identified but were excluded from the analysis because the subjects had not been strictly randomized.)

In this section we illustrate the combining of risk differences for the use of streptokinase in acute MI. The illustration serves to establish notation and display the calculations.

Table 6–1 lays out the counts n_{ti} and n_{ci} for the numbers of treated patients and the numbers of control patients in study i, together with the numbers of deaths d_{ti} and d_{ci} in the treated and control groups, in each of the k studies numbered from $i = 1$ to k. The primary outcome variable y_i is the observed risk difference $p_{ti} - p_{ci}$ in study i. For example, in the first trial ($i = 1$) listed in Table 6–1 (the 1969 European trial), the observed risk difference is

$$\begin{aligned} p_{t1} - p_{c1} &= 20/83 - 15/84 \\ &= 0.241 - 0.179 = 0.062 \end{aligned}$$

Positive differences are unfavorable to streptokinase and negative ones are favorable. The risk differences in the eight trials range from -0.1514 to $+0.0624$; these values suggest that streptokinase may prevent 15 deaths per 100 patients or—at the other extreme—may cause an additional six deaths per 100

TABLE 6–1 • Eight Randomized Trials of Streptokinase (Strepto) in Acute Myocardial Infarction

	No. Randomized		No. of Deaths		Risk Difference			
Trial	*Strepto* n_{ti}	*Control* n_{ci}	*Strepto* d_{ti}	*Control* d_{ci}	$y_i = p_{ti} - p_{ci}$	S_i^2	$w_i = 1/S_i^2$	$W_i = 1/(\sigma_A^2 + S_i^2)$
1st European, 1969	83	84	20	15	+0.0624	.00395	253	188
2nd European, 1971	373	357	69	94	−0.0783	.00095	1055	433
Finnish, 1971	219	207	22	17	+0.0183	.00078	1287	467
Italian, 1971	164	157	19	18	+0.0012	.00127	787	379
2nd Frankfurt, 1972	102	104	13	29	−0.1514	.00302	331	228
Australian, 1973	264	253	21	23	−0.0114	.00060	1656	508
British, 1976	302	293	43	44	−0.0078	.00084	1191	454
European, 1979	156	159	18	30	−0.0733	.00162	618	335
Totals	**1663**	**1614**	**225**	**270**	**−0.2403**	—	**7178**	**2992**

Data from Stampfer M, Goldhaber S, Yusuf S, et al. Effect of intravenous streptokinase on acute myocardial infarction: Pooled results from randomized trials. N Engl J Med 1982; 307:1180–1182.

patients. Only two of the individual trials listed in Table 6–1 (the 2nd European and the 2nd Frankfurt trials) reported statistically significant differences ($P < 0.05$) between treatment and control groups.

One problem that we encounter is how best to combine the results of the trials to estimate a combined (pooled, overall) $p_t - p_c$. A second problem is how to obtain confidence limits for the combined result.

In its simplest form, a pooled summary may be the simple average (equal weighting) of the risk differences from the eight studies. The average risk difference in Table 6–1 is −0.030 (−0.2403/8), representing a reduction of three deaths per 100 patients treated with streptokinase.

More often, a weighted average or mean is estimated using weights that are inversely proportional to the variances of the quantities being combined. This approach often gives larger weights to those studies with larger sample sizes. Provided that all the studies estimate the same true value (according to the homogeneity assumption of the fixed-effects model), this set of weights gives an unbiased estimate of the true risk difference and the estimate with the smallest variance, at least approximately. In the fixed-effects model, we weight the outcome y_i of each study by the reciprocal of the estimated variance S_i^2 of y_i. Here, the variance of the risk difference in study *i* is

$$S_i^2 = p_{ti}(1 - p_{ti})/n_{ti} + p_{ci}(1 - p_{ci})/n_{ci}$$

Thus, the fixed-effects model weights w_i are $1/S_i^2$, and we get the fixed-effects estimate of the effect of treatment by computing

$$y_w = \Sigma w_i y_i / \Sigma w_i$$

For the y_i and w_i in Table 6–1, this estimate is −0.0231, which represents a reduction of 2.3 deaths per 100 persons treated with streptokinase. The variance of y_w is $1/\Sigma w_i$, its standard error (0.0118) is the square root of this, and its 95% confidence interval (CI) is −.046 to 0.00.

The statistic

$$Q = \Sigma w_i (y_i - y_w)^2$$

is a χ^2 statistic with k − 1 degrees of freedom, which can provide a test for heterogeneity. It measures the variability of the treatment effects among studies. Here k = 8, and thus the degrees of freedom are 7. The computed value of Q = 15.25, which is larger than the $P = 0.05$ critical value (14.07) for the χ^2 distribution with 7 degrees of freedom. Our view is that the variation observed among these trials is larger than 0, and we estimate the variance among the true y's of the studies by using the formula

$$\sigma_A^2 = \max 0, \frac{Q - (k - 1)}{\Sigma w_i - (\Sigma w_i^2 / \Sigma w_i)}$$

where the result turns out to be 0.001364. (Although this variance may at first appear to be very small, it is larger than the S_i^2 of five of the eight trials in Table 6–1.) Thus, the standard deviation of treatment effects among studies is 0.037 (= /0.001364).

To include this estimate of variability among study effects in calculating the overall treatment effect, we now use new weights from the random-effects model (denoted by capital W_i),

$$W_i = 1/(\sigma_A^2 + S_i^2)$$

and compute

$$y_W = \Sigma W_i y_i / \Sigma W_i$$

to get a new weighted estimate of the risk difference y_W = −0.0272, whose estimated standard error is $1/\Sigma W_i$ = 0.0183. Thus, the 95% confidence limits on the true risk difference are −.063 to +.009, which includes the null hypothesis of no treatment effect ($P > 0.05$).

Note that the confidence limits on the fixed-effects estimate y_W are narrower (−.046 to .000) because the fixed-effects model does not allow for variation among studies. (Rather, it assumes $\sigma_A^2 = 0$, even though here we estimate that $\sigma_A^2 = 0.0014$.) The point is not that 0.0014 is small but that it is larger than several of the S_i^2 and that therefore the new weights W_i are substantially different from the initial weights w_i, the new random-effects weights of the eight trials are more similar to one another.

Additional Issues in Estimation

Risk differences, risk ratios, and odds ratios are typical measures used in clinical studies. We have some preference for risk differences because they relate directly to deaths, which is what treatment aims to prevent. Stampfer and colleagues' original paper[29] used risk ratios. Other types of studies may have outcomes that are measured in continuous units, such as declines in systolic blood pressure. The methods described here may also be used for continuous outcomes. Further details such as estimation of S_i^2 for risk ratios, odds ratios, and continuous outcomes are provided by Laird and Mosteller.[30]

There are also situations for which specialized methods of meta-analysis have been developed, for example, the meta-analysis of survival curves,[31] of dose-response curves,[32] and of receiver operator characteristic curves in the diagnostic test setting.[33, 34] The meta-analysis of multiple outcomes considered simultaneously, such as systolic and diastolic blood pressure, also may involve specialized methods.[35]

Following the initial research synthesis that provided a quantitative summary of the benefits of streptokinase therapy on survival after MI,[29] correspondence from statistician Marvin Zelen suggested that variation in efficacy could be accounted for through a plot of the observed efficacy, in each trial, against time from onset of chest pain to initiation of therapy. Efficacy was greater when treatment was initiated soon after the onset of symptoms. This example highlights how a systematic synthesis can advance our understanding of the efficacy of therapy and answer questions that cannot be addressed in a single trial.

METHODOLOGIC GUIDELINES FOR RESEARCH SYNTHESIS AND META-ANALYSIS

The Potsdam Consultation outlined a series of methodologic points or guidelines that should be followed in the conduct of a research synthesis or meta-analysis.[3] When reading a report, one should check to see that each of these guidelines has been implemented. The key steps in conducting a meta-analysis, each being described in a subsequent report of the work, include the following:

1. Protocol development
2. Search strategy
3. Study selection
4. Methodologic quality assessment
5. Data extraction
6. Analysis
7. Heterogeneity evaluation
8. Subgroup analysis
9. Sensitivity analysis

When each of these steps is described in the report of a meta-analysis, the reader can follow the methods that have been used and then check that the interpretation of the data is consistent with the material presented in the report. For example, a thorough report specifies *protocol development,* including the question being asked and any specific subgroups that may be of interest. The *search strategy* is defined in sufficient detail that it can, in principle, be replicated by the reader. *Study selection* is detailed. A meta-analysis is often limited to randomized, controlled trials. However, in many settings, observational studies are the only ones available. The study design should be recorded so that the analyses can be stratified according to design (randomized, controlled trial; case control; prospective cohort; cross-sectional study). Ideally, studies that are identified but rejected from the meta-analysis are described along with the reason for rejection. A primary reason for rejection is that the data reported are inadequate for comparison.

Methodologic assessment includes a review of the trials to determine whether they meet the criteria for inclusion: Are they double blind? Do they require laboratory confirmation of diagnoses? Are patients randomized to treatment groups? Sometimes meta-analysts require a minimum sample size for eligibility or impose other conditions.

Data extraction methods should be described, and the data (including individual-study CIs, standard errors, or *P* values) should be summarized in a detailed table. A common approach is to have two independent readers extract the key data as defined in the protocol and then compare the items that have been identified. Discrepancies are resolved by discussion or by a third independent adjudicator. The *analysis* should be described in detail and the results presented in clinically meaningful forms.

Heterogeneity among the results of the studies should be assessed and reported. When substantial heterogeneity is identified, exploratory analyses should attempt to describe factors that account for the heterogeneity.

When *subgroup analyses* have been prespecified,

they should be reported as such. In addition, *sensitivity analyses* to assess the robustness of the findings from the meta-analysis should be described. For example, sensitivity analyses may repeat the analysis omitting those studies of lowest quality or a study that has some unique feature to see if the combined conclusions are altered.

When all these details are present, the reader is in a position to evaluate the meta-analysis and its applicability to the clinical situation at hand.

HETEROGENEITY

Heterogeneity offers an opportunity for the meta-analyst to further analyze the results from the group of studies in hand and to identify features that contribute to the variation among study results. These features may be related, for example, to study design, study implementation, treatment, measures of exposure, or definition of subgroups of patients (e.g., by age, smoking status, gender, or severity of illness). This type of exploration can help the analyst interpret the available results and identify areas for additional research. Consideration of heterogeneity in a meta-analysis may be even more enlightening than the combined point estimate. (See the example at the end of this section.)

The reported mean age of patients in each study or the percentage of male patients in each trial may be useful information regarding why clinical findings differ among trials, though separate subgroup-specific results can more validly and efficiently evaluate associations between patient characteristics and treatment efficacy. The meta-analyst should generally specify a priori a few factors to consider, although data on some of the desired factors may not be available from the published studies. Sometimes factors such as size of dose, length of exposure, duration of treatment, or severity of disease have already been established by previous studies to be important to the outcome. When this is the case, these variables can be used in the analysis without concern for the hazards usually associated with exploratory data analysis, such as an increased chance of reaching false conclusions (the P values that are reported in exploratory analysis may be too small). Because the number of published studies is usually small, apparent associations between study results and study-level covariates are especially vulnerable to confounding by other (possibly unmeasured) factors. Results should therefore be interpreted cautiously.

When information is available on the factors of interest for each of the studies in a meta-analysis, one should use appropriate statistical methods to study the effects of these covariates on the heterogeneous study results. For the analysis of patient-level data arising from a single study, regression methods serve this purpose. Special modifications of regression models adapt the methods for application to the field of meta-analysis.[10, 36] The application of regression methods to meta-analysis can provide answers to new questions as well as describe and adjust or control for covariate differences among studies.

To illustrate the value of identifying sources of heterogeneity among trial results, we go back to the data in Table 6–1 taken from Stampfer and associates,[29] who also provide information on the duration of symptoms in patients before streptokinase was administered. We previously presented the results (risk difference, −0.0231; 95% CI, −0.046 to 0.000) based on the fixed-effects model. However, because of heterogeneity, the random-effects estimates of streptokinase benefit are more appropriate (risk difference, −0.027; 95% CI, −0.063 to +0.009). Both models suggest that between two and three lives are saved per 100 patients treated with streptokinase. However, because we expect patients treated in a more timely manner to benefit more than those treated later, we use a random-effects regression model[36] to estimate the benefit of streptokinase when it is administered within 12 hours of the onset of chest pain. Including duration of symptoms prior to treatment (reported by each study) as a covariate in the model, we estimate that 5.3 lives per 100 patients are saved when streptokinase is administered within 12 hours (risk difference, −0.053; 95% CI, −0.096 to −0.011; $P < 0.05$). Therefore, by explaining the source of heterogeneity among the results of trials, we arrive at an estimate of treatment benefit that is more clinically relevant than the original combined estimate in whose calculation the fact was ignored that patients in some trials were treated 3 days after symptoms began, probably too late to be of benefit.

QUALITY OF ORIGINAL STUDIES

Although many have suggested that the quality of studies be used to adjust their outcomes or to weight them in meta-analysis, these suggestions have not been given a strong statistical basis and are not currently being implemented. Wortman[37] described two methods of rating study quality. One was based on various threats to the validity of studies, as outlined by Campbell and Stanley[38] and by Cook and Campbell,[39] and the other was based on the scoring of features of a clinical trial, as proposed by Chalmers and coworkers.[40] Because judging the quality of studies is subjective, some meta-analysts require that those people who extract the data from published papers and who rate the quality of studies be blinded as to authorship and study results. In other words, certain details are blacked out so that the treatment found to be superior in the study cannot be ascertained. While some advocate the use of such blinding for the assessment of study quality for meta-analysis, as well as for the extraction of study results, such blinding of journal articles is expensive and has not thus far been shown to enhance the objective assessment of study quality. Preliminary data from a comparative evaluation of blind quality assessment versus unblinded assessment by two independent readers show no consistent difference in favor of blinding (J Berlin, personal communication, 1996). Obviously, it is a good idea to avoid bias, but blinding may not be a means to this end.

The investigators compiling the Oxford database on clinical trials in perinatal medicine cited the enormity of the task of assessing quality over many studies and chose to score studies on the following three key dimensions of potential bias[14]:

1. Control of selection bias on entry (quality of random allocation)
2. Control of selection bias after entry (the extent to which the primary analysis included every person entered into the study labeled by intention to treat)
3. Control of bias in assessing outcome (the extent to which the outcome assessment was blinded as to treatment group in the original investigations)

The most commonly used methods for evaluating the effects of study quality on study results are to meta-analyze groups of studies separately by quality (e.g., the highest quality ones) and to determine whether differences in quality are associated with differences in outcome. Attempting to use individual component scores and their summed quality scores for randomized, controlled trials suggested by Chalmers and associates,[40] Emerson and colleagues[41] failed to find quality-related differences in study outcomes, even though the data were adequate over a 30-year period to show a substantial gain in average quality score. On the other hand, a meta-analysis of randomized, controlled trials (each published after 1970) of the efficacy of cognitive behavioral therapies for hypertension showed that estimates of treatment efficacy varied substantially with quality of trial.[42] The five trials that used baseline blood pressure measurements made only on a single day and whose control groups consisted of patients randomly assigned to no therapy (or a waiting list or regular monitoring) reported significant ($P < 0.05$) reductions due to cognitive therapies in both systolic (13.4 mm Hg) and diastolic (9.0 mm Hg) blood pressures. However, either the requirement of baseline blood pressure assessments over 2 or more days or the use of a placebo/sham control group substantially diminished the estimated treatment benefit. Trials with both a longer baseline blood pressure assessment and a credible placebo intervention found no significant benefit of cognitive behavioral therapy (2.8 mm Hg systolic reduction [$P > 0.05$] and 1.3 mm Hg diastolic reduction [$P > 0.05$]).

From studies such as these, we see that quality has improved over time. Detsky and coworkers[43] suggest that the field is not ready to adjust study outcomes for quality or weight analyses by quality score. Greenland[44] argues against using summed or total quality scores because he thinks that this approach mixes up different aspects of quality. He advocates separate analysis of the individual components of the quality rating. Emerson and associates[41] conducted this type of analysis as well but found no effects. Failure to assess quality does not invalidate a meta-analysis but limits our ability to understand sources of heterogeneity when it is present. The average quality in a given field may help identify those fields of research with the best methodologic records and those in which improved methodologic rigor is required. We believe that the emphasis on study quality by the field of meta-analysis is partially responsible for this trend.

PUBLICATION BIAS

The term *publication bias* refers to the phenomenon in which studies with positive (statistically significant) results are more likely to be published than are those with null or negative (nonsignificant) results. This bias can distort the combined results and the interpretation of a meta-analysis. Begg and Berlin summarized much of the work on publication bias and reported their own meta-analysis investigations of its magnitude in medicine.[45] Several approaches to this problem have been suggested, including the "file-drawer" calculation and the creation of registers of clinical trials.

Rosenthal[46] introduced an attractive idea for quantifying the effect of publication bias. He viewed the problem as arising because investigators left studies without statistically significant results (or with negative results) in their file drawers instead of attempting to publish them. He asked how many nonsignificant studies would be required to reduce an observed statistically significant meta-analysis to nonsignificance. If the number was unreasonably large, the observed result would be regarded as good evidence for an effect.

Several approaches to the identification of publication bias have been proposed. Experience with the peer-review process suggests that if unpublished studies are identified for inclusion in a research synthesis, these unpublished studies should be handled separately. We no longer live in a time when articles are accepted without change in peer-reviewed journals. It is commonplace for articles to be rewritten and conclusions changed (or even reversed) before publication. Thus, we cannot regard peer-reviewed articles as coming from the same population as unpublished articles.

A thorough search is the best safeguard against publication bias. A prospective register of all clinical trials initiated would help in some settings, but the costs of establishing such a register and the methods for maintaining it are not clear. Unless well maintained, a register of initiated studies would not add much to the field beyond a thorough search.

JUDGMENT—DOES THE META-ANALYSIS INFORM YOUR CLINICAL PRACTICE?

The issues described earlier, when reported in detail in a published meta-analysis, help the reader interpret the overall body of data addressing a specific clinical question. However, as has been noted by several authors, many meta-analyses fail to report on all these issues,[47] perhaps in part because editors seeking short papers set limits on the space available for methodologic details, description of patient populations, and subgroup results. Even when all the relevant details are available, the reader is still left to make a judgment as to whether the results of the meta-analysis apply to a given clinical situation.

Several factors that may influence the appropriateness of extrapolation include how similar the clinician's patients are to those in the original studies, in terms of both age and underlying disease; whether the treatment described can be administered as effectively in the clinic as in research studies (given issues such as patient compliance); and what quality of research data and of meta-analysis has been used to draw the conclusion. As Richard Peto has asked in several oral presentations: "How sure are we that we can extrapolate results to ages beyond those in the original studies?" Further, when the heterogeneity among the results of different studies is substantial, one must ask whether a sound explanation exists to account for this variation, and if so, how this explanation relates to a given clinician's patients.

SUMMARY

Guidelines for the conduct of meta-analysis offer a framework for the critical reader. However, interpretation and application must go beyond these guidelines. One must make a judgment as to the sharpness of the question addressed, the sources of bias that may distort the evidence, and the generalizability of the results to other clinical settings. Typically, a meta-analysis of randomized, controlled trials provides a suitable estimate of the efficacy of a therapy under study conditions but may exaggerate its efficacy in general practice (outside of the research environment). Application of the tested therapy to individual patients still requires the clinician to weigh the likely benefits against the risks of adverse effects while considering the underlying risk of disease and its complications in the individual patient.[48]

REFERENCES

1. Boushey CJ, Beresford SAS, Omenn GS, et al. A quantitative assessment of plasma homocysteine as a risk factor for vascular disease: Probable benefits of increasing folate intakes. JAMA 1995; 274:1049–1057.
2. Ravnskov U. Cholesterol-lowering trials in coronary heart disease: Frequency of citation and outcome. BMJ 1992; 305:15–19.
3. Cook D, Sackett D, Spitzer W. Methodologic guidelines for systematic reviews of randomized, control trials in health care from the Potsdam Consultation on meta-analysis. J Clin Epidemiol 1995; 48:167–171.
4. Berlin JA, Colditz GA. A meta-analysis of physical activity in the prevention of coronary heart disease. Am J Epidemiol 1990; 132:612–628.
5. Law MR, Wald NJ, Thompson SG. By how much and how quickly does reduction in serum cholesterol concentration lower risk of ischaemic heart disease? BMJ 1994; 308:367–372.
6. Hunter J, Schmidt F. Methods of Meta-Analysis: Correcting Error and Bias in Research Findings. Newbury Park, CA, Sage, 1990.
7. Hedges L, Olkin I. Statistical Methods in Meta-Analysis. Orlando, Academic Press, 1985.
8. National Research Council. On Combining Information: Statistical Issues and Opportunities for Research. Washington, DC, National Academy of Sciences Press, 1992.
9. Cook T, Cooper H, Cordray D, et al. Meta-Analysis for Explanation: A Casebook. New York; Russell Sage Foundation, 1992.
10. Cooper H, Hedges L. The Handbook of Research Synthesis. New York, Russell Sage Foundation, 1994.
11. Light R, Pillemer D. Summing Up: The Science of Reviewing Research. Cambridge, MA; Harvard University Press, 1984.
12. Petitti D. Meta-Analysis, Decision Analysis, and Cost-Effectiveness Analysis in Medicine: Methods for Quantitative Synthesis in Medicine. New York; Oxford University Press, 1994.
13. U.S. Preventive Services Task Force. Guide to Clinical Preventive Services, 2nd ed. Baltimore, Williams & Wilkins, 1996.
14. Chalmers I, Enkin M, Keirse M. Effective Care in Pregnancy and Childbirth. Oxford; Oxford University Press, 1989.
15. Enkin M, Keirse M, Renfrew M, Neilson J. Pregnancy and Childbirth Module: Cochrane Database of Systematic Reviews (Cochrane updates on disk). Oxford; Update Software, 1993 (vol disk issue 2).
16. Olkin I. Statistical and theoretical considerations in meta-analysis. J Clin Epidemiol 1995; 48:133–146.
17. Fisher R. Statistical Methods for Research Workers. Edinburgh; Oliver & Body, 1932.
18. Cochran W. Problems arising in the analysis of a series of similar experiments. J R Stat Soc Suppl 1937; 4:102–118.
19. Cochran W. The combination of estimates from different experiments. Biometrics 1954; 10:101–129.
20. Smith ML, Glass GV. Meta-analysis of psychotherapy outcome studies. Am Psychologist 1977; 32:752–760.
21. Beecher H. The powerful placebo effect. JAMA 1955; 159:1602–1606.
22. Gilbert J, McPeek B, Mosteller F. Progress in surgery and anesthesia: Benefits and risks of innovative therapy. *In* Bunker J, Barnes B, Mosteller F (eds). Costs, Risks, and Benefits of Surgery. Oxford; Oxford University Press, 1977.
23. Sacks H, Berrier J, Reitman D, et al. Meta-analysis of randomized, controlled studies. N Engl J Med 1987; 316:450–455.

24. Louis T, Fineberg H, Mosteller F. Findings for public health from meta-analysis. Annu Rev Public Health 1985; 6:1–20.
25. Sacks HS, Berrier J, Reitman D, et al. Meta-analysis of randomized, control trials: An update of the quality and methodology. *In* Bailar JC, Mosteller F (eds). Medical Uses of Statistics; 2nd ed. Boston; NEJM Books, 1992; pp 427–442.
26. Ingelfinger J, Mosteller F, Thibodeau L, Ware J. Biostatistics in Clinical Medicine; 3rd ed. New York; McGraw-Hill, 1994.
27. Antiplatelet Trialists' Collaboration: Collaborative overview of randomised trials of antiplatelet therapy: I. Prevention of death, myocardial infarction, and stroke by prolonged antiplatelet therapy in various categories of patients. BMJ 1994; 308:81–106.
28. Colditz G, Burdick E, Mosteller F. Heterogeneity in meta-analysis of data from epidemiologic studies: A commentary. Am J Epidemiol 1995; 142:371–382.
29. Stampfer M, Goldhaber S, Yusuf S, et al. Effect of intravenous streptokinase on acute myocardial infarction: Pooled results from randomized trials. N Engl J Med 1982; 307:1180–1182.
30. Laird N, Mosteller F. Some statistical methods for combining experimental results. Int J Technol Assess Health Care 1990; 6:5–30.
31. Dear K. Iterative generalized least squares for meta-analysis of survival data at multiple times. Biometrics 1994; 50:989–1002.
32. Berlin J, Longnecker M, Greenland S. Meta-analysis of epidemiologic dose-response data. Epidemiology 1993; 4:218–228.
33. Irwig L, Tosteson A, Gatsonis C, et al. Guidelines for meta-analyses evaluating diagnostic tests. Ann Intern Med 1994; 120:667–676.
34. Rutter C, Gatsonis C. Regression methods for meta-analysis of diagnostic test data. Acad Radiol 1995; 2:S48–S56.
35. Berkey C, Anderson J, Hoaglin D. Multiple-outcomes meta-analysis of clinical trials. Stat Med 1996; 15:537–557.
36. Berkey CS, Hoaglin D, Mosteller F, Colditz GA. A random-effects regression model for meta-analysis. Stat Med 1995; 14:395–411.
37. Wortman P. Judging research quality. *In* Cooper H, Hedges L (eds). The Handbook of Research Synthesis. New York; Russell Sage Foundation, 1994; pp 97–109.
38. Campbell D, Stanley J. Experimental and Quasi-Experimental Designs for Research. Chicago; Rand McNally, 1966.
39. Cook T, Campbell D. Quasi-Experimentation: Design and Analysis Issues for Field Settings. Boston; Houghton Mifflin, 1979.
40. Chalmers T, Smith HJ, Blackburn B, et al. A method for assessing the quality of a randomized, control trial. Control Clin Trials 1981; 2:31–49.
41. Emerson J, Burdick E, Hoaglin D, Mosteller F. An empirical study of the possible relation of treatment differences to quality scores in controlled, randomized clinical trials. Control Clin Trials 1990; 11:339–352.
42. Eisenberg DM, Delbanco TL, Berkey CS, et al. Cognitive behavioral techniques for hypertension: Are they effective? Ann Intern Med 1993; 118:964–972.
43. Detsky A, Naylor C, O'Rourke K, et al. Incorporating variations in the quality of individual randomized trials into meta-analysis. J Clin Epidemiol 1992; 45:255–265.
44. Greenland S. Invited commentary: A critical look at some popular meta-analytic methods. Am J Epidemiol 1994; 140:290–296.
45. Begg C, Berlin J. Publication bias: A problem in interpreting medical data. J R Stat Soc A 1988; 151:419–463.
46. Rosenthal R. The "file drawer problem" and tolerance for null results. Psychol Bull 1979; 86:638–641.
47. Halvorsen K, Burdick E, Colditz G, et al. Combining results from independent investigations: Meta-analysis in clinical research. *In* Bailar JC, Mosteller F (eds). Medical Uses of Statistics; 2nd ed. Boston; NEJM Books, 1992; pp 413–426.
48. Glasziou PP, Irwig LM. An evidence-based approach to individualising treatment. BMJ 1995; 311:1356–1359.

Section Editor
▶ **Paul Ridker**

SECTION

II TREATMENT TRIALS

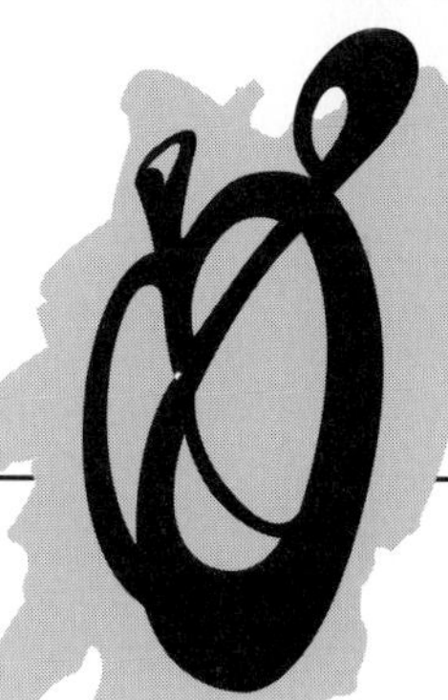

PART

I INTERVENTIONS FOR ACUTE ISCHEMIA

7 Aspirin and Heparin

▶ **Colin Baigent**
▶ **Rory Collins**

This chapter aims to review the available evidence on the clinical effects of aspirin and/or heparin therapy in patients with acute ischemic syndromes (i.e., unstable angina and acute myocardial infarction [MI]). When considering the possible effects of such antithrombotic regimens on major clinical outcomes (such as MI or death), it is important to bear in mind that such effects are likely to be moderate in size, rather than large.[1] That is, risk reductions of 10% to 20% may be plausible, but substantially larger reductions are generally not. Moreover, comparisons of major outcomes between two antithrombotic regimens are likely to yield smaller differences than those between an antithrombotic regimen and no antithrombotic treatment. Hence, the reliable assessment of the effects of antithrombotic regimens is likely to require the consideration of large-scale randomized evidence, either in one or more megatrials or in a large meta-analysis of many smaller trials.[1, 2] Small-scale studies cannot avoid moderate distortion by the play of chance, and nonrandomized methods cannot avoid moderate biases—and, even when large-scale randomized evidence is available, biases may be introduced by undue emphasis on the results from particular trials. Whenever possible, therefore, this chapter aims to consider together *all* of the evidence from relevant randomized trials. (For further discussion of the way in which such issues affect the interpretation of the randomized evidence considered in this chapter, see Chapter 4 [large-scale randomized evidence] and References 1 and 39.)

Within the context of randomized trials, acute ischemic syndromes have generally been divided into "unstable coronary artery disease" (i.e., unstable angina or non–Q wave MI) and transmural (i.e., Q wave) MI. Hence, in this chapter the randomized trials in unstable coronary artery disease are described separately from those in suspected acute MI, with the latter trials chiefly including patients with Q wave MI (although a small percentage had other forms of myocardial ischemia). However, at least during the first few hours or days after the onset of symptoms, when it is often difficult to distinguish these conditions, it may be most appropriate to consider the results from all of these trials together.

ASPIRIN AND HEPARIN FOR UNSTABLE CORONARY ARTERY DISEASE

Both unstable angina and non–Q wave MI are thought to be the result of nonocclusive platelet thrombus at the site of a ruptured atherosclerotic plaque that leads to acute episodes of vascular narrowing and coronary ischemia.[3] A diagnosis of unstable angina is confirmed when, following one or more episodes of chest pain, there is ST segment depression and/or T wave inversion on the electrocardiogram without either significant elevation of cardiac enzymes or the evolution of abnormal Q waves.[4] When these clinical features occur along with significant enzyme changes but without the emergence of abnormal Q waves, a diagnosis of non–Q wave MI is generally considered. The main hazard during the first week or so is the progression of the "culprit" lesion to total occlusion, and early treatment is principally aimed at avoiding this. Thereafter, since an unstable lesion is generally associated with disseminated atherosclerosis, patients are at appreciable risk not just of MI but also of stroke and other occlusive arterial events,[3] and treatment needs to be directed toward reducing these risks.

Aspirin for Unstable Coronary Artery Disease

Aspirin produces a prolonged functional defect in platelets that is due primarily to its irreversible inactivation of the platelet enzyme cyclooxygenase,[5] which in turn inhibits thromboxane A_2 (TxA_2)-mediated platelet aggregation.[6] Aspirin can act on platelets in the portal circulation before the drug reaches the systemic circulation, so that its effects are rapid.[7] The inhibitory effects of aspirin are dose dependent within the range of 5 to 100 mg daily; daily doses of 75 to 100 mg produce almost complete suppression of TxA_2 synthesis within a few days,[8, 9] and higher doses produce this effect within a few hours.[9] Hence, an immediate and complete inhibition of TxA_2-dependent platelet aggregation can generally be achieved in patients with acute ischemic syndromes with an initial dose of a few hundred milligrams of aspirin (but not with lower doses). Since platelets are anucleate, they cannot synthesize new cyclooxygenase enzyme, and the defect induced in a platelet by an aspirin dose lasts for the duration of its lifespan (generally about 8 to 10 days). Consequently, the systemic effect of an aspirin dose on platelet function diminishes only gradually as nucleated megakaryocytes release new intact platelets into the circulation. Complete inhibition can, therefore, be maintained with daily doses as low as 75 mg[10] (or with alternate daily dosing of a few hundred milligrams[9]), thus minimizing any dose-dependent gastrointestinal toxicity that may arise.[11]

In an overview of seven randomized, controlled trials in unstable coronary artery disease,[12–18] prolonged antiplatelet therapy (chiefly aspirin) reduced the risk of a major vascular event (defined as MI, stroke, or vascular death) by about one third during a mean treatment period of 8 months.[19] This corresponded to avoidance of about 50 such events per 1000 patients treated. Major outcomes during the first 5 to 6 days after symptom onset were reported by two trials, comparing 75 mg aspirin daily versus placebo[15] and 650 mg aspirin daily versus placebo[20] among a total of about 1300 patients. Aspirin appeared to halve the risk of MI or death during this early period; however, the selective availability of this information from only these two trials may have led to an overestimate of these early effects. Nevertheless, it would seem that aspirin produces rapid benefit in patients with unstable coronary artery disease, and that continued treatment produces further protection.

In these same two trials, both aspirin versus control and intravenous heparin versus control were compared in 2 × 2 factorial designs, allowing assessment of the early effects of aspirin in the presence and in the absence of heparin. Taken together, the limited evidence available indicated that aspirin reduced the risk of MI or death during the first 5 to 6 days not only among patients who were not receiving inhospital heparin (11/310 [3.5%] aspirin alone vs. 26/317 [8.2%] control; 57% ± 23 odds reduction) but also among those who were (5/332 [1.5%] aspirin plus heparin vs. 12/316 [3.8%] heparin alone; 59% ± 32 odds reduction; test for heterogeneity $\chi^2_1 = 0.01$; NS).

Heparin for Unstable Coronary Artery Disease

Standard unfractionated heparin comprises a heterogeneous mix of sulfated polysaccharide molecules of varying lengths, with a mean molecular weight of 15 kD (range 3 to 30 kD). Some, but not all, heparin molecules are able to form a complex with antithrombin III (ATIII), thereby substantially increasing the ability of ATIII to inactivate certain coagulation enzymes such as thrombin (and, to a lesser extent, factor Xa).[21] The anticoagulant effects of fixed doses of standard heparin may be unpredictable, partly as a result of the neutralizing effects of heparin-binding proteins that are present to varying degrees in the plasma of patients with occlusive vascular disease. Consequently, many treatment regimens with unfractionated heparin have involved continuous intravenous infusions with regular monitoring of the activated partial thromboplastin time (aPTT) and dose modifications according to empirical nomograms.[22] The routine use of such regimens is limited to the early inhospital period when intravenous infusions and regular monitoring are feasible. More recently, however, low-molecular-weight heparin preparations have been developed that comprise fragments of heparin with mean molecular weights in the narrower range of 4 to 6.5 kD. These preparations inactivate factor Xa to a much greater extent than does standard heparin, and they are not neutralized by heparin-binding proteins. Consequently, they may have a more predictable effect on coagulation, even when given in subcutaneous regimens and with little or no monitoring.[23]

Since aspirin has been shown to be effective in patients with unstable coronary artery disease—even in the presence of early heparin—the relevant question to address now is whether the routine addition of heparin to aspirin during the early period produces benefits that outweigh the risks of bleeding. Unfortunately, the randomized trials that have addressed this question are too small to provide a reliable answer, even when they are combined in a systematic overview. Although one meta-analysis of published data from six trials claimed that adding intravenous unfractionated heparin to aspirin reduced the risk of MI or death, the confidence interval for the estimated risk reduction ranged from a 60% reduction to no effect.[24] Moreover, methodologic weaknesses of that meta-analysis (e.g., no attempt to obtain unpublished data and the exclusion of particular trial results) may have resulted in biased-positive estimates of efficacy.[25] Also the limited data available suggested that heparin was associated with an approximately twofold increase in the risk of major bleeding (10/698 [1.4%] heparin plus aspirin vs. 3/655 [0.5%] aspirin alone), which may offset any cardiac benefits.

Larger randomized comparisons of unfractionated heparin plus aspirin versus aspirin alone may demonstrate that heparin adds to the early effects of aspirin, but regimens involving intravenous use are likely to be confined to the early inhospital period. Promising results have recently been reported from a double-blind study that assessed the addition to aspirin of a subcutaneous low-molecular weight heparin regimen (dalteparin 120 units/kg twice daily for 6 days, then 7500 units daily for 35 to 45 days). A substantial reduction in the risk of MI or death was observed within the first 6 days (13/741 [1.8%] of dalteparin plus aspirin vs. 36/757 [4.8%] aspirin alone; 61% ± 19 odds reduction; $2P < 0.001$), and this appeared to be sustained for several months.[26] No excess risk of major bleeding was observed either during the first 6 days (6/746 [0.8%] vs. 4/760 [0.5%]; NS) or during later treatment (2/619 [0.3%] vs. 2/614 [0.3%]; NS), but the trial was still too small to provide a reliable assessment of the balance of benefits and risks.[26]

Preliminary findings are also available from two trials in patients with unstable coronary artery disease[27, 28] that compared low-molecular-weight heparin plus aspirin versus various unfractionated heparin regimens plus aspirin. In the Fragmin in Unstable Coronary Artery Disease Study (FRIC) trial, 1482 patients treated with aspirin were randomized, in an open comparison, to 5 to 8 days of subcutaneous dalteparin (fixed dose of 120 IU/kg twice daily) or of intravenous unfractionated heparin followed by subcutaneous unfractionated heparin (with repeated monitoring and dose adjustment aimed to keep the aPTT between 1.5 and 2.0 × control).[27] At 6 days, there was a slight but nonsignificant increase in the primary endpoint of death, MI, or recurrent angina among patients allocated low-molecular-weight heparin (69/751 [9.2%] dalteparin plus aspirin vs. 55/731 [7.5%] unfractionated heparin plus aspirin; odds ratio, 1.24; 95% confidence interval [CI], 0.86 to 1.79; NS). In the double-blind Efficacy and Safety of Subcutaneous Enoxaparin in Non–Q wave Coronary Events (ESSENCE) trial, 3171 patients treated with aspirin were randomized to 2 to 8 days of subcutaneous enoxaparin (fixed dose of 1 mg/kg twice daily) or of intravenous unfractionated heparin (with frequent monitoring and dose adjustment to keep the aPTT at 2 × control).[28] At 14 days, there was a significant reduction in the primary endpoint of death, MI, or recurrent angina among patients allocated low-molecular-weight heparin (266/1607 [16.6%] enoxaparin plus aspirin vs. 309/1564 [19.8%] unfractionated heparin plus aspirin; odds ratio of 0.80; 95% CI, 0.67 to 0.96; $2P = 0.02$). In both trials, the low-molecular-weight heparin regimens and the unfractionated heparin regimens were associated with similar rates of major bleeding.[27, 28]

Hence, overall, it remains uncertain whether any benefits of adding low-molecular-weight heparin to aspirin outweigh any hazards in comparison with either aspirin alone or aspirin plus unfractionated heparin. Further trials are planned or are in progress (e.g., Thrombolysis in Myocardial Infarction [TIMI]-11B aims to randomize 3500 patients treated with aspirin to up to 43 days of enoxaparin or to up to 8 days of unfractionated heparin[29]), and these may resolve such uncertainties—provided that they are sufficiently large.

Summary

There are clear benefits with aspirin during and after the acute phase of unstable coronary artery disease but uncertain benefits of adding either standard or low-molecular-weight heparin.

Among patients presenting with an episode of unstable coronary artery disease, aspirin reduces the risk of major vascular events during the early period, even in the presence of heparin, and long-term continuation of aspirin produces further benefits. Aspirin should therefore be given to all patients presenting with unstable coronary artery disease, starting with a dose that is sufficient to produce virtually complete inhibition of platelet cyclooxygenase within a few hours (e.g., 160 mg or more)[9, 30] and continuing with a dose sufficient to maintain this inhibition (e.g., about 75 to 80 mg daily)[31] while minimizing gastrotoxicity.

The randomized evidence from comparisons of aspirin plus unfractionated heparin versus aspirin alone has not demonstrated clearly that any advantage of adding heparin to aspirin outweighs any possible excess risks of major bleeding. Similarly, despite promising results from both direct and indirect assessments of low-molecular-weight heparin regimens, there is inadequate evidence to determine whether the routine addition of low-molecular-weight heparin to aspirin produces any worthwhile improvement in net clinical outcome among patients with unstable coronary artery disease.

ASPIRIN AND HEPARIN FOR SUSPECTED ACUTE MYOCARDIAL INFARCTION

Acute MI generally results from the total occlusion of a coronary artery by thrombus, usually at the site of a ruptured atherosclerotic plaque.[3] The randomized trials assessing the effects of antithrombotic therapy after acute MI may be divided into those trials that have examined the early treatment of suspected acute MI, which is the focus of this chapter, and those that have examined the effects of prolonged antithrombotic treatment following MI, which are described more fully in another chapter (see Chapter 20).

Aspirin for Suspected Acute Myocardial Infarction

The Second International Study of Infarct Survival (ISIS-2) provided conclusive evidence for the benefits of starting aspirin early after the onset of suspected acute MI.[32] Allocation to 1 month of 162.5 mg/day of enteric-coated aspirin, with the first tablet crushed or chewed for a rapid antiplatelet effect, produced a highly significant reduction of about one fifth in mortality at 35 days ($2P < 0.00001$; Fig. 7–1). This represents avoidance of about 25 early deaths per 1000 suspected acute MI patients treated with aspirin for 1 month (Table 7–1, right-hand column). Further follow-up showed that this absolute survival advantage of short-term treatment persisted for up to 10 years.[33] ISIS-2 did not assess the additional effects of continuing aspirin therapy after the first month (which would, in such a blinded study, be expected to have occurred to a similar extent among those allocated either aspirin or placebo for the first month). However, the long-term effects of antiplatelet therapy started some months after acute MI have been assessed in an overview of 11 randomized trials, mainly involving aspirin, in which 36 ± 6 major vascular events were avoided per 1000 post-MI patients treated for an average of around 2 years (and the absolute benefits of a somewhat longer period of treatment may be even greater).[19]

In ISIS-2, aspirin produced similar proportional reductions in early mortality among all of the subgroups of patients that were examined. In particular, the early benefits of aspirin were similar irrespective of whether patients had been randomly allocated to receive fibrinolytic therapy or not (see Fig. 7–1), and were similar in the presence or absence of intravenous heparin (see Table 7–1).[34] Hence, the benefits of aspirin in patients with suspected acute MI have been shown to be additional to any benefits of heparin. Likewise, the effects of aspirin on early mortality were similar among those treated early and those treated late after the onset of symptoms: Proportional mortality reductions for those randomized after 0 to 4, 5 to 12, and 13 to 24 hours were 25% ± 7, 21% ± 7, and 21% ± 12, respectively.[32] (This contrasts with

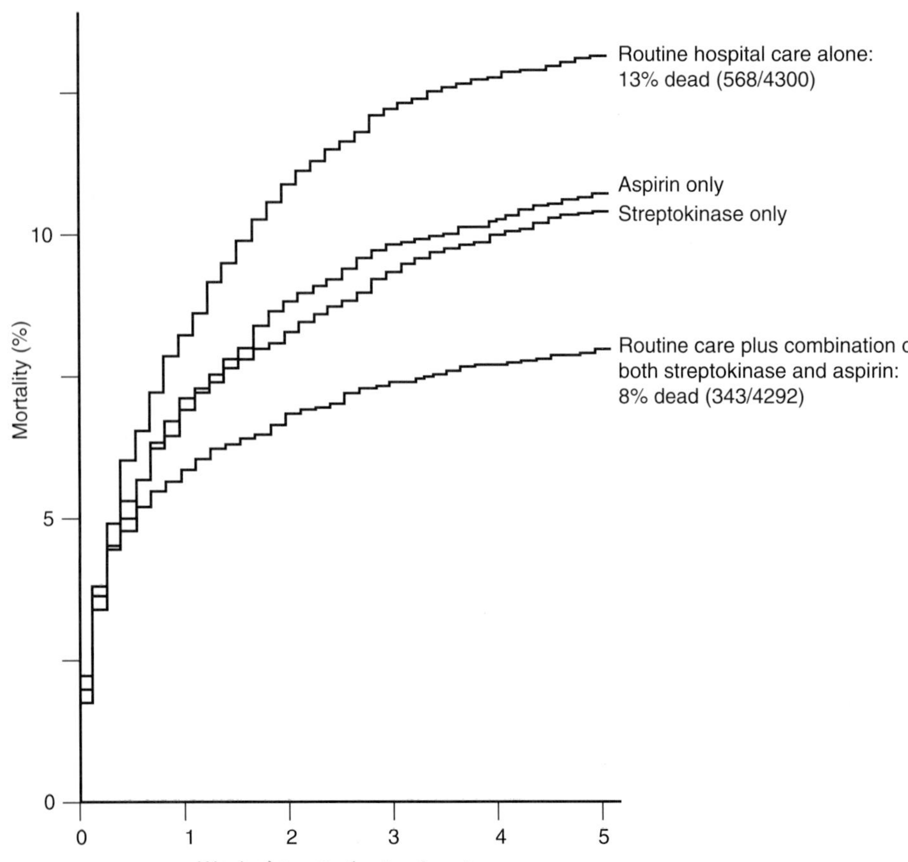

Figure 7–1 Cumulative vascular mortality during the first 35 days in the ISIS-2 trial. In this study, 17,187 patients were randomly assigned within 24 hours of the onset of suspected acute myocardial infarction to receive (1) placebo infusion and placebo tablets; (2) placebo infusion and 162.5 mg of aspirin daily for 1 month (i.e., aspirin only); (3) 1.5 million units of streptokinase infusion over 1 hour and placebo tablets (streptokinase only); or (4) both streptokinase and aspirin. (From ISIS-2 [Second International Study of Infarct Survival] Collaborative Group. Randomised trial of intravenous streptokinase, oral aspirin, both, or neither among 17,187 cases of suspected acute myocardial infarction: ISIS-2. Lancet 1988; 2:349–360.)

TABLE 7–1 • Effects of Aspirin in the Absence and in the Presence of Planned Intravenous Heparin: ISIS-2*

	No IV Heparin Planned (13,000 Patients: 6% Given IV and 56% IV or SC Heparin)			IV Heparin Planned (4000 Patients: 77% Given IV and 91% IV or SC Heparin)			*Effect per 1000 Allocated Aspirin (Irrespective of Heparin Use)*
	Random Allocation		*Effect per 1000 Allocated Aspirin*	*Random Allocation*		*Effect per 1000 Allocated Aspirin*	
	Active Aspirin (6539)	Placebo Aspirin (6547)		Active Aspirin (2048)	Placebo Aspirin (2053)		
Death (5-wk)	9.6% 626	11.9% 778	23 ± 5 less ($2P < 0.0001$)	8.7% 178	11.6% 238	29 ± 9 less ($2P < 0.003$)	25 ± 5 less ($2P < 0.0001$)
Reinfarction	1.6% 104	2.9% 188	13 ± 3 less ($2P < 0.0001$)	2.6% 52	4.7% 96	21 ± 5 less ($2P < 0.0001$)	15 ± 2 less ($2P < 0.0001$)
Stroke	0.6% 42	1.0% 65	4 ± 2 less ($2P < 0.03$)	0.4% 9	1.1% 23	7 ± 3 less ($2P < 0.02$)	4 ± 1 less ($2P < 0.002$)
Stroke, reinfarction, or death	11.0% 710	14.6% 940	36 ± 7 less ($2P < 0.0001$)	10.2% 208	14.9% 302	47 ± 11 less ($2P < 0.0001$)	38 ± 5 less ($2P < 0.0001$)
Major bleed	0.3% 17	0.3% 17	No apparent excess	0.7% 14	0.8% 16	No apparent excess	0 ± 1 (NS)

General note to Tables 7–1 to 7–3: The number of randomized patients is given in parentheses at the top of each column. Each entry within the table is either the number of affected patients and the percentage of those with follow-up or the effect per 1000 ± 1 standard deviation. Reinfarctions, strokes, pulmonary emboli, and bleeds are recorded only if they precede hospital discharge.

*This table should not be used to assess the effects of heparin, since heparin was not randomly allocated. Just before randomizing each patient between aspirin vs. placebo, physicians were asked whether they "planned" to use IV heparin for that individual, and on the discharge form they reported whether they had actually done so. Mortality percentages are based on all randomized patients, and other percentages are based on the 99% with discharge forms (or, for actual heparin use, on those with forms who were discharged alive).[32]

IV, intravenous; SC, subcutaneous.

fibrinolytic therapy, which has not been shown to reduce mortality when given more than approximately 12 hours after the onset of symptoms.[35]) However, neither this finding nor the apparent lack of a survival advantage in the first day or two after MI (which is seen both with aspirin and with fibrinolytic therapy; see Fig. 7–1) means that aspirin therapy can be delayed without loss. Platelet activation and aggregation occur early in patients with acute MI and are further increased by fibrinolytic therapy, with an increased risk of reocclusion and reinfarction.[36–38] Aspirin inhibits this acute platelet activation, and in ISIS-2 appeared to abolish the excess risk of inhospital reinfarction associated with fibrinolytic therapy.[32]

Heparin for Acute Myocardial Infarction

Most individual trials of heparin in patients with acute MI have been too small to detect moderate effects on major outcomes. Taken together, however, the studies of heparin in patients who did not routinely receive aspirin (most of whom also did not receive fibrinolytic therapy) do indicate some net benefit from heparin, despite an excess of major bleeding (Table 7–2, left-hand section).[34] But since ISIS-2 clearly demonstrated that aspirin is effective even in the presence of heparin, these findings are of little direct relevance to current clinical practice. The relevant question now is whether heparin should be added routinely to aspirin in patients with acute MI. Thus far, six trials have compared aspirin plus unfractionated heparin versus aspirin alone in about 68,000 patients (93% of whom had also received fibrinolytic therapy).[34, 39] Any further reductions in mortality or other major vascular events with the heparin regimens in these trials were small (5 ± 2 fewer deaths per 1000 patients treated; see Table 7–2, right-hand section), and there was a small increase in major bleeds.

Two megatrials, ISIS-3[40] and Gruppo Italiano per lo Studio Della Sopravvivenza nell'Infarto Miocardico (GISSI)-2[41] (with its international extension[42]), provided most of these data (Table 7–3, left-hand section). This raises the question as to whether particular aspects of these two trials led to an underestimate of the possible effects of heparin. In both trials, for example, unfractionated heparin was scheduled to begin several hours (12 hours in GISSI-2 and 4 hours in ISIS-3) after the start of any fibrinolytic therapy, and the heparin was given subcutaneously (12,500 IU twice daily for about 1 week), which caused further delay. During the scheduled heparin treatment periods in these two trials, there was some evidence of a reduction in mortality (2071 [6.8%] deaths with heparin plus aspirin plus fibrinolytic therapy vs. 2239 [7.3%] with aspirin plus fibrinolytic therapy), equivalent to 5 ± 2 fewer deaths per 1000 patients allocated heparin. But there was no significant benefit remaining by 35 days (2 ± 2 fewer deaths per 1000; see Table 7–3) or 6 months (1 ± 3 fewer deaths per 1000).[40]

The GISSI-2 and ISIS-3 trials studied high-dose sub-

TABLE 7–2 • Effects of Heparin in the Absence and in the Presence of Aspirin: Overview of 26 Randomized Trials*

	Trials with No Routine Aspirin (5000 Patients: 14% had Fibrinolytic)			Trials with Routine Aspirin (68,000 Patients: 93% also had Fibrinolytic)		
	Random Allocation			*Random Allocation*		
	HEPARIN ONLY (2684†)	NO ANTITHROMBOTIC (2775†)	*Effect per 1000 Allocated Heparin*	ASPIRIN + HEPARIN (34,035)	ASPIRIN ONLY (34,055)	*Effect per 1000 Allocated Heparin*
Death (generally inhospital)	11.4% 284	14.9% 378	35 ± 11 less (2*P* = 0.002)	8.6% 2932	9.1% 3092	5 ± 2 less (2*P* = 0.03)
Reinfarction	6.7% 142	8.2% 176	15 ± 8 less (2*P* = 0.08)	3.0% 1009	3.3% 1103	3 ± 1 less (2*P* = 0.04)
Stroke	1.1% 23	2.1% 44	10 ± 4 less (2*P* = 0.01)	1.2% 397	1.1% 375	1 ± 1 more (NS)
Pulmonary embolism	2.0% 46	3.8% 91	19 ± 5 less (2*P* < 0.001)	0.3% 82	0.4% 117	1 ± 0.4 less (2*P* = 0.01)
Major bleed	1.9% 31	0.9% 14	10 ± 4 more (2*P* = 0.01)	1.0% 342	0.7% 234	3 ± 1 more (2*P* < 0.00001)

*This table should not be used to assess the effects of aspirin or fibrinolytic therapy, since these were not randomly allocated. For the 6 trials (or trial strata) with routine aspirin, mortality and nonfatal events were available from 98–100% of all randomized patients, except pulmonary embolism, which was available from only about 85%. For the 21 trials (or trial strata) with no routine aspirin, mortality was available from about 90% of all randomized patients; reinfarction, stroke, and pulmonary embolism from 75–85%; and major bleeds from only about 60%. A few of the latter trials have 2:1 randomization, and the control group has been counted twice to maintain balance.[38]

†A total of about 100 additional patients were randomized in several of these trials of heparin with no routine aspirin, but their allocated treatment group and outcome are unknown.

See *general note* in Table 7–1 footnote.

cutaneous heparin regimens, whereas an intravenous regimen could have produced more intensive anticoagulation. A total of only about 1300 patients with suspected acute MI have been studied in four small trials[43–46] that compared intravenous unfractionated heparin (24,000 to 25,000 IU per day for two to three days) plus aspirin versus aspirin alone. Even in aggregate, however, there were too few patients in these

TABLE 7–3 • Effects of Adding Heparin to Aspirin and Fibrinolytic Therapy*: Direct and Indirect Randomized Comparisons of (1) Aspirin Plus High-Dose Subcutaneous Heparin Versus Aspirin Alone (GISSI-2 and ISIS-3) and (2) Aspirin Plus Intravenous Heparin Versus Aspirin Plus High-Dose Subcutaneous Heparin (GUSTO-I)

	GISSI-2 and ISIS-3 (Only Those 62,000 Patients Allocated SK, tPA, or APSAC)			GUSTO-I (Only Those 20,000 Patients Allocated SK)			
	Random Allocation			*Random Allocation*			
	ASPIRIN + SC HEPARIN (31,017)	ASPIRIN ALONE (31,054)	*(a) Effect per 1000 Allocated SC Heparin*	ASPIRIN + IV HEPARIN (10,410)	ASPIRIN + SC HEPARIN (9841)	*(b) Effect per 1000 Allocated IV Instead of SC Heparin*	*INDIRECT Assessment of the Effect per 1000 from Adding IV Heparin to Aspirin (Estimated as a + b)*
Death (30–35 d)	9.99% 3100	10.22% 3172	2.2 ± 2.4 less (NS)	7.36% 763	7.27% 712	0.9 ± 3.8 more (NS)	1 ± 4 less (NS)
Reinfarction	3.01% 927	3.28% 1010	2.7 ± 1.4 less (NS)	4.22% 438	3.50% 343	7.2 ± 2.7 more (2*P* < 0.01)	4 ± 3 more (NS)
Any stroke	1.22% 376	1.17% 359	0.6 ± 0.9 more (NS)	1.39% 144	1.19% 117	2.0 ± 1.6 more (NS)	3 ± 2 more (NS)
Hemorrhagic stroke	0.49% 150	0.39% 120	1.0 ± 0.5 more (NS)	0.57% 59	0.46% 45	1.1 ± 1.0 more (NS)	2 ± 1 more (2*P* = 0.08)
Major[38] or severe[45] bleed	1.01% 312	0.69% 213	3.2 ± 0.7 more (2*P* < 0.0001)	1.45% 151	1.19% 117	2.6 ± 1.6 more (2*P* = 0.10)	6 ± 2 more (2*P* < 0.001)

*This table should not be used to make direct comparisons between the absolute event rates in different trials, since the patient populations may differ substantially in age and other characteristics. By contrast with Table 7–2, which involved mortality only in hospital from GISSI-2 and ISIS-3 (and most of the other trials), this table involves 35-day mortality from GISSI-2 and ISIS-3 and 30-day mortality from GUSTO-I. In this table, numbers affected and percentages (based on patients with follow-up) are from References 40 and 71, and numbers randomized and with follow-up are from References 40 and 47 (supplemented by revised GUSTO-I data provided to the National Auxiliary Publications Service).

See *general note* in Table 7–1 footnote.

APSAC, anisoylated plasminogen-streptokinase activator complex; GISSI, Gruppo Italiano per lo Studio Della Sopravvivenza Nell'Infarto Miocardico; GUSTO, Global Use of Strategies to Open Occluded Coronary Arteries; ISIS, International Study of Infarct Survival; IV, intravenous; SC, subcutaneous; SK, streptokinase; tPA, tissue-type plasminogen activator.

trials for the results to be reliable (32/676 [4.7%] deaths with heparin plus aspirin vs. 31/659 [4.7%] deaths with aspirin alone; 23 [3.4%] vs. 22 [3.3%] reinfarctions; 12 [1.8%] vs. 4 [0.6%] strokes).[34]

A more reliable assessment of intravenous heparin may be provided by the large Global Use of Strategies to Open Occluded Coronary Arteries (GUSTO)-I trial, in which—among more than 20,000 patients allocated to receive streptokinase—the effects of aspirin plus the ISIS-3 subcutaneous heparin regimen were compared with aspirin plus at least 48 hours of intravenous unfractionated heparin (see Table 7–3).[47] For the patients allocated intravenous heparin, an initial 5000 IU bolus was to be followed by 1000 IU/h, with monitoring of the aPTT at 6, 12, and 24 hours after initiation of fibrinolytic therapy and adjustment of the heparin infusion rate to aim for an aPTT of 60 to 85 seconds. Intravenous heparin was not associated with any significant reductions in mortality or stroke, and there was a conventionally significant ($2P < 0.01$) excess of reinfarctions with heparin (see Table 7–3, central section). This apparent excess of reinfarctions may be due to chance; but about one third of these reinfarctions occurred within 10 hours of stopping intravenous heparin, and one half within 20 hours,[48] so cessation of intravenous heparin may have produced a rebound increase in thrombin generation[49] and a real excess of reinfarction.

Hence, despite the small improvements in coronary artery patency when intravenous unfractionated heparin is added to adequate doses of aspirin after treatment with tissue plasminogen activator[42] or streptokinase,[50] the intravenous heparin regimen studied in GUSTO-I did not appear to confer any definite clinical advantage over high-dose subcutaneous heparin (see Table 7–3, central section), even if allowance is made for some noncompliance with the allocated heparin regimen—or, indirectly, over aspirin alone (see Table 7–3, right-hand section). Nor was there any good evidence of a difference in clinical outcome in any subgroup of patients, such as those with anterior MI, who might have been at particular risk of thrombotic complications. Intravenous heparin was, however, associated with a small increase in major bleeding.

Higher aPTT values during heparin therapy are associated with higher rates of coronary artery patency a few days after acute MI.[51] Hence, a somewhat more intensive heparin regimen was initially studied in one arm of GUSTO-II[52]—1300 IU/h for patients weighing 80 kg or more, with the upper aPTT limit increased to 90 seconds—and in two other studies.[53, 54] Despite the fact that an average of only 20% more heparin was given, all three of these trials were stopped prematurely because of higher than expected rates of intracerebral bleeding and other major bleeding with the high-dose heparin regimens in patients given fibrinolytic therapy.[52–54] This suggests that more intensive anticoagulation with heparin may not be an appropriate strategy, at least in conjunction with fibrinolytic therapy.

Summary

There are clear benefits with aspirin during and after acute myocardial infarction but no clear evidence of benefit from adding heparin.

As for patients with unstable coronary artery disease, aspirin in a dose of about 160 mg or more reduces the risk of major vascular events during the early period after acute MI, even in the presence of heparin; and the long-term continuation for at least several years of about 75 to 80 mg aspirin daily will produce further benefits. By contrast, there is little evidence of further clinical advantage with the addition of subcutaneous or intravenous unfractionated heparin to aspirin in patients with suspected acute MI receiving any fibrinolytic agent. Further large trials of the effects of adding newer antithrombotic agents (such as low-molecular-weight heparin and thrombin inhibitors) to aspirin, especially among patients not receiving fibrinolytic therapy, could provide valuable information about the balance of benefits and risks of these different antithrombotic regimens.

CONCLUSION

Given the definite and substantial benefits of aspirin during and after acute ischemic events (i.e., unstable angina or MI), aspirin should only be withheld from patients with very clear serious contraindications (e.g., definite evidence of serious allergic reaction to prior aspirin use, or recent severe gastrointestinal or intracerebral bleeding). It should *not* be withheld from those patients with only mild contraindications (e.g., a vague history of allergy, or a history of gastrointestinal bleeding or ulcer that is not recent) for whom the benefits are likely to outweigh the risks. Moreover, in those rare cases of definite aspirin allergy (e.g., a history of aspirin-induced asthma, angioedema, or anaphylaxis), some other effective antiplatelet drug should be considered.

Despite the strength of this evidence, aspirin is still not sufficiently widely used. For example, prospective registries of patients admitted with unstable coronary artery disease from 1993 to 1996[55, 56] found that about one fifth did not receive aspirin during their admission. Likewise, although there appears to have been a gradual increase in the early use of aspirin in patients with acute MI,[57–60] only about 70% of patients in a U.S. registry during the period 1990 to 1993 received aspirin during their admission for acute MI[61];

and in a Medicare study during 1992 to 1993, fewer than half of the patients received aspirin on the day of admission and only two thirds were discharged on it.[62] This underuse appears to be most marked among elderly patients, those with more comorbidity, and those with heart failure,[63] despite clear evidence that such patients derive substantial benefit from aspirin.[32, 33] By contrast, despite the risks of bleeding and the lack of clear evidence of any value, the early use of heparin remains widespread in the treatment of patients with acute ischemic syndromes, albeit with wide international variations.[55, 56, 64] This may be, in part, because intravenous heparin has been particularly recommended for use with "front-loaded" tissue plasminogen activator[65] (although there is also a lack of evidence for this recommendation[39]; see Thrombolytic Therapy, Chapter 8). But, even among patients with suspected acute MI who do not receive any fibrinolytic therapy, surveys in the United States indicate that more than half are treated with intravenous heparin.[61]

During the years following acute MI or unstable angina, long-term aspirin therapy is also not used as widely as the evidence would indicate it should be[58, 66, 67] (although, again, usage may be increasing). In 1992, for example, only about half of the people with a previous MI in the British Regional Heart Survey were taking regular aspirin,[68] and in 1994, only about half of the people with a previous MI or angina in the Scandinavian Simvastatin Survival Study (4S) were taking aspirin.[69] Remarkably, a recent survey of U.S. general internists indicated that only about half believed aspirin definitely improves long-term prognosis after MI.[70] Given the strength of the evidence, physicians should be sufficiently aware of the benefits to ensure that aspirin is used appropriately widely among patients with a high risk of occlusive arterial disease. The opportunities for prevention are especially great among the elderly and other high-risk groups, such as those with heart failure, in which aspirin appears most likely to be inappropriately withheld.

REFERENCES

1. Collins R, Peto R, Gray R, Parish S. Large-scale randomized evidence: Trials and overviews. *In* Weatherall D, Ledingham JGG, Warrell DA, eds. Oxford Textbook of Medicine, vol. 1. Oxford, Oxford University Press, 1996, pp 21–32.
2. Collins R, Gray R, Godwin J, Peto R. Avoidance of large biases and large random errors in the assessment of moderate treatment effects: The need for systematic overviews. Stat Med 1987; 6:245–250.
3. Fuster V, Badimon L, Badimon JJ, Chesebro JH. The pathogenesis of coronary artery disease and the acute coronary syndromes. N Engl J Med 1992; 326:242–250, 310–318.
4. Non-Q wave myocardial infarction [Editorial]. Lancet 1989; 2:899–900.
5. Patrono C. Aspirin as an antiplatelet drug. N Engl J Med 1994; 330:1287–1294.
6. Lefkovits J, Plow EF, Topol EJ. Platelet glycoprotein IIb/IIIa receptors in cardiovascular medicine. N Engl J Med 1995; 332:1553–1559.
7. Pedersen AK, FitzGerald GA. Dose-related kinetics of aspirin: Pre-systemic acetylation of platelet cyclooxygenase. N Engl J Med 1984; 311:1206–1211.
8. Patrignani P, Filabozzi P, Patrono C. Selective cumulative inhibition of platelet thromboxane production by low-dose aspirin in healthy subjects. J Clin Invest 1982; 69:1366–1372.
9. Clarke RJ, Mayo G, Price P, FitzGerald GA. Suppression of thromboxane A_2 but not of systemic prostacyclin by controlled-release aspirin. N Engl J Med 1991; 325:1137–1141.
10. Patrono C, Ciabattoni G, Patrignani P, et al. Clinical pharmacology of platelet cyclooxygenase inhibition. Circulation 1985; 72:1177–1184.
11. Roderick PJ, Wilkes HC, Meade TW. The gastrointestinal toxicity of aspirin: An overview of randomised controlled trials. Br J Clin Pharmacol 1993; 35:219–226.
12. Lewis HD (for the Veterans Administration Cooperative Study Group). Unstable angina: Status of aspirin and other forms of therapy. Circulation 1985; 72(suppl V):155–160.
13. Lewis HD, Davis JW, Archibald DG, et al. Protective effect of aspirin against acute myocardial infarction and death in men with unstable angina: Results of a Veterans Administration cooperative study. N Engl J Med 1983; 309:396–403.
14. Cairns JA, Gent M, Singer J, et al. Aspirin, sulfinpyrazone, or both in unstable angina: Results of a Canadian multicenter trial. N Engl J Med 1985; 313:1369–1375.
15. The RISC Group. Risk of myocardial infarction and death during treatment with low-dose aspirin and intravenous heparin in men with unstable coronary artery disease. Lancet 1990; 336:827–830.
16. Aspirin at Low Dose in Unstable Angina (ALDUSA) pilot study. Report from the coordinating center (Unité de Pharmacologie Clinique, Lyon) 1987. Unpublished.
17. Balsano F, Rizzon P, Violi F, et al (for Studio della Ticlopidina nell'Angina Instabile Group). Antiplatelet treatment with ticlopidine in unstable angina: A controlled multicenter clinical trial. Circulation 1990; 82:17–26.
18. Prandoni P, Milani L, Barbiero M, et al. A combination of dipyridamole with low-dose aspirin in the treatment of unstable angina: A multicenter pilot double-blind study. Minerva Cardioangiol 1991; 39:267–273.
19. Antiplatelet Trialists' Collaboration. Collaborative overview of randomised trials of antiplatelet therapy: I. Prevention of death, myocardial infarction, and stroke by prolonged antiplatelet therapy in various categories of patients. BMJ 1994; 308:81–106.
20. Théroux P, Ouimet H, McCans J, et al. Aspirin, heparin, or both to treat acute unstable angina. N Engl J Med 1988; 319:1105–1111.
21. Hirsh J, Fuster V. Guide to anticoagulant therapy: I. Heparin. Circulation 1994; 89:1449–1468.
22. Cruickshank MK, Levine MN, Hirsh J, et al. A standard heparin nomogram for the management of heparin therapy. Arch Intern Med 1991; 151:333–337.
23. Hirsh J, Levine MN. Low-molecular-weight heparin. Blood 1992; 79:1–17.
24. Oler A, Whooley MA, Oler J, Grady D. Adding heparin to aspirin reduces the incidence of myocardial infarction and death in patients with unstable angina: A meta-analysis. JAMA 1996; 276:811–815.
25. Collins R, Baigent C, Peto R. No significant evidence of clinical benefit with heparin in unstable angina [Letter]. JAMA 1996; 276:1873.
26. Fragmin During Instability in Coronary Artery Disease (FRISC) Study Group. Low-molecular-weight heparin during instability in coronary artery disease. Lancet 1996; 347:561–568.
27. Klein W, Buchwald A, Hillis SE, et al for the FRIC Investigators. Comparison of low-molecular-weight heparin with unfractionated heparin acutely and with placebo for 6 weeks in the management of unstable coronary artery disease: Fragmin in Unstable Coronary Artery Disease (FRIC). Circulation 1997; 96:61–68.
28. Cohen M, Demers C, Gurfinkel E, et al for the ESSENCE Group. A comparison of low-molecular-weight heparin with unfractionated heparin for unstable coronary artery disease. N Engl J Med 1997; 337:447–452.

29. Antman EM, McCabe CH, Marble SJ, et al. Dose-ranging trial of enoxaparin for unstable angina: Results of TIMI-IIA [Abstract]. Circulation 1996; 94(suppl 1):554.
30. Reilley IAG, FitzGerald GA. Inhibition of thromboxane formation in vivo and ex vivo: Implications for therapy with platelet inhibitory drugs. Blood 1987; 69:180–186.
31. Berglund U, Wallentin L. Persistent inhibition of platelet function during long-term treatment with 75 mg acetylsalicylic acid daily in men with unstable coronary artery disease. Eur Heart J 1991; 12:428–433.
32. Second International Study of Infarct Survival (ISIS-2) Collaborative Group. Randomised trial of intravenous streptokinase, oral aspirin, both, or neither among 17,187 cases of suspected acute myocardial infarction: ISIS-2. Lancet 1988; 2:349–360.
33. Baigent C, Collins R, Appleby P, et al on behalf of the ISIS-2 Collaborative Group. ISIS-2: 10-year survival in a randomised comparison of intravenous streptokinase, oral aspirin, both, or neither among patients with suspected acute myocardial infarction. BMJ 1998; in press.
34. Collins R, MacMahon S, Flather M, et al. Clinical effects of anticoagulant therapy in suspected acute myocardial infarction: Systematic overview of randomised trials. BMJ 1996; 313:652–659.
35. Fibrinolytic Therapy Trialists' Collaborative Group. Indications for fibrinolytic therapy in suspected acute myocardial infarction: Collaborative overview of early mortality and major morbidity results from all randomised trials of more than 1000 patients. Lancet 1994; 343:311–322.
36. Fitzgerald DJ, Catalla F, Roy L, FitzGerald GA. Marked platelet activation in vivo after intravenous streptokinase in patients with acute myocardial infarction. Circulation 1988; 77:142–150.
37. Kerins DM, Roy L, FitzGerald GA, et al. Platelet and vascular function during coronary thrombolysis with tissue-type plasminogen activator. Circulation 1989; 80:1718–1725.
38. Fitzgerald DJ, Wright F, FitzGerald GA. Increased thromboxane biosynthesis during coronary thrombolysis: Evidence that platelet activation and thromboxane A_2 modulate the response to tissue-type plasminogen activator in vivo. Circ Res 1989; 65:83–94.
39. Collins R, Peto R, Baigent C, Sleight P. Aspirin, heparin, and fibrinolytic therapy in suspected acute myocardial infarction. N Engl J Med 1997; 336:847–860.
40. Third International Study of Infarct Survival (ISIS-3) Collaborative Group. ISIS-3: A randomised trial of streptokinase vs tissue plasminogen activator versus anistreplase and of aspirin plus heparin versus aspirin alone among 41,299 cases of suspected acute myocardial infarction. Lancet 1992; 339:753–770.
41. Gruppo Italiano per lo Studio della Sopravvivenza nell'Infarto Miocardico. GISSI-2: Randomised trial of intravenous alteplase versus intravenous streptokinase in acute myocardial infarction. Lancet 1990; 336:65–71.
42. The International Study Group. In-hospital mortality and clinical course of 20,891 patients with suspected acute myocardial infarction randomised between tissue plasminogen activator or streptokinase with or without heparin. Lancet 1990; 336:71–75.
43. Collins R, Conway M, Alexopoulos D, et al (for the ISIS pilot study investigators). Randomized factorial trial of high-dose intravenous streptokinase, of oral aspirin, and of intravenous heparin in acute myocardial infarction. Eur Heart J 1987; 8:634–642.
44. de Bono DP, Simoons ML, Tijssen J, et al (for the European Cooperative Study Group). Effect of early intravenous heparin on coronary patency, infarct size, and bleeding complications after alteplase thrombolysis: Results of a randomized double-blind European Cooperative Study Group trial. Br Heart J 1992; 67:122–128.
45. Col J, Decoster O, Hanique G, et al. Infusion of heparin conjunct to streptokinase accelerates reperfusion of acute myocardial infarction: Results of a double-blind randomized study (OSIRIS). Circulation 1992; 86(suppl I):259.
46. O'Connor CM, Meese R, Carney R, et al (for the Duke University Clinical Cardiology Study [DUCCS] Group). A randomized trial of intravenous heparin in conjunction with anistreplase (anisoylated plasminogen streptokinase activator complex) in acute myocardial infarction: The Duke University Clinical Cardiology Study (DUCCS)-1. J Am Coll Cardiol 1994; 23:11–18.
47. The GUSTO Investigators. An international randomized trial comparing four thrombolytic strategies for acute myocardial infarction. N Engl J Med 1993; 329:673–682.
48. Granger CB, Hirsh J, Califf RM, et al for the GUSTO-1 Investigators. Activated partial thromboplastin time and outcome after thrombolytic therapy for acute myocardial infarction. Results from the GUSTO-1 trial. Circulation 1996; 93:870–878.
49. Granger CB, Miller JM, Bovill EG, et al. Rebound increase in thrombin generation and activity after cessation of intravenous heparin in patients with acute coronary syndromes. Circulation 1995; 91:1929–1935.
50. GUSTO Angiographic Investigators. The effects of tissue plasminogen activator, streptokinase, or both in coronary artery patency, ventricular function, and survival after acute myocardial infarction. N Engl J Med 1993; 329:1615–1622.
51. Granger CB, Califf RM, Hirsh J for the GUSTO Investigators. APTTs after thrombolysis and standard intravenous heparin are often low and correlate with body weight, age, and sex: Experience from the GUSTO trial. Circulation 1992; 86(suppl I):258.
52. GUSTO IIa Investigators. Randomized trial of intravenous heparin versus recombinant hirudin for acute coronary syndromes. Circulation 1994; 90:1631–1632.
53. Antman EM for the TIMI-9A Investigators. Hirudin in acute myocardial infarction: Safety report from the thrombolysis and thrombin inhibition in myocardial infarction (TIMI)-9A trial. Circulation 1994; 90:1624–1630.
54. Neuhaus K-L, von Essen R, Tebbe U, et al. Safety observations from the pilot phase of the randomised r-hirudin for improvement of thrombolysis (HIT-III) study. Circulation 1994; 90:1638–1642.
55. Moliterno DJ, Aguirre FV, Cannon CP, et al for the GUARANTEE Investigators. The Global Unstable Angina Registry and Treatment Evaluation (GUARANTEE) Study [Abstract]. Circulation 1996; 94(suppl I):195.
56. Flather M, Pogue J, Avezum A, et al for the OASIS Investigators. Effect of baseline characteristics on outcomes in an international prospective registry of acute myocardial ischemia without ST elevation [Abstract]. Circulation 1996; 94(suppl I):196.
57. Lamas GA, Pfeffer MA, Hamm P for the SAVE investigators. Do the results of randomized clinical trials of cardiovascular drugs influence medical practice? N Engl J Med 1992; 327:241–247.
58. Montague T, Taylor L, Martin S, et al for the Clinical Quality Improvement Network (CQIN) Investigators. Can practice patterns be successfully altered? Examples from cardiovascular medicine. Can J Cardiol 1995; 11:487–492.
59. Chinese Cardiac Study Collaborative Group. Oral captopril versus placebo among 13,634 patients with suspected acute myocardial infarction: Interim report from the Chinese Cardiac Study (CCS-1). Lancet 1995; 345:686–687.
60. Sandoya E. Current treatment habits of AMI in Latin America. Bull Intensive Crit Care 1995; 2:14–16.
61. Rogers WJ, Bowlby LJ, Chandra NC, et al for the Participants in the National Registry of Myocardial Infarction. Treatment of myocardial infarction in the United States (1990 to 1993): Observations from the National Registry of Myocardial Infarction. Circulation 1994; 90:2103–2114.
62. Ellerbeck EF, Jencks SF, Radford MJ, et al. Quality of care for Medicare patients with acute myocardial infarction: A four-state pilot study from the Cooperative Cardiovascular Project. JAMA 1995; 273:1509–1514.
63. Krumholz HM, Radford MJ, Ellerbeck EF, et al. Aspirin in the treatment of acute myocardial infarction in elderly Medicare beneficiaries: Patterns of use and outcomes. Circulation 1995; 92:2841–2847.
64. European Secondary Prevention Study Group. Personal communication, 1997.
65. Ryan TJ, Anderson JL, Antman EM, et al. ACC/AHA Guidelines for the Management of Patients with Acute Myocardial Infarction: Executive Summary. A Report of the American College of Cardiology/American Heart Association Task Force on Practice Guidelines (Committee on Management of Acute Myocardial Infarction). Circulation 1996; 94:2341–2350.
66. Agustí A, Arnau JM, Laporte J-R. Clinical trials versus clinical

practice in the secondary prevention of myocardial infarction. Eur J Clin Pharmacol 1994; 46:95–99.
67. Sides TL, Shahar E, McGovern PG, Luepker RV. Results of a population-based survey documenting aspirin use for the prevention of cardiovascular disease: The Minnesota Heart Survey. Circulation 1995; 92(suppl 1)1:216.
68. MacCallum AK, Whincup PH, Morris RW, Walker M. Aspirin in the prevention of coronary heart disease—are opportunities being missed? Br Heart J 1995; 73(suppl 3):P68.
69. Scandinavian Simvastatin Survival Study Group. Randomised trial of cholesterol lowering in 4444 patients with coronary heart disease: The Scandinavian Simvastatin Survival Study (4S). Lancet 1994; 344:1383–1389.
70. Ayanian JZ, Hauptman PJ, Guadagnoli E, et al. Knowledge and practice of generalist and specialist physicians regarding drug therapy for acute myocardial infarction. N Engl J Med 1994; 331:1136–1142.
71. Van de Werf F, Topol EJ, Lee KL, et al. Variations in patient management and outcome for acute myocardial infarction in the United States and other countries: Results from the GUSTO Trial. JAMA 1995; 273:1586–1591.

8 Thrombolytic Therapy

▶ Colin Baigent
▶ Rory Collins

The aim of this chapter is to review the evidence from all randomized trials that have assessed the effects of thrombolytic therapy on mortality (and other major morbidity, such as strokes) in patients with suspected acute myocardial infarction (MI). When considering the possible effects of thrombolytic therapy on major clinical outcomes, it is important to bear in mind that such effects are likely to be moderate in size, rather than large. That is, risk reductions of 10% to 20% may be plausible, but substantially larger reductions are generally not. Moreover, comparisons of major outcomes between two thrombolytic regimens are likely to yield much smaller differences than those between a thrombolytic regimen and no thrombolytic therapy. Hence, the reliable assessment of the effects of thrombolytic therapy requires consideration of the large-scale randomized evidence available from all relevant trials of thrombolytic therapy, without undue emphasis on the results from particular trials or parts of trials. (For further discussion of how such issues affect the interpretation of the randomized evidence considered in this chapter, see Chapter 20 and References 1 and 2.)

COMPARISONS OF THROMBOLYTIC THERAPY WITH NO SUCH THERAPY

Several randomized trials[3–11] comparing thrombolytic therapy versus no thrombolytic therapy among patients with suspected acute MI have each been large enough to demonstrate that mortality during the first month or so can be reduced substantially by such treatment (see, for example, Fig. 8–1). More recently, long-term follow-up of the 17,187 patients randomized in the Second International Study of Infarct Survival (ISIS-2) has shown that these early benefits are maintained for at least 10 years.[12] To determine more reliably which patients benefit from thrombolytic therapy, the Fibrinolytic Therapy Trialists' (FTT) Collaborative Group conducted combined analyses of death and other major adverse events from the nine largest trials that compared thrombolytic therapy versus no thrombolytic therapy.[13] Altogether, these trials included 58,600 patients, among whom there were 6177 (10.5%) deaths, 564 (1.0%) strokes, and 436 (0.7%) major noncerebral bleeds.

Early Hazard and Later Benefit

Among all patients studied in the FTT analysis, thrombolytic therapy produced an 18% (SD 2) proportional reduction in mortality during the first 35 days, which corresponds to about 18 fewer deaths per 1000 patients treated. During the day of randomization (day 0), however, thrombolytic therapy was associated with a highly significant 26% (SD 6) proportional *increase* in mortality (Table 8–1), which was only partially reversed on the following day (proportional mortality reduction on day 1: 13% [SD 6]). Only subsequently did a definite benefit emerge, with highly significant reductions in mortality during the remainder of the first week (days 2 to 7) and during the subsequent 4 weeks.

Benefit Among Patients with ST Elevation or Bundle Branch Block

Thrombolytic therapy reduced 35-day mortality among patients presenting with either ST elevation or bundle branch block (BBB) up to at least 12 hours after the onset of symptoms (see later). For patients with ST elevation there were similar proportional mortality reductions among those with infarcts in anterior, inferior, or other locations. Thus, although the absolute benefits of thrombolytic therapy appear to be greatest among patients with anterior ST segment elevation, there is good evidence that patients with inferior ST segment elevation, who are at somewhat lower risk, also benefit.

It is not yet clear whether thrombolytic therapy produces worthwhile benefits among certain other types of patients at appreciable risk of early death

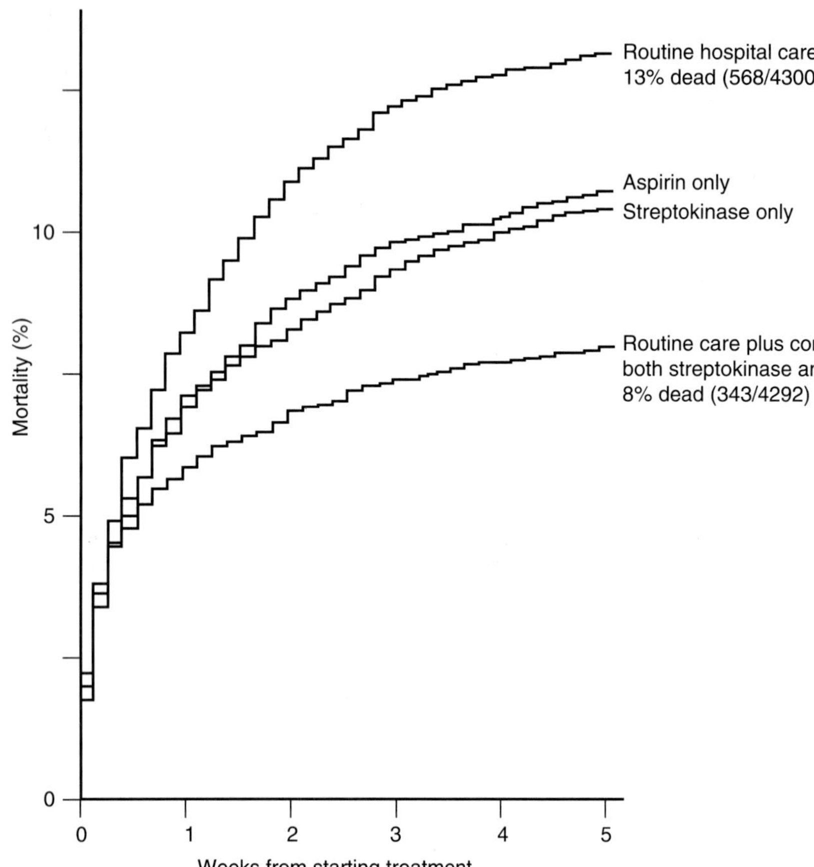

Figure 8–1 Cumulative mortality from vascular causes up to day 35 in the ISIS-2 trial. A total of 17,187 patients were randomly assigned within 24 hours of the onset of suspected acute MI to one of four regimens: (1) placebo infusion and placebo tablets (i.e., routine hospital care); (2) placebo infusion and 162.5 mg of aspirin daily for 1 month (aspirin only); (3) 1.5 million units of streptokinase infusion over 1 hour and placebo tablets (streptokinase only); or (4) both streptokinase and aspirin. (From ISIS-2 [Second International Study of Infarct Survival] Collaborative Group. Randomised trial of intravenous streptokinase, oral aspirin, both, or neither among 17,187 cases of suspected acute myocardial infarction: ISIS-2. Lancet 1988; 2:349–360.)

from cardiac causes who present with other abnormalities on their electrocardiograms (ECGs), such as ST segment depression alone.[14] Further trials of thrombolytic therapy versus control are required to assess whether there are categories of patients with ST depression who might benefit from thrombolytic therapy (or categories for whom thrombolytic therapy should definitely be avoided). Conversely, those patients who present with no or only minor ECG abnormalities (such as isolated T wave inversion) are usually at very low risk of early death, so that any reduction in cardiac deaths may not outweigh the hazards of thrombolytic therapy (notably, early hemorrhagic stroke). Such low-risk patients might best be treated by monitoring their ECGs frequently and giving them thrombolytic therapy only if ST segment elevation or BBB develops. (The effects of thrombolytic therapy among patients with other types of unstable coronary artery disease are not discussed in detail; reported randomized trials in such patients are

TABLE 8–1 • Thrombolytic Therapy: Proportional and Absolute Differences in Mortality During Days 0 to 35

	Deaths During Days 0 to 35			
Day of Death	***Thrombolytic* *(29,315)***	***Control* *(29,285)***	**Proportional Reduction (95% CI)**	**Benefit per 1000 (95% CI)**
Day 0	695 (2.4%)	554 (1.9%)	−26% (SD 6) (−38% to −13%)	−5 (SD 1)** (−7 to −2)
Day 1	475 (1.7%)	549 (1.9%)	13% (SD 6) (2–25%)	3 (SD 1)* (0 to 5)
Days 2 to 7	847 (3.0%)	1100 (3.9%)	23% (SD 4) (16–31%)	9 (SD 2)*** (6–12)
Days 8 to 35	803 (2.9%)	1154 (4.3%)	32% (SD 4) (24–39%)	13 (SD 2)*** (10–16)
Total (days 0–35)	**2820 (9.6%)**	**3357 (11.5%)**	**18% (SD 2) (13–23%)**	**18 (SD 3)*** (13–23%)**

*, **, and *** correspond to $2P < 0.05$, <0.001, and <0.00001, respectively.
CI, confidence interval; SD, standard deviation.

relatively small but they are consistent in suggesting that thrombolytic therapy may be of little benefit, at least among low-risk patients with unstable coronary artery disease.[15, 16])

Greater Benefit from Earlier Treatment, with Clear Benefit Up to 12 Hours from Symptom Onset

The earlier that thrombolytic therapy is started after the onset of symptoms, the greater the benefit (Fig. 8–2). However, in the FTT overview among 46,000 patients with ST elevation or BBB, the slope of absolute benefit plotted against time is fairly gradual and is not significantly steeper in the first few hours after the onset of symptoms than in subsequent hours (see Fig. 8–2). A retrospective subgroup analysis of the Gruppo Italiano per lo Studio della Streptochinasi nell'Infarto Miocardico (GISSI-1) trial suggested that thrombolytic therapy might be especially effective if started within 1 hour of the onset of symptoms[3]—the so-called golden hour.[17] This suggestion is not, however, supported by the overview of large trials,[13] since if the hypothesis-generating GISSI-1 result is excluded, the apparent benefit among those randomized within 1 hour is slightly less than that shown in Figure 8–2. Nor is this conclusion materially altered by a recent reanalysis of selected trials that had published outcome of patients who were randomized during the first hour,[17] because GISSI-1[3] and ISIS-2[4] were the only trials to publish such information, and detailed individual patient data from these and the other trials were included in the more complete FTT analysis. When all of the randomized data are considered, there is no good clinical evidence for a golden hour (although the possibility of a somewhat larger absolute benefit among patients presenting within the first hour cannot be entirely excluded).

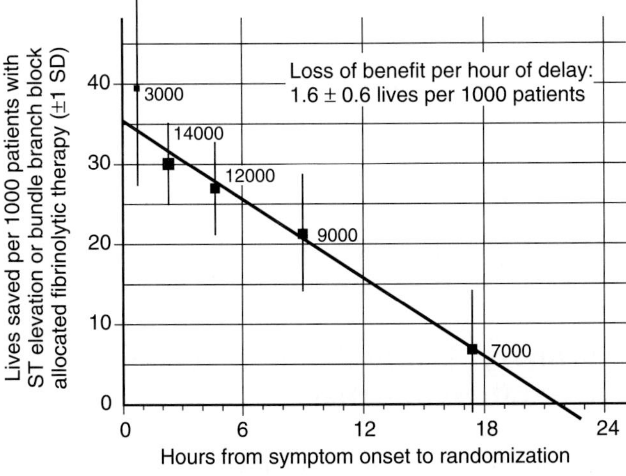

Figure 8–2 Absolute reduction in 35-day mortality with thrombolytic therapy versus delay from symptom onset among 45,000 patients with ST segment elevation or bundle branch block. The figure includes data from all nine randomized trials of thrombolytic therapy versus control with more than 1000 patients (with all patients from ASSET and LATE included, irrespective of electrocardiographic changes).[13] For patients whose delays were recorded as 0–1, 2–3, 4–6, 7–12 and 13–24 h, absolute benefit (±SD) per 1000 patients is plotted against the mean recorded delay time (0.98, 2.50, 4.79, 9.11 and 17.48 h, respectively). The area of each black square and the extent to which it influences the line drawn through the five points is approximately proportional to the number of patients on which it is based. (From Fibrinolytic Therapy Trialists' Collaborative Group. Indications for thrombolytic therapy in suspected acute myocardial infarction: Collaborative overview of early mortality and major morbidity results from all randomised trials of more than 1000 patients. Lancet 1994; 343:311–322.)

Overall, among patients with ST elevation or BBB, thrombolytic therapy produces a definite reduction in mortality, not only among those presenting within 6 hours after the onset of symptoms (about 30 lives saved per 1000 patients treated) but also for those presenting within 7 to 12 hours (about 20 lives saved per 1000 patients treated). Each hour of delay was associated with a mean reduction in the number of lives saved of about 1.6 (SD 0.6) per 1000 patients treated. This estimate may have been somewhat reduced by inaccuracies in assessing the delays[18]; therefore, the real effect of each additional hour of delay may be slightly greater, involving perhaps 2 (or even 3) extra deaths per 1000 patients treated. In principle, a more reliable estimate of the loss of benefit with each hour of delay might be obtainable from randomized trials involving direct comparison of the policy of prehospital administration of thrombolytic therapy versus conventional inhospital administration. Even in aggregate, however, these trials[19–26] have been too small to detect differences of a few per 1000, and selective emphasis on the evidence from one such trial[27] may be misleading.[28]

Too few patients presenting more than 12 hours after the onset of symptoms have been studied to determine whether the benefits of thrombolytic therapy outweigh the risks in such patients. But the general pattern in Figure 8–2 strongly suggests that, at least among patients with ST elevation or BBB who are treated 12 to 18 hours after onset, there may be some net benefit (perhaps about 10 lives saved per 1000 patients treated). The FTT overview indicates that this gradual diminution of benefit may be due to the association between the lateness of starting thrombolytic therapy and the size of the excess of deaths on the day treatment is given and on the following day, whereas the subsequent reduction in mortality with thrombolytic therapy appears to be little affected by the time when patients are treated.[13] The causes of this "early hazard" are unclear,[29–32] but if it could be avoided—perhaps by some adjuvant therapy—then the benefits of thrombolytic therapy might be increased substantially, not just among those treated late after symptom onset but also among those treated early.

Benefits Among the Elderly and Other High-Risk Patients

The absolute survival benefits among patients with ST elevation or BBB were similar among young and old: 15 (SD 4) lives saved per 1000 patients aged less than 55 years; 21 (SD 5) aged 55 to 64 years; 37 (SD 6) aged 65 to 74 years; and 13 (SD 14) aged 75 years and older. Although it had previously been suggested that any benefits of thrombolytic therapy among older patients might be evanescent,[33] the long-term follow-up of ISIS-2 demonstrated that such benefits do persist (survival advantage at the end of 4 years: 23 [SD 7] lives saved per 1000 patients aged <70 years; 41 [SD 19] per 1000 aged ≥70 years) (Fig. 8–3).[12] Hence, age alone should not be considered as a contraindication to thrombolytic treatment.

It has been suggested that thrombolytic therapy may be relatively ineffective among very-high-risk patients, such as those presenting with heart failure or cardiogenic shock.[34] But in the FTT overview, there were particularly large benefits among patients with ST elevation or BBB who presented with systolic blood pressure below 100 mm Hg (64 [SD 21] lives saved per 1000 treated) and among those with a heart rate higher than 100 beats/min (49 [SD 12] lives saved per 1000 treated). Hence, the available evidence suggests that thrombolytic therapy is especially effective among high-risk patients such as those presenting with hypotension or tachycardia, many of whom have experienced heart failure or cardiogenic shock.[13] In GISSI-1, which was the only large trial to record cardiogenic shock and heart failure at entry, the proportional reduction in mortality with streptokinase (SK) among patients with heart failure appeared similar to that seen overall in the study—again suggesting substantial benefit.[3]

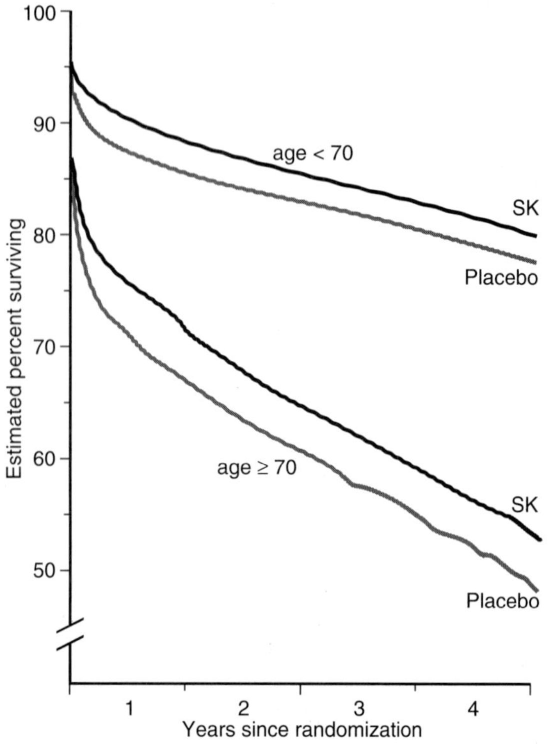

Figure 8–3 Life-table estimates of 4-year survival among patients aged <70 and ≥70 years. Comparisons of patients allocated streptokinase (darker line) versus those allocated matching placebo for patients aged <70 years (upper pair of survival curves) and those patients aged ≥70 years (lower pair). Follow-up to 2 years is 96.0% complete, and 57.7% have been followed to 4 years, with no systematic differences in follow-up between treatment groups.

Strokes and Noncerebral Bleeding with Thrombolytic Therapy

In the FTT overview, thrombolytic therapy was associated with a small but significant excess of approximately 4 extra strokes per 1000 patients treated, with most of this excess appearing on days 0 to 1 and, as far as could be ascertained, chiefly being due to cerebral hemorrhage. Of this early excess, 2 strokes were associated with early death and so were already accounted for in the overall mortality reduction; 1 was moderately or severely disabling; and 1 was not. The excess risk of early stroke associated with thrombolytic therapy increased with age, but there was no significant heterogeneity of this excess risk among the other categories of patient considered. Thrombolytic therapy was also associated with an excess risk of major bleeds (i.e., those that required blood transfusion or were life threatening) of around 7 per 1000 patients treated, but these were rarely fatal.[13]

COMPARISONS BETWEEN DIFFERENT THROMBOLYTIC REGIMENS

Coronary Artery Patency Versus Cerebral Hemorrhage

The first large trials of thrombolytic therapy involved the administration of 1.5 million units of SK in 1 hour. This regimen typically requires a median of 90 minutes from the start of treatment to open the occluded coronary artery.[5] More intensive thrombolytic regimens, generally based on the administration of tissue-type plasminogen activator (t-PA), do not significantly increase the proportion of arteries that is eventually opened within the first few hours, but their action is faster.[5, 35, 36] The exact reduction in the length of time to patency is not known, but the median figure of 90 minutes with SK cannot be reduced by more than about 60 minutes. These transient differences in early patency have not been shown to produce differences in ventricular function.[35, 36] Other things being equal, however, opening the arteries 30 to 60 minutes earlier should be a good thing; Figure 8–2 indicates that it might prevent 1 or 2 deaths from cardiac causes per 1000 patients treated. But other things are not equal because more intensive thrombolytic regimens are associated with a few extra strokes per 1000 patients treated. The fundamental question is whether any cardiovascular advantages of more intensive thrombolytic regimens outweigh any cerebrovascular disadvantages. Because the advantages and disadvantages are both likely to be small (probably involving at most only a few events per 1000 patients treated), any difference between them is likely to be even smaller and hence difficult to measure reliably.

Evidence from Large, Randomized Trials and Avoidance of Selective Emphasis

Two main requirements must be met if differences of only a few adverse events per 1000 treated patients are to be reliably demonstrated or disproved. First, there need to be large-scale randomized trials, and second, the results need to be interpreted as a whole, without undue selective emphasis on parts of the evidence that suit particular conclusions (see Chapter 4).[1, 37, 38]

There have been three large trials of the standard 1.5 million unit SK regimen versus t-PA–based thrombolytic regimens (GISSI-2,[39, 40] ISIS-3,[5] and Global Utilization of Streptokinase and Tissue Plasminogen Activator for Occluded Coronary Arteries [GUSTO-1][41, 42]): stroke and death were the two main clinical endpoints (Table 8–2; see also Fig. 8–3). Patients were randomized at an average of about 2 to 3 hours after the onset of symptoms in the GISSI-2 trial, 4 hours after onset in the ISIS-3 trial, and 2 hours after onset in the GUSTO-1 trial. In each trial, the t-PA–based regimens were designed to ensure appreciably better 90-minute coronary artery patency than the standard SK regimen with which they were compared, and the accompanying aspirin dose was sufficiently large to contribute substantially toward the maintenance of that early patency. Some reviews comparing the effects of SK and t-PA have restricted attention to only one of the trials (GUSTO-1) and, within that trial, to only one of the t-PA–based regimens studied. But the two t-PA–based regimens studied in that trial were actually very similar to each other in terms of the total dose of t-PA delivered within the first hour: 82 mg in the t-PA-alone regimen and 78 mg in the other t-PA–based regimen.[41, 42] Hence, it is appropriate to consider the results from all of the regimens in all three trials together.

Risks of Stroke with Different Thrombolytic Regimens

Compared with SK, an increased risk of stroke was found with the t-PA–based thrombolytic regimens in GISSI-2, ISIS-3, and GUSTO-1 (see Table 8–2). Taking all three trials together, there was a significant excess of 3.3 (SD 0.8) strokes per 1000 patients treated with t-PA ($2P < 0.001$), with an excess of similar size in each trial. Most of this excess risk occurred within the first day or so of giving t-PA and was mainly attributable to cerebral hemorrhage (2.9 [SD 0.5] excess per 1000 treated with t-PA; 95% confidence interval, 2 to 4; $2P < 0.001$). The excess risk associated with these t-PA regimens increased substantially with increasing age and blood pressure.[5, 43, 44] A similar excess of 3 to 4 cerebral hemorrhages per 1000 patients treated—but no significant survival advantage over SK—was observed with anisoylated plasminogen activator complex (APSAC) in ISIS-3,[5] and with reteplase (r-PA)—another recombinant plasminogen activator that produces high rates of early patency[45, 46]—in the 6000-patient International Joint Efficacy Comparison of Thrombolytics (INJECT) trial.[47]

Deaths Not Related to Stroke

For mortality from all causes in the GISSI-2, ISIS-3, and GUSTO-1 trials the evidence of heterogeneity was not statistically significant between treatment effects, and the weighted average of the difference of effect (2.9 [SD 1.9] fewer deaths per 1000 treated with t-PA as compared with SK) in all three trials was not significantly different from zero ($2P > 0.1$; see Table 8–2). Mortality from all causes includes the excess of early deaths after stroke that occurred with the t-PA regimens in all three of these large directly randomized comparisons (an average excess of about 2 deaths after stroke per 1000 patients treated with t-PA). A more sensitive assessment of any cardiac benefits of the t-PA regimens may be obtained by considering separately those deaths not related to stroke (i.e., the deaths of patients in whom no stroke was reported) and those deaths occurring after stroke (most of which were probably due to the stroke). There is some indication of heterogeneity of the results for deaths not related to stroke in the three different trials ($2P = 0.03$; see Table 8–2). Overall, the t-PA–based regimens were associated with 4.9 (SD 1.8) fewer deaths not related to stroke per 1000 patients treated; however, the 95% confidence interval for this estimate spans a wide range, from 1 to 9 fewer such deaths per 1000 patients treated. (This overall result remains about the same when the data from ISIS-3 are restricted to patients randomized within 6 hours after the onset of symptoms,[5] as in the GISSI-2 and GUSTO-1 trials.)

TABLE 8–2 • Direct Randomized Comparisons of the Standard Streptokinase Regimen with Various t-PA–Based Thrombolytic Regimens in Patients with Suspected Acute Myocardial Infarction in the GISSI-2, ISIS-3, and GUSTO-I Trials*

Trial Name and Treatment Regimen	Number of Patients Randomized	Occurrence of Any Stroke		Occurrence of Any Death		Occurrence of Nonstroke Death†		Occurrence of Stroke or Death	
		Percent	*Number*	*Percent*	*Number*	*Percent*	*Number*	*Percent*	*Number*
GISSI-2‡									
SK	10,396	0.94	98	9.22	958	8.81	916	9.75	1014
t-PA	10,372	1.31	136	9.57	993	8.98	931	10.29	1067
Difference/1000 patients		3.7 (SD 1.5) more with t-PA		3.6 (SD 4.0) more with t-PA		1.7 (SD 4.0) more with t-PA		5.3 (SD 4.2) more with t-PA	
ISIS-3‡									
SK	13,780	1.04	141	10.56	1455	10.08	1389	11.10	1530
t-PA	13,746	1.39	188	10.32	1418	9.64	1325	11.01	1513
Difference/1000 patients		3.5 (SD 1.3) more with t-PA		2.4 (SD 3.7) less with t-PA		4.4 (SD 3.6) less with t-PA		1.0 (SD 3.8) less with t-PA	
GUSTO-I‡									
SK (+ subcutaneous heparin)	9841	1.19	117	7.27	712	6.77	666	7.96	783
SK (+ intravenous heparin)	10,410	1.39	144	7.36	763	6.81	709	8.19	853
t-PA alone	10,396	1.55	161	6.31	653	5.63	585	7.18	746
t-PA + SK	10,374	1.64	170	7.01	723	6.24	647	7.88	817
Difference/1000 patients		3.0 (SD 1.2) more with t-PA		6.6 (SD 2.5) less with t-PA		8.6 (SD 2.4) less with t-PA		5.5 (SD 2.6) less with t-PA	
Heterogeneity between the 3 trials		$\chi^2_2 = 0.7$ ($2P = 0.3$)		$\chi^2_2 = 5.6$ ($2P = 0.06$)		$\chi^2_2 = 7.0$ ($2P = 0.03$)		$\chi^2_2 = 5.4$ ($2P = 0.07$)	
Difference/1000 patients in weighted§ average of all 3 trials		**3.3 (SD 0.8) more with t-PA ($2P < 0.0001$)**		**2.9 (SD 1.9) less with t-PA ($2P > 0.1$)**		**4.9 (SD 1.8) less with t-PA ($2P = 0.01$)**		**1.6 (SD 1.9) less with t-PA ($2P = 0.4$)**	

* This table should not be used to make direct, nonrandomized comparisons between the absolute event rates in the different trials, because the patient populations may have differed substantially in age and other characteristics. Deaths recorded throughout the first 35 days are included for GISSI-2 and ISIS-3 and throughout the first 30 days for GUSTO-1. Numbers randomized and numbers with follow-up are from the ISIS-3 report[5] and GUSTO-1[41] (supplemented with revised GUSTO-1 data from the National Auxiliary Publications Service), and numbers with events and the percentages (based on patients with follow-up) are from the ISIS-3 report[5] and Van de Werf and colleagues.[42]

† Nonstroke death denotes death without recorded stroke.

‡ The streptokinase regimen in all three trials involved 1.5 million units infused intravenously over about 1 hour. In the GISSI-2 trial, the t-PA regimen involved 10 mg as an initial bolus, 50 mg in the first hour, and 20 mg in each of the second and third hours. In the ISIS-3 trial, the t-PA regimen involved 40,000 clot lysis units/kg body weight as an initial bolus, 360,000 units/kg in the first hour, and 67,000 units/kg in each of the next three hours. In the GUSTO-I trial, the t-PA alone regimen involved 15 mg as an initial bolus, 0.75 mg/kg (up to 50 mg) in the first 30 minutes, and 0.5 mg/kg (up to 35 mg) in the next hour, whereas the other t-PA–based regimen involved 0.1 mg/kg (up to 9 mg) as an initial bolus and 0.9 mg/kg (up to 81 mg) in the remainder of the first hour, plus 1 million units of SK in the first hour.

§ The weights are proportional to the sizes of the trials, so this average gives the most weight to the GUSTO-I trial and the least to the GISSI-2 trial.

SK, streptokinase; t-PA, tissue-type plasminogen activator.

Each of the t-PA–based regimens studied in these three trials probably opened occluded coronary arteries about 30 to 60 minutes earlier than did the standard SK regimen.[35,36] This would change a delay of about 3 hours between the onset of symptoms and patency into a delay of about 2.5 to 2 hours. Figure 8–2 indicates that this change is likely to reduce mortality from cardiac causes by only about 1 or 2 deaths per 1000 treated (irrespective of what the exact relation between benefit and delay until treatment may be during the so-called first golden hour after the onset of symptoms). Hence, the true cardiac benefit of these t-PA regimens may well be near the lower end of the 95% confidence interval for the overall result presented in Table 8–2; that is, only a few less deaths not related to stroke per 1000 patients treated.

This conclusion is reinforced by the results of studies with newer thrombolytic regimens, such as double-bolus r-PA,[45,46] that produce even higher early patency rates than the so-called front-loaded t-PA regimens. For, despite this higher early patency, no significant improvements were demonstrated when double-bolus r-PA was compared either with SK in over 6000 patients randomized within 12 hours of symptom onset in the INJECT study (270 [9.0%] r-PA vs. 285 [9.5%] SK deaths; $2P > 0.1$)[47] or with front-loaded t-PA in over 15,000 patients randomized within 6 hours in the GUSTO-III trial (7.5% r-PA vs. 7.2% t-PA deaths; $2P > 0.1$).[48] The confidence intervals for these comparisons are wide, however, and it is therefore not possible to determine whether r-PA is associated with a small, although still potentially important, advantage or disadvantage—or, indeed, with no real difference—compared with SK or t-PA. Hence, future studies of novel thrombolytic regimens need to be much larger than INJECT or GUSTO-III to detect reliably the sort of moderate differences in survival (e.g., a few lives per 1000 patients treated) that might plausibly result from such evanescent improvements in patency. (For more detailed discussion of this and other issues related to trial design, see Chapter 20 and References 1 and 2.)

Lack of Difference in Net Clinical Outcome with Different Thrombolytic Regimens

The analyses of stroke or death in Figure 8–4 and Table 8–2 avoid any double counting of patients who had a stroke and also died. These directly randomized comparisons of SK and t-PA again indicate no significant heterogeneity between the results in different trials and no significant difference in net clinical outcome (defined as the occurrence of stroke or death). Taken together, these results suggest that t-PA–based regimens might confer a nonsignificant improvement in net clinical outcome of only 1 or 2 events per 1000 patients. However, the extra hazard with these t-PA regimens is definite (about 3 additional cerebral hem-

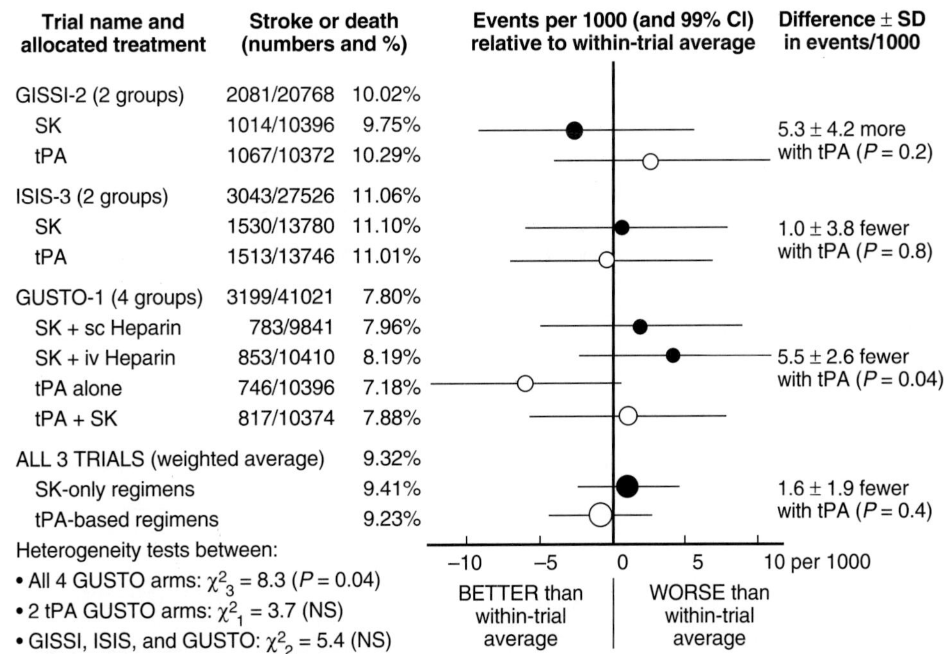

Figure 8–4 Stroke or death in the three large trials of 1.5 million units of streptokinase versus more intensive tissue plasminogen activator (t-PA)-based thrombolytic regimens. For each treatment group the absolute risk per 1000 patients treated (with its 99% confidence interval) is plotted, after subtraction of the overall risk in that trial. Solid symbols denote streptokinase (SK)-only regimens; open symbols denote t-PA–based regimens. (Subtraction of the overall risk does not affect the differences between different groups in one trial but merely centers the results for each trial on the same vertical line.) The SK versus t-PA "ALL 3 TRIALS" result is a weighted average of the results from the three separate trials, with weights proportional to the sizes of those trials. sc, subcutaneous; iv, intravenous.

orrhages per 1000 patients treated; $2P < 0.001$), whereas any excess of benefit over hazard is uncertain (see Fig. 8–4). Indeed, when the definite hazard of 3 extra strokes per 1000 patients treated with t-PA is combined with the indirect evidence of what slightly earlier thrombolytic treatment can achieve (see Fig. 8–2), this suggests a nonsignificant excess of hazard over benefit. Hence, a consideration of all the evidence does not demonstrate any clear differences in net clinical outcome between SK- and t-PA–based regimens—or, indeed, between these regimens and those based on APSAC[5] or r-PA.[47, 48]

Comparisons of Direct Angioplasty and Thrombolytic Therapy for the Routine Treatment of Acute Myocardial Infarction

There has been considerable interest in "direct" (or "primary") *angioplasty* as an alternative reperfusion strategy to thrombolytic therapy. The theoretical advantages include the achievement of Thrombolysis in Myocardial Infarction (TIMI) grade 3 flow in a high proportion of coronary arteries, the avoidance of the excess risk of intracerebral hemorrhage associated with thrombolytic therapy, and the potential treatment of patients with a definite contraindication to thrombolytic therapy.[49, 50] But, the routine use of direct angioplasty is only likely to be available in a small minority of hospitals with experienced operators, and any advantages might be offset by the effects of delays in arranging emergency angioplasty (which might require transfer between hospitals) and by periprocedural risks (including extracranial bleeding).[51]

There is very limited evidence for benefits with direct angioplasty from randomized, controlled trials. A meta-analysis,[52] conducted prior to the completion of the GUSTO-IIb trial,[53] of those randomized trials that had directly compared direct angioplasty versus thrombolytic therapy involved a total of only 58 deaths during the first few weeks. Hence, it was not able to determine reliably whether there was any difference in survival with these different treatment options. The GUSTO-IIb trial approximately doubled the number of early deaths available for analysis, but the 95% confidence interval for the estimated effect in an updated overview of early mortality[53–62] was still wide—ranging from a halving with direct angioplasty to no material difference in survival (Fig. 8–5). Moreover, the existing trials of direct angioplasty versus thrombolytic therapy were generally conducted among low-risk patients—that is, patients for whom mortality during the first few weeks was only about 5% to 10%, compared with about 70% in patients with cardiogenic shock.[63] Consequently, there is no reliable evidence about the effects of direct angioplasty among high-

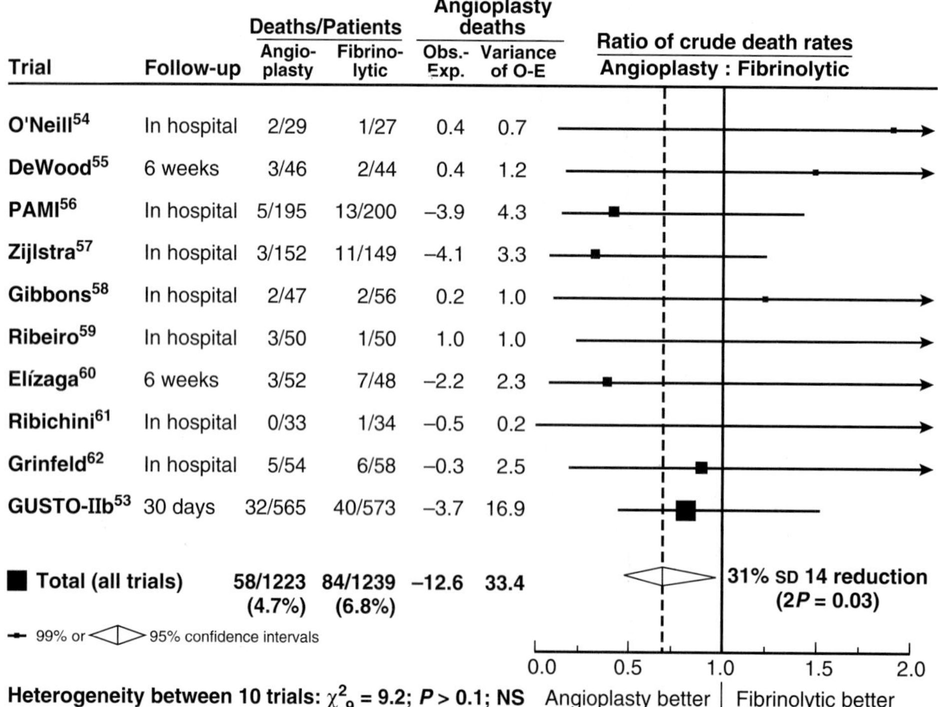

Trial	Follow-up	Deaths/Patients: Angioplasty	Deaths/Patients: Fibrinolytic	Angioplasty deaths: Obs.-Exp.	Angioplasty deaths: Variance of O-E
O'Neill[54]	In hospital	2/29	1/27	0.4	0.7
DeWood[55]	6 weeks	3/46	2/44	0.4	1.2
PAMI[56]	In hospital	5/195	13/200	−3.9	4.3
Zijlstra[57]	In hospital	3/152	11/149	−4.1	3.3
Gibbons[58]	In hospital	2/47	2/56	0.2	1.0
Ribeiro[59]	In hospital	3/50	1/50	1.0	1.0
Elízaga[60]	6 weeks	3/52	7/48	−2.2	2.3
Ribichini[61]	In hospital	0/33	1/34	−0.5	0.2
Grinfeld[62]	In hospital	5/54	6/58	−0.3	2.5
GUSTO-IIb[53]	30 days	32/565	40/573	−3.7	16.9
Total (all trials)		**58/1223 (4.7%)**	**84/1239 (6.8%)**	**−12.6**	**33.4**

Figure 8–5 Proportional effects on early (maximum 6-week) mortality of direct angioplasty compared with fibrinolytic therapy. Proportional reductions are represented by black squares (area proportional to the amount of "statistical information" within each period), with horizontal lines indicating their 99% confidence intervals, and the diamond (a 95% confidence interval) indicating the summary odds ratio. Data for DeWood[55] and Elízaga[60] are from Reference 52, and the data reported by Gibbons[58] excluded 5 randomized patients.

risk patients—even though the American College of Cardiology/American Heart Association Committee on Percutaneous Transluminal Coronary Angioplasty recently recommended direct angioplasty specifically for patients with cardiogenic shock.[64] This emphasizes the need for further, much larger randomized trials of direct angioplasty—including both low-risk and high-risk patients—before its role in routine clinical practice can be determined.

RECOMMENDATIONS FOR THROMBOLYTIC THERAPY

Remaining uncertainties about thrombolytic therapy should not obscure the definite evidence of substantial benefit—irrespective of age, sex, site of infarction, blood pressure, heart rate, heart failure, or history of MI or diabetes—in patients who present with ST elevation or BBB up to at least 12 hours from the onset of symptoms. Among such patients, thrombolytic therapy typically prevents at least 20 to 30 deaths per 1000 patients treated, with the greatest benefits in patients treated earlier and, generally, in those at highest risk of cardiac death. By contrast, thrombolytic therapy was associated, in the large trials with only 4 extra strokes per 1000 patients, of which 2 strokes were associated with early death (and so already accounted for in the reduction of overall mortality). Hence, all such patients should be routinely considered for thrombolytic therapy, and it should be withheld only if there is some extremely clear contraindication (such as a very high risk of intracerebral hemorrhage). Patients who present with no changes, or only minor ones, on their ECGs can be monitored and thrombolytic therapy given only if major changes develop. The choice of thrombolytic regimen appears to make little difference to the overall probability of stroke-free survival because the regimens that dissolve coronary thrombosis more rapidly produce greater risks of cerebral hemorrhage. Nor is there good evidence, as yet, that direct angioplasty produces improved survival compared with thrombolytic therapy.

Despite the strength of the available evidence, there are wide variations in the patterns of thrombolytic therapy use worldwide, and many eligible patients who present with suspected acute MI still do not receive thrombolytic therapy.[65–67] Elderly patients are especially likely to remain untreated: In a recent survey of Medicare patients, about four fifths of patients presenting with acute MI did not receive thrombolytic therapy, and even among those patients considered by the survey's authors to be ideal candidates for thrombolytic therapy, about one third did not receive such therapy (and, moreover, the definition of ideal candidates inappropriately excluded patients presenting 7 to 12 hours after the onset of symptoms).[4] Similarly, an extensive survey conducted throughout Europe in 1993 and 1994 found that more than one third of patients in whom thrombolytic therapy was clearly indicated did not receive it (with the underuse of therapy most marked in women and older patients).[66] Intensive efforts are now required to ensure that all patients who might reasonably be expected to benefit from thrombolytic therapy do actually receive it.

REFERENCES

1. Collins R, Peto R, Gray R, Parish S. Large-scale randomized evidence: Trials and overviews. *In* Weatherall D, Ledingham JGG, Warrell DA, eds. Oxford Textbook of Medicine, vol. 1. Oxford, Oxford University Press, 1996, pp 21–32.
2. Collins R, Peto R, Baigent C, Sleight P. Aspirin, heparin, and fibrinolytic therapy in suspected acute myocardial infarction. N Engl J Med 1997; 336:847–860.
3. GISSI (Gruppo Italiano per lo Studio Della Streptochinasi Nell'Infarto Miocardico). Effectiveness of intravenous thrombolytic treatment in acute myocardial infarction. Lancet 1986; 1:397–401.
4. ISIS-2 (Second International Study of Infarct Survival) Collaborative Group. Randomised trial of intravenous streptokinase, oral aspirin, both, or neither among 17,187 cases of suspected acute myocardial infarction: ISIS-2. Lancet 1988; 2:349–360.
5. ISIS-3 (Third International Study of Infarct Survival) Collaborative Group. ISIS-3: A randomised trial of streptokinase versus tissue plasminogen activator versus anistreplase and of aspirin plus heparin versus aspirin alone among 41,299 cases of suspected acute myocardial infarction. Lancet 1992; 339:753–770.
6. ISAM (Intravenous Streptokinase in Acute Myocardial Infarction) Study Group. A prospective trial of intravenous streptokinase in acute myocardial infarction (ISAM): Mortality, morbidity, and infarct size at 21 days. N Engl J Med 1986; 314:1465–1471.
7. AIMS (APSAC Intervention Mortality Study) Trial Study Group. Effects of intravenous APSAC on mortality after acute myocardial infarction: Preliminary report of a placebo-controlled clinical trial. Lancet 1988; 1:545–549.
8. Wilcox RG, von der Lippe G, Olsson CG, et al for the ASSET (Anglo-Scandinavian Study of Early Thrombosis) Study Group. Trial of tissue plasminogen activator for mortality reduction in acute myocardial infarction (ASSET). Lancet 1988; 2:525–530.
9. Rossi P, Bolognese L on behalf of the Urochinasi per via Sistemica nell'Infarto Miocardico [USIM] Collaborative Group). Comparison of intravenous urokinase plus heparin versus heparin alone in acute myocardial infarction. Am J Cardiol 1991; 68:585–592.
10. EMERAS (Estudio Multicéntrico Estreptoquinasa Repúblicas de América del Sur) Collaborative Group. Randomized trial of late thrombolysis in patients with suspected acute myocardial infarction. Lancet 1993; 342:767–772.
11. LATE (Late Assessment of Thrombolytic Efficacy) Study Group. Late Assessment of Thrombolytic Efficacy (LATE) study with alteplase 6 to 24 hours after onset of acute myocardial infarction. Lancet 1993; 342:759–766.
12. Baigent C, Collins R, Appleby P, et al on behalf of the ISIS-2 (Second International Study of Infarct Survival) Collaborative Group. ISIS-2: 10-year survival in a randomised comparison of intravenous streptokinase, oral aspirin, both, or neither among patients with suspected acute myocardial infarction. BMJ 1998; in press.
13. Fibrinolytic Therapy Trialists' Collaborative Group. Indications for fibrinolytic therapy in suspected acute myocardial infarction: Collaborative overview of early mortality and major morbidity results from all randomised trials of more than 1000 patients. Lancet 1994; 343:311–322.

14. Lee HS, Cross SJ, Rawles JM, et al. Patients with suspected myocardial infarction who present with ST depression. Lancet 1993; 342:1204–1207.
15. Borzak S, Verter J, Bajwa HS, et al. Thrombolytic therapy for unstable angina. Clin Cardiol 1993; 16:637–641.
16. The Thrombolysis in Myocardial Infarction (TIMI)-IIIB Investigators. Effects of tissue plasminogen activator and a comparison of early invasive and conservative strategies in unstable angina and non-Q wave myocardial infarction. Circulation 1994; 89:1545–1556.
17. Boersma E, Maas ACP, Deckers JW, et al. Early thrombolytic treatment in acute myocardial infarction: Reappraisal of the golden hour. Lancet 1996; 348:771–775.
18. Peto R. Two properties of multiple regression analysis; and regression to the mean (and regression from the mean). *In* Fletcher C, Peto R, Tinker C, Speizer FE, eds. The Natural History of Chronic Bronchitis and Emphysema: An Eight-Year Study of Early Chronic Obstructive Lung Disease in Working Men in London. Oxford, Oxford University Press, 1976, pp 218–223.
19. Castaigne AD, Hervé C, Duval-Moulin A-M, et al. Prehospital use of APSAC: Results of a placebo-controlled study. Am J Cardiol 1989; 64:30A–33A.
20. Schofer J, Büttner J, Geng G, et al. Prehospital thrombolysis in acute myocardial infarction. Am J Cardiol 1990; 66:1429–1433.
21. Grampian Region Early Anistreplase Trial (GREAT) Group. Feasibility, safety, and efficacy of domiciliary thrombolysis by general practitioners: Grampian Region Early Anistreplase Trial. BMJ 1992; 305:548–553.
22. The European Myocardial Infarction Project Group. Prehospital thrombolytic therapy in patients with suspected acute myocardial infarction. N Engl J Med 1993; 329:383–389.
23. Weaver WD, Cerqueira M, Hallstrom AP, et al for the Myocardial Infarction Triage and Intervention Project Group. Prehospital-initiated versus hospital-initiated thrombolytic therapy: The Myocardial Infarction Triage and Intervention Trial. JAMA 1993; 270:1211–1216.
24. McNeill AJ, Cunningham SR, Flannery DJ, et al. A double-blind placebo-controlled study of early and late administration of recombinant tissue plasminogen activator in acute myocardial infarction. Br Heart J 1989; 61:316–321.
25. Barbash GI, Roth A, Hod H, et al. Improved survival but not left ventricular function with early and prehospital treatment with tissue plasminogen activator in acute myocardial infarction. Am J Cardiol 1990; 66:261–266.
26. McAleer B, Ruane B, Burke E, et al. Prehospital thrombolysis in a rural community: Short- and long-term survival. Cardiovasc Drugs Ther 1992; 6:369–372.
27. Rawles J. Magnitude of benefit from earlier thrombolytic treatment in acute myocardial infarction: New evidence from Grampian Region Early Anistreplase Trial (GREAT). BMJ 1996; 312:212–216.
28. Leizorovicz A. Benefit from earlier thrombolytic therapy is certain, but what is the magnitude of benefit? BMJ 1996; 312:215–216.
29. Braunwald E. Myocardial reperfusion, limitation of infarct size, reduction of left ventricular dysfunction, and improved survival. Circulation 1989; 79:441–444.
30. Muller DWM, Topol EJ. Selection of patients with acute myocardial infarction for thrombolytic therapy. Ann Intern Med 1990; 113:949–960.
31. Braunwald E, Kloner RA. Myocardial reperfusion: A double-edged sword? J Clin Invest 1985; 76:1713–1719.
32. Honan MB, Harrell FE, Reimer KA, et al. Cardiac rupture, mortality, and the timing of thrombolytic therapy: A meta-analysis. J Am Coll Cardiol 1990; 16:359–367.
33. Gurwitz JH, Goldberg RJ, Gore JM. Coronary thrombolysis for the elderly? JAMA 1991; 265:1720–1723.
34. Bates ER, Topol EJ. Limitations of thrombolytic therapy for acute myocardial infarction complicated by congestive heart failure and cardiogenic shock. J Am Coll Cardiol 1991; 18:1077–1084.
35. The GUSTO Angiographic Investigators. The effects of tissue plasminogen activator, streptokinase, or both on coronary artery patency, ventricular function, and survival after acute myocardial infarction. N Engl J Med 1993; 329:1615–1622.
36. Granger CB, White HD, Bates ER, et al. A pooled analysis of coronary arterial patency and left ventricular function after intravenous thrombolysis for acute myocardial infarction. Am J Cardiol 1994; 74:1220–1228.
37. Peto R, Pike MC, Armitage P, et al. Design and analysis of randomized clinical trials requiring prolonged observation of each patient: II. Analysis and examples. Br J Cancer 1977; 35:1–39.
38. Yusuf S, Collins R, Peto R. Why do we need some large, simple, randomized trials? Stat Med 1984; 3:409–420.
39. Gruppo Italiano per lo Studio della Sopravvivenza nell'Infarto Miocardico. GISSI-2: Randomised trial of intravenous alteplase versus intravenous streptokinase in acute myocardial infarction. Lancet 1990; 336:65–71.
40. The International Study Group. In-hospital mortality and clinical course of 20,891 patients with suspected acute myocardial infarction randomised between tissue plasminogen activator or streptokinase with or without heparin. Lancet 1990; 336:71–75.
41. The GUSTO Investigators. An international randomized trial comparing four thrombolytic strategies for acute myocardial infarction. N Engl J Med 1993; 329:673–682.
42. Van de Werf F, Topol EJ, Lee KL, et al. Variations in patient management and outcomes for acute myocardial infarction in the United States and other countries: Results from the GUSTO trial. JAMA 1995; 273:1586–1591.
43. Gore JM, Granger CB, Simoons ML, et al for the GUSTO investigators. Stroke after thrombolysis: Mortality and functional outcomes in the GUSTO-1 trial. Circulation 1995; 92:2811–2818.
44. Maggioni AP, Franzosi MG, Santoro E, et al. The risk of stroke in patients with acute myocardial infarction after thrombolytic and antithrombotic treatment. N Engl J Med 1992; 327:1–6.
45. Smalling RW, Bode C, Kalbfleisch J, et al and the RAPID Investigators. More rapid, complete and stable coronary thrombolysis with bolus administration of reteplase compared with alteplase infusion in acute myocardial infarction. Circulation 1995; 91:2725–2732.
46. Bode C, Smalling RW, Berg G, et al for the RAPID-2 Investigators. Randomized comparison of coronary thrombolysis achieved with double-bolus reteplase (recombinant plasminogen activator) in front-loaded, accelerated alteplase (recombinant tissue plasminogen activator) in patients with acute myocardial infarction. Circulation 1996; 94:891–898.
47. International Joint Efficacy Comparison of Thrombolytics. Randomised, double-blind comparison of reteplase double-bolus administration with streptokinase in acute myocardial infarction (INJECT): Trial to investigate equivalence. Lancet 1995; 346:329–336.
48. The Global Use of Strategies to Open Occluded Coronary Arteries (GUSTO-III) Investigators. A comparison of reteplase with alteplase for acute myocardial infarction. N Engl J Med 1997; 337:1118–1123.
49. Zijlstra F. Primary angioplasty is the most effective treatment for an acute myocardial infarction. Br Heart J 1995; 5:403–404.
50. Grines CL, O'Neill WW. Primary angioplasty: The optimal reperfusion strategy in the United States? Br Heart J 1995; 5:405–406.
51. Vaitkus PT. Limitations of primary angioplasty in acute myocardial infarction—effectiveness depends on the clinical and operational context. Br Heart J 1995; 5:409–410.
52. Michels KB, Yusuf S. Does PTCA in acute myocardial infarction affect mortality and reinfarction rates? A quantitative overview (meta-analysis) of the randomized clinical trials. Circulation 1995; 91:476–485.
53. The Global Use of Strategies to Open Occluded Arteries in Acute Coronary Syndromes (GUSTO-IIb) Angioplasty Substudy Investigators. A clinical trial comparing primary coronary angioplasty with tissue plasminogen activator for acute myocardial infarction. N Engl J Med 1997; 336:1621–1628.
54. O'Neill W, Timmis GC, Bourdillon PD, et al. A prospective randomized clinical trial of intracoronary streptokinase versus coronary angioplasty for acute myocardial infarction. N Engl J Med 1986; 314:812–818.
55. DeWood MA, Fisher MJ for the Spokane Heart Research Group. Direct PTCA versus intravenous rt-PA in acute myocardial

infarction: Preliminary results from a prospective randomized trial [Abstract]. Circulation 1989; 80 (suppl II):II-418.
56. Grines CL, Browne KF, Marco J, et al for the Primary Angioplasty in Myocardial Infarction Study Group. A comparison of immediate angioplasty with thrombolytic therapy for acute myocardial infarction. N Engl J Med 1993; 328:673–679.
57. Zijlstra F, de Boer MJ, Hoorntje JCA, et al. A comparison of immediate coronary angioplasty with intravenous streptokinase in acute myocardial infarction. N Engl J Med 1993; 328:680–684.
58. Gibbons RJ, Holmes DR, Reeder GS, et al. Immediate angioplasty compared with the administration of a thrombolytic agent followed by conservative treatment for myocardial infarction. N Engl J Med 1993; 328:685–691.
59. Ribeiro EE, Silva LA, Carneiro R, et al. Randomized trial of direct coronary angioplasty versus intravenous streptokinase in acute myocardial infarction. J Am Coll Cardiol 1993; 22:376–380.
60. Elízaga J, García EJ, Delcan JL, et al. Primary coronary angioplasty versus systemic thrombolysis in acute anterior myocardial infarction: In-hospital results from a prospective randomized trial [Abstract]. Circulation 1993; 88 (suppl I):I-411.
61. Ribichini F, Steffenino G, Dellavalle A, et al. Comparison between in-hospital results of primary angioplasty versus thrombolysis in inferior acute myocardial infarction with anterior ST-segment depression: A single-center randomised study [Abstract]. Eur Heart J 1996; 17(suppl):515.
62. Grinfeld L, Berrocal D, Belardi J, et al. Thrombolytics versus primary angioplasty in acute myocardial infarction (FAP): A randomized trial in a community hospital in Argentina [Abstract]. J Am Coll Cardiol 1996; 27(suppl A):222A.
63. Hochman JS, Boland J, Sleeper LA, et al for the Shock Registry Investigators. Current spectrum of cardiogenic shock and effect of early revascularization on mortality: Results of an international registry. Circulation 1995; 91:873–881.
64. Ryan TJ, Bauman WB, Kennedy JW, et al. Guidelines for percutaneous transluminal coronary angioplasty: A report of the American College of Cardiology/American Heart Association Task Force on Assessment of Diagnostic and Therapeutic Cardiovascular Procedures (Committee on Percutaneous Transluminal Coronary Angioplasty). J Am Coll Cardiol 1993; 22:2033–2054.
65. Ellerbeck EF, Jencks SF, Radford MJ, et al. Quality of care for Medicare patients with acute myocardial infarction: A four-state pilot study from the cooperative cardiovascular project. JAMA 1995; 273:1509–1514.
66. European Secondary Prevention Study Group. Translation of clinical trials into practice: A European population-based study of the use of thrombolysis for acute myocardial infarction. Lancet 1996; 347:1203–1207.
67. Pashos CL, Normand S-LT, Garfinkle JB, et al. Trends in the use of drug therapies in patients with acute myocardial infarction: 1988–1992. J Am Coll Cardiol 1994; 23:1023–1030.

9 Beta Blockers

▶ Claudia U. Chae
▶ Charles H. Hennekens

Following the novel concept of α- and β-adrenoreceptors as proposed by Ahlquist,[1] β-adrenoreceptor antagonists were initially developed by Black and colleagues "to find a way of reducing myocardial demand for oxygen in hearts whose oxygen supply was restricted by arterial disease."[2] The benefits of blocking the effects of sympathetic stimulation in the prevention and treatment of cardiovascular disease (CVD) have since been demonstrated in patients with hypertension and myocardial infarction (MI). Evidence is also now accumulating to support the use of beta blockers in patients with heart failure. In this chapter, we review the evidence from randomized trials of beta blockers in hypertension, during and after MI, and in heart failure in the context of the underlying mechanisms by which beta blockers may exert cardioprotective effects.

PHARMACOLOGY

As a class, beta blockers decrease heart rate and myocardial contractility, lower blood pressure, and reduce cardiac work. Beta blockers lower the heart rate by slowing conduction through the sinoatrial and atrioventricular nodes, and blunt the tachycardic response to stressors such as orthostasis and exercise. The decrease in myocardial automaticity also contributes to their class II antiarrhythmic effects. Cardiac output is reduced owing to their negative inotropic and chronotropic properties. Peripheral resistance may initially increase because of unopposed α-receptor–mediated vasoconstriction but tends to normalize over time. The mechanisms by which beta blockers lower blood pressure are unclear. Possibilities include (1) inhibition of norepinephrine release by blockade of presynaptic β-receptors; (2) decreased circulating renin activity; (3) adaptation of vascular resistance to the reduction in cardiac output; and/or (4) decrease in sympathetic outflow from the central nervous system (CNS). However, a central effect appears less likely, given that some beta blockers that poorly penetrate the CNS have equivalent hypotensive effects.

Individual beta blockers differ in their cardioselectivity, intrinsic sympathomimetic activity, and lipid solubility (Table 9–1), which are characteristics that may influence both tolerability and efficacy. *Cardioselective* beta blockers preferentially bind to the cardiac β_1-receptors, rather than to the β_2-receptors, which predominate in the bronchi, peripheral vasculature, and elsewhere. This selectivity is seen at lower doses (e.g., oral metoprolol, 100 mg daily) but not at higher doses. Beta blockers with *intrinsic sympathomimetic activity* (ISA) have partial agonist activity and do not lower heart rate and cardiac output to the same degree as non-ISA agents. Beta blockers with high *lipid solubility* are more likely to be hepatically inactivated, shortening their plasma half-life, and are present in higher concentrations in the CNS.

The major side effects of beta blockers are directly related to antagonism of the β_1- and/or β_2-receptors.[3] To preserve β_2-mediated bronchodilation, β_1-selective

TABLE 9–1 • Pharmacologic Characteristics of Beta Blockers

Beta Blockers	Adrenergic Receptor Selectivity	ISA	Lipid Solubility	Other Properties
Nonselective				
Propranolol	$\beta_1\beta_2$	0	+ + +	
Timolol	$\beta_1\beta_2$	0	0	
Nadolol	$\beta_1\beta_2$	0	0	
Pindolol	$\beta_1\beta_2$	+ +	0	
Oxprenolol	$\beta_1\beta_2$	+ +	+	
Selective				
Atenolol	$+\beta_1$	0	0	
Metoprolol	$+\beta_1$	0	+ +	
Bisopropolol	$++\beta_1$	0	+	
Acebutolol	$+\beta_1$	+	+	
Esmolol	$+\beta_1$	0	0	$t_{1/2}$ = 9 min
Vasodilating				
Labetalol	$\beta_1\beta_2$	0	+ +	Partial α_1 antagonist
Carvedilol	$\beta_1\beta_2$	0	+	Partial α_1 antagonist
Bucindolol	$\beta_1\beta_2$	0	0	Direct vasodilator

ISA = intrinsic sympathomimetic activity, + = mild effect, + + = moderate effect, + + + = marked effect, $t_{1/2}$ = plasma half-life.

Adapted from Braunwald E (ed). Heart Disease: A Textbook of Cardiovascular Medicine, 5th ed. Philadelphia, WB Saunders, 1997.

agents may be safer if beta blockers must be used in patients with asthma or chronic lung disease, although great caution must be exercised in this setting. β_1-Selective agents are preferred in patients with diabetes mellitus because they have less adverse effects on glucose metabolism and the response to hypoglycemia than nonselective agents. Nonselective beta blockers decrease high-density lipoprotein (HDL) by about 10% and increase triglycerides by 20% to 30%; these adverse lipid effects may be less prominent with β_1-selective agents and those with ISA.[3, 4] All beta blockers penetrate the CNS and are associated with side effects (e.g., insomnia, nightmares, and cognitive impairment), but it is unclear if the hydrophilic agents have fewer CNS effects.[3, 5] It is unclear whether beta blockers cause depression[5] because this observation may be related to other confounding factors.[6] β_1-Blockade may exacerbate pre-existing conduction system disease or heart failure, and agents with ISA may be considered in this setting.[7]

As is the case for most drugs that produce small to moderate benefits, rational clinical decision making depends on a totality of evidence, which includes data from randomized trials as to efficacy as well as data on differences in actions and potential side effects of individual drugs within its class. All beta blockers are effective in lowering blood pressure. Whether certain cardioprotective actions of beta blockers are a class effect or are influenced by their other ancillary properties is unclear.[7, 8] In animal models, lipophilic beta blockers such as propranolol and metoprolol[9–11] have antiatherogenic properties, with fewer data available for the hydrophilic beta blockers.[12, 13] It is unclear if preservation of vagal tone by beta blockers, which may contribute to the associated reduction in cardiac death, is related to their degree of lipophilicity.[14–16] There are ample data in support of the use of cardioselective, non-ISA beta blockers such as atenolol[17] and metoprolol[18, 19] during acute MI. However, only beta blockers without ISA (timolol,[20] propranolol,[21] and to a lesser extent, metoprolol[22]) have been definitively demonstrated to reduce the mortality rate in the post-MI population. In heart failure, metoprolol and third-generation beta blockers with ancillary properties such as vasodilation (e.g., carvedilol) are currently being tested.

HYPERTENSION

Based on the totality of evidence, which includes sufficient data from randomized trials, the Joint National Committee (JNC) on Prevention, Detection, Evaluation, and Treatment of High Blood Pressure recommends diuretics and beta blockers as first-line agents in treating patients with uncomplicated essential hypertension.[23] In this section, we review data from the major primary prevention trials that studied the efficacy of beta blockers in reducing the risk of CVD in people with hypertension. The first four trials discussed (Table 9–2)—the Medical Research Council (MRC) trial,[24] the study by Coope and Warrender,[25] the Swedish Trial in Old People with Hypertension (STOP-H),[26] and the MRC trial in older people[27]—used beta blockers in their primary treatment arms. We also review data from other trials that compared the effects of beta blockers and diuretics.[28–30]

Primary Prevention Trials in Hypertension Using Beta Blockers

The single-blind MRC trial of treatment of mild hypertension[24] was conducted in general practices in the United Kingdom among 17,354 subjects (48% women) aged 35 to 64 years, with diastolic blood pressure (DBP) 90 to 109 mm Hg (mean BP 160/98 mm Hg). Randomization was to active treatment (bendrofluazide 10 mg, or propranolol up to 240 mg daily) or placebo. Supplemental therapy with guanethidine or methyldopa was used as needed to reach the goal of reducing DBP below 90 mm Hg. After 4.9 years of average follow-up, systolic blood pressure (SBP) was reduced by 11 mm Hg and DBP reduced by 6 mm Hg in actively treated subjects, compared with those on placebo. Those on active treatment had a 45% reduced risk of stroke (95% CI, 25% to 60%, $P < 0.01$), and a 19% reduced risk of all CVD events (95% CI, 5% to 31%; $P < 0.05$), compared with those on placebo. There were possible small differences in coronary events and total mortality rate, but these differences did not achieve statistical significance. The interpretability was limited by high loss to follow-up (19%) and withdrawals from randomized treatment; in total, 43% of the diuretic group, 42% of the propranolol group, and 47% of the placebo group were not taking the treatment to which they had been assigned at randomization.

In a trial conducted by Coope and Warrender,[25] 884 subjects (70% women) aged 60 to 79 years with SBP above 170 mm Hg or DBP above 105 mm Hg (mean BP 196/99 mm Hg) were randomized to beta-blocker–based treatment (atenolol 100 mg daily) or to an open control group. Two thirds of subjects in the atenolol group needed the addition of a diuretic (bendrofluazide 5 mg daily) to achieve adequate BP control. BP fell by 18/11 mm Hg (SBP/DBP) in those on active treatment compared to the control subjects. Active treatment resulted in a significant 42% reduction in stroke (95% CI, 4% to 65%; $P < 0.03$). There was a nonsignificant 22% reduction in CVD death (95% CI, −20% to 49%), and no significant decrease in coronary heart disease (CHD) events among those assigned to active treatment. Limitations of this trial

TABLE 9–2 • Primary Prevention Trials of Beta Blockers in Hypertension

Trial	*N*	Age (y)	Entry Criteria	Follow-Up (mean)	Study Design	Active Treatment	Stroke*	CHD*	Total CVD*	CVD death*	Death*
MRC[24]	17,354	35–64	DBP 90–109	4.9 y	Single-blind, placebo-controlled	Bendrofluazide or propranolol	45 (25 to 60)	6 (−13 to 21)	19 (5 to 31)	4 (−22 to 24)	2 (−16 to 18)
Coope[25]	884	60–79	SBP >170 or DBP >105	4.4 y	Open, no placebo	Atenolol	42 (4 to 65)	−3 (−63 to 37)		22 (−20 to 40)	3 (−42 to 30)
STOP-H[26]	1627	70–84	SBP >180 and DBP >90, or DBP 105–120	2.1 y	Double-blind, placebo-controlled	Beta Blocker† or HCTZ + amiloride	47 (14 to 67)	13 (−56 to 51)	40‡ (15 to 57)	—	43 (13 to 63)
MCR Trial in Older People[27]	4396	65–74	SBP >160 and DBP <115	5.8 y	Single-blind, placebo-controlled	Atenolol or HCTZ + amiloride	25 (3 to 42)	19 (−2 to 36)	17 (2 to 29)	9 (−12 to 27)	−3 (−14 to 18)

*Results expressed as percent (%) decrease in risk with active treatment compared with placebo or control, with 95% confidence intervals in parentheses.
†Atenolol, metoprolol, or pindolol.
‡Endpoint included any myocardial infarction, any stroke, and other cardiovascular death.
MRC, Medical Research Council; STOP-H, Swedish Trial in Old Patients with Hypertension; SBP, systolic blood pressure (mm Hg); DBP, diastolic blood pressure (mm Hg); CHD, coronary heart disease; CVD, cardiovascular disease; HCTZ, hydrochlorothiazide.

included its relatively small sample size. There was an imbalance of smokers (28% in treatment group vs. 21% in control group), which may account for the apparent increase in noncardiovascular mortality in the treatment group (17 vs. 10) that was due mostly to lung cancer, and may also account in part for the lack of effect on all-cause mortality.

The randomized, double-blind, placebo-controlled STOP-H trial[26] included 1627 subjects (63% women) aged 70 to 84 years with SBP between 180 and 230 mm Hg and DBP at 90 mm Hg or higher, or DBP of 105 to 120 mm Hg regardless of SBP (mean BP 195/102 mm Hg). Randomization was to active therapy (atenolol 50 mg, hydrochlorothiazide 25 mg plus amiloride 2.5 mg, metoprolol 100 mg, or pindolol 5 mg daily) or placebo. Each trial center chose one of the four basic treatment regimens; 71% chose a beta-blocker-based strategy.[31] Two thirds of the active treatment group required combined therapy with diuretics and beta blockers to achieve the target goal of BP below 160/95 mm Hg. The trial was terminated early at 25 months because of the emergence of a statistically extreme benefit on the primary combined CVD endpoint of 40% (95% CI, 15% to 57%; $P = 0.003$), stroke of 47% (95% CI, 14% to 67%, $P = 0.008$), and vascular death of 57% ($P = 0.001$). There was a nonsignificant 13% reduction in risk of MI (95% CI, −56% to 51%). Although not a prespecified endpoint, total mortality was significantly reduced by 43% (95% CI, 13% to 63%; $P = 0.0079$) with active treatment. BP was reduced by 19.5/8.1 mm Hg (mean) in subjects assigned to active treatment compared with placebo. The STOP-H findings demonstrated that the benefits of antihypertensive therapy in reducing the risk of stroke and CVD death previously seen in the "young" elderly also applied to those aged 70 to 84 years.[32]

In the single-blind MRC trial of older adults,[27] 4396 subjects (58% women) aged 65 to 74 years, with SBP 160 mm Hg or higher and DBP below 115 mm Hg (average 185/90 mm Hg), were randomized to active therapy (atenolol 50 mg or a potassium-sparing diuretic regimen of hydrochlorothiazide 25 to 50 mg plus amiloride 2.5 to 5.0 mg daily) or placebo. Over 5.8 years of follow-up (mean), the active treatment group had a significant 25% reduction in stroke (95% CI, 3% to 42%; $P = 0.04$), with a nonsignificant but possible trend to fewer coronary events (19% reduction, 95% CI −2% to 36%; $P = 0.08$), and a significant 17% reduction in total CVD (95% CI, 2% to 29%; $P = 0.03$) compared with the placebo group. There was a possible but nonsignificant 9% reduction in CVD death (95% CI, −12% to 27%). All-cause mortality was similar between the active treatment and placebo groups. As with the prior MRC trial,[24] there was a high proportion of subjects lost to follow-up (25%) or withdrawn from randomized treatment, so that by the end of the trial, 48% in the diuretic group, 63% in the beta-blocker group, and 53% in the placebo group were no longer on randomized assignment.

Overall, the data from these primary prevention trials support the efficacy of beta blockers and diuretics in lowering BP and reducing the risk of stroke and total CVD in middle-aged and older adults with hypertension. These individual trials could not conclusively demonstrate that BP reduction resulted in significant decreases in CHD risk. With the far greater statistical power obtained by pooling data from trials, the benefits of BP reduction in decreasing the risk of CHD, stroke, and cardiovascular morbidity and mortality are clearly demonstrated, as summarized in several recent overviews.[32–35] In an overview of 17 trials, which predominantly used diuretics and beta blockers, involving a total of 23,847 subjects followed for about 3 to 5 years, the average reduction in DBP of 5 to 6 mm Hg was associated with a 16% reduction in CHD (95% CI, 8% to 23%; $P = 0.0001$), 38% reduction in total stroke (95% CI, 31% to 45%; $P < 0.0001$), and 21% reduction in vascular mortality (95% CI, 13% to 28%; $P < 0.0001$).[32] Observational studies had predicted that a 5 to 6 mm Hg reduction in DBP would lead to a 40% to 45% reduction in stroke and 20% to 25% reduction in cardiovascular death, but had predicted a greater reduction in CHD risk of 20% to 25%.[33]

The discrepancy between the observed and predicted magnitude of CHD risk reduction with BP lowering has several plausible explanations. First, this may be a chance finding. Second, beta blockers and diuretics may adversely affect plasma lipids, although the clinical significance of this effect is unclear.[12, 13] Third, the trials were of relatively short duration, and the beneficial effects on stroke may be more immediate and more closely linked to the effects of BP lowering, whereas longer treatment may be needed to fully assess its influence on the longer-term process of atherosclerosis in CHD.[32, 36] This possibility is supported by the findings of the Hypertension Detection and Follow-Up Program[37] and the Multiple Risk Factor Intervention Trial,[38] which demonstrated greater reductions in CHD at 8 and 10 years, respectively, than at 5 and 6 years.

Comparison Between Beta Blockers and Diuretics in Hypertension

In the late 1970s, in the context of emerging data about the benefits of beta blockers after MI, several trials—the two MRC trials,[24, 27] the International Prospective Primary Prevention Study in Hypertension (IPPPSH),[28] and the Heart Attack Primary Prevention in Hypertension (HAPPHY)[29]—were designed to test the hypothesis that beta blockers may confer an additional advantage in primary prevention in hypertension.[39]

Both MRC trials were designed to compare the effects of diuretics versus beta blockers, albeit as secondary analyses. In the MRC trial of mild hypertension,[24] there were no significant differences except for a greater reduction in stroke in those assigned to diuretics compared with the beta-blocker group (0.8 vs. 1.9 events per 1000 person-years, $P = 0.002$). In contrast, in the MRC trial in older people,[27] subgroup analysis by drug type showed no difference in stroke risk. However, those in the diuretic group had a lower risk of CHD (7.7 vs 12.8 events per 1000 person-years; $P = 0.006$) and total CVD (17.4 vs. 24.6 events per 1000 person-years; $P = 0.007$) compared with those in the beta-blocker arm. Total death (21.3 vs. 26.4 per 1000 person-years, $P = 0.07$) was also lower in the diuretic group, owing to a difference in CVD death (10.5 vs. 15 per 1000 person-years; $P = 0.03$).

These data from the MRC trial in older people suggest that a low-dose, potassium-sparing diuretic regimen may be more effective than atenolol in reducing the risk of CHD in hypertensive subjects, a finding that would need to be confirmed. The differences in CHD risk were not seen in the first MRC trial, which used a high-dose, non–potassium-sparing diuretic regimen (which may be associated with an increased risk of sudden death[40, 41]) and propranolol, a nonselective, lipophilic beta blocker known to be beneficial in the post-MI setting in reducing the incidence of recurrent MI, sudden death, and cardiovascular and total mortality.[21] In contrast, the MRC trial in older people used a low-dose, potassium-sparing diuretic regimen in comparison with atenolol, whose shorter duration of action may provide less protection against the circadian pattern of vulnerability to cardiac events,[42] and whose low lipophilicity may confer less long-term protection against sudden death.[16] Diuretics may also offer other benefits beyond BP lowering; for example, diuretics may cause a greater degree of regression of left ventricular hypertrophy, a predictor of CVD risk in hypertensive subjects,[43] than beta blockers.[44, 45] However, the MRC trial data must be interpreted with caution. First, chance is a plausible alternative explanation. Second, because the diuretic group initially had a more rapid reduction in BP than the beta-blocker group, the difference in duration of effective BP reduction is a possible factor. However, the lower risk in the diuretic group persisted even after adjusting for this tendency.[27] Third, the high rates of loss to follow-up and treatment withdrawal are problematic in interpreting these data. In addition, there was overlap in each treatment group due to supplementation with the other therapy (16% in the beta-blocker group and 11% in the diuretic group). Finally, with longer follow-up time, an equal or greater benefit may be seen with beta blockers (as suggested by the Metoprolol Atherosclerosis Prevention in Hypertensives (MAPHY) trial[30] results discussed later), perhaps mediated by longer-term benefits of beta blockers in such areas as atherogenesis.

There are few large trials with the primary aim of directly comparing the effects of diuretics and beta-blocker therapy. In the double-blind IPPPSH,[28] 6357 subjects (50% women), aged 40 to 64 years with DBP of 100 to 125 mm Hg (mean BP 173/108 mm Hg) were randomized to oxprenolol, a nonselective beta blocker with ISA, or to placebo. However, to achieve the target DBP of 95 mm Hg or lower, 85% of subjects in the placebo group were given supplemental therapy with non–beta-blocker drugs (82% diuretics, 48% other agents), and only 30% of the oxprenolol group remained on monotherapy (67% were also on diuretics, 33% on other agents). Over 3 to 5 years of follow-up, there were no statistically significant differences in CHD, CVD, or total mortality. The interpretability of these data, however, is limited by the large overlap in treatment between the two groups.

The HAPPHY trial[29] was an open study which compared beta blockers (atenolol 100 mg or metoprolol 200 mg daily) with diuretics (bendrofluazide 5 mg or hydrochlorothiazide 50 mg daily) in men aged 40 to 64 years, with DBP 100 to 130 mm Hg (mean BP 166/107 mm Hg. Each trial center chose the beta blocker and diuretic it would use. Subjects were stratified by CHD risk factor status. The drug doses were chosen for their equipotent hypotensive effect, so that in contrast to the MRC trials, equal and parallel reductions in BP were achieved in both treatment groups. This increased the likelihood of detecting an effect of the drug itself, independent of the reduction in BP. Crossover or supplementation with the other drug type was not permitted, except in the case of nonfatal MI or CHF. After 3.8 y of average follow-up, both groups had mean BPs of 140/88 mm Hg. About 85% of study subjects were on randomized treatment, with only 4% on the drug in the other group; 62% of the diuretic group and 68% of the beta-blocker group were on monotherapy ($P < 0.001$). The beta-blocker and diuretic groups had no significant differences in risk of CHD (relative risk [RR], 0.88; 95% CI, 0.68 to 1.14) or total mortality (RR, 1.06; 95% CI, 0.80 to 1.41).

The results of HAPPHY did not demonstrate any additional benefit in CHD reduction with diuretics compared with beta blocker, as had been suggested by the MRC trial results. Without a placebo group, it is impossible to know if the HAPPHY data were demonstrating no reduction or an approximately equal reduction in CHD risk with diuretics and beta blocker (the latter being more likely, in the context of other available data). However, the MRC, IPPPSH, and HAPPHY trials were not adequately powered to detect the most plausible small or moderate differences in treatment efficacy between diuretics and beta blockers.[29]

The MAPHY[30] study was essentially extended follow-up of the metoprolol and diuretic arms of the HAPPHY study.[46] After the end of the HAPPHY trial in 1985, the metoprolol centers followed their 3234 participants for 14 more months, for total follow-up time of 4.2 years (median) and 5 years (mean). By the end of MAPHY, 52% and 45% of the beta-blocker and diuretic treatment groups, respectively, were on monotherapy. Of the diuretic group, 11.6% were also taking beta blockers; 6.3% of subjects in the beta-blocker group were also on diuretics. At the time of median follow-up, compared with those in the diuretic group, subjects in the metoprolol group had a significant 48% reduction in total mortality (95% CI 17% to 68%; $P = 0.028$), primarily because of reductions in fatal CHD ($P = 0.048$), fatal stroke ($P = 0.043$), and total CVD ($P = 0.012$). By the end of the study, the reductions in total mortality (22%) and CVD mortality (27%) observed with beta-blocker therapy were lesser in magnitude and no longer statistically significant. The authors suggested that the lack of divergence in survival curves after 4 to 5 years may be due to an increase in treatment crossovers, dropouts from randomized treatment, and noncardiovascular deaths, as well as a delay in events with beta blockade. The CVD mortality benefit from metoprolol was driven primarily by a 30% ($P = 0.017$) reduction in sudden death, which accounted for 78% of total CVD mortality.[47] Metoprolol also reduced CHD events (RR 0.58; 95% CI, 0.41 to 0.80 at median follow-up (RR, 0.76; 95% CI, 0.58 to 0.98 at end of the study).[46]

MAPHY is the only study to have directly demonstrated that a beta blocker, metoprolol, reduced CHD and death and appeared to be more effective than a diuretic in hypertensives. The contrast between the MAPHY findings and those of the MRC and IPPPSH trials may be due to the lack of a class effect with beta blocker, with metoprolol's greater efficacy possibly explained by its higher lipophilicity than atenolol and lack of ISA, unlike oxprenolol. HAPPHY, MAPHY, and subgroup analyses by sex of the MRC trial and IPPPSH[45] suggest that beta blockers are at least similar to diuretics in reducing the risk of CHD in hypertensive men. However, others have argued that the study design of MAPHY was essentially a subgroup analysis of HAPPHY, significantly limiting the interpretability of the data.[48, 49]

In a meta-analysis comparing the relative efficacy of different antihypertensive agents, 18 randomized trials were classified by the type of drug used as first-line therapy (Table 9–3).[50] The beta-blocker category consisted of the beta-blocker arms of the two MRC trials,[24, 27] the study of Coope and Warrender,[25] and STOP-H[26] (which was classified as a beta-blocker trial since 71% of the study centers chose a beta blocker over the diuretic as their first-line therapy). Compared with placebo, beta blockers significantly reduced the risk of stroke (RR, 0.71; 95% CI, 0.59 to 0.86) and CHF (RR, 0.58; 95% CI, 0.40 to 0.84), as did diuretics. However, low-dose diuretics (starting dose 12.5 to 25 mg of chlorthalidone or hydrochlorothiazide daily) significantly reduced the risk of CHD (RR, 0.72; 95% CI, 0.61 to 0.85), whereas beta blockers (RR, 0.93; 95% CI, 0.80 to 1.09) and high-dose diuretics (RR, 0.99; 95% CI, 0.83 to 1.18) did not. CVD death was significantly reduced by low-dose diuretics (RR, 0.76; 95% CI, 0.65 to 0.89) and not by beta blockers (RR, 0.89; 95% CI, 0.76 to 1.05). Similarly, the reduction in total morality among patients assigned to low-dose diuretics achieved significance (RR, 0.90; 95% CI, 0.81 to 0.99), but beta blockers did not (RR, 0.95; 95% CI, 0.84 to 1.07). The results of this meta-analysis are influenced by the strength of the individual data from the four beta-blocker trials. The Coope and Warrender study[25] and STOP-H[26] were not designed to test beta blockers versus diuretics, and in both trials, two thirds of the active treatment groups ended up on combined beta blockers and diuretic therapy. This high degree of overlap makes it difficult to separate the effects of each drug type. The MRC trials,[24, 27] comparing the two drugs as secondary analyses, were further limited by their high rates of loss to follow-up and withdrawal from treatment.

In conclusion, the totality of evidence clearly supports the use of beta blockers and diuretics in the treatment of essential hypertension to reduce the risk of CHD, stroke, and CVD death. However, existing data are insufficient to determine whether there are significant differences in efficacy between beta blockers and diuretics in the treatment of hypertension. In the last decade, there have been increases in the use of newer antihypertensive drugs, predominantly angiotensin-converting enzyme inhibitors and calcium channel blockers. At present, however, data from ongoing randomized trials testing these newer agents against beta blockers and/or diuretics on clinical endpoints are not yet available. In the meantime, the JNC VI guidelines[23] offer a rational basis for the treatment of hypertension, which includes beta blockers and/or diuretics as first-line agents for most patients.

MYOCARDIAL INFARCTION

The cardioprotective effect of beta blockers during MI and in secondary prevention demonstrated in randomized trials[51] may be due to several mechanisms. Beta blockers favorably influence the supply/demand imbalance in the ischemic heart by lowering heart rate and BP and reducing wall stress, cardiac work, and myocardial oxygen demand. In acute MI, this is

TABLE 9–3 • Meta-Analysis of Randomized, Placebo-Controlled Clinical Trials in Hypertension

Outcome Drug Regimen	Dose	No. of Trials	Events, Active Treatment/Control	RR (95% CI)
Stroke				
Diuretics	High	9	88/232	0.49 (0.39–0.62)
Diuretics	Low	4	191/347	0.66 (0.55–0.78)
Beta Blockers		4	147/335	0.71 (0.59–0.86)
HDFP	High	1	102/158	0.64 (0.50–0.82)
Coronary heart disease				
Diuretics	High	11	211/331	0.99 (0.83–1.18)
Diuretics	Low	4	215/363	0.72 (0.61–0.85)
Beta Blockers		4	243/459	0.93 (0.80–1.09)
HDFP	High	1	171/189	0.90 (0.73–1.10)
Congestive heart failure				
Diuretics	High	9	6/35	0.17 (0.07–0.41)
Diuretics	Low	3	81/134	0.58 (0.44–0.76)
Beta Blockers		2	41/175	0.58 (0.40–0.84)
Total mortality				
Diuretics	High	11	224/382	0.88 (0.75–1.03)
Diuretics	Low	4	514/713	0.90 (0.81–0.99)
Beta Blockers		4	383/700	0.95 (0.84–1.07)
HDFP	High	1	349/419	0.83 (0.72–0.95)
Cardiovascular mortality				
Diuretics	High	11	124/230	0.78 (0.62–0.97)
Diuretics	Low	4	237/390	0.76 (0.65–0.89)
Beta Blockers		4	214/410	0.89 (0.76–1.05)
HDFP	High	1	195/240	0.81 (0.67–0.97)

Meta-analysis of randomized, placebo-controlled clinical trials in hypertension according to first-line treatment strategy. Trials indicate number of trials with at least 1 endpoint of interest. RR indicates relative risk; CI, confidence interval; and HDFP, Hypertension Detection and Follow-up Program Study (5484 subjects in stepped care and 5455 in referred care). For these comparisons, the numbers of participants randomized to active therapy and placebo were 7768 and 12,075 for high-dose diuretic therapy; 4305 and 5116 for low-dose diuretic therapy; and 6736 and 12,147 for beta-blocker therapy. Because the Medical Research Council trials included two active arms, the placebo group is included twice in these totals, once for a diuretic comparison and again for a beta-blocker comparison. The total number of participants randomized to active therapy and control therapy were 24,294 and 23,926, respectively.

From Psaty BM, Smith NL, Siscovick DS, et al. Health outcomes associated with antihypertensive therapies used as first-line agents: A systematic review and meta-analysis. JAMA 1997; 277:739–745. Copyright 1997, American Medical Association.

reflected in the reduction in chest pain,[52–54] and possible limitation in infarct size, especially when administered early (<4 hours from onset of symptoms).[55–58] Beta blockers may also favorably affect infarct evolution by redistributing coronary blood flow,[59] shifting the metabolic substrate in ischemic tissue from free fatty acids (which increase myocardial oxygen consumption and may be proarrhythmic) back to glucose and protecting against the direct toxic effects of catechols, which augment cell injury and myocyte necrosis.[60] Beta blockers may decrease the risk of cardiac rupture in the peri-MI period.[61] Beta blockers increase the ventricular fibrillation (VF) threshold in ischemic and nonischemic dogs,[14, 62] and early in MI may reduce the risk of VF by 15%.[17, 63] This may not fully explain the observed early mortality benefit, given that MI patients in coronary care units would be likely to receive prompt defibrillation. Additional benefits with beta blockers may derive from antiplatelet effects,[64, 65] antithrombotic properties,[66] antiatherogenic effects,[12, 13] and reduction in plaque rupture.[67]

Trials of Beta Blockers Early in Myocardial Infarction

In the prethrombolytic era, numerous trials tested the hypothesis that beta blockers had a mortality benefit when given early in MI.[55] The earliest trials of immediate beta blockade were of inadequate power to detect the most plausible small-to-moderate benefits. Other trials tested the effect of immediate intravenous beta blockade followed by oral therapy; for example, in the Goteborg Metoprolol Trial,[68] 1395 patients with acute MI were randomized within 48 hours to metoprolol (15 mg intravenously, followed by 200 mg of oral metoprolol daily for 3 months) or placebo. A significant reduction in mortality was observed at 3 months (5.7% vs. 8.9%; $P < 0.03$). However, this did not clearly address whether beta-blocker treatment early in acute MI was itself of benefit.

The Metoprolol in Acute Myocardial Infarction (MIAMI)[18] trial was the first large study to specifically examine whether immediate beta blockade could reduce short-term (15-day) mortality in acute MI. A total of 5778 patients (77% men, mean age 60 years) with suspected or definite MI who presented within 24 hours of symptom onset (mean time to treatment 6.7 h) were randomized to metoprolol (15 mg of intravenous metoprolol followed by oral therapy, 100 mg twice daily) or placebo for 15 days. There was a nonsignificant 13% reduction in mortality (4.3% vs. 4.9%; 95% CI, −8% to 33%; $P = 0.29$). Based on the Goteborg Metoprolol Study,[68] MIAMI was designed to detect a less plausible, larger benefit of 35%.[69] Furthermore, the eligible MI population was fairly low risk, as reflected in the low event rate in the placebo group. In a post hoc analysis, metoprolol treatment reduced mortality by 29% ($P = 0.033$) in a high-risk subgroup (defined by having three or more of the following: age >60 y, prior MI or angina, CHF, diabetes, or being on diuretics or digitalis), which constituted 30% of the study population.[18]

The First International Study of Infarct Survival (ISIS-1)[17] was designed to test whether beta blockers given early in MI reduced short-term (7-day) mortality. A total of 16,027 subjects (23% women, mean age 59 years) with suspected or definite MI presenting within 12 hours of symptom onset (mean 5 hours) were randomized to atenolol (5 to 10 mg intravenously, followed by 100 mg daily) or to usual care. This was an open study without a placebo control. The 7-day vascular mortality rate in the atenolol group was 3.9% (318 deaths in 8037 subjects) compared with 4.6% (367 deaths in 7990 subjects) in the control group, a significant 15% mortality reduction (95% CI, 1% to 27%; $P < 0.04$). Almost all of the mortality benefit occurred in days 0 to 1 (25% reduction in risk of death, $P < 0.003$), possibly owing to a favorable effect with atenolol on the incidence of cardiac rupture.[61] The mortality benefits of early atenolol treatment appeared to persist at 1 year (10.7% in atenolol group vs. 12% in control group; $P < 0.01$), but those in the treatment group were more likely to be discharged on beta blockers (35% vs. 25%). No significant differences were observed in 7-day rates of nonfatal cardiac arrest (2.4% in atenolol group vs. 2.5% in the control group) and reinfarction (2.5% vs. 2.8%).

In an overview including data from ISIS-1, MIAMI, and 26 earlier trials of early beta-blockers therapy in MI (Fig. 9–1),[17] there was a significant 14% reduction in 7-day mortality (3.7% mortality rate with beta blockers vs. 4.3%; $P < 0.02$). In-hospital rates of reinfarction (18% reduction; $P < 0.02$), cardiac arrest or ventricular fibrillation (15% reduction; $P < 0.05$), and total events (16% reduction; $P < 0.0002$) were also reduced. This suggests that treating 200 acute MI patients with early beta blockade would prevent one reinfarction, one cardiac arrest, and one death in the following 7 days. The risks of beta blockers have been

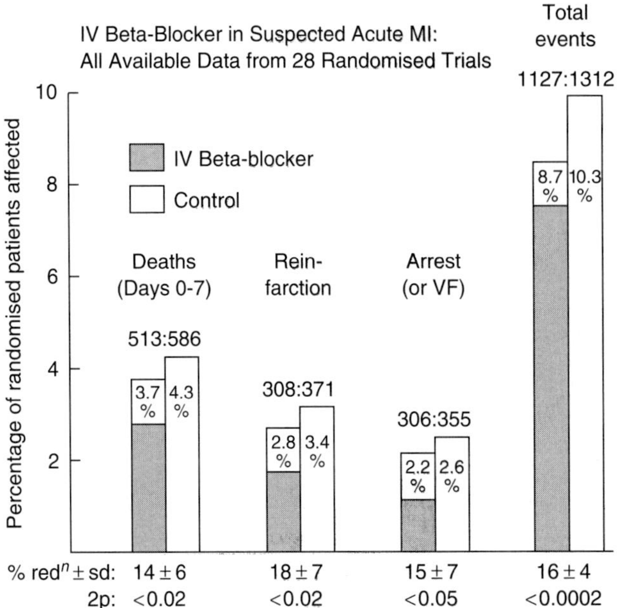

Figure 9–1 Analysis of 28 trials of beta-blocker therapy in myocardial infarction. (From ISIS-1 [First International Study of Infarct Survival] Collaborative Group. Randomised trial of intravenous atenolol among 16,027 cases of suspected acute myocardial infarction: ISIS-1. Lancet 1986; 2:57–65. © by The Lancet Ltd., 1986.)

estimated as 3% for CHF, 3% for complete heart block, and 2% for shock.[70] The mortality benefit early in MI may be greater in high-risk groups such as diabetics, in whom beta-blocker treatment was associated with a 37% mortality reduction.[71]

One trial in the thrombolytic era has evaluated the influence of beta blockers given early in MI. The Thrombolysis in Myocardial Infarction IIB trial (TIMI-IIB)[19] was a substudy of TIMI-II, which tested an invasive versus conservative strategy in MI patients treated with thrombolysis within 4 hours of symptom onset. The primary goal of TIMI-IIB was to assess if immediate versus delayed beta-blocker therapy affected infarct size and cardiac function in the setting of reperfusion, as measured by left ventricular ejection fraction (LVEF) determined by resting radionuclide ventriculography at discharge. There were 1434 patients with acute MI (49% of the TIMI-II population) treated with tissue plasminogen activator (t-PA), heparin, and aspirin, and then randomized to immediate metoprolol (up to 15 mg intravenously given on average 42 min after initiation of t-PA, followed 15 minutes later by 50 mg of oral metoprolol given every 12 hours for the first 24 hours, then 100 mg orally every 12 hours), or delayed oral metoprolol (50 mg twice on day 6, followed by 100 mg twice daily). There was no difference in LVEF at discharge (50.5%) between the immediate and delayed beta-blocker groups, which may reflect the greater effect of thrombolysis in myocardial salvage. In terms of the secondary endpoints, there was no difference in mortality between the beta-blocker groups at 6-day, 42-day, or

TABLE 9–4A • Major Randomized Trials of Beta Blockers in Myocardial Infarction

	Drug	N	Duration	RR of death	95% CI	P value
Early in MI						
ISIS-1[17]	Atenolol	16,027	7 d	0.85	0.73 to 0.99	<0.04
MIAMI[18]	Metoprolol	5,778	15 d	0.87	0.67 to 1.08	0.29
TIMI IIB[19]	Metoprolol	1,434	6 d	1.00	Not reported	0.98
After MI						
Norwegian[20]	Timolol	1,884	33 m	0.61	0.46 to 0.80	<0.001
BHAT[21]	Propranolol	3,837	25 m	0.72	0.74 to 0.80	<0.005

MI, myocardial infarction; RR, relative risk; CI, confidence interval; ISIS-1, First International Study of Infarct Survival; MIAMI, Metoprolol in Acute Myocardial Infarction; TIMI, Thrombolysis in Mycocardial Infarction; BHAT, Beta-Blocker Heart Attack Trial.

Adapted with permission from Hennekens CH, Albert CM, Godfried SL, et al. Adjunctive drug therapy of acute myocardial infarction—evidence from clinical trials. N Engl J Med 1996; 335:1660–1667.

TABLE 9–4B • Overview of Randomized Trials of Beta Blockers in Myocardial Infarction

	Number of Trials	N	Active*	Control*	RR of Death	95% CI	P value
Early in MI	29†	28,970	530/14535	603/14435	0.87	0.77 to 0.98	0.02
After MI	26‡	24,298	934/12438	1124/11860	0.77	0.70 to 0.84	<0.0001
Overall	55	53,268	1464/26973	1727/26295	0.81	0.75 to 0.87	<0.00001

*Expressed as number of deaths per number in treatment group.

†Includes the Thrombolysis in Myocardial Infarction IIB study (TIMI IIB).[19]

‡Includes the Acebutolol et Prévention Secondaire de l'Infarctus study (APSI).[77]

MI, myocardial infarction; RR, relative risk; CI, confidence interval.

Adapted from Teo KK, Yusuf S, Furberg CD. Effects of prophylactic antiarrhythmic drug therapy in acute myocardial infarction: An overview of results from randomized controlled trials. JAMA 1993; 270:1589–1595.

1-year follow-up, although the trial was not powered to detect a mortality difference. Fewer patients in the immediate beta-blocker group had reinfarction at 6 days (2.7% vs. 5.1% in delayed group; $P = 0.02$) and at 42 days (4.5% vs. 7.3%; $P < 0.03$), and were less likely to have recurrent chest pain (18.8% vs. 24.1%; $P < 0.02$) at 6 days. Thus, although early beta-blocker treatment may not enhance myocardial salvage or mortality *in the setting of reperfusion*, it appears to reduce the risk of recurrent ischemia and reinfarction compared with late administration. In more recent overviews[72, 73] that included TIMI-IIB, early use of beta blockers in MI reduced mortality by 13% (95% CI, 2% to 23%; $P = 0.02$) (Table 9–4).

Secondary Prevention After MI

Two major trials showed clear benefits of beta blockers in secondary prevention after MI. The Norwegian Multicenter Study (NMS)[20] and the Beta-Blocker Heart Attack Trial (BHAT)[21] demonstrated that treatment with the nonselective, non-ISA beta blockers timolol and propranolol, started 5 to 28 days after MI, reduced mortality for at least 2 to 3 years. There were also significant reductions in reinfarction and sudden death.

In the NMS,[20] which was double blind, 1884 patients (21% women, mean age 61 years) were randomized to timolol (10 mg twice daily) or placebo, 7 to 28 days after MI (mean 11.5 days). In the first month, there was excess withdrawal in the timolol group (275 vs. 219 in placebo group) mostly because of bradycardia or hypotension. Over an average follow-up of 17 months, mean heart rate fell from 73 to 55 beats/min in the timolol group ($P < 0.001$) using this fixed-dose regimen. There were 250 deaths, of which 93% were cardiac; 77% were defined as sudden. By intention-to-treat analysis, mortality was reduced by 39% in the timolol group compared with the placebo group (13.3% vs. 21.9%; $P = 0.0003$). When analyzed by deaths during treatment or within 28 days of withdrawal, the cumulative mortality rates over 33 months were 10.6% in the timolol versus 17.5% in the placebo group (39% risk reduction; $P = 0.0005$). Sudden death was reduced by 44.6% (7.7% vs. 13.9% in placebo group; $P = 0.0001$), and reinfarction by 28% (14.1% vs. 20.1%; $P = 0.0006$). The survival curves between the timolol and placebo groups showed increasing divergence over 24 months.

In the BHAT,[21] which was double blind, 3837 patients aged 30 to 69 years (14% women, mean age 55 years) were randomized to propranolol (titrated to 180 mg daily in 82% of subjects, and to 240 mg daily in 18%) or placebo, 5 to 21 days after MI (mean 13.8 days). In the propranolol group, mean heart rate fell from 76 to 65 beats/min at 1 year. There were 326 deaths; 90% were cardiac, and 50% were sudden. The trial was terminated after 25 months of mean follow-up owing to the emergence of a statistically extreme

26% reduction in mortality in the propranolol compared with the placebo group (7.2% vs. 9.8%; $P = 0.004$). The propranolol group experienced 27% fewer cardiac deaths (6.2% vs. 8.5%; $P < 0.01$) and 28% fewer sudden deaths (3.3% vs. 4.6%; $P < 0.05$) compared with the placebo group.

In both the Norwegian timolol study and BHAT, the benefits of beta blockers were seen in both high- and low-risk patients (defined by age, prior MI, anterior vs. inferior MI, and MI-related complications). An analysis that pooled the results of these and seven smaller trials also demonstrated the efficacy of beta blockers across a variety of subgroups, with somewhat stronger absolute mortality benefits in high-risk subjects (i.e., prior MI, angina, mechanical or electrical complications, and use of digitalis).[74] A post hoc subgroup analysis from BHAT[75] examined the effect of post-MI beta blocker treatment in the 710 patients with compensated or mild congestive heart failure (CHF) prior to randomization. The overall incidence of subsequent CHF was similar between the beta-blocker and placebo groups (6.7%). In patients with prior CHF, those treated with propranolol were more likely to develop recurrent CHF in the first 30 days than those on placebo (4.3% vs. 1.6%), but there were no cumulative differences over the 3 years of follow-up. The patients with prior CHF, who were at higher risk for all adverse outcomes (Fig. 9–2), had a significant 27% reduction in mortality rate with propranolol, which was similar to the 25% reduction seen in those without heart failure. In further subgroup analyses, there was a 47% reduction in sudden death with propranolol treatment in those with CHF, compared with the 13% reduction seen in those without CHF. Patients with diabetes mellitus constitute another high-risk subgroup that may particularly benefit from long-term beta-blocker treatment after MI, with some analyses suggesting a twofold greater reduction in risk of mortality and reinfarction than in those without diabetes.[71, 76]

There are some data supporting the benefits of cardioselective beta blockers such as metoprolol in secondary prevention. Pooled results of five early trials, including the Goteborg Metoprolol Trial,[68] in which a total of 5474 patients with MI were given immediate intravenous metoprolol and/or oral metoprolol (100 mg twice daily) post MI for 3 months to 3 years, showed a 19.3% reduction in mortality ($P = 0.036$) and a 40% reduction in sudden death ($P = 0.002$).[22]

The Acebutolol et Prévention Secondaire de l'Infarctus (APSI) trial[77] was designed to study the efficacy of acebutolol, a cardioselective beta blocker with moderate ISA, in preventing death in high-risk post-MI patients (defined by clinical criteria as having a 1-year mortality risk of 20% or higher). This randomized, double-blind, placebo-controlled trial used a dose of acebutolol (200 mg twice daily) corresponding to about one third the dose of propranolol used in BHAT. The trial was stopped early after 609 patients had been enrolled and followed for an average of 318 days. The mean heart rate in the acebutolol group had decreased by 9 beats/min. There was a significant 48% reduction in mortality rate in the acebutolol group compared to the placebo group (5.7% vs. 11%; $P = 0.019$) and a 58% decrease in cardiac mortality (4% vs. 9.7%; $P = 0.006$). Thus, the APSI trial was the first to demonstrate a clear mortality benefit for beta blockers with ISA.[55] With the addition of the APSI data, the trend remained in favor of agents without ISA, but there was no longer statistically significant heterogeneity between the trials using non-ISA versus

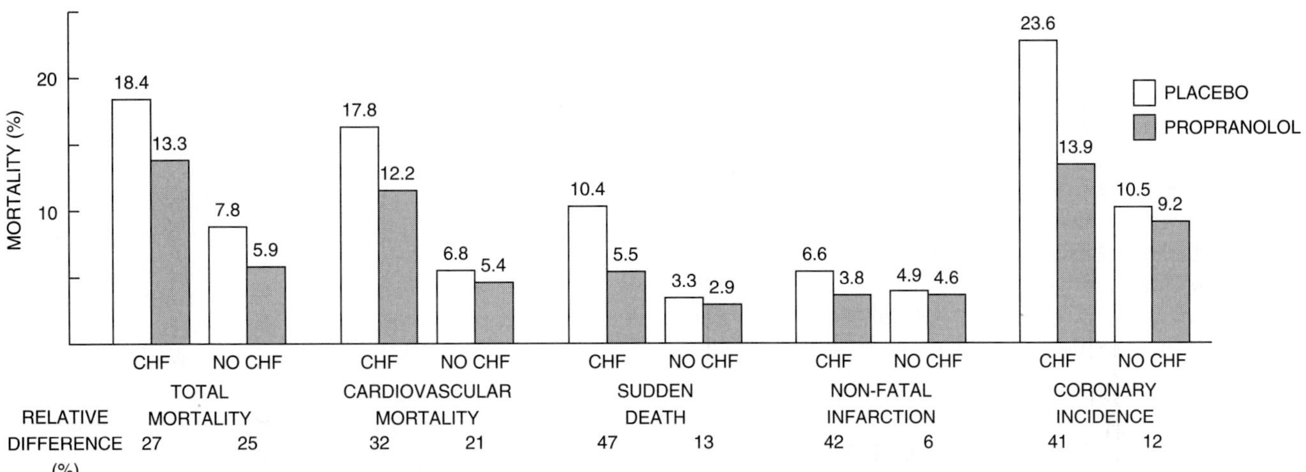

Figure 9–2 Effect of propranolol on morbidity and mortality related to the presence or absence of congestive heart failure (CHF). (From Chadda K, Goldstein S, Byington R, Curb JD. Effect of propranolol after acute myocardial infarction in patients with congestive heart failure. Circulation 1986; 73:503–510.)

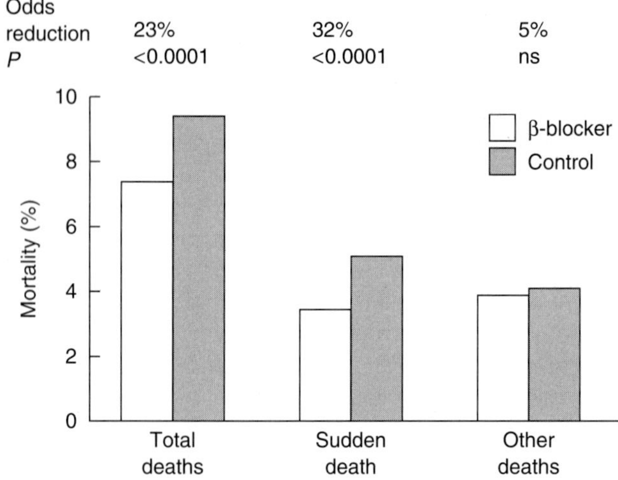

Figure 9–3 Long-term beta blockade after acute MI. Total mortality and cause of death. (From Held PH, Yusuf S. Effects of beta-blockers and calcium channel blockers in acute myocardial infarction. Eur Heart J 1993; 14[suppl F]:18–25.)

ISA beta blockers [mortality reduction 27% ($P < 0.001$) with non-ISA agents vs. 17% ($P < 0.01$) with +ISA agents].[72]

In a meta-analysis of 25 secondary prevention trials, beta blockers resulted in a 23% reduction in mortality (95% CI 16% to 30%; $P < 0.0001$), a 27% reduction in reinfarction (95% CI, 18% to 35%), and a 32% reduction in sudden death ($P < 0.0001$) (Fig. 9–3).[72] Approximately three quarters of the mortality decrease is attributable to a reduction in sudden death, a benefit of beta blockers that contrasts with disappointing results among other antiarrhythmic agents, such as the class I drugs used in the Cardiac Arrhythmia Suppression Trial (CAST).[73] In the context of the shift away from the "arrhythmia suppression hypothesis" since CAST, it is interesting to note that beta blockers only modestly suppress ventricular premature beats.[67, 71] Several mechanisms may contribute to beta-blocker-mediated protection against sudden death: increasing the fibrillatory threshold[62]; attenuating the stress-induced withdrawal of vagal tone that may predispose to malignant ventricular arrhythmias[15, 16]; and modifying sympathetically driven adverse effects on heart rate, BP, local shear forces, platelets and clotting factors that promote the rupture of vulnerable atherosclerotic plaques.[67] The relative importance of the degree of heart-rate lowering, lipophilicity, and cardioselectivity of individual beta blockers in conferring these protective effects is unclear.

Recommendations for Treatment

The data from randomized clinical trials support the recommendation that beta blockers should be given to all patients with acute MI who do not have clear contraindications, such as pulmonary edema, asthma, hypotension, bradycardia, or advanced atrioventricular block.[51] These contraindications are described in detail in the American Heart Association/American College of Cardiology (AHA/ACC) guidelines.[78] However, the benefit-risk profile of beta-blocker treatment must be individualized for each patient. The greatest benefit is seen in patients with the highest baseline mortality risk, such as those with a history of heart failure. For those presenting within 24 hours from the onset of symptoms, intravenous followed by oral therapy is indicated; after 24 hours, initiation of oral therapy is appropriate. The AHA/ACC guidelines do not express a preference regarding selective versus nonselective beta blockers but recommend avoiding those with ISA. Doses used in trials have been relatively high, with no data available about the efficacy of lower doses.

If tolerated, beta blockers should be continued for at least 2 to 3 years and perhaps longer.[51] Some data suggest that the benefits of beta blockade may persist for at least 6 years after MI. After the Norwegian timolol study ended, mortality follow-up continued (median 5 years), at the end of which 28.7% of those randomized to the placebo group were now on beta blockers, whereas 59.5% in the timolol group remained on beta blockers. Intention-to-treat analysis of all 507 deaths in the double-blind and extended follow-up periods demonstrated an 18.3% mortality reduction in those in the timolol group (26.4% vs. 32.3% in the placebo group; $P = 0.0028$).[79] The survival curves diverged until 24 months and then were parallel. Data from the Stockholm Metoprolol Trial also suggested that after 3 years of post-MI beta-blocker treatment, withdrawal of metoprolol was associated with accelerated mortality over 2 to 7 years of subsequent follow-up.[80]

Beta blockers have clearly demonstrated benefits in reducing mortality during and after MI but remain underutilized or are used at lower doses than in the trials in which their efficacy was proved. In the 1990–1993 National Registry of Myocardial Infarction, only 25% and 40% of the 240,989 enrolled patients received intravenous and oral beta blockers, respectively,[81] whereas other studies have reported rates of utilization of 48%[82] and 58%[83] at the time of hospital discharge. In the latter study, only 11% of patients were prescribed doses that were greater than 50% of the doses used in trials.[83] Treatment of MI is evolving rapidly, but data about beta blockers use in MI in the reperfusion era are limited.[19] Finally, carvedilol has additional vasodilatory and antioxidant properties,[84, 85] limits infarct size more effectively than propranolol when given in equivalent beta-blocking doses in animal models,[86, 87] and protects against VF.[88] Benefits on left ventricular function and remodeling have been demonstrated in humans with heart failure treated with carvedilol (see following discussion). These intriguing data suggest that the newer generation of beta blockers are a promising and as yet unexplored possibility in further improving the outcomes of patients with myocardial infarction.

HEART FAILURE

Abnormal neurohormonal activation, which is now understood to play a critical role in the progression of heart failure due to systolic dysfunction,[89–91] has direct cardiotoxic effects and contributes to the hemodynamic abnormalities of heart failure. The current state of knowledge has been described in two recent comprehensive reviews.[90, 91] The adrenergic and renin-angiotensin systems are intimately involved in mechanisms that are activated to support the failing heart (Fig. 9–4), including increases in heart rate, contractility, preload, and the number of contractile elements, as well as myocyte hypertrophy and vasoconstriction.[90, 91] Although initially serving as a compensatory mechanism, chronic neurohormonal activation ultimately contributes to (1) progressive myocyte dysfunction due to increased myocardial oxygen demand, impaired energy utilization, direct cardiac toxicity, abnormal calcium handling, and contractile dysfunction; and (2) cell loss due to direct myocyte toxicity of catechols,[92] apoptosis, and necrosis (Fig. 9–5).[90, 91] These processes contribute to pathologic ventricular remodeling[93] and progressive myocardial failure.

Evidence of adrenergic activation, as reflected in elevated plasma norepinephrine levels, is seen in asymptomatic left ventricular dysfunction and in-

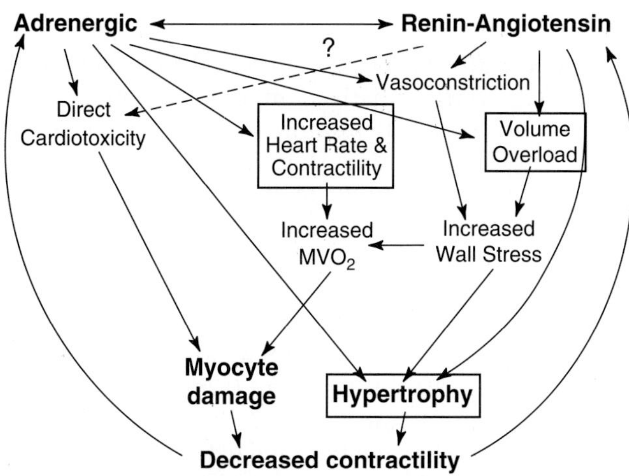

Figure 9–4 Heart failure compensatory mechanisms that are activated to support the failing heart. Boxed areas indicate physiologic mechanisms that stabilize pump function. (From Eichhorn EJ, Bristow MR. Medical therapy can improve the biological properties of the chronically failing heart: A new era in the treatment of heart failure. Circulation 1996; 94:2285–2296.)

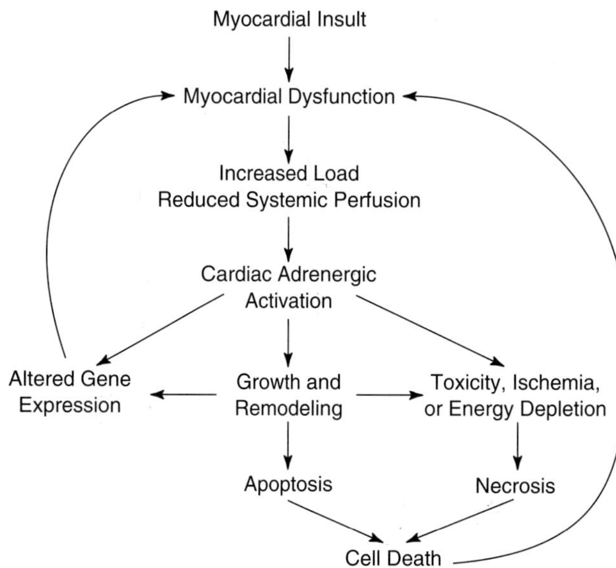

Figure 9–5 Central role of cardiac adrenergic activation in producing adverse biologic effects, which leads to progressive myocardial dysfunction and results in increased adrenergic activation. (Reprinted from Am J Cardiol, vol 80[11A], Bristow MR. Mechanism of action of beta-blocking agents in heart failure, pp 26L–40L, 1997, with permission from Excerpta Medica Inc.)

creases as overt heart failure develops.[94] Prognosis,[95, 96] degree of hemodynamic abnormalities,[97] and impairment of peak oxygen uptake with exercise[98] are also correlated with plasma norepinephrine levels. Recently developed techniques using sympathetic nerve recording and radiolabeled norepinephrine have made it possible to measure sympathetic activity in the heart itself.[99] Preferential cardiac adrenergic activation is the first neurohormonal abnormality detected as asymptomatic left ventricular dysfunction progresses to clinical disease.[100] Norepinephrine spillover from the severely failing human heart occurs at over five times the normal rate[101] owing to increased rates of sympathetic nerve firing and neuronal release of norepinephrine.[102]

The precise cellular mechanisms underlying the myocyte dysfunction seen with chronic adrenergic activation are unknown. Possibilities include abnormal gene expression for proteins involved in regulating myocyte contractility, such as those involved in β-adrenergic signal transduction, calcium handling, energy utilization, and regulation or function of the contractile apparatus and of the cytoskeleton, which are all adrenergically mediated.[91] Downregulation of β-adrenergic receptors has been observed in failing hearts,[91, 103] resulting in decreased contractile reserve[104] and exercise capacity.[105] However, this downregulation may be an adaptive mechanism against long-term sympathetic stimulation[91] and is unlikely to fully explain the effects of adrenergic activation on the failing human heart or its reversal by beta blockade. This is because increases in β-receptor density do not correlate with improved systolic function,[106, 107] and beta blockers such as carvedilol improve myocardial function without upregulating β-receptors, in contrast with metoprolol.[108] Other possible mechanisms of benefit with beta blockers in heart failure are listed in Table 9–5.[109]

Although further research is needed to elucidate the underlying mechanisms, evidence is accumulating as to the potential clinical benefits of chronic beta-blocker therapy in heart failure. In an animal model of cardiomyopathy, beta blockade resulted in normalization of calcium handling by upregulation of calcium uptake proteins, improved energetics, and increased ejection fraction.[110] Others demonstrated improvement in contractility in isolated myocytes as well as in the intact heart with beta-blocker therapy.[111] Although beta blockers initially cause myocardial depression, resulting from withdrawal of adrenergically mediated inotropic and chronotropic support,[107, 112] myocardial function appears to improve with chronic treatment. In randomized trials in patients with heart failure who were treated with beta blockers for at least 1 month, LVEF improved by about 5%, on average.[113] The gain in systolic function appears to be the result of enhanced myocardial contractility and efficiency; treatment with nonselective (bucindolol)[114] and selective (metoprolol, nevibolol)[115, 116] beta blockers resulted in improvement in load-independent measures of left ventricular function, reduced systolic wall stress and end-diastolic pressure, and increased myocardial work, without increasing myocardial oxygen consumption. Decreases in ventricular volume are observed after 3 to 6 months of beta-blocker treatment,[107, 114–116] with improvement or reversal of left ventricular remodeling observed after 12 to 18 months of treatment with metoprolol and carvedilol.[107, 117, 118] The improvements in LVEF and reduction in ventricular volume seen with bucindolol[119] and carvedilol[120] appear to be dose dependent.

It remains unclear whether these improvements in myocardial function and remodeling with beta blockers translate into better clinical outcomes in patients with heart failure. Existing data are promising but not yet conclusive. In terms of functional endpoints, improvement in New York Heart Association (NYHA) class has been observed with metoprolol,[121] bisoprolol,[122] and carvedilol.[123–126] The evidence for improved exercise capacity with beta-blocker treatment is less consistent, with significantly increased exercise capacity shown with metoprolol[121] but not with bucindolol[119, 127] or carvedilol.[120, 126, 128] Exercise capacity may be less useful to measure the efficacy of beta-blocker treatment, because the heart rate response to exercise is limited.[129] However, in contrast with carvedilol and bucindolol, metoprolol does not lower plasma norepinephrine levels or block the β_2-receptor,[108, 115, 127, 130] suggesting that some degree of sympathetic stimulation may explain its observed effect with exercise.[129]

Four large trials have tested the efficacy of beta blockers in reducing the mortality rate in patients with heart failure (Table 9–6). In the Metoprolol in Dilated Cardiomyopathy (MDC) trial,[121] 383 patients (mean age 49 years, 28% women) with nonischemic cardiomyopathy, LVEF less than 0.40 (mean 0.22), and mild to moderate heart failure (94% were NYHA class II or III) were randomized in double-blind fashion to oral metoprolol (up to 150 mg daily, given in two or three divided doses) or placebo for 12 to 18 months. Most patients were on diuretics (75%) and angiotensin-converting enzyme inhibitors (80%). The primary endpoint was the combination of death or need for transplantation, which was reduced by 34% (95% CI, −6% to 62%; $P = 0.058$) in the metoprolol group compared with the placebo group. This benefit was due mostly to fewer patients in the metoprolol group decompensating and needing transplantation (2 vs. 19 in the placebo group). There were 23 deaths in the metoprolol group and 19 in the placebo group and no difference in sudden deaths between groups.

Another trial using a β_1-selective, nonvasodilating agent was the Cardiac Insufficiency Bisoprolol Study (CIBIS).[122] In this study, 641 patients (mean age 60 years, 17% women) with cardiomyopathy (55% ischemic), LVEF less than 0.40 (mean 0.25), and moderate to severe heart failure (95% NYHA class III, 5% NYHA class IV) were randomized in double-blind fashion to bisoprolol (up to 5 mg daily) or placebo. All patients were on diuretics; 90% were on angiotensin-converting enzyme inhibitors. Mean follow-up was 1.9 years. There was a nonsignificant 20% reduction in mortality rate in the bisoprolol group compared with the placebo group (53 vs. 67 deaths; 95% CI,

TABLE 9–5 • Potential Mechanisms of Action of Adrenergic Blockade in Chronic Heart Failure

1. Up-regulation of β receptors
2. Direct myocardial protective effects from toxicity of catecholamines
3. Improved ability of the noradrenergic sympathetic nerves to synthesize norepinephrine
4. Decreased stimulation of other vasoconstrictive neurohormonal systems (renin-angiotensin-aldosterone, vasopressin, endothelin)
5. Antiarrhythmic effects
6. Increased coronary blood flow via coronary vasodilation
7. Negative chronotropic effect lengthens diastolic period, improving subendocardial blood flow
8. Antianginal/anti-ischemic effect
9. Restore normal reflex control of the heart and circulation
10. Prevention of myocyte hypertrophy
11. Antioxidant effects
12. Shift from free fatty acid to carbohydrate metabolism

From Sackner-Bernstein JD, Mancini DM. Rationale for treatment of patients with chronic heart failure with adrenergic blockade. JAMA 1995; 274:1462–1467. Copyright 1995, American Medical Association.

TABLE 9–6 • Effects of Beta Blockade on Mortality in the Large Placebo-Controlled Trials

Trial	Number of Patients		Number of Deaths (Mortality)		Relative Change in Risk	Mean Follow-up (mo)	Lives Saved per 1000 treated	Lives Saved per 1000 treated/year*
	Placebo	*Beta Blockade*	*Placebo*	*Beta Blockade*				
MDC	189	193	19 (10.1%)	23 (11.9%)	+19% (ns)	15	18 excess deaths	14 excess deaths
CIBIS	321	320	67 (20.9%)	53 (16.6%)	−20% (ns)	21	43 saved	25 saved
ANZ	208	207	26 (12.5%)	20 (9.7%)	−23% (ns)	18	28 saved	19 saved
U.S. trials	398	696	31 (7.8%)	22 (3.2%)	−65% (P = 0.0001)	6.5	46 saved	85 saved
Totals	1116	1416	143 (12.8%)	118 (8.3%)	−35% (P = 0.001)	13.3 (approx)	45 saved†	41 saved

*This is a crude adjustment to compensate for different trial durations and assumes constant benefit with time.
†For comparison, about 35 lives would have been saved in the SOLVD treatment study comparing enalapril and placebo over the same duration.
MDC, Metoprolol in Dilated Cardiomyopathy trial; CIBIS, Cardiac Insufficiency Bisoprolol Study; ANZ, Australia–New Zealand Heart Failure Trial.
From Cleland JGF, Bristow MR, Erdmann E, et al. Beta-blocking agents in heart failure: Should they be used and how? Eur Heart J 1996; 17:1629–1639.

−15% to 44%; P = 0.22). There was no difference in sudden death (15 in bisoprolol group, 17 in placebo group). Occurrence of the secondary endpoint of hospitalizations for cardiac decompensation was reduced by 34% in the bisoprolol group (61 vs. 90 in placebo group; $P < 0.01$). In a retrospective subgroup analysis, those with nonischemic cardiomyopathy or no prior history of MI appeared to have greater reductions in mortality (52% and 47%, respectively). The interpretability of the trial is limited by being underpowered to detect a mortality effect, an excess of prior MI patients being randomized to the bisoprolol group, and only half of the bisoprolol group receiving more than 3.75 mg of drug daily.[129]

Two mortality trials in heart failure studied the effects of carvedilol, a nonselective, vasodilating beta blocker. In the U.S. Carvedilol Heart Failure Trial Program,[131] a double-blind trial, 1094 patients (mean age 58 years, 23% women) with cardiomyopathy (48% ischemic), ejection fraction 0.35 or less (mean 0.22), and mild to severe heart failure (97% NYHA class II to III) were randomized to carvedilol (up to 50 or 100 mg daily) or placebo for 7 to 15 months (median 7 months); 95% of patients were on diuretics and angiotensin-converting enzyme inhibitors. Patients were allocated to one of four component studies,[120, 126, 132, 133] based on symptom severity and performance on an exercise test but were pooled for the overall mortality analysis. The trial was stopped early because of a significant 65% reduction in mortality in the carvedilol group (22 vs. 31 deaths, or 3.2% vs. 7.8% in placebo group; 95% CI, 39% to 80%; P = 0.001). A similar mortality benefit was seen across degrees of heart failure severity and for ischemic or nonischemic disease. Sudden death and pump failure death were reduced to the same degree in the carvedilol group. Two of the four component protocols also observed a significant mortality reduction with carvedilol when analyzed individually.[120, 132] The secondary endpoint of hospitalization for cardiovascular reasons was reduced by 27% (14.1% vs. 19.6%; P = 0.036) in the carvedilol group compared with the placebo group, and the combined risk of all-cause mortality and hospitalization was reduced by 38% (15.8% vs. 24.6%; $P < 0.001$) (Fig. 9–6). This trial was the first to demonstrate a significant reduction in mortality rate with beta-blocker treatment in heart failure. However, questions have been raised concerning the pooling of the four component trials, the robustness of the findings based on only 53 deaths and the short duration of follow-up, the high mortality rate (15.5%) in the placebo arm of the component trial that contributed to much of the mortality benefit of carvedilol,[120] and the exclusion from the mortality analysis of patients who died during the open-label run-in period.[134, 134a] If, however, all the run-in deaths are attributed to the carvedilol group, a significant mortality benefit is still observed (48% reduction; P = 0.011).[135]

In the Australia–New Zealand Heart Failure Trial,[128]

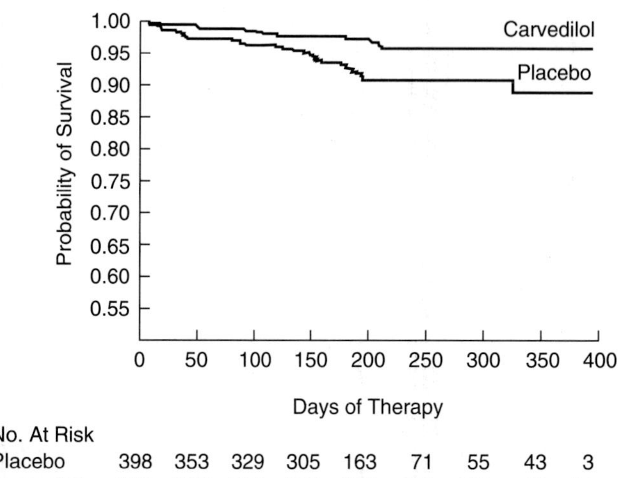

Figure 9–6 U.S. Carvedilol Heart Failure Trial Program results. (From Packer MP, Bristow MR, Cohn JN, et al, for the U.S. Carvedilol Heart Failure Study Group. The effect of carvedilol on morbidity and mortality in patients with chronic heart failure. N Engl J Med 1996; 334:1349–1355. Copyright © 1996, Massachusetts Medical Society. All rights reserved.)

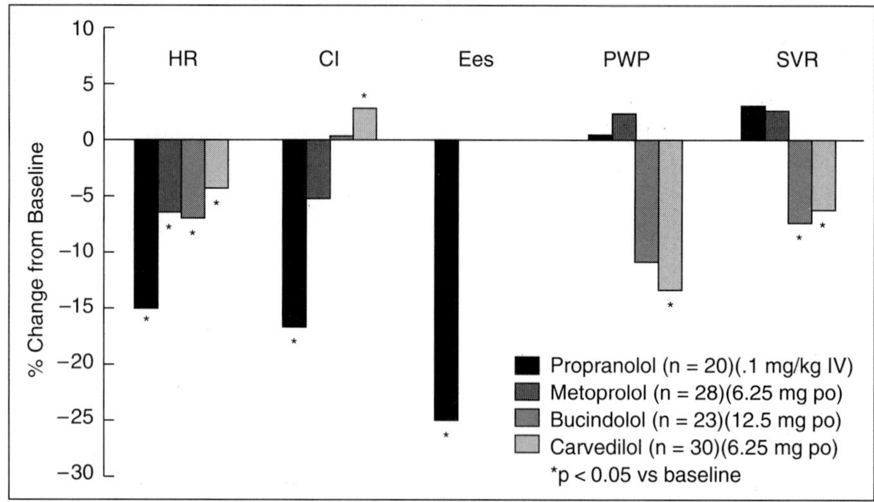

Figure 9–7 Comparative acute hemodynamic effects of first-, second-, and third-generation beta blockers. Response to oral beta blockers was taken from peak effect data obtained at 2 or 4 hours (metoprolol, carvedilol) or at 4 hours after administration (bucindolol). CI, cardiac index; Ees, end systolic elastane, a measure of load independent of systolic function (no data generated for orally administered beta blockers); HR, heart rate; PWP, mean pulmonary artery wedge pressure; SVR, systemic vascular resistance. (Reprinted from Am J Cardiol, vol 80[11A], Bristow MR. Mechanism of action of beta-blocking agents in heart failure, pp 26L–40L, 1997, with permission from Excerpta Medica Inc.)

a double-blind trial, 415 patients (mean age 67 years, 20% women) with mild to moderate heart failure (current NYHA class I to III), ejection fraction less than 0.45 (mean 0.29), and ischemic cardiomyopathy were randomized to carvedilol (up to 25 mg given twice daily) or placebo for 18 to 24 months. Seventy-six percent were on diuretics and 86% were on angiotensin-converting enzyme inhibitors. The primary endpoint was the combined risk of death or hospitalization for any reason, which was reduced by 26% in the carvedilol group (95% CI, 5% to 43%; $P = 0.02$). There was a nonsignificant 24% reduction in mortality alone (20 vs. 26 deaths in placebo group; 95% CI, −36% to 58%; $P > 0.1$), and a 23% reduction in hospitalization of borderline significance (95% CI, 0% to 41%; $P = 0.05$). The difference in mortality results in this trial compared with the U.S. trial may be in part due to the smaller size and lower dose of carvedilol used.[135]

Two recent meta-analyses have been conducted of beta-blocker trials in heart failure. Heidenreich and colleagues[136] examined 17 trials with a total of 3039 patients, followed for 3 to 24 months. Beta blockers were associated with an RR of death of 0.69 (95% CI, 0.54% to 0.88). This effect was similar for ischemic and nonischemic cardiomyopathy. Carvedilol may or may not have a stronger mortality benefit (RR, 0.54; 95% CI, 0.36 to 0.81) than other beta blockers (RR, 0.82; 95% CI, 0.60 to 1.12); the difference did not reach statistical significance ($P = 0.10$). The analysis

TABLE 9–7 • Ongoing Mortality Trials of Beta Blockers in Heart Failure

Trial	Beta Blocker	*N*	Follow-up (mean) (y)	Etiology of Heart Failure	Eligibility Criteria
CIBIS II[143]*	Bisoprololol	2500	3	Ischemic and nonischemic	NYHA III to IV, LVEF ≤0.35
BEST[144]	Bucindolol	2800	3	Ischemic and nonischemic	NYHA III to IV, LVEF ≤0.35
MERIT-HF[145]	Metoprolol CR/XL	3200	2.4	Ischemic and nonischemic	NYHA II to IV, LVEF ≤0.40
COMET	Carvedilol vs. metoprolol	3000	4	Ischemic and nonischemic	NYHA II to IV, LVEF <0.35
COPERNICUS[146]	Carvedilol	2000	3.8	Ischemic and nonischemic	NYHA IIIb to IV, LVEF <0.25
CAPRICORN[146]	Carvedilol	2600	1.8	Ischemic (≤14 days after MI)	LVEF <0.40, with or without symptoms

*Stopped early in March 1998.

¶CIBIS, Cardiac Insufficiency Bisoprolol Study; BEST, β-Blocker Evaluation and Survival Trial; MERIT-HF, Metoprolol CR/XL Randomized Intervention Trial in Heart Failure; COMET, Carvedilol or Metoprolol European Trial; COPERNICUS, Carvedilol Prospective Randomized Cumulative Survival Trial; CAPRICORN, Carvedilol Post-Infarct Survival Control in Left Ventricular Dysfunction; CR/XL, controlled release/extended release; NYHA, New York Heart Association Class; LVEF, left ventricular ejection fraction; MI, myocardial infarction.

suggested a stronger effect of beta blockers in preventing nonsudden death (RR, 0.58; 95% CI, 0.40 to 0.83) than sudden death (RR, 0.84; 95% CI, 0.59 to 1.2). In a meta-analysis by Doughty and associates[137] of 24 trials involving 3141 patients, a similar 31% reduction in death was seen with beta-blocker therapy compared with placebo (95% CI, 11% to 46%; $P = 0.0035$), with a somewhat greater benefit seen with vasodilating beta blockers (mostly carvedilol) compared with nonvasodilating agents (mostly metoprolol), with mortality reductions of 47% versus 18%, respectively ($P = 0.09$).

Based on the known biologic effects of the third-generation beta blockers and the previously discussed trial data, it has been postulated that nonselective beta blockers with ancillary properties may provide greater protection than β_1-selective drugs such as metoprolol.[91, 135] Heart failure is accompanied by an increase in the relative proportion of β_2- and α_1-receptors[138, 139] and is characterized by high-oxidative stress, which may contribute to apoptosis and myocardial dysfunction.[93, 140, 141] By blocking both β_1- and β_2-receptors, the nonselective beta blockers may provide more complete antiadrenergic protection, the degree of which may be correlated with better LVEF and perhaps survival.[91, 119, 120] Carvedilol is also a potent antioxidant.[84] Furthermore, the ancillary vasodilation seen with the third-generation beta blockers offsets the negative cardiodepression seen initially with nonselective beta blockade, so that they are hemodynamically and clinically well tolerated[91] (Fig. 9–7). Whether these nonselective beta blockers provide greater protection against sudden death in heart failure (perhaps via their β_2-antagonist effect)[91, 135, 142] as previously seen in post-MI patients[75] requires further study.

Beta blockers are a promising new therapy in the treatment of heart failure, but more data are needed to answer many remaining questions. Ongoing basic research should help clarify the mechanisms by which systolic function is improved with beta blockers, and trials can demonstrate whether they provide a definite mortality benefit (Table 9–7). Of note, the randomized trial populations in whom beta blockers have been tested thus far were younger and had less ischemic heart disease than those with heart failure in the community[147] and were primarily NYHA class II to III, so that generalizability of the trial results remains to be established, particularly because beta-blocker therapy in heart failure patients requires careful administration and titration.[148] More data are also needed about the optimal dose and duration of therapy, whether beta blockers like carvedilol are more efficacious than others, whether the effect of beta blockers differs depending on the etiology of heart failure, how to select appropriate patients for treatment, and the effects of beta blockers in relation to other therapies for heart failure such as angiotensin-converting enzyme inhibitors and inotropes. The convergence of basic and clinical research in developing and testing the neurohormonal hypothesis has opened a promising new frontier for the use of beta blockers in the treatment of heart failure.

REFERENCES

1. Ahlquist RP. A study of the adrenotropic receptors. Am J Physiol 1948; 153:586–600.
2. Black JW. Ahlquist and the development of beta-adrenoreceptor antagonists. Postgrad Med J 1976; 52(suppl 4):11–13.
3. Lewis RV, Lofthouse C. Adverse reactions with β-adrenoreceptor blocking drugs: An update. Drug Safety 1993; 9:272–279.
4. Cruickshank JM. β-blockers, plasma lipids, and coronary heart disease. Circulation 1990; 82(suppl II):II60–II65.
5. Yudofsky SC. β-blockers and depression: The clinician's dilemma. JAMA 1992; 267:1826–1827.
6. Bright RA, Everitt DE. β-blockers and depression: Evidence against an association. JAMA 1992; 267:1783–1787.
7. Opie LH. Basis for cardiovascular therapy with beta-blocking agents. Am J Cardiol 1983; 52:2D–9D.
8. Harrison DC. Beneficial effects of beta-blockers: A class action or individual pharmacologic spectrum? Circulation 1983; 67(suppl I):I77–I82.
9. Chobanian AV, Brecher P, Chan C. Effects of propranolol on atherogenesis in the cholesterol-fed rabbit. Circ Res 1985; 56:755–762.
10. Östlund-Lindqvist A-M, Lindqvist P, Bräutigam J, et al. Effect of metoprolol on diet-induced atherosclerosis in rabbits. Arteriosclerosis 1988; 8:40–45.
11. Camejo G, Hurt E, Thrubikar M, Bondjers G. Modification of low-density lipoprotein association with the arterial intima. A possible environment for the antiatherogenic action of beta-blockers. Circulation 1991; 84(Suppl VI):VI17–VI22.
12. Kaplan JR, Manuck SB, Adams MR, Clarkson TB. The effects of beta-adrenergic blocking agents on atherosclerosis and its complications. Eur Heart J 1987; 8:928–944.
13. Cruickshank JM, Smith JC. The beta-receptor, atheroma and cardiovascular damage. Pharmac Ther 1989; 42:385–404.
14. Anderson JL, Rodier HE, Green LS. Comparative effects of beta-adrenergic blocking drugs on experimental ventricular fibrillation threshold. Am J Cardiol 1983; 51:1196–1202.
15. Parker GW, Michael LH, Hartley CJ, et al. Central β-adrenergic mechanisms may modulate ischemic ventricular fibrillation in pigs. Circ Res 1990; 66:259–270.
16. Kardos A, Long V, Bryant J, et al. Lipophilic versus hydrophilic $beta_1$ blockers and the cardiac sympathovagal balance during stress and daily activity in patients after acute myocardial infarction. Heart 1998; 79:153–160.
17. ISIS-1 (First International Study of Infarct Survival) Collaborative Group. Randomised trial of intravenous atenolol among 16,027 cases of suspected acute myocardial infarction: ISIS-1. Lancet 1986; 2:57–65.
18. The MIAMI Trial Research Group. Metoprolol in acute myocardial infarction (MIAMI): A randomised placebo-controlled international trial. Eur Heart J 1985; 6:199–226.
19. Roberts R, Rogers WJ, Mueller HS, et al. Immediate versus deferred β-blockade following thrombolytic therapy in patients with acute myocardial infarction: Results of the Thrombolysis in Myocardial Infarction (TIMI) II-B study. Circulation 1991; 83:422–437.
20. The Norwegian Multicenter Study Group. Timolol-induced reduction in mortality and reinfarction in patients surviving acute myocardial infarction. N Engl J Med 1981; 304:801–807.
21. β-Blocker Heart Attack Trial Research Group. A randomized trial of propranolol in patients with acute myocardial infarction: I. Mortality results. JAMA 1982; 247:1707–1714.
22. Olsson G, Wikstrand J, Warnold I, et al. Metoprolol-induced reduction in postinfarction mortality: Pooled results from five double-blind randomized trials. Eur Heart J 1992; 13:28–32.

23. The Sixth Report of the Joint National Committee on Prevention, Detection, Evaluation, and Treatment of High Blood Pressure. Arch Intern Med 1997; 157:2413–2446.
24. Medical Research Council Working Party. MRC trial of treatment of mild hypertension: Principal results. BMJ 1985; 291:97–104.
25. Coope J, Warrender TS. Randomized trial of treatment of hypertension in elderly patients in primary care. BMJ 1986; 293:1145–1151.
26. Dahlöf B, Lindholm LH, Hansson L, et al. Morbidity and mortality in the Swedish Trial of Old Patients with Hypertension (STOP-Hypertension). Lancet 1991; 338:1281–1285.
27. MRC Working Party. Medical Research Council trial of treatment of hypertension in older adults: Principal results. BMJ 1992; 304:405–412.
28. The IPPPSH Collaborative Group. Cardiovascular risk and risk factors in a randomized trial of treatment based on the beta-blocker oxprenolol: the International Prospective Primary Prevention Study in Hypertension (IPPPSH). J Hypertens 1985; 3:379–392.
29. Wilhlemsen L, Berglund G, Elmfeldt D, et al. Beta-blockers versus diuretics in hypertensive men: Main results from the HAPPHY trial. J Hypertens 1987; 5:561–572.
30. Wikstrand J, Warnold I, Olsson G, et al. Primary prevention with metoprolol in patients with hypertension: Mortality results from the MAPHY Study. JAMA 1988; 259:1976–1982.
31. Ekbom T, Dahlöf B, Hansson L, et al. Antihypertensive efficacy and side effects of three beta-blockers and a diuretic in elderly hypertensives: A report from the STOP-Hypertension study. J Hypertens 1992; 10:1525–1530.
32. Hebert PR, Moser M, Mayer J, et al. Recent evidence on drug therapy of mild to moderate hypertension and decreased risk of coronary heart disease. Arch Intern Med 1993; 153:578–581.
33. Collins R, Peto R, MacMahon S, et al. Blood pressure, stroke, and coronary heart disease: II. Short-term reductions in blood pressure: Overview of randomised drug trials in their epidemiological context. Lancet 1990; 335:827–838.
34. Mulrow CD, Cornell JA, Hererra CR, et al. Hypertension in the elderly: Implications and generalizability of randomized trials. JAMA 1994; 272:1932–1938.
35. Cutler JA, Psaty BM, MacMahon S, Furberg CD. Public health issues in hypertension control: What has been learned from clinical trials. *In* Laragh JH, Brenner BM (eds). Hypertension: Pathophysiology, Diagnosis, and Management, 2nd ed. New York, Raven Press, 1995, pp. 253–279.
36. Hennekens CH, Buring JE. Observational evidence. Ann NY Acad Sci 1993; 703:18–24.
37. Hypertension Detection and Follow-up Program Cooperative Group. Persistence of reduction in blood pressure and mortality of participants in the Hypertension Detection and Follow-up Program. JAMA 1988; 259:2113–2122.
38. The Multiple Risk Factor Intervention Trial Research Group. Mortality rates after 10.5 years for participants in the Multiple Risk Factor Intervention Trial. JAMA 1990; 263:1795–1801.
39. Hansson L. Primary prevention against coronary heart disease with β-blockers ruled out by HAPPHY? J Hypertens 1987; 5:573–574.
40. Multiple Risk Factor Intervention Trial Research Group. Multiple Risk Factor Intervention Trial: Risk factor changes and mortality results. JAMA 1982; 248:1465–1477.
41. Siscovick DS, Raghunathan TE, Psaty BM, et al. Diuretic therapy for hypertension and the risk of primary cardiac arrest. N Engl J Med 1994; 330:1852–1857.
42. Kaplan NM. Beta blockade in the primary prevention of hypertensive cardiovascular events with focus on sudden cardiac death. Am J Cardiol 1997; 80(9B):20J–22J.
43. Levy D, Garrison RJ, Savage DD, et al. Prognostic implications of echocardiographically determined left ventricular mass in the Framingham Heart Study. N Engl J Med 1990; 322:1561–1566.
44. Gottdiener JS, Reda DJ, Massie BM, et al. Effect of single-drug therapy on reduction of left ventricular mass in mild to moderate hypertension: Comparison of six antihypertensive agents. Circulation 1997; 95:2007–2014.
45. Devereux RB. Do antihypertensive drugs differ in their ability to regress left ventricular hypertrophy? Circulation 1997; 95:1983–1985.
46. Wikstrand J, Warnold I, Tuomilehto J, et al. Metoprolol versus thiazide diuretics in hypertension: Morbidity results from the MAPHY study. Hypertension 1991; 17:579–588.
47. Olsson G, Tuomilehto J, Berglund G, et al. Primary prevention of sudden cardiovascular death in hypertensive patients. Mortality results from the MAPHY study. Am J Hypertens 1991; 4:151–158.
48. Kaplan NM. Critical comments on recent literature: SCRAAPHY about MAPHY from HAPPHY. Am J Hypertens 1988; 1(4 Pt 1):428–430.
49. Moser M, Sheps S. Confusing messages from the newest of the β-blocker/diuretic hypertension trials: The Metoprolol Atherosclerosis Prevention in Hypertensives trial. Arch Intern Med 1989; 149:2174–2175.
50. Psaty BM, Smith NL, Siscovick DS, et al. Health outcomes associated with antihypertensive therapies used as first-line agents: A systematic review and meta-analysis. JAMA 1997; 277:739–745.
51. Hennekens CH, Albert CM, Godfried SL, et al. Adjunctive drug therapy of acute myocardial infarction—evidence from clinical trials. N Engl J Med 1996; 335:1660–1667.
52. Waagstein F, Hjalmarson ÅC. Double-blind study of the effect of cardioselective beta-blockade on chest pain in acute myocardial infarction. Acta Med Scand 1975; 587(suppl):201–211.
53. Gold HK, Leinbach RC, Maroko PR. Propranolol-induced reduction of signs of ischemic injury during acute myocardial infarction. Am J Cardiol 1976; 38:689–695.
54. Ramsdale DR, Faragher EB, Bennett DH, et al. Ischemic pain relief in patients with acute myocardial infarction by intravenous atenolol. Am Heart J 1982; 103:459–467.
55. Yusuf S, Peto R, Lewis J, et al. Beta-blockade during and after myocardial infarction: An overview of the randomized trials. Prog Cardiovasc Dis 1985; 17:335–371.
56. International Collaborative Study Group. Reduction of infarct size by the early use of intravenous timolol in acute myocardial infarction. Am J Cardiol 1984; 54:14E–15E.
57. Herlitz J, Elmfeldt D, Hjalmarson Å, et al. Effect of metoprolol on indirect signs of the size and severity of acute myocardial infarction. Am J Cardiol 1983; 51:1282–1288.
58. Roberts R, Croft C, Gold HK, et al. Effect of propranolol on myocardial-infarct size in a randomized, blinded, multicenter trial. N Engl J Med 1984; 311:218–225.
59. Buck JD, Hardman HF, Warltier DC, Gross GJ. Changes in ischemic blood flow distribution and dynamic severity of a coronary stenosis induced by beta-blockade in the canine heart. Circulation 1981; 64:708–715.
60. Willerson JT, Buja LM. Short- and long-term influence of beta-adrenergic antagonists after myocardial infarction. Am J Cardiol 1984; 54:16E–20E.
61. ISIS-1 (First International Study of Infarct Survival) Collaborative Group. Mechanisms for the early mortality reduction produced by beta blockade started early in acute myocardial infarction: ISIS-1. Lancet 1988; 1:921–923.
62. Khan MI, Hamilton JT, Manning GW. Protective effect of beta-adrenoreceptor blockade in experimental coronary occlusion in conscious dogs. Am J Cardiol 1972; 30:832–837.
63. Rydén L, Ariniego R, Arnman K, et al. A double-blind trial of metoprolol in acute myocardial infarction: Effects on ventricular tachyarrhythmias. N Engl J Med 1983; 308:614–618.
64. Mehta J, Mehta P. Effects of propranolol therapy on platelet release and prostaglandin generation in patients with coronary heart disease. Circulation 1982; 66:1294–1299.
65. Beckmann ML, Gerber JG, Byyny RL, et al. Propranolol increases prostacyclin synthesis in patients with essential hypertension. Hypertension 1988; 12:582–588.
66. Teger-Nilsson AC, Dahlöf C, Haglund E, et al. Influence of metoprolol CR/ZOK on plasminogen activator inhibitor (PAI-1) in man: A pilot study. J Clin Pharmacol 1990; 30(2 suppl):S132–S137.
67. Kennedy HL. Beta blockade, ventricular arrhythmias, and sudden cardiac death. Am J Cardiol 1997; 80(9B):29J–34J.
68. Hjalmarson Å, Elmfeldt D, Herlitz J, et al. Effect on mortality of metoprolol in acute myocardial infarction: A double-blind randomized trial. Lancet 1981; 2:123–127.

69. Hennekens CH, Buring JE, Hebert P. Implications of overviews for randomized trials. Stat Med 1987; 6:397–402.
70. Yusuf S. The use of beta-blockers in the acute phase of myocardial infarction. *In* Califf RM, Wagner GS (eds). Acute Coronary Care 1986. New York, Kluwer, 1985. p. 73.
71. Kendall MJ, Lynch KP, Hjalmarson Å, Kjekshus J. β-Blockers and sudden cardiac death. Ann Intern Med 1995; 123:358–367.
72. Held PH, Yusuf S. Effects of β-blockers and calcium channel blockers in acute myocardial infarction. Eur Heart J 1993; 14(suppl F):18–25.
73. Teo KK, Yusuf S, Furberg CD. Effects of prophylactic antiarrhythmic drug therapy in acute myocardial infarction: An overview of results from randomized controlled trials. JAMA 1993; 270:1589–1595.
74. The Beta-Blocker Pooling Project Research Group. The Beta-Blocking Pooling Project (BPPP): Subgroup findings from randomized trials in postinfarction patients. Eur Heart J 1988; 9:8–16.
75. Chadda K, Goldstein S, Byington R, Curb JD. Effect of propranolol after acute myocardial infarction in patients with congestive heart failure. Circulation 1986; 73:503–510.
76. Kjekshus J, Gilpin E, Cali G, et al. Diabetic patients and beta-blockers after acute myocardial infarction. Eur Heart J 1990; 11:43–50.
77. Boissel J-P, Leizorovicz A, Picolet H, et al. Secondary prevention after high-risk myocardial infarction with low-dose acebutolol. Am J Cardiol 1990; 66:251–260.
78. Ryan TJ, Anderson JL, Antman EM, et al. ACC/AHA guidelines for the management of patients with acute myocardial infarction: Executive summary: A report of the American College of Cardiology/American Heart Association Task Force on Practice Guidelines (Committee on Management of Acute Myocardial Infarction). J Am Coll Cardiol 1996; 28:1328–1428.
79. Pedersen TR for the Norwegian Multicenter Study Group. Six-year follow-up of the Norwegian Multicenter Study on timolol after acute myocardial infarction. N Engl J Med 1985; 313:1055–1058.
80. Olsson G, Odén A, Johansson L, et al. Prognosis after withdrawal of chronic postinfarction metoprolol treatment: A 2–7 year follow-up. Eur Heart J 1988; 9:365–372.
81. Rogers WB, Bowlby LJ, Chandra NC, et al. Treatment of myocardial infarction in the United States (1990 to 1993): Observations from the National Registry of Myocardial Infarction. Circulation 1994; 90:2103–2114.
82. Brand DA, Newcomer LN, Freiburger A, Tian H. Cardiologists' practices compared with practice guidelines: Use of beta-blockade after acute myocardial infarction. J Am Coll Cardiol 1995; 26:1432–1436.
83. Viskin S, Kitzis I, Lev E, et al. Treatment with beta-adrenergic blocking agents after myocardial infarction: From randomized trials to clinical practice. J Am Coll Cardiol 1995; 25:1327–1332.
84. Yue T-L, Cheng H-Y, Lysko PG et al. Carvedilol, a new vasodilator and beta-adrenoreceptor antagonist, is an antioxidant and free radical scavenger. J Pharmacol Exp Ther 1992; 263:92–98.
85. Feuerstein GZ, Bril A, Ruffolo RR Jr. Protective effects of carvedilol in the myocardium. Am J Cardiol 1997; 80(11A):41L–45L.
86. Feuerstein GZ, Hamburger SA, Smith EF III, et al. Myocardial protection with carvedilol. J Cardiovasc Pharmacol 1992; 19(suppl 1):S138–S141.
87. Bril A, Slivjak MJ, Dimartino MJ, et al. Cardioprotective effects of carvedilol, a novel β adrenoreceptor antagonist with vasodilating properties, in anaesthetized minipigs: Comparison with propranol. Cardiovasc Res 1992; 26:518–525.
88. Brunvand H, Kvitting PM, Rynning SE, et al. Carvedilol protects against lethal reperfusion injury through antiadrenergic mechanisms. J Cardiovasc Pharmacol 1996; 28:409–417.
89. Packer M. The neurohormonal hypothesis: A theory to explain the mechanism of disease progression in heart failure. J Am Coll Cardiol 1992; 20:248–254.
90. Eichhorn EJ, Bristow MR. Medical therapy can improve the biological properties of the chronically failing heart: A new era in the treatment of heart failure. Circulation 1996; 94:2285–2296.
91. Bristow MR. Mechanism of action of beta-blocking agents in heart failure. Am J Cardiol 1997; 80(11A):26L–40L.
92. Mann DL, Kent RL, Parsons B, Cooper G IV. Adrenergic effects on the biology of the adult mammalian cardiocyte. Circulation 1992; 85:790–804.
93. Colucci WS. Molecular and cellular mechanisms of myocardial failure. Am J Cardiol 1997; 80(11A):15L–25L.
94. Francis GS, Benedict C, Johnstone DE, et al. Comparison of neuroendocrine activation in patients with left ventricular dysfunction with and without congestive heart failure: A substudy of the Studies of Left Ventricular Dysfunction (SOLVD). Circulation 1990; 82:1724–1729.
95. Cohn JN, Levine TB, Olivari MT, et al. Plasma norepinephrine as a guide to prognosis in patients with chronic congestive heart failure. N Engl J Med 1984; 311:819–823.
96. Packer M, Lee WH, Kessler PD, et al. Role of neurohormonal mechanisms in determining survival in patients with severe chronic heart failure. Circulation 1987; 75(suppl IV):IV80–IV92.
97. Levine TB, Francis GS, Goldsmith SR, et al. Activity of the sympathetic nervous system and renin-angiotensin system assessed by plasma hormone levels and their relation to hemodynamic abnormalities in congestive heart failure. Am J Cardiol 1982; 49:1659–1666.
98. Francis GS, Goldsmith SR, Cohn JN. Relationship of exercise capacity to resting left ventricular performance and basal plasma norepinephrine levels in patients with congestive heart failure. Am Heart J 1982; 104:725–731.
99. Esler M, Kaye D, Lambert G, et al. Adrenergic nervous system in heart failure. Am J Cardiol 1997; 80(11A):7L–14L.
100. Rundqvist B, Elam M, Bergmann-Sverrirsdottir Y, et al. Increased adrenergic drive precedes generalized sympathetic activation in heart failure. Circulation 1997; 95:169–175.
101. Hasking GJ, Esler MD, Jennings GJ, et al. Norepinephrine spillover to plasma in patients with congestive heart failure: Evidence of increased overall and cardiorenal sympathetic nervous activity. Circulation 1986; 73:615–621.
102. Meredith IT, Eisenhofer G, Lambert GW, et al. Cardiac sympathetic activity in congestive heart failure: Evidence for increased neuronal norepinephrine release and preserved neuronal uptake. Circulation 1993; 88:136–145.
103. Bristow MR, Ginsburg R, Minobe W, et al. Decreased catecholamine sensitivity and β-adrenergic receptor density in failing human hearts. N Engl J Med 1982; 307:205–211.
104. Fowler MB, Laser JA, Hopkins GL, et al. Assessment of the β-adrenergic receptor pathway in the intact failing human heart: Progressive receptor down-regulation and subsensitivity to agonist response. Circulation 1986; 74:1290–1302.
105. White M, Yanowitz F, Gilbert EM, et al. Role of beta-adrenergic receptor downregulation in the peak exercise response in patients with heart failure due to idiopathic dilated cardiomyopathy. Am J Cardiol 1995; 76:1271–1276.
106. Gilbert EM, Olsen SL, Renlund DG, Bristow MR. Beta-adrenergic receptor regulation and left ventricular function in idiopathic dilated cardiomyopathy. Am J Cardiol 1993; 71:23C–29C.
107. Hall SA, Cigarroa CG, Marcoux L, et al. Time course of improvement in left ventricular function, mass, and geometry in patients with congestive heart failure treated with β-adrenergic blockade. J Am Coll Cardiol 1995; 25:1154–1161.
108. Gilbert EM, Abraham WT, Olsen S, et al. Comparative hemodynamic, left ventricular functional, and antiadrenergic effects of chronic treatment with metoprolol versus carvedilol in the failing heart. Circulation 1996; 94:2817–2825.
109. Sackner-Bernstein JD, Mancini DM. Rationale for treatment of patients with chronic heart failure with adrenergic blockade. JAMA 1995; 274:1462–1467.
110. Glass MG, Fueihan F, Liao R, et al. Differences in cardioprotective efficacy of adrenergic receptor antagonists in an animal model of dilated cardiomyopathy: Effects on gross morphology, global cardiac function, and twitch force. Circ Res 1993; 73:1077–1089.
111. Tsutsui H, Spinale FG, Nagatsu M, et al. Effects of chronic β-adrenergic blockade on the left ventricular and cardiocyte abnormalities of chronic canine mitral regurgitation. J Clin Invest 1994; 93:2639–2648.
112. Haber HL, Simek CL, Gimple LW, et al. Why do patients with

congestive heart failure tolerate the initiation of β-blocker therapy? Circulation 1993; 88(part 1):1610–1619.
113. Doughty RN, MacMahon S, Sharpe N. Beta-blockers in heart failure: Promising or proved? J Am Coll Cardiol 1994; 23:814–821.
114. Eichhorn EJ, Bedotto JB, Malloy CR, et al. Effect of β-adrenergic blockade on myocardial function and energetics in congestive heart failure: Improvements in hemodynamic, contractile, and diastolic performance with bucindolol. Circulation 1990; 82:473–483.
115. Eichhorn EJ, Heesch CM, Barnett JH, et al. Effect of metoprolol on myocardial function and energetics in patients with nonischemic dilated cardiomyopathy: A randomized, double-blind, placebo-controlled study. J Am Coll Cardiol 1994; 24:1310–1320.
116. Wisenbaugh T, Katz I, Davis J, et al. Long-term (3 month) effects of a new beta-blocker (nevibolol) on cardiac performance in dilated cardiomyopathy. J Am Coll Cardiol 1993; 21:1094–1100.
117. Doughty RN, Whalley GA, Gamble G, et al. on behalf of the Australian/New Zealand Research Collaborative Group. Left ventricular remodeling with carvedilol in patients with congestive heart failure due to ischemic heart disease. J Am Coll Cardiol 1997; 29:1060–1066.
118. Lowes BD, Gill EA, Rodriguez-Larrain J, et al. Carvedilol is associated with a reversal of remodeling in chronic heart failure. Circulation 1996; 94(suppl I):I–407 (abstract).
119. Bristow MR, O'Connell JB, Gilbert EM, et al. for the Bucindolol Investigators. Dose-response of chronic β-blocker treatment in heart failure from either idiopathic dilated or ischemic cardiomyopathy. Circulation 1994; 89:1632–1642.
120. Bristow MR, Gilbert EM, Abraham WT, et al. for the MOCHA Investigators. Carvedilol produces dose-related improvements in left ventricular function and survival in subjects with chronic heart failure. Circulation 1996; 94:2807–2816.
121. Waagstein F, Bristow MR, Swedberg K, et al. for the Metoprolol in Dilated Cardiomyopathy (MDC) Trial Study Group. Beneficial effects of metoprolol in idiopathic dilated cardiomyopathy. Lancet 1993; 342:1441–1446.
122. CIBIS Investigators and Committees. A randomized trial of β-blockade in heart failure: The Cardiac Insufficiency Bisoprolol Study (CIBIS). Circulation 1994; 90:1765–1773.
123. Metra M, Nardi M, Giubbini R, Dei Cas L. Effects of short- and long-term carvedilol administration on rest and exercise hemodynamic variables, exercise capacity, and clinical conditions in patients with idiopathic dilated cardiomyopathy. J Am Coll Cardiol 1994; 24:1678–1687.
124. Olsen SL, Gilbert EM, Renlund DG, et al. Carvedilol improves left ventricular function and symptoms in chronic heart failure: A double-blind randomized study. J Am Coll Cardiol 1995; 25:1225–1231.
125. Krum H, Sackner-Bernstein JD, Goldsmith RL, et al. Double-blind, placebo-controlled study of the long-term efficacy of carvedilol in patients with severe heart failure. Circulation 1995; 92:1499–1506.
126. Packer M, Colucci WS, Sackner-Bernstein JD, et al, for the PRECISE Study Group. Double-blind, placebo-controlled study of the effects of carvedilol in patients with moderate to severe heart failure: The PRECISE trial. Circulation 1996; 94:2793–2799.
127. Gilbert EM, Anderson JL, Deitchman D, et al. Long-term β-blocker vasodilator therapy improves cardiac function in idiopathic dilated cardiomyopathy: A double-blind, randomized study of bucindolol versus placebo. Am J Med 1990; 88:223–229.
128. Australia/New Zealand Heart Failure Research Collaborative Group. Randomised, placebo-controlled trial of carvedilol in patients with congestive heart failure due to ischaemic heart disease. Lancet 1997; 349:375–380.
129. Eichhorn EJ, Hjalmarson Å. β-blocker treatment for chronic heart failure: The frog prince. Circulation 1994; 90:2153–2156.
130. Woodley SL, Gilbert EM, Anderson JA, et al. Beta-blockade with bucindolol in heart failure caused by ischemic versus idiopathic dilated cardiomyopathy. Circulation 1991; 84:2426–2441.
131. Packer MP, Bristow MR, Cohn JN, et al. for the U.S. Carvedilol Heart Failure Study Group. The effect of carvedilol on morbidity and mortality in patients with chronic heart failure. N Engl J Med 1996; 334:1349–1355.
132. Colucci WS, Packer M, Bristow MR, et al. for the US Carvedilol Heart Failure Study Group. Carvedilol inhibits clinical progression in patients with mild symptoms of heart failure. Circulation 1996; 94:2800–2806.
133. Cohn JN, Fowler MB, Bristow MR, et al. Safety and efficacy of carvedilol in severe heart failure: The U.S. Carvedilol Heart Failure Study Group. J Card Failure 1997; 3:173–179.
134. Pfeffer MA, Stevenson LW. β-adrenergic blockers and survival in heart failure. N Engl J Med 1996; 334:1396–1397.
134a. Goldstein S. Impact of carvedilol on mortality and cardiovascular morbidity in patients with chronic heart failure. Commentary. Evidence-Based Cardiovasc Med 1996; 1:27–28.
135. Packer M. Effects of beta-adrenergic blockade on survival of patients with chronic heart failure. Am J Cardiol 1997; 80(11A):46L–54L.
136. Heidenreich PA, Lee TT, Massie BM. Effect of beta-blockade on mortality in patients with heart failure: A meta-analysis of randomized clinical trials. J Am Coll Cardiol 1997; 30:27–34.
137. Doughty RN, Rodgers A, Sharpe N, MacMahon S. Effects of beta-blocker therapy on mortality in patients with heart failure: A systematic overview of randomized, controlled trials. Eur Heart J 1997; 18:560–565.
138. Bristow MR, Jershberger RE, Port JD, et al. β-adrenergic pathways in nonfailing and failing ventricular myocardium. Circulation 1990; 82(suppl II):112–125.
139. Bristow MR, Minobe W, Rasmussen R, et al. Alpha$_1$-adrenergic receptors in the nonfailing and failing human heart. J Pharmacol Exp Ther 1988; 247:1039–1045.
140. Mallat Z, Philip I, Lebret M, et al. Elevated levels of 8-iso-prostaglandin $F_{2\alpha}$ in pericardial fluid of patients with heart failure. Circulation 1998; 97:1536–1539.
141. Dhalla AK, Hill MF, Singal PK. Role of oxidative stress in transition of hypertrophy to heart failure. J Am Coll Cardiol 1996; 28:506–514.
142. Billman GE, Castillo LC, Hensley J, et al. Beta$_2$-adrenergic recpetor antagonists protect against ventricular fibrillation in vivo and in vitro: Evidence for enhanced sensitivity to β_2-adrenergic stimulation in animals susceptible for sudden death. Circulation 1997; 96:1914–1922.
143. The CIBIS II Scientific Committee. Design of the Cardiac Insufficiency Bisoprolol Study II (CIBIS II). Fundam Clin Pharm 1997; 11:138–142.
144. The BEST Steering Committee. Design of the Beta-Blocker Evaluation Survival Trial (BEST). Am J Cardiol 1995; 75:1220–1223.
145. The International Steering Committee on behalf of the MERIT-HF study group. Rationale, design, and organization of the Metoprolol CR/XL Randomized Intervention Trial in Heart Failure (MERIT-HF). Am J Cardiol 1997; 80(9B):54J–58J.
146. Data on file. SmithKline Beecham Pharmaceuticals.
147. Cleland JGF, Bristow MR, Erdmann E, et al. Beta-blocking agents in heart failure: Should they be used and how? Eur Heart J 1996; 17:1629–1639.
148. Eichhorn EJ, Bristow MR. Practical guidelines for initiation of beta-adrenergic blockade in patients with chronic heart failure. Am J Cardiol 1997; 79:794–798.

10 Angiotensin-Converting Enzyme Inhibitors

▶ Marcus D. Flather
▶ Marc A. Pfeffer

About 15% of all deaths in countries with developed market economies are attributed to myocardial infarction (MI),[1] and survivors face the prospect of decreased life expectancy owing to problems with continuing coronary artery disease or left ventricular (LV) dysfunction. Prevention and treatment of coronary heart disease (CHD) are high priorities in all health systems. Simple and well-recognized public health measures such as decreasing the numbers of smokers,[2, 3] reducing cholesterol through dietary modifications,[4] and increasing physical exercise[5, 6] all have an important role in decreasing CHD rates. Beyond these population-based measures, individual assessment of risk and appropriate use of antiplatelet,[7] antihypertensive,[8] and cholesterol-lowering therapies[9] are the major proven pharmacologic means to reduce CHD. People with manifest CHD are at especially high risk for CHD morbidity and mortality and generally warrant intensive pharmacologic therapy with multiple agents. The management of MI has improved by a succession of clinical trials demonstrating the additive benefits of beta blockers,[10] aspirin,[11] thrombolytic therapy,[12] angiotensin-converting enzyme (ACE) inhibitors,[13] and cholesterol-lowering therapy.[14–16] This chapter reviews the evidence concerning the effects of ACE inhibitors for the treatment of MI, from early experiments to large clinical trials.

THE RENIN-ANGIOTENSIN SYSTEM IN MI

The renin-angiotensin-aldosterone system has both circulating and local tissue hormonal effects.[17, 18] Renin converts an inactive precursor angiotensinogen to an inactive decapeptide angiotensin I in the liver. Renin is secreted from the kidney in response to a number of stimuli, including increased β sympathomimetic activity, low arterial blood pressure, and decreased sodium reabsorption in the distal tubule. Conversion of angiotensin I to an active octapeptide angiotensin II is catalyzed by ACE, a metalloprotease with a zinc group, which also inactivates bradykinin, hence the alternative name *kininase.* ACE activity is chiefly found in the vascular endothelium of the lungs but also occurs in other vascular beds, in the serum, and in other tissues, including the myocardium and coronary arteries. Angiotensin II exerts its powerful vasoconstrictor action by raising cytosolic calcium concentration, but it has other more diverse properties, including modulation of the sympathetic nervous system, modification and stimulation of vascular smooth muscle and myocardial growth, stimulation of aldosterone secretion, and procoagulant effects. ACE inhibitors are a group of compounds based originally on teprotide, a component of the venom of the snake *Bothrops jararaca.*[19] Captopril was synthesized as a result of biochemical analysis of the active carboxypeptidase A site of teprotide.[20] A number of other ACE inhibitors were synthesized shortly after captopril, and many of these have undergone rigorous evaluation to become available for therapeutic use.

The principal action of ACE inhibitors is blockade of the enzyme responsible for conversion of angiotensin I to angiotensin II in the serum as well as in local tissues. It is believed that ACE inhibitors exert each of their beneficial effects primarily through their hemodynamic actions such as arterial and venous dilation, leading to decreased peripheral vascular resistance, and reductions of both cardiac preload and afterload. However, inhibition of local renin-angiotensin systems and decreased sodium retention, as well as other novel mechanisms that are under investigation (including antithrombotic and antiatherogenic effects) and regulation of smooth muscle proliferation may also be important components for their favorable clinical effects.[21]

MI activates the adrenal and renin-angiotensin-aldosterone systems.[22] Levels of catecholamines are highest in the earliest stages of acute MI, whereas angiotensin II and renin usually reach their peaks after 2 to 3 days. In the acute phase of MI, angiotensin II can adversely affect the balance of myocardial oxygen demand and supply by causing coronary vasoconstriction, a decrease in myocardial blood flow, an increase in the inotropic state of the heart, and an increase in ventricular wall stress. In the study by McAlpine and associates, patients with clinical heart failure were noted to have higher levels of all the neurohormones measured (arginine vasopressin, epinephrine, norepinephrine, renin, and angiotensin II), which supports the hypothesis that the neuroendocrine response is greater in patients with larger infarcts.[23] Even 1 to 2 weeks after MI, a substantial proportion of patients may have sustained activation of one or more of these neurohormones.[24] These findings are consistent with elevations of neuroendocrine hormones observed in patients with chronic heart failure.[25, 26] Thus, acute or chronic myocardial damage results in generalized activation of a number of important neurohormones, including arginine vasopressin, epinephrine, norepinephrine, aldosterone, atrial natriuretic factor, angiotensin II, and renin.[25, 27, 28] Several of these markers have been shown to have prognostic implications for patients following MI.[29]

CHANGES IN MYOCARDIAL STRUCTURE AND SHAPE AFTER MI

Prognosis after MI is largely influenced by the occurrence and extent of LV dilation that are associated with an increased risk of congestive heart failure, myocardial aneurysm formation, cardiac rupture, and death.[30, 31] The spectrum of acute and chronic structural changes in the heart after MI is termed *ventricular remodeling*, the nature and extent of which are largely influenced by the size of the MI.[32] The earliest structural change occurring during the first few days after MI is *infarct expansion*, defined as distortion of ventricular topography produced by thinning and dilation of the infarcted segment.[32–34] Extensive MI (i.e., affecting >20% of the left ventricle) causes a reduction in stroke volume and increased LV filling pressures that results in dilation to normalize filling pressures and restore stroke volume, responses that are dependent on Frank-Starling principles.[35] These early shape and volume changes result in increased wall stress, which can become the stimulus for more insidious remodeling of both the infarct and noninfarct areas.[36–38] Ventricular dilation occurs as a result of side-to-side slippage of myocytes in the early phase and cell lengthening in the chronic phase. Thinning of the infarct site and dilation of the ventricle cause compensatory hypertrophy in noninfarcted portions of the ventricle. In summary, infarct expansion occurs in the early stages of MI, whereas ventricular enlargement occurs progressively over the weeks, months, and years after MI.

EXPERIMENTAL STUDIES OF ACE INHIBITORS IN MI

In a classic series of studies using a rat model of MI, Pfeffer and colleagues demonstrated that the progressive pattern of ventricular chamber enlargement in response to the loss of myocytes was favorably modified by ACE inhibitor therapy.[39, 40] In the early post-MI phase, pressure-volume responses were largely unchanged, whereas at 2 to 7 days ventricular dilation, approximately proportional to infarct size, occurred in all groups. In the longer term follow-up phase to 106 days, ventricular dilation was observed, especially in rats with moderate-to-extensive infarcts. Associated with this late dilation was a decrease in LV chamber stiffness and an increase in volume-to-mass ratio.[41] Treatment with captopril added to drinking water started either 2 or 21 days after coronary ligation and continued for 3 months produced a significant attenuation of LV dilation, especially in moderate-sized infarcts.[40] Perhaps most important, a significant improvement in survival was observed in rats treated with captopril. Median survival in captopril-treated rats was 260 days compared with 197 in untreated rats ($P < 0.01$), and the 1-year survival rate in the moderate-sized infarct group was 49% in the captopril group compared with 21% in controls ($P < 0.01$).[42] These and other[43, 44] animal studies laid the foundation for the clinical application of ACE inhibitors for the treatment of MI.

CLINICAL STUDIES

Effects of ACE Inhibitors on the Neuroendocrine System in MI

Several randomized clinical studies have reported on the effects of ACE inhibitors on neuroendocrine activity in the acute and recovery phase of MI.[25, 45–49] In an early study of 28 patients by Kingma and coworkers renin levels in the captopril group were elevated, while noradrenaline levels were significantly reduced by 50% compared with controls.[50] A more comprehensive report by Ray and associates on 99 patients showed significant reductions in angiotensin II by day 3 after MI (10.1 pg/mL in the captopril group compared with 16.8 pg/mL in the placebo group; $P < 0.05$), and levels were still significantly lower 1 week and 2 months after MI in the captopril group compared with placebo.[45] Renin levels were again elevated, as anticipated, in the captopril group compared with placebo (137 μL/mL vs. 67 μL/mL; $P < 0.05$) at day 3 and up to 2 months. No significant differences in plasma adrenaline or noradrenaline levels were detected between the captopril and placebo groups. Other studies have shown similar results for renin, angiotensin II, and aldosterone levels in the first few days after MI for captopril, zofenopril, and enalapril.[46–49, 51]

Long-Term Effects of ACE Inhibitors on Cardiac Structure and Function After MI

Significant reductions in ventricular volumes and pressures, with corresponding improvements in ejection fraction, have been reported in several randomized clinical studies of ACE inhibitors started a few days after acute MI and continued for about a year in patients with LV dysfunction (Table 10–1).[52–58, 81, 82] Pfeffer and coworkers randomized 59 patients with a first anterior MI (ejection fraction < 45%) to either captopril (6.25 mg started about 20 days after MI and titrated to a maintenance dose of 25 to 50 mg tid) or placebo, with treatment continued for 1 year.[53]

TABLE 10–1 • Effects of ACE Inhibitors on Left Ventricular Function and Remodeling After MI: Summary of Results from Randomized, Controlled Trials*

Trial, Year	Eligibility	Treatment	Timing of First Dose After AMI	Total No.	Follow-Up	Method and Main Measurement	Results: ACE-I	Results: Control	P Value
Sharpe, 1988[52]	Q wave MI	Captopril open test 12.5 mg, then 25 mg tid or placebo	8–9 d	40†	12 mo	Echo: change in LVESVI (mL/m²)	−7.24	+5.55	<0.05
Pfeffer, 1988[53]	First Q wave anterior MI	Captopril 6.25 mg titrated to 50 mg tid or placebo	2–4 wk	59	12 mo	Cardiac catheterization: LVEDP (mm Hg)	−7‡	−1‡	NS
Sharpe, 1991[54]	Q wave MI	Captopril open test 12.5 mg, then titrated up to 50 mg bid, or placebo	24–48 h	100	3 mo	Echo: Change LVESVI (mL/m²)	−2.38	+5.58	<0.001
SMILE Pilot, 1991[55]	AMI, no thrombolysis	Zofenopril 7.5 mg up to 30 mg bid or placebo	<24 h	145§	12 mo	Echo: LVES diameter (cm)¶	−0.5	+0.3	NS
Oldroyd, 1991[56]	AMI with ST-elevation small MI excluded	Captopril initial dose 6.25 mg up to 25 mg tid or placebo	<24 h	74**	2 mo	Echo: change in anterior endocardial segment length (mm)	+2.8	+10.4	0.01
Gøtzsche, 1992[57]	AMI <70 yr with heart failure or EF < 45%	Captopril 6.25 mg up to 25 mg bid	7 d	58	6 mo	Echo: change in LVESVI (mL/m²)	−6	+6	<0.05
Pipilis 1993[58]	Suspected AMI	Captopril 6.25 mg test up to 12.5 mg tid or placebo for 4 wk	<36 h	59	6 wk	Echo-Doppler aortic flow velocity: cardiac output (% change)	+22	+7	<0.05
Galcera-Tomas, 1993[81]	Anterior MI, ST-segment elevation, <70 yr	Captopril 6.25 mg then 12.5 mg up to 25 mg tid or placebo	<24 h	40	2 wk	RVG: change in LVESVI (mL/m²)	−1	+9	<0.05
Kyriakidis, 1993[82]	Q wave AMI, no clinical heart failure	Captopril 12.5 mg test then 25 mg tid or control	4th d after MI	78	4 wk	RVG: LVESVI (mL/m²)	−3	+4	NS
CATS Pilot, 1994[66]	First anterior AMI treated with thrombolysis	Captopril 6.25 mg titrated up to 25 mg tid over 24 h or placebo	<6 h	298	3 mo	Echo: LVESVI (mL/m²)	+2.5	+4.5	NS
SAVE Echo Substudy[59]	AMI LVEF < 40%	Captopril 12.5 mg initial dose up to 50 mg tid or placebo	3–16 d after MI	512	1 yr	Echo: LV end-systolic area (cm²)	+1.5	+3.6	0.02
GISSI-3 Echo Substudy[60]	AMI	Lisinopril 5 mg initial dose, 5 mg after 24 h then 10 mg daily or control	<24 h	6405	6 wk	Echo: LVESV (mL)	+0.7	+2.0	<0.02

*Results of randomized, controlled trials of ACE inhibitors vs. control measuring changes in ventricular structure and function after acute MI. All studies have shown either a significant improvement or a trend toward improvement, with ACE inhibitor therapy compared with control.
†Further 20 randomized to furosemide.
‡$P < 0.005$ for change compared to baseline within captopril group, and NS in the placebo group.
§145/204 patients had results available.
¶Approximate values from Figure 5 in Reference 55.
**74/99 patients had results available.
LVESVI, left ventricular end-systolic volume index; RVG, radionuclide ventriculography; LVEDP, left ventricular end-diastolic pressure; LVES, left ventricular end-systolic; EF, ejection fraction; LVESV, left ventricular end-systolic volume; ACE, angiotensin-converting enzyme; MI, myocardial infarction; AMI, acute myocardial infarction.

Changes in baseline LV pressures and volumes measured by angiography were compared with those recorded at 1 year. Captopril treatment resulted in significantly lower LV end-diastolic pressures, wedge pressure, and pulmonary artery pressure compared with controls. Both groups showed an increase in diastolic volume, but this was not significantly different from baseline in the captopril group, whereas the control group showed a significant increase, supporting the hypothesis that ACE inhibitors attenuate ventricular enlargement after a large MI. Similar findings were reported by Sharpe and associates, who randomized patients with ejection fraction less than 45% to captopril, furosemide, or control (60 patients started on study treatment 1 week after MI), or captopril or control (100 patients started on study treatment 24 to 48 hours after MI) in two separate studies.[52, 54] Captopril-treated patients had significantly smaller end-systolic and end-diastolic volumes than controls and about a 5% absolute higher ejection fraction at 3 months ($P < 0.001$). Two larger echocardiographic studies of ventricular structure and function were carried out as substudies of the Survival and Ventricular Enlargement (SAVE) and Gruppo Italiano per lo Studio della Sopravvivenza nell'Infarto Miocardico (GISSI-3) Trials,[59, 60] which are discussed in more detail later. These latter studies confirm previous observations that LV enlargement and impaired function following MI are associated with the development of adverse cardiac events and that ACE inhibitors attenuate ventricular enlargement. A summary of studies that have evaluated the effects of ACE inhibitors compared with control on ventricular volumes, function, and hemodynamics in patients started at varying stages after acute MI is presented in Table 10–1. The overall conclusions from these randomized studies of about 1000 patients in total are that ACE inhibitors reduce progressive ventricular enlargement, systemic blood pressure, and right- and left-sided cardiac pressures. The beneficial effects on ventricular remodeling appear greater in patients with LV dysfunction at the start of treatment.

Hemodynamic Effects of ACE Inhibitors in the Early Phase of Acute MI

The hemodynamic effects of ACE inhibitors were first described in patients with heart failure. Administration of intravenous teprotide, the prototype ACE inhibitor, significantly reduced ventricular afterload and increased cardiac index by about 25% (from a baseline of 2.04 L/min/m^2 to 2.47 L/min/m^2 after infusion of teprotide; $P < 0.001$).[61, 62] One of the first reports of administration of oral ACE inhibitors to patients with acute MI came from Brivet and associates, who gave captopril to eight patients with acute MI and heart failure.[63] One hour after giving 25 mg of oral captopril, they observed significant reductions in mean arterial blood pressure (90 to 76 mm Hg; $P < 0.001$), pulmonary artery wedge pressure, and systemic vascular resistance and an increase in cardiac output (3.2 L/min precaptopril to 4.1 L/min postcaptopril; $P < 0.01$). These findings are consistent with those of the Survival of Myocardial Infarction Long-Term Evaluation (SMILE) Pilot Study, which reported on the effects of oral zofenopril in a randomized trial of 204 patients using an invasive method of monitoring hemodynamic changes.[55] The Internation Study of Infarct Survival-4 (ISIS-4) Pilot Study group also reported an increase in cardiac output by 13% compared with placebo 1 hour after giving oral captopril ($P < 0.01$), 23% at 1 week ($P < 0.001$), and 22% at 6 weeks (2 weeks after treatment had been discontinued; $P < 0.05$) using a noninvasive method.[58] Measures of systemic blood pressure in the GISSI-3 Pilot Study (430 patients on oral lisinopril compared with 442 control patients),[64] the ISIS-4 Pilot Study (370 patients on captopril compared with 371 control),[65] and the SMILE Pilot Study (101 patients on zofenopril compared with 103 controls)[55] showed that systolic and diastolic blood pressures were significantly reduced by about 15% during the first few hours after administration of an ACE inhibitor. Hypotension (generally defined as systolic blood pressure < 90 mm Hg for more than 2 hours) was noted to occur about twice as frequently in the ACE inhibitor groups compared with controls, but in most of these cases hypotension resolved with simple measures without any apparent clinical sequelae. In contrast, the Captopril and Thrombolysis Study (CATS) Group described the effects of intravenous captopril given with streptokinase in acute MI. They observed quite marked early reductions in blood pressure that were not believed to be clinically acceptable,[50] but early oral therapy was well tolerated.[66] On the basis of these and other carefully conducted safety and feasibility studies,[56, 57] it has been concluded that starting oral ACE inhibitors in the early phase of acute MI produces significant, but usually well tolerated, reductions in arterial blood pressure with concomitant reductions in systemic vascular resistance and improvements in cardiac output.

LARGE TRIALS EVALUATING CLINICAL OUTCOMES

Evidence for the safety, feasibility, and beneficial effects of ACE inhibitors in MI generated by the studies described earlier provided the rationale for several large randomized trials using survival as the main

TABLE 10–2 • ACE Inhibitor in MI: Summary of Large Long-Term Trials*

Trial, Year	Design	Eligibility	Timing of First Dose After AMI	Agent and Regimen	Average Follow-Up (mo)	Deaths/Numbers Randomized (%)		Odds Ratio (95% Confidence Interval)	*P* Value
						Treatment	*Control*		
SAVE, 1992[67]	Double-blind	LVEF < 40%	3–16 d	Captopril or placebo 12.5 mg initial dose, titrating up to 25–50 mg tid	42	(228/1115) (20.5%)	275/1116 (24.6%)	0.79 (0.68 to 0.97)	0.019
AIRE, 1993[68]	Double-blind	Clinical heart failure	3–10 d	Ramipril or placebo 2.5 mg bid initial dose, titrating up to 5 mg bid for at least 6 mo	15	170/1004 (16.9%)	222/982 (22.6%)	0.70 (0.60 to 0.89)	0.002
TRACE, 1995[69]	Double-blind	Wall motion index <1.2 (LVEF alt 35%)	3–7 d	Trandolapril or placebo 1 mg od initial dose, titrating up to 4 mg od	36	304/876 (34.7%)	369/873 (42.3%)	0.73 (0.67 to 0.91)	0.001

*See text for complete names of trials. See also Figure 10–1 for additional data.
LVEF, left ventricular ejection fraction; MI, myocardial infarction; ACE, angiotensin-converting enzyme.

outcome measure. The following main trial designs were used in the large clinical outcomes trials:

1. Three large trials selected patients with evidence of LV dysfunction a few days after MI and evaluated the effects of ACE inhibitors on survival after at least 2 years of treatment.[67–69]
2. Five large trials evaluated the effects of ACE inhibitors on survival when started in the acute phase of MI and continued for a few weeks or months in patients with and without LV dysfunction at baseline.[70–74]

Long-Term Trials of ACE Inhibitors Started After MI

Three large long-term randomized, controlled trials have been published: Survival and Ventricular Enlargement (SAVE),[67] Acute Infarction Ramipril Efficacy (AIRE),[68] and Trandolapril in Patients with Reduced Left Ventricular Function After AMI (TRACE).[69] The main design features and results of these trials are summarized in Table 10–2 and Figure 10–1.

The SAVE Study enrolled 2231 patients with an ejection fraction of 40% or less, without clinical evidence of heart failure or ongoing ischemia.[67] Patients were randomized between 3 and 16 days (mean 11 days) after MI to either captopril (titrating up to a maximum dose of 50 mg tid) or matching placebo, and treatment was continued for a mean of 42 months (range, 24 to 60 months). At the last study visit 70% of survivors in the captopril group were taking study treatment compared with 73% in the placebo group, and of these, 79% and 90%, respectively, reached the target dose of 150 mg daily. There were 228 (20.5%) deaths out of 1115 patients in the captopril group compared with 275 (24.6%) deaths out of 1116 patients in the placebo group (odds ratio [OR], 0.79; 95% confidence interval [CI], 0.68 to 0.97; $P = 0.019$). A similar reduction was observed when cardiovascular

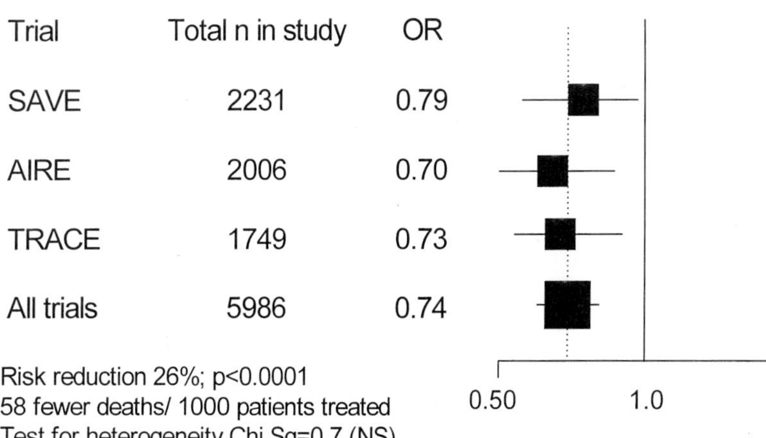

Figure 10–1 Effects of angiotensin-converting enzyme inhibitors on mortality after myocardial infarction: results from the long-term trials. OR, odds ratio; CI, confidence interval. See text for complete names of the trials.

deaths (84% of the total) were compared, and significant benefits of captopril were observed on the incidence of heart failure requiring hospitalization. A 25% risk reduction was also observed in the rate of fatal or nonfatal recurrent MI (133 in the captopril group and 170 in the placebo group; 95% CI, 5% to 40%; $P = 0.015$). This study clearly demonstrates the benefits of long-term ACE inhibition in survivors of MI with reduced ejection fractions (mean ejection fraction, 31%) without clinical heart failure.

The AIRE Study randomized 2006 patients with clinical evidence of heart failure (based on clinical examination or chest x-ray) to ramipril (target dose 5 mg bid) or matching placebo commencing 3 to 10 days after acute MI.[68] Average length of follow-up was 15 months (range 6 to 30 months). All-cause mortality in the ramipril group was 17% (170 deaths out of 1014) compared with 23% in the control group (222 deaths out of 992 patients; OR, 0.70; 95% CI, 0.60 to 0.89; $P = 0.002$). A risk reduction of 19% was observed in the rate of the secondary outcome cluster (first event of death, recurrent heart failure, MI, or stroke) in the ramipril group compared with placebo (95% CI, 5% to 31%; $P = 0.008$). This study clearly showed that ACE inhibitors could be started soon after MI in patients with heart failure and that there were clinically important reductions in mortality in this high-risk group with an average of just 15 months of treatment.

The TRACE Study randomized 1749 patients with echocardiographic wall motion abnormality consistent with an ejection fraction of 35% or lower to either trandolapril (maximum dose of 4 mg daily) or matching placebo 3 to 7 days after MI.[69] Length of follow-up was 24 to 50 months. All-cause mortality in the trandolapril group was 34.7% (304 deaths out of 876 patients) compared with 42.3% in the placebo group (369 deaths out of 873 patients; relative risk of death, 0.74; 95% CI, 0.67 to 0.91; $P = 0.001$). There were similar reductions in the rates of other secondary outcomes, including deaths from cardiovascular causes, sudden death, and progression to severe heart failure. There was no apparent reduction in the rate of fatal or nonfatal recurrent MI. The TRACE Study Group carefully screened 6676 consecutive patients with confirmed MI entering the coronary care units of participating hospitals for entry into the study. Of these, about 25% were entered into the trial, which is a relatively high proportion of patients screened compared with other clinical trials. The TRACE results add to the knowledge base of ACE inhibitors started a few days after MI in patients with LV dysfunction and help confirm the wide generalizability of the results to clinical practice. An important additional feature of these trials was that the benefit of ACE inhibitors was in addition to that of beta blockers, aspirin, and thrombolytic therapy.

Large Trials of ACE Inhibitors Started in the Acute Phase of MI

The design aspects, drug regimens, and mortality results for the five acute-phase, short-term trials are summarized in Table 10–3 and Figure 10–2.

The Cooperative New Scandinavian Enalapril Survival (CONSENSUS) II Study randomized 6090 patients in 103 Scandinavian hospitals to either 2 hours of intravenous enalaprilat followed by oral enalapril, or placebo infusion and tablets, for 6 months.[70] There were 10.2% deaths in the enalapril group and 9.4% deaths in the placebo group (OR, 1.10; 95% CI, 0.93 to 1.29; $P = 0.26$). More deaths were attributed to progressive heart failure (4.3% in the enalapril group vs. 3.4% in the placebo group; NS) and mortality was higher in patients older than 70 years of age who were randomized to enalapril compared with control (17.3% and 14.7%, respectively; $P = 0.07$). The incidence of systolic blood pressure below 90 mm Hg and diastolic blood pressure below 50 mm Hg was 12% in the enalapril group and 3% in the placebo group ($P < 0.001$). The Safety Committee recommended stopping the study early based on safety

Trial	Total n in study	OR
CONSENSUS-II	6090	1.1
GISSI-3	19394	0.88
SMILE	1556	0.67
ISIS-4	58050	0.94
CCS-1	13634	0.94
All trials	98724	0.93

Risk reduction 6.7% P<0.006
4.9 (SD1.7) fewer deaths/1000 patients treated
Test for heterogeneity Chi Sq = 5.7 NS

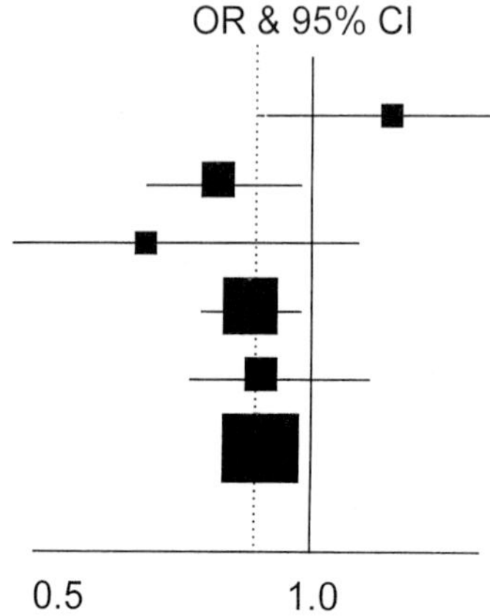

Figure 10–2 Effects of angiotensin-converting enzyme inhibitors on mortality after myocardial infarction: results from the short-term trials. OR, odds ratio; CI, confidence interval. See text for complete names of the trials.

TABLE 10–3 • ACE Inhibitor in AMI: Summary of the Large Short-Term Trials*

Trial, Year	Design	Eligibility	Time of First Dose After AMI (h)	Agent and Regimen and Follow-Up	Average Follow-Up	Deaths/Numbers Randomized (%) Treatment	Control	Odds Ratio (%) (95% Confidence Interval)	P Value
CONSENSUS-II, 1993[70]	Double-blind	ST elevation, Q waves or elevated cardiac enzyme levels	<24	Enalapril or placebo: initial IV infusion of 1 mg enalapril over 2 h, then 2.5 mg oral enalapril titrating up to 10 mg daily	6 mo	312/3044 (10.25%)	286/3046 (9.40%)	1.10 (0.93 to 1.29)	0.26
GISSI-3, 1994[71]	Open	ST elevation or depression	<24	Lisinopril or control 5 mg initial dose, titrating up to 10 mg daily	6 wk	597/9435 (6.33%)	673/9460 (7.11%)	0.88 (0.79 to 0.99)	0.03
SMILE, 1995[74]	Double-blind	Anterior MI, no thrombolysis	<24	Zofenopril or placebo 7.5 mg initial dose, titrating up to 30 mg bid	6 wk	38/772 (4.9%)	51/784 (6.5%)	0.75 (0.40 to 1.11)	0.19
ISIS-4, 1995[72]	Double-blind	Suspected AMI	<24	Captopril or placebo 6.25 mg initial dose, titrating up to target of 50 mg bid	4 wk	2088/29028 (7.19%)	2231/29022 (7.69%)	0.93 (0.87 to 0.99)	0.02
CCS-1, 1995[73]	Double-blind	Suspected AMI	<36	Captopril or placebo 6.25 mg initial dose then 12.5 mg tid	4 wk	617/6814 (9.05%)	654/6820 (9.59%)	0.94 (0.84 to 1.05)	0.3

*See text for complete names of trials. See also Figure 10–2 for additional data.
ACE, angiotensin-converting enzyme; AMI, acute myocardial infarction.

concerns about early hypotension in patients receiving enalapril infusions (particularly elderly patients),[75] and the fact that the effect size was too small for a significant difference to be detected even if the trial went on to the projected sample size of 9000.

The GISSI-3 study, carried out in 200 Italian coronary care units, evaluated the effects of 6 weeks of treatment with oral lisinopril (as well as nitrates in a 2 × 2 factorial design) started within 24 hours of the onset of symptoms of acute MI in an open randomized, controlled study of 19,394 patients.[71] Mortality at 6 weeks was 6.3% in the lisinopril group compared with 7.1% in controls (OR, 0.88; 95% CI, 0.79 to 0.99; $P = 0.03$). For the prespecified combined endpoint of death plus late (beyond day 4) clinical congestive heart failure, or extensive LV damage in the absence of clinical heart failure, the incidence was 15.6% for lisinopril and 17% in control (OR, 0.9; 95% CI, 0.84 to 0.98; $P = 0.009$). The incidence of persistent hypotension (systolic blood pressure below 90 mm Hg for at least 1 hour) was 9% in the lisinopril and 3.7% in the control group ($P < 0.001$). The survival curves of lisinopril-treated patients and controls separated early, suggesting that the benefits of the ACE inhibitor occurred early and persisted throughout the treatment period. There were 76 fewer deaths overall in the lisinopril group compared with placebo, of which on days 0 to 1 (day 0 is the day of randomization) 21 out of 76 deaths were avoided (28% of the overall benefit), 43 in days 2 to 7 (57% of the benefit), and 12 in the subsequent days of treatment.[76]

The ISIS-4 Trial enrolled 58,050 patients within 24 hours (median 8 hours) of the onset of suspected acute MI in 1086 hospitals in 31 countries.[72] Patients were randomized to oral captopril (initial dose of 6.25 mg titrating up to 50 mg twice daily over 24 to 48 hours) or placebo captopril for 28 days (the effects of oral mononitrate and intravenous magnesium were also evaluated in a 2 × 2 × 2 factorial design, but are not discussed here). After 5 weeks of follow-up, there were 2088 (7.19%) deaths in the 29,028 patients allocated captopril compared with 2231 (7.61%) deaths in the 29,022 patients allocated placebo. This represents an OR of 0.93 (95% CI, 0.87 to 0.99; $P = 0.020$) during days 0 to 35 and corresponds to an absolute difference of about 5 fewer deaths per 1000 patients treated with captopril. As in the GISSI Study, there were fewer early deaths in the captopril group (deaths on days 0 to 1, 549 [1.89%] captopril vs. 593 [2.04%] placebo).[76] The benefits of early captopril treatment persisted over about 1 year of follow-up, although little extra gain was observed with time, possibly because treatment was discontinued at 28 days. Cardiogenic shock was reported in 4.6% of patients allocated captopril compared with 4.1% in the control group ($P < 0.01$), but there was no apparent excess of deaths from cardiogenic shock in the captopril group. The incidence of any profound hypotension was 21% in the captopril group compared with 11% in the control group, and hypotension requiring termination of study treatment was 10% versus 5%, respectively (all comparisons, $P < 0.0001$).

The Chinese Cardiac Study (CCS-1) enrolled 13,634 patients who were randomized to either captopril (6.25 mg initial dose followed by 12.5 mg three times daily for 4 weeks) or matching placebo within 36 hours of the onset of suspected acute MI.[73] Captopril was associated with a nonsignificant reduction in 4-week mortality (617 [9.05%] deaths in the captopril group compared with 654 [9.59%] in the control group; $P = 0.3$). As in ISIS-4, there was an excess of hypotension in the captopril group compared with control (16% and 11%, respectively; $P < 0.001$) and a slight excess of cardiogenic shock (4.8% and 4.2%, respectively; P = NS).

The SMILE was a trial of 1556 patients with acute anterior MI who were not receiving thrombolytic therapy (mainly because of late presentation).[74] Patients were randomized within 24 hours from the onset of symptoms to zofenopril (a short-acting ACE inhibitor with a sulfydryl group) 7.5 mg titrated up to 30 mg bid, or placebo control for 6 weeks. The primary outcome of death or severe congestive heart failure during the treatment period occurred in 7.1% of zofenopril-allocated patients compared with 10.6% of placebo patients (OR, 0.66; 95% CI, 0.46 to 0.92; $P = 0.018$). SMILE was a smaller trial than ISIS-4 or GISSI-3 but was studying selected patients with larger MI not treated with thrombolytic therapy. These results are consistent with the hypothesis that the benefits of ACE inhibitor treatment are greater in those patients at highest risk of infarct expansion and ventricular dilation.

SYSTEMATIC OVERVIEWS (META-ANALYSIS) OF THE LARGE TRIALS

A systematic overview of the large trials (both acute trials and long-term trials of >1000 patients) is underway using data from each patient from the original trials. This collaborative project involves all the trial groups, and its main aims are to define more clearly the balance of benefits and risks of ACE inhibitors for MI in the groups overall and in important clinical subgroups. The results of these overviews are still being finalized, but some preliminary data can be reported.[77, 78]

Systematic Overview of the Long-Term Trials

Information was available from the three large trials for a total of 5966 patients.[77] The proportion of deaths in the ACE inhibitor group was 23.4% compared with 29.1% in the control group (OR, 0.74; 95% CI, 0.66 to 0.83; $P < 0.0001$), and the proportion of patients admitted to hospital for heart failure was 11.9% and 15.5%, respectively (OR, 0.73; 95% CI, 0.63 to 0.85: $P < 0.0001$). Recurrent nonfatal MI occurred in 10.8% of the ACE inhibitor group compared with 13.2% of controls (OR, 0.80; 95% CI, 0.69 to 0.94; $P < 0.01$), which supports previous observations of prevention of myocardial ischemic events,[79] while there was no difference in the proportion of strokes which occurred in 4.0% and 3.7%, respectively (OR, 1.10; P = NS). Previous reports had suggested that the beneficial effects of ACE inhibitors could be reduced by the coadministration of aspirin. In the systematic overview, the OR of all-cause mortality among patients taking aspirin at baseline was 0.74 ($P < 0.0001$ for the comparison of ACE inhibitor vs. control), and was 0.73 for patients not taking aspirin at baseline ($P = 0.004$ for the comparison of ACE inhibitor vs. control). These data confirm that the proportional benefits of ACE inhibitors are similar in patients taking aspirin compared with those not taking aspirin at baseline and suggest that coadministration of aspirin and ACE inhibitors at randomization does not significantly attenuate the effects of either beneficial agent. Regression analysis of the OR of mortality in the ACE inhibitor group compared with control and baseline ejection fraction shows a highly significant relationship, with greater benefit accruing in those patients with lower ejection fractions. The long-term trials have shown convincing and consistent risk reductions in mortality (of the order of 20% to 25%) in patients with a history of congestive heart failure or objective evidence of impaired LV function. The estimated number of lives saved per 1000 patients treated for 2 to 3 years is between 40 and 70.

Systematic Overview of the Acute, Short-Term Trials

Data were available for nearly 100,000 patients from four trials.[78] Overall 30-day mortality was 7.1% in the ACE inhibitor group patients and 7.6% in the control group (risk reduction, 7%; 95% CI, 2% to 11%; $P < 0.004$). This represents the avoidance of about 5 deaths for every 1000 patients treated, and most of the benefit was observed in the first week. Overall, 239 deaths were avoided in the first few weeks in the group randomized to ACE inhibitor therapy. Of these, 96 deaths (40% of total benefit) were avoided during days 0 to 1, 104 deaths (44%) avoided during days 2 to 7, and just 39 (16%) during days 8 to 30.[76] Thus, the benefits of starting ACE inhibitors in the early phase of MI are mostly observed in the first week, even in a relatively unselected population. However, most of the benefit appears to be concentrated in patients at greater risk of LV dysfunction at randomization, including anterior MI (11 deaths avoided per 1000 patients treated) compared with other sites of MI (1 death avoided) and patients in Killip class 2 or 3 (14 deaths avoided per 1000 patients) compared with Killip class 1 (3 deaths avoided per 1000 patients). Greater benefits were also observed in patients with higher heart rates and diabetics compared with nondiabetics. Beneficial effects were not apparently observed in elderly patients older than 75 years of age (about 15% of the total) perhaps because of a higher incidence of adverse effects such as hypotension and renal dysfunction. The interpretation that greater benefits occur in patients with more ventricular damage at baseline, although attractive, should be treated with caution since it relies on subgroup analyses in the overview that may be unreliable. Despite early hypotension with the use of ACE inhibitors in the acute phase of MI, the lives saved in GISSI-3 and ISIS-4 during the first few days[71, 72, 76] underscore the importance of this strategy, which is also supported by a more recent mechanistic study in which the Healing and Afterload-Reducing Therapy (HEART) Investigators showed that early use of an ACE inhibitor was associated with prompt improvements in LV function.[80]

SUMMARY AND CONCLUSIONS

ACE inhibitors are of proven benefit for patients who have suffered a recent MI. Starting therapy 3 to 10 days after acute MI in patients with clinical evidence of heart failure or objective evidence of impaired LV function (ejection fraction <40%) and continuing therapy for about 2 years will avoid about 25% of all deaths. Starting ACE inhibitors in the acute phase of MI (i.e., within 24 to 36 hours of symptom onset) and continuing treatment for just 4 to 6 weeks in patients without hypotension or other obvious contraindications is also clearly beneficial. The apparent smaller beneficial effects of ACE inhibitors in the short-term trials (7% overall risk reduction) compared with the longer-term trials (about 25% overall risk reduction) can be largely explained by the shorter treatment duration and use in lower risk patients.

In the first part of this chapter we reviewed the pathophysiologic processes occurring after acute MI and the potential mechanisms of benefit of ACE inhibitors in this setting. In the early post-MI phase, patients with larger infarcts are at greater risk of infarct expansion. Later there is a higher risk of ventricular dilation associated with remodeling of ventricular structure and shape to adapt to a decline in function. The major therapeutic questions are the following:

1. How early after the onset of MI should ACE inhibitor therapy be started?

2. If early therapy is beneficial and safe, should a broad group of patients be treated, or should treatment be targeted to patients who are likely to benefit most?

The large short-term trials have shown convincingly that it is feasible and safe to start low doses of ACE inhibitors in hemodynamically stable patients in the early stages of MI (i.e., within the first 24 hours of symptom onset). Overall there is a modest benefit after a few weeks of treatment, but this benefit is apparent even in the first few days of treatment, during which time patients entered into the long-term trials would not have been started on ACE inhibitors. However, in the short-term trials, the beneficial effects in patients with evidence of LV dysfunction, or those at high risk of developing LV dysfunction (e.g., anterior MI), were more striking than the average, while those in the lower-risk groups (e.g., non-anterior MI) showed little benefit. In contrast, the long-term trials delayed the start of ACE inhibitors for 2 to 3 days, mainly because the safety and feasibility of starting earlier had not yet been established, and showed a clear benefit after prolonged treatment. Evidence of benefit exists for many commonly used ACE inhibitors, suggesting that these benefits are a class effect, but using agents employed in the clinical trials does provide added assurance about dosage.

We believe that the results of the two approaches are complementary. All the available evidence supports the hypothesis that ACE inhibitors primarily benefit patients with LV dysfunction, and there is little evidence that treating patients with small infarcts is helpful. Thus, in our opinion, the optimum strategy is to adopt a targeted approach with the aim of starting treatment in the acute phase of MI in patients with established evidence of LV dysfunction (i.e., patients with clinical heart failure or ejection fraction <40%) or those at high risk of developing LV dysfunction. Identification of the latter group requires clinical judgment but will include patients such as those with anterior MI or large infarcts at other sites, diabetics, patients with prior MI, and patients with tachycardia. Treatment should be started cautiously with low doses of oral ACE inhibitors when patients are hemodynamically stable (if necessary, initiation of treatment can be delayed until the patient is stable) and titrated up to the standard maintenance doses used in the trials over 2 to 3 days. Although there is a greater risk of hypotension if treatment is started in the acute phase of MI, the risk associated with hypotension is offset by early beneficial effects on mortality. Assessment by echocardiography is recommended in post-MI patients to detect and monitor LV dysfunction. Treatment with ACE inhibitors should be continued indefinitely in patients with established LV dysfunction.

REFERENCES

1. Murray C, Lopez A. Global Comparative Assessments in the Health Sector. Geneva, World Health Organization, 1994.
2. Parish S, Collins R, Peto R, et al. Cigarette smoking, tar yields, and nonfatal myocardial infarction: 14000 cases and 32000 controls in the United Kingdom. BMJ 1995; 311:471–477.
3. Doll R, Peto R, Wheatley K, et al. Mortality in relation to smoking: 40 years' observations on male British doctors. BMJ 1994; 309:901–911.
4. Keys A. Coronary heart disease in seven countries. Circulation 1970; 41:I1–I121.
5. Paffenberger RS, Hyde PHR, Wing AL, et al. The association of changes in physical activity level and other lifestyle characteristics with mortality among men. N Engl J Med 1993; 328:538–545.
6. Sandvik L, Erikssen J, Thaulow E, et al. Physical fitness as a predictor of mortality among healthy, middle-aged Norwegian men. N Engl J Med 1993; 328:533–537.
7. Antiplatelet Trialists' Collaboration. Collaborative overview of randomised trials of antiplatelet therapy: I. Prevention of death, myocardial infarction, and stroke by prolonged antiplatelet therapy in various categories of patients. BMJ 1994; 308:81–106.
8. Collins R, Peto R, MacMahon S, et al. Blood pressure, stroke, and coronary heart disease: II. Short-term reductions in blood pressure: Overview of randomised drug trials in their epidemiological context. Lancet 1990; 335:827–838.
9. Prospective Studies Collaboration. Cholesterol, diastolic blood pressure, and stroke: 13000 strokes in 450000 people in 45 prospective cohorts. Lancet 1995; 346:1647–1653.
10. ISIS-1 (First International Study of Infarct Survival) Collaborative Group. Randomised trial of intravenous atenolol among 16027 cases of suspected acute myocardial infarction: ISIS-1. Lancet 1986; 2:57–66.
11. ISIS-2 (Second International Study of Infarct Survival) Collaborative Group. Randomised trial of intravenous streptokinase, oral aspirin, both, or neither among 17187 cases of suspected acute myocardial infarction: ISIS-2. Lancet 1988; 2:349–360.
12. Fibrinolytic Therapy Trialists' Collaboration. Indications for fibrinolytic therapy in suspected acute myocardial infarction: Collaborative overview of early mortality and major morbidity results from all randomised trials of more than 1000 patients. Lancet 1994; 343:311–322.
13. Pfeffer MA. ACE inhibition in acute myocardial infarction. N Engl J Med 1995; 332:118–120.
14. Scandinavian Simvastatin Survival Study Group. Randomised trial of cholesterol lowering in 4444 patients with coronary heart disease: The Scandinavian Simvastatin Survival Study (4S). Lancet 1994; 344:1383–1389.
15. Shepherd J, Cobbe SM, Ford I, et al. Prevention of coronary heart disease with pravastatin in men with hypercholesterolemia. N Engl J Med 1995; 333:1301–1307.
16. Sacks FM, Pfeffer MA, Moyé LA, et al. The effect of pravastatin on coronary events after myocardial infarction in patients with average cholesterol levels. N Eng J Med 1996; 335:1001–1009.
17. Peart WS. The renin-angiotensin system. Pharmacol Rev 1965; 17:143–183.
18. Ertl G. Angiotensin-converting enzyme inhibitors and ischaemic heart disease. Eur Heart J 1988; 9:716–727.
19. Ondetti MA, Williams NJ, Sabo EF, et al. Angiotensin-converting enzyme inhibitors from the venom of *Bothrops jararaca*: Isloation, elucidation of structure, and synthesis. Biochemistry 1971; 10:4033–4039.
20. Ondetti MA, Rubin B, Cushman DW. Design of specific inhibitors of angiotensin-converting enzyme: A new class of orally active antihypertensive agents. Science 1977; 196:441–444.
21. Lonn E, Yusuf S, Jha P, et al. The emerging role of angiotensin-converting enzyme inhibitors in cardiac and vascular protection. Circulation 1994; 90:2056–2069.
22. Ceremuzynski L. Hormonal and metabolic reactions evoked by acute myocardial infarction. Circ Res 1981; 48:767–776.
23. McAlpine HM, Morton JJ, Leckie B, et al. Neuroendocrine activation after acute myocardial infarction. Br Heart J 1988; 60:117–124.
24. Rouleau JL, Moyé LA, deChamplain J, et al. Activation of neurohumoral systems following acute myocardial infarction. Am J Cardiol 1991; 68:80D–86D.
25. Swedberg K, Eneroth P, Kjekshus J, Wilhelmsen L. Hormones regulating cardiovascular function in patients with severe congestive heart failure and their relation to mortality. Circulation 1990; 82:1730–1736.
26. Francis GS, Benedict C, Johnstone DE, et al. Comparsion of neuroendocrine activation in patients with left ventricular dysfunction with and without congestive heart failure. Circulation 1990; 82:1724–1729.
27. Michorowski BL, Ceremuzynski L. The renin-angiotensin-aldosterone system and the clinical course of acute myocardial infarction. Eur Heart J 1983; 4:259–264.
28. Donald RA, Crozier IG, Foy SG, et al. Plasma corticotrophin-releasing hormone, vasopressin, ACTH, and cortisol response to acute myocardial infarction. Clin Endocrinol 1994; 40:499–504.
29. Rouleau JL, Packer M, Lemuel M, et al. Prognostic value of neurohumoral activation in patients with an acute myocardial infarction: Effect on captopril. J Am Coll Cardiol 1994; 24:583–591.
30. White HD, Norris RM, Brown MA, et al. Left ventricular end-systolic volume as the major determinant of survival after recovery from myocardial infarction. Circulation 1987; 76:44–51.
31. The GUSTO Angiographic Investigators. The effects of tissue plasminogen activator, streptokinase, or both on coronary artery patency, ventricular function, and survival after acute myocardial infarction. N Engl J Med 1993; 329:1615–1622.
32. Pfeffer MA, Braunwald E. Ventricular remodeling after myocardial infarction: Experimental observations and clinical implications. Circulation 1990; 81:1161–1172.
33. Hutchins GM, Bulkley BH. Infarct expansion versus extension: Two different complications of acute myocardial infarction. Am J Cardiol 1978; 41:1127–1132.
34. Erlebacher JA, Weiss JL, Bulkley BJ, Weisfeldt ML. Early dilation of the infarcted segment in acute transmural myocardial infarction: Role of infarct expansion in acute left ventricular enlargement. J Am Coll Cardiol 1984; 4:201–208.
35. McKay RG, Pfeffer MA, Pasternak RC, et al. Left ventricular remodeling after myocardial infarction: A corollary to infarct expansion. Circulation 1986; 74:693–702.
36. Mitchell GF, Lamas GA, Vaughan DE, Pfeffer MA. Left ventricular remodeling in the year after first anterior myocardial infarction: A quantitative analysis of contractile segment lengths and ventricular shape. J Am Coll Cardiol 1992; 19:1136–1144.
37. Lamas GA, Pfeffer MA. Left ventricular remodeling after acute myocardial infarction: Clinical course and beneficial effects of angiotensin-converting enzyme inhibition. Am Heart J 1991; 121:1194–1202.
38. Jeremy RW, Allman KC, Bautovitch G, Harris PJ. Patterns of left ventricular dilatation during the six months after myocardial infarction. J Am Coll Cardiol 1989; 13:304–310.
39. Fletcher PJ, Pfeffer JM, Pfeffer MA, Braunwald E. Left ventricular diastolic pressure-volume relations in rats with healed myocardial infarction: Effects on systolic function. Circ Res 1981; 49:618–626.
40. Pfeffer JM, Pfeffer MA, Braunwald E. Influence of chronic captopril therapy on the infarcted left ventricle of the rat. Circulation Research 1985; 57:84–95.
41. Pfeffer JM, Pfeffer MA, Fletcher PJ, Braunwald E. Ventricular performance in rats with myocardial infarction and failure. Am J Med 1984; 76:99–103.
42. Pfeffer MA, Pfeffer JM. Ventricular enlargement and reduced survival after myocardial infarction. Circulation 1987; 75 (Suppl IV):IV93–IV97.
43. Gay RG. Early and late effects of captopril treatment after large myocardial infarction in rats. J Am Coll Cardiol 1990; 16:967–977.
44. Raya TE, Gay RG, Aguirre M, Goldman S. Importance of venodilatation in prevention of left ventricular dilatation after chronic large myocardial infarction in rats: A comparison of captopril and hydralazine. Circ Res 1989; 64:330–337.
45. Ray SG, Pye MP, Oldroyd KG, et al. Early treatment with captopril after acute myocardial infarction. Br Heart J 1993; 69:215–222.
46. Borghi C, Boschi S, Ambrosioni E, et al. Evidence of a partial

escape of renin-angiotensin-aldosterone blockade in patients with acute myocardial infarction treated with ACE inhibitors. J Clin Pharmacol 1993; 33:40–45.
47. Nabel EG, Topol EJ, Galeana A, et al. A randomized placebo-controlled trial of combined early intravenous captopril and recombinant tissue-type plasminogen activator therapy in acute myocardial infarction. J Am Coll Cardiol 1991; 17:467–473.
48. Flather M, Pipilis A, Conway M, et al. Early captopril treatment reduces angiotensin II levels after acute myocardial infarction. J Am Coll Cardiol 1992; 19:380A.
49. Gonzalez-Fernandez RA, Altieri PI, Lugo JE, Fernandez-Martinez J. Effects of enalapril on ventricular volumes and neurohormonal status after inferior wall myocardial infarction. Am J Med Sci 1993; 305:216–221.
50. Kingma JH, van Gilst WH, de Graeff P, et al. Captopril during thrombolysis in myocardial infarction: Feasibility, tolerance, and beneficial neurohumoral effects. *In* Sever P, McGregor G (eds). Current Advances in ACE Inhibition. Edinburgh, Churchill Livingstone, 1989, pp 291–295.
51. Vaughan DE, Lamas GA, Pfeffer MA. Role of ventricular dysfunction in selective neurohumoral activation in the recovery phase of anterior wall acute myocardial infarction. Am J Cardiol 1990; 66:529–532.
52. Sharpe N, Murphy J, Smith H, Hannan S. Treatment of patients with symptomless left ventricular dysfunction after myocardial infarction. Lancet 1988; 1:255–259.
53. Pfeffer MA, Lamas GA, Vaughan DE, et al. Effect of captopril on progressive ventricular dilatation after anterior myocardial infarction. N Engl J Med 1988; 319:80–86.
54. Sharpe N, Smith H, Murphy J, et al. Early prevention of left ventricular dysfunction after myocardial infarction with angiotensin-converting enzyme inhibition. Lancet 1991; 337:872–876.
55. Ambrosioni E, Borghi C, Magnani B. Early treatment of acute myocardial infarction with angiotensin-converting enzyme inhibition: Safety considerations. Am J Cardiol 1991; 68:101D–110D.
56. Oldroyd KG, Pye MP, Ray SG, et al. Effects of early captopril administration on infarct expansion, left ventricular remodeling, and exercise capacity after acute myocardial infarction. Am J Cardiol 1991; 68:713–718.
57. Gøtzsche C, Sogaard P, Ravkilde J, Thygesen K. Effects of captopril on left ventricular systolic and diastolic function after acute myocardial infarction. Am J Cardiol 1992; 70:156–160.
58. Pipilis A, Flather M, Collins R, et al. Hemodynamic effects of captopril and isosorbide mononitrate started early in acute myocardial infarction: A randomized placebo-controlled study. J Am Coll Cardiol 1993; 22:73–79.
59. Sutton MGSJ, Pfeffer M, Plappert T, et al. Quantitative two-dimensional echocardiographic measurements are major predictors of adverse cardiovascular events after acute myocardial infarction: The protective effects of captopril. Circulation 1994; 89:68–75.
60. Nicolosi GL, Latini R, Marino P, et al. The prognostic value of predischarge quantitative two-dimensional echocardiographic measurements and the effects of early lisinopril treatment of left ventricular structure and function after acute myocardial infarction in the GISSI-3 Trial. Eur Heart J 1996; 17:1646–1656.
61. Faxon DP, Creager MA, Halperin JL, et al. Central and peripheral hemodynamic effects of angiotensin inhibition in patients with refractory congestive heart failure. Circulation 1980; 61:925–930.
62. Dzau VJ, Colucci WS, Williams GH, et al. Sustained effectiveness of converting-enzyme inhibition in patients with severe congestive heart failure. N Engl J Med 1980; 302:1373–1379.
63. Brivet F, Delfraissy J, Giudicelli J, et al. Immediate effects of captopril in acute left ventricular failure secondary to myocardial infarction. Eur J Clin Invest 1981; 11:369–373.
64. Latini R, Avanzini F, De Nicolao A, et al, and GISSI-3 Investigators. Effects of lisinopril and nitroglycerin on blood pressure early after myocardial infarction: The GISSI-3 pilot study. Clin Trials Ther 1995; 56:680–692.
65. Flather M, Pipilis A, Collins R, et al. Randomised controlled trial of oral captopril, of oral isosorbide mononitrate, and of intravenous magnesium sulphate started early in acute myocardial infarction: Safety and haemodynamic effects. Eur Heart J 1994; 15:608–619.
66. Kingma JH, Van Gilst WH, Peels CH, et al. Acute intervention with captopril during thrombolysis in patients with first anterior myocardial infarction: Results from the Captopril and Thrombolysis Study (CATS). Eur Heart J 1994; 15:898–907.
67. Pfeffer MA, Braunwald E, Moyé LA, et al. Effect of captopril on mortality and morbidity in patients with left ventricular dysfunction after myocardial infarction (Survival and Ventriclar Enlargement [SAVE] Study). N Engl J Med 1992; 327:669–677.
68. The Acute Infarction Ramipril Efficacy (AIRE) Study Investigators. Effects of ramipril on mortality and morbidity of survivors of acute myocardial infarction with clinical evidence of heart failure. Lancet 1993; 342:821–828.
69. Kober L, Torp-Pedersen C, Carlsen JE, et al. A clinical trial of the angiotensin-converting enzyme inhibitor trandolapril in patients with left ventricular dysfunction after myocardial infarction. N Engl J Med 1995; 333:1670–1676.
70. Swedberg K, Held P, Kjekshus J, et al. Effects of the early administration of enalapril on mortality in patients with acute myocardial infarction: Results of the Cooperative New Scandinavian Enalapril Survival Study II (CONSENSUS II). N Engl J Med 1992; 327:678–684.
71. Gruppo Italiano per lo Studio della Sopravvivenza nell'Infarto Miocardico. GISSI-3: Effects of lisinopril and transdermal glyceryl trinitrate singly and together on 6-week mortality and ventricular function after acute myocardial infarction. Lancet 1994; 343:1115–1121.
72. ISIS-4 (Fourth International Study of Infarct Survival) Collaborative Group. ISIS-4: A randomised factorial trial assessing early oral captopril, oral mononitrate, and intravenous magnesium sulphate in 58,050 patients with suspected acute myocardial infarction. Lancet 1995; 345:669–685.
73. Chinese Cardiac Study Collaborative Group. Oral captopril versus placebo among 13,634 patients with suspected acute myocardial infarction: Interim report from the Chinese Cardiac Study (CCS-1). Lancet 1995; 345:686–687.
74. Ambrosioni E, Borghi C, Magnani B. The effect of the angiotensin-converting enzyme inhibitor zofenopril on mortality and morbidity after anterior myocardial infarction. N Engl J Med 1995; 332:80–85.
75. Furberg CD, Campbell RW, Pitt B. ACE inhibitors after myocardial infarction [Letter]. N Engl J Med 1993; 328:967–969.
76. Latini R, Maggioni A, Flather M, et al. ACE inhibitor use in patients with myocardial infarction. Circulation 1995; 92:3132–3137.
77. Flather MD, Kober L, Pfeffer MA, et al. Meta-analysis of individual patient data from trials of long-term ACE-inhibitor treatment after acute myocardial infarction. Circulation 1997; 96(Suppl):I-597.
78. ACE Inhibitor Myocardial Infarction Collaborative Group: Indications for ACE inhibitors in the early treatment of acute myocardial infarction: Systematic overview of individual data from 100,000 patients in randomized trials. Circulation 1998; in press.
79. Yusuf S, Pepine CJ, Garces C, et al. Effect of enalapril on myocardial infarction and unstable angina in patients with low ejection fraction. Lancet 1992; 340:1173–1178.
80. Pfeffer MA, Greaves SC, Arnold JM, et al. Early versus delayed angiotensin-converting enzyme inhibition therapy in acute myocardial infarction: The Healing and Afterload-Reducing Therapy Trial. Circulation 1997; 95:2643–2651.
81. Galcera-Tomas J, Antonio Nuno de la Rosa J, Torres-Martinez G, et al. Effects of early captopril use on haemodynamics and short-term ventricular remodelling in acute anterior myocardial infarction. Eur Heart J 1993; 14:259–266.
82. Kyriakidis MK, Petropoulakis PN, Georgiou EK, et al. The effects of early captopril treatment on left ventricular volumes and function in patients with and without depressed global ejection fraction after acute myocardial infarction. Eur Heart J 1993; 14:1692–1700.

11 Calcium Channel Blockers

▶ **David Waters**

Calcium channel blockers are a diverse group of compounds that act primarily on the L-type plasma membrane calcium channel.[1] Although more than 35 calcium channel blockers are available for clinical use in various parts of the world, the most widely used ones are verapamil, a phenylalkylamine; diltiazem, a benzothiazepine; and a large number of dihydropyridines, including nifedipine, nicardipine, nimodipine, nitrendipine, nisoldipine, amlodipine, isradipine, and felodipine.[2, 3] The chemical structures of these three classes differ substantially, as illustrated in Figure 11–1; however, the dihydropyridines all share the same basic structure, as shown in Figure 11–2. The physiologic effects of calcium channel blockade include coronary and peripheral vasodilation and reduced myocardial contractility. Verapamil and diltiazem share electrophysiologic effects such as atrioventricular nodal blockade and slowing of the heart rate, while some dihydropyridines induce a reflex increase in heart rate. These physiologic differences among various drugs of this class may account for some of the differences among them observed in clinical trials.

The two main indications for calcium channel blockers are the treatment of angina and hypertension. For angina, many short-term studies have demonstrated that these drugs prolong treadmill exercise time and reduce episodes of myocardial ischemia during daily life.[4–9] Diltiazem and verapamil accomplish these objectives more effectively than do the dihydropyridines.[10] For hypertension, calcium channel blockers are attractive therapy because they are perceived as having a better side effect profile than alternative drugs, and because they lack the adverse metabolic consequences of diuretics and most beta blockers. However, controlled trials to demonstrate that calcium channel blockers reduce mortality or prevent stroke and myocardial infarction (MI) in hypertensive patients are almost entirely lacking.

Calcium channel blockers have been evaluated in controlled clinical trials for the prevention of coronary events post-MI; unstable angina; prevention of progression of coronary and carotid atherosclerosis; heart failure; and preservation of neurologic function during stroke, cardiac arrest, and open heart surgery. These trials are reviewed in this chapter.

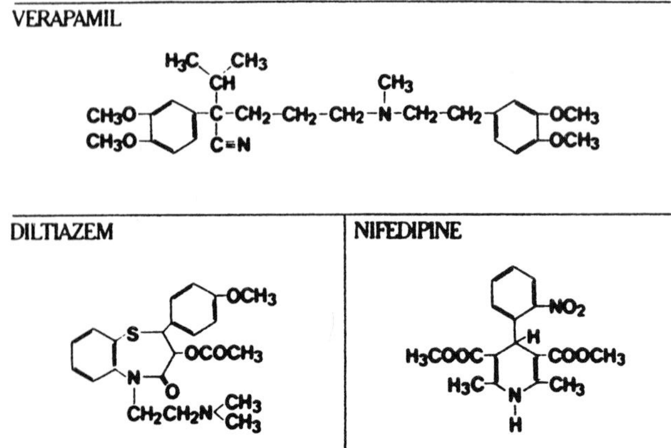

Figure 11–1 Chemical structures of verapamil (a phenylalkylamine), diltiazem (a benzothiazepine), and nifedipine (a dihydropyridine).

TRIALS DURING AND AFTER MYOCARDIAL INFARCTION

When calcium channel blockers became available in the early 1980s, clinical trials were launched in an attempt to demonstrate that these drugs reduced post-MI mortality and reinfarction rates, as had been shown for beta blockers in the preceding 5 years. Several lines of reasoning suggested that calcium channel blockers would be effective in this circumstance. Coronary spasm was then considered to be a major pathophysiologic mechanism responsible for MI,[11] and these drugs effectively blocked spasm.[12] They also decreased myocardial oxygen consumption as beta blockers did, and they had the added advantage of being coronary vasodilators.[12] In animal models, calcium channel blockers reduced myocardial ischemic injury, and they were thus called *cardioprotective*.[13]

By 1989, 22 randomized trials of calcium channel blockers after MI had been published, involving 18,000 patients.[14] Verapamil was used in three trials

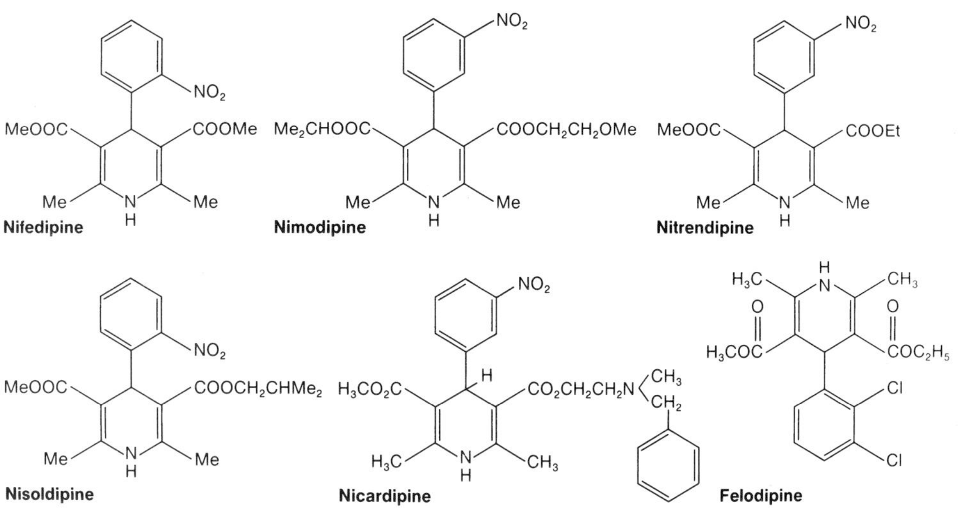

Figure 11–2 Basic chemical structures of the dihydropyridines.

with 3500 patients, nifedipine in 13 trials with 9700 patients, diltiazem in 4 trials with 3100 patients, and lidoflazine and tiapamil in 1 trial each.[14] The duration of these studies ranged from 24 hours to 6 weeks in 17 trials, and from 6 months to 5 years in the other 5 trials. Held and associates[14] concluded in their overview of these data that calcium channel blockers did not reduce the risk of recurrent infarction or death when routinely given to patients with acute MI. The more important of these trials are described in the following sections.

Secondary Prevention Reinfarction Israeli Nifedipine Trials (SPRINT 1 and 2)

SPRINT 1 enrolled 2276 men and women in 14 Israeli hospitals between 7 and 21 days after MI to nifedipine 30 mg per day or placebo.[15] The average follow-up was 10 months, and the endpoints were total mortality and recurrent infarction. The mortality rate was 5.7% in the placebo group and 5.8% in the nifedipine group; reinfarction rates were 4.8% and 4.4%, respectively. The authors concluded that the drug as used in this trial had no effect on cardiac events.

SPRINT 2 was undertaken to test the hypothesis that nifedipine would reduce mortality and recurrent infarction if given in the early hours of infarction in higher doses to high-risk patients.[16] Treatment was usually begun within 3 hours of admission, and the dose was titrated up to 60 mg per day within the first 6 days. Of 1358 men and women initially enrolled, treatment was discontinued in 352 who did not develop the criteria for high-risk infarction. The trial was stopped prematurely because of an excess mortality in the nifedipine group: 18.7% versus 15.6% overall and 7.8% versus 5.5% during the first 6 days (adjusted odds ratio, 1.60; 95% confidence interval, 0.86 to 3.00). Nonfatal reinfarction occurred in 5.1% of nifedipine-treated patients and in 4.2% of controls, a nonsignificant (NS) difference. The authors concluded that nifedipine "may be hazardous and seems to be contraindicated" early after MI.

Diltiazem Reinfarction Study

The Diltiazem Reinfarction Study was designed to assess whether diltiazem reduced the early risk of reinfarction when administered beginning 24 to 72 hours after the onset of a non–Q wave MI.[17] The trial enrolled 576 men and women, employed a diltiazem dose of 360 mg per day, and defined reinfarction as an abnormal re-elevation of CK-MB within 14 days of the initial event. Blood samples were drawn every 12 hours to measure CK-MB levels, and the average duration of follow-up was 10.5 days. Reinfarction was detected in 9.3% of placebo patients and 5.2% of diltiazem patients, a difference that was statistically significant ($P = 0.0297$), but with a one-sided test. Mortality was slightly but not significantly higher in the diltiazem group (3.8% vs. 3.1%).

Multicenter Diltiazem Postinfarction Trial (MDPIT)

The primary objective of MDPIT was to determine whether long-term therapy with diltiazem in patients with previous infarction would reduce the rates of mortality and reinfarction.[18] In 38 hospitals in the United States and Canada, 2466 men and women were randomized to placebo or diltiazem 240 mg per day, 3 to 15 days after MI. Patients were followed for a minimum of 12 months and a mean of 25 months. Total mortality rates (13.5%) were nearly identical in the two groups. There were 11% fewer first recurrent cardiac events (cardiac death or nonfatal reinfarction) in the diltiazem group (Cox hazard ratio, 0.90; 95% confidence intervals, 0.74 to 1.08). The authors reported an important interaction between treatment assignment and the presence or absence of pulmonary congestion on the baseline chest x-ray, one of 12 preselected covariates. In 490 patients with pulmonary congestion, diltiazem was associated with an increased number of cardiac events (hazard ratio, 1.41; 95% confidence intervals, 1.01 to 1.96), but in 1909 patients without this finding, the hazard ratio was 0.77 (95% confidence intervals, 0.61 to 0.98). The authors concluded that the overall effect of diltiazem on cardiac events after MI was neutral, reflecting a reduction of such events in patients with good left ventricular function, counterbalanced by an increase in events in patients with left ventricular dysfunction.

In a follow-up report, the effects of diltiazem in MDPIT patients with signs of left ventricular dysfunction were explored in greater detail.[19] In patients with anterolateral Q wave infarctions, pulmonary congestion on x-ray or an ejection fraction below 0.40 at baseline, heart failure developed during follow-up in 21% of diltiazem-treated patients versus 12% of controls ($P = 0.004$). The cardiac mortality rate was 34 (35%) of 96 in diltiazem-treated patients who developed heart failure and 18 (22%) of 81 in placebo-treated patients developing failure ($P = 0.055$). Among patients with an ejection fraction above 0.40, heart failure was not more common in diltiazem-treated patients than in controls. The authors recommended that diltiazem not be used in postinfarction patients with left ventricular dysfunction.

Danish Study Group on Verapamil in Myocardial Infarction (DAVIT-I and DAVIT-II)

DAVIT-I randomized 1436 MI patients to verapamil 120 mg tid or placebo as soon as possible after admission and followed them for 6 months.[20] The primary endpoints were total mortality and reinfarction rates. The differences in mortality (12.8% in verapamil-treated vs. 13.8% in placebo patients) and in reinfarction (7.0% vs. 8.3%, respectively) were not statistically significant, but a retrospective analysis of the data showed a survival and a reinfarction advantage favoring verapamil between days 22 and 180 of follow-up. This finding inspired DAVIT-II.

The purpose of DAVIT-II was to ascertain whether verapamil given from the second week after acute infarction for 12 to 18 months might reduce total mortality and the combined endpoint of death or reinfarction.[21] A total of 1775 patients were randomized to placebo or the same dose of verapamil used in DAVIT-I. The mortality rate was 11.1% in the verapamil group and 13.8% in the control group (hazard ratio, 0.80; 95% confidence intervals, 0.61 to 1.05). Death or reinfarction occurred in 18.0% of verapamil patients and in 21.6% of placebo patients (hazard ratio, 0.80; 95% confidence intervals, 0.64 to 0.99). Nine subgroups were selected before the data were analyzed, and differences were seen for one of them: in patients without heart failure in the coronary care unit, the verapamil group had a significantly lower mortality, 7.7% compared with 11.8% ($P = 0.02$). In this respect, the results of DAVIT-II are congruent with those of MDPIT.

Current Overview of Postinfarction Trials

The overview of Held and associates[14] in 1989 pooled data for all calcium channel blockers. An updated overview published in 1991 distinguished between the calcium channel blockers that slow heart rate—diltiazem and verapamil—and those that tend to increase heart rate—the dihydropyridines.[22] Following the publication of another verapamil postinfarction trial in 1996,[23] Yusuf recalculated the odds ratios for the major endpoints for this drug.[24] A composite of the data for the three main drugs is presented in Table 11–1.

A 13% increase in mortality and a 14% increase in reinfarction are seen with nifedipine. For neither of these endpoints is the difference significant; however, as discussed later, similar trends have been seen with nifedipine and with other dihydropyridines when these drugs were used in other circumstances. Diltiazem and verapamil had no effect on overall mortality, but both drugs tended to reduce reinfarction, with odds ratios of 0.79 and 0.81, respectively. The reduction in reinfarction rates was of borderline statistical significance for both diltiazem and verapamil. Borderline significance for clinical benefit from pooled data should be interpreted with great caution.

How should this information be applied to clinical practice? Calcium channel blockers should not be used routinely in patients who survive MI, and a dihydropyridine should be used only when a compelling indication exists, such as documented coronary spasm uncontrolled by other drugs. Diltiazem and verapamil are contraindicated in postinfarction patients with moderate or severe left ventricular dysfunction.

TRIALS IN UNSTABLE ANGINA

Calcium channel blockers were expected to be beneficial for the treatment of unstable angina for many of the same reasons they were expected to be useful

TABLE 11–1 • Current Overview of Postinfaction Trials

	Drug	Placebo	Odds Ratio	95% Confidence Interval
Diltiazem				
Death	180/1574 (11.4%)	181/1577 (11.5%)	0.99	0.80 to 1.24
Reinfarction	113/1557 (7.3%)	142/1560 (9.1%)	0.79	0.61 to 1.02
Nifedipine				
Death	365/4731 (7.7%)	330/4733 (7.0%)	1.13	0.97 to 1.32
Reinfarction	124/3645 (3.4%)	111/3680 (3.0%)	1.14	0.68 to 1.92
Verapamil				
Death	274/3175 (8.6%)	295/3191 (9.2%)	0.93	0.78 to 1.10
Reinfarction	179/3137 (5.7%)	222/3166 (7.0%)	0.81	0.67 to 0.98

Adapted from Held et al,[14] Yusuf et al,[15] and Yusuf.[16]

after MI. These drugs proved to be extremely effective in preventing angina[12] and improving the long-term outcome of patients with variant angina.[25] Coronary spasm, the cause of variant angina, was assumed to play a major role in other coronary syndromes, including unstable angina.[26, 27] The dominant role of plaque rupture with overlying thrombus formation was not appreciated in the late 1970s and early 1980s when calcium channel blockers became available for clinical investigation.

The clinical trials of calcium channel blockers for unstable angina are of limited value for several reasons. First, the primary purpose of these trials was usually to ascertain whether calcium channel blockers controlled symptoms, either compared to placebo or to a beta blocker. Thus, the studies lacked the power to show differences in less common but more important endpoints such as MI or death. Compared with the postinfarction trials, the number of patients enrolled in all of the unstable angina trials of calcium channel blockers is small indeed. The duration of follow-up ranged from only 48 hours to less than 6 months, and in some of the studies an unusually high proportion of the patients had evidence of coronary spasm, a factor favoring the calcium channel blocker. Aspirin and heparin—treatments now known to decrease substantially the infarct rate in unstable angina—were not routinely used in these trials. Their applicability to current practice is thus somewhat questionable.

Table 11–2 lists the main trials of calcium channel blockers for unstable angina, with the MI rate and mortality rate for the active treatment and control groups. Gerstenblith and colleagues[28] added nifedipine or placebo to standard medical treatment in 138 patients with unstable angina and followed them for 4 months. They concluded that the drug was "safe and effective" because it reduced the combined endpoint of death, MI, or need for coronary bypass surgery. The benefit was particularly marked in patients with transient ST elevation, where coronary spasm was likely to be the cause. The MI and mortality rates did not differ between the nifedipine and placebo groups, as shown in Table 11–2.

The largest unstable angina trial was the Holland Interuniversity Nifedipine/Metoprolol Trial (HINT).[29] HINT was discontinued after an interim analysis of the first 593 randomized patients showed an increased MI rate in the nifedipine group (relative risk, 2.0; 95% confidence interval, 1.1 to 3.6). Overall, 668 patients were enrolled, but results were not reported for the 153 patients who had protocol violations or

TABLE 11–2 • Randomized Trials of Calcium Channel Blockers (CCBs) in Unstable Angina

				MI Rate		Mortality Rate	
Study, Year	CCB	Comparison Treatment	Duration of Follow-Up	*CCB*	*Control*	*CCB*	*Control*
Gerstenblith, 1982[28]	Nifedipine	Placebo	4 mo	11/68 (16%)	12/70 (17%)	7/68 (10%)	5/70 (7%)
HINT, 1986[29]	Nifedipine	Placebo	48 h	38/185 (21%)	29/165 (18%)	—	—
Muller, 1984[30]	Nifedipine	Propranolol/nitrates	14 d	9/63 (14%)	9/63 (14%)	4/63 (6%)	0/63 (0%)
Theroux, 1985[31]	Diltiazem	Propranolol	5.1 mo	5/50 (10%)	4/50 (8%)	2/50 (4%)	2/50 (4%)
Andre-Fouer, 1983[32]	Diltiazem	Propranolol	48 h	3/34 (9%)	1/36 (3%)	0/34 (0%)	0/36 (0%)
Totals				**66/400 (16.5%)**	**55/384 (14.3%)**	**13/215 (6.0%)**	**7/219 (3.2%)**

MI, myocardial infarction.

MI prerandomization. Among evaluated patients not previously taking a beta blocker, the adjusted odds ratio for MI for nifedipine compared with placebo was 1.51 (95% confidence interval, 0.87 to 2.74); however, the combination of nifedipine and metoprolol, or the addition of nifedipine in patients already taking a beta blocker, was not associated with an increased rate of infarction. Most of the infarctions in HINT occurred within the first few hours after enrollment, and the duration of follow-up for this event was only 48 hours.

Muller and coworkers[30] randomized 126 unstable angina patients to nifedipine or isosorbide dinitrate plus propranolol and followed them for 14 days. Both treatments relieved angina equally well, and in each group 9 of 63 patients developed MI. Although not highlighted in the paper, 4 deaths occurred, all in patients randomized to nifedipine.

Data from controlled trials in unstable angina are sparse for other calcium channel blockers. As shown in Table 11–2, diltiazem was compared with propranolol in two trials. Theroux and associates[31] randomized 100 patients and followed them for 5.1 months; Andre-Fouet and colleagues[32] enrolled 70 patients and evaluated them over 48 hours. Neither study revealed differences between the two drugs.

Taken together, the studies in unstable angina demonstrate that while calcium channel blockers may be helpful to control symptoms, they do not prevent MI or reduce mortality. Used alone, nifedipine increases the risk of MI. This increased risk appears to be attenuated if a beta blocker is given with nifedipine. The trials comparing diltiazem with propranolol lack the power to detect differences in important endpoints. No trial data are available for other calcium channel blockers in unstable angina.

ANGIOGRAPHIC TRIALS OF CORONARY PROGRESSION

A large body of experimental evidence from animal models suggests that calcium channel blockers should favorably influence the development and progression of human atherosclerosis.[33, 34] The model that has been used most extensively in these experiments is the cholesterol-fed rabbit. Rabbits fed a 1% to 2% cholesterol diet for 8 to 12 weeks develop serum cholesterol levels in the range of 2000 mg/dL, massive hepatic lipid accumulation, and diffuse aortic atherosclerosis characterized by an abundance of lipid-laden foam cells. The features of this type of atherosclerosis and the time course of its development obviously differ greatly from human atherosclerosis. In this model, many dihydropyridines, diltiazem, and verapamil all have been shown to retard the evolution of atherosclerosis.[33, 34] Nifedipine and amlodipine also suppress atherogenesis in monkeys, a model more relevant to human atherosclerosis. Table 11–3 lists the mechanisms that have been proposed to explain the antiatherogenic effect of calcium channel blockers.

TABLE 11–3 • Potential Explanations for the Antiatherogenic Effect of Calcium Channel Blockers

Reduction of arterial pressure
Antithrombotic and antiplatelet activity
Preservation of endothelial function
Antioxidant activity
Reduction of intracellular lipid accumulation by stimulating cholesteryl ester hydrolase activity
Inhibition of smooth muscle cell proliferation in response to growth factors
Inhibition of smooth muscle cell migration
Promotion of cholesterol efflux and preventing cholesteryl ester deposition in macrophages

International Nifedipine Trial on Antiatherosclerotic Therapy (INTACT)

The primary purpose of INTACT was to determine whether nifedipine retarded the progression of coronary atherosclerosis; a secondary objective was to determine whether this drug prevented the formation of new coronary lesions.[35] Among 425 patients with "mild coronary disease" at angiography, randomized to placebo or nifedipine 20 mg qid, 348 (82%) underwent repeat coronary arteriography 3 years later, with lesions measured by a computerized quantitative system, as shown in Figure 11–3. Nifedipine had no effect on progression or regression of established coronary lesions, the main aim of the trial, and the proportion of patients who developed new lesions was not significantly different between the two groups. However, the number of new lesions per patient was 0.59 in the nifedipine group and 0.82 in controls ($P = 0.034$). Figure 11–4 illustrates a new coronary lesion. The authors concluded that "nifedipine substantially suppresses disease progression as shown by the appearance of new lesions."[35]

Montreal Heart Institute Trial

Waters and coworkers[36] randomized 383 patients with diffuse but not necessarily severe coronary disease at angiography to placebo or nicardipine 30 mg tid. In 335 patients (87%), coronary arteriography was repeated after 2 years, and the angiograms were analyzed using a quantitative system. Nicardipine had

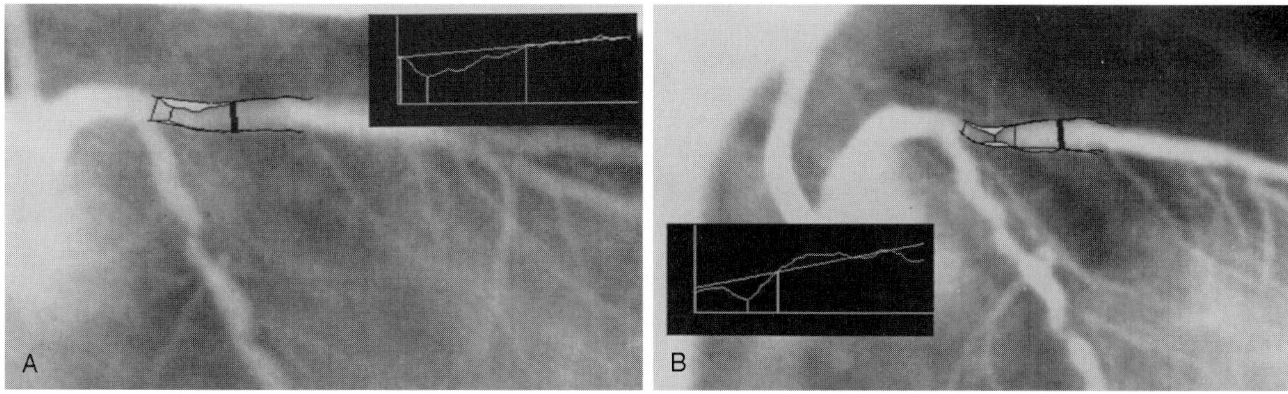

Figure 11–3 Example of progression of a coronary atherosclerotic lesion as demonstrated by quantitative coronary arteriography. At baseline *(A)*, a moderated stenosis is seen in the proximal left anterior descending coronary artery. The black panel in the top right corner of the illustration shows the diameter of the artery on the vertical axis and distance down the vessel on the horizontal axis. The minimum luminal diameter is 1.26 mm and the diameter stenosis is 52.5%. Follow-up angiography 2 years later *(B)* shows that the minimum luminal diameter is now 0.58 mm and the diameter stenosis is 77.3%. Patients with progression are at increased risk for future coronary events.

no effect on progression or regression of coronary atherosclerosis, the primary endpoint of the trial. However, for minimal coronary lesions (those 20% diameter stenosis at baseline), an effect similar to the results of INTACT was seen. Minimal lesions progressed in 15 of 99 nicardipine patients with such lesions at baseline, compared with 32 of 118 placebo patients ($P = 0.046$). On a per-lesion basis, 16 of 178 nicardipine and 38 of 233 placebo minimal lesions progressed ($P = 0.038$). The authors concluded that nicardipine has no effect on advanced coronary atherosclerosis but may retard the progression of minimal lesions.

Diltiazem and Coronary Atherosclerosis After Cardiac Transplantation

Schroeder and associates[37] randomly assigned 104 cardiac transplant recipients to diltiazem 60 to 90 mg tid or to no calcium channel blocker and reported the angiographic results on the 57 patients who had angiograms at baseline plus 1 and 2 years later. Coronary arterial diameters decreased in untreated patients ($P < 0.001$) but not in patients who received diltiazem; the differences between the groups was statistically significant ($P < 0.001$). Limitations of this trial include its unblinded nature, the incomplete angiographic follow-up, and the fact that diltiazem, a coronary vasodilator, was discontinued only 24 hours before angiography.

Multicenter Isradipine/Diuretic Atherosclerosis Study (MIDAS)

MIDAS randomized 883 men and women with hypertension and a carotid intimal-medial thickness between 1.3 and 3.5 mm to isradipine 5 or 10 mg per day or to hydrochlorthiazide 25 or 50 mg per day.[38]

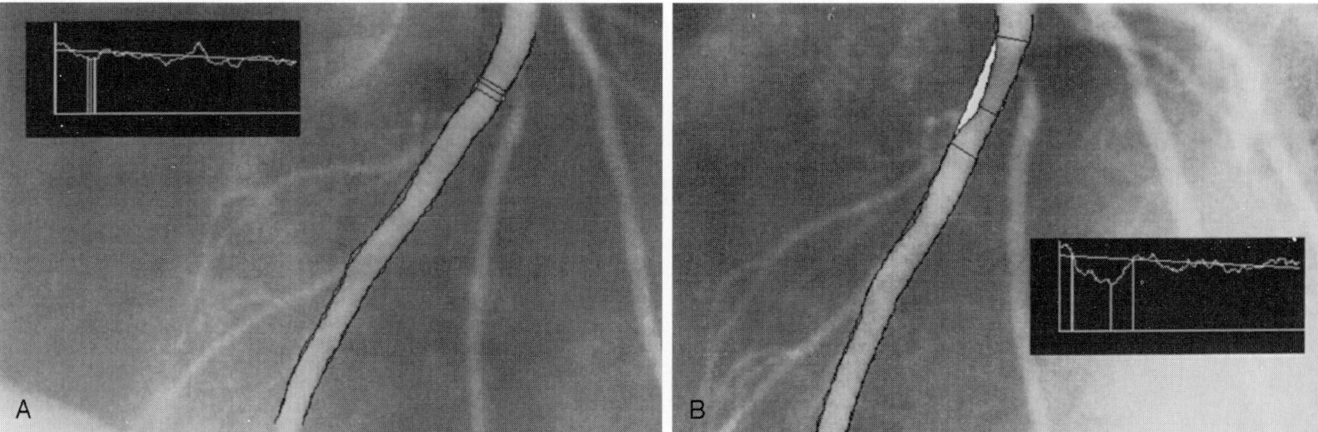

Figure 11–4 Example of the development of a new coronary lesion as assessed by quantitative coronary arteriography. At baseline *(A)*, the edges of the left anterior descending coronary artery are relatively smooth. At follow-up angiography *(B)*, a narrowing reduces the minimum luminal diameter from 2.41 to 1.55 mm, producing a 36% diameter stenosis. New coronary lesions are important because they have the potential to progress by means of plaque rupture to produce clinical coronary events.

The endpoint of MIDAS was based on changes in carotid intimal-medial thickness over 36 months as measured by B-mode echo. This parameter changed erratically over the course of the trial: at 6 months a large increase was observed in the hydrochlorthiazide group but not in the isradipine group. Between 24 and 36 months, intimal-medial thickness steeply increased in both groups. The difference at 6 months is unlikely to be due to a difference in the rate of progression of carotid atherosclerosis, and the late increase in both groups is perhaps best explained by a variation in the measurement technique.

Cardiovascular Events in Angiographic Trials

Table 11–4 summarizes the mortality, MI, and cardiovascular event rates in the four angiographic trials. All-cause mortality was increased in the nifedipine group in INTACT[35] ($P < 0.01$). A trend toward more MIs was seen in the nicardipine group in the trial of Waters and associates,[36] and the increased cardiovascular event rate in the isradipine group in MIDAS[38] was of borderline statistical significance ($P = 0.07$). Viewed in isolation, these findings suggest that the dihydropyridine calcium channel blockers increase risk in patients with documented coronary disease or peripheral atherosclerosis. Taken together with the results of the postinfarction and unstable angina trials discussed earlier, the case against the dihydropyridines becomes strong and consistent.

TRIALS IN STABLE ANGINA

The Angina Prognosis Study in Stockholm (APSIS) randomized 809 men and women with stable angina pectoris to metoprolol 200 mg daily or to verapamil 240 mg bid and followed them for a mean of 3.4 years.[39] The primary endpoints were death, cardiovascular events, and psychological variables reflecting quality of life. The mortality rate was 5.4% in the metoprolol group and 6.2% in the verapamil group; the rates of nonfatal cardiovascular events were 26.1% and 24.3%, respectively. Neither of these differences approached statistical significance. The quality of life assessments also did not differ between the two groups.

The Total Ischemic Burden European Trial (TIBET)[40] was a double-blind, randomized comparison of atenolol 50 mg bid, nifedipine SR 20 or 40 mg bid, and the combination in 682 patients, with a follow-up of 2 years. For the endpoints of the trial, the respective results for the 226 atenolol and 232 nifedipine SR were 3 and 6 patients for cardiac death, 14 and 15 for nonfatal infarction, 12 and 4 for unstable angina, 7 and 6 for coronary bypass surgery, and 1 and 0 for coronary angioplasty. None of these differences approached statistical significance; however, a trend was seen in favor of patients treated with the combination.

Most studies of calcium channel blockers in stable angina used endpoints derived from exercise testing or ambulatory electrocardiographic monitoring, and thus rarely exposed patients to drug for more than a few weeks or months. Patients who experienced coronary events during these studies were often reported as dropouts, and in some studies no mention at all was made of coronary events. In 1991, Glasser and colleagues[41] surveyed all dropouts in the angina trials reported to the U.S. Food and Drug Administration in support of new drug applications. Cardiovascular events were defined as death, MI, ventricular tachycardia, other serious arrhythmia causing the patient to discontinue drug, and other cardiovascular signs or symptoms causing the patient to drop out. The odds ratio for these events for calcium channel blockers compared with placebo was 1.63 (95% confidence interval, 1.02 to 2.59). The drugs included in these trials were bepredil, diltiazem, lidoflazine, nicardipine, and verapamil.

Nisoldipine was also associated with an increased cardiovascular event rate in a study of stable angina patients reported later in 1991.[42] During only 2 weeks

TABLE 11–4 • Cardiovascular Events and Mortality in Angiographic Trials

		Mortality		Myocardial Infarction		Cardiovascular Events*	
Study, Year	**Drug**	*Drug*	*Control*	*Drug*	*Control*	*Drug*	*Control*
INTACT, 1990[35]	Nifedipine	12 (6.9%)	2 (1.1%)†	11 (6.4%)	9 (5.1%)	52 (30%)	44 (25%)
Waters, 1990[36]	Nicardipine	2 (1.0%)	3 (1.6%)	14 (7.3%)	8 (4.2%)	28 (14.6%)	23 (12%)
Schroeder, 1993[37]	Diltiazem	16 (30%)	11 (21%)	NA	NA	NA	NA
MIDAS, 1996[38]	Isradipine	NA	NA	6 (1.4%)	5 (1.1%)	25 (5.7%)‡	14 (3.2%)‡

*Cardiovascular events defined differently among trials.
†$P < 0.02$.
‡$P < 0.07$.
NA, data not available.

of treatment with nisoldipine in 137 patients, 2 died suddenly, 4 developed unstable angina, and 4 others experienced worsening angina. In 48 placebo patients, the only event was worsening angina in one patient. Both deaths occurred at the highest nisoldipine dose, 10 mg bid, and the authors suggested that a dose-response relationship might be present for coronary events. As discussed in the accompanying editorial,[43] proischemic complications with nisoldipine were not reported in the limited number of other stable angina studies. Drug-induced reflex tachycardia associated with a decrease in coronary perfusion pressure was proposed as the most likely cause of proischemic complications. Other investigators have reported that nifedipine worsens exercise-induced ischemia in patients with coronary collaterals and have concluded that a coronary steal is the mechanism involved.[44, 45]

TRIALS IN HEART FAILURE

Vasodilator therapy has become a key component in the management of patients with symptomatic left ventricular failure. Furthermore, as discussed in Chapter 10, angiotensin-converting enzyme inhibitors not only improve symptoms and survival in congestive heart failure but also prevent deterioration of ventricular function in patients with depressed ejection fractions. Calcium channel blockers initially held enormous appeal as therapy for heart failure, in part because the side effect profile of this class of drugs is relatively benign, and in part because many patients with heart failure also have symptoms of myocardial ischemia that could also benefit from this treatment.

By the late 1980s it was apparent that calcium channel blockers had not fulfilled their promise in heart failure.[46] Dramatic deterioration occurred in some heart failure patients with the first dose of nifedipine, the first-generation calcium channel blocker most likely to provide benefit. Most patients experienced short-term hemodynamic improvement; however, this proved illusory: Elkayam and coworkers[47] found that clinical deterioration occurred significantly more often in heart failure patients randomized to nifedipine compared with controls. The inherent negative inotropic effects of calcium channel blockade best explained then why these drugs fail in heart failure.[48, 49]

Second-generation calcium channel blockers, such as nicardipine, nisoldipine, nitrendipine, felodipine, amlodipine, and isradipine, were designed to exert less negative inotropic effect than drugs from the first generation, but to exhibit similar or even enhanced coronary and systemic vasodilator activity.[49] Initial hemodynamic improvement is seen in nearly all heart failure patients treated with these newer drugs, but even when sustained, hemodynamic improvement is not associated with better exercise tolerance.[49–51] Instead, long-term therapy has been associated with fluid retention and clinical deterioration.[49–51] The reason why newer calcium channel blockers fail to improve patients with heart failure may not be their negative inotropic effects, since beta blockers often result in long-term improvement in such cases, but rather stimulation of the release of vasoconstrictor neurohormones.[50]

Prospective Randomized Amlodipine Survival Evaluation (PRAISE)

The PRAISE Trial randomized 1153 patients with New York Heart Association Class 3 or 4 heart failure to placebo or amlodipine, with continuation of other standard heart failure therapy.[52] For the primary endpoint, death from any cause plus hospitalization for major cardiovascular events, there was a 9% reduction with amlodipine (95% confidence intervals, −24% to +10%; $P = 0.31$). Similarly, for total mortality, a secondary endpoint, the 16% reduction in favor of amlodipine, 33% versus 38% (95% confidence intervals, −31% to +2%; $P = 0.07$), did not attain statistical significance. The predefined hypothesis that a mortality benefit might be seen in patients with coronary disease and heart failure was not confirmed. In fact, a 46% mortality reduction, from 31% to 18%, was seen in patients with heart failure without coronary disease (95% confidence intervals, 21% to 63% reduction; $P < 0.001$). These results suggest that amlodipine exerts a beneficial effect on survival in heart failure, but that the benefit may be mitigated in coronary patients by the same increased mortality risk seen with earlier dihydropyridines.

Trials in Specific Types of Heart Failure

The results of the PRAISE Trial raise the possibility that calcium channel blockers might improve outcomes in heart failure caused by specific etiologies, such as cardiomyopathy. The Diltiazem in Dilated Cardiomyopathy Trial[53] provides supportive evidence: 186 patients with this condition were randomized to diltiazem 60 to 90 mg tid or placebo and followed for 24 months. The short-term improvement in hemodynamic measures and exercise capacity persisted long term, and a trend was seen toward better survival without being listed for transplant.

Another specific niche where a calcium channel blocker has been reported to be effective is the asymptomatic patient with severe aortic regurgitation. Scognamiglio and associates[54] randomized 143 such patients without blinding to nifedipine 20 mg bid or to

TABLE 11–5 • New Trials of Calcium Channel Blockers (CCBs) in Hypertension

Trial Acronym	CCB	Other Drug	N
ALLHAT	Amlodipine	Diuretic, lisopril, doxazosin	40,000
CONVINCE	Verapamil	Thiazide, beta blocker	15,000
HOT	Felodipine	Diuretic, ACE inhibitor, beta blocker	18,000
INSIGHT	Nifedipine	Amiloride, hydrochlorthiazide	6,600
NORDIC	Nifedipine	Conventional therapy	12,000
STOP	CCBs	Diuretic, ACE inhibitor	6,600

digoxin 0.25 mg daily. After 6 years, 15% of the nifedipine patients and 34% of the digoxin patients had undergone aortic valve replacement ($P < 0.001$). The indication for valve replacement was left ventricular dysfunction, defined as an ejection fraction by echocardiography of less than 50%. The benefit of nifedipine in this trial was attributed to its ability to decrease systolic and diastolic blood pressures and left ventricular mass and volume in severe aortic regurgitation, a situation perhaps analogous to severe hypertension but not to other usual causes of heart failure.

TRIALS IN HYPERTENSION

A large body of evidence from clinical trials clearly indicates that treatment of hypertension reduces total mortality, stroke, and to a lesser extent, MI.[55] Treatment also has a favorable effect on progression to severe hypertension, progression of left ventricular hypertrophy, and progression to heart failure, three powerful predictors of adverse outcomes.[56] The drugs used in these trials were diuretics, beta blockers, and older agents such as methyldopa, hydralazine, and reserpine. In the mid-1980s, calcium channel blockers (and angiotensin-converting enzyme inhibitors) were approved for the treatment of hypertension, based on their demonstrated ability to lower blood pressure safely and effectively in short-term studies. Calcium channel blockers have been shown to produce other benefits in hypertensives, such as a reduction in left ventricular mass. But they have not yet been evaluated in large, long-term clinical trials powered to prove that they reduce mortality, stroke, and MI or are equivalent to the drugs that have been proven to do so. In spite of this limitation, calcium channel blockers have been widely prescribed for hypertension.

The Systolic Hypertension in Europe (Syst-Eur) Trial is the first to address these long-term concerns.[57] A total of 4695 patients aged 60 years or older, with systolic blood pressures 160 mm Hg or higher and diastolic pressures lower than 95 mm Hg, were randomized to nitrendipine 10 to 40 mg/day or placebo. At 2 years of follow-up, active treatment was associated with a 44% (95% CI 14 to 63%) reduction in stroke, a 33% (95% CI 3 to 53%) reduction in cardiac endpoints (heart failure, myocardial infarction), but no significant reduction in all-cause mortality.

In 1995, Psaty and coworkers[58] published a case-control study that found an increased risk of MI in hypertensive patients taking a calcium channel blocker (nifedipine, diltiazem, or verapamil) compared with a beta blocker (relative risk, 1.57; 95% confidence intervals, 1.21 to 2.04). This report raised a storm of controversy and editorial comment.

As listed in Table 11–5, at least six large, randomized trials have been launched to compare calcium channel blockers with other forms of therapy for hypertension.[59, 60] These trials are scheduled to enroll nearly 100,000 patients but will mostly not be completed until after the year 2000.

CEREBROVASCULAR TRIALS

Cell death caused by ischemic injury is associated with an influx of calcium, and calcium channel blockers have been shown to prevent this influx and reduce ischemic injury in animal models. A limitation of this form of therapy is that much of the potential benefit is lost if the drug cannot be administered before the ischemic insult. Calcium channel blockers have been assessed in stroke, in subarachnoid hemorrhage, in comatose survivors of cardiac arrest, and for "neuroprotection" during cardiopulmonary bypass. Nimodipine was the drug used in most of these trials because of its comparative selectivity for the cerebral circulation.[3]

Gelmers and associates[61] randomized 168 patients with acute ischemic stroke to nimodipine 30 mg every 6 hours or placebo, with total mortality and neurologic outcome at 28 days as the primary endpoints. Fewer nimodipine patients died: at the end of 1 month when treatment was stopped, 8 of 93 nimodipine and 19 of 93 placebo patients had died, and this difference persisted to 6 months ($P = 0.046$). Neurologic outcome as assessed by the Matthew scale was also significantly better in the active treatment group.

Ohman and Heiskanen[62] randomized 213 patients with aneurysmal subarachnoid hemorrhage to nimodipine or placebo. Overall mortality was not significantly reduced in the nimodipine group, but in the subset of those undergoing early or subacute surgery, a mortality advantage in favor of nimodipine was reported. Pickard and colleagues[63] enrolled 554 patients with subarachnoid hemorrhage into a double-blind, randomized trial comparing nimodipine 60 mg every 4 hours to placebo, with cerebral infarction and a poor neurologic outcome as endpoints. The incidence of cerebral infarction was lower in the nimodipine group (61 [22%] of 278 compared with 92 [33%] of 276 control patients) (risk reduction, 34%; 95% confidence interval, 13% to 50%). Poor outcomes were also significantly reduced, from 33% in controls to 20% in the nimodipine group.

Roine and coworkers[64] randomized 155 consecutive patients resuscitated from out-of-hospital ventricular fibrillation to intravenous nimodipine or placebo, with survival and overall outcome at 1 year as the primary endpoint. No significant differences were found between the groups. However, 10 of 75 nimodipine and 2 of 80 placebo patients died during the 24 hours of treatment ($P = 0.01$). In a similar trial, 522 patients with cardiac arrest who remained comatose after restoration of spontaneous circulation were randomized to lidoflazine, an experimental calcium channel blocker, or placebo.[65] Lidoflazine was not beneficial with respect to the primary endpoint and recovery of cerebral function, and the mortality rate at 6 months was the same in both groups. However, the incidence of any cardiovascular complication, hypotension, or another nonfatal arrest was higher in the lidoflazine group during the 24 hours of treatment, 69% versus 60% ($P = 0.02$).

Wagenknecht and associates[66] performed a randomized, double-blind, placebo-controlled trial among patients undergoing cardiac valve replacement to determine whether nimodipine reduced the combined incidence of neurologic, neuro-ophthalmologic, and neuropsycological deficits at 6 months. The trial was discontinued after the enrollment of 149 patients owing to an excess mortality in the nimodipine group: 8 of 75 compared with 1 of 74. Major bleeding had occurred more often in the nimodipine group ($P = 0.03$) and accounted for the excess mortality. The authors postulated that the vasodilator and mild antiplatelet effects of the drug interacted in the platelet-depleted patient after cardiopulmonary bypass to increase the risk from hemorrhage.

In summary, this group of trials indicates that nimodipine may improve outcome in specific circumstances such as subarachnoid hemorrhage. However, in the hemodynamically unstable survivor of cardiac arrest, the risk of calcium channel blockers is again apparent. The unexpected increased risk from hemorrhage after cardiac surgery should stimulate further investigation.

CONCERNS AND CONTROVERSY

Calcium channel blockers are widely used in patients with hypertension and coronary disease and have been clearly shown to reduce blood pressure and control angina with acceptable side effect profiles. However, as reviewed in this chapter, the results of clinical trials with these drugs have been uniformly disappointing. Calcium channel blockers do not reduce mortality after MI or prevent MI in patients with unstable angina. They do not reduce overall mortality in heart failure, although they may prove to be beneficial when heart failure is not related to coronary disease. The effect of calcium channel blockers on the important outcomes of hypertension has not yet been well defined by clinical trials.

Furthermore, evidence that calcium channel blockers may have major, unanticipated adverse effects continues to accumulate. In a recent reanalysis of the nifedipine trials, Furberg and colleagues[67] drew attention to the dose-response relationship for total mortality. In trials using 80 mg per day of nifedipine, the relative risk is 2.69 (95% confidence interval, 1.16 to 6.26); in trials using more than 100 mg per day, the relative risk is 2.58 (95% confidence intervals, 1.03 to 6.47).[68] An increase in mortality was not seen in trials at lower doses.

This risk may not apply to other calcium channel blockers, to long-acting formulations that do not induce abrupt fluctuations in blood pressure and heart rate, or to nifedipine when used in combination with a beta blocker.[43] Insufficient clinical trial data are available to permit informed judgments for these conditions. Nevertheless, some of the adverse effects linked to calcium channel blockers are unlikely to be limited to only nifedipine. Pahor and coworkers[69] have recently reported that in an elderly population, calcium channel blockers were associated with an increased risk of gastrointestinal hemorrhage compared with beta blockers (relative risk, 1.86; 95% confidence interval, 1.22 to 2.82). The risks for verapamil, diltiazem, and nifedipine did not differ significantly. Vasodilation and mild platelet inhibition were postulated by the authors to be the reason for this finding.

Lastly, an increased incidence of cancer has been reported in patients taking calcium channel blockers in a prospective cohort study in the elderly.[70] The relative risk was 1.72 (95% confidence interval, 1.27 to 2.34) after adjustment for confounding factors. A significant dose-response gradient was found ($P = 0.0094$), but the hazard ratios associated with verapamil, diltiazem, and nifedipine did not differ significantly from one another.

It has been hypothesized, based on data that are rather sparse, that calcium channel blockers interfere with apoptosis (programmed cell death).[70] Apoptosis appears to be an important mechanism whereby older cells with higher neoplastic potential are eliminated. Apoptosis also limits growth of established cancers, so that calcium channel blockers might not only facilitate the appearance of cancer but also promote the growth of established tumors.[70]

An informed judgment on the clinical implications of this potential risk, and other risks with these drugs, is not possible until results from clinical trials of long-term calcium channel blocker treatment become available. In the interim, these drugs should be used cautiously; beta blockers and angiotensin-converting enzyme inhibitors may be better drugs for many patients.

REFERENCES

1. Katz AM. Calcium channel diversity in the cardiovascular system. J Am Coll Cardiol 1996; 28:522–529.
2. Godfraind T. Classification of calcium antagonists. Am J Cardiol 1987; 59:11B–23B.
3. Freedman DD, Waters DD. "Second generation" dihydropyridine calcium antagonists: Greater vascular selectivity and some unique applications. Drugs 1987; 34:578–598.
4. Pine MB, Citron PD, Bailly DJ, et al. Verapamil versus placebo in relieving stable angina pectoris. Circulation 1982; 65:17–22.
5. Sadick NN, Tan ATH, Fletcher PJ, et al. A double-blind randomized trial of propranolol and verapamil in the treatment of effort angina. Circulation 1982; 66:574–579.
6. Wagniart P, Ferguson RJ, Chaitman BR, et al. Increased exercise tolerance and reduced electrocardiographic ischemia with diltiazem in patients with stable angina pectoris. Circulation 1982; 66:23–28.
7. Theroux P, Baird M, Juneau M, et al. Effect of diltiazem on symptomatic and asymptomatic episode of ST segment depression occurring during daily life and during exercise. Circulation 1991; 84:15–22.
8. Glasser SP, West TW. Clinical safety and efficacy of once-a-day amlodipine for chronic stable angina pectoris. Am J Cardiol 1988; 62:518–522.
9. Deanfield JE, Detry JMRG, Lichtlen PR, et al. Amlodipine reduces transient myocardial ischemia in patients with coronary artery disease: Double-blind circadian anti-ischemia program in Europe (CAPE Trial). J Am Coll Cardiol 1994; 24:1460–1467.
10. Leon MB, Rosing DR, Bonow RO, et al. Combination therapy with calcium-channel blockers and beta blockers for chronic stable angina pectoris. Am J Cardiol 1985; 55:69B–80B.
11. Oliva PB, Breckenridge JC. Arteriographic evidence of coronary arterial spasm in acute myocardial infarction. Circulation 1977; 56:366–374.
12. Theroux P, Waters DD, Latour JG. Clinical manifestations and pathophysiology of myocardial ischemia with special reference to coronary artery spasm and the role of slow channel calcium blockers. Prog Cardiovasc Dis 1982; 25:157–180.
13. Messerli FH. "Cardioprotection"—not all calcium antagonists are created equal. Am J Cardiol 1990; 66:855–856.
14. Held PH, Yusuf S, Furberg CD. Calcium channel blockers in acute myocardial infarction and unstable angina: An overview. BMJ 1989; 299:1187–1192.
15. The Israeli SPRINT Study Group. Secondary Prevention Reinfarction Israeli Nifedipine Trial (SPRINT): A randomized intervention trial of nifedipine in patients with acute myocardial infarction. Eur Heart J 1988; 9:354–364.
16. Goulbourt U, Behar S, Reicher-Reiss H, et al. Early administration of nifedipine in suspected acute myocardial infarction: The Secondary Prevention Reinfarction Israel Nifedipine Trial 2 Study. Arch Intern Med 1993; 153:345–353.
17. Gibson RS, Boden WE, Theroux P, et al. Diltiazem and reinfarction in patients with non–Q wave myocardial infarction: Results of a double-blind, randomized, multicenter trial. N Engl J Med 1986; 315:423–429.
18. The Multicenter Diltiazem Postinfarction Trial Research Group. The effect of diltiazem on mortality and reinfarction after myocardial infarction. N Engl J Med 1988; 319:385–392.
19. Goldstein RE, Bocuzzi SJ, Cruess D, et al. Diltiazem increases late-onset congestive heart failure in postinfarction patients with early reduction in ejection fraction. Circulation 1991; 83:52–60.
20. The Danish Study Group on Verapamil in Myocardial Infarction. Verapamil in acute myocardial infarction. Eur Heart J 1984; 5:516–528.
21. The Danish Study Group on Verapamil in Myocardial Infarction. Effect of verapamil on mortality and major events after acute myocardial infarction (The Danish Verapamil Infarction Trial II–DAVIT II). Am J Cardiol 1990; 66:779–785.
22. Yusuf S, Held P, Furberg C. Update of effects of calcium antagonists in myocardial infarction or angina in light of the second Danish Verapamil Infarction Trial (DAVIT-II) and other recent studies. Am J Cardiol 1991; 67:1295–1297.
23. Rengo F, Carbonin P, Pahor M, et al. A controlled trial of verapamil in patients after acute myocardial infarction: Results of the Calcium Antagonist Reinfarction Italian Study (CRIS). Am J Cardiol 1996; 77:365–369.
24. Yusuf S. Verapamil following myocardial infarction—promising, but not proven. Am J Cardiol 1996; 77:421–422.
25. Waters DD, Miller DD, Szlachcic J, et al. Factors influencing the long-term prognosis of treated patients with variant angina. Circulation 1983; 68:258–265.
26. Hillis LD, Braunwald E. Coronary-artery spasm. N Engl J Med 1978; 299:695–702.
27. Maseri A. The revival of coronary artery spasm. Am J Med 1981; 79:752–754.
28. Gerstenblith G, Ouyang P, Achuff S, et al. Nifedipine in unstable angina: A double-blind, randomized trial. N Engl J Med 1982; 306:885–889.
29. Report of the Holland Interuniversity Nifedipine/metoprolol Trial (HINT) Research Group. Early treatment of unstable angina in the coronary care unit: A randomised, double-blind, placebo-controlled comparison of recurrent ischemia in patients treated with nifedipine or metoprolol or both. Br Heart J 1986; 56:400–413.
30. Muller JE, Turi ZG, Pearle DL, et al. Nifedipine and conventional therapy for unstable angina pectoris: A randomized, double-blind comparison. Circulation 1984; 69:728–739.
31. Theroux P, Taeymans Y, Morissette D, et al. A randomized study comparing propranolol and diltiazem in the treatment of unstable angina. J Am Coll Cardiol 1985; 5:717–722.
32. Andre-Fouet X, Usdin JP, Gayet C, et al. Comparison of short-term efficacy of diltiazem and propranolol in unstable angina at rest—a randomized trial in 70 patients. Eur Heart J 1983; 4:691–698.
33. Waters D, Lesperance J. Interventions that beneficially influence the evolution of coronary atherosclerosis: The case for calcium channel blockers. Circulation 1992; 86(Suppl III):III-111–III-116.
34. Waters D, Lesperance J. Calcium channel blockers and coronary atherosclerosis: From the rabbit to the real world. Am Heart J 1994; 128:1309–1316.
35. Lichtlen PR, Hugenholtz PG, Rafflenbeul W, et al. Retardation of angiographic progression of coronary artery disease by nifedipine: Results of the International Nifedipine Trial on Antiatherosclerotic Therapy (INTACT). Lancet 1990; 335:1109–1113.
36. Waters D, Lesperance J, Francetich M, et al. A controlled clinical trial to assess the effect of a calcium channel blocker on the progression of coronary atherosclerosis. Circulation 1990; 82:1940–1953.
37. Schroeder JS, Gao SZ, Alderman E, et al. A preliminary study

of diltiazem in the prevention of coronary artery disease in heart transplant recipients. N Engl J Med 1993; 328:164–170.
38. Borhani N, Mercuri M, Borhani PA, et al. Final outcome results of the Multicenter Isradipine Diuretic Atherosclerosis Study (MIDAS): A randomized controlled trial. JAMA 1996; 276:785–791.
39. Rehnqvist N, Hjemdahl P, Billing E, et al. Effects of metoprolol versus verapamil in patients with stable angina pectoris: The Angina Prognosis Study in Stockholm (APSIS). Eur Heart J 1996; 17:76–81.
40. Dargie HJ, Ford I, Fox KM, et al. Total Ischemic Burden European Trial (TIBET): Effects of ischemia and treatment with atenolol, nifedipine SR, and their combination on outcome in patients with chronic stable angina. Eur Heart J 1996; 17:104–112.
41. Glasser SP, Clark PI, Lipicky RJ et al. Exposing patients with chronic, stable, exertional angina to placebo periods in drug trials. JAMA 1991; 265:1550–1554.
42. Thadani U, Zellner SR, Glasser S, et al. Double-blind, dose-response, placebo-controlled multicenter study of nisoldipine: A new second-generation calcium channel blocker in angina pectoris. Circulation 1991; 84:2398–2408.
43. Waters D. Proischemic complications of dihydropyridine calcium channel blockers. Circulation 1991; 84:2598–2600.
44. Schulz W, Jost S, Kober G, et al. Relation of antianginal efficacy of nifedipine to degree of coronary arterial narrowing and to presence of coronary collateral vessels. Am J Cardiol 1985; 55:26–32.
45. Egstrup K, Andersen PE. Transient myocardial ischemia during nifedipine therapy in stable angina pectoris, and its relation to coronary collateral flow and comparison with metoprolol. Am J Cardiol 1993; 71:177–183.
46. Packer M, Kessler PD, Lee WH. Calcium-channel blockade in the management of severe chronic congestive heart failure: A bridge too far. Circulation 1987; (Suppl V):V-56–V-64.
47. Elkayam U, Amin J, Mehra A, et al. A prospective, randomized, double-blind, crossover study to compare the efficacy and safety of chronic nifedipine therapy with that of isosorbide dinitrate and their combination in the treatment of chronic congestive heart failure. Circulation 1990; 82:1954–1961.
48. Packer M. Calcium channel blockers in chronic heart failure: The risks of "physiologically rational" therapy. Circulation 1990; 82:2254–2257.
49. Packer M. Second generation calcium channel blockers in the treatment of chronic heart failure: Are they any better than their predecessors? J Am Coll Cardiol 1989; 14:1339–1342.
50. Barjon JN, Rouleau JL, Bichet D, et al. Chronic renal and neurohumoral effects of the calcium entry blocker nisoldipine in patients with congestive heart failure. J Am Coll Cardiol 1987; 9:622–630.
51. Littler WA, Sheridan DJ. Placebo-controlled trial of felodipine in patients with mild to moderate heart failure. Br Heart J 1995; 73:428–433.
52. Packer M, O'Connor CM, Ghali JK, et al. Effect of amlodipine on morbidity and mortality in severe chronic heart failure. N Engl J Med 1996; 335:1107–1114.
53. Figulla HR, Gietzen F, Zeymer F, et al. Diltiazem improves cardiac function and exercise capacity in patients with idiopathic dilated cardiomyopathy: Results of the Diltiazem in Dilated Cardiomyopathy Trial. Circulation 1996; 94:346–352.
54. Scognamiglio R, Rahimtoola S, Fasoli G, et al. Nifedipine in asymptomatic patients with severe aortic regurgitation and normal left ventricular function. N Engl J Med 1994; 331:689–694.
55. Collins R, Peto R, MacMahon S, et al. Blood pressure, stroke, and coronary heart disease: II. Short-term reductions in blood pressure: Overview of randomised drug trials in their epidemiological context. Lancet 1990; 335:827–838.
56. Moser M, Hebert PR. Prevention of disease progression, left ventricular hypertrophy, and congestive heart failure in hypertension treatment trials. J Am Coll Cardiol 1996; 27:1214–1218.
57. Staessen JA, Fagard R, Thijs L, et al: Randomized double-blind comparison of placebo and active treatment for older patients with isolated systolic hypertension. Lancet 1997; 350:757–764.
58. Psaty BM, Heckbert SR, Koepsell TD, et al. The risk of myocardial infarction associated with antihypertensive drug therapies. JAMA 1995; 274:620–625.
59. Yusuf S. Calcium antagonists in coronary artery disease and hypertension: Time for reevaluation? Circulation 1995; 92:1079–1082.
60. Parmley WW. A delayed answer to the calcium channel blocker question. J Am Coll Cardiol 1996; 27:510–511.
61. Gelmers HJ, Gorter K, De Weerdt CJ, et al. A controlled trial of nimodipine in acute ischemic stroke. N Engl J Med 1988; 318:203–207.
62. Ohman J, Heiskanen O. Effect of nimodipine on the outcome of patients after aneurysmal subarachnoid hemorrhage and surgery. J Neurosurg 1988; 69:683–686.
63. Pickard JD, Murray GD, Illingworth R, et al. Effect of oral nimodipine on cerebral infarction and outcome after subarachnoid hemorrhage: British aneurysm nimodipine trial. BMJ 1989; 298:636–642.
64. Roine RO, Kaste M, Kinnunen A, et al. Nimodipine after resuscitation from out-of-hospital ventricular fibrillation: A placebo-controlled, double-blind, randomized trial. JAMA 1990; 264:3171–3177.
65. Brain Resuscitation Clinical Trial II Study Group. A randomized clinical study of a calcium-entry blocker (lidoflazine) in the treatment of comatose survivors of cardiac arrest. N Engl J Med 1991; 324:1225–1231.
66. Wagenknecht LE, Furberg CD, Hammon JW, et al. Surgical bleeding: Unexpected effect of a calcium antagonist. BMJ 1995; 310:776–777.
67. Furberg CD, Psaty BM, Meyer JV. Dose-related increase in mortality in patients with coronary heart disease. Circulation 1995; 92:1326–1331.
68. Furberg CD, Psaty BM. Corrections to the nifedipine meta-analysis [Letter]. Circulation 1996; 93:1475–1476.
69. Pahor M, Guralnik JM, Furberg CD, et al. Risk of gastrointestinal hemorrhage with calcium antagonists in hypertensive persons over 67 years old. Lancet 1996; 347:1061–1065.
70. Pahor M, Guralnik JM, Ferrucci L, et al. Calcium-channel blockade and the incidence of cancer in aged populations. Lancet 1996; 348:493–497.

12 Magnesium

▶ Kent L. Woods
▶ Hanne Berg Ravn

The therapeutic use of intravenous magnesium salts in the management of acute myocardial infarction (AMI) has been progressively explored over the past 40 years. Early reports of uncontrolled case series were followed in the 1980s by several unpowered, randomized controlled trials.[1–7] Although individually too small to provide convincing evidence of efficacy, when combined by meta-analysis[8] these randomized studies indicated a substantial reduction in early mortality among patients receiving an intravenous magnesium salt (sulfate or chloride) early in the course of AMI.

These findings prompted two hypothesis-testing trials differing in design of a 24-hour infusion of magnesium sulfate in patients with AMI. The first trial, the Second Leicester Intravenous Magnesium Intervention Trial (LIMIT-2), was a conventional double-blind, placebo-controlled, randomized trial[9] whose size was determined by power calculations based on the lower limit of the treatment effect suggested by a meta-analysis of preceding trials. Approximately 2300 patients were recruited between September 1987 and February 1992. Significantly lower mortality was observed in magnesium-treated patients than control subjects at 28 days[9] and during follow-up over several years.[10] The second study, the Fourth International Study of Infarct Survival (ISIS-4), compared intravenous magnesium sulfate with an open control group as one of three treatments tested in a factorially designed megatrial.[11] Patients from more than 1000 hospitals worldwide participated between July 1991 and August 1993. No significant difference in mortality was observed between the magnesium and control groups either at 35 days or during 12 months of follow-up.

A meta-analysis, an adequately powered conventional trial, and a megatrial have given substantially different estimates of the treatment effect for intravenous Mg^{2+} in patients with AMI. Two broad possibilities should be considered. The first is that Mg^{2+} has no effect on mortality in patients with AMI and that the meta-analysis and the conventionally powered trial each generated false-positive results. If so, then the megatrial becomes the necessary standard for evaluating new treatments, with all the resource implications that entails. Alternatively, the differing results may reflect true differences in treatment effect dependent on the exact conditions under which intravenous Mg^{2+} was used. Resolution of this issue extends beyond the therapeutic role of Mg^{2+} in patients with AMI; it more generally influences the interpretation of evidence from these trials.

This chapter considers the strength and generalizability of the Mg^{2+} data from the various published trials. In establishing whether the results can be reconciled, it considers the candidate mechanisms by which Mg^{2+} might modify the outcome of AMI, reviewing first the cardiovascular pharmacology of intravenous Mg^{2+} and then examining the effects of Mg^{2+} in relevant laboratory models.

CARDIOVASCULAR PHARMACOLOGY OF Mg^{2+}

Many of the cardiovascular effects of Mg^{2+} reflect an antagonism of Ca^{2+}-initiated processes, which has led to the characterization of magnesium as "nature's physiological calcium blocker."[12] This summary is restricted to effects obtained with an elevation of serum Mg^{2+} concentrations higher than the physiologic range (0.75 to 1.00 mmol).

Antiarrhythmic Effects of Mg^{2+}

Magnesium infusion lengthens the PR interval, prolongs the sinoatrial and atrioventricular conduction time, and increases the atrioventricular nodal refractory period, but it has no effect on atrial or ventricular refractoriness or conduction.[13, 14] *Torsades de pointes* (polymorphic ventricular tachycardia) is the arrhythmia most consistently responsive to intravenous magnesium,[15] although lesser degrees of effectiveness against monomorphic ventricular tachycardia,[16] reentrant supraventricular tachycardia,[17–19] and multifocal atrial tachycardia[20] have also been reported.

Hemodynamic Effects and Coronary Circulation

The impact of intravenous infusion of magnesium on systemic and coronary circulation has been studied in healthy volunteers and in patients with normal coronary arteries. A decrease in systolic blood pressure and systemic resistance was observed.[21] The reduction in afterload and the rise in heart rate was followed by an increased cardiac output without any increase in myocardial oxygen consumption. The rise in heart rate may be secondary to hypotension-induced baroreceptor activation overcoming the direct depressor effect of magnesium on the sinus node. Coronary resistance fell, accompanied by a significant increase in coronary blood flow.

Mg^{2+} is known to reduce coronary vascular tone both in isolated coronary strips[22] and in patients with Prinzmetal's angina.[23, 24] Mg^{2+}-induced coronary and systemic vasodilatation may therefore be entirely due to the calcium-antagonist effect of magnesium at the level of vascular smooth muscle cells,[25] although it may in part be mediated by the release of prostacyclin or nitric oxide from the vessel wall.[26–28]

Protection of the Ischemic Myocardium

A protective effect of magnesium on the ischemic myocardium has been observed in a range of experimental models that are reviewed later. Proposed mechanisms of cellular protection include a reduction of calcium influx,[29] an inhibition of mitochondrial calcium overload,[30] a conservation of intracellular adenosine triphosphate (ATP),[31] and a reduced generation of oxygen-derived free radicals during reperfusion.[32]

Antiplatelet Effect

Antiplatelet therapy has been shown to reduce mortality in patients with AMI.[33] An antiplatelet effect of magnesium has been demonstrated in vitro[34–37] and ex vivo.[36, 38] Furthermore, a substantial reduction in thrombus formation has been demonstrated in several experimental studies. The importance of the observed platelet inhibition is discussed later.

EARLY AND UNPOWERED TRIALS OF Mg^{2+} IN ACUTE MYOCARDIAL INFARCTION

Three published meta-analyses of randomized trials of Mg^{2+} in patients with AMI[8, 9, 39] each identified the same seven studies.[1–7] Given the evidence of an Mg^{2+} effect modification by reperfusion (see later), it is notable that all these trials predated the use of thrombolytic therapy. Each trial was small, the largest having randomized fewer than 400 patients. With one exception (in which magnesium chloride was used),[2] the treatment tested was magnesium sulfate. Dose regimens varied; a total of 30 to 90 mmol of Mg^{2+} was infused during the 24- to 96-hour period following admission. Meta-analysis of the seven trials indicated a highly significant reduction in short-term mortality ($P < 0.001$). A meta-analysis including an additional trial[40] is shown in Figure 12–1.

It is well recognized that the technique of meta-analysis has several limitations.[41] First, a judgment has to be made that the trials included are sufficiently similar in design to be testing a single biologically plausible hypothesis. It must be assumed that differences in dose, the timing of treatment, or the characteristics of patients randomized do not substantially modify the observed treatment effect. Such assumptions, however, may or may not be justified and must be evaluated in the light of all evidence on mechanism. Second, the validity of the analysis rests on a complete ascertainment (or at least an unbiased sampling) of all the relevant trials performed. Trials showing an adverse effect or a lack of effect of the treatment being tested may be less likely to enter the accessible literature (publication bias). Third, small trials undertaken without prior power calculations may also have other design weaknesses affecting the validity of the final results. For all these reasons, meta-analysis is best considered as a hypothesis-generating technique to extract additional information from a group of trials that are individually of inadequate power. Conclusions drawn from meta-analysis must be considered tentative and subjected to corroboration in properly powered studies; this was the motivation for the design of the LIMIT-2 and the ISIS-4 trials.

During the wide debate that has arisen around the magnesium trials, only two small studies[42, 43] came to light that were overlooked in the meta-analyses; these studies were reported in 1990 and contributed too few cases to have influenced the interpretation of the meta-analysis. Therefore, no positive evidence exists

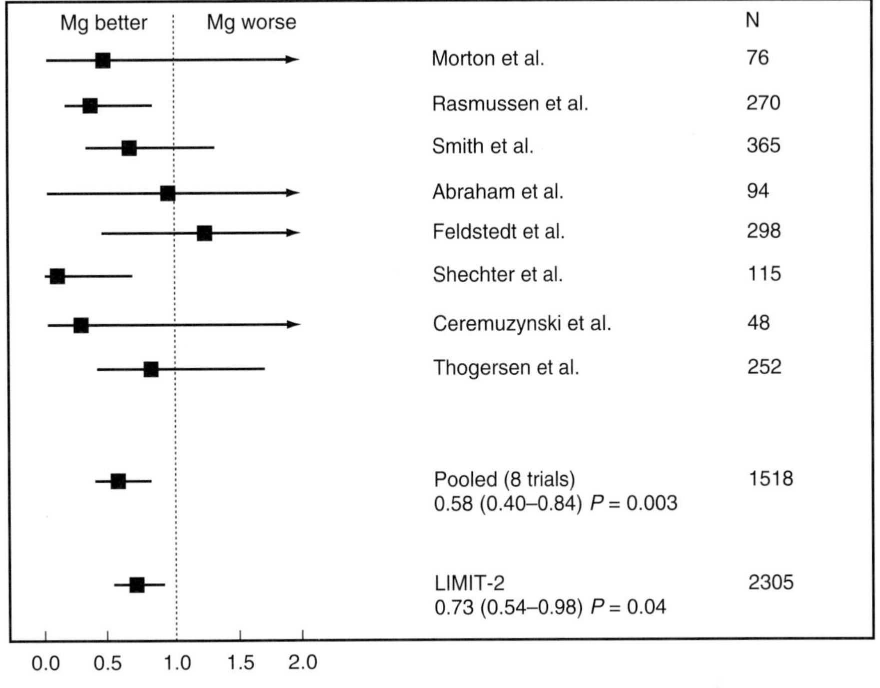

Figure 12–1 Pooled analysis of unpowered early randomized trials of intravenous Mg^{2+} in patients with acute myocardial infarction. Second Leicester Intravenous Magnesium Intervention Trial (LIMIT-2) result for 28-day mortality shown for comparison. (Adapted from Woods KL, Fletcher S, Roffe C, et al. Intravenous magnesium sulphate in suspected acute myocardial infarction: Results of the second Leicester Intravenous Magnesium Intervention Trial [LIMIT-2]. Lancet 1992; 339:1553–1558, © by The Lancet Ltd., 1992; see original source for references cited.)

of publication bias, although such bias is impossible to exclude.

HYPOTHESIS-TESTING TRIALS

LIMIT-2

The LIMIT-2 study was a double-blind, placebo-controlled trial of intravenous magnesium sulfate given immediately on admission to patients with suspected AMI.[9, 10] The Mg^{2+} regimen consisted of an initial loading injection of 8 mmol of magnesium sulfate given over 5 minutes followed by 65 mmol given by constant infusion over the following 24 hours. Placebo treatment was equal volumes of saline. The power calculation assumed (1) that there was a treatment effect on 28-day mortality at the lower 95% confidence limit of a pooled analysis of earlier published trials and (2) that AMI would be confirmed in 60% of patients. The number of patients entering the study was 2316, of whom 65% had AMI confirmed. The median time from symptom onset to randomization was 3 hours. Thrombolytic therapy and early aspirin were introduced into routine care during the study. Thrombolytic therapy, when given, was infused after the loading injection of a trial drug and concurrently with the first part of the trial infusion. Thirty-five percent of randomized patients (48% of those with subsequently confirmed AMI) received thrombolytic treatment, which was nearly always streptokinase, and 65% were given aspirin. The groups were well balanced for prognostic factors, and follow-up was more than 99% complete.

According to an intention-to-treat analysis, the 28-day mortality from all causes was 7.8% in the magnesium group and 10.3% in the placebo group (P = 0.04), a relative reduction of 24% (95% confidence interval, 1 to 43). The incidence of left ventricular failure while in the coronary care unit was reduced by 25% (7% to 39%) in the magnesium group (P = 0.009). There were no differences between the groups in the frequency of any class of arrhythmia, although sinus bradycardia was noted slightly more commonly in the magnesium group (10% vs. 8%; P = 0.02). Long-term mortality follow-up (mean 4.5 years) by certified cause of death has shown a sustained reduction in mortality from ischemic heart disease (P = 0.01) in magnesium-treated patients (Fig. 12–2).

The pattern of morbidity and mortality in the magnesium group was consistent: Early impairment of left ventricular function is strongly predictive of both early and long-term mortality. The predefined study size, placebo-controlled, double-blind randomization, and virtually complete follow-up and mortality endpoints effectively excluded bias. There was no evidence of a prognostic imbalance of the groups' baseline characteristics. The comparability of the two groups at baseline with respect to left ventricular function was supported by the near identity of their systolic blood pressure distributions before the start of trial treatment (Fig. 12–3). The trial therefore gives strong evidence for the protection of myocardial function with the early infusion of magnesium continued for the first 24 hours.

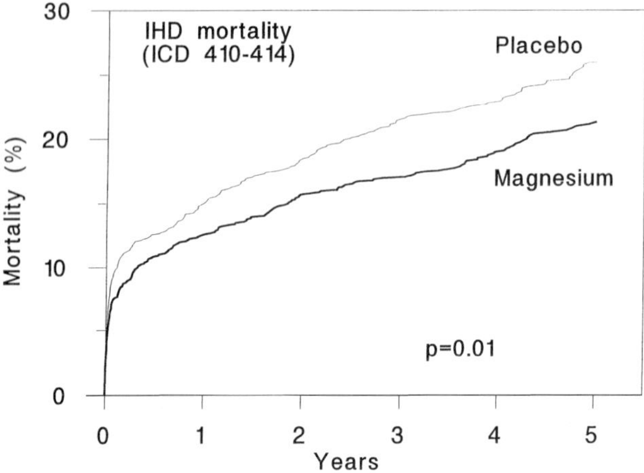

Figure 12–2 Cumulative mortality from ischemic heart disease during long-term follow-up of patients randomized in the LIMIT-2 study. ICD, International Classification of Diseases; IHD, ischemic heart disease. (Adapted from Woods KL, Fletcher S. Long-term outcome after magnesium sulphate in suspected acute myocardial infarction: The second Leicester Intravenous Magnesium Intervention Trial [LIMIT-2]. Lancet 1994; 343:816–819. © by The Lancet Ltd., 1994.)

ISIS-4

The ISIS-4 Trial was a large, simple study of factorial design carried out in 1086 hospitals worldwide.[11] A total of 58,050 patients were randomized. The three treatment comparisons were as follows:

1. Oral captopril for 1 month (vs. matched placebo)
2. Oral isosorbide mononitrate for 1 month (vs. matched placebo)
3. Intravenous magnesium sulfate 8 mmol over 15 minutes followed by 72 mmol over 24 hours (vs. open control)

Participating centers were encouraged to use thrombolytic therapy when appropriate. Since one in eight of randomized patients were to receive all three trial drugs—each a vasodilator—there was a perceived risk of hypotension with the simultaneous use of streptokinase. The protocol therefore recommended that thrombolytic treatment be carried out *before* trial randomization. The use of nonstudy treatments among all randomized patients included antiplatelet therapy (94%), thrombolytic medication (70%), intravenous nitrate (54%), other nonprotocol nitrate (6%), and nonprotocol converting enzyme inhibitor (5%).

Intention-to-treat analysis of the ISIS-4 data showed no significant difference in mortality between magnesium-treated patients and their control group, either at 35 days (7.64% vs. 7.24%, respectively) or during 12 months of follow-up. Reported small excesses of cardiogenic shock (4.6% vs. 4.1%), profound hypotension (4.4% vs. 3.3%), and heart failure (10.8% vs. 9.4%) on days 0 to 1 in the magnesium group were not accompanied by any excess mortality during these same days. The low incidence of these complications in an AMI population suggests underreporting that would be subject to bias by the open-study design.

The mononitrate comparison showed no significant differences in 35-day mortality or survival over 12 months. For the captopril comparison, there was a small reduction in 35-day mortality among patients allocated to captopril (7.19% vs. 7.69%; $P = 0.02$). There was a marginal treatment effect of captopril as well as a lack of any significant mortality reduction by captopril in the 8000 patients with heart failure at entry. These results contrast with the evidence from large conventional trials[44, 45] that angiotensin-converting enzyme inhibitors are of particular benefit in patients with impaired left ventricular function post-AMI. These observations raise questions about the ability of a large, simple trial design with an unrestrictive protocol to maximize the contrast between treatment and control groups and between clinically important subgroups,[46] as is discussed later.

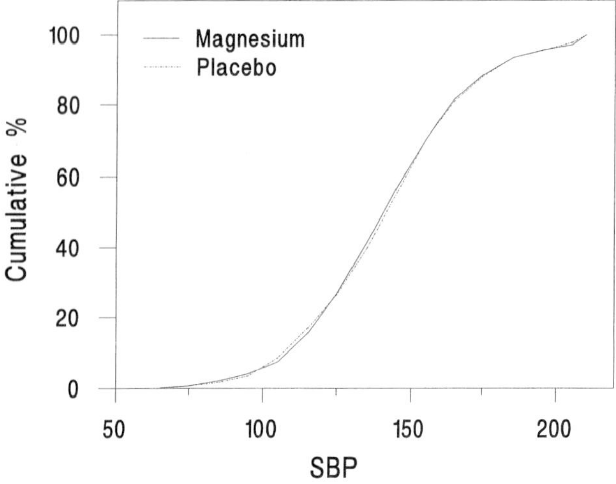

Figure 12–3 Cumulative distribution of systolic blood pressure (SBP) at baseline by randomization group before the initiation of trial treatment in the LIMIT-2 study.

Other Trials' Evidence

Since the publication of the meta-analyses, Shechter and coworkers[47] published the results of an unpowered double-blind, placebo-controlled trial of intravenous magnesium sulfate (91.6 mmol over 48 hours) in patients with AMI considered unsuitable for thrombolytic therapy. Compared with control subjects, inhospital mortality was lower in the magnesium-treated group (4% vs. 17%; $P < 0.01$) and left ventricular ejection fraction significantly higher ($P < 0.01$) at 72 hours and at 1 to 2 months after admission.

Several randomized trials have examined the effect of using intravenous magnesium salts during cardiac surgery under bypass, when hypomagnesemia is common and can be profound. This surgical intervention represents a human model of myocardial ischemia and reperfusion, and investigators have tested the hypothesis that supplementary intravenous Mg^{2+} reduces postoperative cardiac morbidity. England and colleagues[48] demonstrated a significantly higher postoperative cardiac index (2.8 L/min vs. 2.5 L/min) in 50 patients randomized to receive intravenous magnesium chloride at the end of bypass compared with 50 saline-treated control subjects. Ventricular arrhythmias were significantly less common in the magnesium group. In patients undergoing coronary artery bypass grafting for unstable angina, a randomized trial reported similar findings for both postoperative left ventricular stroke work index and ventricular arrhythmias; in this trial, intravenous magnesium sulfate was given before aortic cross-clamping and was continued for 24 hours after the removal of the aortic clamp.[49] In a placebo-controlled trial of intravenous magnesium sulfate given for 24 hours from the end of bypass,[50] which raised serum Mg^{2+} to a mean of 1.49 ± 0.34 mmol/L, there was a highly significant ($P = 0.001$) reduction in creatine kinase-MB isoenzyme postoperatively. This result suggests that myocardial protection is the mechanism of reduction in ventricular arrhythmias after bypass.

RECONCILING THE TRIALS' EVIDENCE

Potential Bias in Meta-Analysis

The results of meta-analysis, corroborated by the findings of the LIMIT-2, gave strong support for the addition of Mg^{2+} to the standard treatment of patients with AMI.[51] The ISIS-4 result, in contrast, gave no support for such a policy and was interpreted as undermining the value of the meta-analytic approach.[52, 53] The potential biases in meta-analysis are recognized, although it was previously thought unlikely that a *qualitatively* incorrect effect estimate would be generated. Three observations are relevant to the validity of meta-analyzing the results of the early magnesium trials.

1. No overlooked datasets have emerged that would alter the results of the published meta-analyses.
2. The results of the LIMIT-2 study for early mortality show no significant heterogeneity with the pooled effect estimate of the meta-analysis of earlier trials (see Fig. 12–1). Clear heterogeneity is evident between the meta-analysis and the LIMIT-2 on the one hand and the ISIS-4 result on the other ($P < 0.0001$).
3. Reliance on the ISIS-4 magnesium result as a gold standard against which to judge the meta-analysis assumes that there was no real difference in the treatments tested (i.e., that there was no effect modification by concurrent treatments such as thrombolysis, aspirin, or vasodilators) and that the megatrial design is exempt from bias. These assumptions are discussed subsequently.

Random Variation Between Trials

If evidence from the meta-analyses is disregarded, a more fundamental question than their validity remains: Why should two hypothesis-testing trials—one an adequately powered conventional trial; the other of megatrial design—produce substantially different answers when each ostensibly tested the same treatment regimen in the same clinical population? Can the difference be attributed to a type 1 error in LIMIT-2 or a type 2 error in ISIS-4? The probabilities of the differences in mortality and morbidity seen in LIMIT-2 arising by chance under the null hypothesis are each about 1%; the P values observed are as predicted in the power calculations used to set study size; and the pattern of morbidity and mortality differences are internally consistent and corroborated by models of Mg^{2+} effect in experimental myocardial ischemia and reperfusion. Conversely, the probability of ISIS-4 failing by a type 2 error to detect a treatment effect as large as that suggested by meta-analysis (and by LIMIT-2) is vanishingly small for the main analysis (although this cannot be assumed for subgroup analyses). It is therefore necessary to examine the trial conditions in LIMIT-2 and in ISIS-4 to establish whether they were in fact replicate experiments. This can only be done with insight into the *mechanism(s)* by which Mg^{2+} might modify the outcome of patients with AMI, drawing on the current experimental literature.

Potential Bias and Nongeneralizability in Megatrials

The motivation for large-scale recruitment (tens of thousands rather than thousands) is to achieve sufficient statistical power to detect small treatment effects.[54] Small, true effects are intrinsically vulnerable to small biases. To achieve very large recruitment, the amount of information collected on each patient is restricted, but physicians also retain clinical freedom in their choice of nontrial treatments. There are several mechanisms by which these design features might produce either a bias toward the null (obscuring a true treatment effect) or a true null result of limited generalizability.[46] First, frequent use outside the trial protocol of the treatment under test blunts the contrast between the randomized groups. This may have occurred in the nitrate comparison of ISIS-

4, in which 60% of patients received nontrial nitrates. However, only 5% of the patients allocated to the open control group of the magnesium comparison received intravenous magnesium.

Second, a similar mechanism could arise from high nonprotocol use of a treatment with an effect that overlaps that of the treatment being tested. For instance, a therapeutic effect of magnesium resulting from an antiplatelet action might have been concealed by a 94% use of antiplatelet therapy; however, there is now experimental evidence that Mg^{2+} produces substantial inhibition of platelet function at the concentrations achieved in the trials even in the presence of aspirin (see later).

A third mechanism could arise whereby a large simple trial might fail to detect a true treatment effect in which the timing of treatment substantially alters its efficacy. (This is not a source of *bias*, since the measured treatment effect is a valid estimate under the actual conditions of use; it is, however, a result that cannot be *generalized* to more favorable conditions of use.) A large, simple trial lacks a highly prescriptive protocol and presents difficulties in defining retrospectively the actual conditions of use from a limited dataset. The major controversy of the ISIS-4 magnesium study is the possibility that treatment was given too late to modify myocardial injury occurring during reperfusion of the infarct-related artery.[55, 56] The key questions are (1) What were the differences in the timing of treatment in the different trials and (2) How strong is the experimental evidence that a treatment effect of magnesium is likely to be highly time dependent? These issues are explored in the next two sections.

Differences Between the Trials

PATIENT POPULATION

Control group mortality in ISIS-4 was 7.2% (at 35 days)[11] compared with 10.3% for the placebo group of LIMIT-2 (at 28 days).[9] At least two factors appear to have contributed to the low-risk sample in ISIS-4: (1) selective nonrecruitment of hypotensive patients who might be intolerant of vasodilators and (2) late randomization excluding patients dying early after admission.[11]

MAGNESIUM TREATMENT IN RELATION TO LIKELY REPERFUSION

The randomization of patients into ISIS-4 occurred relatively late, at a median of 8 hours after symptom onset compared with 3 hours in LIMIT-2. Possibly more important—given the experimental evidence that Mg^{2+} protects against reperfusion injury (see later)—70% of ISIS-4 patients received thrombolytic treatment before randomization. Are any of these patients likely to have received Mg^{2+} before reperfusion of the infarct-related artery occurred? The time delay between starting thrombolytic treatment and starting trial treatment was not recorded, but indirect evidence suggests that the delay was on average 3 hours or more. For trial patients given thrombolysis, the time lapse from symptom onset to trial randomization was 7 hours; by extrapolation from ISIS-3, the typical time from symptom onset to thrombolytic administration would have been 3 to 4 hours. It must be concluded that reperfusion in response to the thrombolytic drug is highly likely to have occurred *before* the level of plasma Mg^{2+} was raised.

Without thrombolytic treatment, spontaneous reperfusion occurs in at least a third of patients during the first 12 to 24 hours after AMI.[57] The true proportion is likely to be higher than this figure, however, because the frequency of intermittent reperfusion is underestimated by angiography. In the 30% of ISIS-4 patients not given a thrombolytic drug, the average delay from symptom onset to randomization was 12 hours. Therefore, any spontaneous reperfusion of viable myocardium is likely to have already occurred before beginning trial treatment. In addition, the amount of viable myocardium at this time is likely to be reduced, and thus the benefit of late Mg^{2+} infusion limited by the restricted number of myocytes with reversible ischemic injury.

To assess the importance of these timing differences in relation to reperfusion, experimental evidence is required to establish the potential mechanism of benefit of Mg^{2+} in patients with AMI and whether it is likely to be highly time dependent, particularly in relation to reperfusion.

EXPERIMENTAL EVIDENCE FOR THE MODE OF ACTION AND TIME DEPENDENCY OF AN Mg^{2+} EFFECT

Ischemia/Reperfusion Injury

Reperfusion of the artery, although beneficial in terms of myocardial salvage, may come at the cost of reperfusion injury.[58] Four aspects of reperfusion injury have been recognized[59]:

1. *Lethal reperfusion injury*—reperfusion-induced death of cells still viable at the time blood flow is restored
2. *Vascular reperfusion injury*—progressive damage to the vasculature that results in an expanding zone of *no-reflow* and a loss of vasodilatory reserve

3. *Stunned myocardium*—prolonged postischemic contractile dysfunction
4. *Reperfusion arrhythmias*—ventricular fibrillation or tachycardia occurring within seconds to minutes after the restoration of coronary flow

Substantial experimental data have shown that Mg^{2+} therapy can reduce myocardial injury during ischemia and reperfusion.[30, 60–65] The importance of correct timing of Mg^{2+} therapy has been demonstrated recently in two studies. In a canine model, Mg^{2+} was given after 15 or 45 minutes of coronary occlusion or after 15 minutes of reperfusion.[66] Infarct size divided by area at risk (IS/AR) was significantly reduced by more than 60% in the two groups given Mg^{2+} starting during coronary occlusion. A nonsignificant decrease in IS/AR was observed in the group receiving Mg^{2+} after 15 minutes of reperfusion. Similar results were obtained in a swine model by Herzog and colleagues, who evaluated the effect of intracoronary infusion of Mg^{2+} initiated immediately with the onset of reperfusion or after 1 hour of reperfusion.[67] Infarct size was significantly reduced by more than 50% in the early Mg^{2+} group but not in the late Mg^{2+} group. Contractile impairment of the heart (termed *stunning*) after reperfusion can also be mitigated by elevating Mg^{2+} in the perfusate, but the time window for therapeutic effect appears to be within 1 to 2 minutes of the onset of reperfusion.[62, 64, 68, 69] This is consistent with the rapid time course of reperfusion injury.[70]

The concentration-effect relationship may also be nonlinear. In a canine model of reperfusion after 60 minutes of regional myocardial ischemia, an elevation of regional perfusate Mg^{2+} to around 5 mmol before and during the first 60 minutes of reperfusion significantly increased regional coronary blood flow and oxygen consumption; however, contractile dysfunction was unaffected, and the infarct size at 6 hours was nonsignificantly reduced.[71] In the major trials, peak plasma Mg^{2+} was around 1.5 mmol/L. These data indicate that Mg^{2+} can reduce both myocardial necrosis and stunning associated with reperfusion but that benefit is lost when therapy is started after the onset of reperfusion. Mg^{2+} is also likely to be ineffective when reperfusion occurs too late to rescue a useful amount of viable myocardium.[66, 67, 72] The concentration-effect relationship requires further study.

MECHANISMS OF PROTECTIVE ACTION BY Mg^{2+} DURING ISCHEMIA AND REPERFUSION

The role of Mg^{2+} during ischemia and reperfusion seems to be multifactorial, which is unsurprising given the numerous functions of the ion. Table 12–1 summarizes several factors that may influence pathophysiologic events during ischemia and reperfusion injury. Some of these mechanisms have been documented in experimental studies, whereas others are hypothetical.

TABLE 12–1 • Possible Mechanisms of Action of Mg^{2+} as a Myocardial Protective Agent During Ischemia and Reperfusion

Reduced cardiac work
Negative chronotropy
Reduced systolic blood pressure
Increase in coronary flow
Mg^{2+}-Ca^{2+} antagonism–induced smooth muscle relaxation
Release of vasodilating agents from the endothelium (e.g., nitric oxide, epoprostenol)
Reduced intracellular ionic alterations
Reduced mitochondrial Ca^{2+} overload
Conservation of intracellular K^+ concentration
Oxygen-derived free radicals
Reduced generation of free radicals
Reduced oxidative endothelial cell damage
Improvement in recovery of metabolism
Conservation of intracellular Mg^{2+}
Enhanced replenishment of adenosine triphosphate and creatine phosphate

A reduction in systolic blood pressure and a reduced heart rate have been observed in some experimental studies, which may contribute to a reduction in cardiac work[65, 72] (see Table 12–1). Although these changes in hemodynamics cannot be disregarded, they do not give a satisfactory explanation of the protection of the myocardium noted in experiments by Christensen and colleagues[66] and Herzog and coworkers,[67] since no hemodynamic differences were observed between the treatment groups in these studies. Furthermore, in the former study[66] no significant differences were observed in transmural blood flow during coronary occlusion or at 60 minutes of reperfusion, suggesting that the observed myocardial protective effect is not likely to result from differences in collateral blood flow.

During early reperfusion, intracellular Ca^{2+} overload occurs, together with a reduced myofibrillar sensitivity to Ca^{2+} transients.[70, 73] Mg^{2+} can inhibit Ca^{2+} flux across the sarcolemma[74] and reduce mitochondrial Ca^{2+} overload.[30] The loss of Mg^{2+} during ischemia may restrict the replenishment of ATP during reperfusion and thus impair the return of normal contractile function.[61, 75] Elevated extracellular levels of Mg^{2+} were found to improve the recovery of energy metabolism as assessed by ATP, creatine phosphate, and intracellular pH, resulting in improved myocardial contractility.[76] The study of Lareau and colleagues,[63] in which atrial trabeculae from cardiac surgery patients demonstrated an enhanced contractile force and adenylate concentration with high extracellular Mg^{2+} concentrations, suggests that these observations may also be valid in humans. Experimentally induced Mg^{2+} deficiency in a swine model prolonged myocardial stunning, which could be restricted by pretreatment with Mg^{2+}.[68, 77]

An increase in oxygen-derived free radicals occurs at the time of reperfusion after coronary occlusion and may mediate reperfusion injury.[78] Several agents that block the generation and release of free radicals have been shown to limit infarct size when administered prior to reperfusion.[79, 80] The time-dependent effect of Mg^{2+} in relation to experimental reperfusion damage may be explained by a blockade of free radical formation. In cell cultures, the formation of free radicals has been shown to depend on Mg^{2+} content, and oxidative endothelial injury has been shown to be more extensive in Mg^{2+}-deficient cells.[32]

The reduction in ischemia-reperfusion injury by Mg^{2+} demonstrated in several experimental studies in four different animal species has important clinical implications. In the laboratory models, correct timing is essential to achieve the cardioprotective effect of Mg^{2+}. In patients with AMI, reperfusion (obtained either with thrombolysis or spontaneously) is characterized by an intermittent reocclusion of the artery resulting from a variable combination of thrombosis and vasoconstriction during the early phase. An optimal Mg^{2+} regimen for clinical trial thus includes (1) early bolus administration of Mg^{2+} before any thrombolytic therapy has taken effect and (2) continuous infusion to protect the myocardium against stunning and enhanced necrosis during the time when either spontaneous reperfusion of viable myocardium or intermittent occlusion-reperfusion after thrombolysis might occur.

Mg^{2+} and Platelet Function

Platelets are intimately involved in thrombus formation at the site of coronary occlusion. Even following successful thrombolysis or percutaneous transluminal coronary angioplasty, the underlying stimulus to platelet-related rethrombosis persists for many hours or longer.[81] Platelet activation can be initiated by several pathways through specific platelet membrane receptors and secondary messengers to stimulate the intracellular Ca^{2+} mobilization and degranulation of platelets.[82, 83] Binding of fibrinogen to the glycoprotein IIb/IIIa enables platelets to form microaggregates via interplatelet fibrinogen binding.[36] The platelet plug is further stabilized by an activation of the coagulation cascade in which thrombin generation reinforces platelet aggregation and induces fibrin polymerization.[83]

Following thrombolytic therapy with streptokinase[84] or a tissue-type plasminogen activator,[85] the urinary excretion of thromboxane metabolites increases. Streptokinase can promote platelet aggregation, perhaps through the formation of immune complexes with antistreptokinase antibodies.[86, 87] Experimental studies indicate that platelet aggregation limits the response to thrombolysis[84] and that the

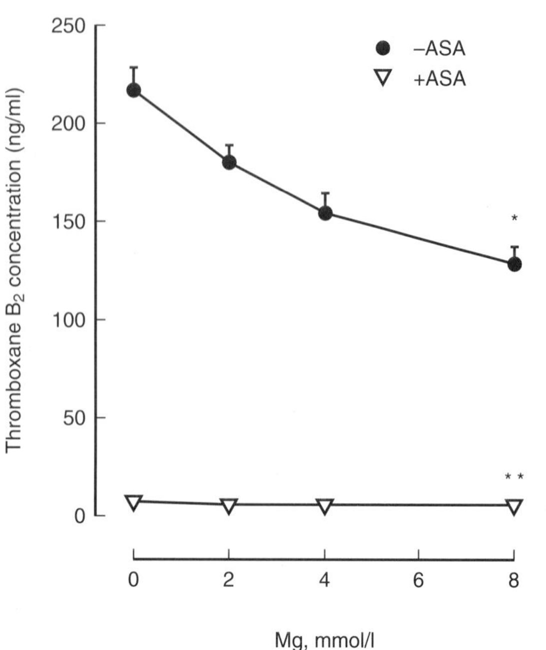

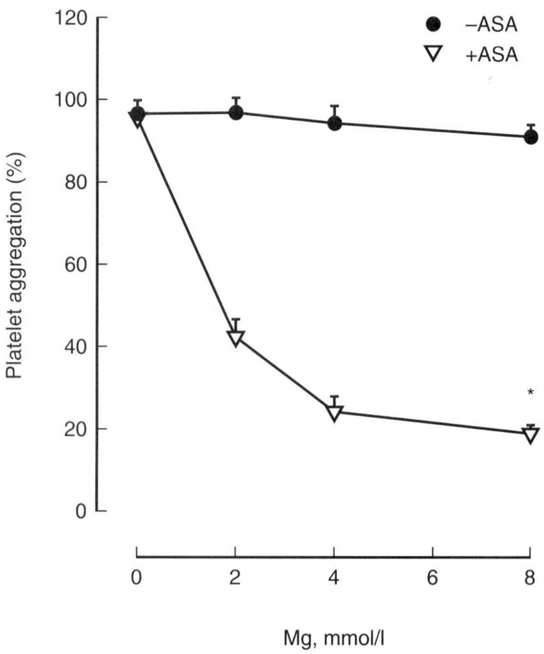

Figure 12–4 Thromboxane B_2 (TxB2) concentration in the supernatant of platelet-rich plasma following collagen-induced (5 µg/mL) platelet aggregation before and after aspirin (ASA) pretreatment *(left panel)*. Platelet aggregation response following this strong collagen induction shows that neither Mg^{2+} nor aspirin alone was able to reduce platelet reactivity. However, concomitant administration of these two drugs causes a synergistic inhibition of platelet aggregation *(right panel)*. (From Ravn HB, Vissinger H, Kristensen SD, et al. Magnesium inhibits platelet activity—an in vitro study. Thromb Haemost 1996; 76:88–93.)

clinical efficacies of thrombolytic therapy and aspirin are additive.[33]

A dose-dependent inhibition of platelet reactivity by Mg^{2+} has been demonstrated in several in vitro and ex vivo studies.[35, 36, 38, 77, 88] Platelet inhibition is consistent following stimulation with both strong (e.g., collagen and thrombin) and weak agonists (e.g., adenosine diphosphate, arachidonic acid, and adrenaline). The degranulation of platelets and thromboxane A_2 (TxA_2) synthesis is inhibited in a dose-dependent manner following the in vitro addition of Mg^{2+}. However, granule release reaction and TxA_2 synthesis induced by many agonists has an aggregation-dependent component.[89] The reduction of α-granule release and TxA_2 synthesis may therefore reflect only a surface-mediated inhibition of platelet aggregation. The reduction in TxA_2 synthesis is minimal in comparison to that obtained with aspirin ingestion (Fig. 12–4).

The consistent inhibitory effect of Mg^{2+} with different agonists suggests either that inhibition is due to blockage of a common pathway or that Mg^{2+} induces a general increase in threshold for the activation of platelets. Increments of intracellular free Ca^{2+} play a pivotal role in signal transduction in platelets. Mg^{2+} dose-dependently inhibits Ca^{2+} influx in platelets across the plasma membrane.[35, 88] A blockage of the glycoprotein receptor IIb/IIIa that makes it inaccessible for fibrinogen binding may be another mechanism of surface-mediated platelet inhibition.[36]

In the LIMIT-2 study, the beneficial effect of Mg^{2+} was not modified by concomitant aspirin therapy.[9] A recent in vitro study demonstrated that the platelet inhibitory effect of Mg^{2+} was also present after pretreatment with aspirin and, moreover, that a synergistic effect was found when platelets were pretreated with both Mg^{2+} and aspirin following collagen stimulation[37] (see Fig. 12–4).

Significantly reduced ex vivo platelet aggregation has been demonstrated following intravenous Mg^{2+} infusion in humans.[38] The Mg^{2+} regimens used have attained plasma Mg^{2+} levels comparable to clinical studies in patients with AMI (1.50–1.76 mmol/L). A significant increase in bleeding time from 7.9 ± 0.5 minutes to 11.8 ± 0.9 minutes was observed during the Mg^{2+} infusion period.[38]

In vivo inhibition of platelet aggregation, thrombus formation, and embolization by intravenous Mg^{2+} has been shown in several models of arterial injury, including rabbit cerebral and carotid artery, dog left anterior descending coronary artery, and rat femoral artery.[90–92] A recent study evaluated the possible time dependency of this antithrombotic effect of Mg^{2+} in relation to arterial reperfusion by inducing arterial thrombus formation in the femoral artery in rats. Intravenous Mg^{2+} was given in the Mg-early group during occlusion and preparation of the arterial injury, whereas in the Mg-late group Mg^{2+} infusion was not initiated until 10 minutes after reperfusion of the artery. Thrombus area (measured dynamically using in vivo microscopy) was significantly reduced by 75% in the Mg-early group, whereas no effect on thrombus formation was observed in the Mg-late group (Fig. 12–5).[92] Five out of 15 animals in the Mg-early group did not develop any thrombus, whereas all animals in the Mg-late group developed thrombus, thus demonstrating the importance of pretreatment. It is not known why Mg^{2+} is so effective in reducing thrombus formation when given prior to but not after reperfusion. One explanation may be that platelets are more easily inhibited when pretreated before exposure to thrombogenic stimuli. Platelet aggregation involves a cascade reaction in which the initial reaction between a single platelet and the thrombogenic subendothelial tissue leads to an exponential activation of other platelets through several pathways. Reducing the initial platelet–vessel wall interaction would thus dampen the whole cascade reaction. Another possible explanation may be that the platelet–vessel wall interaction is more susceptible to Mg^{2+} than is the platelet-platelet interaction.[92]

In ISIS-4, by protocol, patients given thrombolytic therapy were not randomized to study drug until after the completion of the early lytic phase. This delay may be important, since two of the plausible

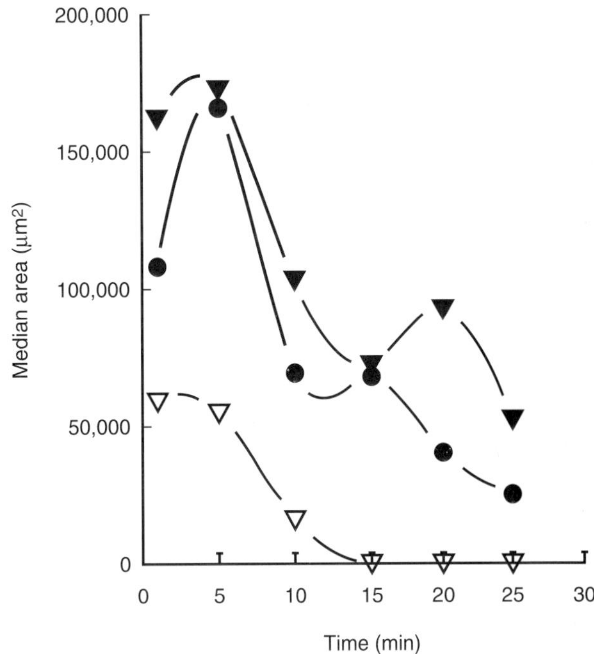

Figure 12–5 Median area of thrombus over time in each treatment group; rat femoral arteriotomy model. A significant reduction in thrombus area was observed in the Mg-early group ($P < 0.005$), whereas no difference in thrombus size was observed in the Mg-late group compared to placebo. Clear triangle, Mg-early group; solid circle, Mg-late group; solid triangle, placebo group; data given as median values. (From Ravn HB, Kristensen SD, Hjortdal VE, et al. Early administration of intravenous magnesium inhibits arterial thrombus formation. Arterioscler Thromb Vasc Biol 1997; 17:3620–3625.)

mechanisms by which Mg^{2+} exerts its effect depend on the correct timing of Mg^{2+} therapy. In LIMIT-2, Mg^{2+} was initiated immediately at arrival and prior to any thrombolytic therapy. It has been suggested that the nonthrombolyzed subgroup in ISIS-4 (30%; approximately 17,000 patients) provided an adequate test of the efficacy of Mg^{2+}.[11] Late randomization of these patients, at a median of 12 hours from symptom onset, casts doubt on such an assertion. The statistical power of this subgroup analysis is too low to reliably detect even a treatment effect as large as that attributable to thrombolytic therapy, assuming the same time dependence (10% mortality reduction at 12 hours[93]; control mortality 9.3%; $2\alpha = 0.05$; power = 57%).[46] If, as the laboratory evidence suggests, the time dependence of Mg^{2+} is much steeper than that of thrombolytic treatment, this calculation will overestimate the power of the subgroup analysis.

CURRENT STATUS OF Mg^{2+} IN ACUTE MYOCARDIAL INFARCTION

ISIS-4 has clearly shown that Mg^{2+} infusion is without benefit when given after thrombolysis or late after symptom onset. LIMIT-2 gives strong evidence that Mg^{2+} given early and before any thrombolytic treatment has acted protects the myocardium and improves long-term survival. Laboratory evidence now supports the view that doubling plasma Mg^{2+} concentration moderates myocardial reperfusion injury and inhibits platelet function to a degree that has therapeutic potential in patients with AMI. It also clearly indicates, however, that these effects of Mg^{2+} are likely to operate only in a brief time window around coronary reperfusion and the exposure of the thrombogenic arterial wall to blood. There is no valid evidence to suggest that Mg^{2+} is hazardous at the doses used in the clinical trials and this treatment is cheap and simple to administer.[51] If the mortality benefit in the Mg^{2+} group of LIMIT-2 (persisting absolute reduction of 4.5% in ischemic heart disease mortality at 3 years) represents the true treatment effect, the potential health gain from routine use of Mg^{2+} may be substantial. However, the unexpected findings of ISIS-4 justify additional trials. These must be designed and implemented using the laboratory evidence now available.

To this end, a multicenter double-blind, placebo-controlled trial (Magnesium in Coronaries [MAGIC]) has recently been approved for funding by the U.S. National Institutes of Health (EM Antman, MD, personal communication, 1997). This will enroll predominantly high-risk patients, including those older than 65 years of age and those considered unsuitable for thrombolytic treatment. Treatment will be started before or concurrent with any reperfusion therapy and within 6 hours of symptom onset. The primary endpoint will be 30-day mortality. A sample size of 10,200 offers greater than 90% power to detect a 20% difference in mortality, assuming a 10.5% placebo group mortality.

At present, no consensus exists on the therapeutic role of Mg^{2+} in patients with AMI, despite continuing debate on the interpretation of the trial results.[94, 95] Resolution of the issue is essential, not only to guide the management of this large group of patients but also to increase our understanding of the strengths and weaknesses of trial designs and analyses used widely in therapeutic research. The debate also highlights the importance of mechanistic knowledge in the planning and interpretation of clinical trials. Had it been available, the recent laboratory evidence on Mg^{2+} effects in myocardial ischemia-reperfusion would undoubtedly have influenced the design of these previous Mg^{2+} trials.

REFERENCES

1. Morton BC, Nair RC, Smith FM, et al. Magnesium therapy in acute myocardial infarction—a double-blind study. Magnesium 1984; 3:346–352.
2. Rasmussen HS, Norregard P, Lindeneg O, et al. Intravenous magnesium in acute myocardial infarction. Lancet 1986; 1:234–236.
3. Smith LF, Heagarty AM, Bing RF, et al. Intravenous infusion of magnesium sulphate after acute myocardial infarction: Effects on arrhythmias and mortality. Int J Cardiol 1986; 12:175–180.
4. Abraham AS, Rosenmann D, Kramer M, et al. Magnesium in the prevention of lethal arrhythmias in acute myocardial infarction. Arch Intern Med 1987; 147:753–755.
5. Feldstedt M, Bouchelouche P, Svenningsen A, et al. Failing effect of magnesium-substitution in acute myocardial infarction. Eur Heart J 1988; 9:226.
6. Shechter M, Hod H, Marks N, et al. Beneficial effect of magnesium sulfate in acute myocardial infarction. Am J Cardiol 1990; 66:271–274.
7. Ceremuzynski L, Jurgiel R, Kulakowski P, et al. Threatening arrhythmias in acute myocardial infarction are prevented by intravenous magnesium sulphate. Am Heart J 1989; 118:1333–1334.
8. Teo KK, Yusuf S, Collins R, et al. Effects of intravenous magnesium in suspected acute myocardial infarction: An overview of the randomized trials. BMJ 1991; 303:1499–1503.
9. Woods KL, Fletcher S, Roffe C, et al. Intravenous magnesium sulphate in suspected acute myocardial infarction: Results of the second Leicester Intravenous Magnesium Intervention Trial (LIMIT-2). Lancet 1992; 339:1553–1558.
10. Woods KL, Fletcher S. Long-term outcome after magnesium sulphate in suspected acute myocardial infarction: The Second Leicester Intravenous Magnesium Intervention Trial (LIMIT-2). Lancet 1994; 343:816–819.
11. ISIS-4 (Fourth International Study of Infarct Survival) Collaborative Group. ISIS-4: A randomised factorial trial assessing early oral captopril, oral mononitrate, and intravenous magnesium sulphate in 58,050 patients with suspected acute myocardial infarction. Lancet 1995; 345:669–685.
12. Iseri LT, French JH. Magnesium: Nature's physiologic calcium blocker. Am Heart J 1984; 108(1):188–193.
13. DiCarlo LA, Morady F, De Buitleir M, et al. Effects of magnesium sulfate on cardiac conduction and refractoriness in humans. J Am Coll Cardiol 1986; 7(6):1356–1362.
14. Kulick DL, Hong R, Ryzen E, et al. Electrophysiologic effects

of intravenous magnesium in patients with normal conduction systems and no clinical evidence of significant cardiac disease. Am Heart J 1988; 115(2):367–373.

15. Tzivoni D, Banai S, Schuger C, et al. Treatment of torsade de pointes with magnesium sulphate. Circulation 1988; 77(2):392–397.
16. Allen BJ, Brodsky MA, Capparelli EV, et al. Magnesium sulphate therapy for sustained monomorphic ventricular tachycardia. Am J Cardiol 1989; 64:1202–1204.
17. Etienne Y, Blanc JJ, Boschat J, et al. Effets antiarythmiques du sulphate de magnesium intraveineux dans les tachycardies supraventriculaires paroxystiques. Ann Cardiol Angeiol 1988; 37(9):535–538.
18. Wesley RC, Haines DE, Lermon BB, et al. Effect of intravenous magnesium sulphate on supraventricular tachycardia. Am J Cardiol 1989; 63:1129–1131.
19. Sager PT, Widerhorn J, Petersen R, et al. Prospective evaluation of parenteral magnesium sulphate in the treatment of patients with reentrant AV supraventricular tachycardia. Am Heart J 1990; 119:308–316.
20. Iseri LT, Fairshter RD, Hardemann JL, et al. Magnesium and potassium therapy in multifocal atrial tachycardia. Am Heart J 1985; 110:789–794.
21. Vigorito C, Giordano A, Ferraro P, et al. Haemodynamic effects of magnesium sulphate on the normal human heart. Am J Cardiol 1991; 67:1435–1437.
22. Kimura T, Yasue H, Sakaino N, et al. Effects of magnesium on the tone of isolated human coronary arteries: Comparison with diltiazem and nitroglycerin. Circulation 1989; 79(5):1118–1124.
23. Kugiyama K, Yasue H, Okumura K, et al. Supression of exercise-induced angina by magnesium sulphate in patients with variant angina. J Am Coll Cardiol 1988; 12(5):1177–1183.
24. Miyagi H, Yasue H, Okumura K, et al. Effect of magnesium on anginal attack induced by hyperventilation in patients with variant angina. Circulation 1989; 79:597–602.
25. Altura BM, Altura BT, Carella A, et al. Mg^{2+}-Ca^{2+} interaction in contractility of vascular smooth muscle: Mg^{2+} versus organic calcium channel blockers on myogenic tone and agonist-induced responsiveness of blood vessels. Can J Physiol Pharmacol 1987; 65:729–745.
26. Watson KV, Moldow CF, Ogburn PL, et al. Magnesium sulphate: Rationale for its use in preeclampsia. Proc Natl Acad Sci U S A 1986; 83:1075–1078.
27. Briel RC, Lippert TH, Zahradnik HP. Veranderungen von Blutgerinnung, Thrombozytenfunktion und vaskularer Prostazyklinsynthese durch Magnesiumsulfat. Gerburt Frauen 1987; 47:332–336.
28. Kemp PA, Gardiner SM, March JE, et al. Hindquarters vasodilator effect of $MgSO_4$ in conscious rats: Possible involvement of nitric oxide. Br J Pharmacol 1992; 107:403P.
29. White RE, Hartzell HC. Effects of intracellular free magnesium on calcium current in isolated cardiac myocytes. Science 1988; 239:778–780.
30. Ferrari R, Curello AS, Ceconi C, et al. Myocardial recovery during post-ischaemic reperfusion: Effects of nifedipine, calcium, and magnesium. J Mol Cell Cardiol 1986; 18:487–498.
31. Hearse DJ, Stewart DA, Braimbridge MV, et al. Cellular protection during myocardial ischemia. Circulation 1976; 54:193–202.
32. Dickens BF, Weglicki WB, Li YS, et al. Magnesium deficiency in vitro enhances free radical-induced intracellular oxidation and cytotoxicity in endothelial cells. FEBS Lett 1992; 311:187–191.
33. ISIS-2 (Second International Study of Infarct Survival) Collaborative Group. Randomised trial of intravenous streptokinase, oral aspirin, both, or neither among 17,187 cases of suspected acute myocardial infarction: ISIS-2. Lancet 1988; 2:349–360.
34. Heptinstall S. The use of a chelating ion exchange resin to evaluate the effects of extracellular calcium concentration on adenosine diphosphate–induced aggregation of human blood platelets. Thromb Haemost 1976; 36:208–220.
35. Hwang DL, Yen CF, Nadler JL. Effect of extracellular magnesium on platelet activation and intracellular calcium mobilization. Am J Hypertens 1992; 5:700–706.
36. Gawaz M, Ott I, Reininger AJ, Neumann FJ. Effects of magnesium on platelet aggregation and adhesion. Thromb Haemost 1994; 72(6):912–918.
37. Ravn HB, Vissinger H, Kristensen SD, et al. Magnesium inhibits platelet activity—an in vitro study. Thromb Haemost 1996; 76:88–93.
38. Ravn HB, Vissinger H, Kristensen SD, et al. Magnesium inhibits platelet activity—an infusion study in healthy volunteers. Thromb Haemost 1996; 75:939–944.
39. Horner SM. Efficacy of intravenous magnesium in acute myocardial infarction in reducing arrhythmias and mortality. Circulation 1992; 86:774–779.
40. Thögersen AM, Johnson O, Wester PO. Effects of intravenous magnesium sulphate in suspected acute myocardial infarction on acute arrhythmias and long-term outcome. Int J Cardiol 1995; 49:143–151.
41. Borzak S, Ridker PM. Discordance between meta-analysis and large-scale randomized controlled trials. Examples from the management of acute myocardial infarction. Ann Intern Med 1995; 123:873–877.
42. Singh RB, Sircar AR, Rastogi SS, et al. Magnesium and potassium administration in acute myocardial infarction. Magnes Trace Elem 1990; 9:198–204.
43. Pereira D, Pereira TG, Rabaçal C, et al. Efeito da administração de SO_4Mg por via intra-venosa na fase aguada do enfarte do miocárdio. Rev Portug Cardiol 1990; 9:205–210.
44. The Acute Infarction Ramipril Efficacy (AIRE) Study Investigators. Effect of ramipril on mortality and morbidity of survivors of acute myocardial infarction with clinical evidence of heart failure. Lancet 1993; 342:821–827.
45. Pfeffer MA, Braunwald E, Moye LA, et al. Effect of captopril on mortality and morbidity in patients with left ventricular dysfunction after myocardial infarction. N Engl J Med 1992; 327:669–677.
46. Woods KL. Mega-trials and the management of acute myocardial infarction. Lancet 1995; 346:611–614.
47. Shechter M, Hod H, Chouraqui P, et al. Magnesium therapy in acute myocardial infarction when patients are not candidates for thrombolytic therapy. Am J Cardiol 1995; 75:321–323.
48. England MR, Gordon G, Salem M, et al. Magnesium administration and dysrhythmias after cardiac surgery: A placebo-controlled, double-blind, randomized trial. JAMA 1992; 268(17):2395–2402.
49. Caspi J, Rudis E, Bar I, et al. Effects of magnesium on myocardial function after coronary artery bypass grafting. Ann Thorac Surg 1995; 59:942–947.
50. Karmy-Jones R, Hamilton A, Dzavik V, et al. Magnesium sulfate prophylaxis after cardiac operations. Ann Thorac Surg 1995; 59:502–507.
51. Yusuf S, Teo KK, Woods KL. Intravenous magnesium in acute myocardial infarction. Circulation 1993; 87(6):2043–2046.
52. Yusuf S, Flather M. Magnesium in acute myocardial infarction: ISIS-4 provides no ground for its routine use. BMJ 1995; 310:751–752.
53. Egger M, Smith GD. Misleading meta-analysis. BMJ 1995; 310:752–754.
54. Yusuf S, Collins R, Peto R. Why do we need some large, simple randomized trials? Stat Med 1984; 3:409–420.
55. Woods KL, Fletcher S. Magnesium and myocardial infarction. Lancet 1994; 343:1565–1566.
56. Antman EM. Magnesium in acute MI: Timing is critical. Circulation 1995; 92:2367–2372.
57. de Wood MA, Spores J, Notske R, et al. Prevalence of total coronary occlusion during the early hours of transmural myocardial infarction. N Engl J Med 1980; 303(16):897–902.
58. Braunwald E, Kloner RA. Myocardial reperfusion: A double-edged sword? J Clin Invest 1985; 76:1713–1719.
59. Kloner RA. Does reperfusion injury exist in humans? J Am Coll Cardiol 1993; 21:537–545.
60. Hearse DJ, Stewart DA, Braimbridge MV. Myocardial protection during ischaemic cardiac arrest. J Thorac Cardiovasc Surg 1978; 75(6):877–885.
61. Borchgrevink PC, Bergan AS, Bakoy OE, et al. Magnesium and reperfusion of ischaemic rat heart as assessed by 31P-NMR. Am J Physiol 1989; 256:H195–H204.
62. Hara A, Matsumura H, Abiko Y. Beneficial effect of magnesium on the isolated perfused rat heart during reperfusion after ischaemia: Comparison between pre-ischaemic and post-ischae-

mic administration of magnesium. Naunyn Schmiedebergs Arch Pharmacol 1990; 342:100–106.
63. Lareau S, Boyle A, Deslauriers R, et al. Magnesium enhances function of postischaemic human myocardial tissue. Cardiovasc Res 1993; 27:1009–1014.
64. du Toit EF, Opie LH. Modulation of severity of reperfusion stunning in the isolated rat heart by agents altering calcium flux at onset of reperfusion. Circ Res 1992; 70:960–967.
65. Barros LFM, Chagas ACP, da Luz PL, et al. Magnesium treatment of acute myocardial infarction: Effects on necrosis in an occlusion/reperfusion dog model. Int J Cardiol 1995; 48:3–9.
66. Christensen CW, Rieder MA, Silverstein EL, et al. Magnesium sulfate reduces myocardial infarct size when administered before but not after coronary reperfusion in a canine model. Circulation 1995; 92:2617–2621.
67. Herzog WR, Schlossberg ML, MacMurdy KS, et al. Timing of magnesium therapy affects experimental infarct size. Circulation 1995; 92:2622–2626.
68. Atar D, Serebruany V, Poulton J, et al. Effects of magnesium supplementation in a porcine model of myocardial ischemia and reperfusion. J Cardiovasc Pharmacol 1994; 24:603–611.
69. Herzog WR, Atar D. Magnesium and myocardial infarction. Lancet 1994; 343:1285–1286.
70. Bolli R. Mechanism of myocardial "stunning." Circulation 1990; 82(3):723–738.
71. Schlack W, Bier F, Schäfer M, et al. Intracoronary magnesium is not protective against acute reperfusion injury in the regional ischaemic-reperfused dog heart. Eur J Clin Invest 1995; 25:501–509.
72. Leor J, Kloner RA. Does magnesium have a place in the therapy of acute myocardial infarction? Significance of early vs. late reperfusion. Presented at the American College of Cardiology 44th Annual Scientific Session, New Orleans, LA, 1995.
73. Marban E, Koretsune Y, Corretti M, et al. Calcium and its role in myocardial cell injury during ischemia and reperfusion. Circulation 1989; 80:1V.17–1V.22.
74. White RE, Hartzell HC. Magnesium ions in cardiac function: Regulator of ion channels and second messengers. Biochem Pharmacol 1989; 38(6):859–867.
75. Shattock MJ, Hearse DJ, Fry CH. The ionic basis of the anti-ischemic and anti-arrhythmic properties of magnesium in the heart. J Am Coll Nutr 1987; 6:27–33.
76. Steenbergen C, Perlman ME, London RE, et al. Mechanisms of preconditioning: Ionic alterations. Circ Res 1993; 72:112–125.
77. Herzog WR, Atar D, Gurbel PA, et al. Effect of magnesium sulphate infusion on ex vivo platelet aggregation in swine. Magnes Res 1993; 6:349–353.
78. Bolli R. Oxygen-derived free radicals and postischemic myocardial dysfunction ("stunned myocardium"). J Am Coll Cardiol 1988; 12:239–249.
79. Jolly SR, Kane WJ, Bailie MB, et al. Canine myocardial reperfusion injury: Its reduction by the combined administration of superoxide dismutase and catalase. Circ Res 1984; 54:277–285.
80. Myers ML, Bolli R, Lekich RF, et al. Enhancement of recovery of myocardial function by oxygen free radical scavengers after reversible regional ischemia. Circulation 1985; 72:915–921.
81. Anderson HV, Willerson JT. Thrombolysis in acute myocardial infarction. N Engl J Med 1993; 329:703–725.
82. Lefkovits J, Plow EF, Topol EJ. Platelet glycoprotein IIb/IIIa receptors in cardiovascular medicine. N Engl J Med 1995; 332:1553–1559.
83. Wu K. Platelet activation mechanisms and markers in arterial thrombosis. J Intern Med 1996; 239:17–34.
84. Fitzgerald DJ, Catella F, Roy L, et al. Marked platelet activation in vivo after intravenous streptokinase in patients with acute myocardial infarction. Circulation 1988; 77:142–150.
85. Kerins DM, Roy L, Fitzgerald DJ. Platelet and vascular function during coronary thrombolysis with tissue-type plasminogen activator. Circulation 1989; 80:1718–1725.
86. Vaughan DE, Kirschenbaum JM, Loscalzo J. Streptokinase-induced, antibody-mediated platelet aggregation: A potential cause of clot propagation in vivo. J Am Coll Cardiol 1988; 11:1343–1348.
87. Heptinstall S, Sanderson HM, Fox S, et al. Factors that potentiate or inhibit platelet activation by streptokinase. Thromb Haemost 1993; 69:1074.
88. Hardy E, Heptinstall S, Rubin PC, et al. Effects of raised extracellular magnesium on platelet reactivity. Platelets 1995; 6:346–353.
89. Crawford N, Scrutton MC. Biochemistry of the blood platelets. *In* Bloom AL, Thomas DP, eds. Haemostasis and Thrombosis. New York, Churchill-Livingstone, 1987, pp 47–77.
90. Adams JH, Mitchell JRA. The effect of agents which modify platelet behaviour and of magnesium ions on thrombus formation in vivo. Thromb Haemost 1979; 42:603–610.
91. Gertz SD, Wajnberg RS, Kurgan A, et al. Effect of magnesium sulfate on thrombus formation following partial arterial constriction: Implications for coronary vasospasm. Magnesium 1987; 6:225–235.
92. Ravn HB, Kristensen SD, Hjortdal VE, et al. Early administration of intravenous magnesium inhibits arterial thrombus formation. Circulation 1996; 94(suppl):I-461.
93. Fibrinolytic Trialists' Collaborative Group. Indications for fibrinolytic therapy in suspected acute myocardial infarction: Collaborative overview of early mortality and major morbidity results from all randomised trials of more than 1000 patients. Lancet 1994; 343:311–322.
94. Hennekens CH, Albert CM, Godfried SL, et al. Adjunctive drug therapy of acute myocardial infarction—evidence from clinical trials. N Engl J Med 1996; 335:1660–1667.
95. Baxter GF, Summeray MS, Walker JM. Infarct size and magnesium: Insights into LIMIT-2 and ISIS-4 from experimental studies. Lancet 1996; 348:1424–1426.

13 Nitrates

▶ Ari D. Levinson
▶ James L. Velianou
▶ Salim Yusuf

Nitrates have been an integral part of the treatment of ischemic heart disease for more than 130 years, with the first use of amyl nitrate reported in 1867.[1] Use of nitroglycerin (NTG) followed in 1879.[2] Although the effects of both preparations were noted to be short acting, it was not until 1946 that use of the longer-acting isosorbide dinitrate (ISDN) was reported. Use of intravenous (IV) NTG has become widespread since it was first approved by the U.S. Food and Drug Administration in 1979 for unstable angina pectoris (UAP).[3–5] Although the use of nitrates in myocardial infarction was considered contraindicated until the late 1960s, much work was done evaluating their impact on physiologic outcomes in the early 1970s that provided justification for the small clinical trials of the 1980s and the large trials of the 1990s.[6] This chapter briefly outlines the important biochemical and hemodynamic effects of nitrates before discussing in detail the relevant clinical trials.

MECHANISMS OF ACTION

Biochemical Effects

Nitric oxide (NO) has been shown to be the endothelial-derived relaxing factor (EDRF) that activates the vascular smooth muscle enzyme guanylate cyclase. This process increases intracellular cyclic guanosine monophosphate, which plays a major role in vascular smooth muscle relaxation by phosphorylation of the myosin light chain, blocking its interaction with myosin.[7] Normal endothelium usually releases EDRF (NO), which modulates vascular tone locally by diffusing back into the underlying smooth muscle. Impaired EDRF (NO) release has been documented in endothelial dysfunction caused by coronary atherosclerosis and is believed to account for the abnormal vasomotor responses seen in patients with coronary artery disease (CAD).[8, 9]

NTG and the organic nitrates are now known to be NO donors and are believed to replenish NO in vascular smooth muscle cells, thus inducing vasodilation (Fig. 13–1).[10] Emerging data also suggest that nitrates are more potent coronary arterial vasodilators in the presence of endothelial dysfunction, possibly owing to lack of availability of physiologic NO produced by healthy endothelium.[11] Thus, in the setting of CAD and its resultant endothelial dysfunction, there is a clear biochemical rationale for the use of nitrates. NO donation is most likely its major antianginal mechanism in acute ischemic syndromes.

Nitrates may also have significant antiplatelet effects. Although the clinical importance of this hypothesis is still the subject of debate, several studies suggest that platelet activation may be suppressed by nitrates at conventional clinical doses.[10] In vitro, nitrates increase the platelet concentrations of guanylate cyclase, which increases platelet cyclic guanosine monophosphate, inhibiting calcium flux, and, in turn, decreasing glycoprotein IIb/IIIa receptor binding to fibrinogen.[12]

Hemodynamic Effects

NTG induces nonuniform, dose-related vasodilation in several vascular beds. Venodilation occurs at low concentrations and results in pooling of blood in the venous capacitance vessels, decreasing venous return to the heart, thereby decreasing both cardiac output and myocardial oxygen demand. At higher concentrations, nitrates induce epicardial, coronary arteriolar, and coronary collateral dilation, thereby increasing myocardial oxygen supply. Peripheral arterial dilation decreases afterload, further decreasing myocardial ox-

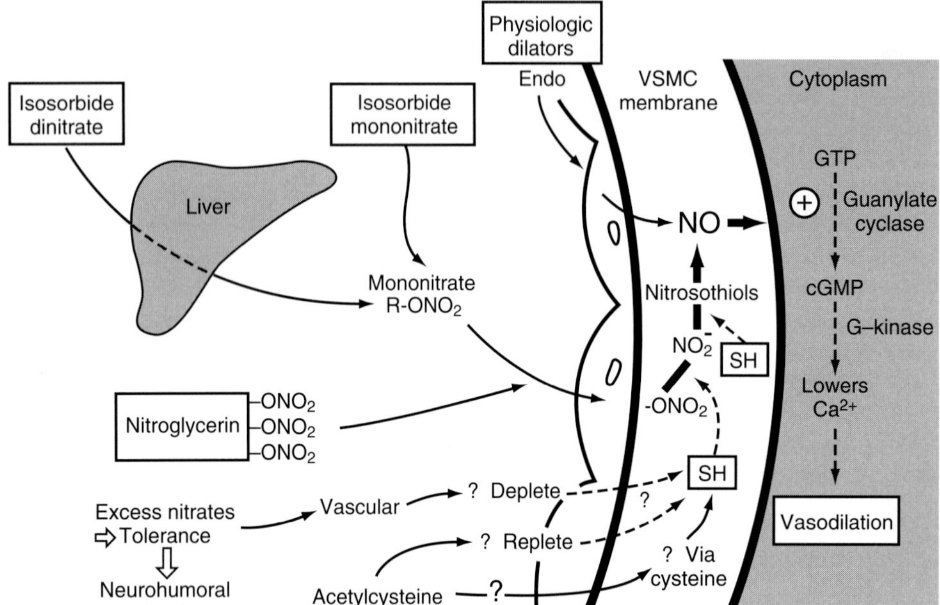

Figure 13–1 *Mechanisms of action of nitrates.* Effects of nitrates in generating nitric oxide (NO) and stimulating guanylase cyclase to produce cyclic guanosine monophosphate (cGMP)-mediated vasodilation. Sulfhydryl (SH) groups are required for the formation of NO and the stimulation of guanylate cyclase. Isosorbide dinitrate is metabolized by the liver, whereas this is bypassed by the mononitrates. GTP, guanosine triphosphate; VSMC, vascular smooth muscle cell; G-kinase, kinase dependent on cGMP. (Copyright 1996, L.H. Opie.)

ygen demands.[13] The need for cautious upward titration of IV nitrates has been emphasized to prevent hypotension and reflex tachycardia. Common infusion protocols start at 5 to 10 μg/min IV followed by upward titration every 5 to 10 minutes until pain is relieved or the systolic blood pressure reaches 90 to 100 mm Hg.[14]

In both animal and human studies, nitroprusside has been shown to induce a coronary steal phenomenon, thereby redistributing flow away from ischemic areas of the myocardium.[10, 15] This concern, together with the need to shield the compound from light, the risk of thiocyanate toxicity, and the need for closer monitoring, makes IV nitroprusside a less attractive alternative to IV NTG in acute ischemic syndromes.[16]

Nitrate Tolerance

Continuous high doses of chronic oral ISDN, transdermal ISDN, and continuous high-dose IV NTG induces tolerance to the anti-ischemic, antianginal, and hemodynamic effects.[5] Continuous high-dose IV NTG produces progressive attentuation starting within 24 hours despite high plasma concentrations.[17] In contrast, low-dose IV NTG (mean dose of 45 ± 34 μg/min) was found to be associated with only partial tolerance in 24% of patients.[18] In several animal models, tolerance has been found to affect different vascular beds in a nonuniform manner, but the implications of this observation are unclear in humans.[5, 13]

Several mechanisms are believed to account for tolerance to high-dose nitrates. Biochemical, or "true," tolerance is believed to be a result of depletion of intracellular sulfhydryl groups (nitrothiols) in vascular smooth muscle, which may be necessary for conversion of nitrates into the active NO compound that is able to function as a vasodilator.[19, 20] However, prevention or reversal of tolerance with IV *N*-acetylcysteine (NAC) or methionine infusions (both thiol donors) have not been consistently reported in acute ischemic syndromes.[13] NAC has been consistently shown to reverse nitrate tolerance in patients with heart failure in several studies.[17] Tolerance can be overridden in the short term by dose escalation. This may also cast some doubt on the depletion of sulfhydryls being the primary mechanism for tolerance.[14]

Emerging data suggest that neurohormonal activation during nitrate therapy may play an important role in the development of nitrate tolerance. These changes would theoretically counteract nitrate-induced vasodilation and induce sodium and water retention, resulting in increased plasma volume. Preliminary studies suggest that angiotensin-converting enzyme (ACE) inhibitors and diuretics may counteract these effects and reduce tolerance[21, 22] (see section on prevention of nitrate tolerance with ACE inhibitors).

Tolerance clearly presents more of a problem in patients with unstable ischemic syndromes requiring high, continuous doses of IV NTG for longer than 24 to 48 hours. In chronic stable angina or in the stable post-infarct patient, it can be prevented by allowing for daily adequate nitrate-free intervals.[5] This was the rationale behind the use of daily topical nitrate that was removed at night in the Gruppo Italiano per lo Studio della Sopravvivenza nell'Infarto Miocardico–3 (GISSI-3) trial, and daily oral single-dose mononitrate in the International Study of Infarct Survival–4 (ISIS-4) trial[23, 24] (see sections on the GISSI-3 and ISIS-4 trials).

NITRATES IN ACUTE MYOCARDIAL INFARCTION

Rationale

Early studies in dogs demonstrated that low-dose IV nitrates, given soon after coronary occlusion, improved regional perfusion and limited both infarct size and remodeling.[25] Several human studies demonstrated reduced creatine kinase peaks, smaller thallium-201 perfusion defects, and reduced overall ischemic injury in acute myocardial infarction with early use of nitrates.[6, 26, 27] In a more recent randomized study of 310 patients with acute myocardial infarction comparing low-dose IV NTG with placebo, treated patients had less regional left ventricular (LV) dysfunction, less infarct expansion and thinning, and less alteration in hemodynamics at 10 days.[26] There are also some reasons to believe that vasodilators may have adverse effects in patients with acute myocardial infarction. These include reflex tachycardia (with an increase in myocardial oxygen demand), coronary steal (with diversion of blood flow from ischemic to nonischemic areas), and hypotension (with resultant decreased epicardial blood flow).[5, 26, 27] Despite the systemic fall in blood pressure with nitrates, several, but not all, studies have demonstrated favorable redistribution of flow from nonischemic to ischemic areas.[28–31]

Two recent small trials that randomized patients receiving recombinant thromboplastin activator (rTPA) to concurrent IV NTG or a control group suggest that NTG decreases plasma rTPA concentrations.[32, 33] In one of these studies, plasminogen activator inhibitor-1 levels were also higher in the nitrate group.[32] The clinical implications of these observations are unclear.

Overview of the Smaller Trials

ORAL NITRATES IN ACUTE MYOCARDIAL INFARCTION

Five small trials of oral nitrates or placebo started soon after myocardial infarction have been reported.[34–38] These involved a total of 1110 patients. Most were reported from 1964 to 1970, preceding the common use of thrombolytics, aspirin, beta blockers, or IV heparin.[34–37] Four of the trials used pentaerythritol tetranitrate, a long-acting nitrate available in Europe. One of the trials used isosorbide mononitrate.[39] The pooled data of these trials demonstrated a statistically nonsignificant trend toward lower mortality rates in the nitrate group. The overall mortality was 68 (11.9%) of 576 patients in the nitrate-treated group as compared with 71 (13.3%) of 534 control subjects (odds ratio [OR], 0.88; 95% confidence interval [CI], 0.53 to 1.88).[39]

IV NITRATES IN ACUTE MYOCARDIAL INFARCTION

Ten small trials of IV nitrates were reported between 1981 and 1985 (IV nitrates: seven trials; IV nitroprusside: three trials).[40–49] In 1988 an overview of these 10 randomized, controlled trials of IV organic nitrates in acute myocardial infarction was published.[50] A total of 2041 patients were randomized, 851 to NTG or placebo. Only one NTG trial involved more than 200 patients,[49] with the others each having fewer than 100 patients.[43–48] In an additional three trials, 1190 patients were randomized to nitroprusside or placebo.[40–42] Therefore, most of these trials were individually too small to adequately assess plausible effects of nitrates on mortality.

All patients were randomized within 24 hours of symptom onset. In general patients were excluded if they were older than 70 to 75 years, in cardiogenic shock, or had severe congestive heart failure (CHF), uncontrolled hypertension, chronic obstructive pulmonary disease or other life-threatening disease. In the NTG trials, low doses were initiated and gradually titrated up to reduce mean arterial blood pressure by 10 mm/Hg[45, 46, 49] or the systolic blood pressure by 10% to 30%, depending on initial blood pressure.[43, 47, 48] In the nitroprusside trials initial doses ranged from 10 to 33 μg/kg per minute. The infusions were continued 24 to 48 hours in most of the studies.[41–49] Although seven of the studies (five in the NTG trials,[41, 42] two in the nitroprusside trials[43, 45–48]) used a placebo, because of the blood pressure drop in the patients on active treatment, none of the trials were likely to have been fully blinded. This lack of full blinding was unlikely to have been a major source of bias because of the use of major endpoints (such as mortality) requiring little clinical judgment in their assessment.

The results of this meta-analysis are summarized in Figure 13–2. In eight of the trials the mortality rate was lower in the treatment arms.[40–45, 48, 49] There were no deaths in one trial[46] and an excess of deaths in another.[47] Of the total of 426 patients randomized to IV NTG, there were 51 deaths (12.0%) as compared with 87 deaths (20.5%) in the 425 control subjects, giving a risk reduction of 49%. In the nitroprusside trials, there were 85 deaths (14.3%) in the 595 patients randomized to active treatment as compared with 106 deaths (17.8%) in the 595 control subjects, giving a risk reduction of 24% that did not reach statistical significance.

Although the duration of follow-up varied substantially, treatment with either agent appeared to reduce early mortality significantly (5.5% versus 9.6%, 2*P*

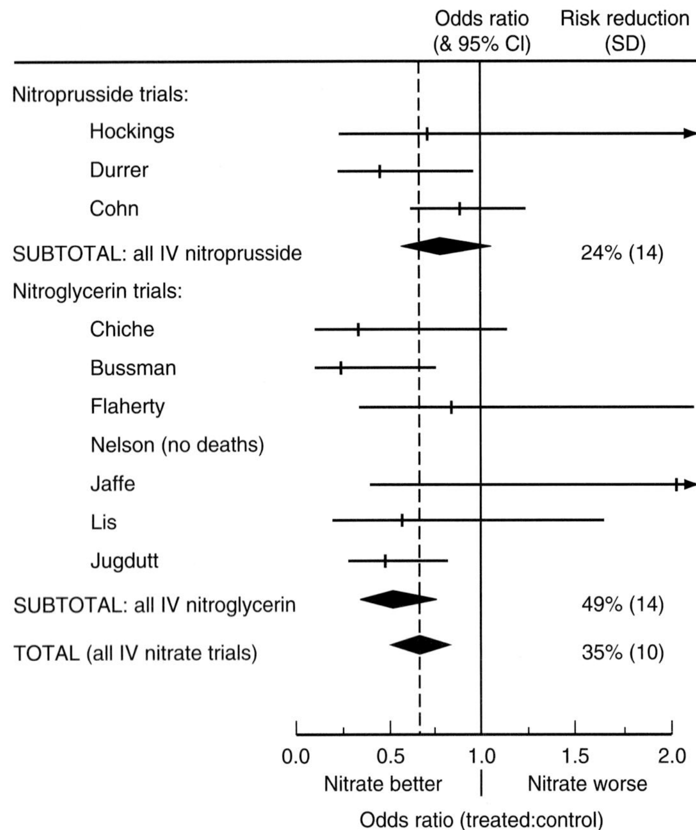

Figure 13–2 Apparent effects of intravenous (IV) nitroprusside and nitroglycerin on mortality in the randomized trials of the treatment of acute myocardial infarction. Vertical line, odds ratio; horizontal line, 95% confidence interval (CI); a 95% CI that does not include 1.0 indicates a statistically significant difference ($2P = 0.05$) in mortality between the treatment groups. Broken line, "typical" odds ratios indicated by an overview of all IV nitrate trials. For complete citation information of trials, see the original source. (From Yusuf S, Collins R, MacMahon S, et al. Effect of intravenous nitrates on mortality in acute myocardial infarction: An overview of the randomized trials. Lancet 1988; 1:1088–1092. © by The Lancet Ltd., 1988.)

<0.001) with a nonsignificant trend toward benefit seen later (9.4% late deaths in the treatment arm vs. 11.6% in the control arm, $2P = 0.1$). In the largest trial included in the meta-analysis, 310 high-risk patients with acute myocardial infarction were randomized to IV NTG or placebo. NTG was titrated to reduce the mean arterial blood pressure by 10% in normotensive patients and 30% in hypertensive patients. As well as the benefits on remodeling and infarct size (described earlier), there was a significant survival advantage in those patients with anterior myocardial infarction receiving NTG as compared with placebo (inhospital mortality 14% vs. 26% [$P < 0.01$], 3-month mortality 16% vs. 28% [$P < 0.025$], and 12-month mortality 21% vs. 31% [$P < 0.05$]).[27]

The overview of all 10 studies included suggested that treatment reduced mortality by 30% to 35%, with 95% confidence limits between one half and one sixth. Because of the potential limitations of meta-analysis and the relatively modest numbers of patients randomized (<2000), the authors cautioned that any real benefits would likely be much more moderate, that is, closer to one sixth than to one half. No consistent patterns emerged with respect to variations in treatment effect by infarct location or timing of nitrate therapy.[50]

Few of these trials used aspirin, beta blockers, or thrombolytics routinely as standard therapy, and the control group patients experienced high mortality rates. Therefore, these results, although strongly suggestive of a benefit in the 1980s, are difficult to extrapolate to the latter half of the 1990s. However, on the basis of this meta-analysis, routine IV nitrate therapy was recommended by Task Forces of the American Heart Association and the American College of Cardiology in 1990. Based on these data, the GISSI and ISIS investigators evaluated nitrates in two large randomized trials.[23, 24]

The Large Trials

THE GISSI-3 TRIAL

The GISSI-3 investigators randomized 19,394 patients with acute myocardial infarction to glyceryl trinitrate (GTN) or open control, and the ACE inhibitor lisinopril or open control in a 2 × 2 factorial design. The four treatment arms were GTN alone, lisinopril alone, combined GTN and lisinopril, or no trial therapy. Patients were randomized between 1991 and 1993 from approximately 200 coronary care units in Italy.[23] Patients were included if they presented within 24 hours of symptoms and were excluded if there were clear clinical indications for the study medications. The main endpoints were a prespecified combined outcome measure of 6-week mortality and severe LV dysfunction (the latter manifested by clinical heart failure, ejection fraction, ≤ 35%, or the presence of substantial LV dysfunction on echocardiography). Thrombolytics, aspirin, and beta blockers were used in 72%, 84%, and 31% of patients, respectively.

Those patients randomized to GTN received a 24-hour infusion of IV NTG, followed by 6 weeks' treatment with topical NTG 10 mg daily (removed at night to avoid tolerance). The IV NTG infusion was started at 5 μg per minute and titrated up until a 10% reduction in the systolic blood pressure was achieved.

The results indicated a small, nonsignificant reduction in deaths at 6 weeks in the group randomized to NTG (6.52%) as compared with the control group (6.92%) (OR, 0.94; CI, 0.84 to 1.05; $2P = 0.28$). There was a similar small, nonsignificant reduction in the combined endpoints of death or LV dysfunction as compared with control (15.9% vs. 16.73%; OR, 0.94; CI, 0.87 to 1.02).

The patients randomized to lisinopril experienced a significant reduction in the combined endpoint (15.6% vs. 17%; OR, 0.90 [CI, 0.84–0.95]; $2P = 0.009$) and mortality (6.3% vs. 7.1%; OR, 0.88 [CI, 0.79–0.99]; $2P = 0.03$). Both mortality and combined endpoints suggested an additive effect for the combination of NTG and lisinopril (mortality 6.0%) as compared with control (mortality in the group with neither treatment 7.2%) (OR, 0.83; CI, 0.70 to 0.97).

The absence of a statistically significant effect of the overall NTG group compared with placebo needs to be interpreted with some caution. It should be noted that 57.1% of patients in the control group received nonstudy NTG. Although most received short-term treatment (24 hours) only, 11.3% of the control group did receive long-term NTG treatment. (The precise mode of administration is not stated.) Such extensive use of nitrates in the control group could have obscured additional small, but significant, beneficial effects of NTG.

Use of NTG in this trial was associated with few side effects. Nitrate treatment was discontinued mainly because of hypotension (2.6%) or headache (3.0%), but there were no significant differences in persistent hypotension between treatment and control groups (6.6% vs. 6.2%; OR, 1.07; CI, 0.95 to 1.20). The nitrate group had a significantly lower frequency of cardiogenic shock (2.1% vs. 2.6%; OR, 0.78; CI, 0.64 to 0.94), although this may well have been owing to chance, because a similar benefit was not observed in the ISIS-4 trial (see later). The nitrate group did have a slightly lower incidence of postinfarction angina (20.0% vs. 21.2%; OR, 0.93; CI, 0.86 to 0.99).[23]

THE ISIS-4 TRIAL

Between 1991 and 1993, ISIS-4 investigators[24] randomized 58,050 patients with suspected myocardial infarction to oral isosorbide mononitrate or placebo control. (The 2 × 2 × 2 factorial design also involved randomizing patients to IV magnesium vs. control and the ACE inhibitor captopril vs. control.) This trial involved 1086 hospitals in 31 countries. Inclusion criteria included presentation within 24 hours of symptom onset. Contraindications included persistent severe hypotension, cardiogenic shock, and high risk of death from noncardiac disease. Myocardial infarction was subsequently confirmed in 92% of randomized patients. In keeping with current practice, 94% of patients received antiplatelet therapy and 70% received thrombolytic therapy. Only 9% received IV beta blockers. Seventy-four percent of patients were male and 28% of patients were older than 70 years of age.

Patients received 1 month of controlled-release mononitrate orally, starting at a dose of 30 mg initially and titrated up to 60 mg daily versus matching placebo. The prespecified primary outcome measure was mortality at 5 weeks.

The results of ISIS-4 study were consistent with GISSI-3 and did not demonstrate a significant reduction in 5-week mortality with use of nitrates as compared with control (7.3% vs. 7.5%; $2P = 0.30$). Furthermore, follow-up to 12 months showed no additional adverse or detrimental effect (at 1 year, 1.8 fewer deaths in the nitrate group/1000, P = NS). Subgroup analysis also showed no survival benefit, in particular, in subgroups with heart failure and/or early randomization. Although there was an increase in hypotension in the mononitrate group (8.1% vs. 6.7%), this was not associated with a higher mortality rate and suggests no persisting adverse impact of transient hypotension induced by nitrates. Unlike in GISSI-3 there was no decrease in postinfarction angina, reinfarction rates, or cardiogenic shock in the nitrate arm.

Additional treatments (IV magnesium or oral captopril) conferred neither benefit, nor risk, when added to mononitrate, in contrast with GISSI-3 in which the addition of the ACE inhibitor lisinopril to nitrates conferred a small, but statistically significant, survival advantage. The ISIS-4 trial also had a high rate of nonstudy nitrate use: 55% of patients were treated with nonstudy IV nitrates on randomization (47% IV and 8% oral or transdermal). As in GISSI-3, this high rate of nonstudy nitrate use may have been a confounder obscuring small but significant effects of mononitrate. (The use of nonstudy nitrates varied substantially between countries, with no overall treatment benefit shown in those countries where their use was more common. Nonstudy IV nitrates were used in approximately 75% of patients in the United States, Germany, Poland, and Norway as compared with 25% or less in the United Kingdom, Sweden, Brazil, and New Zealand.[24])

THE ESPRIM TRIAL

Between 1990 and 1992, the European Study of Prevention of Infarct with Molsidomine (ESPRIM) investigators[51] randomized 4017 patients with acute myocardial infarction to linsidomine followed by molsidomine or placebo. Although molsidomine is not a true organic nitrate, its active metabolite linsidomine is a nitric oxide donor and has vasodilating properties similar to NTG.[52] Because NO is released by spontaneous hydrolysis of linsidomine (rather than by the enzymatic steps required for its generation from NTG and nitroprusside), studies have shown a lack of tolerance to this agent.[53] The ESPRIM trial involved 117 centers in Europe.

Patients presenting within 24 hours of symptom onset, but without Killip class III/IV heart failure, were randomly assigned to IV linsidomine 1 mg per hour for 48 hours, followed by 16 mg of oral molsidomine daily for a further 12 days versus matching placebo control. The primary outcome measure was all-cause 35-day mortality. Although only 50% of patients received thrombolytics, 86% of patients received concomitant aspirin, 75% IV heparin, and 65% beta blockers. Thirty-nine percent of patients in the molsidomine group and 40% of patients in the placebo group received IV NTG during the hospitalization.[51]

In keeping with the results of GISSI-3 and ISIS-4, the ESPRIM trial did not demonstrate significant differences in 35-day all-cause mortality between molsidomine and placebo (8.4% vs. 8.8% deaths; $P = 0.66$). Similarly, there was no difference in long-term mortality at a mean of 13 months' follow-up (14.7% vs. 14.2% deaths; $P = 0.67$). This agent was well tolerated with no increase in significant side effects as compared with placebo, except for an increase in the risk of hemorrhagic stroke in the subgroup receiving molsidomine as well as heparin, aspirin, and thrombolytics (10 vs. 2 events; $P = 0.021$).[51] Although it is possible that the additive antithrombotic effects of all four agents combined may have increased the risk of hemorrhagic stroke, such a subgroup effect should be interpreted with considerable skepticism.[51]

The ESPRIM trial therefore also did not support the routine treatment of myocardial infarction with an NO donor.

THE RECENT MEGATRIALS VERSUS THE META-ANALYSIS OF OLD TRIALS

Despite the combined enrollment of nearly 80,000 patients, the GISSI-3 and ISIS-4 trials individually failed to show a clear survival advantage for routine nitrates started early in acute myocardial infarction. Furthermore, no survival advantage was shown in any subgroup analyzed individually.[23, 24] That the ISIS-4 trial found no benefits in the addition of nitrates to ACE inhibition suggests that the very small advantage of this combination in GISSI-3 may have been a chance finding.[23, 24] The ESPRIM trial of 4000 patients also failed to show mortality benefits from the NO donor molsidomine.[51]

A combined meta-analysis of *all trials* reveals a just statistically significant 5.4% reduction for mortality in myocardial infarct patients assigned to nitrates (7.4% mortality with nitrates vs. 7.78% mortality without nitrates; $2P = 0.033$; OR, 0.90–0.99). This translates to 3.8 fewer deaths per 1000 patients treated with nitrates (Fig. 13–3*A*). However, meta-analysis of the nitrate arms of the *three largest and most recent trials* (GISSI-3, ISIS-4, and ESPRIM) shows a nonsignificant mortality reduction of 3.7% (7.2% mortality with nitrates vs. 7.46% mortality without nitrates; OR, 0.91–1.01; $2P = 0.16$), or 2.6 fewer deaths per 1000 patients (Fig. 13–3*B*).

The *combined day 0–1 mortality data for the ISIS-4 and GISSI-3 trials* shows a highly statistically significant 17% ± 5 odds reduction ($2P < 0.001$) in the nitrate group versus placebo (1.7% vs. 2.1% day 0–1 mortality in ISIS-4 and 1.5% vs. 1.7% day 0–1 mortality in the GISSI-3). No further benefit beyond 24 hours was observed for the combined mortality data of these trials (OR, −2% ± 3; P = NS) (R Collins, personal communication, 1997).

The discrepancy in results between the large trials (which overall demonstrated a nonstatistically significant risk reduction of 3.7%) and the meta-analysis of older but smaller trials (which demonstrated a statistically significant 31% risk reduction) warrants close consideration. There were important differences with regard to nontrial treatment. There was little or no use of thrombolytic and antiplatelet agents in the early trials summarized by the meta-analysis, as compared with relatively high rates of thrombolytic and

Figure 13–3 *A* and *B*, Meta-analysis of effects on short-term mortality (average 5 weeks) of starting nitrates early after acute myocardial infarction: *A* shows the updated meta-analysis of the smaller intravenous (IV) and oral trials as well as the three large trials; and *B* indicates the updated meta-analysis of the three larger trials only (GISSI-3, ISIS-4, and ESPRIM). In both *A* and *B*, squares denote the point estimate for the odds ratio (OR), and the horizontal lines denote 99% confidence intervals (CI). Size of the squares is proportional to the amount of "statistical information" available (related to the number and proportion of events) for each trial or set of trials. The overall result and 95% CI are shown by the diamond, with the overall proportional reduction (or increase) and statistical significance given alongside. Squares or diamonds to the left of the vertical solid line indicate benefit (significant at $P < 0.01$) when the entire horizontal line is to the left of the vertical line and at $P < 0.05$ when the diamond does not overlap the vertical line. Dotted vertical line denotes pooled OR for all studies. For the GISSI and ISIS studies, subgroup comparisons are presented for the effects of nitrates in the presence and absence of angiotensin-converting enzyme inhibitor (ACE-I). (Adapted from Flather MD, Avezum A, Yusuf S. General approach to management of acute myocardial infarction. *In* Fuster V, Ross R, Topol E (eds). Atherosclerosis and Coronary Artery Disease. Philadelphia, Lippincott-Raven, 1996, pp 942–943.)

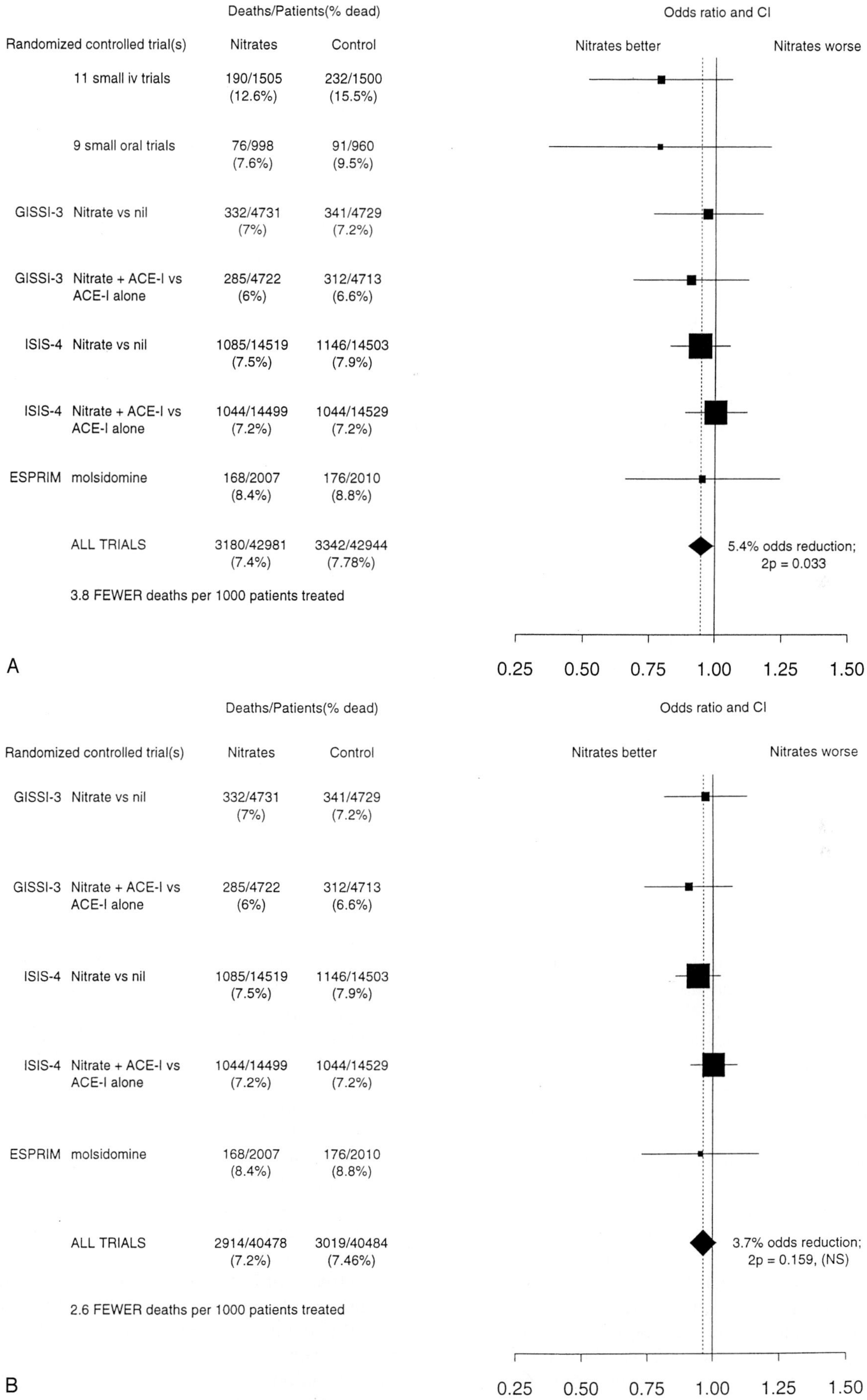

Figure 13–3 *See legend on opposite page.*

antiplatelet drugs in the large trials. Further, the mortality rates were 18.9% in the control group in the meta-analysis of old trials compared with 7.8%, 7.2%, and 8.8% in the ISIS-4, GISSI-3, and ESPRIM control groups, respectively.[23, 24, 50, 51] The markedly different mortality rates suggest that the types of patients enrolled in the recent large trials were at lower risk. It is possible that treatment with nitrates may be less beneficial in low-risk patients.

The high rates of nontrial nitrate use in the placebo groups (57% in GISSI-3 and 55% in ISIS-4) are a significant confounder.[24, 51] Although no apparent benefit was observed in those not receiving nontrial nitrates, such analyses are confounded by postrandomization changes in clinical status influencing the use of these agents. Therefore, such subgroup analysis cannot be considered "proper" because of substantial risk of confounding.

In the 1988 meta-analysis,[50] IV nitrates were generally given for 48 hours and titrated to keep the blood pressure between 90 and 100 mm Hg. The GISSI-3 patients only received IV nitrates for 24 hours followed by topical nitrates for 6 weeks. The ISIS-4 patients received oral daily mononitrate in a regimen where the dose was not adjusted in response to blood pressure changes. It is possible that these differences in administration, the type of nitrate used, and the substantial use of nontrial nitrates may have had some confounding effect on the results in the large trials. On the other hand, some of the discrepancies in results may have been due to the inherent limitations of the meta-analysis itself. As was mentioned in the section presenting an overview of smaller trials, the individual trials had small patient numbers and were not individually of sufficient size to provide reliable results on mortality. Other concerns about some of the individual small trials included high numbers of withdrawals following randomization and the essentially open design in most trials. The major limitation of the 1988 meta-analysis, however, is the potential for publication bias. The possibility cannot be excluded that some trials with unpromising results were not known, despite extensive attempts made by the authors to seek unpublished randomized data.[50] Even if one or two unpublished trials of a few hundred patients with unpromising results were missed, the meta-analysis could have been substantially affected.

In summary, the combined ISIS-4 and GISSI-3 data suggest a significant 17% odds reduction for routine use of nitrates in the first 24-hour period after myocardial infarction. Although these data do not support the use of nitrates beyond 24 hours, this approach cannot be completely discarded for the reasons discussed earlier. Further, nitrates were safe and well tolerated in both the older and the more recent large randomized trials. This provides the clinician with reassurance about the safety of nitrates in myocardial infarction; therefore, it would be reasonable also to use nitrates beyond 24 hours for the symptomatic relief of angina, hypertension, or heart failure where clinically indicated.[54]

NITRATES IN UNSTABLE ANGINA

Clinical Studies

The major goals of therapy of patients presenting with UAP are relief or prevention of anginal symptoms and prevention of progression to acute myocardial infarction. UAP is usually caused by fissuring of an atherosclerotic plaque with superimposed platelet deposition. Although severe coronary spasm is no longer believed to be a common primary cause of UAP, inappropriate increases in coronary tone are believed to be a contributing factor.[55] IV nitrates are widely used in UAP as vasodilators, despite the paucity of randomized, controlled data.[56] Indeed, there are no placebo-controlled studies evaluating the usefulness of nitrates in UAP.[14]

Most of the available studies are small observational series that were uncontrolled and unblinded. Those series with 16 or more patients[57–61] are summarized in Table 13–1. These data indicate consistent symptomatic relief with IV NTG. Several studies also showed a significant decrease in the need for narcotic analgesic requirements.[59, 61] Although both topical and oral nitrates have been shown to reduce chest pain in UAP, IV nitrate infusions are used most commonly because of their rapid onset of action and prompt reversibility.[62, 63] IV nitrates in UAP are now frequently used in combination with beta blockers or rate-limiting calcium channel blockers.[55]

In most of the small studies tabulated in Table 13–1, the dose of IV NTG was adjusted to keep the systolic blood pressure between 90 and 100 mm Hg.[56, 58, 60] Although optimal infusion rates for IV NTG are still unresolved,[64] there is evidence that the NTG infusion should not reduce the mean arterial pressure by more than 15% in normotensive patients.[18]

In one of the few randomized, controlled trials in this area, Curfman and associates[85] randomized 40 patients with UAP to IV NTG or a combination of oral and topical nitrates. The dosage of these agents was titrated up to reduce the systolic blood pressure by 15% ± 3% or, in the case of IV NTG, to a maximum infusion of 200 μg per minute. IV NTG reduced the number of spontaneous ischemic episodes from 3.3 ± 0.8 to 1.0 ± 0.3 per 24 hours ($P < 0.01$). The effect was similar to the effect of oral or transdermal NTG (reduction in ischemic episodes from 3.1 ± 0.4 to 1.4 ± 0.3 per 24 hours; $P < 0.01$). The data did suggest a trend toward more consistent control of

TABLE 13–1 • Nitrate Therapy in Unstable Angina Pectoris (UAP): Summary of the Larger Uncontrolled Case Series of 16 or More Patients

Study (Reference)	Year	No. of Patients	Entry Criteria	Design	Results	Discussion
Roubin GS, et al (57)	1982	16	UAP despite oral nitrates, beta blockers, calcium channel blockers	Open-label IV NTG (12–960 μg/min)	Complete (38%) or partial (62%) resolution of CP	Observational; uncontrolled
DePace NL, et al (58)	1982	20	UAP despite beta blockers, oral nitrate, and nifedipine	Open-label IV NTG (15–226 μg/min)	Complete (70%) resolution of CP	Observational; uncontrolled
Heinsimer JA, et al (68)	1981	32	UAP; background medications not stated	Open-label IV NTG (82 ± 23 μg/min) vs. oral or transdermal nitrates	70% initial reduction of CP (IV NTG) vs. 55% (oral or transdermal nitrates). P = NS	Randomized; open label; no nonnitrate group
Curfman GD, et al (85)	1983	40	UAP despite beta blockers and fixed-dose oral or transdermal nitrates	Open-label IV NTG (10–200 μg/min) vs. oral or transdermal nitrates	Complete or partial resolution of CP in ~70% in each group (see text)	Randomized; open label; no nonnitrate group
Kaplan K, et al (59)	1983	27	UAP refractory to oral treatment, including oral or topical NTG	Open-label IV NTG (50–350 μg/min)	Complete (71%) or partial (23%) resolution of CP	Observational; uncontrolled
Page A, et al (60)	1981	67	UAP refractory to beta blockers and oral nitrates	Open-label IV NTG (12.5–50 μg/min)	Complete (63%) or partial (32%) resolution of CP	Observational; uncontrolled
Mikolich JR, et al (61)	1980	45	UAP refractory to usual treatment of beta blockers and sublingual NTG	Open-label IV NTG (5–267 μg/min)	Complete (0%) or partial (89%) resolution of CP	Observational; uncontrolled
Squire A, et al (67)	1982	42	UAP despite beta blockers and sublingual NTG q 2 h	Open-label IV NTG (<393 μg/min)	Complete (45%) resolution of CP	Observational; uncontrolled

NTG, nitroglycerin; CP, chest pain.
Data from Conti RG. Use of nitrates in unstable angina pectoris. Am J Cardiol 1987; 60:31H–34H; Horowitz JD: Role of nitrates in unstable angina pectoris. Am J Cardiol 1992; 70:64B–71B; and Thadani U, Opie LH. Nitrates for unstable angina. Cardiovasc Drugs Ther 1994; 8:719–726.

ischemic episodes in the first 24-hour period of this 72-hour trial, but this did not reach statistical significance. There was no placebo comparison group.

In another small trial, Dellborg and colleagues[65] randomized 29 patients with UAP to continuous IV NTG or to buccal NTG given every 4 hours. (Buccal NTG has a rapid onset of action with a sustained effect of 3 to 5 hours.) No significant difference in outcome was noted, but fewer adverse effects (less hypotension and less headache) were noted in the group receiving buccal therapy. This trial also did not have a placebo comparison group.

Figueras and coworkers[66] reported a prospective, uncontrolled withdrawal trial in which IV NTG was abruptly discontinued at between 24 and 72 hours in 46 consecutive patients with UAP. Twenty-six (55%) of these patients developed chest discomfort and ischemic ST changes on continuous electrocardiographic (ECG) monitoring 10 ± 6 minutes after nitrate withdrawal. There were no significant early changes in the double product (heart rate × systolic blood pressure), suggesting rebound coronary vasoconstriction as the underlying mechanism for the withdrawal-associated ischemia. The study was seriously flawed by lack of a control group and also by the exclusion of patients treated with other antianginal agents. However, the large proportion of patients experiencing clinical or ECG evidence of ischemia indicates the possibility of rebound ischemia on nitrate withdrawal. Little other clinical data exist on how best to prevent possible rebound ischemia associated with nitrate withdrawal.

The evidence for the efficacy of IV nitrates in relieving pain in UAP is good despite the nonrandomized nature of most of the studies and the lack of placebo control groups. Most of the studies listed earlier were also conducted before the routine use of aspirin, IV heparin, and beta blockers, and there is an urgent need therefore for trials of nitrates in the context of these agents. Remaining questions include the efficacy of adding IV rate-limiting calcium channel blockers (see later) to IV nitrates in UAP, the optimal duration of therapy, and the best protocols for discontinuation of IV nitrates.

IV Nitroglycerin Versus IV Calcium Channel Blockers in Unstable Angina Pectoris

In a recent randomized, double-blind, open-label study, Gobel and associates[69] compared the calcium channel blocker diltiazem with NTG in 129 patients with UAP associated with ECG changes. Both agents were infused IV in standard doses. All patients received IV heparin. The principal endpoints were persistent angina despite study medications, new myocardial infarction, or both, at 48 hours. Intention-to-treat analysis revealed a statistically significant reduction in combined endpoint of persistent angina and myocardial infarction (20% in the IV diltiazem group vs. 41% in the IV nitrates group; OR, 0.49; 95% CI, 0.27 to 0.88; $P = 0.02$). Atrioventricular conduction delay occurred more frequently in the diltiazem arm (8% vs. 0%; $P = 0.03$). No patients required pacing. Headache occurred more frequently in the NTG arm (5% vs 25%; $P < 0.004$).[69]

These results need to be interpreted cautiously. First, the open-label design raises the possibility of bias. Second, the higher rates of myocardial infarction and/or death at 48 hours in this trial (13% and 25% in the diltiazem and nitrate arms, respectively) compared with other trials of UAP (4% and 16%) are a concern.[69, 86] Third, calcium channel blockers used by the patient prior to admission were discontinued. More patients were on prior calcium channel blockers in the group assigned to diltiazem (33% vs. 21%; $P =$ NS). Fourth, beta blockers were not used except in the few patients in whom they were used prior to randomization (37% and 23% in the patients assigned diltiazem and nitrates, respectively; $P =$ NS). The results of this trial are therefore difficult to generalize to current practice.[55] However, they raise questions regarding the value of IV NTG in UAP in the context of modern treatment.

In a small, open, randomized study of 18 patients with UAP, Fang and coworkers[70] compared IV diltiazem to IV NTG. All patients received aspirin and heparin. Although patients randomized to diltiazem had significantly fewer episodes of silent ischemia (55% vs. 100%; $P = 0.05$), the study was not designed to assess other clinical endpoints.

Few other data exist that directly compare the use of IV NTG to IV calcium channel blockers in UAP.[82] Thus, the available data from the earlier discussed two trials suggest that IV NTG may be less effective than IV diltiazem (a rate-limiting calcium antagonist) in the first few days of UAP. However, until additional comparative studies become available in which beta blockers, aspirin, and heparin are given to all patients, IV NTG still remains a first-line treatment for UAP together with heparin and aspirin.[55]

IV Nitroglycerin Versus IV Nitroprusside in Unstable Angina Pectoris

In a combined clinical and hemodynamic study, Breisblatt and colleagues[72] randomized 40 patients with UAP to IV NTG ($n = 22$) or IV nitroprusside ($n = 18$). There was a high rate of symptomatic clinical response in each group (82% vs. 83%; $P =$ NS). Swan-Ganz catheterization revealed similar changes in mean arterial pressure (decreases of 10% to 15%), no alteration of heart rate in either group, and similar decreases in mean pulmonary capillary wedge pressure (7 to 8 mm Hg). Serial radionuclide angiographic studies revealed a similar increase in ejection fraction for each group (average increases of 17% and 13%, respectively; $P =$ NS). Thus, in this trial, both agents had similar short-term efficacy.

Heparin-Nitroglycerin Interaction

The combined use of IV heparin and IV NTG is almost universal in the management of UAP today. Several initial reports suggested an interaction between NTG and heparin with impairment of activated partial thromboplastin time (aPTT) prolongation.[56, 72, 73] One study linked this interaction to the propylene glycol diluent used to stabilize the otherwise potentially explosive IV NTG solution.[74] These concerns have not been confirmed by more recent clinical studies. Gonzalez and associates[75] found no significant differences in aPTT values in 22 patients before and after discontinuation of NTG. Nottestad and Maxcette[76] found no overall differences in the heparin doses required to achieve therapeutic anticoagulation in 58 patients receiving low- or high-dose IV NTG. Other studies have also showed no interaction between these two agents.[77]

Combined Nitrate–*N*-Acetylcysteine Therapy

As outlined earlier in the section on biochemical effects, the vasodilator effects of NTG are mediated by the activation of guanylate cyclase in a process that is believed to require availability of free sulfhydryl groups. NAC is a sulfhydryl donor that has been shown to potentiate NTG-induced coronary and systemic vasodilation.[78, 79] The combination of NAC and NTG also results in *S*-nitroso–NAC, an inhibitor of platelet aggregation.[80]

Horowitz and coworkers,[81] in a double-blind, placebo-controlled trial of refractory UAP, randomized 46 patients to IV NTG alone (24 patients), or IV NTG combined with IV NAC boluses of 5 g every 6 hours (22 patients). Patients did not receive heparin. Although there was no significant difference in the frequency of chest discomfort or the need to increase the NTG infusion rates, patients assigned NTG plus NAC did have a lower incidence of acute myocardial infarction (3 vs. 10 patients; $P = 0.013$). Symptomatic hypotension, however, developed in 30% of the patients in the NTG plus NAC group as compared with none in the control group (7/24 vs. 0/22; $P = 0.006$). In a subsequent case series of 20 patients reported in the same paper,[81] NAC administration in a lower dose as a continuous infusion (10 g per 24 hours) eliminated the hypotensive episodes in all patients. Lack of controls in the second series limits interpretation of the results regarding the combined use of IV NTG with IV NAC. Furthermore, lack of use of IV heparin makes it difficult to apply these data to current treatment protocols.

A small recent study[82] of 27 patients presenting with acute myocardial infarction investigated the use of NAC. All patients received streptokinase and IV NTG. Randomization was in a 3:1 ratio: 20 patients received NAC (15 g per 24 hours continuous infusion) and 7 patients were controls. There were trends toward better preservation of LV function and earlier reperfusion in the NAC group.[82] These results require confirmation in much larger randomized trials.

Prevention of Nitrate Tolerance with ACE Inhibitors

Data are accumulating that ACE inhibitors may have a role in preventing tolerance to continuous longer-term (>24- to 48-hour) use of IV NTG. Pizzulli and coworkers[87] randomized 26 patients with stable CAD to captopril (25 mg twice daily) or placebo for 7 days. Hemodynamic responses to 0.8 mg sublingual NTG were then assessed at the beginning and end of a 48-hour infusion of IV NTG with right and left heart catheterization. No differences were observed between the captopril and placebo groups in baseline hemodynamics and in the response to sublingual NTG on the first day of the IV NTG infusion. The response to sublingual NTG, however, was markedly diminished in the placebo group at 48 hours, whereas persistent significant hemodynamic responses to sublingual NTG were still seen in the captopril group. The lack of increased vasodilation in the captopril group at baseline and the persistent vasodilation at 48 hours compared with placebo does suggest that captopril prevented the onset of nitrate tolerance as opposed to simply augmenting the vasodilatory responses of nitrates.[87] Captopril is a thiol-containing ACE inhibitor.[88] Because its effect in reducing tolerance could theoretically be explained by sulfhydryl donation, other groups have studied the effect of the non–thiol-containing ACE inhibitor benazepril. This agent has been found to reduce nitrate tolerance in the dog model, suggesting a mechanism independent of sulfhydryl donation.[89] In a randomized, double-blind, placebo-controlled, 2 × 2 factorial study of 24 patients with chronic stable angina, Muiesan and colleagues[90] found that benazepril (10 mg twice daily) significantly increased the exercise duration as compared with placebo in patients assigned continuous transdermal NTG. Although these studies need to be confirmed in larger trials with clinical endpoints, they do suggest that ACE inhibitors may attenuate or prevent nitrate tolerance with continuous administration of IV or transdermal NTG. The mechanism is likely independent of sulfhydryl donation and possibly relates to a decrease in neurohormonal activation and/or alterations in properties intrinsic to the vascular endothelium.[89, 90]

CONCLUSIONS

Nitrates in Acute Myocardial Infarction

The GISSI-3, ISIS-4, and ESPRIM trials, despite a combined enrollment of almost 82,000 patients with acute myocardial infarction, failed to show an *overall* statistically significant mortality benefit in patients treated routinely with nitrates. *Combined subgroup analysis* of the GISSI-3 and ISIS-4 day 0–1 mortality data show an odds reduction of 17% in the nitrate group with no additional benefit beyond this period. These results are in contrast with the 1988 meta-analysis of 10 small earlier trials (3 IV nitrate, 3 IV nitroprusside) involving 2041 patients that showed an overall risk reduction of 30% to 35%.

The lack of benefit of routine postmyocardial infarction nitrates beyond 24 hours in the recent large trials may be explained by the following factors:

1. The lower overall mortality in the GISSI-3, ISIS-4, and ESPRIM trials as a result of the routine use of thrombolytic therapy, aspirin, and beta blockers.
2. The possibility of reduced power and confounding that obscured any real benefits of nitrates in GISSI-3 and ISIS-4 beyond day 1 because of extensive and early use of nonstudy nitrates (>50% use in GISSI-3 and ISIS-4). Further, the use of *oral mononitrate* in ISIS-4 and *short-term IV nitrate* use (<24 hours) in GISSI-3 may have limited the efficacy of the nitrate regimen.
3. The results of the GISSI-3, ISIS-4, and ESPRIM trials may reflect a real lack of efficacy of routine postmyocardial infarction nitrate therapy in the context of other current treatments. However, the GISSI-

3 and ISIS-4 trials confirm the safety of IV, oral, and transdermal nitrates in the immediate postmyocardial infarction period.

Routine IV NTG may therefore be considered in the first 24 hours following acute myocardial infarction. It is not recommended for routine post–acute myocardial infarction management beyond the first 24 hours. IV NTG is also a safe and reasonable option for specific indications in the post–acute myocardial infarction setting; these include persistent or recurrent ischemia, uncontrolled hypertension, or CHF.

Nitrates in Unstable Angina Pectoris

There are *no randomized, placebo-controlled studies* of IV nitrates in UAP. Several small uncontrolled case series and a large clinical experience suggest that nitrates are effective in symptomatic management of UAP. However, most of these small studies (<300 patients in total) were conducted at a time when heparin, aspirin, beta blockers, and calcium channel blockers were used infrequently. No data showing efficacy of nitrates in preventing progression to myocardial infarction, need for revascularization, or death are available in the context of modern therapies.

Although IV nitrates continue to be widely used in patients with UAP, there are no good data to support its routine use in patients who receive heparin, aspirin, beta blockers, and a rate-limiting calcium channel blocker. Further, because of the potential for tolerance with 24 hours of IV administration, the optimal dose and duration of use of IV NTG are yet to be elucidated. The possible clinical usefulness of ACE inhibitors in preventing tolerance awaits confirmation. Although difficult to conduct, a well-designed, placebo-controlled, randomized trial of the routine use of IV nitrates in UAP in the context of modern therapy is urgently required.

REFERENCES

1. Brunton TL. Lectures on the Actions of Medicines. New York, Macmillan, 1867.
2. Murrel W. Nitro-glycerine as a remedy for angina pectoris. Lancet 1879; I:80–81.
3. Goldberg L, Porje IG. En studie over sorbid-nitratets karleffekt. Nordisk Medicin 1946; 29:190–193.
4. Sorkin EM, Brogden RN, Romankiewicz JA. Intravenous glyceryl trinitrate (nitroglycerin): A review of its pharmacocological properties and therapeutic efficacy. Drugs 1984; 27:45–80.
5. Jugdutt BI. Nitrates in unstable angina and acute myocardial infarction. *In* Rezakovic DE, Alpert JS (eds). Nitrate Therapy and Nitrate Tolerance. Basel, Karger, 1993, pp 111–167.
6. Flaherty JT. Role of nitrates in acute myocardial infarction. Am J Cardiol 1987; 60:35H–38H.
7. Wilhelmen L. Nitrates. *In* Julian D, Braunwald E (eds). Management of Acute Myocardial Infarction, 4th ed. Philadelphia, WB Saunders, 1992.
8. Ganz P, Ludmer PL, Leopold JA, et al. Endothelial dysfunction in vivo: Studies in animals and in patients with coronary atherosclerosis. *In* Vanhoutte PM (ed). Vasodilation: Vascular Smooth Muscle, Peptides, Autonomic Nerves, and Endothelium. New York, Raven Press, 1988, p 543.
9. Ludmer PL, Selwyn AP, Shook TL, et al. Paradoxical vasoconstriction induced by acetylcholine in atherosclerotic arteries. N Engl J Med 1986; 315:1046–1051.
10. Abrams J. Mechanisms of action of the organic nitrates in the treatment of myocardial ischemia. Am J Cardiol 1992; 70:30B–42B.
11. Dinerman JL, Lawson DL, Mehta JL. Interactions between nitroglycerin and endothelium in vascular smooth muscle relaxation. Am J Physiol 1991; 260:H698–H701.
12. Loscalzo J. Antiplatelet and antithrombotic effects of organic nitrates. Am J Cardiol 1992; 70:18B–22B.
13. Bassenge E, Zanzinger J. Nitrates in different vascular beds, nitrate tolerance, and interactions with endothelial function. Am J Cardiol 1992; 70:23B–29B.
14. Thadani U, Opie LH. Nitrates for unstable angina. Cardiovasc Drugs Ther 1994; 8:719–726.
15. Chiarello M, Gold K, Leinbach RC, et al. Comparison between the effects of nitroprusside and nitroglycerin in ischemic injury during acute myocardial infarction. Circulation 1976; 54:766–773.
16. Opie LH. Angiotensin-converting enzyme inhibitors and conventional vasodilators. *In* Opie LH (ed). Drugs for the Heart, 3rd ed. Philadelphia, WB Saunders, 1991, p 117.
17. Zimrin D, Reichek N, Bogin K, et al. Antianginal effects of IV nitroglycerin over 24 hours. Circulation 1988; 77:1376–1384.
18. Jugdutt BI, Warnica WJ. Tolerance with low-dose intravenous nitroglycerin therapy in acute myocardial infarction. Am J Cardiol 1989; 64:481–587.
19. Fung H-L, Chung S-J, Bauer JA, et al. Biochemical mechanism of organic nitrate action. Am J Cardiol 1992; 70:4B–10B.
20. Elkayam U, Mehra A, Shotan A, Ostrzega E. Nitrate resistance and tolerance: Potential limitations in the treatment of congestive heart failure. Am J Cardiol 1992; 70:98B–104B.
21. Parker JO, Parker JD. Neurohormonal activation during nitrate therapy: A possible mechanism of tolerance. Am J Cardiol 1992; 70:93B–97B.
22. Fung HL, Bauer JA. Mechanisms of nitrate tolerance. Cardiovasc Drugs Ther 1994; 8(3):489–499.
23. GISSI-3 Investigators. Effects of lisinopril and transdermal glyceryl trinitrate singly and together on 6-week mortality and ventricular function after acute myocardial infarction. Lancet 1994; 343:1115–1122.
24. ISIS-4 Investigators. A randomized factorial trial assessing early oral captopril, oral mononitrate, and intravenous magnesium sulphate in 58,050 patients with suspected acute myocardial infarction. Lancet 1995; 345:669–685.
25. Jugdutt BI. Nitrates in myocardial infarction. Cardiovasc Drugs Ther 1994; 8:635–646.
26. Jugdutt BI. Role of nitrates after acute myocardial infarction. Am J Cardiol 1992; 70:82B–87B.
27. Jugdutt BI, Warnica JW. Intravenous nitroglycerin therapy to limit myocardial infarct size, expansion, and complications: Effect of timing, dosage, and infarct location. Circulation 1988; 78:906–919.
28. Horowitz LD, Gorlin R, Taylor WJ, et al. Effects of nitroglycerin on regional myocardial blood flow in coronary artery disease. J Clin Invest 1971; 50:1578–1584.
29. Passamani ER. Nitroprusside in myocardial infarction. N Engl J Med 1982; 306:1168–1170.
30. Hillis LD, Davis C, Khuri SF. The effect of nitroglycerin and nitroprusside on ischemic injury during acute myocardial infarction. Circulation 1976; 54:766–773.
31. Jugdutt BI. Myocardial salvage by intravenous nitroglycerin in conscious dogs: Loss of beneficial effect with marked nitroglycerin-induced hypotension. Circulation 1983; 68:673–684.
32. Romeo F, Rosano GM, Martuscelli E, et al. Concurrent nitroglycerin administration reduces the efficacy of recombinant tissue-type plasminogen activator in patients with acute anterior wall myocardial infarction. Am Heart J 1995; 130:692–697.
33. Nicolini FA, Ferrini D, Ottani F, et al. Concurrent nitroglycerin therapy impairs tissue-type plasminogen activator–induced

thrombolysis in patients with acute myocardial infarction. Am J Cardiol 1994; 74:662–667.
34. Mellen HS, Goldberg HS, Friedman HF. Therapeutic effects of pentaerythritol tetranitrate in the immediate postmyocardial infarction period. N Engl J Med 1967; 276:319–322.
35. Newell DJ. Pentaerythritol tetranitrate (sustained action) in acute myocardial infarction. Br Heart J 1970; 32:16–20.
36. Oscharoff A. Pentaerythritol tetranitrate as adjunctive therapy in the immediate postinfarction period. Angiology 1964; 15:505–514.
37. Ryan TJ, Schnee M. Pentaerythritol tetranitrate in acute myocardial infarction [Abstract]. Circulation 1965; 32:Suppl II-105.
38. Fitzgerald LJ, Bennett ED. The effects of oral isosorbide 5-mononitrate on mortality following acute myocardial infarction: A multicenter study. Eur Heart J 1990; 11:121–126.
39. Held P, Teo KK, Yusuf S. Effects of beta-blockers, calcium channel blockers, and nitrates in acute myocardial infarction and unstable angina pectoris. *In* Topol E (ed). Interventional Cardiology. Philadelphia, WB Saunders, 1989, pp 49–65.
40. Hockings BEF, Cope GD, Clarke GM, Taylor RR. Randomized, controlled trial of vasodilator therapy after myocardial infarction. Am J Cardiol 1981; 48:245–251.
41. Durrer JD, Lie KI, van Capelle FJL, Durrer D. Effect of sodium nitroprusside on mortality in acute myocardial infarction. N Engl J Med 1982; 306:1121–1128.
42. Cohn JN, Franciosa JA, Francis GS, et al. Effect of short-term infusion of sodium nitroprusside on mortality rate in acute myocardial infarction complicated by left ventricular failure: Results of a VA Cooperative Study. N Engl J Med 1982; 306:1129–1136.
43. Chiche P, Baligaadoo SH, Derrida JP. A randomized trial of prolonged nitroglycerin infusion in acute myocardial infarction [Abstract]. Circulation 1979; 59, 60:Suppl II-165.
44. Bussman WD, Passek D, Seidel W, Kaltenbach M. Reduction of CK and CK-MB indexes of infarct size by intravenous nitroglycerin. Circulation 1981; 63:615–622.
45. Flahery JT, Becker LC, Bulkley BH, et al. A randomized prospective trial of IV nitroglycerin in patients with acute myocardial infarction. Circulation 1983; 68:576–588.
46. Nelson GIC, Silke B, Ahuha RC, et al. Haemodynamic advantages of isosorbide dinitrate over furosemide in acute heart failure following myocardial infarction. Lancet 1983; 1:730–733.
47. Jaffe AS, Geltman EM, Tiefenbrunn AJ, et al. Reduction of infarct size in patients with inferior infarction with IV glyceryl trinitrate: A randomized study. Br Heart J 1983; 49:452–460.
48. Lis Y, Bennett D, Lambert G, Robson D. A preliminary double-blind study of IV nitroglycerin in acute myocardial infarction. Intensive Care Med 1984; 10:179–184.
49. Jugdutt BI, Wortman C, Warcica WJ. Does nitroglycerin therapy in acute myocardial infarction reduce the incidence of infarct expansion [Abstract]? J Am Coll Cardiol 1985; 5:447.
50. Yusuf S, Collins R, MacMahon S, Peto R. Effect of intravenous nitrates on mortality in acute myocardial infarction: An overview of the randomized trials. Lancet 1988; 1:1088–1092.
51. ESPRIM Investigators: The ESPRIM trial: Short-term treatment of acute myocardial infarction with molsidomine. Lancet 1994; 344:91–97.
52. Aptecar M, Otero y Garzon C, Vasquez A, et al. Hemodynamic effects of molsidomine vasodilator therapy in acute myocardial infarction. Am Heart J 1981; 101:369–373.
53. Meinertz T, Brandstatter A, Trenk D, et al. Relationship between pharmacokinetics and pharmacodynamics of molsidomine and its metabolites in humans. Am Heart J 1985; 109:644–648.
54. Flather MD, Avezum A, Yusuf Y. General approach to management of acute myocardial infarction. *In* Fuster V, Ross R, Topol EJ (eds). Atherosclerosis and Coronary Artery Disease. Philadelphia, Lippincott-Raven, 1996, pp 942–943.
55. Cairns JA. Medical management of unstable angina [Editorial]. Lancet 1995; 346:1644–1645.
56. Jaffrani NA, Ehrenpreis S, Laddu A, Somberg MD. Therapeutic approach to unstable angina: Nitroglycerin, heparin, and combined therapy. Am Heart J 1993; 126:1239–1242.
57. Roubin GS, Harris PJ, Eckhardt I, et al. Intravenous nitroglycerin in refractory unstable angina pectoris. Aust NZ J Med 1982; 12:598–602.
58. DePace NL, Herling IH, Kotler MN, et al. Intravenous nitroglycerin for rest angina: Potential pathophysiologic mechanisms of action. Arch Intern Med 1982; 142:1806–1809.
59. Kaplan K, Davison R, Parker M, et al. Intravenous nitroglycerin for the treatment of angina at rest unresponsive to standard nitrate therapy. Am J Cardiol 1983; 51:694–698.
60. Page A, Gateau P, Ohayon J, et al. Intravenous nitroglycerin in unstable angina. *In* Lechtlen PR, Engel H (eds). Nitrates III: Cardiovascular Effects. Berlin, Springer-Verlag, 1981, pp 371–376.
61. Mikolich JR, Nicoloff NB, Robinson RH, Logue RB. Relief of refractory angina with continuous intravenous infusion of nitroglycerin. Chest 1980; 77:375–379.
62. Conti RG. Use of nitrates in unstable angina pectoris. Am J Cardiol 1987; 60:31H–34H.
63. Conti CR, Hill JA, Mayfield WR. Unstable angina pectoris: Pathogenesis and management. Curr Prob Cardiol 1989; 14:459–624.
64. Horowitz JD. Thiol-containing agents in the management of unstable angina pectoris and acute myocardial infarction. Am J Cardiol 1991; 91:113S–117S.
65. Dellborg M, Gustafsson G, Swedberg K. Buccal versus intravenous nitroglycerin in unstable angina pectoris. Eur J Clin Pharmacol 1991; 41:5–9.
66. Figueras J, Lidon R, Cortadellos J. Rebound myocardial ischemia following abrupt interruption of intravenous nitroglycerin infusion in patients with unstable angina at rest. Eur Heart J 1991; 12:405–411.
67. Squire A, Cantor R, Packer M. Limitations of continous intravenous nitroglycerin in patients with refractory angina at rest. Circulation 1982; 66(Suppl):II-120.
68. Heinsimer JA, Curfman GD, Fung HL, et al. Intravenous nitroglycerin for spontaneous angina: A short-term, prospective, randomized trial [Abstract]. Circulation 1981; 64:IV-10.
69. Gobel EJAM, Hautvast RWM, van Gilst WH, et al. Randomized, double-blind trial of intravenous diltiazem versus glyceryl trinitrate for unstable angina pectoris. Lancet 1995; 346:1653–1657.
70. Fang ZY, Picart N, Abramowicz M, et al. Intravenous diltiazem versus nitroglycerin for silent and symptomatic myocardial ischemia in unstable angina pectoris. Am J Cardiol 1991; 68:42C–46C.
71. Habbab MA, Haft JI. Heparin resistance induced by intravenous nitroglycerin: A word of caution when both drugs are used concomitantly. Arch Intern Med 1987; 147:857–860.
72. Breisblatt WM, Navratil DL, Burns MJ, Spaccavento LJ. Comparable effects of intravenous nitroglycerin and intravenous nitroprusside in acute ischemia. Am Heart J 1988; 116:465–472.
73. Pye M, Oldroyd KG, Conkie JA, et al. A clinical and in vitro study on the possible interaction of intravenous nitrates with heparin anticoagulation. Clin Cardiol 1994; 17:658–661.
74. Col J, Col-Debeys C, Lavenne-Pardonge E, et al. Propylene glycol–induced heparin resistance during nitroglycerin infusion. Am Heart J 1985; 110:171–173.
75. Gonzalez ER, Jones HD, Graham S, Elswick RK. Assessment of the drug interaction between intravenous nitroglycerin and heparin. Ann Pharmacother 1992; 26(12):1512–1514.
76. Nottestad SY, Maxcette AM. Nitroglycerin-induced heparin resistance: Absence of interaction at clinically relevant doses. Mil Med 1994; 159:569–571.
77. Bode V, Welzel D, Franz G, Polensy U. Absence of drug interaction between heparin and nitroglycerin. Arch Intern Med 1990; 150:2117–2119.
78. Horowitz JD, Antman EM, Lorell BH, et al. Potentiation of the cardiovascular effects of nitroglycerin by *N*-acetylcysteine. Circulation 1983; 68:1247.
79. Winniford MD, Kennedy PL, Wels PJ, Hillis LD. Potentiation of nitroglycerin-induced coronary dilation by *N*-acetylcysteine. Circulation 1986; 73:138.
80. Loscalzo J. *N*-acetylcysteine potentiates inhibition of platelet aggregation by nitroglycerin. J Clin Invest 1985; 76:103.
81. Horowitz JD, Henry CA, Syrjanen ML, et al. Combined use of nitroglycerin and *N*-acetylcysteine in the management of unstable angina pectoris. Circulation 1988; 77:787–794.
82. Arstall MA, Yang J, Stafford I, et al. *N*-acetylcysteine in combination with nitroglycerin and streptokinase for the treatment

of evolving acute myocardial infarction: Safety and biochemical effects. Circulation 1995; 92:2855–2862.
83. Held PH, Yusuf S, Furberg CD. Calcium channel blockers in acute myocardial infarction and unstable angina: An overview. BMJ 1995; 299:1187–1192.
84. Horowitz JD. Role of nitrates in unstable angina pectoris. Am J Cardiol 1992; 70:64B–71B.
85. Curfman GD, Heinsimer JA, Lozner EC, Fung H. Intravenous nitroglycerin in the treatment of spontaneous angina pectoris: A prospective, randomized trial. Circulation 1983; 67:276–282.
86. Wales, Lam J, Theroux P. Newer concepts in the management of unstable angina pectoris. Am J Cardiol 1991; 68:340.
87. Pizzulli L, Hagendorff A, Zirbes M, et al. Influence of captopril on nitroglycerin-mediated vasodilation and development of nitrate tolerance in arterial and venous circulation. Am Heart J 1996; 131:342–349.
88. Opie LH. Ace inhibitors—specific agents: Pharmacokinetics. *In* Opie LH (ed). Angiotensin-Converting Enzyme Inhibitors: Scientific Basis for Clinical Use, 2nd ed. New York, John Wiley & Sons, 1992, pp 177–179.
89. Munzel T, Bassenge E. Long-term angiotensin-converting enzyme inhibition with high-dose enalapril retards nitrate tolerance in large epicardial arteries and prevents rebound coronary vasoconstriction in vivo. Circulation 1996; 93:2052–2058.
90. Muiesan ML, Boni E, Castellano M. Effects of transdermal nitroglycerin in combination with an ACE inhibitor in patients with chronic stable angina pectoris. Eur Heart J 1993; 14:1701–1708.

14 Direct Thrombin Inhibitors

▶ Elliott M. Antman
▶ John A. Bittl

DIRECT THROMBIN INHIBITORS FOR UNSTABLE ANGINA AND ACUTE MYOCARDIAL INFARCTION

Pathophysiology of Acute Coronary Syndromes

A coronary artery plaque that is moderately stenotic and relatively soft, has a central core that is rich in lipids, and is covered by a fibrous cap that is poor in connective tissue and smooth muscle cells is referred to as a "vulnerable" plaque.[1] When it ruptures and exposes its contents to the blood stream, platelets adhere to the subendothelial matrix, release adenosine diphosphate and thromboxane A_2, and amplify the generation of thrombin. As a result, a platelet aggregate begins to develop.[2, 3] In addition, the coagulation cascade is activated and fibrin strands are formed. The culprit coronary artery becomes occluded by a thrombus containing a fibrin mesh and platelet aggregates.

When coronary blood flow is reduced sufficiently, patients experience ischemic discomfort. Complete occlusion of the culprit vessel produces ST-segment elevation, and most of these patients ultimately evolve a Q wave myocardial infarction (MI).[4] A small proportion may sustain only a non–Q wave MI. When the obstructing thrombus is subtotally occlusive, obstruction is transient, or a rich collateral network is present, no ST-segment elevation is seen. Most such patients are diagnosed as having unstable angina, or if a serum cardiac marker indicative of myocardial necrosis is detected, as having a non–Q wave MI. A few patients may actually develop a Q wave MI. The spectrum of presentations ranging from unstable angina through non–Q wave MI and Q wave MI is referred to as the *acute coronary syndromes*.[5]

Antithrombotic Therapy for the Acute Coronary Syndromes

Thrombolytic therapy exerts a highly significant, 21% proportional reduction in 35-day mortality among patients with acute MI who present with ST-segment elevation.[6] However, the available evidence suggests that thrombolytic therapy is not effective and may actually be harmful in patients presenting without ST-segment elevation and it is therefore not recommended for those groups of patients.[7] In contrast, antiplatelet and antithrombin therapies are applicable across the entire spectrum of acute coronary syndromes and have been the subject of intensive clinical investigation.[2, 3]

Antithrombin Agents

The standard antithrombin agent used in clinical practice is heparin.[8] Although familiar to most clinicians, unfractionated heparin has the disadvantages of

1. A variable anticoagulant effect, necessitating frequent activated partial thromboplastin time (aPTT) monitoring
2. Sensitivity to platelet factor 4
3. A relative inability to inhibit clot-bound thrombin
4. The potential to cause thrombocytopenia

In an attempt to circumvent some of the difficulties with heparin, direct antithrombins (antithrombin III independent) have been developed.[3, 9, 10] When sufficient quantities of direct antithrombins were made available (in many cases, by recombinant technology), clinical trials were undertaken to evaluate their efficacy and safety in acute coronary syndromes.

While several direct antithrombins have been developed, those that have undergone the most clinical investigation are hirudin, bivalirudin (Hirulog), argatroban, efegatran, and inogatran.[3, 9, 11] All four agents exhibit a concentration-dependent anticoagulant effect. Hirudin and bivalirudin are irreversible inhibitors of thrombin, whereas argatroban, efegatran, and inogatran are reversible inhibitors. Although all the agents are capable of antithrombin III–independent inhibition of thrombin, available data suggest that their mechanism of inhibition may vary.[12] On a weight basis, hirudin appears to be the most potent of the group. However, in vitro studies suggest hirudin and the other irreversible direct antithrombin, bivalirudin, have a limited capacity to block generation of thrombin, while this process appears to be inhibited to a somewhat greater degree by the reversible thrombin inhibitors[12]; the clinical significance of such distinctions remains to be elucidated.

Mechanism of Action of Antithrombin Agents

Figure 14–1 compares the antithrombotic action of heparin with hirudin, the prototypical direct antithrombin.[3, 13] Thrombin exists both in the fluid phase and the clot-bound phase. Heparin binds to the heparin-binding domains of both thrombin and antithrombin III, amplifying antithrombin III's ability to block the catalytic center of thrombin. The carboxy terminus of hirudin binds to the substrate recognition site on thrombin, while the amino terminus inhibits the active catalytic center of thrombin. (The smaller, reversible antithrombins bind directly to the catalytic center of thrombin.)

Clot-bound thrombin is less effectively inhibited by heparin because the attachment of fibrin to the fibrin-binding domain makes the heparin-binding domain inaccessible.[14] In contrast, direct antithrombins have a greater ability to block both fluid-phase and clot-bound thrombin. The notion that more complete and consistent inhibition of thrombin activity could be achieved by direct antithrombins has been referred to as the *thrombin hypothesis* and was the inspiration for several randomized, controlled trials.

Phase II Clinical Trials of Direct Antithrombins in Acute Coronary Syndromes

ST-SEGMENT ELEVATION MYOCARDIAL INFARCTION—ADJUNCTIVE THERAPY TO THROMBOLYSIS

Trials of Hirudin

Inadequate initial reperfusion of infarct-related arteries and reocclusion of successfully reperfused vessels continue to be important limitations of thrombolytic regimens for ST-segment MI. In an effort to develop

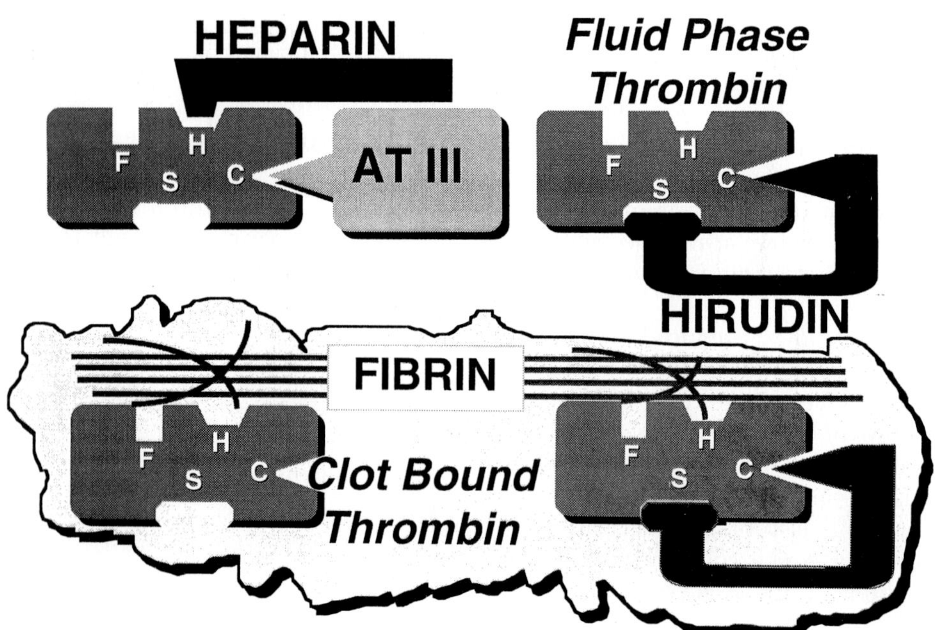

Figure 14–1 Mechanism of action of antithrombin agents heparin and hirudin. Thrombin exists both in the fluid phase (top portion) and in the clot-bound phase (bottom portion). Heparin binds simultaneously to the heparin-binding domain (H) of thrombin and antithrombin III (ATIII), amplifying ATIII's ability to block the catalytic center (C) of thrombin. In contrast, hirudin binds simultaneously to the substrate recognition domain (S) of thrombin and to the catalytic center of thrombin. Clot-bound thrombin is not effectively inhibited by heparin, because the attachment of fibrin to the fibrin-binding domain of thrombin (F) makes the heparin-binding domain inaccessible. In contrast, a direct antithrombin such as hirudin is capable of inhibiting thrombin in both the fluid phase and clot-bound phase (see text for further discussion).

improved adjunctive regimens to thrombolysis, direct antithrombins were evaluated in a number of Phase II trials.

The Thrombolysis in Myocardial Infarction (TIMI) 5 trial enrolled 246 patients with ST-segment elevation MI who were treated with front-loaded tissue plasminogen activator (t-PA) and were randomized to receive one of four ascending doses of recombinant desulfatohirudin (from an initial bolus of 0.15 mg/kg and infusion of 0.05 mg/kg per hour up to a bolus of 0.6 mg/kg and infusion of 0.2 mg/kg per hour) versus heparin (bolus of 5000 U and initial infusion of 1000 U per hour titrated to an aPTT of 65 to 90 seconds).[15] Figure 14–2 shows the proportion of patients achieving TIMI grade 3 flow in the heparin and hirudin groups. A slightly higher proportion of patients treated with hirudin achieved TIMI grade 3 flow compared with heparin. In addition, infarct-related artery patency was significantly higher in the hirudin-treated patients who underwent follow-up angiography (18 to 36 hours) compared with heparin. Reocclusion by 18 to 36 hours was seen in only 1.6% of hirudin patients compared with 6.7% of heparin patients ($P = 0.07$). No intracranial hemorrhages occurred in any of the hirudin-dose groups; a single intracranial hemorrhage occurred in the heparin group (1 [1.2%] of 86 patients). Major hemorrhage occurred predominantly at an instrumented site and ranged from 11.5% at the lowest dose of hirudin (0.05 mg/kg per hour infusion) to 29.4% at the highest dose of hirudin (0.2 mg/kg per hour infusion), as compared with 18.6% in heparin-treated patients. Analysis of the characteristics of the patients experiencing major hemorrhage suggested that an aPTT in excess of 100 seconds was associated with an increased risk of bleeding.

The Hirudin for the Improvement of Thrombolysis (HIT) Investigators conducted a series of angiographic trials with recombinant hirudin (HBW 023).[16] An initial pilot study (HIT-I) in 40 patients presenting within 6 hours of the onset of symptoms evaluated a bolus of hirudin of 0.07 mg/kg and infusion of 0.05 mg/kg per hour for 48 hours in conjunction with front-loaded t-PA. TIMI grade 3 flow was observed in 71% of patients; early, complete, and sustained patency (i.e., TIMI 3 flows at 60 and 90 minutes and at 24 to 48 hours) was observed in 55% of patients. The HIT-II sequential dose-escalation study examined three doses of hirudin (boluses of 0.1, 0.2, and 0.4 mg/kg followed, respectively, by infusions of 0.06, 0.1, and 0.15 mg/kg per hour) in 143 patients receiving front-loaded t-PA. TIMI grade 3 flow at 60 minutes was observed in 50%, 58%, and 63% of the three-dose groups, respectively. Major bleeding was seen in 0, 7%, and 11% of the three-dose groups.

The TIMI 6 Trial consisted of 193 patients treated with streptokinase for ST-segment elevation MI.[17] Patients were randomized to three doses of hirudin (boluses of 0.15, 0.3, and 0.6 mg/kg followed, respectively, by infusion rates of 0.05, 0.1, and 0.2 mg/kg per hour) versus heparin (bolus 5000 U, initial infusion 1000 U per hour). Major hemorrhage, either spontaneous or at an instrumented site, occurred during the initial hospitalization in 5.5%, 6.5%, and 5.6% of patients treated with hirudin with the regimens described earlier and 5.6% of heparin-treated patients. Death or nonfatal reinfarction occurred by hospital discharge in 8.8% of heparin patients and 13.7%, 9.7%, and 5.7% of the three ascending dose groups for hirudin. The trend toward a reduction in events with higher doses of hirudin persisted at 6 weeks following enrollment.

Of note, despite careful designs to efficiently select an optimal dose, experience in HIT-II, TIMI 5, and

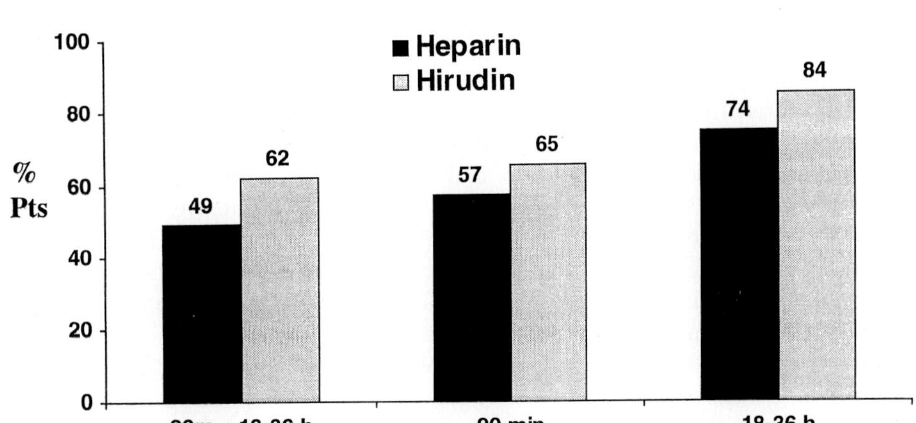

Figure 14–2 Results from a trend toward a higher proportion of patients achieving TIMI grade 3 flow was observed in the combined hirudin group versus the heparin group. A greater proportion of patients in the combined hirudin group showed TIMI grade 3 flow both at 90 minutes and at 18 to 36 hours. (Adapted from Cannon CP, McCabe CH, Henry TD, et al. A pilot trial of recombinant desulfatohirudin compared with heparin in conjunction with tissue-type plasminogen activator and aspirin for acute myocardial infarction: Results of the Thrombolysis in Myocardial Infarction [TIMI] 5 trial. J Am Coll Cardiol 1994; 23:993–1003. Reprinted with permission from the American College of Cardiology (**Journal of the American College of Cardiology**, 1994, vol 23, pp 993–1003.)

TIMI 6 did not adequately predict the safety concerns observed in large Phase III trials (see discussion later).

Trials of Bivalirudin

Bivalirudin has been evaluated as adjunctive therapy to streptokinase for MI by several investigators. Lidón and associates compared low-dose bivalirudin (0.5 mg/kg per hour) and high-dose bivalirudin (1.0 mg/kg per hour) with heparin (bolus 5000 U; infusion 1000 U per hour).[18] At 90 minutes, 85% (P = 0.008) of patients had TIMI grade 3 flow in the low-dose bivalirudin group compared with 61% in the high-dose bivalirudin group and 31% in the heparin group. The suggestion that a low dose of a direct thrombin inhibitor may be more effective than a high dose has been hypothesized as being due to the "thrombin paradox," which states that low doses of antithrombins allow sufficient thrombin activity to persist, leading to stimulation of the inhibitory thrombomodulin and protein C pathway. However, inconsistent observations have been reported with doses of bivalirudin and TIMI flow in streptokinase-treated patients. White and coworkers in the Hirulog Early Reperfusion/Occlusion (HERO) Trial reported a TIMI grade 3 flow rate at 90 to 120 minutes of 48% of patients receiving high-dose bivalirudin (bolus 0.25 mg/kg; infusion 0.5 mg/kg per hour for 12 hours and then 0.25 mg/kg per hour) compared with 46% in patients receiving low-dose bivalirudin (bolus 0.125 mg/kg; infusion 0.25 mg/kg per hour for 12 hours and then 0.125 mg/kg per hour) and 100 patients receiving heparin (bolus 5000 U; infusion 1000 to 2000 U per hour).[19]

Trials with Other Agents

Dose-ranging clinical trials with angiographic endpoints have been performed with several other direct antithrombins in patients with ST-elevation MI. The Promotion of Reperfusion in Myocardial Infarction (PRIME) Investigators compared efegatran (0.3 to 1.2 mg/kg per hour) with heparin (bolus 5000 U; infusion 1000 U per hour) as adjunctive therapy to accelerated t-PA and aspirin.[20] The expected dose-dependent prolongation of the aPTT was observed with efegatran, but the rate of TIMI grade 3 flow at 90 minutes was similar in patients receiving efegatran in doses that were considered therapeutic but were not associated with excessive prolongation of the aPTT (0.6 to 1.0 mg/kg per hour; 56% to 57% TIMI 3 flow) versus heparin (54% TIMI 3 flow). The Efagatran and Streptokinase to Canalize Arteries Like Accelerated t-PA (ESCALAT) Investigators compared four doses of efegatran (0.3 to 1.0 mg/kg per hour) as adjunctive therapy to streptokinase with heparin as adjunctive therapy to accelerated t-PA.[21] Again, a dose-dependent prolongation of the aPTT was observed with efegatran, but no evidence of superiority of the efegatran-streptokinase combination was seen as compared with the heparin–t-PA combination.

Argatroban (bolus 100 μg/kg; infusion 3.0 μg/kg per minute for 72 hours) was compared with heparin (bolus 5000 U; infusion 1000 U per hour) in patients receiving accelerated t-PA in the Argatroban in Myocardial Infarction (ARGAMI) Trial.[22] The proportion of patients exhibiting TIMI grade 3 flow at 90 minutes was slightly higher in the heparin group (67%) versus the argatroban group (57%). Ongoing clinical trials with argatroban in thrombolytic-treated MI patients include (1) Myocardial Infarction using Novastan and t-PA (MINT)—a comparison of two doses of argatroban (infusions of 1.0 and 3.0 μg/kg per minute) with heparin (bolus 70 U/kg; infusion 15 U/kg per hour) in conjunction with accelerated t-PA; and (2) a comparison of two doses of argatroban (infusions of 1.0 and 3.0 μg/kg per minute) with placebo in conjunction with streptokinase (1.5 million U) (an angiographic evaluation at 90 minutes is being obtained in a subgroup of patients).

UNSTABLE ANGINA/NON–Q WAVE MYOCARDIAL INFARCTION

Trials of Hirudin

The Organization to Assess Strategies for Ischemia Syndromes (OASIS) Investigators randomized 909 patients with unstable angina or suspected acute MI without ST elevation to receive either heparin (bolus 5000 U; infusion 1000 to 1200 U per hour), low-dose hirudin (bolus 0.2 mg/kg; infusion 1.0 mg/kg per hour), or medium-dose hirudin (bolus 0.4 mg/kg; infusion 0.15 mg/kg per hour) for 72 hours.[23] Randomization to heparin versus hirudin was performed in an open-label fashion, but randomization to the two different doses of hirudin was blinded. Events were adjudicated by an independent committee, blinded to treatment allocation. The primary follow-up period was 7 days, at which point the treatment regimens were compared using four different cluster endpoints, including combinations of cardiovascular death, MI, refractory angina, severe angina, and severe angina requiring revascularization. Figure 14–3 summarizes the main findings. There was no significant difference among the treatment groups for the endpoint of cardiovascular death or MI. Use of composite endpoints including varying definitions of angina (see Fig. 14–3) showed a consistent pattern of the lowest rate of events in the medium-dose hirudin group. Of note, a rebound increase in adverse clinical events occurred following discontinuation of antithrombotic therapy so that the differences in event rates narrowed by 35 and 180 days of follow-up, although patients receiving the medium dose of hirudin appeared to continue to have the lowest rate of events over long-term follow-up.

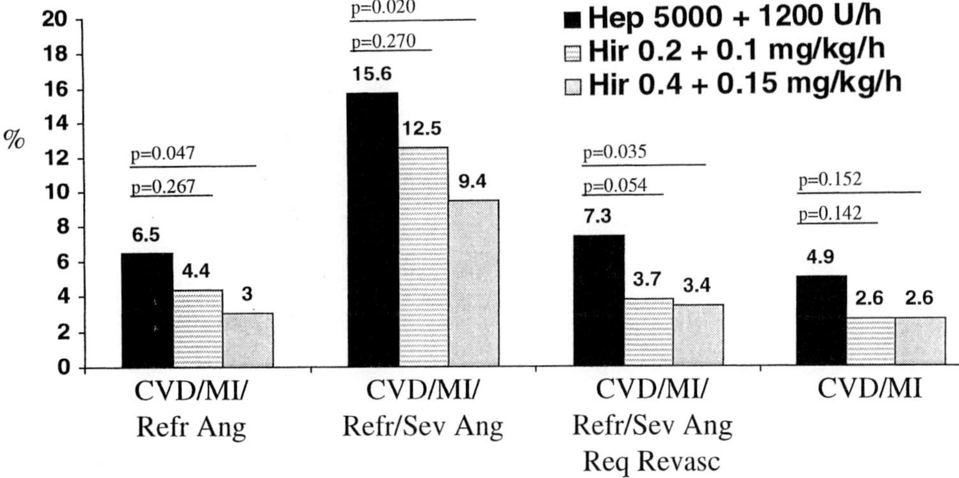

Figure 14–3 Clinical events in OASIS pilot studies. The proportion of patients experiencing a variety of composite cluster endpoints of cardiovascular events (shown on the y axis) by 7 days is shown for the heparin group (black bars), low-dose hirudin group (middle bars), and medium-dose hirudin group (gray bars). CVD, cardiovascular disease; MI, myocardial infarction. (Adapted from the OASIS Investigators. Comparison of the effects of two doses of recombinant hirudin compared with heparin in patients with acute myocardial ischemia without ST elevation: A pilot study. Circulation 1997; 96:769–777.)

Trials of Bivalirudin

Sharma and colleagues[24] and Lidón and associates[25] collectively treated 75 patients with unstable angina with bivalirudin (0.02 to 1.0 mg/kg per hour) and observed a dose-dependent prolongation of the aPTT and no major hemorrhagic events. Subsequently, the TIMI 7 Trial evaluated the safety and efficacy of 72 hours of treatment with four doses of bivalirudin: 0.02, 0.25, 0.5, and 1.0 mg/kg per hour.[26] The 160 patients who were treated with the lowest dose of bivalirudin experienced death or MI at hospital discharge at a rate of 10.0% compared with 3.2% in the 250 patients who received one of the higher doses of bivalirudin ($P < 0.008$). This beneficial treatment effect of the higher dose of bivalirudin compared with the lower dose was sustained at 6 weeks where the rate of death or MI was 12.5% in the low-dose group compared with 5.2% in the high-dose group ($P = 0.009$). Of note, the patients receiving one of the three higher doses of bivalirudin exhibited a stable aPTT pattern, with 93% having values within a 30-second range throughout the study drug infusion. No intracranial hemorrhages occurred, and major spontaneous hemorrhage occurred in two (0.5%) patients.

Trials with Other Agents

The Thrombin Inhibition in Myocardial Ischemia (TRIM) study group performed a dose-finding study of inogatran in unstable angina/non–Q wave MI.[27] A total of 1209 patients were randomized to receive 72 hours of treatment with a low (bolus 1.10 mg; infusion 2.0 mg per hour), medium (bolus 2.75 mg; infusion 5.0 mg per hour), or high (bolus 5.50 mg; infusion 10.0 mg per hour) dose of inogatran versus heparin (bolus 5000 U; infusion 1200 U per hour). There was a dose-dependent prolongation of the aPTT in inogatran-treated patients with greater stability of the anticoagulant effect compared with heparin—fewer than 5% of inogatran patients required adjustment of the infusion to maintain the aPTT less than three times control compared with 41.3% of heparin-treated patients. The primary endpoint of death, recurrent infarction, and refractory or recurrent ischemia was ascertained at 7 days and occurred in 45% to 46% of inogatran-treated patients ($N = 902$) versus 41% of heparin-treated patients ($N = 305$). The rate of death or recurrent infarction tended to be lower in the heparin group compared with the combined inogatran groups at 3 days (0.7% vs. 3.2%), 7 days (2.6% vs. 5.1%), and 30 days (5.9% vs. 8.3%). The rate of major hemorrhage was 1.1% by 7 days, and no differences were observed among the treatment groups.

Phase III Trials of Direct Antithrombins in Acute Coronary Syndromes

SAFETY OBSERVATIONS IN INITIAL PHASE III TRIALS WITH HIRUDIN

The TIMI 9A,[28] Global Use of Strategies to Open Occluded Coronary Arteries (GUSTO) IIa,[29] and HIT-III[30] Trials (Table 14–1) were the initial Phase III trials

TABLE 14–1 • Initial Phase III Trials Testing Hirudin Versus Heparin

	TIMI 9A	GUSTO IIa	HIT III
Trial Design			
Profile of patients	ST-segment elevation MI	ACS	ST-segment elevation MI
Planned sample size	3000	12,000	7000
Age limit	None	None	None
Treatment window since chest pain	12 h	12 h	6 h
Creatinine limit	2.5–2.0	2.5	"Renal Insuff"
Lytic	t-PA, SK	t-PA, SK	t-PA
HEPARIN			
Bolus	5000 U	5000 U	70 U/kg
Initial infusion	1000 U/h <80 kg 1300 U/h ≥80 kg	1000 U/h <80 kg 1300 U/h ≥80 kg	15 U/kg/h
Infusion adjusted?	Yes	Yes	Yes
HIRUDIN			
Source or r-hirudin	CGP	CGP	HBW
Bolus (mg/kg)	0.6	0.6	0.4
Infusion (mg/kg/h)	0.2	0.2	0.15
Infusion adjusted?	No	No	No
APTT TARGET	60–90 s	60–90 s	2.0–3.5 × control
Trial Results			
Number of patients enrolled when trial stopped	757	2564	302
ICH			
Lytic Patients			
Heparin	7/368 = 1.9%	9/620 = 1.5%	0/154 = 0%
Hirudin	6/345 = 1.7%	14/644 = 1.7%	4/148 = 2.7%
Nonlytic Patients			
Heparin	—	0/599 = 0%	—
Hirudin	—	3/569 = 0.5%	—

ACS, acute coronary syndrome; aPTT, activated partial thromboplastin time; CGP, Ciba-Geigy Pharmaceuticals; HBW, Hoechst Behringwerke; r-hirudin, recombinant hirudin; SK, streptokinase; t-PA, tissue plasminogen activator; ICH, intracranial hemorrhage.

testing the direct antithrombin hirudin versus heparin. TIMI 9A and HIT-III focused on patients with ST-segment elevation MI, and GUSTO IIa enrolled patients with clinical presentations across the acute coronary syndrome spectrum. A feature common to all three trials was that they were stopped prematurely because of unacceptable rates of serious bleeding, particularly intracranial hemorrhage. This excessive rate of bleeding appeared to be attributable to high levels of anticoagulation in both the heparin and hirudin groups in TIMI 9A and GUSTO IIa. Although a slightly lower dose of hirudin was used in HIT-III, it also was associated with an unacceptable rate of major hemorrhage. Possible explanations for the unexpectedly high rates of bleeding observed in these Phase III trials include (1) low estimates of the hemorrhagic risk at the doses of hirudin infused owing to the relatively small number of patients receiving that dose in earlier studies and (2) attempts to push the heparin dose to achieve higher aPTT levels in an effort to prevent reocclusion of successfully reperfused vessels.[28] In addition, patients at higher risk of hemorrhage (advanced age, renal dysfunction) were enrolled in these Phase III trials compared with the earlier Phase II dose-ranging studies.

Since the high rates of hemorrhage in these initial Phase III trials led to permanent discontinuation of the study drug in a substantial number of patients, it appeared premature to derive any definitive conclusions about the relative efficacy of hirudin versus heparin based on TIMI 9A, GUSTO IIa, and HIT-III. After downward modification of the dose of antithrombins, additional Phase III trials were undertaken.

RESULTS OF PHASE III TRIALS WITH HIRUDIN USING REVISED DOSING

The TIMI 9B Trial incorporated reduction of the doses of both heparin and hirudin along with additional safety measures, including titration of both antithrombins to a reduced target aPTT range of 55 to 85 seconds.[31] Patients randomized to hirudin were significantly more likely to have an aPTT measurement in the target range over the first 96 hours of the trial. Importantly, only 15% of hirudin-treated patients compared with 34% of heparin-treated patients had aPTT values below the target range within the first 24 hours. However, the primary endpoint (death, recurrent nonfatal MI, or development of severe congestive heart failure or cardiogenic shock by 30 days) occurred in 11.9% of the 1491 patients in the heparin group and 12.9% of the 1511 patients in the hirudin group (*P* = NS) (Fig. 14–4). In addition, there was no statistically significant difference in the development rate of the important secondary endpoint of death plus recurrent nonfatal MI (see Fig. 14–4). No significant difference in the odds of unsatisfactory outcome was observed for any of the prespecified patient subgroups (Fig. 14–5). The rates of percutaneous revascularization procedures and coronary artery bypass graft surgery were not different between the two treatment groups either during the initial hospitalization or within 30 days of randomization. After adjustment for statistically significant baseline variables (age, sex, weight, systolic blood pressure, heart rate, location of infarction, and history of prior infarction), there was no significant incremental contribution to a multivariate model when terms for the antithrombin to which the patient was randomized or the time from symptoms to thrombolytic or thrombolytic to initiation of antithrombin therapy were introduced in the model. The rate of major hemorrhage was similar in the heparin (5.3%) and hirudin (4.6%) groups. Intracranial hemorrhage occurred in 0.9% of the heparin and 0.4% of the hirudin patients. These rates of bleeding compared favorably with the major hemorrhage and intracranial hemorrhage rates for the heparin (10.1% and 1.9%) and hirudin (13.9% and 1.7%) groups in TIMI 9A.

The GUSTO IIb Trial stratified patients with an acute coronary syndrome into those that presented with ST-segment elevation (*N* = 4131) or without ST-segment elevation (*N* = 8011).[32] Patients in each of the electrocardiogram strata were randomized to receive either heparin or hirudin. Study drug was infused for a minimum of 3 days and a maximum of 5 days. Hirudin was administered as a bolus of 0.1 mg/kg and then as an initial infusion of 0.1 mg/kg per hour. Heparin was administered as a bolus of 5000 U followed by an initial infusion of 1000 U per hour. Both antithrombins were titrated to maintain the aPTT in the range of 60 to 85 seconds. At 24 hours, the rate of death or MI was significantly lower in the group assigned to hirudin therapy (1.3%) versus the group assigned to heparin therapy (2.1%; *P* = 0.001). However, the primary endpoint of the trial, death or nonfatal MI or reinfarction at 30 days, occurred in 9.8% of the heparin group and 8.9% of the hirudin group (odds ratio [OR], 0.89; 95% confidence interval, 0.79 to 1.00; *P* = 0.06) (Fig. 14–6). As summarized in Table 14–2, the main effect of hirudin was a reduction in MI by about 14%; the magnitude of the treatment effect was similar in patients presenting with or without ST-segment elevation. The incidence of bleeding complications and stroke in GUSTO IIb is summarized in Table 14–3. Although the rates of intracranial hemorrhage were similar for the hirudin and heparin patients across the entire trial, a trend toward a higher rate of intracranial hemorrhage was observed in the hirudin-treated patients compared with heparin-treated patients and the cohort without ST-segment elevation (0.2% vs. 0.02%; *P* = 0.06).

The results of a prospectively planned meta-analysis of the TIMI 9B and GUSTO IIb data are summarized in Tables 14–4 and 14–5.[33] Heterogeneity was observed between TIMI 9B and GUSTO IIb with respect to mortality at 24 hours with discordant trends favoring heparin in TIMI 9B and hirudin in GUSTO IIb, although neither trial observed a statistically significant difference at that early time (see Table 14–4). Mortality rates were similar at 30 days in both treatment arms across the various patient groups. A generally consistent reduction in the rate of reinfarction of about 14% was observed in the data set by 30 days (see Table 14–5). The OR for the primary endpoint of death and reinfarction by 30 days was 0.91 (0.82 to 1.02) with no evidence of heterogeneity between the trials or across patient strata.

DIRECT THROMBIN INHIBITORS DURING CORONARY ANGIOPLASTY

Although heparin is the mainstay of anticoagulation therapy for percutaneous transluminal coronary an-

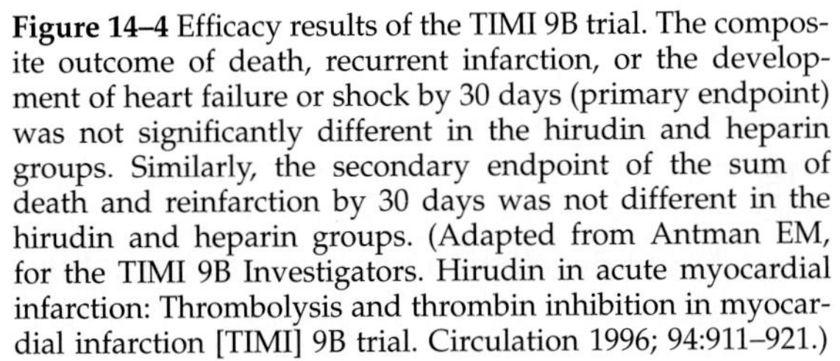

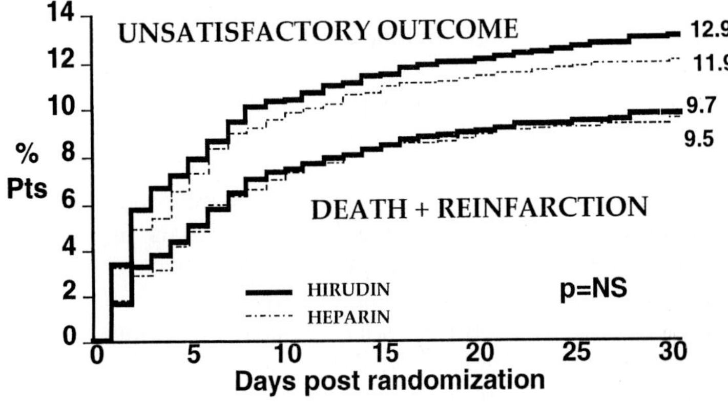

Figure 14–4 Efficacy results of the TIMI 9B trial. The composite outcome of death, recurrent infarction, or the development of heart failure or shock by 30 days (primary endpoint) was not significantly different in the hirudin and heparin groups. Similarly, the secondary endpoint of the sum of death and reinfarction by 30 days was not different in the hirudin and heparin groups. (Adapted from Antman EM, for the TIMI 9B Investigators. Hirudin in acute myocardial infarction: Thrombolysis and thrombin inhibition in myocardial infarction [TIMI] 9B trial. Circulation 1996; 94:911–921.)

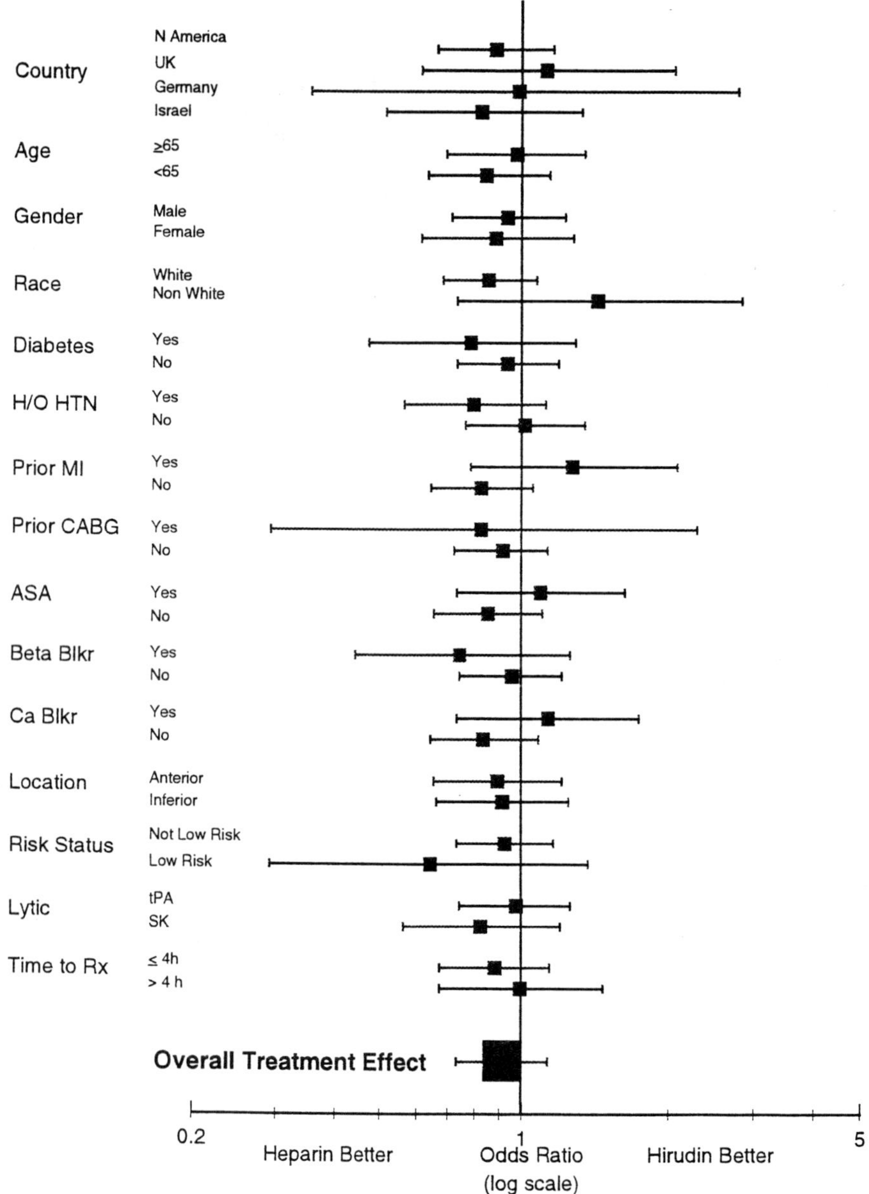

Figure 14–5 Subgroup analyses in the TIMI 9B trial. The odds ratio for development of the primary endpoint (death, reinfarction, or heart failure or shock by 30 days) was similar in the prespecified patient subgroups. The odds ratio was either near unity or the confidence intervals overlapped unity so that no subgroup showed a particularly beneficial response to one of the antithrombins. HTN, hypertension; ASA, aspirin; CABG, coronary artery bypass graft; MI, myocardial infarction. (Adapted from Antman EM, for the TIMI 9B Investigators. Hirudin in acute myocardial infarction: Thrombolysis and thrombin inhibition in myocardial infarction [TIMI] 9B trial. Circulation 1996; 94:911–921.)

gioplasty (PTCA), this treatment has several shortcomings. Major ischemic complications such as death, MI, or need for emergency bypass surgery occur in 5% to 10% of patients,[34–38] and restenosis often requiring repeat angioplasty or bypass surgery appears in 30% to 50% of patients.[35–39] Recently, direct thrombin inhibitors have been evaluated in clinical trials as substitutes for heparin to reduce the likelihood of acute complications and restenosis. The purpose of this section is to present the scientific basis for using direct thrombin inhibitors in PTCA, to review the epidemiologic background for designing clinical trials of direct thrombin inhibitors, and to define the magnitude of their treatment effects.

Thrombin Activation and Activity During PTCA

The rationale for developing direct thrombin inhibitors as anticoagulants for PTCA is based on several experimental and clinical studies of balloon injury of atherosclerotic arteries. Arterial thrombus formation is a high-shear, platelet-dependent process whose

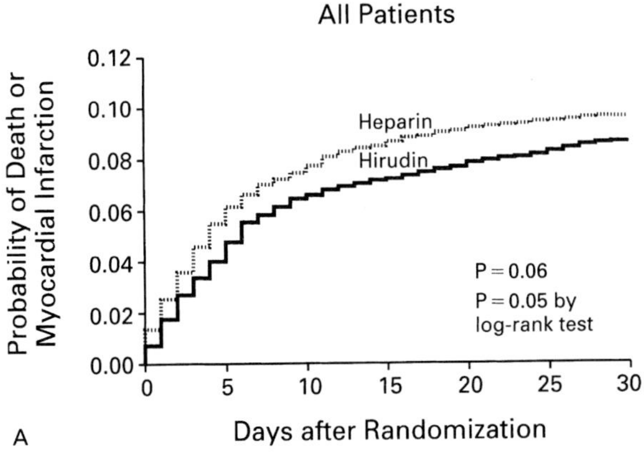

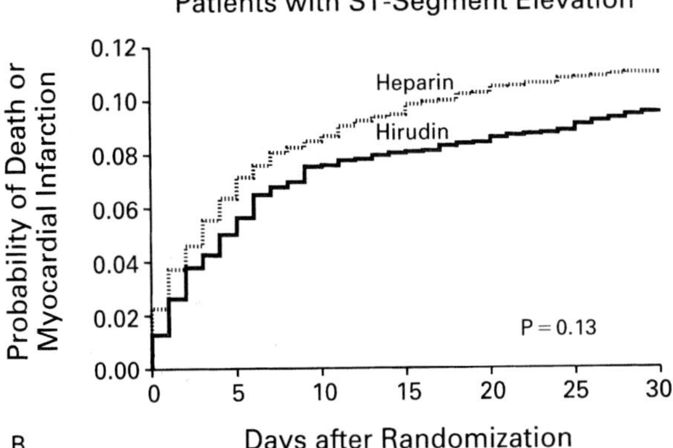

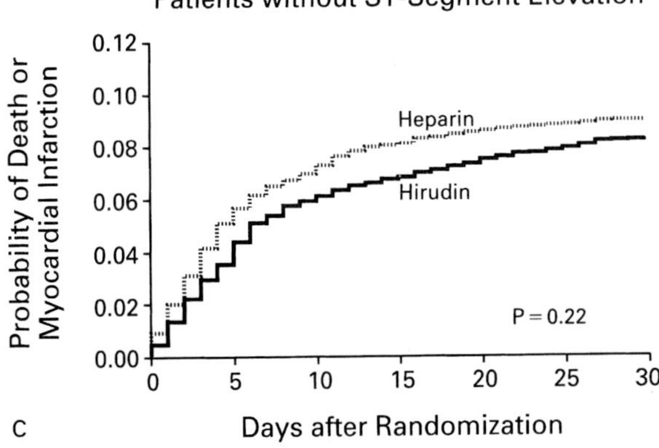

Figure 14–6 Efficacy results of the GUSTO IIb Trial in *(A)* all patients, *(B)* patients with ST-segment elevation, and *(C)* patients without ST-segment elevation. (From The Global Use of Strategies to Open Occluded Coronary Arteries [GUSTO] IIb Investigators. A comparison of recombinant hirudin with heparin for the treatment of acute coronary syndromes. N Engl J Med 1996; 335:775–782. Copyright 1996, Massachusetts Medical Society. All rights reserved.)

magnitude is determined by the thrombogenicity of the underlying substrate,[40] the deviation of shear rates outside the normal range,[41] and the activity or inhibition of coagulation factors and platelets.[5]

Balloon dilation during PTCA denudes the vascular endothelium and frequently ruptures atherosclerotic plaque, which contains a high content of tissue factor protein.[42] Tissue factor protein combines with factors VIIa and Xa to form the prothrombinase complex,[43] which converts prothrombin to thrombin by splitting off prothrombin fragment F_{1+2}, the concentration of which reflects the extent of local thrombin generation. In addition to generating fibrin from the cleavage of fibrinogen from its fragment fibrinopeptide A, thrombin potently activates platelets through the specialized thrombin receptor present on platelet surface.[44] Platelet activation leads to externalization of glycoprotein IIb/IIIa receptors for crosslinking adhesive macromolecules such as fibrinogen for the process of platelet aggregation.[45] Of several platelet-activating factors (including subintimal collagen, fibronectin, and von Willebrand factor), thrombin is considered to be the strongest agonist of platelet activation and exerts its effects independent of pathways inhibited by aspirin.

The importance of shear on thrombus formation during PTCA has been studied in several experimental models. It has been observed that balloon injury of canine carotid artery increases platelet deposition significantly, but the presence of a constriction induced by a vascular ring to mimic the presence of a superimposed stenosis causes an additional threefold increase in platelet deposition.[46]

Clinical evidence for thrombin generation during PTCA has been reported by Marmur and colleagues,[47] who measured both the intracoronary concentration of prothrombin fragment F_{1+2} as a marker of thrombin activation and also the content of fibrinopeptide A to assess thrombin activity. They observed that concentrations of prothrombin fragment F_{1+2} rose from 0.47 nM (95% confidence interval, 0.40 to 0.50) before balloon dilation to 0.55 nM (95% confidence interval, 0.46 to 0.72) after balloon dilation (P = 0.001). In the presence of heparin anticoagulation, evidence for thrombin-mediated conversion of fibrinogen to fibrin, as determined by the appearance of fibrinopeptide A, did not increase in response to balloon dilation for the entire study group of 26 patients: 2.0 ng/mL (95% confidence interval, 1.3 to 2.2) before dilation versus 1.8 ng/mL (95% confidence interval, 1.3 to 3.0) after dilation (P = NS). Increases in fibrinopeptide A, however, were seen in five of seven patients undergoing high-risk PTCA for ulcerated or thrombus-containing lesions.[47]

Inhibition of Arterial Thrombus Formation During PTCA

HEPARIN

Grüntzig performed the first PTCA procedures in 1977 using heparin, aspirin, dextran, and long-term anticoagulation with warfarin to prevent arterial thrombus formation.[48] By 1980, the anticoagulation

TABLE 14–2 • Incidence of Primary Clinical Endpoints at 30 Days in Patients with Acute Coronary Syndromes: GUSTO IIb

Group	Hirudin		Heparin			
	No. of Patients	*Percentage*	*No. of Patients*	*Percentage*	Odds Ratio (95% CI)	*P* Value
ALL PATIENTS	6069		6073			
Death		4.5		4.7	0.95 (0.80–1.13)	0.58
Myocardial infarction		5.4		6.3	0.86 (0.74–1.00)	0.04
Death or myocardial infarction		8.9		9.8	0.89 (0.79–1.00)	0.058
PATIENTS WITH ST-SEGMENT ELEVATION	2075		2056			
Death		5.9		6.2	0.94 (0.73–1.2)	0.64
Myocardial infarction		5.0		6.0	0.82 (0.63–1.07)	0.15
Death or myocardial infarction		9.9		11.3	0.86 (0.70–1.05)	0.13
PATIENTS WITHOUT ST-SEGMENT ELEVATION	3994		4017			
Death		3.7		3.9	0.96 (0.76–1.21)	0.72
Myocardial infarction		5.6		6.4	0.87 (0.73–1.05)	0.152
Death or myocardial infarction		8.3		9.1	0.90 (0.78–1.06)	0.22

CI, confidence interval.
Modified from The Global Use of Strategies to Open Occluded Coronary Arteries (GUSTO) IIb Investigators. A comparison of recombinant hirudin with heparin for the treatment of acute coronary syndromes. N Engl J Med 1996; 335:775–782.

regimen for routine PTCA was simplified to heparin and aspirin. The gradual adoption of activated clotting time (ACT) measurements after 1990 refined heparin dosing. In spite of its ubiquitous use as an anticoagulant for coronary angioplasty, heparin has several theoretical limitations.

DIRECT THROMBIN INHIBITORS

Antiproliferative Effects. Because thrombin has been reported to be a potent smooth muscle mitogen, enhanced thrombin inhibition may abrogate the process of intimal proliferation after balloon injury. This was tested by Sarembock and colleagues[49] who showed that hirudin reduced the extent of neointima formation in a balloon overstretch injury model involving the rabbit femoral arteries.[49] This finding was confirmed by Gallo and colleagues[50] in an experimental study involving balloon overstretch injury of porcine coronary arteries, in which heparin was administered as a bolus compared with hirudin given for 14

TABLE 14–3 • Incidence of Bleeding Complications and Stroke in Patients with Acute Coronary Syndromes: GUSTO IIb

Group	Hirudin		Heparin		
	No. of Patients	*Percentage*	*No. of Patients*	*Percentage*	*P* Value
ALL PATIENTS	6069		6073		
Severe bleeding		1.2		1.1	0.49
Moderate bleeding		8.8		7.7	0.03
Transfusion		9.7		8.6	0.04
Intracranial hemorrhage		0.3		0.2	0.24
Stroke*		0.9		0.8	0.43
PATIENTS WITH ST-SEGMENT ELEVATION	2075		2056		
Severe bleeding		1.1		1.5	0.20
Moderate bleeding		8.6		7.8	0.32
Transfusion		9.0		8.9	0.93
Intracranial hemorrhage		0.5		0.4	0.84
Stroke*		1.3		0.8	0.14
PATIENTS WITHOUT ST-SEGMENT ELEVATION	3994		4017		
Severe bleeding		1.3		0.9	0.06
Moderate bleeding		8.9		7.7	0.06
Transfusion		10.2		8.4	0.01
Intracranial hemorrhage		0.2		0.02	0.06
Stroke*		0.8		0.7	0.72

*This category includes stroke from any cause.
Modified from The Global Use of Strategies to Open Occluded Coronary Arteries (GUSTO) IIb Investigators. A comparison of recombinant hirudin with heparin for the treatment of acute coronary syndromes. N Engl J Med 1996; 335:775–782.

TABLE 14–4 • GUSTO-TIMI Meta-Analysis: Events Within 24 Hours

		Mortality			Reinfarction			Death + Reinfarction		
Group	*N*	*Heparin (%)*	*Hirudin (%)*	*OR (95% CI)*	*Heparin (%)*	*Hirudin (%)*	*OR (95% CI)*	*Heparin (%)*	*Hirudin (%)*	*OR (95% CI)*
TIMI 9	3002	1.5	2.3	1.58 (0.92–2.71)	0.9	0.6	0.68 (0.29–1.60)	2.3	2.8	1.23 (0.78–1.94)
GUSTO II Lytic	3052	2.9	2.0	0.70 (0.44–1.11)	0.9	0.5	0.61 (0.25–1.48)	3.7	2.6	0.68 (0.45–1.02)
Combined	6054			0.99 (0.70–1.40)			0.65 (0.35–1.20)			0.88 (0.65–1.19)
GUSTO II other ST	1078	2.5	0.7	0.29 (0.09–0.90)	0.2	0.8	3.89 (0.43–34.5)	2.5	1.5	0.60 (0.24–1.43)
GUSTO II non-ST	8009	0.6	0.3	0.57 (0.29–1.12)	1.1	0.6	0.51 (0.31–0.86)	1.6	0.9	0.56 (0.37–0.84)
Total	**15,141**			**0.81 (0.61–1.08)**			**0.61 (0.42–0.89)**			**0.74 (0.58–0.93)**
P for combined lytic group				*P* = 0.97			*P* = 0.16			*P* = 0.41
P overall				*P* = 0.16			*P* = 0.011			*P* = 0.011
Tests for heterogeneity										
TIMI 9 vs. GUSTO II lytic				*P* = 0.024			*P* = 0.87			*P* = 0.059
Lytic vs. nonlytic				*P* = 0.03			*P* = 0.82			*P* = 0.069
ST-segment elevation vs. non–ST-segment elevation				*P* = 0.26			*P* = 0.30			*P* = 0.11

OR, odds ratio; CI, confidence interval.
Modified from Simes RJ, Granger CB, Antman EM, et al. Impact of hirudin versus heparin on mortality and (re)infarction in patients with acute coronary syndromes: A prospective meta-analysis of the GUSTO-IIb and TIMI 9B trials. Circulation 1996; 94:I-430.

TABLE 14–5 • GUSTO-TIMI Meta-Analysis: Events Within 30 Days

		Mortality			Reinfarction			Death + Reinfarction		
Group	*N*	*Heparin (%)*	*Hirudin (%)*	*OR (95% CI)*	*Heparin (%)*	*Hirudin (%)*	*OR (95% CI)*	*Heparin (%)*	*Hirudin (%)*	*OR (95% CI)*
TIMI 9	3002	5.1	6.1	1.21 (0.88–1.65)	5.2	4.5	0.85 (0.61–1.18)	9.5	9.7	1.02 (0.80–1.31)
GUSTO II Lytic	3052	6.5	6.0	0.91 (0.68–1.23)	6.8	5.3	0.77 (0.58–1.04)	12.1	10.2	0.84 (0.66–1.03)
Combined	6054			1.04 (0.84–1.29)			0.81 (0.65–1.00)			0.91 (0.77–1.08)
GUSTO II other ST	1078	5.5	5.7	1.04 (0.62–1.75)	4.5	4.6	1.05 (0.60–1.86)	9.3	9.1	0.99 (0.65–1.49)
GUSTO II non-ST	8009	3.9	3.7	0.95 (0.76–1.22)	6.4	5.7	0.87 (0.73–1.05)	9.1	8.3	0.91 (0.78–1.06)
Total	**15,141**			**1.00 (0.87–1.17)**			**0.86 (0.75–0.98)**			**0.91 (0.82–1.02)**
P for combined lytic group										*P* = 0.055
P overall										*P* = 0.024
Tests for heterogeneity										
TIMI 9 vs. GUSTO II lytic				*P* = 0.20			*P* = 0.20			*P* = 0.66
Lytic vs. nonlytic				*P* = 0.63			*P* = 0.95			*P* = 0.52
ST-segment elevation vs. non-ST-segment elevation				*P* = 0.57			*P* = 0.90			*P* = 0.77

OR, odds ratio; CI, confidence interval.
Modified from Simes RJ, Granger CB, Antman EM, et al. Impact of hirudin versus heparin on mortality and (re)infarction in patients with acute coronary syndromes: A prospective meta-analysis of the GUSTO-IIb and TIMI 9B trials. Circulation 1996; 94:I-430.

days. At 28 days after initial injury, the percent diameter stenosis was 61% in the heparin-treated animals but only 38% in the hirudin-treated animals.[50]

In an experimental study involving balloon angioplasty in hypercholesterolemic rabbits,[51] a 2-hour infusion of hirudin failed to reduce evidence of cellular proliferation, which peaked at 72 hours as shown by incorporation of ^{3}H-thymidine. Hirudin treatment, however, reduced the degree of luminal cross-sectional narrowing at 28 days. Thus, inhibition of cellular proliferation within the first 7 days after angioplasty is not the mechanism by which hirudin exerts its beneficial effects. It is possible that hirudin reduces restenosis after balloon injury by affecting cell migration rather than proliferation, reducing the magnitude of mural thrombosis formation or its incorporation into plaque, or by regulating the extent of matrix production.[51]

High-Risk Coronary Angioplasty

The development of new antithrombotic regimens to improve the results of high-risk angioplasty is based on the assertions that thrombin is generated during high-risk coronary angioplasty, most of the complications of high-risk coronary angioplasty are related to thrombus formation, and direct thrombin inhibitors are superior to heparin in preventing thrombin-mediated ischemic complications of angioplasty.

Several clinical studies have established that the outcome of angioplasty performed with heparin anticoagulation is related to the severity and acuity of the clinical presentation.[52] Pooled analyses reveal that rates of acute MI after angioplasty are approximately 6.3% for patients with postinfarction angina,[53–60] 6.3% for patients with refractory unstable angina,[61–68] 5.1% for patients with unstable angina stabilized on medical therapy,[53, 66, 69–71] 1.6% for patients with stable angina,[72–78] and 1.0% for patients undergoing angioplasty for symptomatic restenosis.[79–82] Although the acute ischemic syndromes are commonly linked together because of common pathogenic features involving plaque rupture and arterial thrombus formation, each syndrome is associated with a different degree of thrombus burden accounting for the range of angioplasty-related complications that spans almost an order of magnitude.

To identify the predictors and rates of acute ischemic complications during conventional PTCA carried out with heparin dosing guided by ACTs, a pilot study was carried out in 1992.[34] The study involved 591 consecutive patients with a mean age of 61 years undergoing conventional balloon angioplasty at nine medical centers in North America. The peak ACT achieved during the PTCA was 363 ± 92 seconds. Angioplasty was performed for unstable angina in 386 patients (65%), after recent MI in 115 patients (19%), and in the presence of a filling defect in 21 patients (3.6%). Forty-five patients (7.6%) experienced at least one major complication during hospitalization. Nine patients (1.5%) died, 9 patients (1.5%) had Q wave MI, 16 patients (2.7%) experienced non–Q wave MI, and 19 patients (3.2%) required emergency bypass surgery within 24 hours of the PTCA procedure. Ninety-one patients (15.4%) experienced a major ischemic complication, abrupt vessel closure, or both. Complications were found to be associated with several baseline clinical and angiographic variables on multivariable logistic regression analysis (Fig. 14–7). The presence of a filling defect before PTCA, as detected in the core angiographic laboratory, increased the likelihood of any complication (complication rate, 38.1%; OR, 3.1; 95% confidence interval, 1.2 to 8.4; $P = 0.02$). Other variables associated with an increased risk of major or minor complications included multivessel coronary artery disease (complication rate, 19.8%, OR, 1.9; 95% confidence interval, 1.1 to 3.3; $P = 0.02$), unstable angina (complication rate, 18.4%; OR, 1.9; 95% confidence interval, 1.1 to 3.3; $P = 0.03$), lesion complexity (OR, 1.6; 95% confidence interval, 1.1 to 2.2, for an additional increase in grade; $P = 0.01$), and patient age (OR, 1.4; 95% confidence interval, 1.1 to 1.8, per additional decade; $P = 0.002$). ACT (median value, 350 seconds; range, 280 to 1032), female sex, and diabetes were not related to PTCA complications on univariable analysis. Thus, this study showed that complications of PTCA carried out with heparin anticoagulation increased in the setting of unstable angina.

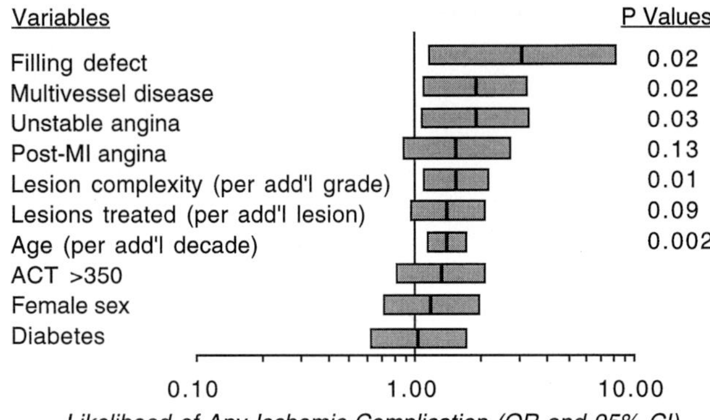

Figure 14–7 Predictors of percutaneous transluminal coronary angioplasty (PTCA) complications. The likelihood of complications for a series of clinical and angiographic variables in 591 patients who had 756 lesions treated with PTCA is given by the odds ratios (OR) and multivariable *P* values obtained by logistic regression analysis. The statistical reliability of the OR is given by the 95% confidence intervals. ACT, activated clotting time; CI, confidence interval; MI, myocardial infarction; lesion complexity, American College of Cardiology/American Heart Association classification of lesion complexity in which the OR refers to the average likelihood of complication for an increase in complexity from grade A to B or from B to C.[106] (From Wolfe MW, Roubin GS, Schweiger M, et al. Length of hospital stay and complications after percutaneous transluminal coronary angioplasty: Clinical and procedural predictors. Circulation 1995; 92:311–319.)

Studies of Hirudin in PTCA

ACUTE RESULTS

The effect of hirudin on angiographic findings has been compared with heparin in 166 patients with ischemic rest pain, abnormal electrocardiogram, and abnormal coronary arteriograms showing evidence of thrombus. The patients treated with hirudin tended to show greater improvement in cross-sectional area of the culprit lesion than the patients treated with heparin, suggesting that the direct thrombin inhibitor was more effective than heparin in reducing the extent of coronary thrombus burden associated with the syndrome of unstable angina.[83]

In the study entitled Hirudin in a European Trial Versus Heparin in the Prevention of Restenosis after PTCA (HELVETICA),[84] 1141 patients with unstable angina scheduled for PTCA were treated with aspirin randomized to one of three anticoagulation regimens. Patients were randomized to treatment with either heparin 10,000-U bolus plus 15 U/kg per hour for 24 hours, hirudin 40-mg bolus plus 0.2 mg/kg per hour for 24 hours, or the identical hirudin regimen plus additional hirudin 40 mg administered subcutaneously twice daily for an additional 3 days. The incidence of death, MI, or coronary artery bypass graft at 96 hours was 11.0% in the control group and 5.6% in the subcutaneous hirudin group (Fig. 14–8).

RESTENOSIS

In the HELVETICA Trial, the differences in major ischemic complications or need for repeated revascularization 6 months after treatment with heparin or hirudin narrowed to 32.0% and 33.7% because of a "catch-up" phenomenon seen at 3 months in the hirudin-treated patients.[84] Quantitative angiography showed no reduction in late loss in the hirudin-treated patients. Hirudin appeared to rescue patients from immediate ischemic complications associated with what would have otherwise been considered borderline angioplasty results but could not reduce the risk of ischemic complications or need for repeated revascularization during the 6 months after angioplasty.

Studies of Bivalirudin in PTCA

PHASE II STUDY

Topol and colleagues[85] evaluated the safety and efficacy of bivalirudin as a substitute for heparin in an open-label, dose-escalation study involving 258 patients undergoing elective angioplasty. Five successive bolus doses (0.15, 0.25, 0.35, 0.45, and 0.55 mg/kg body weight) matched with five successive infusion doses (0.6, 1.0, 1.4, 1.8, and 2.2 mg/kg per hour) were evaluated in five groups of approximately 50 patients each. Bivalirudin produced a dose-dependent anticoagulant effect without an increase in bleeding complications. The incidence of major and minor angioplasty complications (including abrupt vessel closure, MI, or the need for emergency bypass surgery) was reduced in patients treated with the highest two doses compared with the lower doses. This study[85] suggested that a dose-response curve for bivalirudin exists at the lower end of the dosing range, demonstrated for the first time that coronary angioplasty could be performed with a direct thrombin inhibitor in place of heparin, and provided the basis for a controlled comparison of bivalirudin with heparin in patients undergoing coronary angioplasty.

PHASE III STUDY

Bivalirudin was compared directly with heparin in the Hirulog Angioplasty Study,[86] a double-blind, randomized study involving 4098 patients with postinfarction or unstable angina scheduled for PTCA. All patients enrolled in the study were given aspirin in an oral dose of 300 to 325 mg. Patients assigned to heparin therapy were given a bolus of 175 U/kg, followed by an 18- to 24-hour infusion of 15 U/kg per hour. The dosing of heparin was based on several factors. Consensus was reached among investigators in 1992 that the minimum ACT should be 350 seconds

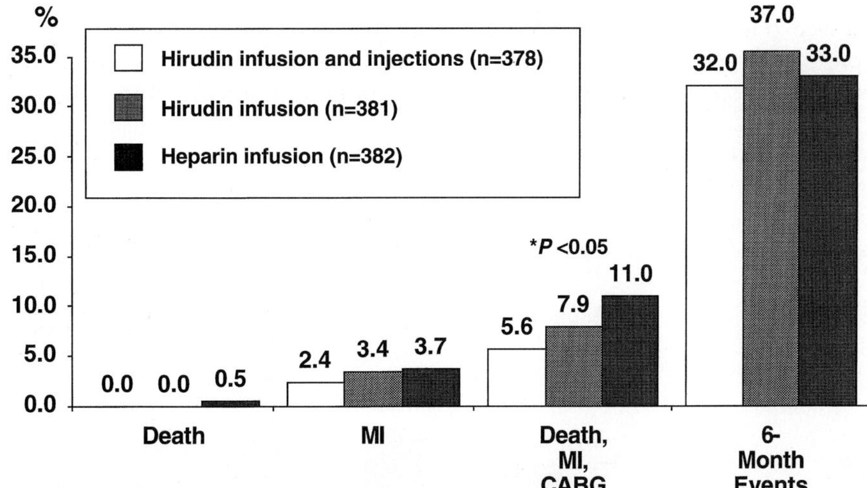

Figure 14–8 Major ischemic complications in patients receiving hirudin or heparin during angioplasty. The incidence of death, myocardial infarction (MI), emergency bypass surgery (coronary artery bypass graft [CABG]), or the composite endpoint at 96 hours is shown. The cumulative incidence of any major complication or need for revascularization at 6 months is presented. The dosing of anticoagulants involved either heparin infusion (10,000 IU intravenous [IV] bolus plus 15 IU/kg IV per hour for 24 hours), hirudin infusion alone (40 mg IV bolus plus 0.2 mg/kg IV per hour for 24 hours), or hirudin infusion plus prolonged subcutaneous therapy (40 mg IV bolus plus 0.2 mg/kg IV per hour for 24 hours plus 40 mg subcutaneously twice daily for 72 hours). *$P < 0.05$. (Data from Serruys PW, Herrman J-PR, Simon R, et al. A comparison of hirudin with heparin in the prevention of restenosis after coronary angioplasty. N Engl J Med 1995; 333:757–763.)

during angioplasty and that weight-adjusted and overnight heparin dosing should parallel that for bivalirudin for high-risk patients with unstable or postinfarction angina. Observations made in the Heparin Registry[34, 87] in patients with unstable angina suggested that the standard practice with heparin was to achieve a median ACT of 375 seconds with a median 24-hour dose of 41,100 U of heparin, which was equivalent to 178 U/kg bolus plus 15 U/kg per hour for 24 hours.

Patients randomly assigned to bivalirudin therapy were given a bolus of 1.0 mg/kg, followed by a 4-hour infusion of 2.5 mg/kg per hour and a 14- to 20-hour infusion of 0.2 mg/kg per hour. The dosing of bivalirudin was based on observations in the Phase II study[85] that a bolus of 0.55 mg/kg followed by 2.2 mg/kg per hour resulted in a median ACT of 352 seconds. The bivalirudin concentrations associated with the highest doses in this study resulted in systemic concentrations of drug (10 μM)[85] that exceeded the expected concentrations of thrombin measured in coronary arterial blood during coronary angioplasty (0.5 nM)[47] as well as the inhibition constant of bivalirudin (2 nM)[88] by more than three orders of magnitude.

During the study, blinding of personnel was achieved by having the research pharmacist prepare three syringes for bolus administration and two infusion bags for the 4-hour and 14- to 20-hour infusions of study drug. No labeling information revealed whether the syringes or bags contained heparin or bivalirudin. Patients randomized to heparin or to bivalirudin had an infusion bag change at 4 hours, even though no change in dose was made for the heparin-treated patients. ACTs were measured at 5 minutes and 45 minutes after the first bolus of study drug with the same type of device (Hemochron, International Technidyne) at all participating centers. If the value was less than 350 seconds, a saline bolus was given to bivalirudin-assigned patients, and a heparin bolus of 60 U/kg was given to heparin-assigned patients.

As compared with heparin therapy in the entire cohort of patients, bivalirudin did not reduce the likelihood of inhospital death (OR, 2.2; 95% confidence interval, 0.7 to 2.2; $P = 0.27$), Q wave or non–Q wave MI (OR, 0.8; 95% confidence interval, 0.6 to 1.1; $P = 0.20$), or emergency bypass surgery (OR, 1.0; 95% confidence interval, 0.6 to 1.6; $P = 1.00$) (Fig. 14–9). The use of bivalirudin was not associated with a significant reduction in the incidence of abrupt vessel closure, which was defined nonrestrictively as either *established closure* in the presence of total or subtotal occlusion with TIMI grade 0 to 1 flow,[89, 90] or *threatened closure* in the presence of greater than 50% diameter stenosis and reduced TIMI flow, requiring additional therapy with intracoronary stenting, thrombolytic therapy, or return to the cardiac catheterization laboratory.[34, 91] No differences in the cumulative incidence of death, MI, or need for revascularization were seen at 6-month follow-up (see Fig. 14–9).

Limitations of Direct Thrombin Inhibitors in PTCA

THROMBIN REBOUND

Although the direct thrombin inhibitors potently block the action of activated thrombin, they do not inhibit the generation of thrombin. Thus, several experts have raised the possibility that discontinuation of direct thrombin inhibitors could be associated with the sudden onset of acute ischemic syndromes precipitated by elevated local concentrations of uninhibited thrombin accompanied by persistence of the underlying thrombogenic substrate, dissociation of thrombin-antithrombin complexes, or a reduced clearance of thrombin. Chesebro and others predicted a higher

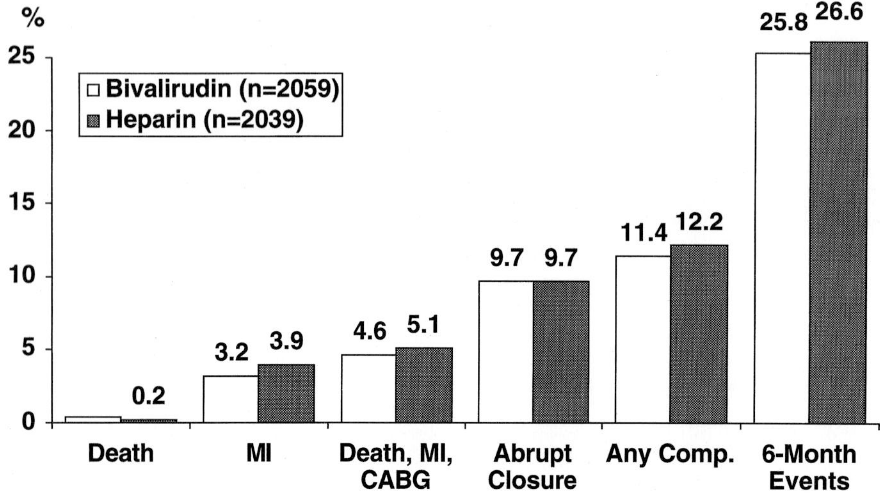

Figure 14–9 Major and minor ischemic complications in patients receiving bivalirudin or heparin during angioplasty performed for unstable angina. The incidence of death, Q wave or non–Q wave myocardial infarction (MI), emergency bypass surgery (coronary artery bypass graft [CABG]), abrupt vessel closure, or the composite during hospitalization is shown. The cumulative incidence of any major complication or need for revascularization at 6 months is also shown. (Data from Bittl JA, Strony J, Brinker JA, et al. Treatment with bivalirudin [Hirulog] as compared with heparin during coronary angioplasty for unstable or postinfarction angina. N Engl J Med 1995; 333:764–769.)

incidence of ischemic events after stopping a direct thrombin inhibitor than after stopping heparin.[92] Because hirudin does not inhibit the activation of thrombin, evidence of persistent thrombin generation is often seen during treatment with direct thrombin inhibitors.[92] This concern was also raised in a study of the inhibition and generation of thrombin in the presence of thrombin inhibitors carried out in plasma. Activation of citrated plasma was accompanied by the sudden onset of thrombin generation after a delay of about 2 minutes. Addition of 50 ng of hirudin per milliliter or 0.1 U heparin per milliliter prolonged the clotting time to 3 minues. Thrombin generation and F_{1+2} was significantly lower in heparinized plasma than in hirudinized plasma, suggesting that heparin was more effective than hirudin in inhibiting the action of factor Xa.[93]

Analogous clinical results observed in the biochemical substudy in HELVETICA[84] provided interesting insights into the comparison of the actions of heparin and hirudin. Heparin therapy was associated with a reduction in the generation of thrombin, as determined by the levels of prothrombin fragment F_{1+2} (1.0 nM before balloon dilation vs. 0.9 nM after dilation), whereas hirudin administered intravenously and subcutaneously was associated with a slight increase in levels of F_{1+2} (1.0 nM vs. 1.3 nM). Although hirudin was at least as effective as heparin in inhibiting activated thrombin, increased thrombin generation at the time of discontinuation of anticoagulant therapy theoretically increased the risk of "thrombin rebound," but this was not observed in the study.[84]

The possibility of ischemic rebound was directly evaluated in the Hirulog Angioplasty Study.[86] In the Hirulog Angioplasty Study, the timing of major complications such as death, MI, or emergency bypass was carefully reported by blinded study personnel. After discontinuation of either heparin or bivalirudin at 18 to 24 hours, 25 (1.2%) of 2039 patients who had received heparin therapy experienced a major complication, whereas only 7 (0.3%) of 2059 patients treated with bivalirudin experienced a complication.[94] These clinical results are consistent with the absence of ischemic rebound reported after discontinuation of hirudin in TIMI 5.[15]

INFLUENCE OF BASELINE RISK ON APPARENT TREATMENT EFFECT

In the Hirulog Angioplasty Study, the overall rates of ischemic complications were lower than anticipated from the pilot study using heparin anticoagulation.[34] The overall rate of major complications of 4.8% seen in the Hirulog Angioplasty Study was lower than the rate of 7.6% seen in the Heparin Registry using identical definitions and methods for data quality assurance[34] and lower than the rates reported in several other studies of patients with unstable angina.[52] Of the 2039 heparin-treated patients in the Hirulog Angioplasty Study, 0.2% of the patients died, 1.7% required bypass surgery, and 3.9% experienced Q wave or non–Q wave MI. Because the heparin dosing used in the Hirulog Angioplasty Study was associated with a low incidence of MI, the comparison treatment would have to result in an MI rate of less than 2% for statistical significance. It is unlikely that any new antithrombotic therapy could achieve this goal.

The profile of patients enrolled in the Hirulog Angioplasty Study may not have reflected the real-life case mix of patients undergoing PTCA. This possibility has been tested by comparing the baseline characteristics and outcomes for patients enrolled in the Heparin Registry, which provided a cross-sectional view of PTCA practice in 1992, with those of patients enrolled at the same sites in the Hirulog Angioplasty Study. Patients evaluated in the Heparin Registry[34, 87] with unstable or postinfarction angina were more likely than those in the Hirulog Angioplasty Study[86] to have multivessel coronary artery disease or complex lesions targeted for angioplasty. The patients in the Heparin Registry had higher event rates than those in the randomized study.

In the Hirulog Angioplasty Study, the higher-risk subgroup of patients with postinfarction angina was prespecified by the protocol for separate analysis. A single trial might need to randomize thousands of patients to assess the overall benefit of direct thrombin inhibitors for the heterogeneous group of patients with unstable angina. It may nonetheless fail to yield statistically reliable evidence for a benefit in certain subgroups. For this reason, one subgroup of relatively homogenous patients with postinfarction angina was prospectively defined. In the group of patients with postinfarction angina, a significant treatment effect of bivalirudin was noted. For patients with postinfarction angina, however, bivalirudin produced a significant reduction in the incidence of MI (OR, 0.4; 95% confidence interval, 0.2 to 0.9; $P = 0.04$) or any complication of death, MI, or emergency bypass surgery (OR, 0.4; 95% confidence interval, 0.2 to 0.9; $P = 0.03$). This difference, however, had disappeared at 6-month follow-up evaluation (Fig. 14–10). One concern of this study design involving the lumping of patients with unstable angina and postinfarction angina is that the two treatment groups may be so different based on their pathogeneses and response to treatment with direct thrombin inhibitors that the analysis of safety and efficacy provides conclusions that in fact are applicable to neither group.

Bivalirudin and heparin treatment resulted in identical rates of abrupt vessel closure, an ischemic complication predominantly ascribed to thrombus formation currently attributed to intimal dissection or extrusion of atheromatous plaque in about 80% of

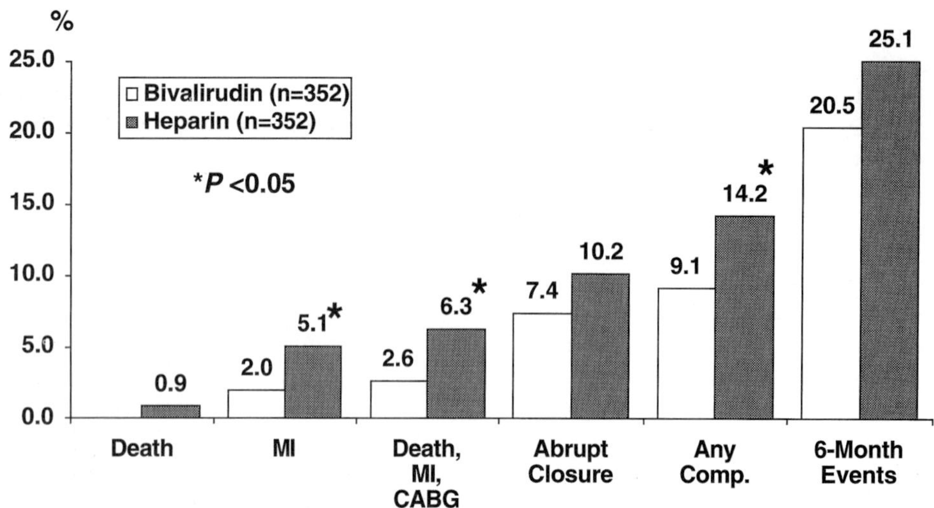

Figure 14–10 Major and minor ischemic complications in patients receiving bivalirudin or heparin during angioplasty performed for postinfarction angina. The incidence of death, Q wave or non–Q wave myocardial infarction (MI), emergency bypass surgery (coronary artery bypass graft [CABG]), abrupt vessel closure, or the composite during hospitalization is shown. The cumulative incidence of any major complication or need for revascularization at 6 months is presented. *$P < 0.05$. (Data from Bittl JA, Strony J, Brinker JA, et al. Treatment with bivalirudin [Hirulog] as compared with heparin during coronary angioplasty for unstable or postinfarction angina. N Engl J Med 1995; 333:764–769.)

cases.[34, 95–97] Such mechanical disruption is unlikely to respond to improved anticoagulation regimens but may improve with coronary stenting.

Advantages of Direct Thrombin Inhibitors over Heparin for PTCA

HEMORRHAGIC COMPLICATIONS DURING PTCA

The large studies evaluating the safety of direct thrombin inhibitors as substitutes for heparin during PTCA indicate that these new agents can be used without an increased risk of bleeding. In the HELVETICA study, the incidence of hemorrhagic complications was equivalent among the three treatment groups. The rate of overt bleeding associated with a decrease in hemoglobin of 2 g/dL or more, transfusion, and intracranial or retroperitoneal bleeding was 6.2% in patients treated with heparin, 5.5% in patients treated with intravenous hirudin, and 7.7% in patients treated with intravenous and subcutaneous hirudin.[84]

The large randomized, double-blind studies of bivalirudin versus high-dose heparin showed substantial reductions in bleeding rates for patients treated with bivalirudin. As compared with heparin, the use of bivalirudin was associated with lower odds of major bleeding complications such as intracranial hemorrhage (OR, 0.5; 95% confidence interval, 0.0 to 5.5; $P = 0.62$), retroperitoneal bleeding (OR, 0.3; 95% confidence interval, 0.1 to 0.9; $P = 0.02$), or red blood cell transfusion (OR, 0.4; 95% confidence interval, 0.3 to 0.6; $P < 0.001$).[86] Bivalirudin therapy was associated with no increase in complications involving pulmonary, neurologic, or other organ systems in the 4098-patient study.[98] Lower levels of systemic anticoagulation in the bivalirudin-treated patients than in the heparin-treated patients may have explained the difference in bleeding risk (median ACT of 346 seconds [interquartile range, 305 to 405] for bivalirudin-treated patients vs. 383 seconds [332 to 450] for heparin-treated patients; $P < 0.001$).

HEPARIN-INDUCED THROMBOCYTOPENIA

Mediated by the action of heparin, platelet factor 4, and immunoglobulin G, the syndrome of heparin-induced thrombocytopenia is a complex illness that frequently leads to arterial thrombosis, venous thrombosis, or both. Although the syndrome can be prevented by the use of low-molecular-weight heparin,[99] once it appears low molecular weight is no longer recommended. Several studies have suggested that direct thrombin inhibitors are safe in the treatment of patients with this syndrome. Chamberlin and colleagues[100] successfully treated three patients with bivalirudin without ischemic or bleeding complications. Bivalirudin has also been used for heparin-associated thrombocytopenia and deep venous thrombosis.[101]

COMBINATION OF DIRECT THROMBIN INHIBITORS AND PLATELET GLYCOPROTEIN IIB/IIIA RECEPTOR BLOCKERS

Because of the possibility that multiple redundant pathways may lead to platelet activation during coronary angioplasty, arterial thrombus formation may nonetheless proceed in the presence of complete thrombin inhibition. The final common pathway for platelet aggregation is mediated by the exposure of the platelet glycoprotein IIb/IIIa fibrinogen receptor. It is thus reasonable to evaluate the combination of a thrombin inhibitor and simultaneous inhibition of the more distal steps in platelet aggregation mediated by the IIb/IIIa receptor to provide an optimal approach in preventing arterial thrombus formation. In a canine model of intracoronary thrombosis, the combination of t-PA (1 mg/kg over 20 minutes) together with the platelet glycoprotein IIb/IIIa receptor inhibitor Integrelin (2.5 μg/kg per minute for 90 minutes) and the direct thrombin inhibitor hirudin (10 μg/kg per minute for 90 minutes) was associated with more complete restoration of coronary flow and reduction in the reocclusion rate than the use of either Integrelin or hirudin alone.[102]

CRITIQUE OF DIRECT ANTITHROMBINS IN ACUTE CORONARY SYNDROMES AND ANGIOPLASTY

By inhibiting the coagulation cascade upstream from thrombin, heparin has an advantage over the direct antithrombins because of its additional ability to decrease thrombin generation, along with its ability to inhibit thrombin activity. Hirudin has a greater ability than heparin to decrease thrombin activity, but once the thrombin inhibitory capacity is exceeded (by virtue of the local concentration of hirudin), free thrombin may be generated in an explosive fashion.[103, 104] The net result of this balance of actions is that use of heparin or the direct antithrombins results in an equivalent decrement in thrombus formation in the culprit coronary artery.

Data from the classic experiments by Weitz and colleagues show the percent inhibition of fluid-phase thrombin and clot-bound thrombin, respectively (Fig. 14–11).[14] Although it is true that hirudin is more effective at inhibiting clot-bound thrombin than is heparin, this relative difference between the antithrombins is most marked at the left of the concentration-effect relationship and diminishes at higher concentrations. It is noteworthy that in the range of concentrations that would not be associated with excessive bleeding and therefore would be acceptable clinically, hirudin's ability to inhibit clot-bound thrombin is only about 50% as potent as its ability to inhibit fluid-phase thrombin. Also, as emphasized by Loscalzo,[104] the concentration of hirudin required to inhibit thrombin-induced platelet activation is 10-fold that required to inhibit fibrin formation.[105] These facts minimize hirudin's potential advantage over heparin in the clinically relevant dose range.

Finally, another important difference between heparin and hirudin is illustrated in the revised model of their inhibitory effects on thrombin as shown in Figure 14–12. Each molecule of hirudin binds tightly in a 1:1 stoichiometric fashion to thrombin in the fluid phase and clot-bound phase. It is possible to "exhaust" the available supply of hirudin, allowing thrombin molecules to remain enzymatically active. Increasing the concentration of hirudin would be associated with unacceptable bleeding rates, as was

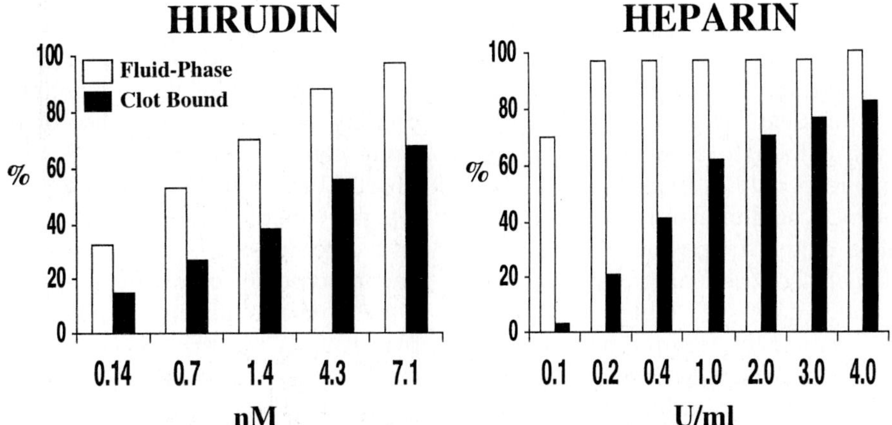

Figure 14–11 Comparison of the inhibition of fluid-phase and clot-bound thrombin by hirudin and heparin. These data from the classic experiments of Weitz and colleagues show the percentage of thrombin inhibition in the fluid-phase and clot-bound phase in an in vitro system. The relative difference between the ability of hirudin and heparin to inhibit fluid-phase (open bars) versus clot-bound (dark bars) thrombin is most marked at the left of the dose-response relationship. The concentration of antithrombins shown toward the left and the dose-response relationship are similar to those obtained when the drugs are exhibited in doses that would not be associated with unacceptable levels of bleeding. Note that the ability of hirudin to inhibit clot-bound thrombin at concentrations that would be clinically acceptable is only 50% of its ability to inhibit fluid-phase thrombin. (Adapted from Weitz JI, Hudoba M, Massel D, et al. Clot-bound thrombin is protected from inhibition by heparin–antithrombin III but is susceptible to inactivation by antithrombin III–independent inhibitors. The Journal of Clinical Investigation, 1990, vol 86, pp 385–391, by copyright permission of The American Society for Clinical Investigation.)

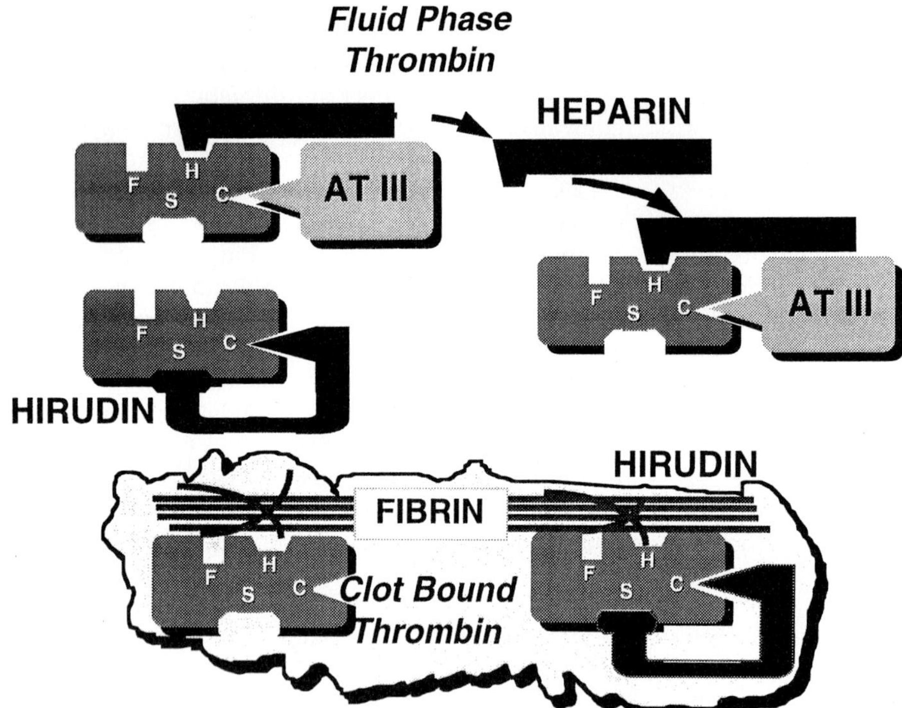

Figure 14–12 Revised model of antithrombin activity. Hirudin binds in a stoichiometric 1:1 relationship such that a single molecule of hirudin inhibits a single molecule of thrombin in the fluid phase (top portion) or clot-bound phase (bottom portion). In contrast, heparin is a catalytic inhibitor of thrombin so that a single molecule of heparin may catalyze the action of multiple molecules of antithrombin III (ATIII) (see text for further discussion). See Figure 14–1 for additional abbreviations. (Adapted from Giugliano RP, Antman EM, Braunwald E. Reexamination of the thrombin hypothesis: What we have learned from TIMI 9B and GUSTO IIB [editorial]. J Thromb Thrombolys 1997; 4:321–323; with kind permission from Kluwer Academic Publishers.)

seen in TIMI 9A and GUSTO IIa. In contrast, heparin is a catalytic inhibitor capable of dissociating from the complex of antithrombin III and thrombin, so that a single molecule of heparin may serve to catalyze the action of multiple molecules of antithrombin III.[8] In this way, antithrombin III works as a "suicide substrate," liberating heparin for further action against activated thrombin.

Based on the results of the clinical trials described earlier, it can be concluded that direct antithrombins have the advantage of a more consistent anticoagulant effect and fewer adjustments of the infusion rate. The therapeutic range appears to be much narrower than originally appreciated; within the clinically acceptable dose range, hirudin and heparin appear to be therapeutically equivalent for patients with acute coronary syndromes. Although an early benefit favoring hirudin with respect to reduction in MI was seen, this was observed predominantly while therapeutic concentrations of the drug were present, but loss of this early benefit occurred progressively over short-term follow-up (30 days) (see Table 14–4).

The angiographic trials with efegatran and clinical findings with inogatran showed a generally consistent pattern to that observed with hirudin. Dose-dependent prolongation of the anticoagulant effect was seen, but efficacy findings were not superior to heparin. Whether important differences will emerge with argatroban must await the results of the MINT and AMI Trials. Additional data on the combination of streptokinase and direct antithrombins will be forthcoming from the HIT-IV (hirudin) and HERO-2 (Hirulog) Trials.

Both the GUSTO IIb and OASIS pilot trials observed that in patients without ST-segment elevation, a marginally significant reduction in nonfatal recurrent ischemic events was observed during infusion of hirudin compared with heparin, but the difference in event rates between groups receiving a direct and indirect antithrombin progressively narrowed following discontinuation of the infusion of antithrombotic therapy. These results suggest that antithrombin therapy administered intravenously is useful for reducing the rate of events in the acute phase of treatment, but the culprit coronary vessel does not appear to be sufficiently "passivated," resulting in recurrent ischemic events over the intermediate and long term. The concept of administering continued antithrombotic therapy in the chronic phase of management of an acute coronary syndrome is being tested in several Phase III trials: in TIMI 11B where the low-molecular-weight heparin, enoxaparin, is administered acutely and chronically (vs. unfractionated heparin acutely and placebo injections in the chronic phase) and in OASIS where hirudin is infused during the acute phase and warfarin is administered during the chronic phase (vs. unfractionated heparin in the acute phase and vs. no anticoagulation in the chronic phase).

Results from several randomized, controlled studies establish the principle that the direct thrombin inhibitors hirudin and bivalirudin are safe substitutes for heparin during coronary angioplasty. Hirudin therapy is associated with a lower risk of inhospital complications in patients undergoing angioplasty for unstable angina. Bivalirudin therapy is associated with a lower risk of ischemic complications than is heparin in patients undergoing angioplasty for postinfarction angina, suggesting that the complications of angioplasty performed in this setting are thrombin mediated. Therapy with these agents results in at least an efficacy equivalent as heparin but with a lower risk of bleeding in patients who undergo angioplasty for unstable angina. Although the apparent treatment effect of the direct thrombin inhibitors appears to be weaker than that for the platelet glycoprotein IIb/IIIa receptor inhibitors, it is also possible that the profile of risk in patients enrolled in the clinical trials of thrombin inhibitors did not replicate that for patients undergoing PTCA in routine clinical practice to provide a reasonable opportunity to demonstrate adequate treatment effect.

The major obstacle to further development of direct thrombin inhibitors is financial. The costs of treatment and the ability to pay for them by a third party will govern the ultimate acceptance or rejection of direct thrombin inhibitors as anticoagulants in PTCA. In an earlier era when the cost of new treatments was not as important as it is now, the direct thrombin inhibitors would have had greater appeal because of their ease of use, trends toward reduced ischemic complications, and significant reduced bleeding risk. In the current atmosphere of managed care, the direct thrombin inhibitors must be viewed guardedly. Further areas of development will involve direct thrombin inhibitors in angioplasty in settings where the consequences of increased thrombus burden are substantial, or where the risk of heparin is unacceptable, as in the syndrome of heparin-associated thrombocytopenia and thrombosis.

REFERENCES

1. Libby P. Molecular basis of the acute coronary syndromes. Circulation 1995; 91:2844–2850.
2. Cairns J, Lewis HD Jr, Meade TW, et al. Antithrombotic agents in coronary artery disease. Circulation 1995; 95:380S–400S.
3. Weitz JI, Califf RM, Ginsberg JS, et al. New antithrombotics. Chest 1995; 108:471S–485S.
4. Ryan T, Anderson J, Antman E, et al. ACC/AHA guidelines for the management of patients with acute myocardial infarction: A report of the American College of Cardiology/American Heart Association Task Force on Practice Guidelines (Committee on Management of Acute Myocardial Infarction). J Am Coll Cardiol 1996; 28:1328–1428.
5. Fuster V, Badimon L, Badimon JJ, et al. The pathophysiology of coronary artery disease and the acute coronary syndromes. N Engl J Med 1992; 326:242–250, 310–318.
6. Fibrinolytic Therapy Trialists' (FTT) Collaborative Group. Indications for fibrinolytic therapy in suspected acute myocardial infarction: Collaborative overview of mortality and major morbidity results from all randomised trials of more than 1000 patients. Lancet 1994; 343:311–322.
7. The TIMI IIIB Investigators. Effects of tissue plasminogen activator and a comparison of early invasive and conservative strategies in unstable angina and non–Q wave myocardial infarction. Circulation 1994; 89:1545–1556.
8. Hirsh J, Fuster V. Guide to anticoagulant therapy: I. Heparin. Circulation 1994; 89:1449–1468.
9. Markwardt F. The development of hirudin as an antithrombotic drug. Thromb Res 1994; 74:1–23.
10. Maraganore JM. Pre-clinical and clinical studies on Hirulog: A potent and specific direct thrombin inhibitor. *In* Claeson G, Scully MF, Kakkar VV, Deadman J (eds). Design of Synthetic Inhibitors of Thrombin. New York, Plenum Press, 1993, pp 227–236.
11. Cannon CP, Maraganore JM, Loscalzo J, et al. Anticoagulant effects of Hirulog, a novel thrombin inhibitor, in patients with coronary artery disease. Am J Cardiol 1993; 71:778–782.
12. Callas DD, Hoppensteadt D, Fareed J. Comparative studies on the anticoagulant and protease generation inhibitory actions of newly developed site-directed thrombin inhibitory drugs. Semin Thromb Hemost 1995; 21:177–183.
13. Weitz JI. Activation of blood coagulation by plaque rupture: Mechanisms and prevention. Am J Cardiol 1995; 75:188–228.
14. Weitz JI, Hudoba M, Massel D, et al. Clot-bound thrombin is protected from inhibition by heparin–antithrombin III but is susceptible to inactivation by antithrombin III–independent inhibitors. J Clin Invest 1990; 86:385–391.
15. Cannon CP, McCabe CH, Henry TD, et al. A pilot trial of recombinant desulfatohirudin compared with heparin in conjunction with tissue-type plasminogen activator and aspirin for acute myocardial infarction: Results of the Thrombolysis in Mycardial Infarction (TIMI) 5 Trial. J Am Coll Cardiol 1994; 23:993–1003.
16. Zeymer U, von Essen R, Tebbe U, et al. Recombinant hirudin and front-loaded alteplase in acute myocardial infarction: Final results of a pilot study. Eur Heart J 1995; 16(Suppl D):22–27.
17. Lee LV, for the TIMI 6 Investigators. Initial experience with hirudin and streptokinase in acute myocardial infarction: Results of the Thrombolysis in Myocardial Infarction (TIMI) 6 trial. Am J Cardiol 1995; 75:7–13.
18. Lidón RM, Théroux P, Lespérance J, et al. A pilot, early angiographic patency study using a direct thrombin inhibitor as adjunctive therapy to streptokinase in acute myocardial infarction. Circulation 1994; 89:1567–1572.
19. White HD, Aylward PE, Frey MJ, et al. Randomized, double-blind comparison of Hirulog versus heparin in patients receiving streptokinase and aspirin for acute myocardial infarction (HERO). Circulation 1997; 96:2155–2161.
20. Ohman EM, Slovak JP, Anderson RL, et al. Potent inhibition of thrombin with Efegatran in combination with tPA in acute myocardial infarction: Results of a multicenter randomized dose-ranging trial. Circulation 1996; 94:I-430.
21. Weaver WD, Fung A, Lorch G, et al. Efegatran and streptokinase vs tPA and heparin for treatment of acute MI. Circulation 1996; 94:I-430.
22. Vermeer F, Vahanian A, Fels PW, et al. Intravenous argatroban versus heparin as co-medication to alteplase in the treatment of acute myocardial infarction: Preliminary results of the ARGAMI pilot study. J Am Coll Cardiol 1997; 29:185A.
23. Organization to Assess Strategies for Ischemic Syndromes (OASIS) Investigators. Comparison of the effects of two doses of recombinant hirudin compared with heparin in patients with acute myocardial ischemia without ST elevation: A pilot study. Circulation 1997; 96:769–777.
24. Sharma GV, Lapsley D, Vita JA, et al. Usefulness and tolerability of Hirulog, a direct thrombin inhibitor, in unstable angina pectoris. Am J Cardiol 1993; 72:1357–1360.
25. Lidón RM, Théroux P, Juneau M, et al. Initial experience with a direct antithrombin, Hirulog, in unstable angina: Anticoagulant, antithrombotic, and clinical effects. Circulation 1993; 88:1495–1501.
26. Fuchs J, Cannon CP, and the TIMI 7 Investigators. Hirulog in the treatment of unstable angina: Results of the Thrombin Inhibition in Myocardial Ischemia (TIMI) 7 Trial. Circulation 1995; 92:727–733.
27. Grip L, Wallentin L, Dellborg M, et al. A low-molecular-weight, specific thrombin inhibitor, inogatran, versus heparin, in unstable coronary artery disease. Circulation 1996; 94:I-430.
28. Antman E, for the TIMI 9A Investigators. Hirudin in acute myocardial infarction: Safety report from the Thrombolysis

and Thrombin Inhibition in Myocardial Infarction (TIMI) 9A Trial. Circulation 1994; 90:1624–1630.

29. The Global Use of Strategies to Open Occluded Coronary Arteries (GUSTO) IIa Investigators. Randomized trial of intravenous heparin versus recombinant hirudin for acute coronary syndromes. Circulation 1994; 90:1631–1637.
30. Neuhaus KL, von Essen R, Tebbe U, et al. Safety observations from the pilot phase of the randomized r-Hirudin for Improvement of Thrombolysis (HIT-III) Study: A study of the Arbeitsgemeinschaft Leitender Kardiologischer Krankenhausärzte (ALK). Circulation 1994; 90:1638–1642.
31. Antman EM, for the TIMI 9B Investigators. Hirudin in acute myocardial infarction: Thrombolysis and Thrombin Inhibition in Myocardial Infarction (TIMI) 9B trial. Circulation 1996; 94:911–921.
32. The Global Use of Strategies to Open Occluded Coronary Arteries (GUSTO) IIb Investigators. A comparison of recombinant hirudin with heparin for the treatment of acute coronary syndromes. N Engl J Med 1996; 335:775–782.
33. Simes RJ, Granger CB, Antman EM, et al. Impact of hirudin versus heparin on mortality and (re)infarction in patients with acute coronary syndromes: A prospective meta-analysis of the GUSTO-IIb and TIMI 9B trials. Circulation 1996; 94:I-430.
34. Wolfe MW, Roubin GS, Schweiger M, et al. Length of hospital stay and complications after percutaneous transluminal coronary angioplasty: Clinical and procedural predictors. Circulation 1995; 92:311–319.
35. Topol EJ, Leya F, Pinkerton CA, et al. A comparison of balloon angioplasty with directional atherectomy in patients with coronary artery disease. N Engl J Med 1993; 329:221–227.
36. Adelman AG, Cohen EA, Kimball BP, et al. A comparison of coronary atherectomy with coronary angioplasty for lesions of the proximal left anterior descending coronary artery. N Engl J Med 1993; 329:228–233.
37. Serruys P, de Jaegere P, Kiemeneij F, et al. A comparison of balloon–expandable-stent implantation with balloon angioplasty in patients with coronary artery disease. N Engl J Med 1994; 331:489–495.
38. Fischman DL, Leon MB, Baim DS, et al. A randomized comparison of coronary stent placement and balloon angioplasty in the treatment of coronary artery disease. N Engl J Med 1994; 331:496–501.
39. Nobuyoshi M, Kimura T, Nosaka H, et al. Restenosis after successful percutaneous transluminal coronary angioplasty: Serial angiographic follow-up of 229 patients. J Am Coll Cardiol 1988; 12:616–623.
40. Fernández-Ortiz A, Badimon JJ, Falk E, et al. Characterization of the relative thrombogenicity of atherosclerotic plaque components: Implications for consequences of plaque rupture. J Am Coll Cardiol 1994; 23:1562–1569.
41. Strony J, Beaudoin A, Brands D, et al. Analysis of shear stress and hemodynamic factors in a model of coronary artery stenosis and thrombosis. Am J Physiol 1993; 265:H1787–H1796.
42. Annex BH, Denning SM, Channon KM, et al. Differential expression of tissue factor protein in directional atherectomy specimens from patients with stable and unstable coronary syndromes. Circulation 1995; 91:619–622.
43. Banner DW, D'Arcy A, Chene C, et al. The crystal structure of the complex of blood coagulation factor VIIa with soluble tissue factor. Nature 1996; 380:41–46.
44. Coughlin SR, Vu THH, Hung DR, et al. Characterization of a functional thrombin receptor. J Clin Invest 1992; 89:351–355.
45. Coller BS, Peerschke EI, Scudder LE, et al. A murine monoclonal antibody that completely blocks the binding of fibrinogen to platelets produces a thrombasthenic-like state in normal platelets and binds to glycoprotein IIb and/or IIIa. J Clin Invest 1983; 72:325–338.
46. Merino A, Cohen M, Badimon JJ, et al. Synergistic action of severe wall injury and shear forces on thrombus formation in arterial stenosis: Definition of a thrombotic shear rate threshold. J Am Coll Cardiol 1994; 24:1091–1094.
47. Marmur JD, Merlinie PA, Sharma SK, et al. Thrombin generation in human coronary arteries after percutaneous transluminal balloon angioplasty. J Am Coll Cardiol 1994; 24:1484–1491.
48. Grüntzig AR, Senning A, Siegenthaler WE. Nonoperative dilatation for coronary artery stenosis—percutaneous transluminal coronary angioplasty. N Engl J Med 1979; 301:61–68.
49. Sarembock IJ, Gertz SD, Gimple L, et al. Effectiveness of recombinant desulphatohirudin in reducing restenosis after balloon angioplasty of atherosclerotic femoral arteries in rabbits. Circulation 1991; 84:232–243.
50. Gallo R, Toschi V, Fallon JT, et al. Prolonged thrombin inhibition reduces restenosis after balloon angioplasty in porcine coronary arteries [Abstract]. J Am Coll Cardiol 1996; 27:320A.
51. Ragosta M, Barry WL, Gimple LW, et al. Effect of thrombin inhibition with desulfatohirudin on early kinetics of cellular proliferation after balloon angioplasty in atherosclerotic rabbits. Circulation 1996; 93:1194–1200.
52. de Feyter PJ, Serruys PW. Percutaneous transluminal coronary angioplasty for unstable angina. *In* Topol EJ (ed). Textbook of Inteventional Cardiology. Philadelphia, WB Saunders, 1994, pp 274–291.
53. de Feyter PJ, Serruys PW, Soward A, et al. Coronary angioplasty for early postinfarction unstable angina. Circulation 1986; 74:1365–1370.
54. Holt GW, Sugrue DD, Bresnahan JF, et al. Results of percutaneous transluminal coronary angioplasty for unstable angina pectoris in patients 70 years of age and older. Am J Cardiol 1988; 61:994–997.
55. Gottlieb SO, Walford GD, Ouyang P, et al. Initial and late results of coronary angioplasty for early postinfarction unstable angina. Cathet Cardiovasc Diagn 1987; 13:93–99.
56. Safian RD, Snyder LD, Snyder BA, et al. Usefulness of percutaneous transluminal coronary angioplasty for unstable angina pectoris after non–Q-wave acute myocardial infarction. Am J Cardiol 1987; 59:263–266.
57. Hopkins J, Savage M, Zalewski A, et al. Recurrent ischemia in the zone of prior myocardial infarction: Result of coronary angioplasty of the infarct-related artery. Am Heart J 1988; 115:14–19.
58. Suryapranata H, Beatt K, de Feyter PJ, et al. Percutaneous transluminal coronary angioplasty for angina pectoris after a non–Q-wave acute myocardial infarction. Am J Cardiol 1988; 61:240–243.
59. Morrison DA. Coronary angioplasty for medically refractory unstable angina in patients with prior coronary bypass surgery. Cathet Cardiovasc Diagn 1990; 20:174–181.
60. TIMI Study Group Phase II Trial. Comparison of invasive and conservative strategies after treatment with intravenous tissue plasminogen activator in acute myocardial infarction. N Engl J Med 1989; 320:618–627.
61. Timmis AD, Griffin B, Crick JC, et al. Early percutaneous transluminal coronary angioplasty in the management of unstable angina. Int J Cardiol 1987; 14:25–31.
62. de Feyter PJ, Suryapranata H, Serruys PW, et al. Coronary angioplasty for unstable angina: Immediate and late results in 200 consecutive patients with identification of risk factors for unfavorable early and late outcome. J Am Coll Cardiol 1988; 12:324–333.
63. Thijs Plokker HW, Ernst SM, Bal ET, et al. Percutaneous transluminal coronary angioplasty in patients with unstable angina pectoris refractory to medical therapy: Long-term clinical and angiographic results. Cathet Cardiovasc Diagn 1988; 14:15–18.
64. Sharma B, Wyeth RP, Kilath GS, et al. Percutaneous transluminal coronary angioplasty of one-vessel for refractory unstable angina pectoris: Efficacy in single and multivessel disease. Br Heart J 1988; 59:280–286.
65. Perry RA, Seth A, Hunt A, et al. Coronary angioplasty in unstable angina and stable angina: A comparison of success and complications. Br Heart J 1988; 60:367–372.
66. Myler RK, Shaw RE, Stertzer SH, et al. Unstable angina and coronary angioplasty [Review]. Circulation 1990; 82:II-88–II-95.
67. Morrison DA. Percutaneous transluminal coronary angioplasty for rest angina pectoris requiring intravenous nitroglycerin and intra-aortic balloon counterpulsation. Am J Cardiol 1990; 66:168–172.
68. Rupprecht HJ, Brennecke R, Kottmeyer M, et al. Short- and long-term outcome after percutaneous transluminal coronary angioplasty in patients with stable and unstable angina. Eur Heart J 1990; 11:964–969.

69. Quigley PJ, Erwin J, Maurer BJ, et al. Percutaneous transluminal coronary angioplasty in unstable angina. Br Heart J 1986; 55:227–230.
70. Steffenino G, Meier B, Finci L, et al. Follow-up results of treatment of unstable angina by coronary angioplasty. Br Heart J 1987; 57:416–419.
71. Stammen F, de Scheerder I, Glazier JJ, et al. Immediate and follow-up results of the conservative coronary angioplasty strategy for unstable angina pectoris. Am J Cardiol 1992; 69:1533–1537.
72. Bredlau CE, Roubin G, Leimgruber P, et al. In-hospital morbidity and mortality in patients undergoing elective coronary angioplasty. Circulation 1985; 72:1044–1052.
73. Hartzler G. Complex coronary angioplasty: Multivessel/multilesion dilatation. *In* Ischinger T (ed). Practice of Coronary Angioplasty. New York, Springer-Verlag, 1986, pp 250–267.
74. Holmes DR Jr, Holubkov R, Vlietstra RE, et al. Comparison of complications during percutaneous transluminal angioplasty from 1977 to 1981 and from 1985 to 1986: The National Heart, Lung, and Blood Institute Percutaneous Transluminal Coronary Angioplasty Registry. J Am Coll Cardiol 1988; 12:1149–1155.
75. Tuzcu EM, Simpfendorfer C, Badhwar K, et al. Determinants of primary success in elective percutaneous transluminal coronary angioplasty for significant narrowing of a single major coronary artery. Am J Cardiol 1988; 62:873–875.
76. de Feyter PJ, van den Brand M, Serruys PW. Increase of initial success and safety of single-vessel PTCA in 1371 patients: A seven-years' experience. J Intervent Cardiol 1988; 1:1–10.
77. O'Keefe JH Jr, Reeder GS, Miller GA, et al. Safety and efficacy of percutaneous transluminal coronary angioplasty performed at time of diagnostic catheterization compared with that performed at other times. Am J Cardiol 1989; 63:27–29.
78. Myler RK, Shaw RE, Stertzer SH, et al. Lesion morphology and coronary angioplasty: Current experience and analysis. J Am Coll Cardiol 1992; 19:1641–1652.
79. Dimas AP, Grigera F, Arora RR, et al. Repeat coronary angioplasty as treatment for restenosis. J Am Coll Cardiol 1992; 19:1310–1314.
80. Weintraub WS, Ghazzal ZMB, Douglas JS, et al. Initial management and long-term clinical outcome of restenosis after initially successful percutaneous transluminal coronary angioplasty. Am J Cardiol 1992; 70:47–55.
81. Alfonso R, Macaya C, Iniquez A, et al. Repeat coronary angioplasty during the same angiographic diagnosis of coronary restenosis. Am Heart J 1990; 119:237–241.
82. Meier B, King SB III, Gruentzig AR, et al. Repeat coronary angioplasty. J Am Coll Cardiol 1984; 4:463–466.
83. Topol EJ, Fuster V, Harrington RA, et al. Recombinant hirudin for unstable angina pectoris: A multicenter, randomized angiographic trial. Circulation 1994; 89:1557–1566.
84. Serruys PW, Herrman JPR, Simon R, et al. A comparison of hirudin with heparin in the prevention of restenosis after coronary angioplasty. N Engl J Med 1995; 333:757–763.
85. Topol EJ, Bonan R, Jewitt D, et al. Use of a direct antithrombin, Hirulog, in place of heparin during coronary angioplasty. Circulation 1993; 87:1622–1629.
86. Bittl JA, Strony J, Brinker JA, et al. Treatment with bivalirudin (Hirulog) as compared with heparin during coronary angioplasty for unstable or postinfarction angina. N Engl J Med 1995; 333:764–769.
87. Grassman ED, Leya F, Johnson SA, et al. Percutaneous transluminal coronary angioplasty for unstable angina: Predictors of outcome in a multicenter study. J Thromb Thrombolys 1994; 1:73–78.
88. Maraganore JM, Bourdon P, Jablonski J, et al. Design and characterization of Hirulogs: A novel class of bivalent peptide inhibitors of thrombin. Biochemistry 1990; 29:7095–7101.
89. The TIMI Research Group. Immediate versus delayed catheterization and angioplasty following thrombolytic therapy for acute myocardial infarction: TIMI II A results. JAMA 1988; 260:2849–2858.
90. Detre KM, Holmes DR Jr, Holubkov R, et al. Incidence and consequences of periprocedural occlusion: The 1985–1986 National Heart, Lung, and Blood Institute Percutaneous Transluminal Coronary Angioplasty Registry. Circulation 1990; 82:739–750.
91. Roubin GS, Cannon AD, Agrawal SK, et al. Intracoronary stenting for acute and threatened closure complicating percutaneous transluminal coronary angioplasty. Circulation 1992; 85:916–927.
92. Zoldhelyi P, Bichler J, Owen WG, et al. Persistent thrombin generation in humans during specific thrombin inhibition with hirudin. Circulation 1994; 90:2671–2678.
93. Gallistl S, Muntean W. Thrombin-hirudin complex formation, thrombin–antithrombin III complex formation, and thrombin generation after intrinsic activation of plasma. Thromb Haemost 1994; 72:387–392.
94. Strony J, Ahmed WH, Meckel CR, et al. Clinical evidence for thrombin rebound after stopping heparin but not Hirulog [Abstract]. Circulation 1995; 92:I-609.
95. Lincoff AM, Popma JJ, Ellis SG, et al. Abrupt vessel closure complicating coronary angioplasty: Clinical, angiographic, and therapeutic profile. J Am Coll Cardiol 1992; 19:926–935.
96. White CJ, Ramee SR, Collins TJ, et al. Coronary angioscopy of abrupt occlusion after angioplasty. J Am Coll Cardiol 1995; 25:1681–1684.
97. Sassower MA, Abela GS, Koch JM, et al. Angioscopic evaluation of periprocedural and postprocedural abrupt closure after percutaneous coronary angioplasty. Am Heart J 1993; 126:444–450.
98. Bittl JA, on behalf of the Hirulog Angioplasty Study Investigators. Comparative safety profiles of Hirulog and heparin in patients undergoing coronary angioplasty. Am Heart J 1995; 130:658–665.
99. Warkentin TE, Levine MN, Hirsh J, et al. Heparin-induced thrombocytopenia in patients treated with low-molecular-weight heparin or unfractionated heparin. N Engl J Med 1995; 332:1330–1335.
100. Chamberlin JR, Lewis B, Leya F, et al. Successful treatment of heparin-associated thrombocytopenia and thrombosis using Hirulog. Can J Cardiol 1995; 11:511–514.
101. Reid T III. Hirulog therapy for heparin-associated thrombocytopenia and deep venous thrombosis [Letter]. Am J Hematol 1994; 45:352–353.
102. Nicolini FA, Lee P, Rios G, et al. Combination of platelet fibrinogen receptor antagonist and direct thrombin inhibitor at low doses markedly improves thrombolysis. Circulation 1994; 89:1802–1809.
103. Gallistl S, Muntean W, Leis HJ. Effects of heparin and hirudin on thrombin generation and platelet aggregation after intrinsic acivation of platelet rich plasma. Thromb Haemost 1995; 74:1163–1168.
104. Loscalzo J. Thrombin inhibitors in fibrinolysis: A Hobson's choice of alternatives. Circulation 1996; 94:863–865.
105. Liu L, Freedman J, Hornstein A, et al. Thrombin binding to platelets and their activation in plasma. Br J Haematol 1994; 88:592–600.
106. Ryan TJ, Bauman WB, Kennedy JW, et al. Guidelines for percutaneous transluminal coronary angioplasty: A report of the American Heart Association/American College of Cardiology Task Force on Assessment of Diagnostic and Therapeutic Cardiovascular Procedures (Subcommittee on Percutaneous Transluminal Coronary Angioplasty). Circulation 1993; 88:2987–3007.

15 Platelet Glycoprotein IIb/IIIa Receptor Inhibitors

▶ **Keaven M. Anderson***
▶ **Harlan F. Weisman***
▶ **Barry S. Coller†**

Thrombotic cardiovascular disease is the leading cause of death and disability throughout the world.[1] The underlying pathogenesis of this disorder involves progressive coronary atherosclerosis, but most acute events involve thrombotic occlusion at the site of plaque fissure, erosion, or rupture.[2] Platelets are primarily responsible for the occlusive thrombus, with leukocytes, fibrin, and entrapped erythrocytes also contributing. Because plaque fissure, erosion, or rupture does not always lead to a thrombotic event, other factors affect the final result, including the nature of the exposed material, the geometry of the blood vessel, rheologic factors, and the predisposition of the individual's platelets and coagulation system to initiate and sustain thrombus formation.[3, 4] There has probably been considerable evolutionary pressure favoring an active hemostatic system in humans because people with such systems were less likely to die from traumatic hemorrhage before passing on their genes. In contrast, there probably has been little evolutionary pressure against thrombosis because it primarily affects people who are beyond their reproductive years. Thus, the current hemostatic system of humans is poorly adapted to modern culture, which is characterized by longer life and progressive atherosclerosis.

PLATELET PHYSIOLOGY AND CORONARY THROMBOSIS

The nearly immediate deposition of platelets on a damaged, atherosclerotic blood vessel is the first observable event leading to thrombus formation. Two different mechanisms may be responsible for this phenomenon: (1) exposure of tissue factor in the lipid-rich region of the plaque,[5] resulting in thrombin generation, fibrin deposition, and binding of von Willebrand factor (and perhaps other adhesive glycoproteins) to fibrin; or (2) exposure of collagen, von Willebrand factor, fibronectin, and perhaps other adhesive glycoproteins that are either present in the subendothelial region or deposited from plasma.[6–9] In either scenario, platelets can then adhere to the damaged surface via their receptors for these glycoproteins (GP), including GPIb, GPIIb/IIIa, GPIa/IIa ($\alpha_2\beta_1$), GPIc*/IIa ($\alpha_5\beta_1$), GPIc/IIa ($\alpha_6\beta_1$), and perhaps GPIV and GPVI.[9] The GPIIb/IIIa receptors on the luminal side of the adherent platelets then undergo an activation-dependent change in conformation that results in the high-affinity binding of fibrinogen or von Willebrand factor (or both).[10] Additional platelets are recruited to the adherent platelets via bridging by fibrinogen or von Willebrand factor (or both), resulting in platelet thrombus formation, release of vasoactive agents such as thromboxane A_2 and serotonin,[11] and generation of thrombin,[12] which leads to additional fibrin formation. Thromboxane A_2, serotonin, and thrombin all can also result in activation of the GPIIb/IIIa receptors on circulating platelets, resulting in further recruitment of platelets to the thrombi.

GPIIb/IIIa RECEPTOR

The GPIIb/IIIa receptor, which is made up of two different subunits (α_{IIb} and β_3), is a member of the integrin receptor superfamily, whose members include more than 20 receptors involved in cell adhesion and related phenomena in many organ systems.[13, 14] GPIIb/IIIa and several other integrin receptors bind some glycoproteins via an arginine-glycine-aspartic acid sequence in the ligand.[15] This

*Drs. Anderson and Weisman are employed by Centocor, Inc., Malvern, Pennsylvania, the manufacturer of abciximab.
†Dr. Coller is an inventor of abciximab. In compliance with federal law and the patent policy of the Research Foundation of the State University of New York, he shares in the royalties received by the Foundation from sales of abciximab.

Supported in part by Grant 19278 from the National Heart, Lung, and Blood Institute.

observation led to the remarkable observation that low-molecular-weight peptides and peptidomimetic agents patterned on this arginine-glycine-aspartic acid motif can block the binding of adhesive glycoproteins to the GPIIb/IIIa receptor.[16, 17] These data have been exploited in the preparation of a variety of new agents designed to block the GPIIb/IIIa receptor.

Some integrin β subunits can combine with more than one α subunit, and this is true for the β_3 subunit, which can combine with GPIIb to form GPIIb/IIIa or α_v to form the $\alpha_v\beta_3$ vitronectin receptor. The $\alpha_v\beta_3$ vitronectin receptor has been implicated in a wide variety of different functions, including bone resorption, angiogenesis, metastasis formation, and development of intimal hyperplasia after vascular injury.[18] Intimal hyperplasia is one of the processes believed to contribute to *restenosis* after balloon angioplasty of coronary arteries, and thus it has been postulated, but not established, that blockade of $\alpha_v\beta_3$ vitronectin receptors may help prevent restenosis after balloon angioplasty. Inhibitors of the GPIIb/IIIa receptor vary significantly in their ability to inhibit $\alpha_v\beta_3$ vitronectin receptors.

GPIIb/IIIa ANTAGONISTS

The central role of the GPIIb/IIIa receptor in platelet thrombus formation makes it a logical target for antithrombotic therapy. Thus, all physiologic and pathologic platelet activating agents rely on the GPIIb/IIIa receptor to mediate platelet aggregation. Moreover, selective blockade of GPIIb/IIIa receptors should leave platelet adhesion relatively intact, and platelet adhesion (which produces a monolayer of platelets) may contribute to hemostasis while posing only a minimal risk of causing vaso-occlusive thrombosis. Finally, patients who lack GPIIb/IIIa receptors on an inherited basis (Glanzmann thrombasthenia) have a moderate to severe mucocutaneous hemorrhagic diathesis but rarely have spontaneous central nervous system hemorrhage,[19, 20] despite having no functional GPIIb/IIIa receptors and extremely long bleeding times. These observations provide hope that GPIIb/IIIa receptor blockade for relatively short periods may not produce an unacceptable risk of hemorrhage.

GPIIb/IIIa ANTAGONISTS STUDIED IN RANDOMIZED CLINICAL TRIALS

Abciximab

Abciximab (c7E3 Fab; ReoPro, Centocor/Lilly) is the Fab fragment of the murine/human chimeric monoclonal antibody 7E3,[21, 22] which was derived from the original murine 7E3 monoclonal antibody[23] by recombinant DNA techniques. The antithrombotic efficacy of abciximab and the prototype 7E3 antibodies (murine 7E3 F[ab′]$_2$ and Fab) were variably evaluated in dog, monkey, and baboon models of coronary, carotid, and femoral artery thrombosis.[24] Doses of the antibodies that produced high-grade (>80%) GPIIb/IIIa receptor blockade uniformly prevented acute arterial thrombosis. When used in combination with a thrombolytic agent (with and without conjunctive heparin therapy), abciximab and the prototype 7E3 antibody augmented the effects of low doses of thrombolytic agents, facilitated the lysis of resistant thrombi, speeded reperfusion, prevented reocclusion, and decreased infarct size.[25, 26]

Although inhibition of platelet aggregation and thus platelet thrombus formation as a result of GPIIb/IIIa receptor blockade is probably the dominant mechanism of action of abciximab, other mechanisms of action may contribute to its effects. Thus, abciximab may also (1) decrease thrombin generation by both decreasing the number of platelets in a thrombus and inhibiting platelets from undergoing activation-dependent enhancement of their surface catalytic efficiency in supporting thrombin generation, thus ultimately reducing clot-bound thrombin[27]; (2) decrease the release from platelets of fibrinolysis inhibitors (α_2-plasmin inhibitor and plasminogen activator inhibitor-1), thus facilitating thrombolysis,[28, 29] as well as agents implicated in inducing intimal hyperplasia (platelet-derived growth factor, serotonin, adenosine diphosphate [ADP]); (3) inhibit factor XIIIa binding to platelets and release of platelet factor XIII, thus inhibiting fibrin crosslinking and the crosslinking of α_2-plasmin inhibitor to fibrin[30]; (4) inhibit clot retraction, which has been implicated in conferring resistance to thrombolysis[31, 32]; and (5) inhibit $\alpha_v\beta_3$ vitronectin receptors on platelets, endothelial cells, or smooth muscle cells, which may be involved in platelet function or the development of intimal hyperplasia (or both).[18, 33]

Pharmacokinetic data on abciximab indicate that after intravenous bolus administration, free plasma concentrations decrease rapidly (initial half-life of about 30 minutes) as a result of rapid binding to platelet GPIIb/IIIa receptors, with approximately 65% of the injected antibody becoming attached to platelets in the circulation and spleen.[34] In most patients, intravenous administration of a 0.25 mg/kg bolus of abciximab followed by continuous infusion of 10 μg per minute produces sustained high-grade receptor blockade (>80%) and marked inhibition of platelet function (ex vivo platelet aggregation in response to ADP <20% of baseline and bleeding time >30 minutes) for the duration of the infusion.[22, 35] Bleeding time returns to normal within 12 hours after the end of the infusion in most patients and within 24 hours in nearly all patients. Platelet aggregation in response to 20 μM ADP returns to 50% or greater of baseline within 24 hours in most patients and within 48 hours in nearly all patients. Small amounts of abciximab can be detected on circulating platelets as late as 14 days after administration, presumably as a result of antibody redistribution from platelet to platelet.[22]

Side effects of abciximab treatment include the following:

1. Hemorrhage, which is discussed in the context of the individual trials.
2. Thrombocytopenia, with approximately 1% to 2% of patients treated with abciximab developing platelet counts less than 50,000/μL, of which approximately 0.5% to 1% reflects rapid decreases (beginning within 2 hours of administration) owing to abciximab.[36–38] Thus far, all reports indicate that the thrombocytopenia can be treated effectively with platelet transfusions and is reversible, with recovery occurring over several days.[37, 38]

In the Evaluation of c7E3 for Prevention of Ischemic Complications (EPIC) Trial, approximately 6% of patients treated with abciximab developed antibodies to the variable regions of abciximab (human antichimeric antibody).[36] Few data are currently available to assess the potential risks of reinjecting abciximab, which theoretically include anaphylaxis, neutralization of injected abciximab, and thrombocytopenia.

Tirofiban

Tirofiban (MK-383; Aggrastat, Merck) (L-tyrosine,*N*-[n-butylsulfonyl]-*0*-{4-butyl-4-piperidinyl}], monohydrochloride, monohydrate) is a nonpeptide derivative of tyrosine that selectively inhibits the GPIIb/IIIa receptor, with minimal effects on the $\alpha_v\beta_3$ vitronectin receptor.[39, 40] Thus, it inhibits platelet aggregation of gel-filtered platelets induced by 10 μM ADP with an inhibitory concentration of 50% (IC_{50}) of 9 nM, but the IC_{50} for inhibition of human umbilical vein adhesion to vitronectin, which depends on $\alpha_v\beta_3$ vitronectin receptors, is almost four orders of magnitude greater (62 μM).[40] Infusion of tirofiban into dogs at 10 μg/kg per minute produced nearly complete inhibition of ADP-induced platelet aggregation, with the aggregation response returning to approximately 70% of normal within 30 minutes of discontinuing the therapy.[41] Tirofiban demonstrated potent antithrombotic effects in animal models.[41]

When administered to humans at 0.15 μg/kg per minute for 4 hours, tirofiban produced a 2.5 ± 1.1-fold increase in bleeding time and 97.4% ± 4.7% inhibition of 3.4 μM ADP-induced platelet aggregation.[42, 43] The mean plasma clearance was 329 mL per minute and the half-life in plasma was 1.6 hours. Bleeding times returned to normal within 4 hours after stopping tirofiban, and the inhibition of platelet aggregation declined to approximately 20% over the same period. When administered with aspirin, the bleeding time increased 4.1 ± 1.5 fold, even though aspirin did not affect tirofiban plasma levels. The plasma concentration of tirofiban needed to inhibit platelet aggregation by 50% decreased, however, from approximately 12 ng/mL to approximately 9 ng/mL when aspirin was coadministered. Peak plasma concentrations were approximately 40 ng/mL, and the plasma levels decreased to less than 2 ng/mL within 6 hours after discontinuing therapy.

Seventy-three patients undergoing coronary artery balloon angioplasty in a pilot study were treated with aspirin, heparin, and bolus doses of tirofiban of 5, 10, or 10 μg/kg followed by tirofiban infusions of 0.05, 0.10, or 0.15 μg/kg per minute.[44] The onset of platelet inhibition was rapid, with platelet aggregation in response to 5 μM ADP inhibited by 93% and 96% within 5 minutes of administering the two higher dose regimens. Median bleeding times at 2 hours after starting the infusions were 19.5, greater than 30, and greater than 30 minutes. At the end of the infusion (16 to 24 hours), platelet aggregation was inhibited by 57%, 87%, and 95%. After discontinuing the infusion, platelet aggregation began to return toward normal within 1.5 hours in all groups, and by 4 hours platelet aggregation inhibition decreased to less than 50%, even in the group receiving the highest dose.

The hemorrhagic risk associated with tirofiban is discussed in the individual trials. Severe but reversible thrombocytopenia has been reported in a small percentage of patients treated with tirofiban; an immunologic mechanism has been proposed in which patients have preformed antibodies to a conformation of the GPIIb/IIIa receptor induced by the binding of tirofiban to the receptor.[45] Severe thrombocytopenia was more common in patients treated with tirofiban in the Platelet Receptor Inhibition for Ischemic Syndrome (PRISM) Trial (n = 3231) (1.2% vs. 0.4%). No published data are available yet on the treatment of thrombocytopenia or the safety of reinfusing tirofiban.

Eptifibatide

Eptifibatide (Integrilin, COR Therapeutics/Schering Plough) is a synthetic disulfide-linked cyclic heptapeptide whose precise structure has not been disclosed by the manufacturer. It is said to be patterned after the lysine-glycine-aspartic acid (KGD) sequence found in the snake venom disintegrin obtained from *Sistrurus m. barbouri* (barbourin), which confers high specificity for inhibition of GPIIb/IIIa compared with inhibition of the $\alpha_v\beta_3$ vitronectin receptor.[46, 47] In animal studies, eptifibatide was shown to be a potent inhibitor of platelet aggregation and platelet thrombus formation. Preliminary reports indicated that eptifibatide produced less prolongation of the bleeding time than other GPIIb/IIIa inhibitors at doses producing comparable inhibition of platelet aggregation. More recent studies indicate that the citrate anticoagulation used for aggregation studies may result in an overestimation of eptifibatide's inhibition of platelet aggregation,[47a] so it is unclear whether there is a differential effect of eptifibatide on the bleeding time. The clearance of eptifibatide depends principally on plasma clearance rather than drug metabolism. Patients treated with heparin plus eptifibatide had longer activated clotting times (393 seconds and 407 seconds for 4- and 12-hour eptifibatide infusion groups) than patients treated with heparin alone (368 seconds),[48] indicating that eptifibatide can inhibit thrombin generation in vitro. As noted earlier, a similar phenomenon was observed with abciximab treatment.

In 21 patients undergoing elective percutaneous coronary artery balloon angioplasty or directorial coronary atherectomy treated with aspirin, heparin (10,000 U bolus plus additional doses to maintain an activated clotting time at 300 to 350 seconds), and a bolus dose of 90 μg/kg of eptifibatide followed by a 1 μg/kg per minute infusion for 4 or 12 hours, platelet aggregation was measured before, 1 hour after the bolus, at the end of the infusion, and 4 hours after the end of the infusion.[48] On average, platelet aggregation in response to 20 μM ADP decreased from approximately 80% before eptifibatide to approximately 15% both at 1 hour after the bolus dose and at the end of the infusion. There was, however, significant interindividual variation in the inhibitory responses, with the 95% confidence limits extending from 0% to approximately 30% and 0% to approximately 40% at the two time points tested. Four hours after stopping the infusion, the average aggregation response was approximately 55%, but there was marked individual variation, with the 95% confidence interval between approximately 10% and 90%. Median bleeding times were prolonged with eptifibatide therapy from approximately 6 minutes before treatment to approximately 26 minutes both at 1 hour after beginning the infusion and at the end of the infusion. The bleeding times returned toward normal (median 15 minutes) within 15 minutes of stopping eptifibatide and declined to approximately 12 minutes after stopping the drug for 1 hour. At each time point, however, there were considerable interindividual differences.

In a subsequent study,[49] four eptifibatide regimens were tested in 54 patients undergoing coronary interventions who were also treated with aspirin and heparin: (1) 180 μg/kg bolus plus 1 μg/kg per minute infusion for 18 to 24 hours ($n = 4$); (2) 135 μg/kg bolus plus 0.5 μg/kg per minute infusion for 18 to 24 hours ($n = 16$); (3) 90 μg/kg bolus plus 0.75 μg/kg per minute infusion for 18 to 24 hours ($n = 6$); and (4) 135 μg/kg bolus plus 0.75 μg/kg per minute for 18 to 24 hours ($n = 28$). Fifteen minutes after the 180 μg/kg bolus dose, platelet aggregation in response to 20 μM ADP was inhibited by greater than 95%, with virtually no interindividual variation, whereas the 135 μg/kg bolus dose resulted in 80% to 90% inhibition in 75% of the patients, and the 90 μg/kg bolus produced only slightly less inhibition than the 135 μg/kg dose. The high-grade inhibition of platelet aggregation achieved with the 180 μg/kg bolus dose was sustained throughout the infusion by the 1 μg/kg per minute dose, but there was a tendency for the platelet aggregation response to return toward normal during the infusion in some patients given the 0.75 μg/kg per minute dose; the return of the platelet aggregation response toward normal was more marked in those given the 0.5 μg/kg per minute infusion dose. There was substantial return of platelet aggregation function 2 hours after discontinuing the eptifibatide infusion in all groups and return of more than half of the baseline aggregation response in all groups after 4 hours. Median bleeding times were prolonged in all groups at the time the infusion was terminated (22, 12, 12, and 17 minutes compared with control values of 7 to 8 minutes), and the bleeding times returned toward normal after 1 hour (9, 10, 9, and 11 minutes). As in the previous study, activated clotting times were longer in patients treated with eptifibatide plus heparin than in those treated with placebo plus heparin.

The hemorrhage risks of eptifibade therapy are discussed in the individual trials. In the Integrilin to Minimize Platelet Aggregation and Coronary Thrombosis (IMPACT) II study ($n = 4010$), eptifibatide treatment was not associated with an increased frequency of thrombocytopenia. In the 10,948-patient Platelet IIb/IIIa in Unstable Angina: Receptor Suppression Using Integrilin Trial (PURSUIT), there was no difference in thrombocytopenia between treatment groups, but there was a greater incidence of severe thrombocytopenia (< 20,000 platelets per microliter) in the eptifibatide group (10 cases; 0.2%) than in the placebo group (2 cases; < 0.1%).[49a] No data are available concerning the safety of reinfusing eptifibatide.

Lamifiban

Lamifiban (Ro 44-9883, Roche) ([[1-[*N*-(*p*-amidinobenzoyl)-L-tyrosyl]-4-piperidinyl]oxy] acetic acid) is a nonpeptide compound that inhibits platelet aggregation of platelet-rich plasma induced by 10 μM ADP with an IC_{50} of 25 nM and binds to gel-filtered platelets with a dissociation constant (K_D) of 5 nM; it has little or no effect on $\alpha_v\beta_3$.[50, 51] Of note, binding of lamifiban to GPIIb/IIIa does not induce the ligand binding conformation of the receptor as does the binding of other peptides and peptidomimetics[52]; similarly, binding of lamifiban does not expose at least some ligand-induced binding sites on GPIIb/IIIa.[53] Pharmacokinetic data were obtained from ascending doses of 30-minute continuous infusions.[54] A free plasma concentration of 6.1 nM produced 50% inhibition of ADP-induced platelet aggregation. The bleeding time doubled when platelet aggregation inhibition reached nearly 100%. Using a one-compartment model, the volume of distribution was 22 L, the half-life (free drug) was 40 minutes, the half-life (bound drug) was 9.5 hours, and plasma clearance was 417 mL per minute.

In a dose-ranging study,[55] patients with unstable angina were given either placebo or one of four different lamifiban regimens: (1) 150 μg bolus plus 1 μg per minute infusion; (2) 300 μg bolus plus 2 μg per minute infusion; (3) 600 μg bolus plus 4 μg per minute infusion; and (4) 750 μg bolus plus 5 μg per minute infusion. The infusion rate was decreased by 10%, 20%, and 30% for patients weighing less than 70, 60, and 50 kg, respectively. The infusions were maintained for 72 to 120 hours (mean duration, 84 hours). All patients received aspirin, but heparin treatment was left to the discretion of the physician. Platelet aggregation studies and bleeding times were performed on 58 patients while on steady-state drug infusion at 2 and 72 hours and 2 to 6 hours after stopping the drug.

At steady-state, the 4 and 5 μg per minute infusion regimens nearly abolished platelet aggregation induced by 10 μM ADP, whereas the 1 and 2 μg per minute infusions produced approximately 60% and 75% inhibition. Platelet aggregation induced by 100 μM thrombin receptor activating peptide was inhibited to a lesser extent than that induced by ADP, but at 5 μg per minute lamifiban infusion, it too was nearly abolished. Bleeding time prolongation demonstrated a dose-response relationship, increasing to a median of approximately 23 minutes with the 5 μg per minute lamifiban infusion.

The hemorrhagic risks associated with lamifiban treatment are discussed with the individual studies. No data on the frequency of thrombocytopenia or the safety of reinfusing lamifiban are currently available.

TRIALS IN PERCUTANEOUS CORONARY INTERVENTION

Percutaneous coronary intervention (PCI) was chosen as the first indication to demonstrate the potential clinical utility of inhibiting platelet aggregation by blocking the platelet GPIIb/IIIa receptor. A vessel undergoing PCI invariably undergoes plaque rupture and arterial damage, leading to platelet adhesion and platelet thrombus formation. Platelet thrombi and subsequent fibrin deposition can lead to partial or complete vessel occlusion resulting in ischemic complications, including angina or myocardial infarction (MI). These processes can result in death or the need for an urgent intervention, such as a repeat PCI or emergency coronary artery bypass surgery (CABS). Moreover, several different studies indicate that suffering an MI as a complication of a PCI, as judged by elevations in serum cardiac creatine kinase levels, results in both higher inhospital mortality and long-term (3- to 4-year) mortality.[56, 57] Even relatively small increases in creatine kinase appear to increase long-term mortality. The healing process after the arterial injury and plaque rupture produced by PCI can result in a narrowing of the arterial lumen, a process generally termed *restenosis*. This problem is especially common in the first 3 to 8 months after PCI.

This set of trials includes protocols studying platelet GPIIb/IIIa receptor inhibition immediately before and after PCI. More than 15,000 patients have been enrolled in the seven studies that have been completed. Three compounds have been studied in this setting: abciximab, eptifibatide, and tirofiban. The first of the phase III trials conducted, the EPIC Trial, resulted in marketing approval of abciximab for high-risk PCI patients in many countries around the world. Eptifibatide and tirofiban have been studied in the Integrilin to Manage Platelet Aggregation to Prevent Coronary Thrombosis (IMPACT) II and Randomized Efficacy of Tirofiban for Outcomes and Restenosis (RESTORE) Trials, respectively. Although neither of these trials achieved their predefined efficacy endpoints, there was a suggestion in each case that the compound was active. The c7E3 Antiplatelet Therapy in Unstable Refractory Angina (CAPTURE) Trial demonstrated the efficacy of an 18- to 24-hour abciximab treatment before PCI in patients with unstable angina refractory to aspirin, heparin, and nitrates. The Evaluation of PTCA to Improve Long-term Outcome by c7E3 GPIIb/IIIa Receptor Blockade (EPILOG) Trial demonstrated the efficacy of abciximab in a broad patient population undergoing PCI, not just patients judged to be at high risk as in the EPIC and CAPTURE Trials. In addition, EPILOG demonstrated that the hemorrhagic risk associated with abciximab could be reduced dramatically by decreasing and weight adjusting the heparin dose. The ReoPro in Acute Myocardial Infarction and Primary PTCA Organization and Randomized Trial (RAPPORT) demonstrated results in patients with acute MI that were consistent with larger trials. The EPISTENT Trial demonstrated the efficacy of abciximab plus either balloon angioplasty on stenting compared with stenting without abciximab.

Abciximab

EPIC

Phase I and II Trials of abciximab[34] and its precursor, m7E3 Fab,[58] established the bolus and infusion doses of abciximab needed to achieve consistently the goals of 80% or greater platelet blockade and 80% or greater inhibition of aggregation. These trials gave preliminary indications of acceptable clinical safety in the setting of PCI.

The EPIC Trial[36, 59] was the first trial to establish the clinical efficacy of a GPIIb/IIIa inhibitor. EPIC was a randomized, double-blind, placebo-controlled trial that studied the use of abciximab either as a bolus or as a bolus plus 12-hour infusion in patients judged to be at high risk of ischemic complications based on their having an acute MI or unstable angina at the time of study entry or by virtue of having a combination of angiographic and clinical criteria previously noted to confer high risk of ischemic complications.[60] The objectives of the trial were to examine the safety and efficacy of two abciximab regimens. A total of 2099 patients were enrolled in three arms: (1) an abciximab bolus of 0.25 mg/kg and a 12-hour abciximab infusion of 10 μg per minute (bolus plus infusion, $n = 708$); (2) an abciximab bolus and a 12-hour placebo infusion (bolus, $n = 695$); and (3) a placebo bolus and a 12-hour placebo infusion (placebo, $n = 696$). The infusion dose of 10 μg per minute totals 7.2 mg over 12 hours. This compares to 20 mg in the bolus dose for an 80-kg individual. The pharmacodynamics of abciximab suggest that the bolus dose provides substantial inhibition of aggregation (>80%) for 4 to 6 hours, whereas the bolus plus infusion provides substantial inhibition of aggregation for 16 to 18 hours, with an extended tapering of receptor blockade thereafter.[22, 34]

The primary endpoint of the EPIC Trial was a composite 30-day endpoint comprising death, MI, and urgent intervention (CABS, repeat PCI, urgent stent placement during the index PCI, and urgent intra-aortic balloon pump for ischemia). No significant differences were found between the placebo and the bolus alone group for either the primary 30-day endpoint or the 6-month endpoint. In contrast, the primary 30-day endpoint was reduced by 35% (4.5% absolute)—from 12.8% in the placebo group to 8.3% in the bolus plus infusion group ($P = 0.008$).[36] A composite 6-month endpoint of death, MI, and any intervention was reduced by 23% (8% absolute)—from 35% in the placebo group to 27% in the bolus plus infusion group ($P = 0.001$).[59] Through 3 years of follow-up, the bolus plus infusion group continued to enjoy an absolute benefit similar to that observed at 6 months (47.2% placebo, 41.1% bolus plus infusion; $P = 0.009$).[61]

In the 30-day follow-up, no excess in mortality (1.7% placebo, 1.7% bolus plus infusion, by intention to treat; 1.7% placebo, 1.4% bolus plus infusion by actual treatment received), hemorrhagic stroke (0.3% placebo, 0.4% bolus plus infusion by intention to treat; 0.3% placebo, 0.1% bolus plus infusion by actual treatment received), or other irreversible safety events were observed in patients in the bolus plus infusion group compared with patients in the placebo group. Treated patients experienced an increase in major bleeding events—from 7% in the placebo group to 14% in the bolus plus infusion group ($P < 0.001$). These events were primarily localized to the groin access site. There were also increases in the percentages of patients receiving red blood cell transfusions, from 7.1% to 15.4% ($P < 0.001$), and experiencing severe thrombocytopenia (platelet count <50,000/μL), from 0.7% to 1.6% ($P = 0.09$).

Examination of bleeding events in relationship to patient weight and heparin dosing suggested that lowering and weight adjusting the heparin dose might improve the safety of the bolus plus infusion regimen without loss of efficacy.[62] Figure 15–1 shows rates of the primary endpoint and major bleeding events not associated with CABS for patients in EPIC by treatment group and weight. Among patients under 75 kg of body weight, there was less efficacy and a greater risk of bleeding. The rate of major bleeding decreased with increasing weight, however, in the bolus plus infusion group to the point that little excess major bleeding was observed compared with placebo among patients weighing 90 kg or more. Because the heparin bolus dose was not weight adjusted in the EPIC Trial, it was hypothesized that excess bleeding among lighter-weight patients might primarily be due to the combination of abciximab plus high-dose heparin. It was further hypothesized that the high primary endpoint rate in the bolus plus infusion group among lightweight patients might actually be caused by high heparin dosing through either the platelet activating effect of heparin[63] or through hypotension related to excess bleeding.

PROLOG, EPILOG, RAPPORT, AND EPISTENT

The PROLOG Trial[64] was a 103-patient, randomized, double-blind, 2 × 2 factorial pilot trial for the EPILOG Trial.[65] All patients undergoing PCI, not just those at high risk of suffering ischemic complications, were eligible for entry into the trial. The protocol treatment consisted of a 0.25 mg/kg bolus plus a 12-hour 10 μg/kg per minute infusion of abciximab. All

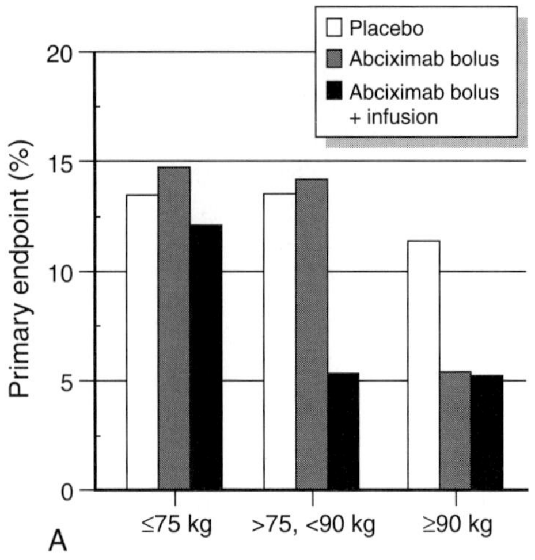

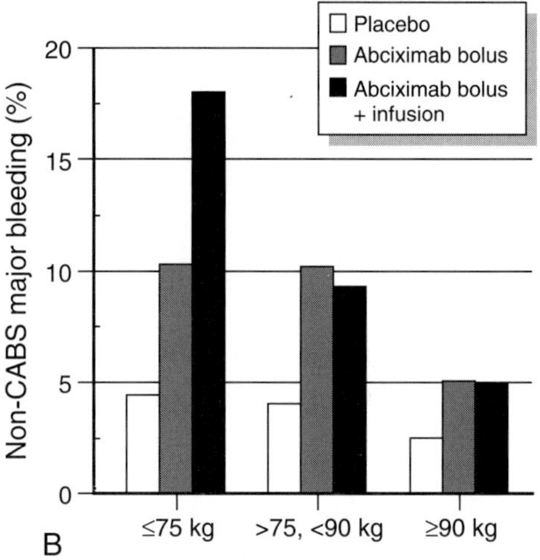

Figure 15–1 Primary endpoint *(A)* and major bleeding other than that associated with coronary artery bypass surgery (non-CABS) *(B)* in EPIC.

patients also received aspirin and heparin. The results of the EPIC Trial suggested that the increased bleeding with abciximab might be due to the conjoint use of abciximab with a relatively high (10,000 U), non–weight-adjusted dose of heparin. Thus, two lower-dose, weight-adjusted heparin regimens were tested in PROLOG: *standard* (100 U/kg initial bolus before PCI with a target activated clotting time of at least 300 seconds), and low dose (70 U/kg bolus with no activated clotting time target). Early discontinuation of heparin and sheath removal 4 hours later, even if during infusion of abciximab, was compared with a 12-hour infusion of heparin and sheath removal at least 6 hours after discontinuation of abciximab and at least 4 hours after discontinuation of heparin. Guidelines for controlling bleeding at the sheath access site were recommended for all patients.[66, 67] The composite efficacy endpoint of death, MI, and urgent intervention was observed in eight patients (7.8%), which was a result comparable to that observed in EPIC, whereas major bleeding was reported in only two patients (1.9%), which was much lower than the rate observed in EPIC (7%). The sheath/patient management guidelines and weight adjustment of heparin thus appeared successful in lowering the bleeding risk. Both the lower dose of heparin and the early sheath removal compared with EPIC appeared to contribute to the reduced bleeding.

EPILOG was designed to enroll 4800 patients in a randomized, three-arm, double-blind, placebo-controlled trial. Patients who might be at high risk of bleeding were excluded, as were patients meeting EPIC criteria for unstable angina or MI, because it was judged that it would be unethical to withhold abciximab treatment from these groups based on the data from EPIC. All other patients undergoing PCI were eligible for entry into EPILOG. The EPILOG Trial was designed to test three hypotheses: (1) reducing the heparin dose would reduce the excess bleeding observed with abciximab treatment in the EPIC Trial; (2) the efficacy benefit observed from abciximab treatment in high-risk patients in EPIC would be maintained despite the reduction in the heparin dose; and (3) patients undergoing PCI who did not meet the EPIC criteria for being at high risk of suffering acute ischemic events would benefit from abciximab therapy.

All patients in the trial received aspirin and weight-adjusted heparin. In the placebo group, a bolus of 100 U/kg was given before PCI with a target activated clotting time of 300 seconds or more. Discontinuation of heparin immediately after PCI was recommended for all patients unless contraindicated. Early sheath removal, 2 to 6 hours after heparin discontinuation (activated partial thromboplastin time ≤50 seconds or activated clotting time ≤175 seconds), during placebo or abciximab infusion, was also recommended. Patients in each of the two abciximab treatment arms received a 0.25 mg/kg bolus of abciximab followed by a 0.125 μg/kg per minute infusion. The infusion dosing was limited to a maximum of 10 μg per minute for patients weighing 80 kg or more. Patients in one of the two abciximab treatment arms received the same, *standard* weight-adjusted heparin regimen as the placebo group. Patients in the other abciximab arm received a 70 U/kg bolus of heparin with a target activated clotting time of 200 seconds or more.

A single interim analysis of the first 1500 patients enrolled was planned. The analysis of the composite, 30-day endpoint of death or MI reached the criteria for a positive efficacy result. The pairwise comparison of the placebo group with the abciximab plus low-dose heparin group had a P value of 0.00008. At the time the interim analysis was performed, 2792 patients had been enrolled. Final analysis of the 30-day composite of death or MI demonstrated a rate of 9.1% in the placebo group, with a 59% reduction in the abciximab plus low-dose heparin group to 3.8% (P <

0.0001) (5.3% absolute reduction) and a 54% reduction to 4.2% in the abciximab plus standard-dose heparin group ($P < 0.0001$) (4.9% absolute reduction).[68] The event rate for the composite of death, MI, or urgent intervention was 11.7% in the placebo group, with a 56% reduction to 5.2% in the abciximab plus low-dose heparin group ($P < 0.0001$) (6.5% absolute reduction) and a 54% reduction to 5.4% in the abciximab plus standard-dose heparin group ($P < 0.0001$) (6.3% absolute reduction). Mortality was low in all three groups (0.8% placebo, 0.3% abciximab plus low-dose heparin, 0.4% abciximab plus standard-dose heparin). MI was observed in 8.7% of placebo patients, with a 58% reduction to 3.7% in the abciximab plus low-dose heparin group ($P < 0.001$) (5.0% absolute reduction) and a 56% reduction to 3.8% in the abciximab plus standard-dose heparin group ($P < 0.001$) (4.9% absolute reduction). Urgent intervention was observed in 5.2% of placebo patients, with a 68% reduction to 1.6% in the abciximab plus low-dose heparin group ($P < 0.001$) (3.6% absolute reduction) and a 55% reduction to 2.3% in the abciximab plus standard-dose heparin group ($P \leq 0.001$) (2.9% absolute reduction).

A 6-month efficacy endpoint was prespecified as part of the primary analysis of the EPILOG Trial. The composite endpoint of death and MI through 6 months was reduced by 45% from 11.1% in the placebo group to 6.1% in the combined abxicimab groups ($P < 0.001$, one-sided). The composite of death, MI, and urgent intervention through 6 months was reduced by 43% from 14.7% in the placebo group to 8.4% in the combined abciximab groups ($P < 0.001$, one-sided). The event rate for the composite endpoint of death, MI, or repeat revascularization through 6 months was 25.8% in the placebo treatment group, 22.8% in the abciximab plus low-dose heparin group (11.7% reduction, 3% absolute reduction, $P = 0.034$, one-sided), and 22.3% in the abciximab plus standard-dose heparin group (13.7% reduction, 3.5% absolute reduction; $P = 0.020$, one-sided). When the abciximab groups were combined, the event rate was 22.5%, a 12.6% reduction ($P = 0.011$, one-sided). These results met prespecified criteria for statistical significance, which required a reduction in the combined abciximab treatment groups compared with placebo before each individual abciximab group could be compared with placebo. The rate of 25.8% in the placebo group was substantially lower than the EPIC placebo rate of 35.1%. This difference between the trials may be partially attributable to differences in the patient population and the more common use of provisional stenting during the EPILOG Trial.

No intracranial hemorrhage was observed in the placebo group compared with one (0.1%) in the abciximab plus low-dose heparin group and four (0.4%) in the abciximab plus standard-dose heparin group. Major bleeding was observed in 3.1% of placebo patients, with a 34% reduction to 2.0% ($P = 0.2$) in the abciximab plus low-dose heparin group and a 13% increase to 3.5% ($P = 0.7$) in the abciximab plus standard-dose heparin group. Red blood cells were transfused in 3.9% of placebo patients, 1.9% of abciximab plus low-dose heparin patients, and 3.3% of abciximab plus standard-dose heparin patients. Severe thrombocytopenia (platelet count <50,000/μL) occurred in 0.4% of placebo patients, 0.4% of abciximab plus low-dose heparin patients, and 0.9% of abciximab plus standard-dose heparin patients.

The adjustments in heparin therapy or sheath management made between EPIC and EPILOG apparently improved the effectiveness and reduced the bleeding risk associated with abciximab bolus plus infusion therapy. Primary endpoint and major non-CABS bleeding rates were similar in all weight groups in EPILOG (Fig. 15–2), similar to the results observed among the heaviest patients in EPIC (see Fig. 15–1).[69] Patients receiving directional atherectomy benefited from abciximab therapy, with a 55% reduction in the EPIC Trial compared with placebo treatment.[70] In EPI-

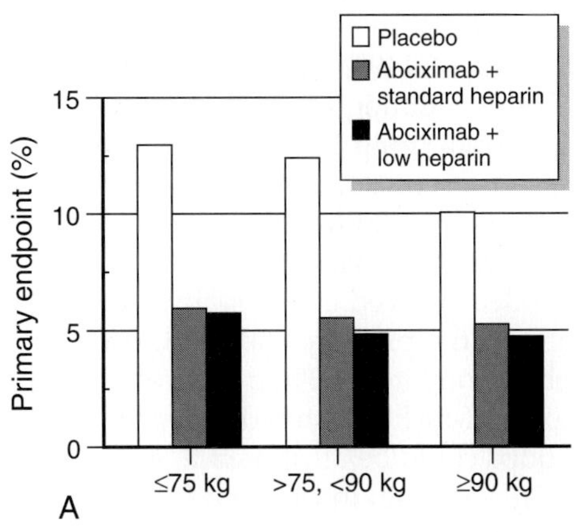

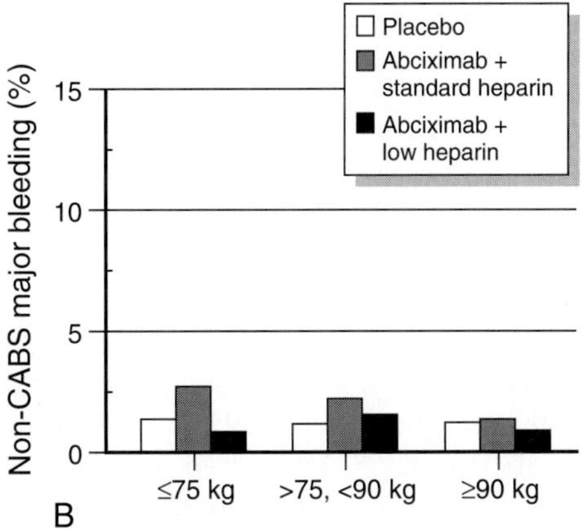

Figure 15–2 Primary endpoint *(A)* and major bleeding other than that associated with coronary artery bypass surgery (non-CABS) *(B)* in EPILOG.

LOG, the composite of death or MI at 30 days was reduced to a similar degree among patients undergoing balloon angioplasty (6.9% in the placebo group vs. 2.8% in the combined abciximab groups; $P <$ 0.001); stent implantation (19.5% in the placebo group vs. 7.1% in the combined abciximab groups; $P <$ 0.001); or directional coronary atherectomy, transluminal extraction catheter atherectomy, or laser atherectomy (19.2% in the placebo group vs. 8.2% in the combined abciximab groups; $P = 0.027$).

Endpoint event rates were somewhat higher in the high-risk placebo group than the low-risk placebo group in EPILOG, but both groups achieved similar reductions in endpoint events with abciximab treatment.[71] In the high-risk patients, a reduction was seen in the composite endpoint event rate from 13.1% in placebo-treated patients to 6.2% in abciximab-treated patients (52.9% reduction, 6.9% absolute; $P < 0.001$). In low-risk patients, a composite endpoint event rate reduction from 9.2% in placebo-treated patients to 3.7% in abciximab-treated patients was observed (60.3% reduction, 5.5% absolute; $P < 0.001$). These data indicate that patients judged by conventional criteria to be at low risk of ischemic complications of PCI are benefited by treatment with abciximab.

The RAPPORT was a 483-patient, randomized, double-blind trial in patients with balloon angioplasty planned within 12 hours of onset of a myocardial infarction.[71a] Patients were randomized to receive placebo or abciximab in addition to standard therapy. The incidence of the primary endpoint of death, MI, or target vessel revascularization through 6 months of follow-up was nearly identical in the placebo (28.1%) and abciximab (28.2%) treatment groups. However, the 30-day endpoint of death, MI, and urgent target vessel revascularization was reduced by 48% from 11.2% in the placebo group to 5.8% in the abciximab group (4.4% absolute reduction; $P = 0.04$). There were no patients who had intracranial hemorrhage in the trial. Heparin was given as a 100-U/kg bolus in both treatment groups, with a heparin infusion following intervention. This strategy was undertaken to simplify blinding but may have been the cause of excess major bleeding in both the abciximab group (16.6%) and the placebo group (9.5%; $P =$ 0.02). This is in contrast to EPILOG and EPILOG stent, where reduced heparin doses and a recommendation of early discontinuation of heparin and sheath removal resulted in very low major bleeding rates in both the placebo and abciximab groups.

In the EPISTENT trial patients, undergoing PCI were randomized to one of three strategies: stenting plus placebo, stenting plus abciximab, or balloon angioplasty plus abciximab.[71b] Abciximab and heparin were administered as in the EPILOG trial. Early heparin discontinuation and sheath removal following PCI were recommended in all groups, also as in the EPILOG trial. The primary endpoint of death, MI, or the need for urgent revascularization in the first 30 days was reduced by 51.0% from 10.8% in the stent and placebo group to 5.3% for the stent plus abciximab group (5.5% absolute reduction; $P < 0.001$) and reduced by 35.8% to 6.9% for the balloon angioplasty and abciximab group (3.9% absolute reduction; $P =$ 0.007). No intracranial hemorrhages were reported in the trial. Major bleeding occurred in 2.2% of patients in the stent and placebo group, 1.5% of the stent and abciximab group, and 1.4% of the balloon angioplasty and abciximab group.

CAPTURE

The CAPTURE Trial was a randomized, double-blind, placebo-controlled trial designed to enroll 1400 patients in two treatment groups.[72] It included patients with unstable angina that was refractory to medical therapy with aspirin, heparin, and nitrates. Patients had to have chest pain associated with electrocardiogram changes within 24 hours of entry and had to have coronary angiography within 48 hours before study entry indicating a single lesion in a native artery amenable to PCI. Patients entered into the abciximab treatment group received a bolus of 0.25 mg/kg, a 10 μg per minute infusion for 18 to 24 hours before PCI, and continuation of the infusion for 1 hour after the PCI. Patients enrolled in the placebo group received comparable placebo bolus and infusion therapy. All patients were treated with heparin, nitrates, and aspirin. Before PCI, patients were to receive a weight-adjusted, 100 U/kg bolus of heparin. Discontinuation of heparin immediately after the procedure was encouraged to allow early sheath removal.

The primary endpoint for the CAPTURE Trial was a 30-day composite comprising death, MI, urgent CABS, urgent stent placement either during or after the initial PCI, or urgent repeat PCI after completion of the planned study PCI. A secondary 6-month efficacy endpoint comprised death, MI, CABS, and repeat PCI after the planned study PCI.

CAPTURE enrolled patients from early 1993 until the end of 1995, when the trial was stopped at the recommendation of the Independent Safety and Efficacy Monitoring Committee of the trial in response to a positive efficacy result at an interim analysis of 1050 patients. A total of 1266 patients were enrolled at the time the trial was stopped. Analysis of all patients enrolled showed a 29% relative reduction (4.6% absolute) in the primary endpoint, from 15.9% in the placebo group to 11.3% in the abciximab group ($P =$ 0.012). Much of the difference between treatment groups could be attributed to a 50% relative reduction (4.1% absolute) in MI from 8.2% in the placebo group to 4.1% in the abciximab group ($P = 0.002$). During the medical therapy period before PCI, the MI rate was reduced from 2.0% in the placebo group to 0.6% in the abciximab group (*P* = 0.029) (Fig. 15–3). Another benefit of pretreatment with abciximab was a reduction in the PCI failure rate as judged by angiography, from 11.2% in the placebo group to 6.0% in the abciximab group (*P* = 0.001). Figure 15–3 also shows that abciximab provided protection against the sharp increase in the MI rate immediately after the PCI; the high rate of MI post-PCI persisted for approximately 12 to 14 hours post-PCI, however, and so the protection by abciximab was incomplete, with the rate of MI in the 24 hours after PCI 5.3% in the placebo group and 2.5% in the abciximab group (*P* = 0.009). Collectively, these data suggest that continuing the abciximab infusion for more than 1 hour after PCI, as was done in the EPIC and EPILOG Trials, may be an appropriate strategy to try to improve abciximab's antithrombotic efficacy. Mortality was not different in the two groups with treatment (1.3% placebo, 1.0% abciximab, *P* = 0.6), but urgent interventions were reduced by 28% (3.1% absolute reduction) from 10.9% placebo to 7.8% abciximab (*P* = 0.054). Many of the urgent interventions were stents (6.6% placebo, 5.6% abciximab, *P* = 0.408). There was one stroke of unknown type (0.2%) observed in the abciximab group 15 days after study entry; there were three strokes (0.5%) in the placebo group, one of which (0.2%) was hemorrhagic. Major bleeding other than that associated with CABS was reported for 1.9% of patients in the placebo group compared with 3.8% in the abciximab group (*P* = 0.043).

Six-month follow-up of the CAPTURE Trial showed no difference in the number of patients reaching the composite endpoint of death, MI, or repeat revascularization (30.8% placebo, 31.0% abciximab). Abciximab-treated patients, however, tended to have fewer endpoint events per patient (0.43 per patient in the placebo group, 0.38 in the abciximab group, *P* = 0.067). The MI benefit observed at 30 days was preserved at 6 months (9.3% placebo, 6.6% abciximab, *P* = 0.055), whereas mortality (2.2% placebo, 2.8% abciximab) and repeat revascularization (24.9% placebo, 25.9% abciximab) showed no differences.

Eptifibatide

IMPACT I AND II

The IMPACT I Trial[48] was a 150-patient, randomized, double-blind study of two dosing regimens of eptifibatide and a control arm in patients undergoing elective PCI. A bolus of 90 μg/kg of eptifibatide with an infusion of 1 μg/kg per minute was studied. In one eptifibatide arm, the infusion duration was 4 hours; in the other, the infusion duration was 12 hours. The primary efficacy endpoint for the study was the same as for EPIC: a composite of death, MI, or urgent intervention (CABS or repeat PCI). Six events occurred in the placebo group, compared with five in the 4-hour infusion group and two in the 12-hour infusion group. One patient in the 4-hour infusion group died after an intracerebral hemorrhage, with clinical onset 8.5 hours after eptifibatide was discontinued. No increase in the rate of major bleeding was seen in the eptifibatide groups as defined by Thrombolysis in Myocardial Infarction (TIMI) Study Group criteria.[73]

The IMPACT II Trial was a phase III, randomized, placebo-controlled, double-blind study enrolling 4010 patients to test the clinical efficacy and safety of eptifibatide in patients undergoing PCI.[74] In contrast with EPIC, the population was not restricted to patients judged to be at high risk of ischemic complications. Dosing was modified from IMPACT I, with the eptifibatide bolus increased from 90 μg/kg to 135 μg/kg. Two 24-hour infusion regimens were studied: 0.5 μg/kg per minute and 0.75 μg/kg per minute,

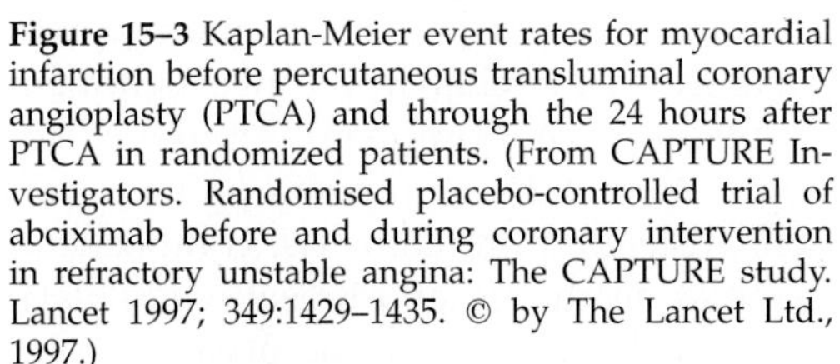

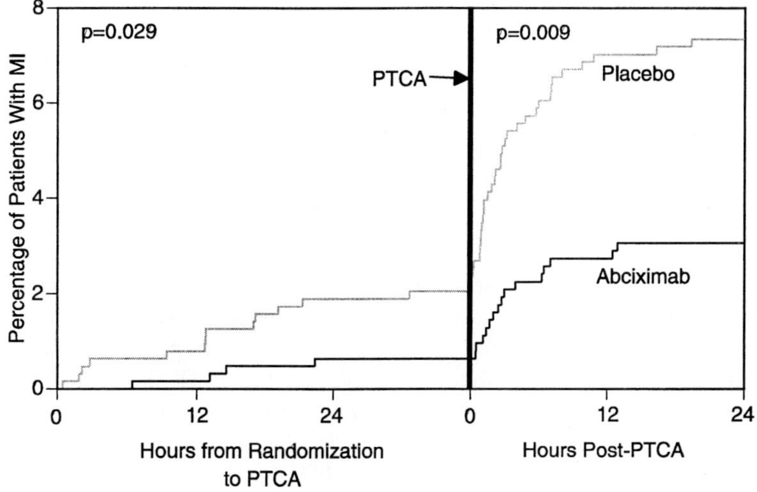

Figure 15–3 Kaplan-Meier event rates for myocardial infarction before percutaneous transluminal coronary angioplasty (PTCA) and through the 24 hours after PTCA in randomized patients. (From CAPTURE Investigators. Randomised placebo-controlled trial of abciximab before and during coronary intervention in refractory unstable angina: The CAPTURE study. Lancet 1997; 349:1429–1435. © by The Lancet Ltd., 1997.)

compared with the 1 μg/kg per minute infusion rate in IMPACT I. The total bolus plus infusion dose in this trial was thus specified as 855 μg/kg in the low-dose group and 1215 μg/kg in the high-dose group. All patients also received aspirin and heparin. The pharmacodynamics of eptifibatide would suggest similar, high-grade receptor blockade for the two experimental arms during the initial hours of treatment but subsequent variable tapering of the effect. A 100 U/kg bolus dose of heparin during PCI was used, but the target activated clotting time of 300 to 350 seconds was the same as in the EPIC Trial, in which patients received a non–weight-adjusted bolus of 10,000 to 12,000 units. Eptifibatide-treated patients demonstrated longer activated clotting times than did controls, suggesting that eptifibatide, similar to abciximab, can decrease thrombin generation in the activated clotting time. Heparin discontinuation was encouraged immediately after completion of the PCI, with vascular sheath removal 4 to 6 hours later, when the activated clotting time had decreased to less than 150 seconds.

The primary endpoint for the IMPACT II Trial was a composite 30-day endpoint comprising death, MI, emergency repeat PCI, emergency CABS, or stent placement for abrupt closure. The primary efficacy analysis of the IMPACT II Trial showed no statistically significant difference between treatment arms, although there was a trend toward improvement in the low-dose eptifibatide group.[74] Observed primary endpoint event rates were 11.4% in the placebo group, 9.2% (19% relative reduction from placebo, 2.2% absolute reduction; $P = 0.06$) in the low-dose eptifibatide infusion arm, and 9.9% (13% relative reduction from placebo, 1.5% absolute reduction; $P = 0.22$) in the high-dose eptifibatide infusion arm. Even though the EPIC Trial attempted to enroll only patients at high risk of ischemic complications, the primary endpoint rate was only slightly higher in the EPIC placebo group than that in the IMPACT II placebo group (12.8% vs. 11.4%). Death rates during the 30-day follow-up were 1.1% in the placebo group, 0.5% in the low-dose eptifibatide group, and 0.8% in the high-dose eptifibatide group.

The percentage of patients experiencing major bleeding events was not statistically different between the treatment arms: 4.8% in the placebo group compared with 5.1% in the low-dose infusion arm and 5.2% in the high-dose infusion arm. In the placebo group of the EPIC Trial, the major bleeding rate was 6.6% compared with 4.8% in IMPACT II. Although the trials were not concurrent, this finding suggests that the reduction and weight adjustment of the heparin dose or the early sheath removal in IMPACT II had some effect on bleeding risk, and this is consistent with the even greater reduction in bleeding rates observed in the EPILOG and EPISTENT Trials.

In a substudy of 617 patients who underwent angiography at 6 months after PCI in IMPACT II, no treatment effect was found on angiographic outcomes. Among all treated patients in the overall study, no significant difference was found in the 6-month composite clinical endpoint of death, MI, or repeat revascularization (32.1% placebo, 30.6% low-dose eptifibatide, 29.5% high-dose eptifibatide). The 6-month composite of death or MI was also not significantly different among treated patients (11.8% placebo, 10.6% low-dose eptifibatide, 10.1% high-dose eptifibatide).

Tirofiban

RESTORE

The RESTORE Trial was a 2139-patient, two-arm, randomized, double-blind, placebo-controlled trial in high-risk patients undergoing PCI with standard therapy plus a 36-hour infusion of tirofiban or placebo.[75] Patients presenting within 72 hours of onset of an acute coronary syndrome (MI or unstable angina) qualified for study entry. Heparin and aspirin were given in both treatment arms. The protocol specified a 334 μg/kg dose of tirofiban given as a 10 μg/kg bolus plus an infusion of 0.15 μg/kg per minute for 36 hours. The pharmacodynamics of this compound suggest that a high degree of GPIIb/IIIa receptor blockade was achieved during the infusion of tirofiban, with a quick recovery of platelet function after discontinuation.

The primary endpoint of the RESTORE Trial was a 30-day composite of death, MI, and repeat revascularization (PCI or CABS) for ischemia related to a vessel treated in the study PCI. Repeat revascularization did not have to be urgent to be an endpoint in RESTORE as was required in EPIC and IMPACT II. Although the primary endpoint was reduced by 16%, from 12.2% in the placebo group to 10.3% in the tirofiban group (1.9% absolute reduction), this difference was not statistically significant ($P = 0.16$). Major bleeding was observed in 4.5% of patients in the placebo group and 6.0% of patients randomized to tirofiban. Mortality was similar in the two treatment groups (0.7% placebo, 0.8% tirofiban). Thrombocytopenia was reported in 1.2% of placebo patients and 1.5% of patients receiving tirofiban. The composite 6-month endpoint of death, MI, and repeat revascularization was reduced from 27.1% in the placebo group to 24.1% in the tirofiban group (11% reduction, $P = 0.108$). MI event rates through 6 months were 7.6% in the placebo group and 6.3% in the tirofiban group (17% reduction; $P = 0.226$).

Subgroup and Secondary Analyses from Percutaneous Coronary Intervention Trials

Although primary analyses were negative for the IMPACT II and RESTORE Trials, secondary analyses suggested early differences in the composite primary endpoints after the first 48 hours. Similar analyses have been presented for EPIC and EPILOG. These results are presented in Table 15–1. The ability to compare these trials directly is limited because of variations in the entry criteria and the assessment of endpoints in the trials. In particular, in RESTORE, cardiac enzymes were measured less frequently during the early time period after PCI, and the definition of an intervention endpoint was different. Despite this caveat, however, the improvements in efficacy appear similar at 48 hours for all the trials except the EPILOG and EPISTENT (abciximab plus stent) Trials, in which larger relative reductions in events were observed. At 30 days, the three trials with abciximab showed significant differences between GPIIb/IIIa inhibition compared with placebo, whereas the other two trials did not.

Risk stratification was incorporated into several trials with GPIIb/IIIa inhibitors. EPIC and RESTORE were specifically designed to enroll patients thought to be at high risk of primary endpoints after PCI. IMPACT II, EPILOG, and EPISTENT enrolled broad-based populations, including patients who were believed to be both at low risk and at high risk. Patients with acute coronary syndromes at the time of enrollment into EPIC appeared to have particular benefit from abciximab treatment. Thus, among 489 patients with unstable angina in the EPIC Trial, Lincoff and colleagues[76] reported a 62% reduction in the 30-day primary endpoint, from 12.8% in the placebo group to 4.8% in the abciximab bolus plus infusion group (8.0% absolute benefit; $P = 0.012$); at 6 months, both MI (11.1% placebo, 2.4% abciximab bolus plus infusion; $P = 0.002$) and mortality (6.6% placebo, 1.8% abciximab bolus plus infusion; $P = 0.018$) were substantially reduced with abciximab therapy; and at 3 years, the benefits for MI (13.4% placebo, 7.7% abciximab bolus plus infusion; $P = 0.065$) and mortality (11.4% placebo, 5.1% abciximab bolus plus infusion; $P = 0.032$) were maintained. Among 65 patients with MI within 12 hours before entry in the EPIC Trial, an 83% reduction in the 30-day primary endpoint was observed, from 26.1% in the placebo group to 4.5% in the abciximab bolus plus infusion group; at 6 months, the composite endpoint of death, MI, and repeat revascularization was reduced by 91%, from 47.8% in the placebo group to 4.5% in the abciximab bolus plus infusion group ($P = 0.002$).[77] As noted earlier, this reduction was not replicated in the primary analysis of the RAPPORT Trial. Patients treated with atherectomy in the EPIC Trial[78] and stent in IMPACT II[79] also received particular benefit from GPIIb/IIIa blockade.

TRIALS OF GPIIb/IIIa ANTAGONISTS AS MEDICAL THERAPY FOR UNSTABLE ANGINA

Eptifibatide

PURSUIT

The PURSUIT Trial was a randomized, double-blind, placebo-controlled trial in 10,948 patients with unstable angina or non–Q wave MI treating patients with eptifibatide or placebo for 72 to 96 hours. The initial part of the study was a dose-selection trial. Two dose groups were studied, each treated with a bolus of 180 μg/kg of eptifibatide. The low-dose-infusion group received 1.3 μg/kg per minute of eptifibatide, and the high-dose infusion group received 2.0 μg/kg per minute. All patients received aspirin, and heparin was optional. The low-dose eptifibatide treatment group was discontinued early when the higher-dose eptifibatide group was judged to be safe at an interim analysis. The final analysis compared 4722 eptifibatide patients randomized to the high-dose infusion and 4739 placebo patients. The incidence of the primary endpoint of death or MI through 30 days was reduced by 9% from 15.7% in the placebo group to 14.2% in the eptifibatide group (1.5% absolute reduction; $P = 0.042$).[78a] Moderate or severe bleeding, other than CABS-related bleeding, was observed in 2.0% of placebo patients compared with 5.2% of eptifibatide patients.[78b]

Tirofiban

PRISM PLUS

PRISM Plus was a phase III randomized, double-blind, placebo-controlled trial in the setting of unstable angina or non–Q wave MI.[79a] Unstable angina or non–Q wave MI was defined as one of the following: (1) accelerating pattern of angina, (2) prolonged (>20 minutes) chest pain, or (3) postinfarction angina. In the PRISM Plus study, 773 patients received tirofiban (bolus of 0.4 μg/kg bolus over 30 minutes and infusion of 10 μg/kg per minute) plus heparin (5000 U bolus, 1000 U per hour infusion), compared with 797 patients who received the same heparin regimen but not tirofiban. A third arm of the study, in which no concomitant heparin was given, was discontinued after it had enrolled 345 patients on the recommenda-

TABLE 15–1 • Event Rate—48-Hour and 30-Day—of the Composite Endpoint for EPIC, IMPACT II, RESTORE, CAPTURE, and EPILOG Trials

Trial	Treatment Group	48-Hour Event Rate (%)*	*P* Value vs. Placebo	30-Day Event Rate (%)	*P* Value vs. Placebo
EPIC	Placebo	9.8		12.8	
	Abciximab bolus	9.1	0.66	11.5	0.43
	Abciximab bolus + infusion	6.6	0.039	8.3	0.008
IMPACT II	Placebo	10.2		11.4	
	Low-dose Eptifibatide	7.6	0.021	9.2	0.06
	High-dose Eptifibatide	7.9	0.045	9.9	0.22
RESTORE	Placebo	8.7		12.2	
	Tirofiban	5.4	0.005	10.3	0.16
CAPTURE	Placebo	13.4		15.9	
	Abciximab	8.2	0.005	11.3	0.012
EPILOG	Placebo	9.2		11.7	
	Abciximab + low-dose heparin	4.0	<0.001	5.2	<0.001
	Abciximab + standard-dose heparin	4.7	<0.001	5.4	<0.001
EPISTENT	Placebo + stent	10.1		10.8	
	Abciximab + stent	4.9	<0.001	5.3	<0.001
	Abciximab + balloon	6.3	0.005	6.9	0.007

*48-hour analysis includes only patients treated with study agent for the IMPACT II Trial.

tion of the study's Data Safety Monitoring Board as a result of an unacceptably high incidence of death and MI.

Coronary angiography was recommended in the PRISM Plus trial, with PCI to be performed if indicated. An important distinction from the CAPTURE Trial was that catheterization was performed after therapy was initiated rather than before qualification. Medical therapy was given for 48 to 96 hours, including 12 hours after any PCI. Of the total patients enrolled in the two arms that were completed, 30.5% went on to PCI, 23.4% went on to CABS, and 46.1% were continued on medical therapy only. The overall average duration of therapy was 72 hours.

The primary endpoint of the trial was the occurrence of death, MI, or refractory ischemia within 7 days after enrollment. The primary endpoint event rate was reduced by 28% from 17.9% in the standard therapy group to 12.9% in the tirofiban plus heparin group ($P = 0.004$). This reduction was maintained at 30 days (22.3% event rate in the standard therapy group compared with 18.5% in the tirofiban plus heparin group, a 17% relative reduction and a 3.8% absolute reduction; $P = 0.039$). Mortality at 30 days was 4.5% in the standard therapy group compared with 3.6% in the tirofiban plus heparin group ($P = 0.35$). MI through 30 days occurred in 9.2% of patients in the standard therapy group compared with 6.6% in the tirofiban plus heparin group (28% relative reduction and 2.6% absolute reduction; $P = 0.057$). Major bleeding occurred in 1.2% of patients in the standard therapy group compared with 1.8% in the tirofiban group ($P = 0.42$).

PRISM

The PRISM Trial was a phase III, 3231-patient, two-arm, randomized, double-blind, placebo-controlled trial of medical therapy for patients with unstable angina.[79a] To qualify, patients had to have either accelerated symptoms with electrocardiogram changes or chest pain at rest within 24 hours before study entry. Patients in the tirofiban arm received a 0.6 μg/kg bolus over 30 minutes plus a 0.15 μg/kg per minute infusion, along with a placebo heparin infusion. Patients in the control arm received a placebo bolus and infusion comparable to the tirofiban treatment in the experimental arm, plus a 5000 U heparin bolus followed by a 1000 U per hour heparin infusion. The primary endpoint was a composite of death, MI, and refractory ischemia (pain with electrocardiogram changes on optimal medical therapy or hemodynamic instability related to ischemia) at the end of the infusion at 48 hours. The primary endpoint event rate was reduced by 28%, from 5.3% in the heparin group to 3.8% in the tirofiban group (absolute reduction 1.5%; $P = 0.007$). Each of the components of the primary endpoint was reduced in the tirofiban group compared with the heparin group at 48 hours (death 0.6% vs. 0.4%, P = NS; MI 1.3% vs. 0.9%, P = NS; refractory ischemia 5.3% vs. 3.6%; $P = 0.01$). Although the rate of MI was nearly identical at 30 days (4.2% in the heparin group vs. 4.0% in the tirofiban group; P = NS), there was a suggestion of reduced mortality at 30 days (3.6% in the heparin group vs. 2.3% in the tirofiban group; $P = 0.02$). Major bleeding occurred in 0.1% of patients in the heparin group compared with 0.2% in the tirofiban group (P = NS).

Severe thrombocytopenia occurred in 0.4% of patients in the heparin group compared with 1.2% in the tirofiban group.

The dosing of tirofiban and heparin differs in the arms of PRISM (higher-dose tirofiban, no heparin) and PRISM Plus (lower-dose tirofiban plus heparin) that provided positive efficacy results. The apparent inconsistency in results between the PRISM Plus and PRISM studies with regard to the relative efficacy of tirofiban alone versus heparin alone for the treatment of unstable angina remains to be resolved.

Lamifiban

Théroux and colleagues[55] performed a randomized, double-blind, dose-ranging study of medical therapy with lamifiban in 365 patients with unstable angina. Infusions of placebo or 1, 2, 4, or 5 μg per minute of lamifiban for 72 to 120 hours were studied. All patients received aspirin, and 28% received heparin. The rate of death or MI through 30 days in the two highest dose groups was 2.5% compared with 8.1% in the placebo group (P = 0.03). The composite endpoint of death, MI, or need for urgent revascularization during the infusion period was reduced from 8.1% in the placebo group to 3.3% (P = 0.04) in the combined lamifiban groups (2.5%, 4.9%, 3.3%, and 2.4% in the 1, 2, 4, and 5 μg per minute groups, respectively).

PARAGON

PARAGON enrolled 2282 patients with unstable angina or non–Q wave MI. The study tested medical therapy using a factorial design randomizing patients to heparin or no heparin and to one of two doses of lamifiban (1 or 5 μg per minute). A control arm in which patients received heparin and no lamifiban was also included. All patients received aspirin. Preliminary results from the PARAGON Trial have been presented by the PARAGON investigators.[80] No reduction in the primary endpoint of death or MI through 30 days was found using lamifiban therapy.

TRIALS OF GPIIb/IIIa ANTAGONISTS AS MEDICAL THERAPY FOR MYOCARDIAL INFARCTION

Randomized studies of GPIIb/IIIa antagonists as either adjuncts to or replacement for thrombolytic therapy have been conducted or are being conducted with lamifiban, eptifibatide, and abciximab. The PARADIGM Trial studied the addition of lamifiban to a thrombolytic agent (tissue-type plasminogen activator or streptokinase) to test the hypothesis that lamifiban would improve reperfusion results.[81] A total of 150 patients were randomized in a 2:1 ratio to receive lamifiban (400 μg bolus and 1.5 μg per minute infusion for 24 hours) or placebo. Time to steady-state reperfusion was reduced from 167 minutes in the placebo group to 87 minutes in the lamifiban group (P = 0.002). More patients achieved steady-state reperfusion within 2 hours in the lamifiban group (69%) than in the placebo group (33%; P = 0.001). No strokes were observed, and major bleeding rates were 4% in the lamifiban group compared with 2% in the placebo group. An additional 220 patients will be studied in this trial.

IMPACT AMI was a randomized, placebo-controlled trial that sought to find an adjunctive dose of eptifibatide that would increase the vessel patency (TIMI 3 flow 90 minutes after start of reperfusion therapy) achieved with standard accelerated alteplase therapy.[82] A total of 180 patients were enrolled (125 in six eptifibatide plus alteplase groups and 55 patients randomized to alteplase without eptifibatide). Some suggestion of a higher rate of TIMI 3 flow at 90 minutes was seen with the highest eptifibatide dose (66% TIMI 3 flow with a 180 μg/kg bolus plus 0.75 μg/kg per minute infusion for 24 hours) compared with alteplase alone (39%), but the controls were not all randomized simultaneously with the eptifibatide patients. A suggestion of earlier reperfusion (recovery of ST segment deviation) was observed in the high-dose eptifibatide group (median of 65 minutes) compared with patients receiving alteplase alone (116 minutes). The prespecified composite clinical endpoint of death, reinfarction, stroke, revascularization, heart failure, or pulmonary edema did not differ between treatment groups. One of 51 patients randomized to the highest eptifibatide dose was the only patient in the trial to experience an intracranial hemorrhage.

Eptifibatide has also been studied with streptokinase in 181 myocardial infarction patients.[82a] A standard 1.5 million U dose of streptokinase was studied with placebo and three doses of eptifibatide. Each of the eptifibatide groups used a 180 μg/kg bolus. The infusion levels were 0.75, 1.33, and 2.0 μg/kg per minute. Results from 171 patients showed a TIMI 3 flow of 38% in the streptokinase alone group. This compared with 53% in the 0.75 μg/kg group, 44% in the 1.33 μg/kg group, and 52% in the 2.0 μg/kg group. The highest-dose eptifibatide arm was discontinued because of excess bleeding complications. Moderate to severe bleeding was observed in 3% of the streptokinase alone group, 16% in the 0.75 μg/kg group, 40% in the 1.33 μg/kg group, and 40% in the 2.0 μg/kg group.

In April 1998, the TIMI 14 Trial was randomizing patients with MIs associated with ST segment elevations presenting within 12 hours of symptom onset to one of four treatment reperfusion strategies: (1) standard front-loaded alteplase, (2) low-dose alteplase plus abciximab (0.25 mg bolus plus 0.125 μg/kg per minute to a maximum of 10 μg per minute), (3) low-dose streptokinase plus abciximab, and (4) abciximab with no thrombolytic agent. The rationale for including abciximab therapy without a thrombolytic agent comes from animal studies and a nonrandomized trial by Gold and coworkers[83] wherein 7 of 13 patients treated with abciximab, heparin, and aspirin achieved TIMI 2 or 3 flow within 10 minutes. The primary endpoint for TIMI 14 is TIMI 3 flow at 90 minutes after the initiation of therapy. The trial may test several different doses of both alteplase and streptokinase in combination with standard-dose abciximab in an attempt to find a regimen that produces a high rate of TIMI 3 flow at 90 minutes with acceptable toxicity.

Preliminary results on the first 681 patients enrolled[83a] suggest that a 1-hour treatment of reduced-dose (15 mg bolus plus 35 to 50 mg infusion over 1 hour) alteplase with abciximab (0.25 mg/kg bolus plus 0.125 μg/kg per hour infusion to a maximum of 10 μg per minute) yields TIMI 3 flow in 73% of patients compared with 58% with standard, front-loaded alteplase without abciximab. TIMI 3 flow was achieved in 32% of patients with abciximab alone, comparable to historical rates for streptokinase from TIMI 1[83b] and GUSTO 1.[83c] There was no apparent dose-response in TIMI 3 flow with abciximab plus increasing doses of streptokinase ranging from 500,000 to 1.5 million U (36% to 49% TIMI 3 flow in groups with 35 or more patients); there was unacceptably high bleeding risk at higher doses of streptokinase, however.

The Strategies for Patency Enhancement in the Emergency Department (SPEED) Trial is an angiographic study of therapy with abciximab alone or abciximab with reduced doses of reteplase in patients with myocardial infarction. A 60-minute angiographic endpoint is being studied. Enrollment is under way, and doses of up to 10 U of reteplase have been studied as of this writing (April 1998).

CONCLUSIONS

The EPIC and EPILOG Trials demonstrated that GPIIb/IIIa receptor blockade with abciximab is effective in the prevention of ischemic complications of PCI for patients judged to be either at low or high risk of suffering such complications based on conventional criteria. Although no other GPIIb/IIIa blocking agent has achieved statistically significant reductions in the primary endpoints in phase III trials of PCI, short-term benefits were suggested with eptifibatide and tirofiban. The PRISM, PRISM Plus, and PURSUIT Trials suggest the usefulness of GPIIb/IIIa receptor blockade with tirofiban as medical therapy for unstable angina. Food and Drug Administration review for regulatory approval of eptifibatide and tirofiban in this indication is expected to be finished in 1998. The CAPTURE Trial also showed the utility of GPIIb/IIIa blockade with abciximab as medical therapy among unstable angina patients who were candidates for PCI. Phase II trials in MI with abciximab, eptifibatide, and lamifiban have suggested potential benefit using GPIIb/IIIa blockade as an adjunct to thrombolysis. TIMI 14 is currently investigating the use of abciximab with or without reduced doses of a thrombolytic agent in the setting of acute MI.

Although it is possible that all GPIIb/IIIa antagonists will be equally effective with optimal dosing, differences in the pharmacokinetics and pharmacodynamics of these agents may explain the apparent differences in effectiveness observed to date in the large PCI trials. For example, because abciximab has a slower off-rate from platelets than the other agents, a relatively low infusion rate is adequate to maintain high-grade receptor blockade. The platelet off-rates for small molecules are higher, and thus higher infusion rates are required to maintain high-grade receptor blockade; as a result, variations in plasma clearance of these agents from patient to patient may result in considerable interindividual variation in the extent of GPIIb/IIIa blockade. As a possible reflection of this concern PARAGON B, a placebo-controlled Phase III study in unstable angina beginning in 1998, will adjust lamifiban dosage by creatinine clearance. In addition, the antiplatelet effect of abciximab lasts longer after discontinuing the infusion than does the effect of the small molecules. The extent of GPIIb/IIIa blockade by abciximab may be more affected by severe thrombocytosis because the ratio of abciximab to GPIIb/IIIa receptors is less than with the low-molecular-weight molecules.

The relatively short time to reversal of GPIIb/IIIa blockade after discontinuation of small molecule inhibitors compared with abciximab was believed by some to be a possible safety advantage. For instance, this may be of some value in patients who require urgent CABS. Animal models, however, demonstrate that much of the platelet function inhibition produced by abciximab can be reversed immediately by platelet transfusion.[84] The ability to reverse the effects of the small molecule inhibitors by platelet transfusion is less clear, especially if renal or hepatic insufficiency prolongs the drug's intravascular survival.[85] The slow tapering of GPIIb/IIIa blockade after discontinuation of abciximab therapy may provide a partial explanation for the better 30-day results with abciximab in the EPIC, CAPTURE, EPILOG, and EPISTENT studies than with small molecules in the IMPACT II and RESTORE Trials. The results of EPILOG, EPISTENT,

IMPACT II, and RESTORE indicate a low rate of bleeding events relative to placebo with all three agents. Finally, it remains possible, but unproved, that the longer-term benefit with abciximab may arise because of blockade of the $\alpha_v\beta_3$ vitronectin receptor in addition to the GPIIb/IIIa receptor.

The CAPTURE Trial proved the short-term effectiveness of GPIIb/IIIa blockade with abciximab as medical therapy in patients with unstable angina who are candidates for PCI, and the PRISM and PRISM Plus Trials provide support for the use of GPIIb/IIIa receptor blockade with tirofiban as medical therapy in a broader group of patients with unstable angina. Phase II trials in MI with abciximab, eptifibatide, and lamifiban have suggested potential benefit of GPIIb/IIIa blockade as an adjunct to thrombolysis. Ongoing trials in patients with MI and unstable angina will further clarify the role of GPIIb/IIIa blockade in these disorders.

Taken together, the randomized trials of GPIIb/IIIa antagonists for PCI, unstable angina, and MI support a powerful therapeutic role for these agents. Thus, there appears to be considerable reason to be optimistic that after further studies refine their optimal use, GPIIb/IIIa antagonists will have a major impact on the management of patients with ischemic thrombotic cardiovascular disease.

REFERENCES

1. Murray CJL, Lopez AD. Alternative projections of mortality and disability by cause 1990–2020: Global Burden of Disease Study. Lancet 1997; 349:1498–1504.
2. Davies MJ. Pathology of arterial thrombosis. Br Med Bull 1994; 50:789–802.
3. Thompson SG, Kienast J, Pyke SD, et al. Hemostatic factors and the risk of myocardial infarction or sudden death in patients with angina pectoris. N Engl J Med 1995; 332:635–641.
4. Weiss HJ, Turitto VT, Baumgartner HR. The role of shear rate and platelets in promoting fibrin formation on rabbit subendothelium: Studies utilizing patients with quantitative and qualitative platelet defects. J Clin Invest 1986; 78:1072–1082.
5. Fernandez Ortiz A, Badimon JJ, Falk E, et al. Characterization of the relative thrombogenicity of atherosclerotic plaque components: Implications for consequences of plaque rupture. J Am Coll Cardiol 1994; 23:1562–1569.
6. Coller BS. Platelets in cardiovascular thrombosis and thrombolysis. *In* Fozzard HA, Jennings RB, Katz AM, et al (eds). The Heart and Cardiovascular System. New York, Raven Press, 1992, pp 219–273.
7. Coller BS. Platelets and thrombolytic therapy. N Engl J Med 1990; 322:33–42.
8. van Zanten GH, de Graaf S, Slootweg PJ, et al. Increased platelet deposition on atherosclerotic coronary arteries. J Clin Invest 1994; 93:615–632.
9. Ware AJ, Coller BS. Platelet morphology, biochemistry and function. *In* Beutler E, Lichtman MA, Coller BS, et al (eds). Williams Hematology. New York, McGraw-Hill, 1995, pp 1161–1201.
10. Coller BS, Kutok JL, Scudder LE, et al. Studies of activated GPIIb/IIIa receptors on the luminal surface of adherent platelets: Paradoxical loss of luminal receptors when platelets adhere to high density fibrinogen. J Clin Invest 1993; 92:2796–2806.
11. Willerson JT, Eidt JF, McNatt J, et al. Role of thromboxane and serotonin as mediators in the development of spontaneous alterations in coronary blood flow and neointimal proliferation in canine models with chronic coronary artery stenoses and endothelial injury. J Am Coll Cardiol 1991; 17:101B–110B.
12. Walsh PN, Schmaier AH. Platelet-coagulant protein interactions. *In* Colman RW, Hirsh J, Marder VJ, et al (eds). Hemostasis and Thrombosis: Basic Principles and Clinical Practice. Philadelphia, JB Lippincott, 1993, pp 629–651.
13. Phillips DR, Charo IF, Parise LV, et al. The platelet membrane glycoprotein IIb-IIIa complex. Blood 1988; 71:831–843.
14. Hynes RO. Integrins: Versatility, modulation and signalling in cell adhesion. Cell 1994; 69:11–25.
15. Pytela R, Pierschbacher MD, Ginsberg MH, et al. Platelet membrane glycoprotein IIb/IIIa: Member of a family of Arg-Gly-Asp-specific adhesion receptors. Science 1986; 231:1559–1562.
16. Cook NS, Kottirsch G, Zerwes H. Platelet glycoprotein IIb/IIIa antagonists. Drugs of Future 1994; 19:135–159.
17. Cox D, Aoki T, Seki J, et al. The pharmacology of integrins. Med Res Rev 1994; 14:195–228.
18. Felding-Habermann B, Cheresh DA. Vitronectin and its receptors. Curr Opin Cell Biol 1993; 5:864–868.
19. George JN, Caen JP, Nurden AT. Glanzmann's thrombasthenia: The spectrum of clinical disease. Blood 1990; 75:1383–1395.
20. Coller BS. Hereditary qualitative platelet disorders. *In* Beutler E, Lichtman MA, Coller BS, et al (eds). Williams Hematology. New York, McGraw-Hill, 1995, pp 1364–1385.
21. Knight DM, Wagner C, Jordan R, et al. The immunogenicity of the 7E3 murine monoclonal Fab antibody fragment variable region is dramatically reduced in humans by substitution of human for murine constant regions. Mol Immunol 1995; 32:1271–1281.
22. Jordan RE, Wagner CL, Mascelli M, et al. Preclinical development of c7E3 Fab; a mouse/human chimeric monoclonal antibody fragment that inhibits platelet function by blockade of GPIIb/IIIa receptors with observations on the immunogenicity of c7E3 Fab in humans. *In* Horton MA (ed). Adhesion Receptors as Therapeutic Targets. Boca Raton, CRC Press, 1996, pp 281–305.
23. Coller BS. A new murine monoclonal antibody reports an activation-dependent change in the conformation and/or microenvironment of the platelet GPIIb/IIIa complex. J Clin Invest 1985; 76:101–108.
24. Coller BS, Scudder LE, Beer J, et al. Monoclonal antibodies to platelet GPIIb/IIIa as antithrombotic agents. Ann N Y Acad Sci 1991; 614:193–213.
25. Coller BS. Inhibitors of the platelet glycoprotein IIb/IIIa receptor as conjunctive therapy for coronary artery thrombolysis. Coron Artery Dis 1992; 3:1016–1029.
26. Kohmura C, Gold HK, Yasuda T, et al. A chimeric murine/human antibody Fab fragment directed against the platelet GPIIb/IIIa receptor enhances and sustains arterial thrombolysis with recombinant tissue-type plasminogen activator in baboons. Arterioscler Thromb 1993; 13:1837–1842.
27. Reverter JC, Beguin S, Kessels H, et al. Inhibition of platelet-mediated, tissue factor-induced, thrombin generation by the mouse/human chimeric 7E3 antibody: Potential implications for the effect of c7E3 Fab treatment on acute thrombosis and "clinical restenosis." J Clin Invest 1996; 98:863–874.
28. Fay WP, Eitzman DT, Shapiro AD, et al. Platelets inhibit fibrinolysis in vitro by both plasminogen activator inhibitor-1 dependent and independent mechanisms. Blood 1994; 83:351–356.
29. Coller BS. Augmentation of thrombolysis with antiplatelet drugs: Overview. Coron Artery Dis 1995; 6:911–914.
30. Cox AD, Devine DV. Factor XIIIa binding to activated platelets is mediated through activation of glycoprotein IIb-IIIa. Blood 1994; 83:1006–1016.
31. Cohen I, Burk DL, White JG. The effect of peptides and monoclonal antibodies that bind to platelet glycoprotein IIb-IIIa complex on the development of clot tension. Blood 1989; 73:1880–1887.
32. Carr ME Jr, Carr SL, Hantgan RR, et al. Glycoprotein IIb/IIIa blockade inhibits platelet-mediated force development and reduces gel elastic modulus. Thromb Haemost 1995; 73:499–505.
33. Coller BS, Cheresh DA, Asch E, et al. Platelet vitronectin recep-

tor expression differentiates Iraqi-Jewish from Arab patients with Glanzmann thrombasthenia in Israel. Blood 1991; 77:75–83.

34. Tcheng JE, Ellis SG, George BS, et al. Pharmacodynamics of chimeric glycoprotein IIb/IIIa integrin antiplatelet antibody Fab 7E3 in high-risk coronary angioplasty. Circulation 1994; 90:1757–1764.
35. Abciximab (ReoPro) package insert. Centocor/Lilly, Malvern, PA, 1995.
36. EPIC Investigators. Use of a monoclonal antibody directed against the platelet glycoprotein IIb/IIIa receptor in high-risk coronary angioplasty. N Engl J Med 1994; 330:956–961.
37. Kereiakes DJ, Essell JH, Abbottsmith CW, et al. Abciximab-associated profound thrombocytopenia: Therapy with immunoglobulin and platelet transfusion. Am J Cardiol 1996; 78:1161–1166.
38. Berkowitz SD, Harrington RA, Rund MM, et al. Acute profound thrombocytopenia following c7E3 Fab (abciximab) therapy. Circulation 1997; 95:809–813.
39. Hartman GD, Egbertson MS, Halczenko W, et al. Non-peptide fibrinogen receptor antagonists: 1. Discovery and design of exosite inhibitors. J Med Chem 1992; 35:4640–4642.
40. Egbertson MS, Chang CT, Duggan ME, et al. Non-peptide fibrinogen receptor antagonists: 2. Optimization of a tyrosine template as a mimic for Arg-Gly-Asp. J Med Chem 1994; 37:2537–2551.
41. Lynch JJ Jr, Cook JJ, Sitko GR, et al. Nonpeptide glycoprotein IIb/IIIa inhibitors: 5. Antithrombotic effects of MK-0383. J Pharmacol Exp Ther 1995; 272:20–32.
42. Barrett JS, Murphy G, Peerlinck K, et al. Pharmacokinetics and pharmacodynamics of MK-383, a selective non-peptide platelet glycoprotein-IIb/IIIa receptor antagonist, in healthy men. Clin Pharmacol Ther 1994; 56:377–388.
43. Peerlinck K, De Lepeleire I, Goldberg M, et al. MK-383 (L-700,462), a selective nonpeptide platelet glycoprotein IIb/IIIa antagonist, is active in man. Circulation 1993; 88:1512–1517.
44. Kereiakes DJ, Kleiman NS, Ambrose J, et al. Randomized, double-blind, placebo-controlled dose-ranging study of tirofiban (MK-383) platelet IIb/IIIa blockade in high risk patients undergoing coronary angioplasty. J Am Coll Cardiol 1996; 27:536–542.
45. Bednar B, Bednar RA, Cook JJ, et al. Drug-dependent antibodies against GPIIb/IIIa induce thrombocytopenia. Circulation 1996; 94:I-99.
46. Uthoff K, Zehr KJ, Geerling R, et al. Inhibition of platelet adhesion during cardiopulmonary bypass reduces postoperative bleeding. Circulation 1994; 90:II269–II274.
47. Scarborough RM, Naughton MA, Teng W, et al. Design of potent and specific integrin antagonists: Peptide antagonists with high specificity for glycoprotein IIb-IIIa. J Biol Chem 1993; 268:1066–1073.
47a. Phillips DR, Teng W, Arfsten A, et al. Effect of Ca^{2+} on GP IIb-IIIa interactions with integrilin: Enhanced GP IIb-IIIa binding and inhibition of platelet aggregation by reductions in the concentration of ionized calcium in plasma anticoagulated with citrate. Circulation 1997; 96:1488–1494.
48. Tcheng JE, Harrington RA, Kottke Marchant K, et al. Multicenter, randomized, double-blind, placebo-controlled trial of the platelet integrin glycoprotein IIb/IIIa blocker Integrelin in elective coronary intervention. Circulation 1995; 91:2151–2157.
49. Harrington RA, Kleiman NS, Kottke Marchant K, et al. Immediate and reversible platelet inhibition after intravenous administration of a peptide glycoprotein IIb/IIIa inhibitor during percutaneous coronary intervention. Am J Cardiol 1995; 76:1222–1227.
49a. McClure M, Kleiman NS, Berdan LG, et al. Thrombocytopenia in a large, international trial of the GP IIb/IIIa inhibitor eptifibatide in patients with acute coronary syndromes [Abstract]. J Am Coll Cardiol 1998; 31:93A.
50. Alig L, Edenhofer A, Hadvary P, et al. Low molecular weight, non-peptide fibrinogen receptor antagonists. J Med Chem 1992; 35:4393–4407.
51. Carteaux JP, Steiner B, Roux S. Ro 44-9883, a new non-peptidic GPIIb/GPIIIa antagonist prevents platelet loss in a guinea pig model of extracorporeal circulation. Thromb Haemost 1993; 70:817–821.
52. Carroll RC, Steiner B, Kouns WC. The effects of Ro 43-5054 and Ro 44-9883, peptidomimetic inhibitors of the GPIIb-IIIa fibrinogen binding site on platelet stimulus-response coupling [Abstract]. Thromb Haemost 1993; 69:785.
53. Steiner B, Haring P, Jennings L, et al. Five independent neo-epitopes on GPIIb-IIIa are differentially exposed by two potent peptidomimetic platelet inhibitors [Abstract]. Thromb Haemost 1993; 69:782.
54. Jones CR, Ambros RJ, Rapold HJ, et al. A novel non peptide GPIIb/IIIa antagonist in man [Abstract]. Thromb Haemost 1993; 69:560.
55. Théroux P, Kouz S, Roy L, et al. Platelet membrane receptor GPIIb/IIIa antagonism in unstable angina: The Canadian lamifiban study. Circulation 1996; 94:899–905.
56. Kong TQ, Davidson CJ, Meyers SN, et al. Prognostic implication of creatine kinase elevation following elective coronary artery interventions. JAMA 1997; 277:461–466.
57. Ohman EM, Tardiff BE. Periprocedural cardiac marker elevation after percutaneous coronary artery revascularization: Importance and implications. JAMA 1997; 277:495–497.
58. Ellis SG, Tcheng JE, Navetta FI, et al. Safety and antiplatelet effect of murine monoclonal antibody 7E3 Fab directed against platelet glycoprotein IIb/IIIa in patients undergoing elective coronary angioplasty. Coron Artery Dis 1993; 4:167–175.
59. Topol EJ, Califf RM, Weismann HF, et al. Randomized trial of coronary intervention with antibody against platelet IIb/IIIa integrin for reduction of clinical restenosis: Results at six months. Lancet 1994; 343:881–886.
60. Ryan TJ, Faxon DP, Gunnar RM, et al. Guidelines for percutaneous transluminal coronary angioplasty: A report of the American College of Cardiology/American Heart Association Task Force on Assessment of Diagnostic and Therapeutic Cardiovascular Procedures (Subcommittee on Percutaneous Transluminal Coronary Angioplasty). Circulation 1988; 78:486–502.
61. Topol EJ, Ferguson JJ, Weisman HF, et al. Long-term protection from myocardial ischemic events in a randomized trial of brief integrin β3 blockade with percutaneous coronary intervention. JAMA 1997; 278:479–484.
62. Aguirre FV, Topol EJ, Ferguson JJ, et al. Bleeding complications with the chimeric antibody to platelet glycoprotein IIb/IIIa integrin in patients undergoing percutaneous coronary intervention. Circulation 1995; 91:2882–2890.
63. Salzman EW, Rosenberg RD, Smith MH, et al. Effect of heparin and heparin fractions on platelet aggregation. J Clin Invest 1980; 65:64–73.
64. Lincoff AM, Tcheng JE, Califf RM, et al. Standard versus low dose weight-adjusted heparin in patients treated with the platelet GPIIb/IIIa receptor antibody fragment abciximab (c7E3 Fab) during percutaneous coronary revascularization. Am J Cardiol 1997; 79:286–291.
65. EPILOG Investigators. Platelet glycoprotein IIb/IIIa receptor blockade and low-dose heparin during percutaneous coronary revascularization. N Engl J Med 1997; 336:1689–1696.
66. Aguirre F. Post-procedural patient management: Prevention and management of bleeding complications. J Invas Cardiol 1994; 6:34a–37a.
67. Brezina K, Murphy M, Stonner T. Care of the patient receiving ReoPro following angioplasty. J Invas Cardiol 1994; 6:38a–42a.
68. Lincoff AM, Tcheng JE, Miller DP, et al. Marked enhancement of clinical efficacy of platelet GPIIb/IIIa blockade with c7E3 Fab (abciximab) linked to reduction in bleeding complication: Outcome in the EPILOG and EPIC trials [Abstract]. Circulation 1996; 94:I-375.
69. Aguirre FA, Talley DJ, Ferguson JJ III, et al. Efficacy of abciximab, despite patient weight, using lower heparin dosing during percutaneous coronary intervention [Abstract]. Circulation 1996; 94:I-198.
70. Ghaffari S, Kereiakes DJ, Kelly T, et al. Platelet GPIIb/IIIa receptor blockade reduces ischemic complications in patients undergoing directional coronary atherectomy [Abstract]. Circulation 1996; 94:I-98.
71. Ward SR, Lincoff AM, Miller DP, et al. Clinical outcome is improved at 30 days regardless of pre-treatment clinical and angiographic risk in patients receiving abciximab for angioplasty: Results from the EPILOG study [Abstract]. Circulation 1996; 94:I-198.
71a. Brener SJ, Barr LA, Burchenal JEB, et al. A randomized, pla-

cebo-controlled trial of platelet glycoprotein IIb/IIIa blockade with primary angioplasty for acute myocardial infarction. Submitted for publication.

71b. Topol EJ, for the EPISTENT Investigators. Primary results from the EPISTENT Trial. Presented at the American College of Cardiology Scientific Sessions, Atlanta, GA, March 31, 1998.

72. CAPTURE Investigators. Randomised placebo-controlled trial of abciximab before and during coronary intervention in refractory unstable angina: The CAPTURE study. Lancet 1997; 349:1429–1435.

73. Rao AK, Pratt C, Berke A, et al. Thrombolysis in myocardial infarction (TIMI) trial—Phase I: Hemorrhagic manifestations and changes in plasma fibrinogen and the fibrinolytic system in patients treated with recombinant tissue plasminogen activator and streptokinase. J Am Coll Cardiol 1988; 11:1–11.

74. IMPACT-II Investigators. Randomised placebo-controlled trial of effect of eptifibatide on complications of percutaneous coronary intervention: IMPACT-II. Lancet 1997; 349:1422–1428.

75. The RESTORE Investigators. Effects of platelet glycoprotein IIb/IIIa blockade with tirofiban on adverse cardiac events in patients with unstable angina or acute myocardial infarction undergoing coronary angioplasty. Circulation 1997; 96:1445–1453.

76. Lincoff AM, Califf RM, Anderson KM, et al. Evidence for prevention of death and myocardial infarction with platelet membrane glycoprotein IIb/IIIa receptor blockade by abciximab (c7E3 Fab) among patients with unstable angina undergoing percutaneous coronary revascularization. J Am Coll Cardiol 1997; 30:149–156.

77. Lefkovits J, Ivanhoe RJ, Califf RM, et al. Effects of platelet glycoprotein IIb/IIIa receptor blockade by a chimeric monoclonal antibody (abciximab) on acute and six-month outcomes after percutaneous transluminal coronary angioplasty for acute myocardial infarction: EPIC investigators. Am J Cardiol 1996; 77:1045–1051.

78. Lefkovits J, Blankenship JC, Anderson KM, et al. Increased risk of non-Q wave myocardial infarction after directional atherectomy is platelet dependent: Evidence from the EPIC trial: Evaluation of c7E3 for the Prevention of Ischemic Complications. J Am Coll Cardiol 1996; 28:849–855.

78a. Simoons ML, for the PURSUIT Investigators. Platelet IIb/IIIa in Unstable Angina: Receptor Suppression Using Integrilin Trial (PURSUIT). Presented at the European Meeting of Cardiology, Stockholm, August 25, 1997.

78b. Lincoff AM, Harrington RA, Califf RM, et al. Clinical efficacy of integrilin in unstable angina is accompanied by a modest increase in hemorrhagic risk: The PURSUIT Trial [Abstract]. J Am Coll Cardiol 1998; 31:185A.

79. Zidar JP, Kruse KR, Thel MC, et al. Integrelin for emergency coronary artery stenting [Abstract]. J Am Coll Cardiol 1996; 27:138A.

79a. Ferguson JJ. Meeting Highlights. 46th Annual Scientific Sessions of the American College of Cardiology. Circulation 1997; 96:367–371.

80. PARAGON Investigators. A randomized trial of potent platelet IIb/IIIa antagonism, heparin, or both in patients with unstable angina: The PARAGON Study [Abstract]. Circulation 1996; 94:I-553.

81. Moliterno DJ, Harrington RA, Krucoof MW, et al. More complete and stable reperfusion with platelet IIb/IIIa antagonism plus thrombolysis for AMI: The PARADIGM Trial [Abstract]. Circulation 1996; 94:I-553.

82. Ohman EM, Kleiman NS, Gacioch G, et al. Combined accelerated tissue-plasminogen activator and platelet glycoprotein IIb/IIIa integrin receptor blockade with Integrelin in acute myocardial infarction: Results of a randomized, placebo-controlled, dose-ranging trial. Circulation 1997; 95:846–854.

82a. Ronner E, van Kesteren HAM, Zijnen P, et al. Combined therapy with streptokinase and integrilin [Abstract]. J Am Coll Cardiol 1998; 31:191A.

83. Gold HK, Garabedian HD, Dinsmore RL, et al. Restoration of coronary flow in myocardial infarction by intravenous chimeric 7E3 antibody without exogenous plasminogen activators: Observations in animals and man. Circulation 1997; 95:1755–1759.

83a. Antman EM, Giugliano RP, McCabe CH, et al. Abciximab (ReoPro) potentiates thrombolysis in ST elevation myocardial infarction: Results of the TIMI 14 Trial [Abstract]. J Am Coll Cardiol 1998; 31:191A.

83b. The TIMI Study Group. Special Report: The Thrombolysis in Myocardial Infarction (TIMI) Trial. Phase I Findings. N Engl J Med 1985; 312:932–936.

83c. The GUSTO Angiographic Investigators. The effects of tissue plasminogen activator, streptokinase, or both on coronary artery patency, ventricular function, and survival after acute myocardial infarction. N Engl J Med 1993; 329:1615–1622.

84. Wagner CL, Cunningham MR, Wyand MS, et al. Reversal of the anti-platelet effects of chimeric 7E3 Fab treatment by platelet transfusion in cynomolgus monkeys [Abstract]. Thromb Haemost 1995; 73:1313.

85. Simpfendorfer C, Kottke-Marchant K, Lowrie M, et al. First chronic platelet glycoprotein IIb/IIIa integrin blockade: A randomized placebo-controlled pilot study of xemilofiban in unstable angina with percutaneous coronary interventions. Circulation 1997; 96:76–81.

16 Primary Angioplasty, Rescue Angioplasty, and New Devices

▶ C. Michael Gibson

HISTORICAL PERSPECTIVE

The open artery hypothesis and likewise the strategies used to open acutely occluded vessels have evolved over the past two decades. Initial efforts to restore antegrade flow to occluded vessels began with the administration of intracoronary thrombolytic agents in the late 1970s and the early 1980s.[1–3] These recanalization trials and the intracoronary route of thrombolytic administration were logistically demanding, and they were soon replaced by trials involving the simpler, more rapid intravenous route of thrombolytic administration in 90-minute patency trials in the mid-1980s.[4, 5] The original open artery hypothesis—that early and full reperfusion would lead to improved clinical outcomes—has subsequently been confirmed by large-scale megatrials with angiographic substudies that have linked improved 90-minute patency profiles to improved left ventricular function and, in turn, to improved mortality.[6, 7]

Up to the mid-1980s, the cardiac catheterization laboratory had served predominantly as a diagnostic tool in the setting of acute myocardial infarction. In more recent years, however, its role as a therapeutic modality has been rapidly expanding. Initially the potential therapeutic role of the cardiac catheterization laboratory was perceived as only supplementary to a pharmacologic approach. It was anticipated that adjunctive angioplasty would improve on the suboptimal 90-minute patency rates, the tight residual stenosis, and the risk of reocclusion that resulted from the lone use of available thrombolytic agents. Somewhat surprisingly, in several randomized, prospective trials undertaken in the late 1980s, the combination of intravenous thrombolysis coupled with immediate angioplasty did not confer any clinical benefit over thrombolysis alone with deferred angioplasty.[8–10] Although the combination of thrombolysis and angioplasty was not beneficial, an expanding group of nonrandomized, observational studies suggested that primary angioplasty as a lone strategy might be effective. The potential benefits included achieving high rates of patency, minimal residual stenoses, a lower rate of intracranial hemorrhage, and the early definition of coronary anatomy that would aid in the identification of patients who would benefit from coronary artery bypass grafting or early hospital discharge. Several randomized, prospective trials have subsequently compared the efficacy of thrombolysis and primary angioplasty as separate reperfusion strategies.

The data from these trials quickly become obsolete given the incredibly rapid expansion in the scope of both mechanical and pharmacologic methods to achieve acute coronary revascularization. For instance, the potential role of new device technologies, such as intracoronary stenting, is an emerging focus of research in this area. Likewise, more potent and more fibrin-specific thrombolytic agents have now been developed as well as newer antithrombotic and antiplatelet agents. Thus, research in this area is a rapidly moving target, and the numerous permutations of mechanical and pharmacologic strategies require ongoing reevaluation.

This chapter reviews trial data pertaining to (1) the use of routine adjunctive angioplasty in conjunction with thrombolytic agents, (2) primary angioplasty versus thrombolysis, (3) the use of new devices in acute myocardial infarction, and (4) the role of rescue angioplasty after failed thrombolysis. Whenever appropriate, the limitations of existing data and the critical need for future research in these rapidly evolving fields are discussed.

CONVENTIONAL PERCUTANEOUS CORONARY ANGIOPLASTY AS ROUTINE ADJUNCTIVE THERAPY TO THROMBOLYSIS IN THE SETTING OF ACUTE MYOCARDIAL INFARCTION

Several randomized, prospective trials have failed to demonstrate improved outcomes for a strategy of thrombolysis coupled with immediate routine adjunctive angioplasty when compared with a strategy of thrombolysis alone coupled with deferred angioplasty.[8–10] These trials differed in the dosing of recombinant tissue-plasminogen activator (rt-PA), the inclusion criteria for randomization to angioplasty, and the frequency as well as timing with which angioplasty was undertaken.[11] In the Thrombolysis and Angioplasty in Myocardial Infarction (TAMI) trial, patients were treated with 150 mg of rt-PA, and only patients with a patent artery and a residual stenosis were randomized to receive angioplasty either immediately or 7 days later if clinically indicated.[8] In contrast, in the European Cooperative Study Group trial (ECSG) and in the Thrombolysis in Myocardial Infarction (TIMI)-2A trial, patients were assigned to an angioplasty strategy before cardiac catheterization, and consequently patients with both patent and occluded vessels were randomized.[9, 10] In the ECSG trial, patients underwent either immediate angioplasty or cardiac catheterization 10 to 20 days later, and in TIMI-2A, patients were randomized to either immediate angioplasty or cardiac catheterization with angioplasty if appropriate at an earlier time of 18 to 48 hours.

Despite these differences in trial design and differences in the patency status of the culprit artery, the results of these trials were fairly uniform (Table 16–1). The primary endpoint of all three trials was the left ventricular function at hospital discharge, which did not differ between the two strategies. Although it was not a predefined primary endpoint of these studies, mortality was higher in the immediate angioplasty group than in the deferred group in the ECSG trial (7% [12 of 183] vs. 3% [5 of 184]) and tended to be higher in the TAMI trial (4% [4 of 99] vs. 1% [1 of 98]) and the TIMI-2A trial (8% [15 of 195] vs. 5% [10 of 194]). The higher mortality rate in the ECSG trial may be due to the fact that a large proportion (92%) of patients randomized to immediate angioplasty actually underwent angioplasty, whereas only 68% of TAMI patients and 70% of TIMI-2A patients underwent an angioplasty. Thus, the ECSG dataset may be enriched with higher-risk multivessel disease patients who underwent angioplasty.[11] When data from these trials are pooled, the mortality rate was higher in the immediate angioplasty group (31 of 477, 6.5%) than in the deferred angioplasty group (16 of 476, 3.4%) ($P = 0.04$) (see Table 16–1).[12] In addition, these trials showed higher rates of vascular complications and three times the control group transfusion and coronary artery bypass grafting rates in the immediate angioplasty group.[8–11]

Although the above-mentioned trials were prospective and randomized, they were fairly small by today's standards of randomized, controlled trials (197 to 389 randomized patients per trial, a total of 953 randomized patients available for pooled analysis from three trials),[8–10] and their sample sizes stand in stark contrast to more recent thrombolytic megatrials.[6, 7] In the TAMI trial, for instance, the difference in the number of deaths in the two strategies was small (four vs. one patient),[8] and the power of this study to detect a mortality difference is only 12%. Despite the limited statistical power of these individual trials in assessing mortality, the relatively high doses of rt-PA used in some studies, and the absence of new device use, the consensus in the cardiology community at this time is that there does not appear to be a role for routine adjunctive *conventional* angioplasty in *all* patients after thrombolysis. Certain important unanswered questions remain, however, such

TABLE 16–1 • Pooled Data from Randomized Prospective Trials Evaluating the Effectiveness of Thrombolysis Followed Immediately by Routine Adjunctive PTCA Versus Thrombolysis Alone with Deferred PTCA

	Pre-Discharge LVEF		30-Day Mortality	
	Immediate PTCA (%)	*Deferred PTCA (%)*	*Immediate PTCA*	*Deferred PTCA*
TAMI 1[8]	53	56	4/99 (4%)	1/98 (1%)
ECSG[9]	51	51	12/183 (7%)	5/184 (3%)
TIMI-2A[10]	50	49	15/195 (8%)	10/194 (5%)
Total experience	50*	51*	31/477 (6.5%)†	16/476 (3.4%)

*These values represent weighted averages for the respective columns of trial data.
†$P = 0.04$ for mortality of immediate PTCA vs. deferred PTCA.
PTCA, percutaneous transluminal coronary angioplasty; LVEF, left ventricular ejection fraction.

as whether there are potential subgroups that may derive benefit from adjunctive angioplasty. Although the role of rescue angioplasty for *failed* thrombolysis (TIMI grade 0/1 flow) has been investigated on a limited randomized trial basis as discussed later, a randomized trial of adjunctive angioplasty in patients with what could be termed *suboptimal* thrombolysis (i.e., TIMI grade 2 flow) has not been undertaken. Another unresolved question is whether lower doses of rt-PA (a bolus of 20 to 50 mg) administered while the patient is being prepared for angioplasty might result in meaningful early patency without exposing the patient to undue risk from either extensive intramural plaque hemorrhage after angioplasty[13] or intracranial hemorrhage. Although the use of conventional angioplasty techniques after thrombolysis does not appear to be beneficial, the routine adjunctive use of new device strategies, such as intracoronary stenting, has not been evaluated in the immediate postthrombolytic setting. If intramural hemorrhage after the combination of thrombolytic administration and angioplasty is an important cause of abrupt closure,[13] the risk of this complication might be reduced with the use of intracoronary stents. In addition, the use of newer antiplatelet agents might also be effective in reducing the risk of abrupt closure.

THROMBOLYSIS AS ROUTINE ADJUNCTIVE THERAPY TO CONVENTIONAL PERCUTANEOUS CORONARY ANGIOPLASTY IN THE SETTING OF ACUTE MYOCARDIAL INFARCTION

Although many investigators initially interpreted the results of the above-mentioned three trials as showing no additional benefit of immediate conventional balloon angioplasty techniques when routinely added to thrombolysis, other trialists approached this question from the opposite perspective: If thrombolysis was instead added to angioplasty, would this confer any benefit over angioplasty alone?[12] Again the pathophysiologic basis for the suboptimal outcomes in the immediate angioplasty arm in the above-mentioned studies[8–10] was hypothesized to be a heightened risk of bleeding into the vessel wall after thrombolytic administration.[13] Meanwhile, an increasing body of observational evidence suggested high rates of patency and favorable mortality rates for primary angioplasty as a lone strategy. This led Meier[14] to raise a provocative question in the title of his 1992 *Circulation* article "Balloon Angioplasty for Acute Myocardial Infarction: Was It Buried Alive?"[15] To begin to answer this question, O'Neill and others[16] from William Beaumont Hospital undertook a randomized trial of streptokinase and angioplasty versus lone angioplasty therapy in acute myocardial infarction. The strategy of angioplasty alone resulted in a shorter length of stay (9.3 vs. 7.7 days, $P = 0.046$), lower costs ($25,200 vs. $19,600, $P = 0.02$), lower rates of vascular complications (29% vs. 5%, $P = 0.004$), lower transfusion rates (39% vs. 8%, $P = 0.0001$), and lower coronary artery bypass grafting rates (10.3% vs. 1.6%, $P = 0.03$).[16] This counterposing perspective played an important role in setting the stage for randomized trials that have focused on the comparison of angioplasty alone versus an up-front approach of thrombolysis alone.

NONRANDOMIZED OBSERVATIONAL DATA PERTAINING TO PRIMARY PERCUTANEOUS TRANSLUMINAL CORONARY ANGIOPLASTY

Over the past 10 years, numerous observational series of primary angioplasty in acute myocardial infarction have been reported, and the pooled results are arranged chronologically in Table 16–2.[17–40] All attempts have been made to exclude duplicate reporting of patients by the same study group in this table, and where duplicate data do exist, the most recent or the largest reporting of data by a trialist is listed. Citations are for full-length manuscripts when they exist. The pooled mortality in 10,591 patients is 8.7% (919 of 10,591), with a range in individual series of 2.7%[36] to 16%.[37] Of note, these two widely divergent mortality rates were reported from two community hospital series, highlighting the potential variability in results particularly from smaller studies. These mortality data are not necessarily comparable to that from thrombolytic trials for the following reasons: (1) Many of these patients may have been ineligible for thrombolytic therapy and may be at higher risk for adverse outcomes; (2) likewise, these primary angioplasty series often include patients who were in cardiogenic shock at the time of the procedure; (3) substantial numbers of these patients were enrolled in the mid to late 1980s, and technical advances such as intracoronary stenting have been made since this time; and (4) it is only relatively recently that operators have had the capacity to monitor the activated clotting time and have appreciated the importance of maintaining the activated clotting time of approximately 300 to 350 seconds. These limitations of the data derived from observational studies of primary angioplasty underscore the need for randomized, prospective trials in this rapidly changing field.

Despite these limitations, there are several noteworthy observations from these pooled data. Although data from only 5 of the 24 studies are available, the

TABLE 16–2 • Pooled Data from Nonrandomized Studies of Primary PTCA

Trialist	Number of Patients	30-Day or In-Hospital Mortality (%)	Reinfarction (%)	Stroke (%)	CABG (%)
Rothbaum, 1987[17]	151	9.0	—	—	—
Marco, 1987[18]	43	14.0	—	—	—
Flaker, 1989[19]	93	14.0	—	—	—
Ellis, 1989[20]	271	13.3	—	—	—
Bittl, 1991[21]	20	10.0	—	—	—
Williams, 1991[22]	226	4.9	—	—	—
Grines, 1991[23]	58	5.0	—	—	—
Jaski, 1992[24]	151	3.1	—	—	6.7
Rogers, 1993[25]	107	9.4	—	0.9	—
Himbert, 1993[26]	45	9.0	0.0	0.0	—
O'Keefe, 1993[27]	1000	7.8	—	0.5	—
Nakagawa, 1993[28]	160	4.0	—	—	—
Dussaillant, 1994[29]	21	5.0	—	—	—
Sarkis, 1994[30]	12	16.0	—	—	—
Helmreich, 1994[31]	44	9.0	2.0	0.0	—
Chamorro, 1995[32]	64	6.0	3.0	—	3.0
MITI, 1995[33]	1010	5.9	—	—	8.0
Brodie, 1995[34]	907	8.6	0.7	—	—
Wharton, 1995[35]	186	5.9	3.1	1.1	0.0
Jhangiani, 1996[36]	37	2.7	—	—	24.3
Patel, 1996[37]	42	16.0	—	—	18.0
Caputo, 1996[38]	62	12.9	—	—	—
German Multicenter Registry, 1996[39]	2957	11.3	—	—	—
NRMI 2, 1996[40]	2924	7.6	—	—	—
Total experience	10,591	8.7 (919/10,591)	1.3 (16/1246)	0.36 (5/1382)	7.4 (110/1490)

PTCA, percutaneous transluminal coronary angioplasty; CABG, coronary artery bypass grafting.

pooled rate of reinfarction after primary angioplasty appears to be fairly low at 1.3% (16 of 1246) (see Table 16–2). Again, in the five studies with reported data, the potentially low risk of intracranial hemorrhage after primary angioplasty appears to be borne out by the low pooled stroke rate of 0.36% (5 of 1382 patients) with a range of 0.0% in several series to a high of 1.1% in one series.[35] In the six studies in which data are available, the pooled rate of emergency coronary artery bypass grafting was 7.4% (110 of 1490), which approximates that reported for primary angioplasty in the randomized trials discussed subsequently. This not infrequent need for emergency coronary artery bypass surgery raises an important question as to whether it is appropriate to perform primary angioplasty in the community hospital setting where emergency coronary bypass surgery may not be immediately available on site. Although data from moderate-sized studies have been reported, it is not clear that these results could be applied widely to all community hospitals that might offer primary angioplasty for acute myocardial infarction. Thus, the need for provision of immediate emergency bypass surgery remains unanswered, and large randomized trials involving operators from cardiac catheterization laboratories with a heterogeneous range of experience in geographically disparate locations (urban and rural) with varying proximity to operative suites (a building away versus a helicopter ride away) are sorely needed to answer this question. Only limited observational data are available regarding primary angioplasty in the elderly.[41–43]

RANDOMIZED, PROSPECTIVE TRIALS OF PRIMARY ANGIOPLASTY VERSUS THROMBOLYSIS IN THE SETTING OF ACUTE MYOCARDIAL INFARCTION

Mechanical and pharmacologic revascularization strategies offer different advantages. Thrombolytic administration has no learning curve, and consistent results should be obtainable by many physicians and centers. Thrombolytics may be effective in three-vessel disease or left main disease, whereas a mechanical approach may not be applicable in these situations. An interventional approach does offer the advantage of early triage of patients with either left main or extensive disease to immediate coronary artery bypass grafting. Thrombolytics, if stored and administered in the emergency department, may be given rapidly 24 hours a day in the majority of hospitals, whereas there may be enormous institutional costs encountered in having an in-hospital on-call team prepared to perform primary angioplasty quickly at all times. There is a trend toward a lower rate of intracranial bleeding with a mechanical approach, but this comes at the cost of a higher rate of instrumented site bleeding.[47]

Despite a slight but statistically significantly lower inhospital mortality rate compared with other first-generation thrombolytic agents,[6, 7] rt-PA still has the following limitations: failure to achieve patency by 90 minutes in 15% to 20% of patients, a 0.72% risk of hemorrhagic stroke (which may be fatal, disabling, or nondisabling) that is higher than streptokinase (0.52%, $P = 0.03$),[6] a 10% to 15% risk of reocclusion and reinfarction, and the potential for residual ischemia given that a tight stenosis often remains. Streptokinase has the limitations of a lower rate of 90-minute patency and a slightly higher mortality rate compared with rt-PA[6, 7] and the potential for allergic reaction with readministration.

Direct or primary angioplasty in acute myocardial infarction has been demonstrated to achieve high patency rates and high rates of the desirable TIMI grade 3 flow (normal flow) in angiographic trials.[44–49] The Primary Angioplasty in Myocardial Infarction (PAMI) investigators have reported a 97.1% success rate (TIMI grade 2 or 3 flow with a residual stenosis <50%) for primary angioplasty in acute myocardial infarction.[47] Among the 195 patients randomized to primary angioplasty, 20 patients (10.3%) did not undergo the procedure. Ten of these patients were considered to be at high risk associated with angioplasty, and the majority (nine) of these patients underwent emergency coronary bypass grafting. Some of the benefits reported in this study may be due to the fact that candidates for coronary artery bypass grafting were identified and revascularized (without being treated by angioplasty it might be added), whereas patients randomized to thrombolysis who did not undergo angiography may not have accrued the benefits of triage to coronary artery bypass grafting. In eight of the remaining patients, a minimal residual stenosis was present on angiography, making it unlikely that these patients would derive benefit from angioplasty. Compared with the older 3-hour dosing strategy of rt-PA, there was a trend for patients treated with primary angioplasty to have a lower mortality than patients treated with thrombolysis alone (6.5% vs. 2.6%, $P = 0.06$) in this trial of 395 patients (Table 16–3).[47] Hemorrhagic strokes occurred more commonly in rt-PA–treated patients (2.0% vs. 0.0%, $P = 0.05$).

Three additional randomized trials involving fewer than 100 patients for each treatment arm (angioplasty versus thrombolysis) have demonstrated a nonsignificant trend toward higher mortality but lower rates of reinfarction in patients randomized to primary angioplasty (see Table 16–3).[44–46] The larger trial of de Boer (301 patients),[48] however, paralleled the results of PAMI and demonstrated reduced mortality in the primary angioplasty arm (1.9% vs. 7.4%, $P = 0.024$) (see Table 16–3). Patients randomized to primary angioplasty also had a lower incidence of recurrent

TABLE 16–3 • Pooled Data from Randomized Prospective Trials Evaluating the Effectiveness of Primary PTCA Versus Thrombolysis in Acute Myocardial Infarction

Trialist	Number of Patients	30-Day Mortality	Reinfarction	CABG
O'Neill, 1986[44]				
Angioplasty	29	2 (6.8%)	2 (7%)	—
Thrombolysis (IC SK)	27	1 (3.7%)	4 (15%)	—
Ribeiro, 1993[45]				
Angioplasty	50	3 (6.0%)	4 (8.0%)	1 (2.0%)
Thrombolysis (IV SK)	50	1 (2.0%)	5 (10.0%)	6 (15.0%)
Gibbons, 1993[46]				
Angioplasty	47	2 (4.3%)	0 (0.0%)	6 (13.0%)
Thrombolysis (Duteplase)	56	2 (3.6%)	2 (3.6%)	7 (13.0%)
Grines, 1993[47]				
Angioplasty	195	5 (2.6%)	5 (2.6%)	16 (8.0%)
Thrombolysis (3-h tPA)	200	13 (6.5%)	13 (6.5%)	24 (12.0%)
de Boer, 1994[48]*				
Angioplasty	152	3 (1.9%)	2 (1.3%)	—
Thrombolysis (IV SK)	149	11 (7.4%)	15 (10.1%)	—
GUSTO-II, 1997[50]				
Angioplasty	565	32 (5.7%)	25 (4.4%)	47 (7.5%)
Thrombolysis (90-min tPA)	573	40 (7.0%)	37 (6.5%)	47 (8.2%)
Total experience				
Angioplasty	1038	47 (4.5%)†	38 (3.7%)‡	65 (6.3%)§
Thrombolysis	1055	68 (6.4%)	76 (7.2%)	84 (8.0%)

*Includes 142 patients previously reported by Zijlstra F, de Boer MJ, Hoorntje JCA, et al: A comparison of immediate coronary angioplasty with intravenous streptokinase in acute myocardial infarction. N Engl J Med 1993; 328:680–684.

†$P = 0.056$ for angioplasty vs. thrombolysis.

‡$P = 0.001$ for angioplasty vs. thrombolysis.

§$P = 0.15$ for angioplasty vs. thrombolysis.

infarction (15 patients [10%] vs. 2 patients [1%], $P < 0.001$) as well as improved left ventricular function (left ventricular ejection fraction of 44% ± 11% vs. 50% ± 11%, $P < 0.001$).

Early randomized comparisons of primary percutaneous transluminal coronary angioplasty (PTCA) with thrombolysis, however, have been limited by either the use of older dosing regimens of rt-PA or the use of streptokinase rather than using the more efficacious regimen of front-loaded rt-PA.[44–49] The trials also involved relatively small numbers of patients, and, likewise, the trials did not involve large numbers of centers or operators, which might limit the generalizability of the results.[44–49] The most recent randomized trial in this field (Global Use of Strategies to Open Occluded Coronary Arteries [GUSTO]-2B) overcomes some of these limitations in its comparison of direct angioplasty to front-loaded rt-PA in a large series of 1138 patients drawn from multiple international centers. The primary endpoint of the trial was the incidence of death, reinfarction, or stroke, and these adverse events were significantly less frequent in the primary angioplasty group compared with the front-loaded rt-PA group (9.6% vs. 13.7%, $P = 0.033$). The mortality rates were slightly lower for primary angioplasty (5.7% vs. 7%, P = NS), and the discrepancy in mortality was not as great as that reported in the previous smaller studies (PAMI[47] and de Boer et al[48]) with limited multicenter enrollment. A stroke occurred in 0.9% of rt-PA patients, whereas there was one stroke (0.2%) in the PTCA arm ($P = 0.11$).

Another advantage of the GUSTO-2B trial lies in its use of an independent angiographic core laboratory to compare TIMI flow grades rather than relying on the angioplasty operator's assessment. In contrast to the rates of TIMI grade 3 flow that have previously been reported to be in the upper 80% to 90% range by angioplasty operators, only 73% of patients achieved TIMI grade 3 flow after primary angioplasty in GUSTO-2B when the TIMI flow was assessed by an independent angiographic core laboratory. Nonetheless, this 73% rate of normal TIMI grade 3 flow in the artery still compares favorably with the 53% and 60% rates of TIMI grade 3 flow reported in the GUSTO-1 and the TIMI-4 angiographic studies for front-loaded rt-PA.[7]

REGISTRY DATA COMPARING THROMBOLYTIC THERAPY TO PRIMARY PERCUTANEOUS TRANSLUMINAL CORONARY ANGIOPLASTY

The outcomes among 1050 patients treated with primary angioplasty versus 2095 patients treated with thrombolysis in a community setting were compared in the Myocardial Infarction Triage and Intervention (MITI) Project Registry.[51] There was no difference in the baseline characteristics of patients treated with thrombolysis versus those treated with primary PTCA, and, likewise, there was no difference in mortality during hospitalization or long-term follow-up (in-hospital mortality 5.6% and 5.5%, $P = 0.93$; adjusted hazard ratio of death within 3 years after primary PTCA, 0.95; 95% confidence interval, 0.8 to 1.2).[51] Patients in the thrombolytic therapy group were hospitalized a mean of 1.1 days longer than patients in the primary angioplasty group (7.9 ± 5.3 vs. 6.8 ± 4.4 days, $P < 0.001$), but their mean total hospital costs were lower ($16,838 ± 12,480 vs. $19,702 ± 12,175, $P < 0.001$). Subgroup analyses of patients with no contraindications to thrombolytic therapy, patients admitted to centers with higher volumes of primary angioplasty, and *high-risk* subgroups of patients all showed similar rates of short-term and long-term mortality. After 3 years of follow-up, in the thrombolysis group there were 30% fewer coronary angiograms, 15% fewer PTCAs, and 13% lower costs.[51]

Although these data are provocative, the authors acknowledge that this is not a randomized, controlled trial, and although the authors adjusted for potential differences in baseline characteristics in the dataset, there may still exist unmeasured differences that may have influenced both the choice of reperfusion strategy and the outcomes.[51] The fact that primary PTCA patients tended to return for procedures more frequently may not be due to a problem with the PTCA procedure itself but may instead reflect the more aggressive or catheterization-oriented style of interventionalists. There are several potential reasons why the mortality rate for PTCA patients in the MITI registry was higher and the mortality rate of thrombolytic-treated patients lower than those previously reported in smaller randomized trials.[51] The PTCA success rate in the community setting of the MITI registry was 89%, which is lower than the 98% rate observed in the PAMI trials, and this may result in less optimal outcomes compared with those observed in highly specialized centers. Operators in the MITI registry may not have maintained an activated clotting time above 350 seconds, and they may not have avoided nonionic contrast media, in contrast to clinical practices at centers conducting randomized trials. With respect to the lower mortality rate observed for thrombolytic-treated patients, the time to treatment in the MITI registry was faster for thrombolytic-treated patients than had been reported in the PAMI study (198 vs. 230 minutes). The fact that 32% of those patients treated with thrombolysis crossed over to treatment with PTCA may have also minimized the differences in outcomes.

NEW DEVICE STRATEGIES IN THE SETTING OF ACUTE MYOCARDIAL INFARCTION

Although previous trials have examined the utility of conventional angioplasty techniques, intracoronary stenting is an emerging new device technology that has thus far produced favorable results. In the analysis, all attempts were made to include only those trials in which primary stenting was performed early (within the first 24 hours) in the setting of acute myocardial infarction. Those trials in which stents were placed only for PTCA failure (i.e., bailout situations—*conditional* stenting) were excluded. With 1357 patients enrolled in 20 trials to date,[52–70] mortality rates range from 0.0% in several trials to 7.0% in the relatively small U.S. multicenter experience of only 44 patients (Table 16–4).[56] Pooled data from 1357 patients show a favorable 30-day mortality rate of 2.4% (33 of 1357). Despite fears of an increased risk of stent thrombosis, the pooled incidence of stent thrombosis appears to be low at 1.5% (17 of 1163). Also of particular note is the low pooled rate of coronary artery bypass grafting of 1.3% (11 of 816). A nonrandomized analysis of these pooled stent data shows that this 1.3% rate of emergency coronary artery bypass grafting is lower than the 7.4% (110 of 1490) (see Table 16–2) reported in the observational studies of conventional primary angioplasty ($P < 0.001$), and it is lower than the pooled data from randomized trials of primary angioplasty versus thrombolysis (70 of 1129 or 6.2% for primary angioplasty, $P < 0.001$, and 84 of 1055 or 8.0% for thrombolysis, $P < 0.001$). The pooled mortality rate of 2.4% for primary stenting (see Table 16–4) is lower than the 4.5% pooled mortality rate in primary PTCA trials (see Table 16–3) ($P = 0.007$) and lower than the 6.4% pooled mortality rate for medical therapy (see Table 16–3) ($P < 0.0001$). These comparisons are nonrandomized, and the efficacy of intracoronary stenting must obviously be directly compared with conventional PTCA techniques, newer thrombolytic agents, or both in a randomized, prospective fashion. Whether these favorable results from experienced centers can be widely reproduced in large multicenter trials involving less experienced operators also remains to be determined. Finally, whether these low rates of emergency coronary artery bypass surgery can be achieved in the community hospital setting also remains to be determined.

RESCUE ANGIOPLASTY

If thrombolytic therapy is not effective in the setting of acute myocardial infarction (i.e., if TIMI grade 0 or 1 flow is present), a *rescue* or *salvage* angioplasty may be performed to restore flow. The angiographic sub-

TABLE 16–4 • Pooled Data of Intracoronary Stenting as Primary Therapy in Acute Myocardial Infarction

Trial	30-Day Mortality	Reinfarction	Emergency CABG	Rethrombosis
Spaulding et al, 1996[52]*	4.4% (2/45)	—	—	0.0% (0/45)
French Registry, 1996[53]*	5.9% (5/85)	2.4% (2/85)	1.2% (1/85)	1.2% (1/85)
LeMay et al, 1996[54]*	4.3% (1/23)	0.0% (0/23)	0.0% (0/23)	—
Monassier et al, 1996[55]*	4.5% (6/134)	—	1.5% (2/134)	3.0% (4/134)
U.S. Multicenter, 1996[56]†	7.0% (3/44)	—	5.0% (2/44)	5.0% (2/44)
Rodriguez et al, 1996[57]‡	3.0% (1/30)	—	0.0% (0/30)	3.0% (1/30)
ESCOBAR, 1996[58]	0.0% (0/46)	0.0% (0/46)	—	0.0% (0/46)
Katz et al, 1996[59]	2.6% (3/117)	0.0% (0/117)	—	0.0% (0/117)
Medina et al, 1996[60]	0.0% (0/59)	0.0% (0/59)	0.0% (0/59)	0.0% (0/59)
Glatt et al, 1996[61]§	3.3% (4/120)	0.8% (1/120)	0.8% (1/120)	1.6% (2/120)
Valeix et al, 1996[62]	1.5% (1/67)	3.0% (2/67)	—	3.0% (2/67)
Schomig et al, 1977[63]‖	0.0% (0/61)	0.0% (0/61)	0.0% (0/61)	0.0% (0/61)
Siegel et al, 1997[64]	2.7% (1/54)	—	—	—
GRAMI, 1997[65]§	0.0% (0/40)	0.0% (0/40)	—	0.0% (0/40)
PAMI Stent Pilot, 1997[66]§	0.4% (1/230)	1.3% (3/230)	1.7% (4/230)	1.3% (3/230)
Wright et al, 1997[66a]	0.0% (0/41)	—	—	—
PASTA, 1997[67]	4.9% (2/41)	—	—	—
STAMI, 1997[68]	3.3% (1/30)	—	3.3% (1/30)	0.0% (0/30)
Ganim, 1997[69]	3.6% (2/55)	—	—	3.6% (2/55)
FRESCO, 1997[70]	0.0% (0/35)	2.8% (1/35)	—	—
Total experience	2.4% (33/1357)	1.1% (10/883)	1.3% (11/816)	1.5% (17/1163)

*Postimplantation therapy included ticlopidine 250 mg PO qd, aspirin, low-molecular-weight heparin for 7 days to 1 month.
†Postimplantation therapy included aspirin and 19% of patients were treated with ticlopidine, 19% of patients were treated with ReoPro.
‡23 patients were treated with dextran, dipyridamole, warfarin, and ASA; 7 patients received ticlopidine 250 mg PO bid and ASA 325 mg PO qd for 1 month and IV heparin for 2 days, with subcutaneous low-molecular-weight heparin for 2 weeks. High-pressure balloon inflations with ultrasound were used.
§Patients treated with aspirin and ticlopidine. No warfarin or low-molecular-weight heparinoids were administered.
‖Includes only the 61 patients treated with ticlopidine (current management), which had superior outcomes compared with those patients treated with warfarin.
CABG, coronary artery bypass grafting; ASA, acetyl salicylic acid; GRAMI, GR II stent in Acute Myocardial Infarction trial; PASTA, Primary Angioplasty versus STent Implantation in Acute myocardial infarction trial; STAMI, STenting in Acute Myocardial Infarction trial; FRESCO, Florence Randomized Elective Stenting in acute Coronary Occlusion trial.

study of the GUSTO trial linked full reperfusion to improved clinical outcomes, and consequently an aggressive approach to restore flow to a persistently occluded vessel mechanically appears quite reasonable.[6, 7] A major obstacle encountered in evaluating the efficacy of rescue angioplasty has been the inherent belief among angioplasty operators that rescue angioplasty after failed thrombolysis would clearly be beneficial given the open artery paradigm. This inherent bias in favor of performing rescue angioplasty is reflected by the fact that nearly 80% of operators approached to participate in the Randomized Evaluation of Salvage Angioplasty with Combined Utilization of Endpoints (RESCUE) study declined because they thought that it would be unethical to randomize patients to a strategy that withheld attempted revascularization for an occluded vessel immediately after failed thrombolysis.[71, 72] The benefits of intuitive strategies such as this are not always substantiated, however, when evaluated in a randomized, prospective clinical trial. For example, as was discussed previously, despite the intuitive belief that immediate adjunctive angioplasty would improve clinical outcomes in patients with a patent but narrowed artery after successful thrombolysis, several large trials have shown no benefit to immediate adjunctive angioplasty in this setting.[8–10] Although rescue angioplasty has been used to establish reperfusion after failed thrombolysis, a high incidence of complications has left its overall benefit in question.

RESCUE Trial

The RESCUE trial is currently the only randomized, prospective trial to examine the benefits of angioplasty after failed thrombolysis.[71, 72] This trial enrolled 151 patients from 20 centers with TIMI grade 0 or 1 flow a mean of 4.5 hours after myocardial infarction. Generalization of results from this trial are somewhat limited because enrollment was restricted to patients with their first anterior wall myocardial infarction. Patients in this trial were hemodynamically stable, and 134 eligible patients were not randomized, raising a question as to whether the study population was enriched with healthier patients.[71, 72] In addition, the 92% success rate is higher than that reported in other series. There was no difference in outcome for the prespecified primary endpoint of the trial, the resting left ventricular ejection fraction at 30 days after myocardial infarction (40% in the rescue angioplasty group vs. 39% in the conservative group, P = NS). The mortality rate in patients treated with rescue angioplasty was 5.1%, which did not differ significantly from the 9.6% for those not treated with rescue angioplasty. As a secondary endpoint, death and congestive heart failure were analyzed together, and there was a trend for a reduced incidence in the rescue angioplasty group (6.4%) compared with the group not treated with rescue angioplasty (16.6%, $P = 0.055$).

TIMI Experience

In contrast to the RESCUE trial, patients were enrolled in the TIMI-4 trial *regardless* of infarct location or prior history of myocardial infarction.[73] Rescue angioplasty in the TIMI-4 trial was performed at the discretion of the operator in a nonrandomized fashion for an occluded vessel at 90 minutes after thrombolysis. In the TIMI-4 trial, although successful rescue angioplasty for an occluded artery at 90 minutes resulted in restoration of TIMI grade 3 flow at a rate that was superior to that of successful thrombolysis (86.5% vs. 64.8%, $P = 0.002$), the incidence of adverse events (death, recurrent myocardial infarction, severe congestive heart failure, cardiogenic shock, or an ejection fraction <40%) for rescue angioplasty was slightly worse than that of successful thrombolysis.[73] Although improved flow velocities *and full* reperfusion were more frequently achieved after successful rescue angioplasty, it was achieved *later*, as the angioplasty was performed at 120 minutes. In keeping with the fact that the *early and full* reperfusion paradigm of thrombolytic success was only partially fulfilled in the successful rescue angioplasty patients, the *delayed* and often *full* reperfusion achieved in successful rescue angioplasty patients resulted in an overall adverse event rate (28.8%) that was intermediate between that of patients with immediate thrombolytic success (22.8%) and that of patients treated with no rescue angioplasty for an occluded vessel (35.1%) who frequently achieved reperfusion later. Among all patients in whom rescue angioplasty was performed (successes and failures combined), 34.5% of patients experienced an adverse outcome, which was similar to the 35.1% incidence observed in patients not undergoing rescue angioplasty (P = NS) and tended to be higher than the 22.8% incidence observed in patients with patent arteries ($P = 0.07$). Although rescue angioplasty patients were demonstrated to have superior flow compared with patients with successful thrombolysis in TIMI-4, this finding is important because it underscores the time-dependent nature of the open artery hypothesis in that the flow after rescue angioplasty, which albeit was superior, was achieved later than the inferior flow achieved in patients after successful thrombolysis, and this may explain in part the less optimal outcomes for this strategy.[73] Thus, it would appear to be incumbent on any institution routinely performing primary or rescue angioplasty to ensure that the restoration of flow is achieved quickly, with a door-to-balloon time approximating that in the PAMI trial of about 60 minutes for primary angioplasty.

The outcomes of 100 consecutive patients not treated with rescue angioplasty in the TIMI phase 1 trial (angioplasty was prohibited in this trial) have been compared with the outcomes of 33 consecutive patients treated with rescue angioplasty in the TIMI phase 2A trial, in which mechanical intervention was required as part of the protocol.[74] Twenty-one-day mortality in patients treated with no rescue angioplasty was 7%, which did not differ from the 12% mortality in patients treated with rescue angioplasty.[74] There was also no difference in the left ventricular ejection fraction between the two groups.

Other Nonrandomized Trial Experience

Several other trials have evaluated the strategy of rescue angioplasty for an occluded artery in a nonrandomized fashion.[75–83] Overall success rates have varied (71%[77] to 100%[78]) and, on the whole, have been lower than those reported for primary angioplasty, which has been postulated to be due to either a larger or more pharmacologically resistant thrombus burden or more extensive plaque rupture.[15, 72] Pooled analyses have shown a high overall mortality rate of 10.6%, no improvement in left ventricular function between the time of the rescue angioplasty and 7 days, and a higher rate of reocclusion in patients treated with rt-PA (24%) compared with nonspecific plasminogen activators (14%) possibly owing to the adherence of generated fibrinogen fragments that would bind to glycoprotein IIb/IIIa (fibrinogen) receptor.[15, 72]

Several studies have shown higher rates of intraprocedural complications such as ventricular fibrillation, hypotension, severe bradycardia, abrupt closure, and reocclusion for the right coronary artery compared with the left anterior descending artery.[81–83] The risk of mortality in patients with a failed rescue angioplasty is extremely high. In the TIMI-2A trial, mortality after failed rescue angioplasty was 33%,[80] 33.3% in the TIMI-4,[73] and 39% in the TAMI experience.[81] It is unclear whether this high mortality rate reflects the selection of a disproportionate number of high-risk patients for the procedure or if performing a rescue angioplasty may itself pose major risks.

Limitations and Future Directions in Rescue Angioplasty Trials

In the aforementioned nonrandomized trials, patients with occluded arteries at 90 minutes were not prospectively randomized to the strategies of rescue angioplasty versus no rescue angioplasty. Consequently, there might have been the potential for selection bias toward performing a rescue angioplasty as a last-ditch effort in patients who were sicker. Another problem in these analyses is the fact that a substantial number of patients managed noninvasively early in their course may eventually cross over to the angioplasty strategy during their hospitalization. In many trials, rescue angioplasty may not have been performed early enough to optimize myocardial salvage. It is possible, but as yet untested, that earlier intervention before the traditional 90-minute endpoint after failed thrombolysis might result in improved clinical outcomes. Another potential advantage of rescue angioplasty is the larger minimum diameters and reduced percent diameter stenoses obtained at the completion of the procedure. It is possible that these patients would have a lower incidence of recurrent ischemic events if the follow-up period were to extend beyond the usual 30-day period in reported studies.

A potential problem in implementing a rescue angioplasty strategy lies in identifying patients who would be appropriate candidates for intervention because reliable clinical and noninvasive markers of reperfusion have not been validated for widespread use. Clinical symptoms, the electrocardiogram, and reperfusion arrhythmias are somewhat poor markers of the status of the culprit artery.[84] Other newer potential modalities include technetium 99m sestamibi, continuous ST-segment monitoring, and troponin or myoglobin assays.[85, 86] Other disadvantages of a rescue angioplasty strategy include the fact that a minority of U.S. hospitals have a cardiac catheterization laboratory equipped to perform angioplasty and the high costs of round-the-clock staffing of a cardiac catheterization laboratory.

RELATIONSHIP BETWEEN CORONARY BLOOD FLOW AND ADVERSE OUTCOMES

TIMI grade 3 flow after thrombolysis has been shown to be associated with improved mortality after thrombolysis.[7] TIMI grade 3 flow is more often observed in right coronary arteries, however, and TIMI grade 2 flow is more often seen in left anterior descending arteries. Given these complex interrelationships between flow, infarct artery location, and myocardium at risk, analyses comparing the clinical, enzymatic, ventriculographic, or electrocardiographic outcomes of the various TIMI flow grades should correct for the fact that left anterior descending location is associated with a higher incidence of TIMI grade 2 flow.[87] The TIMI frame count is a new, more objective method to assess coronary blood flow in which the number of

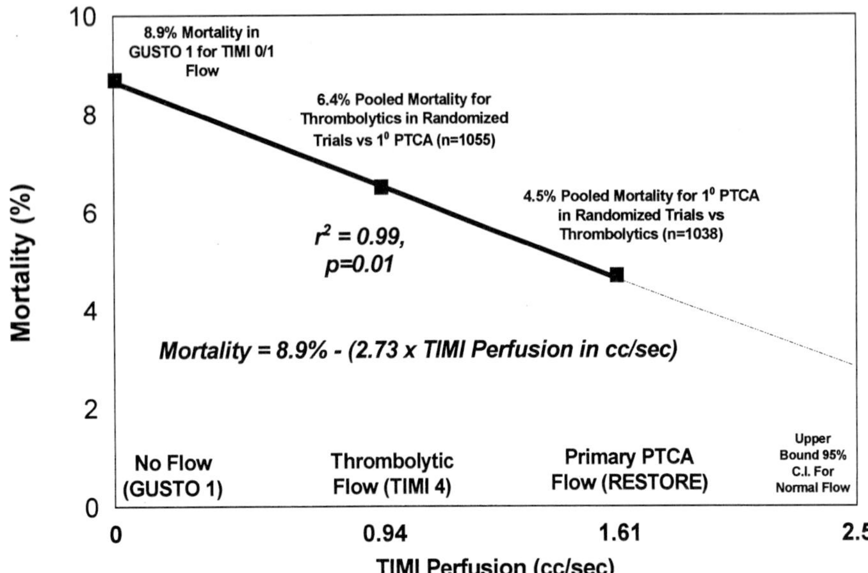

Figure 16–1 Relationship between coronary blood flow and mortality in acute myocardial infarction.

frames required for dye to arrive at standardized distal landmarks is counted.[87] Higher TIMI frame counts (i.e., slower flow) after thrombolysis and after PTCA are associated with higher rates of mortality.[88, 89] This new method may provide a more sensitive metric in assessing flow after different reperfusion strategies.

Figure 16–1 shows the relationship between coronary perfusion and the pooled mortality for either primary PTCA or thrombolysis (see Table 16–3). The TIMI perfusion is the coronary flow (cm^3 per second), which is calculated as the 21/(observed corrected TIMI frame count) × 1.7 (based on Doppler velocity wire data showing normal flow = 1.7 cm^3 per second, which is proportional to 21 frames). Occluded arteries (TIMI grades 0, 1) obviously have a TIMI perfusion of 0 cm^3 per second, and the mortality rate in these patients has been reported as 8.9% in GUSTO-1.[7] Based on pooled data from the TIMI trials, the TIMI perfusion after treatment with current thrombolytic agents can be calculated as 0.94 cm^3 per second,[87] and the pooled mortality in these patients is 6.4% (see Table 16–3). The TIMI perfusion after primary PTCA in the Randomized Efficacy Study of Tirofiban for Outcomes and REstenosis (RESTORE) trial was nearly normal at 1.61 cm^3 per second,[90] and the pooled mortality for primary PTCA is 4.5% (see Table 16–3). Figure 16–1 shows a linear relationship between improved perfusion and improved mortality (r^2, 0.99; P = 0.011). Linear regression shows that in acute myocardial infarction, mortality = 8.9% − (2.73% × TIMI perfusion in cm^3 per second). For every 1 frame improvement in flow, there is a 0.12% improvement in mortality. In other words, flow must improve by 8.3 frames (an improvement in dye transit of 0.28 second) to improve mortality by 1.0%.

FUTURE DIRECTIONS IN THE ASSESSMENT OF PRIMARY ANGIOPLASTY AND THROMBOLYSIS

The choice of whether to use a pharmacologic or a mechanical reperfusion strategy in a given patient is quite complex. Both mechanical and pharmacologic strategies are evolving rapidly, and their relative efficacy will need to be reassessed periodically. Newer thrombolytic agents are under development (rPA, nPA, TNK, staphylokinase), and the rates of intracranial hemorrhage, reocclusion, patency, and mortality associated with these agents remain to be defined.[91–93] If new device strategies are found to be superior to conventional angioplasty techniques, they will need to be compared with these newer thrombolytic agents. The potential adjunctive role of new antiplatelet agents in the setting of primary angioplasty also remains to be determined. The Evaluation of c7E3 for Prevention of Ischemic Complications (EPIC) investigators have demonstrated a trend for c7E3-treated patients to have a lower incidence of the composite endpoint of death, reinfarction, repeat intervention, or bypass surgery in the setting of primary angioplasty (26.1% in placebo patients to 4.5% in c7E3 patients, P = 0.06).[94] At 6 months, ischemic events were reduced from 47.8% in placebo-treated patients to 4.5% in c7E3-treated patients (P = 0.002).[94]

REFERENCES

1. Rentrop KP, Blanke H, Karsch KR, et al. Initial experience with transluminal recanalization of the occluded infarct related

artery in acute myocardial infarction: Comparison with conventionally treated patients. Clin Cardiol 1979; 2:92–102.
2. Khaja F, Walton JA, Brymer JF, et al. Intracoronary fibrinolytic therapy in acute myocardial infarction: Report of a prospective randomized trial. N Engl J Med 1983; 308:1305–1311.
3. Kennedy JW, Ritchie JL, Davis KB, et al. Western Washington randomized trial of intracoronary streptokinase in acute myocardial infarction. N Engl J Med 1983; 390:1477–1482.
4. TIMI Study Group. The thrombolysis in myocardial infarction (TIMI) trial. N Engl J Med 1985; 31:932–936.
5. Verstraete M, Bernard R, Bory M. Randomized trial of intravenous streptokinase in acute myocardial infarction: Report from the European Cooperative Study Group for recombinant tissue type plasminogen activator. Lancet 1985; 1:842–847.
6. GUSTO Investigators. An international randomized trial comparing four thrombolytic strategies for acute myocardial infarction. N Engl J Med 1993; 329:673–682.
7. GUSTO Angiographic Investigators. The effects of tissue plasminogen activator, streptokinase, or both on coronary artery patency, ventricular function, and survival after acute myocardial infarction. N Engl J Med 1993; 329:1615–1622.
8. Topol EJ, Califf RM, George BS, et al. A randomized trial of immediate versus delayed elective angioplasty after intravenous tissue plasminogen activator in acute myocardial infarction. N Engl J Med 1987; 317:581–588.
9. Simons ML, Col J, Betriu A, et al. Thrombolysis with tissue plasminogen activator in acute myocardial infarction: No additional benefit from immediate percutaneous coronary angioplasty. Lancet 1988; 1:197–203.
10. TIMI Research Group. Immediate versus delayed catheterization and angioplasty following thrombolytic therapy for acute myocardial infarction. JAMA 1988; 260:2849–2858.
11. Topol EJ. Coronary angioplasty for acute myocardial infarction. Ann Intern Med 1988; 109:970–980.
12. O'Neill WW. The evolution of primary PTCA therapy of acute myocardial infarction: A personal perspective. J Invas Cardiol 1995; 7(suppl F):2–11.
13. Waller B, Rothbaum D, Pinkerton C, et al. Status of the myocardium and infarct-related coronary artery in 19 necropsy patients with acute recanalization using pharmacologic (streptokinase, r-tissue plasminogen activator), mechanical (percutaneous transluminal coronary angioplasty) or combined types of reperfusion therapy. J Am Coll Cardiol 1987; 9:785–801.
14. Meier B. Balloon angioplasty for acute myocardial infarction: Was it buried alive? Circulation 1990; 82:2243–2245.
15. Topol E (ed). Textbook of Interventional Cardiology, 2nd ed. Philadelphia, WB Saunders, 1994, pp 292–317.
16. O'Neill WW, Weintraub R, Grines CL, et al. A prospective, placebo-controlled, randomized trial of intravenous streptokinase and angioplasty versus lone angioplasty therapy of acute myocardial infarction. Circulation 1992; 86:1710–1717.
17. Rothbaum DA, Linnemeier TJ, Landin RJ, et al. Emergency percutaneous transluminal coronary angioplasty in acute myocardial infarction: A 3 year experience. J Am Coll Cardiol 1987; 10:264–272.
18. Marco J, Caster L, Szatmary IJ, et al. Emergency percutaneous transluminal coronary angioplasty without thrombolysis as initial therapy in acute myocardial infarction. Int J Cardiol 1987; 15:55–63.
19. Flaker GC, Webel RR, Meinhardt S, et al. Emergency angioplasty in acute myocardial infarction. Am Heart J 1989; 118:1154–1160.
20. Ellis SG, O'Neill WW, Bates ER, et al. Coronary angioplasty as primary therapy for acute myocardial infarction 6 to 48 hours after symptom onset: Report of an initial experience. J Am Coll Cardiol 1989; 13:1122–1126.
21. Bittl JA. Indications, timing, and optimal technique for diagnostic angiography and angioplasty in acute myocardial infarction. Chest 1991; 99:150S–156S.
22. Williams DO, Holubkov AL, Detre KM, et al. Impact of pretreatment by thrombolytic therapy upon outcome of emergency direct angioplasty for patients with acute myocardial infarction (abstract). J Am Coll Cardiol 1991; 17:337A.
23. Grines CK, Meany TB, Weintraub R, et al. Streptokinase angioplasty myocardial infarction trial: Early and late results (abstract). J Am Coll Cardiol 1991; 17:336A.
24. Jaski BE, Cohen JD, Trausch J, et al. Outcome of urgent percutaneous transluminal coronary angioplasty in acute myocardial infarction: Comparison of single vessel versus multivessel coronary artery disease. Am Heart J 1992; 124:1427–1433.
25. Rogers WJ, Dean LS, Moore PB, et al. Outcome of patients managed with primary PTCA versus lytic therapy in a multicenter registry (abstract). J Am Coll Cardiol 1993; 21:330A.
26. Himbert D, Juliard JM, Steg PG, et al. Primary coronary angioplasty for acute myocardial infarction with contraindication to thrombolysis. Am J Cardiol 1993; 71:377–381.
27. O'Keefe JH Jr, Bailey WL, Rutherford BD, et al. Primary angioplasty for acute myocardial infarction in 1,000 consecutive patients: Results in an unselected population and high risk subgroups. Am J Cardiol 1993; 72:107G–115G.
28. Nakagawa Y, Iwasaki Y, Nosaka H, et al. Serial angiographic follow-up after successful direct angioplasty for acute myocardial infarction: Single-center experience (abstract). Circulation 1993; 88:I-106.
29. Dussaillant G, Martinez A, Marchant E, et al. Primary coronary angioplasty as early reperfusion treatment of acute myocardial infarction. Rev Med Chil 1994; 122:401–407.
30. Sarkis A, Badaoui G, Kassab R, et al. Primary angioplasty at the stage of acute myocardial infarction. J Med Liban 1994; 42:100–104.
31. Helmreich G, Kratzer H, Baumgartner H, et al. Primary angioplasty in acute myocardial infarction. Wien Klin Wochenschr 1994; 106:507–512.
32. Chamorro H, Ducci H, Methei R, et al. Primary coronary angioplasty as a treatment choice in the 1st 6 hours following acute myocardial infarction. Rev Med Chil 1995; 1123:727–734.
33. Every N, Douglas W, Parsons L, et al. Direct PTCA vs. thrombolysis: Immediate and one year outcome and procedure utilization for the two treatment strategies. Circulation 1995; 92:I-138 (abstract).
34. Brodie B, Stuckey T, Weintraub R, et al. Timing and mechanism of death after direct angioplasty for acute myocardial infarction (abstract). J Am Coll Cardiol 1995; 27:295A.
35. Wharton TP, Schmitz JM, Fedele FA, et al. Primary angioplasty in acute myocardial infarction at community hospitals without cardiac surgery: Experience in 195 cases (abstract). Circulation 1995; 92:I-138.
36. Jhangiani AH, Jorgensen MB, Mansukhani PW, et al. Community practice of primary angioplasty for myocardial infarction (abstract). J Am Coll Cardiol 1996; 27:61A.
37. Patel S, Reese C, O'Connor RE, et al. Adverse outcomes accompanying primary angioplasty (PTCA) for acute myocardial infarction (AMI)—dangers of delay. J Am Coll Cardiol 1996; 27:62A.
38. Caputo RP, Lopez JJ, Stoler RC, et al. The effect of institutional experience on the outcome of primary angioplasty for acute MI. J Am Coll Cardiol 1996; 27:62A.
39. Neuhaus KL, Vogel A, Harmjanz D, et al. Primary PTCA in acute myocardial infarction: Results from a German multicenter registry (abstract). J Am Coll Cardiol 1996; 27:62A.
40. Cannon CP, Costas TL, Tiefenbrunn AG, et al. Influence of door to balloon time on mortality in 3,648 patients in the second national registry of myocardial infarction (NRMI 2) (abstract). J Am Coll Cardiol 1996; 27:61A.
41. Mattos LA, Cano MN, Maldonado G, et al. The use of primary coronary angioplasty in acute myocardial infarction in patients over 70 years of age. Arq Bras Cardiol 1992; 58:181–187.
42. Moulichon ME, Mossard JM, Arbogast R, et al. Acute myocardial infarction in patients over 70 years of age treated by immediate primary angioplasty. Ann Cardiol Angeiol 1993; 42:73–78.
43. Laster SB, Rutherford BD, McConahay DR, et al. Is direct angioplasty the preferred reperfusion therapy in octogenarians? (abstract) Circulation 1994; 90:I-169.
44. O'Neill WW, Timmis G, Bourdillon P, et al. A prospective randomized clinical trial of intracoronary streptokinase versus coronary angioplasty for acute myocardial infarction. N Engl J Med 1986; 314:812–818.
45. Ribeiro EE, Silva LA, Carneiro R, et al. Randomized trial of direct coronary angioplasty versus intravenous streptokinase in acute myocardial infarction. J Am Coll Cardiol 1993; 22:376–380.

46. Gibbons RJ, Holmes DR, Reeder GS, et al. Immediate angioplasty compared with the administration of a thrombolytic agent followed by conservative treatment for myocardial infarction. N Engl J Med 1993; 328:685–691.
47. Grines CL, Browne KF, Marco J, et al. A comparison of immediate angioplasty with thrombolytic therapy for acute myocardial infarction. N Engl J Med 1993; 328:673–679.
48. de Boer MJ, Hoorntje JCA, Ottervanger JP, et al. Immediate coronary angioplasty versus intravenous streptokinase in acute myocardial infarction: Left ventricular ejection fraction, hospital mortality and reinfarction. J Am Coll Cardiol 1994; 23:1004–1008.
49. Zijlstra F, De Boer MJ, Hoorntje JCA, et al. A comparison of immediate coronary angioplasty with intravenous streptokinase in acute myocardial infarction. N Engl J Med 1993; 328:680–684.
50. GUSTO IIb Investigators: A clinical trial comparing primary coronary angioplasty with tissue plasminogen activator for acute myocardial infarction. N Engl J Med 1997; 336:1621–1628.
51. Every NR, Parsons LS, Hlatky M, et al, for the Myocardial Infarct Triage and Intervention Investigators. A comparison of thrombolytic therapy with primary coronary angioplasty for acute myocardial infarction. N Engl J Med 1996; 335:1253–1260.
52. Spaulding C, Hamda KB, Roussel L, et al. One week and six months angiographic controls of coronary stent implantation during primary angioplasties for acute myocardial infarction. J Am Coll Cardiol 1996; 27(suppl A):68A.
53. Lefèvre T, Morice MC, Karrillon G, et al. Coronary stenting during acute myocardial infarction: Results from the Stent Without Coumadin French registry. J Am Coll Cardiol 1996; 27(suppl A):69A.
54. LeMay MR, Labinaz M, Beanlands RSB, et al. Intracoronary stenting in the setting of myocardial infarction. J Am Coll Cardiol 1996; 27(suppl A):69A.
55. Monassier JP, Elias J, Meyer P, et al. STENTIM I: The French registry of stenting at acute myocardial infarction. J Am Coll Cardiol 1996; 27(suppl A):68A.
56. Steinhubl SR, Moliterno DJ, Teirstein PS, et al. Stenting for acute myocardial infarction: The early United States multicenter experience. J Am Coll Cardiol 1996; 27(suppl A):279A.
57. Rodriguez AE, Fernandez M, Santaera O, et al. Coronary stenting in patients undergoing percutaneous transluminal coronary angioplasty during acute myocardial infarction. Am J Cardiol 1996; 77:685–689.
58. Hoorntje JC, Suryapranata H, de Boer MK, et al, for the ESCOBAR study group: Primary stenting for acute myocardial infarction: Preliminary results of a randomized trial. Circulation 1996; 94:I-570.
59. Katz S, Chepurko L, Ong LY, et al. Is stent deployment during acute myocardial infarction superior to balloon angioplasty? Circulation 1996; 94:I-576.
60. Medina A, Hernandez J, Suarez J, et al. Primary stent treatment for acute evolving myocardial infarction. Circulation 1996; 94:I-576.
61. Glatt B, Diab N, Chevalier B, et al. Prospective primary stenting in acute myocardial infarction. Circulation 1996; 94:I-577.
62. Valeix BH, Labrune PJ, Massiani PF. Systematic coronary stenting in the first eight hours of acute myocardial infarction. Circulation 1996; 94:I-577.
63. Schomig A, Neumann FJ, Walter H, et al. Coronary stent placement in patients with acute myocardial infarction: Comparison of clinical and angiographic outcome after randomization to antiplatelet or anticoagulant therapy. J Am Coll Cardiol 1997; 29:28–34.
64. Siegel RM, Underwood P, Barker B, et al. Stenting in acute myocardial infarction may improve procedural and long-term outcomes. J Am Coll Cardiol 1997; 29(suppl A):72A.
65. Rodriguez A, Fernandez V, Bernardi C, et al. Coronary stents improved hospital results during coronary angioplasty in acute myocardial infarction: Preliminary results of a randomized controlled study (GRAMI Trial). J Am Coll Cardiol 1997; 29(suppl A):221A.
66. Stone GW, Brodie B, Griffin J, et al. Safety and feasibility of primary stenting in acute myocardial infarction—in-hospital and 30 day results of the PAMI stent pilot trial. J Am Coll Cardiol 1997; 29(suppl A):389A.
66a. Wright RS, Nunez GS, Reeder SL, et al: Intracoronary stent therapy enhances luminal diameter and reduces residual stenosis in a subset of patients with acute myocardial infarction. J Am Coll Cardiol 1997; 29(Suppl A):236A.
67. Saito S, Hosokawa G, Suzuki S. Primary stent implantation is superior to balloon angioplasty in acute myocardial infarction—the result of Japanese PASTA (Primary Angioplasty Versus Stent Implantation in Acute Myocardial Infarction) Trial. J Am Coll Cardiol 1997; 29(suppl A):390A.
68. Benzuly KH, O'Neill WW, Gangadharan V. Stenting in acute myocardial infarction (STAMI): Bailout, conditional and planned stents. J Am Coll Cardiol 1997; 29(suppl A):456A.
69. Ganim M, Wong P, Grover R, et al. Superiority of coronary stenting compared to balloon angioplasty in acute myocardial infarction. J Am Coll Cardiol 1997; 29(suppl A):456A.
70. Antoniucci D, Santoro GM, Bolognese L, et al. Elective stenting in acute myocardial infarction: Preliminary results of the Florence randomized elective stenting in acute coronary occlusion (FRESCO) study. J Am Coll Cardiol 1997; 29(suppl A):456A.
71. Ellis SG, Ribeiro da Silva E, Heyndrickx GR, et al, for the RESCUE Investigators. Randomized comparison of rescue angioplasty with conservative management of patients with early failure of thrombolysis for acute anterior myocardial infarction. Circulation 1994; 90:2280–2284.
72. Ellis SG, Van De Werf F, Ribeiro da Silva E, et al. Present status of rescue coronary angioplasty: Current polarization of opinion and randomized trials. J Am Coll Cardiol 1992; 19:681.
73. Gibson CM, Cannon CP, Greene RM, et al. Rescue angioplasty in the TIMI 4 Trial. Am J Cardiol 1997; 80:21–26.
74. McKendall GR, Forman S, Sopko G, et al, and the Thrombolysis in Myocardial Infarction Investigators: Value of rescue percutaneous transluminal coronary angioplasty following unsuccessful thrombolytic therapy in patients with acute myocardial infarction. Am J Cardiol 1995; 76:1108–1111.
75. Califf RM, Topol EJ, Stack RS, et al, for the TAMI Study Group. Evaluation of combination thrombolytic therapy and timing of cardiac catheterization in acute myocardial infarction. Circulation 1991; 83:1543.
76. Fung AY, Lai P, Topol EJ, et al. Value of percutaneous transluminal coronary angioplasty after unsuccessful intravenous streptokinase therapy in acute myocardial infarction. Am J Cardiol 1986; 58:686.
77. Holmes DR, Gersh BJ, Bailey KR, et al. Emergency "rescue" percutaneous transluminal coronary angioplasty after failed thrombolysis with streptokinase. Circulation 1990; 81:IV-51.
78. Grines CL, Nissen SE, Booth DC, et al. Efficacy, safety and cost effectiveness of a new thrombolytic regimen for acute myocardial infarction using half dose tPA with full dose streptokinase. Circulation 1988; 78:II-304.
79. Muller DW, Topol EJ, Ellis SG, et al. Determinants of the need for early acute intervention in patients treated conservatively after thrombolytic therapy for acute myocardial infarction. J Am Coll Cardiol 1991; 18:1594.
80. Baim DS, Diver DJ, Knatterud GL, and the TIMI II-A Investigators. PTCA "salvage" for thrombolytic failures—implications from TIMI 2A. Circulation 1988; 78:II-112.
81. Abbottsmith CW, Topol EJ, George BS, et al. Fate of patients with acute myocardial infarction with patency of the infarct-related vessel achieved with successful thrombolysis versus rescue angioplasty. J Am Coll Cardiol 1990; 16:770–778.
82. Muller DW, Topol EJ, Ellis SG, et al. Determinants of the need for early acute intervention in patients treated conservatively after thrombolytic therapy for acute myocardial infarction. J Am Coll Cardiol 1991; 18:1594–1601.
83. Gacioch GM, Topol EJ. Sudden paradoxical clinical deterioration during angioplasty of the occluded right coronary artery in acute myocardial infarction. J Am Coll Cardiol 1989; 14:1202–1209.
84. Califf RM, O'Neill W, Stack RS, et al. Failure of simple clinical measurements to predict perfusion status after intravenous thrombolysis. Ann Intern Med 1988; 108:658–662.
85. Kwon K, Freedman B, Wilcox I, et al. The unstable ST segment early after thrombolysis for acute myocardial infarction and its usefulness as a marker of recurrent coronary occlusion. Am J Cardiol 1991; 67:109–115.
86. Laperche T, Steg PG, Hanssen M, et al. A study of biochemical

markers of reperfusion early after thrombolysis for acute myocardial infarction: The PERM study group: Prospective evaluation of reperfusion markers. Circulation 1995; 92:2079–2086.

87. Gibson CM, Cannon CP, Daley WL, et al, for the TIMI 4 Investigators. The TIMI Frame Count: A quantitative method of assessing coronary artery flow. Circulation 1996; 93:879–888.
88. Gibson CM, Cannon CP, Marble SJ, et al. The Corrected TIMI Frame Count (CTFC) predicts clinical outcomes in acute MI. Circulation 1996; 94:I-441.
89. Gibson CM, Goel M, Dotani I, et al. The Post-PTCA TIMI Frame Count and Mortality in RESTORE. Circulation 1996; 94:I-85.
90. Gibson CM, Daley WL, Rizzo MJ, et al. Flow following primary PTCA for acute MI. Circulation 1996; 94:I-670.
91. Smalling RW, Bode C, Kalbfleisch J, et al. More rapid, complete, and stable coronary thrombolysis with bolus administration of reteplase compared with alteplase infusion in acute myocardial infarction: RAPID investigators. Circulation 1995; 91:2725–2732.
92. Cannon CP, McCabe CH, Gibson CM, et al, and the TIMI 10A Investigators. TNK-tissue plasminogen activator in acute myocardial infarction: Results of the Thrombolysis in Myocardial Infarction (TIMI) 10A dose-ranging trial. Circulation 1997; 95:351–356.
93. Vanderschueren S, Stockx L, Wilms G, et al. Thrombolytic therapy of peripheral arterial occlusion with recombinant staphylokinase. Circulation 1995; 92:2050–2057.
94. Lefkovits J, Ivanhoe RJ, Califf RM, et al, for the EPIC Investigators. Effects of platelet glycoprotein IIb/IIIa receptor blockade by a chimeric monoclonal antibody (abciximab) on acute and six month outcomes after percutaneous transluminal coronary angioplasty for acute myocardial infarction. Am J Cardiol 1996; 77:1045–1051.

PART

II INTERVENTIONS FOR SECONDARY PREVENTION

17 Lipid-Lowering Therapy

▶ B. Greg Brown
▶ Xue-Qiao Zhao

There have been important recent advances in the understanding of the vascular biology of atherogenesis in terms of the dynamic interplay between atherosclerotic plaque size, vasomotor tone, blood flow, thrombosis, and, most recently, the pathologic processes that lead to plaque disruption and clinical ischemic events. This chapter reviews a series of angiographic *regression* trials completed in the past decade in patients with established coronary artery disease (CAD). It also reviews larger clinical endpoint trials of secondary prevention for CAD. This chapter interprets these studies from the perspective of the underlying pathologic processes, the treatment of which appears to contribute to enhanced perfusion, plaque stability, or both in this clinical setting. It summarizes the evidence supporting the unifying hypothesis that lipid depletion from two important plaque pools results in plaque stability and reduced clinical events.

CLINICAL TREATMENT GOALS FOR PATIENTS WITH CORONARY ARTERY DISEASE

Comprehensive management of CAD has two fundamental clinical goals. The first goal is to reduce the severity of ischemic symptoms. The presence of ischemia indicates an impairment of the capacity of the vascular bed to meet fully the varying oxygen demands of the myocardium. This impairment is usually due to a flow-limiting coronary stenosis,[1, 2] the physiologic impact of which may be modulated by abnormal epicardial vessel tone,[3, 4] by intermittent arterial vasospasm,[5] by inadequate vasodilatory reserve[6] in its distal bed, or by insufficient collateral development.

A variety of medical approaches are now used to relieve symptoms by favorably altering this oxygen supply-demand imbalance. Alternatively, this objective of symptom relief may be accomplished through more direct structural or physiologic (or both) changes favorably affecting the diminished vascular perfusion capacity. These include development of collaterals, relaxation of excess vasoconstrictor tone, or improvement in the severity of flow-limiting stenosis (*regression*). Regression has been debated as a possible mechanism for symptom relief. This chapter reviews evidence for the occurrence of regression, together with the role of lipid-lowering therapy in achieving it; mechanisms contributing to regression are also discussed.

The second fundamental clinical goal in CAD is to prevent the anticipated worsening of symptoms or progression to a clinical event such as cardiac death, myocardial infarction (MI), or worsening angina requiring bypass surgery or angioplasty. This chapter reviews briefly the mechanisms of gradually progressive arterial obstruction and mechanisms of plaque disruption resulting in abrupt worsening of arterial obstruction. Evidence is presented that indicates a linkage between lipid lowering and stabilization of the plaque structure. This set of observations supports the idea that lipid-lowering therapy prevents clinical events by selectively lipid depleting or *regressing* a relatively small subgroup of lipid-rich plaques that are at high risk of plaque disruption, ulceration, and hemorrhage and that account for the great majority of clinical events.

EVIDENCE FOR REGRESSION OR DELAYED PROGRESSION OF CORONARY ARTERY DISEASE

Understanding of atherosclerosis regression comes from animal experiments and from clinical arteriographic studies. There are important biologic and methodologic differences between the various experimental models of atherosclerosis and the human disease. Accordingly, concepts emerging from these two views are not always equivalent. Even the basic term *regression* means something quite different to the experimental pathologist than to the clinician, as can be seen in terms of the histologic sections of Figure 17–1. To the pathologist, *regression* means shrinkage of intimal plaque through a reduction in its major components—smooth muscle, macrophages, connective tissues, and lipid. To the clinician interpreting human disease from its arteriographic appearance, *regression* has traditionally been defined as an enlargement in the caliber of the narrowed arterial lumen. Such enlargement occurs only occasionally in the natural course of the disease.[7] Regression may occur by plaque shrinkage but also, as discussed subsequently, by a variety of other possible mechanisms. For example, relaxation of arterial vasomotor tone can similarly improve lumen caliber.[3, 4] Lysis of fully or partially occlusive thrombi is observed commonly in the course of unstable ischemic syndromes.[8, 9] Wound healing may favorably alter an acutely disrupted plaque.[10] Remodeling of the underlying arterial architecture can improve arteriographic lumen caliber independently of changes in plaque size.[11–14] Understanding of the principal process(es) by which arteriographic regression occurs in patients is limited because these images do not permit an easy distinction among the aforementioned mechanisms.

Thus, the key question is not does arteriographic regression occur in patients (it does), but can such regression be promoted with a sufficiently great *magnitude* and *frequency* to justify a major therapeutic strategy? Important related questions are what are its mechanisms, and does regression provide clinical benefits and if so how? Although there is not yet a consensus, the emerging evidence is encouraging.

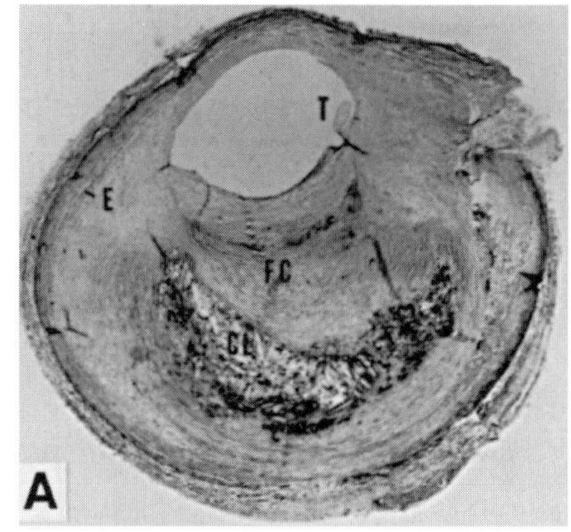

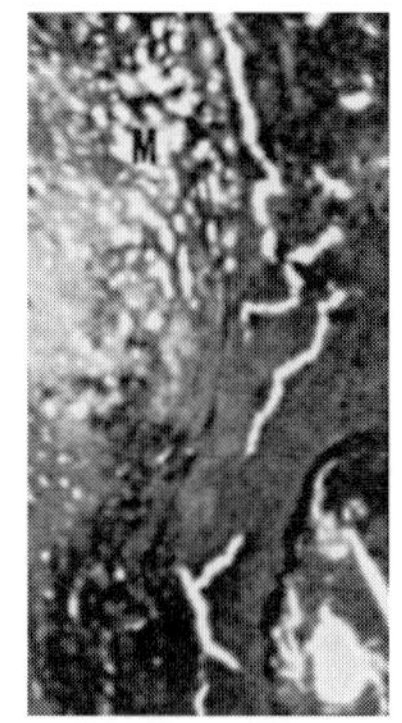

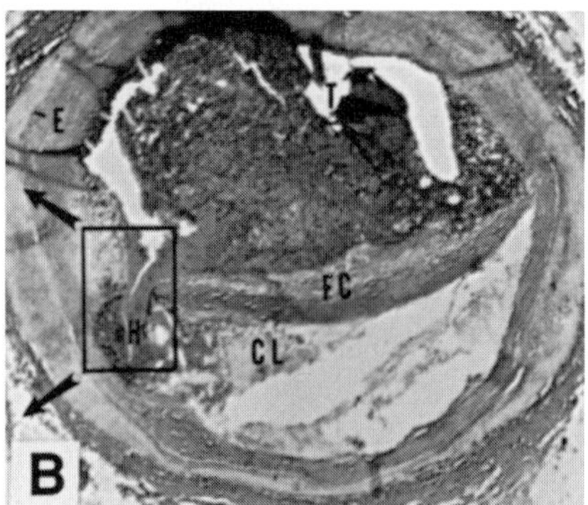

Figure 17–1 *A,* Histologic section through a structurally stable coronary plaque in a patient with vasospastic angina. Morphologic features include internal elastic lamina (E); a thick fibrous cap (FC) composed largely of collagen and smooth muscle cells (SMC); core lipid (CL), here largely crystalline; and a small tag of thrombus (T). *B,* Section through a structurally unstable coronary plaque in a patient dying from myocardial infarction. The lumen, only moderately narrowed by the plaque, is acutely occluded by thrombus (T). There are many features in common with the section in *A.* In the unstable plaque, core lipid (some dislodged by sectioning artifact) composes a much larger fraction of the plaque. The fibrous cap is much thinner than in *A* and is fissured (or vented) at its left shoulder, permitting a small pocket of hemorrhage (H) in the plaque. This fissure, the associated hemorrhagic pocket, and the plaque shoulder, here rich in lipid-laden macrophages (M) (round, bright spots), are shown at increased magnification in the *inset.* Also at higher magnification (not shown), the fibrous cap has few SMC but many M. (*B* from Brown BG, Zhao X-Q, Sacco DE, et al: Lipid lowering and plaque regression: New insights into prevention of plaque disruption and clinical events in coronary disease. Circulation 1993; 87:1781–1791.)

Evidence for Regression in Experimental Models

Atherosclerosis has been shown convincingly to regress with dietary cholesterol lowering in the nonhuman primate studies of Wissler, Armstrong, Clarkson, and Small and their colleagues.[15–19] In the typical regression experiment, the amount and composition of intimal disease among cholesterol-fed animals is assessed at specified times, using group-averaged chemical and histologic endpoints. During sustained consumption of an *atherogenic* diet, plasma cholesterol may increase to more than 600 mg/dL, and there are substantial rises in coronary artery content of collagen (three times), elastin (four times), and cholesterol (seven times, mostly esterified). On return to a native vegetarian *regression* diet, plasma cholesterol falls quickly to normal (140 mg/dL), and the arterial lipid and connective tissue accumulations partially regress over 20 to 40 months. Collagen content does not decline much from its peak value (−20%), but elastin (−50%) and cholesterol (−60%) do,[17, 19] and there is a fibrous transformation that atrophies the myointimal cellular response.[20] Not all forms of cholesterol are readily depleted from these lipid-rich intimal deposits. The more mobile forms, including cholesteryl esters in foam cells, lipoproteins, and cholesteryl ester droplets, are depleted in response to lowered plasma cholesterol,[18] but the cholesterol monohydrate crystals of the core lipid region are resistant to mobilization.[18, 20] By histologic morphometry, plaque mass is reduced during regression therapy.[16, 18, 21]

Evidence for Regression in the Patient with Coronary Artery Disease

As late as 1987, there was only anecdotal evidence from pioneering angiographic studies[22] that the observations of regression in animals could be extended to patients with atherosclerotic disease. A series of randomized clinical arteriographic trials has provided a perspective on the magnitude of, frequency of, and conditions under which regression can occur in patients.[22–41] These trials have incorporated more powerful therapeutic regimens to modify lipids and more objective methods for analysis of the arteriogram. The most recent trials have examined the effect of *monotherapy*, frequently using one of the hydroxymethylglutaryl–coenzyme A (HMG-CoA) reductase inhibitors, on angiographic disease. These trials and their lipid response data are summarized in Table 17–1. Their results, based on arteriographic and clinical outcomes, are summarized in Table 17–2 and Figures 17–2 through 17–5.

Despite the diversity among these trials in clinical presentation, lipid entry requirements, treatment regimens, duration, and methods for arteriographic analysis, the outcomes (see Table 17–2) are surprisingly consistent. Most studies demonstrated a benefit from treatment, whether by diet or by diet supplemented by other lifestyle changes or by lipid-lowering drugs. As a generalization of the composite of results (not a meta-analysis), 8% of the *control* group patients were found to regress during the study period, and more than 50% progressed. By contrast, about 25% of *treated* patients regressed and 25% progressed. This type of comparison is illustrated using Familial Atherosclerosis Treatment Study (FATS) data in Figure 17–2.

As a generalization from Table 17–2, averaged estimates of disease severity, per patient, worsened (progressed) by about 3% stenosis among the controls. Disease actually improved (regressed) by 1% to 2% stenosis among the patients treated with *combination therapy*. In the *monotherapy* studies, with somewhat less pronounced low-density lipoprotein (LDL) cholesterol and high-density lipoprotein (HDL) cholesterol treatment changes, net regression did not occur. Nevertheless, the delays in progression were usually statistically significant because the group variance of these estimates of disease change were also quite small—a testament to the precision of the quantitative coronary arteriographic (QCA) methods (Fig. 17–3).

Disease progression in saphenous vein coronary bypass grafts was examined in the Post Coronary Artery Bypass Graft Trial.[40] LDL cholesterol, averaging 155 mg/dL at baseline, fell 39% with aggressive therapy (lovastatin 76 mg per day, mean, with or without cholestyramine) and fell 14% with moderate therapy (lovastatin 4 mg per day). After 4.3 years of follow-up, progression was seen on adjusted average in 27% of grafts per patient among the aggressive therapy group and in 39% among the moderate therapy group ($P < 0.001$); repeat revascularization was required in 6.5% and 9.2% of patients ($P = 0.03$). An inadequate dosage of warfarin in this trial had no effect on graft obstruction.

Correlates of Progression and Regression

Multivariate statistical analysis has been used to identify those factors correlated with change in disease severity. Such change was usually characterized, per patient, either as the mean difference (final-baseline) in percent stenosis (%S) or minimum lumen diameter (MLD) among all lesions measured. These analyses have found that reduction of LDL cholesterol or its components (apolipoprotein B [apo B]) or reduction of the LDL cholesterol-to-HDL cholesterol ratio[22] has been a frequently observed correlate of arterial benefit. The percent change from baseline levels in risk variables has often shown better correlation with disease change than the in-treatment levels of those same variables (see Fig. 17–3).[26] Despite clear evidence that LDLs are atherogenic, the exact mechanisms are yet to be determined. Proposed modifications of LDLs that appear to increase their atherogenicity include oxidation, aggregation, glycation, enzymatic degradation, and delipidation with diminished particle size—possibly as a result of increased hepatic lipase activity. The importance of small dense LDL particles (metabolically linked to high triglycerides, low HDL-cholesterol, hypertension, insulin resistance syndrome, diabetes, and increased hepatic lipase activity) is becoming increasingly evident.[42–48]

Blood pressure reduction,[26] apo C-III distribution,[49] Lp(a) levels,[50] and compliance with lifestyle changes have also emerged in one or more studies. In the National Heart, Lung and Blood Institute Type II (NHLBI-II), FATS, University of California–SCOR (UC-SCOR), Lifestyle Heart Study, and St. Thomas'

TABLE 17–1 • Summary Descriptions for 16 Reported Arteriographic Lipid-Lowering Trials: Lipid Response to Treatments

Study*	*n*	Entry Requirements	Control Regimen†	Treatment Regimen	Treatment Response LDL (%)	Treatment Response HDL (%)	Years
Combination Therapy Studies							
CLAS	188	CABG	D (−)	D + R + N	−43	+37	2
POSCH	838	MI, CHOL	D	D + PIB ± R	−42	+5	9.7
LIFESTYLE	48	CAD	U	V + M + E	−37	−3	1
FATS (N + C)	146	CAD, APO B	D ± R	D + R + N	−32	+43	2.5
FATS (L + C)	146	CAD, APO B	D ± R	D + R + L	−46	+15	2.5
CLAS II	138	CABG	D	D + R + N	−40	+37	4
STARS (D + R)	90	CAD, CHOL	U	D + R	−36	−4	3
SCRIP	300	CAD	U	D + (R/N/L/F) + E, BP	−22	+12	4
HEIDELBERG	113	CAD	U	D + Ex	−8	+3	1
HARP	91	CAD, normal Lipids	D ± R	P ± N ± R ± F	−41	+13	2.5
Monotherapy Studies							
NHLBI	143	CAD, LDL	D	D + R	−31	+8	5
STARS (D)	90	CAD, CHOL	U	D	−16	0	3
MARS	270	CAD	D	D + L	−38	+9	2
CCAIT	331	CAD, CHOL	D	D + L	−29	+7	2
PLAC I	408	CAD, LDL	D	D + P	−28	+9	3
MAAS	381	CAD	D	D + S	−31	+9	4
REGRESS	885	CAD	D	D + P	−29	+10	2
BECAIT	92	MI, CHOL	D	D + B	−3	+9	5
LCAS	429	CAD	D	D + Fl ± R	−24	+4	−2.5

*See text for the details and full name of these studies.
†Mean response to control regimen: LDL cholesterol = −7%, HDL cholesterol = 0%.
CAD, coronary artery disease; LDL, low-density lipoprotein >90th percentile; CABG, coronary artery bypass graft surgery; MI, myocardial infarction; apo B, apolipoprotein B ≤125 mg/dL; FH, familial hypercholesterolemia; CHOL, cholesterol >220 mg/dL; D, diet; U, usual care; R, resin (colestipol or cholestyramine); N, nicotinic acid; PIB, partial ileal bypass; V, vegetarian diet <10% fat; M, relaxation techniques; Ex, exercise program; L, lovastatin; S, simvastatin; C, colestipol; F, fibrate-type drugs; Fl, fluvastatin; B, bezafibrate; BP, blood pressure therapy.

Atherosclerosis Regression Study (STARS), the insertion of these predictive variables in the analysis abolished the association of benefit with treatment group, implying that the effect of therapy on arterial disease was mediated by its effect on the risk variable(s) identified. It would appear from the more recent *monotherapy* studies that the magnitude of arterial and clinical benefit is somewhat reduced when LDL cholesterol, HDL cholesterol, or both are less intensively altered. The Howard Atherosclerosis Reversibility Project (HARP)[32] and the Canadian Coronary Atherosclerosis Intervention Trial (CCAIT)[34] call into question the merits of treating patients with more normal lipid levels, although CLAS[23] and FATS[26] tend to support treatment of such patients. The HARP results are difficult to interpret because they combine lesion change data from vessels treated with bypass and angioplasty as well as untreated native vessels. When clinical outcomes and native disease only are considered, HARP tends to be consistent with other angiographic trials, with a nonsignificant ($P = 0.19$) 33% reduction in ischemic events and a tendency toward delayed progression ($P = 0.07$). When women are included in these studies,[30, 51] the arterial treatment benefits appear comparable to those of men.

Figure 17–4 provides examples of lesion regression seen in intensively treated FATS patients over a 2.5-year period. As Figures 17–4 and 17–5 indicate, regression may occur in mild, moderate, and severe lesions. Although regression was somewhat more frequent among the more severe lesions, the relative benefit from therapy was roughly uniform over the spectrum of disease severity. Lesions that did regress improved by an average of 19 ± 12(SD)%S or by an average of 16 ± 5%S after excluding regression owing to recanalization of 12 initially occluded arteries. Thus, only a few lesions (about 5%) undergo natural or spontaneous regression by the criterion amount of 10%S or less (see Fig. 17–5). Although this number can be significantly increased (to about 12%) by lipid-lowering therapy, the great majority of stenoses do not improve even with *intensive* regimens that result in marked alterations in the lipid and lipoprotein profile. Yet these regimens are commonly associated with much more substantial reductions in clinical event rate (see Table 17–2). This apparent paradox is discussed later.

Figure 17–5 shows that the likelihood of a lesion's *progression* is, in part, determined by its baseline severity. Intensive lipid-lowering therapy decreases, by about fourfold, the likelihood of definite lesion progression among mild (10% to 40%) and moderate (40% to 70%) lesions but does not appear to benefit the small number of severe (70% to 98%) lesions studied.

TABLE 17–2 • Summary of Arteriographic Outcomes, Treatment Lipid Response, and Frequencies of Reported Clinical Events in 16 Lipid-Lowering Coronary Arteriographic Trials

	Control Patients				Changes Among Treated Patients				% Event§
Study*	*Progression*	*Regression*	Δ%S†	ΔMLD (mm)†	*Progression*	*Regression*	Δ%S (P)‡	ΔMLD (P)‡	*Reduction*
Combination Therapy Studies									
CLAS	61%	2%	—	—	39%	16%	—	—	25%
POSCH (10 y)	65%	6%	—	—	37%	14%	—	—	35% (62%¶)**
LIFESTYLE	32%	32%	+3.4%	—	14%	41%	−2.2 (.001)‖	—	0 vs. 1
FATS (N + C)	46%	11%	+2.1%	−0.05	25%	39%	−0.9 (.005)	+0.035 (0.005)	80%**
FATS (L + C)	46%	11%	+2.1%	−0.05	22%	32%	−0.7 (.02)	+0.012 (0.06)	70%
CLAS II	83%	6%	—	—	30%	18%	—	—	43%
STARS (D + R)	46%	4%	+5.8%	−0.23	12%	33%	−1.9 (.01)	+0.12 (0.001)	89%**
SCRIP	50%	10%	+3.2%	−0.20	50%	20%	+1.2 (.02)	−0.08 (.003)	39%**
HEIDELBERG	42%	4%	+3.0%	−0.13	20%	30%	−1.0 (.05)‖	0.00 (0.05)	−27%††
HARP	38%	15%	+2.4%	−0.17	33%	13%	+2.1 (NS)	−0.12 (NS)	33%
Monotherapy Studies									
NHLBI	49%	7%	—	—	32%	7%	—	—	33%
STARS (D)	46%	4%	+5.8%	−0.23	15%	38%	−1.1 (NS)	+0.03 (0.05)	69%**
MARS	41%	12%	+2.2%	−0.06	29%	23%	+1.6% (0.2)	−0.03 (0.2)	29%
CCAIT	50%	7%	+2.9%	−0.09	33%	10%	+1.7% (0.04)	−0.05 (0.01)	22%
PLAC I	38%	14%	+3.4	−0.15	26%	14%	+2.1% (0.13)	−0.09 (0.04)	13% (54%)‡‡
MAAS	32%	12%	3.6%	−0.13	23%	19%	1.0 (0.006)	−0.04 (0.007)	22%
REGRESS	NA	NA	NA	−0.09	NA	NA	NA	−0.03 (0.001)	39%**
BECAIT	NA	NA	+4.3	−0.17	NA	NA	+1.7 (0.07)	−0.06 (0.049)	77%**
LCAS	39	8	+2.8	−0.10	29	15	+0.6 (0.01)	−0.3 (0.005)	20%

* See text for the details, abbreviations, and full name of these studies. Progression and regression are variably defined, per patient, in each study.

§ Events are variably defined in these studies; in general, the frequency of cardiovascular events (death, myocardial infarction, unstable ischemia requiring revascularization or hospitalization, or both) in control and treated groups are compared using the sometimes sketchy details and definitions provided.

† Δ(%S) is usually reported as the average change in percent stenosis over all the lesions measured per patient. A positive (+) value represents *progression;* (−), *regression.* ΔMLD is a similar estimate for change in minimum lumen diameter, averaged for all lesions.

‡ *P*-value for comparison of Δ%S or ΔMLD in control vs. treated groups.

‖ Statistical comparison in Lifestyle uses a lesion-based method.

** Studies for which the reduction in cardiovascular clinical events was statistically significant.

†† A reduction of −27% means 27% increase (NS).

‡‡ 54% reduction in coronary heart disease death and nonfatal myocardial infarction.

¶ 62% reduction in coronary bypass surgery.

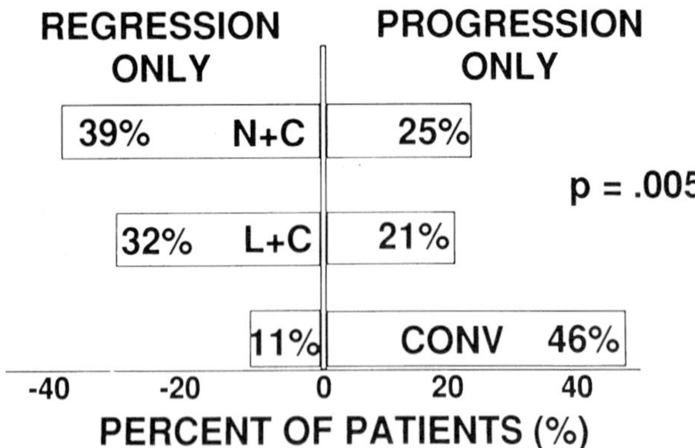

Figure 17–2 Effect of therapy in FATS on the per-patient frequency of proximal lesion progression (worsening by ≥10% of at least one of nine lesions without any improving by that much) or of regression (converse of above). In comparison with conventional treatment, the frequency of per-patient progression is halved, and regression is tripled with the two more intensive lipid-altering strategies. See Table 17–2 for comparable data in other studies.

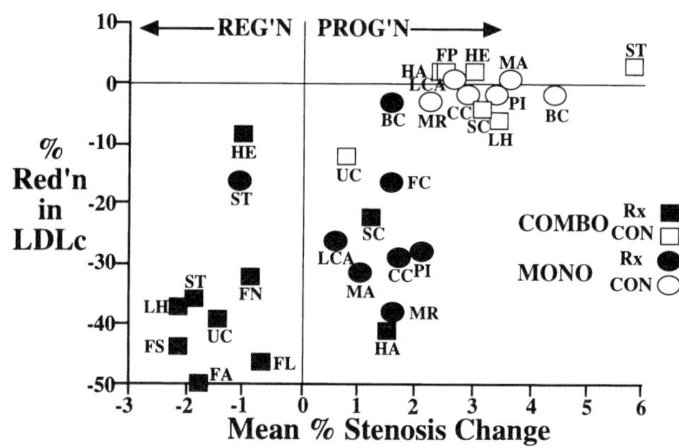

Figure 17–3 Data from reported angiographic trials relating the percentage of low-density lipoprotein lowering, from baseline, with the average change in coronary percent stenosis, per patient, in each treatment group. Comparisons are made between the therapy (Rx) and control (CON) groups for studies using drug combinations (combo) and single drugs (mono). See Tables 17–1 and 17–2 for details. Codes—LH: Lifestyle[25]; FN, FL, FC, FP: FATS (niacin, lovastatin, colestipol, placebo)[26]; ST: STARS[29]; SC: SCRIP[30]; HE: Heidelberg[31]; HA: HARP[32]; MR: MARS[33]; CC: CCAIT[34]; PI: PLAC I[35]; MA: MAAS[36]; BC: BCCAIT[38]; LCA: LCAS[39]; FS, FA: FHRS.[41]

EVIDENCE FOR REDUCED ISCHEMIA

In its natural history, angina pectoris may worsen gradually or abruptly. It may also improve (even completely disappear) in many cases. Independent of physiologic adaptations, angina may vary in frequency and severity based simply on changes in medication, climate, altitude, and level of activity. As a consequence, demonstrating an independent contribution to improvement in angina from lipid-lowering therapy is difficult. Angina-related variables are therefore considered *soft* endpoints; as such, their change has not been measured or reported in most trials. Nonetheless, most physicians have the sense that patients often experience a substantial reduction, or disappearance, of angina after 3 to 12 months of effective lipid treatment. Angina frequency, severity, and duration were reported in the Lifestyle Heart Study,[25] in which physicians and patients were not blinded to intervention. Disregarding this potential bias, patients on the program of strict vegetarian diet, exercise, and relaxation techniques had reductions in angina frequency (91%), in duration (42%), and in

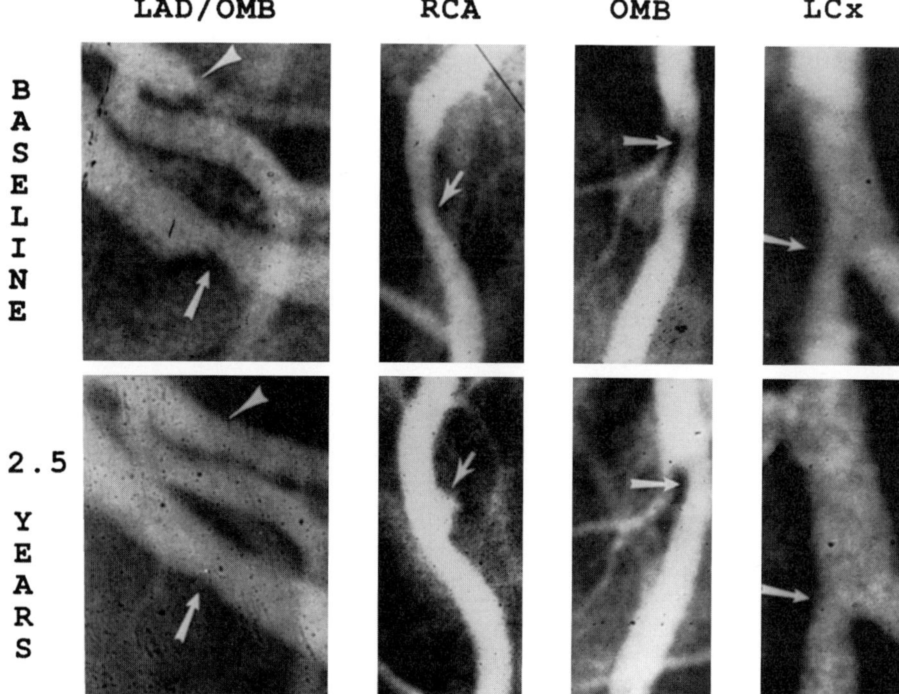

Figure 17–4 Examples of definite regression in intensively treated patients in FATS. *Top row,* Baseline. *Bottom row,* 2.5 years later. left anterior descending artery (LAD) (top arrow), (100→20%S); obtuse marginal branch (OMB) (bottom arrow), (39→18%S); right coronary artery (RCA) (48→30%S) (note plaque ulcer at 2.5 years); OMB (69%→37%); left circumflex artery (LCx) (44→30%S). (Modified with permission from Brown BG, Albers JJ, Fisher LD, et al: Regression of coronary artery disease as a result of intensive lipid-lowering therapy in men with high levels of apolipoprotein B. N Engl J Med 1990; 323:1289–1298. Copyright 1990, Massachusetts Medical Society. All rights reserved.)

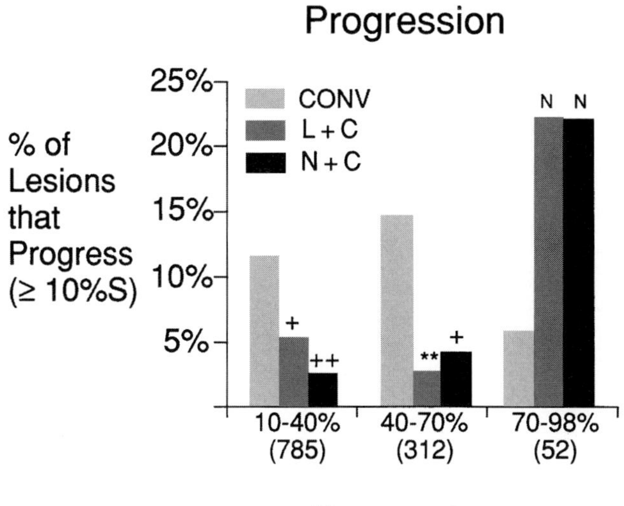

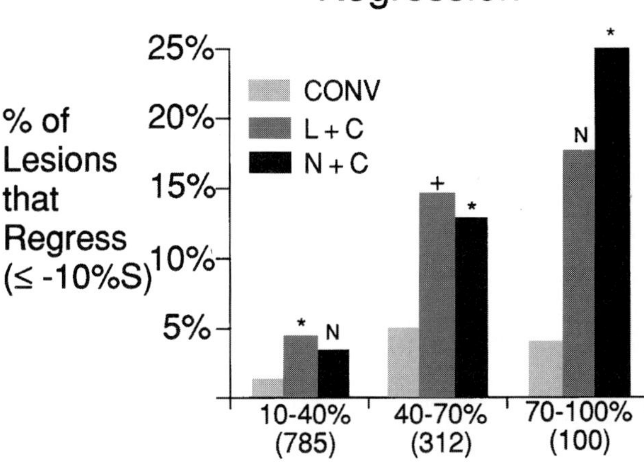

Figure 17–5 Frequency of definite lesion change in FATS, expressed as the percentage of lesions that decrease in severity (regress) by a measured 10% stenosis or more. Lesions from 120 patients are subgrouped into 785 mild stenoses (10→40%S), 312 moderate stenoses (40→70%S), and 52 severe stenoses (70→98%S). Also, 48 lesions, initially totally occluded, are added to the severe lesion regression analysis because these may *regress* by recanalization. In general, change is relatively infrequent. The more severe the lesion at baseline, the more likely its change. Intensive lipid-lowering therapy increases regression frequency at all levels of severity. See Table 17–1 for abbreviations. χ^2 statistical comparisons versus control group (CONV) frequency: $^{*}P < 0.05$; $^{+}P < 0.02$; $^{**}P < 0.005$; $^{++}P < 0.001$; N, not significant. (From Brown BG, Zhao X-Q, Sacco DE, et al: Lipid lowering and plaque regression: New insights into prevention of plaque disruption and clinical events in coronary disease. Circulation 1993; 87:1781–1791.)

severity (28%), whereas control group patients experienced worsening.

Perfusion imaging (positron-emission tomography) in the Lifestyle patients showed consistent improvement in the treated group and evenly mixed changes in the control group.[52] Similarly, in the Heidelberg trial, exercise-rest thallium studies demonstrated significant improvement in balance of regional perfusion in the group receiving American Heart Association (AHA) phase III diet counseling and regular exercise, whereas the control group was unchanged.[53] The Scandinavian Simvastatin Survival Study (4S) investigators have reported that in patients with angina at entry, simvastatin treatment does not improve angina but significantly reduces its likelihood of worsening, relative to control.[54]

Ambulatory monitoring has been used to demonstrate a substantial reduction in ischemic ST-segment changes during daily living in patients with known CAD who were given diet counseling and 20 to 40 mg per day of lovastatin versus its placebo. Previously documented, silent ST-segment depression completely resolved after 4 to 6 months in 13 of 20 treated patients, as compared with 2 of 20 in the placebo group ($P < 0.001$).[55] Further studies are needed to determine the frequency, magnitude, and time course of angina relief attributable to lipid alteration.

EVIDENCE FOR REDUCED CLINICAL EVENTS

Angiographic Trials

Table 17–2 provides evidence that clinical cardiac events are decreased by lipid-lowering therapy. The majority of these smaller studies report event reductions, although each trial reports events somewhat differently. In general, when reported, the authors have classified as clinical events *cardiac death, confirmed MI, and progressive or unstable ischemia requiring revascularization.* In nearly every study, the frequency of clinical cardiovascular events was reduced substantially by treatment, although the reductions achieved statistical significance in only 7 of 16 studies. Failure to confirm a significant clinical treatment benefit is not unexpected because the trials using arteriographic endpoints were powered to demonstrate arteriographic effects, using patient samples with marginal power to detect clinical benefits. The data from FATS in Table 17–2 demonstrate a 70% to 80% reduction in event rate ($P < 0.01$), compared with control, among intensively treated patients. In the angiographic trials, taken as a whole, clinical cardiovascular events are consistently and substantially reduced by lipid-lowering therapy.

Clinical Endpoint Trials

A number of secondary prevention trials addressing the effect of lipid therapy have been published. Four informative examples are presented here (Table 17–3).

Table 17–3 • Summary of Large, Long Randomized Secondary Prevention Trials of Lipid-Lowering Therapy, 1975–1996

									Effects of Treatment					
												% Reduction in Clinical Events†		
					Baseline				% Change in Lipids†					
Study	*n*	%F‡	Entry Requirement	Duration (ys)	*Age (y)*	*LDLc*	*HDLc (mg/dL)*	*Cholesterol*	LDLc	HDLc (%)	Cholesterol	Coronary Death + Nonfatal MI	PTCA or CABG	All-Cause Mortality
CDP-Niacin	3908	0	MI	6.2	45	NA	NA	252	NA	NA	−10%	15%*	67%*	4%[ns]
				15							NA			11%**
CDP-Clofibrate	3892	0	MI	6.2	45	NA	NA	251	NA	NA	−7%	7%[ns]	41%[ns]	0%
				15							NA			1%[ns]
POSCH	838	9	MI	9.7	51	178	40	250	−38%	+4%	−23%	35%**	62%***	21%[ns]
4S	4444	19	MI or AP	5.5	59	188	46	260	−35%	+8%	−25%	34%****	37%****	30%**
CARE	4159	14	MI	5.0	59	139	39	209	−28%	+5%	−20%	24%*	27%**	9%[ns]

Statistical confidence: NS, not significant. *$P < 0.01$, **$P < 0.001$, ***$P < 0.0001$, ****$P < 0.00001$.
†Mean in-treatment changes, relative to control group. Intention-to-treat analysis.
‡Percent female participants.
LDLc, low-density lipoprotein cholesterol; HDLc, high-density lipoprotein; MI, myocardial infarction; AP, angina pectoris; PTCA, percutaneous transluminal coronary angioplasty; CABG, coronary artery bypass grafting.

CORONARY DRUG PROJECT—NIACIN AND CLOFIBRATE

One of the earliest randomized studies reported in secondary prevention of CAD, the Coronary Drug Project, compared niacin (3 g per day), clofibrate (1.8 g per day), D-thyroxine (6 grains per day) and two doses of estrogen (5 and 2.5 mg per day) with a placebo-treated control group in more than 8000 men with prior MI.[56] The D-thyroxine and both of the estrogen groups were discontinued because of adverse effects. The clofibrate group experienced clinical cardiovascular outcomes comparable with the control group (see Table 17–3). The niacin group had a significant 15% reduction in the composite endpoint (cardiac death and nonfatal MI) ($P = 0.01$) after 6.2 years' mean follow-up. Of great interest was the observation, after 15 years of total follow-up, of an 11% reduction in all-cause mortality ($P = 0.0004$) among men originally assigned to niacin relative to those originally assigned to placebo, despite niacin's discontinuation for 9 years after completion of the planned 6-year follow-up (see Table 17–3).[57]

PROGRAM FOR SURGICAL CONTROL OF THE HYPERLIPIDEMIAS

Partial ilial bypass, an intestinal diversion procedure, was developed by Buchwald[58] as a surgical means for cholesterol lowering. He subsequently evaluated this operation as a means for CAD prevention in the Program for Surgical Control of the Hyperlipidemias (POSCH). A total of 838 patients with cholesterol greater than 220 mg/dL who had survived a first MI were randomly assigned to surgery or to medical management in a *usual care* strategy in the pre-statin era.[24] The surgical group averaged 42% reduction in LDL cholesterol, relative to control. After 9.7 years' mean follow-up, the surgical group had a 35% reduction in the composite endpoint, death plus nonfatal MI, and a 65% reduction in the need for *coronary* bypass surgery (see Tables 17–1 through 17–3). Progression of disease by angiogram in years 0 to 3 in the POSCH control group predicted a fourfold greater mortality risk over the subsequent 7 years,[59] supporting the utility of angiographic trials as surrogates for larger clinical trials.[60]

SCANDINAVIAN SIMVASTATIN SURVIVAL STUDY TRIAL

The 4S trial[61] adds to the now-irrefutable evidence that secondary prevention with lipid-lowering therapy provides major clinical benefit. In this group of 4444 men and women with a history of MI, angina pectoris, or both, a 38% LDL cholesterol reduction with simvastatin in the treated group was associated with a 42% reduction, relative to the control group, in cardiac death ($P < 0.00001$) and a 30% reduction in all-cause mortality ($P = 0.003$) (see Table 17–3). This is the first randomized trial of lipid therapy in which all-cause mortality was significantly reduced.

Subgroup analyses of 4S have been reported. In terms of the variable *major coronary events* (coronary death or nonfatal MI, 34% overall risk reduction with simvastatin), there is a similar benefit from treatment for women; those over 65 years old (small subgroup); and those taking acetylsalicylic acid, beta blockers, and calcium channel antagonists, as compared with their respective counterparts. There was a modest treatment advantage for those younger than 60 years old (39% risk reduction versus 29% for those ≥60 years old), for those with hypertension (37% vs. 32%), and for never-smokers (41% versus 31% for ex- and current smokers). The small subgroup with diabetes (5% of total patients) achieved striking reductions in major coronary events (55% vs. 32% for those without diabetes). A cost-effectiveness evaluation of the 4S results, applied to the U.S. health care system, suggests that the cost of treatment with simvastatin (wholesale acquisition cost, excluding monitoring costs) would be nearly completely (88%) offset by the drug-induced reduction in hospitalization and revascularization expenses.[62]

CHOLESTEROL AND RECURRENT EVENTS TRIAL

The Cholesterol and Recurrent Events (CARE) Trial[63] was designed to address the efficacy of monotherapy with pravastatin among patients with *typical* cholesterol levels after MI. Entry criteria included cholesterol less than 240 mg/dL, LDL cholesterol 115 to 174 mg/dL, and fasting triglycerides less than 350 mg/dL at least 5 weeks post MI. At baseline, cholesterol averaged 209 mg/dL, triglycerides 155 mg/dL, LDL 139 mg/dL, and HDL 39 mg/dL. More than half of these patients had prior percutaneous transluminal coronary angioplasty or coronary artery bypass grafting. See Table 17–3 for results. The primary endpoint, coronary heart disease death or nonfatal MI, was reduced 24% by treatment; fatal MI was reduced by 37% and revascularization by 27%. Subgroup analyses showed patients with hypertension, those with diabetes, those previously revascularized, or those with low left ventricular ejection fraction fared as well as their respective counterparts without these features. There were modest treatment advantages to those older than 60 or with prior Q wave MIs or with HDL cholesterol 37 mg/dL or less. Striking treatment advantages were found for women (46% risk reduction vs. 20% for men (P = NS), for current smokers (33% vs. 22% for ex-smokers or nonsmokers), for those with triglycerides less than the median, 144 mg/dL (32% vs. 15% for ≥144 mg/dL), and particularly for those with the highest baseline LDL cholesterol levels (3% risk *increase* for those with LDL cholesterol <125 mg/dL, 26% risk reduction when LDL cholesterol >125 to 150 mg/dL, and 35% reduction when LDL cholesterol >150 to 175 mg/dL). This finding calls into question the National Cholesterol Education Program guideline of target LDL cholesterol 100 mg/dL or less in patients with CAD. The substantial difference between 4S and CARE in characteristics predicting an increased treatment benefit, however, is a reminder that subgroup analyses may be misleading in trials powered only to address the primary outcome. In this regard, the lack of treatment benefit to those with LDL cholesterol less than 125 mg/dL in CARE requires further confirmation.

WEST OF SCOTLAND CORONARY PREVENTION STUDY

Although not technically a secondary prevention study, the West of Scotland Coronary Prevention Study (WOSCOPS)[64] is another study demonstrating reduced coronary events and drug safety among 6595 patients treated with either 40 mg daily of pravastatin or its placebo. The endpoint, *coronary death* or *nonfatal MI,* was reduced by 31% with pravastatin and all-cause mortality by 22% ($P = 0.051$).

SUMMARY

The five examples presented provide convincing evidence that lipid-lowering therapy reduces clinical cardiovascular events without important toxicity. Women, diabetics, older patients (>65 years old), and those with other cardiovascular risk factors appear to fare at least as well as their counterpart groups in terms of relative risk reduction. The amount of risk reduction in all the trials seems disproportionate to the average 1 to 2%S regression in lesion severity seen in the angiographic trials and with the fact that only about 12% of all intensively treated lesions actually regress (see Fig. 17–5). In the following section, this apparent paradox is addressed.

Trials Pending Completion

Three important larger clinical trials and two angiographic trials may shed further light on issues that are not completely resolved. The results of two of these have been reported at national meetings; these preliminary results are briefly summarized here.

LIPID

LIPID is an Australian trial among 9014 men and women with baseline LDL cholesterol ranging between 131 and 167 mg/dL and with HDL averaging 36 mg/dL with a history of acute MI or unstable angina.[65] Randomized therapy is 40 mg daily of pravastatin or placebo. An initial report indicates a 24% reduction ($P < 0.001$) in coronary death and nonfatal MI, and a 23% reduction in all-cause mortality ($P < 0.001$).

AIR FORCE/TEXAS CORONARY ATHEROSCLEROSIS PREVENTION STUDY

The Air Force/Texas Coronary Atherosclerosis Prevention Study (AFCAPS/TexCAPS) primary prevention trial has enrolled 6605 men and women without prior cardiovascular disease and LDL cholesterol ranging between 130 and 160 mg/dL with HDL cholesterol 45 mg/dL (47 in women).[66] Randomized therapy is 20–40 mg daily of lovastatin or placebo. An initial report indicates a 35% reduction with lovastatin in coronary death and nonfatal MI but identical total mortality rates in the two treatment groups in this relatively low-risk population.

HDL-ATHEROSCLEROSIS TREATMENT STUDY

HDL-Atherosclerosis Treatment Study (HATS), a double-blind angiographic trial, will study the effect of lipid-altering therapy (simvastatin 10 to 20 mg daily plus niacin 2 to 4 g daily) or antioxidant vitamins (E, C, and β-carotene combined) on the progression of CAD and on defined clinical events.[67] Therapy is randomized in a factorial design. Baseline LDL cholesterol averages 125 mg/dL and HDL cholesterol 31 mg/dL. All patients have established CAD. Additional studies examining therapy for low HDL cholesterol include the Air Force Regression Study (AFREGS), a quantitative angiographic study, and HDL Intervention Trial (HIT), a Department of Veterans' Affairs cooperative trial, for which details are not obtainable.

MECHANISMS OF BENEFIT

Pathologic Processes in Dyslipidemia and Their Alteration with Lipid Therapy

This section focuses briefly on several clinically important aspects of plaque biology that are adversely affected in dyslipidemia. In addition, current understanding of the effects of lipid-altering therapy on these atherogenic processes is briefly reviewed.

ENDOTHELIUM-DEPENDENT PROCESSES

At the critical interface between flowing blood and the vessel wall, the endothelial monolayer mediates important short-term and long-term homeostatic responses. In certain atherogenic states, specific forms of endothelial dysfunction have been clearly documented. Clinicians are likely to find, when the endothelium is better understood, that its generalized dysfunction in atherogenic states broadly diminishes vascular homeostatic capacity.

Vasodilatory Dysfunction

The epicardial coronary arteries and the coronary microvascular bed normally dilate in response to increased flow demands. One mechanism is the flow-dependent endothelial production of endothelium-derived relaxing factor,[68] which is nitric oxide.[69] Atherosclerosis risk factors, including hypercholesterolemia,[70] diabetes mellitus,[71] estrogen deficiency,[72] low HDL cholesterol,[73] elevated Lp(a),[74] small dense LDL particles,[75] and hypertension,[76] all impair endothelium-dependent vascular relaxation. Absent this vasodilatory mechanism, the circulating vasoconstrictors dominate vascular response at loci of such endothelial dysfunction. This imbalance appears to account for the apparently paradoxic epicardial coronary vasoconstriction effects of isometric[77] and aerobic[78] exercise in patients with CAD. Vasodilatory dysfunction is experimentally reversed by reducing dietary cholesterol,[79] despite persistence of intimal thickening. Furthermore, vascular smooth muscle responsiveness to direct dilators is largely unaltered by atherosclerosis. Vasodilatory dysfunction is therefore believed to be a direct effect of these risk factors on the local availability of nitric oxide, owing to either inhibition of constitutive nitric oxide synthesis[80] or quenching of released nitric oxide by superoxide ion.[81] Evidence has accumulated that therapy of these risk factors reverses the associated vasodilatory dysfunction.[72, 82–87] The effects of estrogen and of LDL apheresis are almost immediate.[72, 86] Restoration of flow-mediated vasodilation would raise the angina threshold, perhaps accounting for diminished ambulatory ischemia within 4 to 6 months among lovastatin-treated patients.[55]

Enhanced Thrombogenesis

Thrombus formation at sites of plaque rupture is the final step in the process leading to the acute ischemic syndromes. Although this chapter cannot detail the spectrum of prothrombotic processes, the reader is referred to related reviews.[88, 89] There are some intriguing links to hyperlipidemia that are discussed briefly. Risk of arterial thrombosis is determined by a complex interplay among factors leading to disruption of atherosclerotic plaque, to activation of fibrinogen, and to impaired fibrinolysis. The last-mentioned depends on a balance between the cellular synthesis and release of plasminogen activators (tissue- and urokinase-type plasminogen activator) and of plasminogen activator inhibitors, principally PAI-1.[90] The procoagulant state associated with elevated fibrinogen levels has been epidemiologically linked to clinical CAD.[91] Furthermore, platelet aggregability is increased in hypercholesterolemia,[92] possibly related to inhibition of platelet nitric oxide release.[93] Lp(a), an LDL particle complexed to a protein with high sequence homology to plasminogen,[94] has been associated with increased risk of MI,[95] has been shown experimentally to interfere with fibrinolysis,[96] and is linked with the stuttering course of acute MI.[97]

Cells of the vessel wall may also contribute to a procoagulant state. Endothelial dysfunction may impair the cellular production or release of tissue plasminogen activator. Macrophages and smooth muscle cells colocalize with tissue factor in atherectomy specimens from patients with unstable (but not stable) angina.[98]

Healing and Remodeling

The processes involved in the homeostatic regulation of arterial lumen size are not yet fully deciphered. Evidence indicates that flow and fluid shear stress at the endothelial interface play important roles. By developmental regulation of vessel size in the branching epicardial coronary tree, basal blood flow velocity is held relatively constant at about 10 to 20 cm per second in branches ranging from large to small. This implies a relatively constant basal shear stress. In conditions of high basal flow, such as arteriovenous fistulas, coronary segments can grow to four times normal diameter, stabilizing size at diameters that result in subturbulent Reynold's numbers ($Re = 4\rho / \pi\mu D < 2000$).[14] This capacity for flow-dependent remodeling appears to require a functioning endothelium.[13] Glagov and colleagues[11] and Clarkson and associates[12] have shown for humans and for nonhuman primates that overall vessel size increases in concert with the growth of intimal atherosclerosis to maintain a constant lumen size. This adaptive remodeling fails when plaque area approaches 40% of area circumscribed by the internal elastica. Flow-dependent remodeling, although incompletely understood, almost certainly stands as another example of normal endothelial function. States of endothelial dysfunction are likely to interfere with this process.

PLAQUE LIPID ACCUMULATION

LDL and more recently Lp(a) have been localized in the intimal extracellular space. Intimal lipid also accumulates intracellularly in subendothelial monocyte-derived macrophages.[99, 100] Such *foam cell* formation is thought to occur by unregulated scavenger receptor uptake of modified LDL[101, 102] and possibly of Lp(a)[103, 104] by macrophages. Smooth muscle cells may also become foam cells. Foam cells are abundant in precursor fatty streak lesions[105]; in the cap of early fibrous plaques; and in the shoulders, cap, and basilar neovascular complex of advanced plaques.[106] Lipid may enter the core region of the fibrous plaque by transmural flux[107] of its more mobile forms (lipoprotein particles, perifibrous droplets, and vesicles[108–110]), or it may be deposited there as a result of foam cell necrosis.[105] There, lipids coalesce into lower energy phases dictated by the local cholesterol, phospholipid, and cholesteryl ester concentrations.[18] Cholesteryl ester droplets and vesicles and cholesterol monohydrate crystals are the dominant core lipids.[18, 106]

Roberts and others[111–114] have studied plaque composition as it relates to certain aspects of the spectrum of clinical atherosclerosis. Briefly, by quantitative morphometry of the histologic section, they have determined the proportion of intimal area that is contributed by each of the principal plaque components: (1) dense fibrous tissue, (2) cellular fibrous tissue, (3) calcific deposits, (4) inflammatory infiltrates, (5) extracellular core lipid (as *pultaceous debris*), and (6) foam cell lipid.[111] They separated serially sampled arterial sections into four ranges of lumen area reduction. They found, on average, that early intimal involvement is almost entirely fibrocellular, but at the stage of severe arterial obstruction, the cellular contribution has declined to about 25% of total intimal area, whereas dense fibrous tissue occupies about 50%. Foam cells appear in some numbers when intimal involvement is moderate; their fraction increases to 10% of area in the more severe stages, then declines in the most severe. Calcific deposits and extracellular lipid become relatively abundant in the more severe stages; each increases progressively to contribute, on average, about 10% of intimal area in the most severe. Younger women (<40 years old) with CAD were found to have significantly less dense fibrous tissue and more cellular connective tissue and lipid-rich foam cells than their older male counterparts, suggesting a greater potential for reversibility.[112] Conversely the very elderly showed a tendency toward a more fibrotic disease and had significantly fewer foam cells than younger men and women.[113] The above-mentioned reports describe *average plaque morphology*. Some plaques in this spectrum have considerably greater lipid deposits and, as seen later, greater risk of plaque disruption. It is unclear why certain arterial segments develop lipid-rich plaques, whereas adjacent segments have the more stable fibrous intimal involvement.

PLAQUE DISRUPTION IN ACUTE ISCHEMIC SYNDROMES

Acute ischemic syndromes are most commonly precipitated when sites of mild or moderate atherosclerotic narrowing become disruptively transformed into severely obstructive culprit lesions. As illustrated in Figure 17–1*B*, such a transformation usually involves fissuring of the fibrous cap of the atheroma, often with intramural hemorrhage and mural or occlusive thrombus. The plaque at high risk for such fissuring and subsequent hemorrhage or thrombosis usually has a large core lipid pool and a structurally weakened fibrous cap. The cap can be weakened by the migration or death of its smooth muscle cells, by an accumulation of lipid-laden macrophages, or by proteolytic or mechanical damage to its collagen. Evolving insights into three major aspects of atherosclerosis have greatly altered understanding of the precipitation of plaque events leading to acute clinical events.

First, *mild* and *moderate* coronary lesions (<70% stenosis) may progress abruptly to severe obstruction, with resulting unstable angina, MI, or death. In fact, a majority of clinical events occur under these circumstances.[8, 115–117] When the lesion precipitating an MI has, by chance, been seen on a recent angiogram, its preinfarct severity averages 50% stenosis, and its morphology does not usually suggest that it is destined soon to become occluded.[8, 115–117] Although a given severe (≥70%) lesion is more likely to progress or totally occlude than a less severe lesion, clinical events are more frequently triggered by lesions that are initially mild or moderate because (1) these are much more numerous in the patient's anatomy[118] and (2) because the majority of occlusions of *severe* stenoses occur without an event.[119] The plaque mass of a 30% angiographic stenosis exceeds 50% of normal lumen area and often substantially more in the setting of arterial remodeling. Thus, it is inappropriate to refer to these as *small* plaques.[120]

A second insight was originally brought into focus by Constantinides[121] but has received renewed attention.[10, 122–128] For the great majority of ischemic coronary events, a culprit lesion can be identified with variations of the following disruptive morphologic features at histologic examination, as illustrated in Figure 17–1*B*: (1) a fissure, tear, or vent in the fibrous cap overlying the core lipid pool; (2) thrombus adherent at the site of the fissure; (3) bleeding into the core lipid region; and (4) severe arterial obstruction by the composite mass of expanded plaque and thrombus. Angiographic examples of plaques that have become unstable and caused a clinical event are shown in Figure 17–6.

A third insight is that there are features of plaque structure and lipid composition that predict the risk of fissuring.[124–132] Fissures of the arterial intima rarely

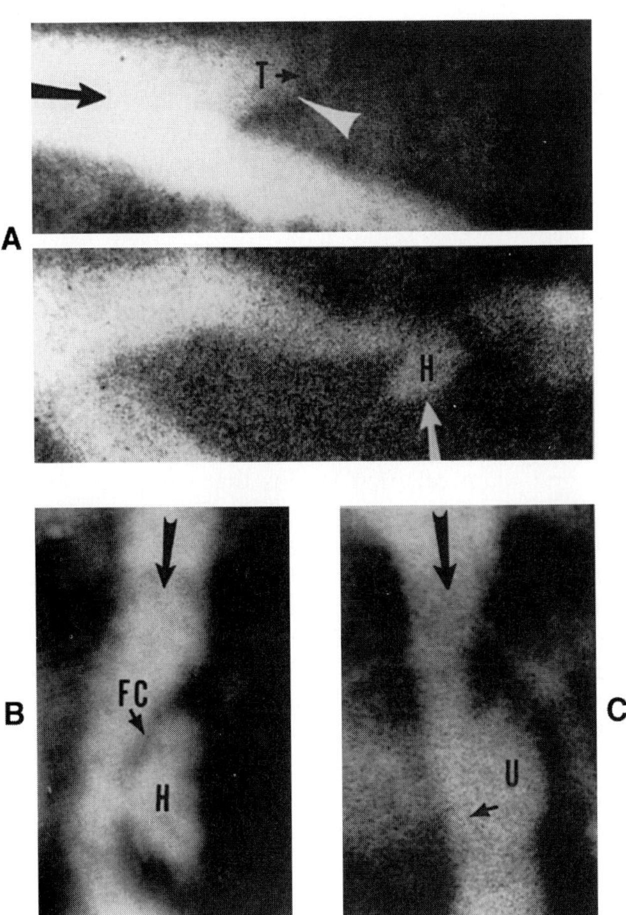

Figure 17–6 Highly magnified arteriographic images of structurally unstable plaques causing unstable angina or myocardial infarction. *A,* This left anterior descending artery is acutely occluded; 24 hours after intravenous tissue plasminogen activator, the thrombotic component (T) of the obstruction is lysed, revealing a pocket of contrast (H) protruding beyond the lumen boundaries into presumed plaque and fed through a narrow-necked fissure. This appears to be the arteriographic counterpart of the hemorrhagic pocket (H) in Figure 17–1*B*. *B,* Angiographically visualized plaque hemorrhage. Bleeding into the lipid-rich core of the plaque appears to have formed a hemorrhagic pocket (H), which has driven the thin fibrous cap (FC) into the lumen, progressively obstructing it. The opposite wall has been remodeled, curving outward to preserve lumen size in the face of the expanding plaque. On cine, contrast material enters this pocket from the lumen via small breaks or channels at its upstream shoulder and exits via a mid-FC vent. *C,* A large ulcer (U) is seen after tissue plasminogen activator for unstable angina. This image appears to have been created by full-length erosion or eruption of the FC, of which only a thin arteriographic vestige remains (arrow). (From Brown BG, Zhao X-Q, Sacco DE, et al: Lipid lowering and plaque regression: New insights into prevention of plaque disruption and clinical events in coronary disease. Circulation 1993; 87:1781–1791.)

occur in the absence of atheroma. The greater the plaque core lipid content, the greater the likelihood of its disruption,[111, 125, 126] as illustrated in Figure 17–1*B*. Yet in any given patient, only a small subgroup of all plaques (perhaps one in eight) has a substantial core lipid accumulation. Certain aspects of fibrous cap composition also heighten the risk of fissuring. The macrophage density in disrupted caps is greater than that in intact caps.[124] Fissuring occurs most commonly at the shoulder of an eccentric lipid-rich plaque (see Fig. 17–1*B*), a location of high macrophage density[125] and also of high circumferential stress,[125 126] when there is significant core lipid. Finally, the fibrous cap is thinned and weakened by the cytotoxic decline of smooth muscle cells[133, 134] and by lysis of collagen.[131, 135] The perception of plaque disruption as a *passive* process related to the softness and size of the core lipid pool and the strength of the fibrous cap is being refined as understanding of the *active* macrophage inflammatory mechanisms evolves.[128–132, 136] Atherectomy specimens from culprit lesions for unstable angina have a significantly higher macrophage content than those from stable angina lesions.[129] Macrophages release metalloproteinases such as interstitial collagenase, gelatinase, and stromalysin, all of which have been identified in atherosclerotic plaques[130] and in cultured macrophages.[131] The inflammatory aspect of macrophages and T cells is emphasized by Van der Wal and colleagues,[128] who uniformly identified increased macrophage density at focal sites of plaque erosion or disruption, colocalizing with focal expression of HLA-DR inflammatory antigens.

Therapy directed at reduction of plasma LDL would be expected to reduce the likelihood of plaque disruption because of the experimentally documented favorable effects of LDL lowering on macrophage foam cell density, core lipid pool size, and intimal LDL concentration.[18] As a clinical consequence, LDL-lowering therapy ought to decrease the frequency of abrupt progression to clinical events. This has been the case. Analysis of 13 coronary events among 146 FATS patients reveals that the events each were precipitated by a culprit coronary lesion in the distribution of worsening ischemia that had progressed significantly in severity from the baseline stenosis measurement to that at the time of the event.[26] As seen in Figure 17–7, the *culprit* lesions causing the great majority (eight of nine) of cardiac events among the *conventionally* treated patients arose from a pool of 414 lesions that were mild or moderate at baseline. By comparison, only 1 of 683 such lesions progressed to an event in the two *intensively* treated patient groups ($P < 0.004$, per patient or per lesion). The few lesions that were severe ($\geq$70%S) at baseline, however, did not appear to benefit from lipid-lowering therapy.

Lipid Depletion for Plaque and Clinical Stability: Hypothesis that Fits the Facts

OBSERVATIONS

- Of unstable clinical episodes (e.g., MI), 60% to 90% are due to disruption and thrombosis of lipid-rich plaques.[121, 122, 124, 127–129]

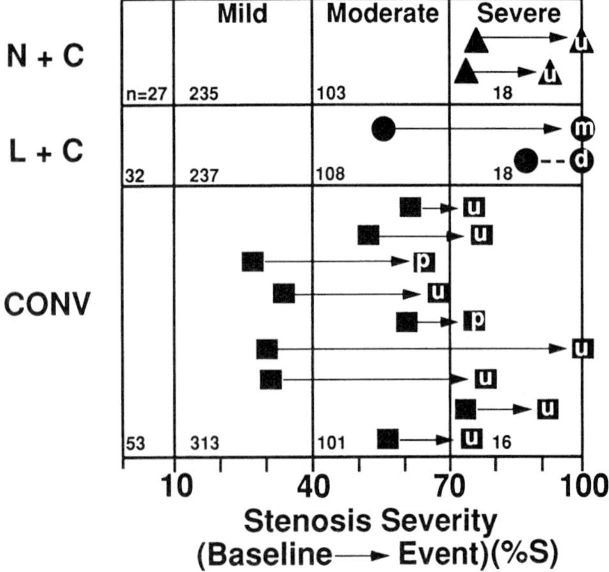

Figure 17–7 Lesion changes associated with the 13 coronary events as measured from 1316 lesions in 120 FATS patients. Among lesions exposed to intensive lipid-lowering therapy, only 1 of 683 mild or moderate lesions, at baseline, among 74 such patients progressed to a clinical event (see Fig. 17–5 for definitions), whereas 8 of 414 such lesions among 46 conventionally treated patients did so (per patient or per lesion, $P < 0.004$). By this standard, severe lesions did not appear to benefit from therapy. N, niacin; C, colestipol; L, lovastatin; CONV, conventional therapy; u, unstable angina event; m, myocardial infarction; d, death; p, progressive angina; %S, percentage diameter stenosis. The number in each panel represents the number of lesions at risk, at baseline, in each subgroup. (From Brown BG, Zhao X-Q, Sacco DE, et al: Lipid lowering and plaque regression: New insights into prevention of plaque disruption and clinical events in coronary disease. Circulation 1993; 87:1781–1791.)

- Plaque lipid may be depleted by normalizing elevated plasma cholesterol.[15–19]
  - Lipid-laden macrophages (foam cells) disappear within 6 months.[16–18]
  - Core lipid volume begins to diminish after 6 months.[18]
  - After 2 years, 60% of plaque cholesterol depleted.[16]
  - Plaque shrinkage primarily due to cholesteryl ester depletion.[16, 18]
- Plaque instability is predicted by its lipid-related features.[122]
  - Area of the core lipid region as a percent of total plaque area.[132]
  - Foam cell number in fibrous cap and shoulder regions.[121, 122, 124, 127–129]
  - Foam cell stromalysin, one of a family of inflammatory metalloproteinases that can weaken the fibrous cap.[130, 131]
- Only about 15% of human coronary lesions are lipid-rich plaques (>50% lipid, by volume).[132]
- Only about 12% of all coronary lesions visibly regress (≥10% stenosis change) with intensive lipid-lowering therapy.[26]
- Clinical benefits from intensive lipid-lowering therapy are associated with a 10-fold reduction in the frequency of abrupt progression of mild or moderate coronary lesions to become severe lesions (see Fig. 17–7).[26]

UNIFYING HYPOTHESIS

Angiographic coronary stenosis regression, seen in 12% of all coronary lesions during intensive lipid-lowering therapy, reflects depletion of cholesteryl esters selectively from the *vulnerable* subgroup of lipid-rich and foam cell–rich lesions that comprise about 15% of all visible coronary lesions. Such lipid depletion typically reduces stenosis severity by 10% to 20% but, more importantly, stabilizes the plaque in terms of its mechanical strength, inflammatory activity, and endothelial functional integrity. The plaque fibrous cap is strengthened by favorable geometric changes and by a marked reduction in the number of intimal inflammatory cells (macrophages and T lymphocytes), which secrete proteolytic enzymes. Plaque stabilization by these mechanisms appears to explain the substantial reduction of clinical events associated with intensive lipid-lowering therapy.

SUMMARY

The consensus of evidence from angiographic trials demonstrates both coronary artery and clinical benefits from lipid-lowering therapy, using any of a variety of treatment regimens. The findings of decreased arterial disease progression and increased regression have been convincing but, at best, modest in their magnitude. For example, among those treated intensively in FATS, the mean improvement in proximal stenosis severity was less than 1%S per patient; only 12% of all lesions showed convincing regression. In view of these modest arterial benefits, the associated reductions in major cardiovascular events have been surprisingly great (24% to 35% in three large trials [see Table 17–3]). Coronary events were reduced 75% with more intensive lipid-lowering therapy in FATS; this was entirely explained by a 93% reduction in the likelihood that a mildly or moderately diseased arterial segment would experience substantial progression to become the severe lesion that triggered the clinical event. The authors believe the magnitude of the clinical benefit is best explained in terms of this observation, using the following lines of reasoning. Clinical events most commonly spring from lesions that are initially of mild or moderate severity and that abruptly undergo a disruptive transformation to a severe *culprit* lesion. The process of *plaque fissuring* leading to plaque disruption and thrombosis triggers most clinical coronary events. Fissuring is predicted by a large accumulation of core lipid in the plaque and by a high density of lipid-laden macrophages in its thinned fibrous cap. Lesions with these characteristics compose only 10% to 20% of the overall lesion population but account for 80% to 90% of the acute clinical events. In the experimental setting, normalization of an atherogenic lipid profile substantially decreases the number of lipid-laden intimal macrophages (foam cells) and gradually depletes cholesterol from the core lipid pool. In the clinical setting, intensive lipid-lowering therapy virtually halts the progression of mild and moderate lesions to severe obstructions precipitating clinical events.

The reduction in clinical events observed in these trials appears to be best explained by the relationship of the lipid and foam cell content of the plaque to its likelihood of fissuring and by the effects of lipid-lowering therapy on these *high-risk* features of plaque morphology. The composite of data presented here supports the hypothesis that lipid-lowering therapy selectively lipid depletes (regresses) that relatively small but dangerous subgroup of fatty lesions containing a large lipid core and dense clusters of intimal macrophages. By doing so, these lesions are effectively stabilized, and clinical event rate is accordingly decreased.

Acknowledgments

The efforts of Brad Sousa in preparing this manuscript are greatly appreciated. This chapter has been extensively modified from an article published previously.[27]

REFERENCES

1. Demer LL, Gould KL, Goldstein RA, et al. Assessment of coronary artery disease severity by positron emission tomography: Comparison with quantitative arteriography in 193 patients. Circulation 1989; 79:825–835.
2. Klocke FJ. Measurements of coronary flow reserve: Defining pathophysiology versus making decisions about patient care. Circulation 1987; 76:1183–1189.
3. Ludmer PL, Selwyn AP, Shook TL, et al. Paradoxical vasoconstriction induced by acetylcholine in atherosclerotic coronary arteries. N Engl J Med 1986; 315:1046–1051.
4. Nabel EG, Selwyn AP, Ganz P. Large coronary arteries in humans are responsive to changing blood flow: An endothelium-dependent mechanism that fails in patients with atherosclerosis. J Am Coll Cardiol 1990; 16:349–356.
5. Kaski JC, Crea F, Meran DO, et al. Local coronary super sensitivity to diverse vasoconstrictive stimuli in patients with variant angina. Circulation 1986; 74:1255–1265.
6. Cannon RO, Camici PG, Epstein SE. Pathophysiological dilemma of syndrome x. Circulation 1992; 85:883–892.
7. Brown BG, Bolson EL, Pierce CD, et al. Regression of atherosclerosis in man: Current data and their methodological limitations. *In* Malinow MR, Blaton VH (eds): Regression of Atherosclerotic Lesions. New York, Plenum Press, 1984, pp 289–310.
8. Brown BG, Gallery CA, Badger RS, et al. Incomplete lysis of thrombus in the moderate underlying atherosclerotic lesion during intracoronary infusion of streptokinase for acute myocardial infarction: Quantitative angiographic observations. Circulation 1986; 73:653–661.
9. TIMI IIIA Investigators. Early effects of tissue-type plasminogen activator added to conventional therapy on the culprit coronary lesion in patients presenting with ischemic cardiac pain at rest: Results of the Thrombolysis in Myocardial Ischemia (TIMI IIIA) trial. Circulation 1993; 87:1–14.
10. Fuster V, Badimon L, Badimon JJ, et al. The pathogenesis of coronary artery disease and the acute coronary syndromes. N Engl J Med 1992; 326:242–250, 310–318.
11. Glagov S, Weisenberg E, Zarins CK, et al: Compensatory enlargement of human atherosclerotic coronary arteries. N Engl J Med 1987; 316:1371–1375.
12. Clarkson TB, Pritchard RW, Morgan TM, et al. Remodeling of coronary arteries in human and non-human primates. JAMA 1994; 271:317–318.
13. Langille BL, O'Donnell F. Reductions in arterial diameter produced by chronic decreases in blood flow are endothelium dependent. Science 1986; 231:405–407.
14. Jaffe RB, Glancy DC, Epstein SE, et al. Coronary arterial–right heart fistulae: Long-term observations in seven patients. Circulation 1973; 47:133–143.
15. Wissler RW, Vesselinovitch D. Can atherosclerotic plaques regress? Anatomic and biochemical evidence from nonhuman animal models. Am J Cardiol 1990; 65:33–40.
16. Armstrong ML, Megan MB. Lipid depletion in atheromatous coronary arteries in rhesus monkeys after regression diets. Circ Res 1972; 30:675–680.
17. Clarkson TB, Bond MG, Bullock BC, et al. A study of atherosclerosis regression in Macaca mulatta: IV. Changes in coronary arteries from animals with atherosclerosis induced for 19 months and then regressed for 24 or 48 months at plasma cholesterol concentrations of 300 or 200 mg/dL. Exp Mol Pathol 1981; 34:345–368.
18. Small DM, Bond MG, Waugh D, et al. Physiochemical and histological changes in the arterial wall of nonhuman primates during progression and regression of atherosclerosis. J Clin Invest 1984; 73:1590–1605.
19. Armstrong MC, Megan MB. Arterial fibrous protein in cynomolgus monkeys after atherogenic and regression diets. Circ Res 1975; 36:256–261.
20. Brown BG, Fry DL. The fate and fibrogenic potential of subintimal implants of crystalline lipid in the canine aorta: Quantitative histological and autoradiographic studies. Circ Res 1978; 43:261–273.
21. Carew TE, Schwenke DC, Steinberg D. An antiatherogenic effect of probucol unrelated to its hypocholesterolemic effect: Evidence that antioxidants in vivo can selectively inhibit low density lipoprotein degradation in macrophage-rich streaks slowing the progression of atherosclerosis in the WHHL rabbit. Proc Natl Acad Sci U S A 1987; 84:7725–7729.
22. Levy RI, Brensike JF, Epstein SE, et al. The influence of changes in lipid values induced by cholestyramine and diet on progression of coronary artery disease: Results of the NHLBI Type II Coronary Intervention Study. Circulation 1984; 69:325–337.
23. Blankenhorn DH, Nessim SA, Johnson RL, et al. Beneficial effects of colestipol niacin therapy on coronary atherosclerosis and coronary venous bypass grafts. JAMA 1987; 257:3233–3240.
24. Buchwald H, et al. Effect of partial ileal bypass on mortality and morbidity from coronary heart disease in patients with hypercholesterolemia: Report of the Program on Surgical Control of the Hyperlipidemias (POSCH). N Engl J Med 1990; 323:946.
25. Ornish D. Can lifestyle changes reverse coronary heart disease? Lancet 1990; 336:129–133.
26. Brown BG, Albers JJ, Fisher LD, et al. Regression of coronary artery disease as a result of intensive lipid-lowering therapy in men with high levels of apolipoprotein B. N Engl J Med 1990; 323:1289–1298.

27. Brown BG, Zhao X-Q, Sacco DE, et al. Lipid lowering and plaque regression: New insights into prevention of plaque disruption and clinical events in coronary disease. Circulation 1993; 87:1781–1791.
28. Cashin-Hemphill L, Mack WJ, Pogoda MJ, et al. Beneficial effects of colestipol-niacin on coronary atherosclerosis. JAMA 1990; 264:3013–3017.
29. Watts GF, Lewis B, Brunt JNH, et al. Effects on coronary artery disease of lipid-lowering diet, or diet plus cholestyramine, in the St. Thomas' Atherosclerosis Regression Study (STARS). Lancet 1992; 339:563–569.
30. Alderman E, Haskell WL, Fain JM, et al. Beneficial angiographic and clinical response to multifactor modification in the Stanford Coronary Risk Intervention Project (SCRIP) (abstract). Circulation 1991; 84(suppl II):II-140.
31. Schuler G, Hambrecht R, Schlierf G, et al. Regular physical exercise and low-fat diet: Effects on progression of coronary artery disease. Circulation 1992; 86:1–11.
32. Sacks, F, Pasternak RC, Gibson CM, et al. Effect on coronary atherosclerosis of decrease in plasma cholesterol concentrations in normocholesterolemic patients. Lancet 1994; 344:1182–1186.
33. Blankenhorn DH, Azen SP, Kramsch DM, et al. Coronary angiographic changes with lovastatin therapy: The Monitored Atherosclerosis Regression Study (MARS). Ann Intern Med 1993; 119:967–976.
34. Waters D, Higginson L, Gladstone P, et al. Effects of monotherapy with an HMG-CoA reductase inhibitor on the progression of coronary atherosclerosis as assessed by serial quantitative arteriography: The Canadian Coronary Atherosclerosis Intervention Trial. Circulation 1994; 89:959–968.
35. Pitt B, Mancini GBJ, Ellis SG, et al. Pravastatin limitation of atherosclerosis in the coronary arteries (PLAC I): Reduction in atherosclerosis progression and clinical events. J Am Coll Cardiol 1995; 26:1133–1139.
36. MAAS Investigators. Effect of simvastatin on coronary atheroma: The Multicenter Anti-Atheroma Study (MAAS). Lancet 1994; 344:633–638.
37. Jukema JW, Bruschke AVG, van Boren AJ, et al. Effects of lipid-lowering by pravastatin on progression and regression of coronary artery disease in symptomatic men with normal or moderately elevated cholesterol levels: The Regression Growth Evaluation Statin Study (REGRESS). Circulation 1995; 91:2528–2540.
38. Ericsson C-G, Hamsten A, Nilsson J, et al. Angiographic assessment of effects of bezafibrate on progression of coronary artery disease in young male post infarction patients. Lancet 1996; 347:849–853.
39. Herd JA, Ballantyne CM, Farmer JA, et al. The effect of fluvastatin on coronary atherosclerosis in patients with mild-to-moderate cholesterol elevations: The Lipoprotein and Coronary Atherosclerosis Study (LCAS). Am J Cardiol 1997; 80:278–286.
40. Post Coronary Artery Bypass Graft Trial Investigators. The effect of aggressive lowering of low density lipoprotein cholesterol and low dose anticoagulation of obstructive changes in saphenous vein coronary artery bypass grafts. N Engl J Med 1997; 336:153–162.
41. Thompson GR, Maher VMG, Matthews S, et al. The Familial Hypercholesterolemia Regression Study: A randomized comparison of bi-weekly LDL apheresis plus simvastatin versus colestipol plus simvastatin. Lancet 1995; 345:811–816.
42. Miller BD, Alderman EL, Haskell WL, et al. Predominance of dense low-density lipoprotein particles predicts angiographic benefit of therapy in Stanford Coronary Risk Intervention Project. Circulation 1996; 94:2146–2153.
43. Stamfer MJ, Krauss RM, Blanche PJ, et al. A prospective study on triglyceride level, low density lipoprotein particle diameter, and risk of myocardial infarction. JAMA 1996; 276:882–888.
44. Lamarche B, Tchernof A, Moorjani S, et al. Small, dense low density lipoprotein particles as a predictor of the risk of ischemic heart disease in men: Prospective results from the Quebec Cardiovascular Study. Circulation 1997; 95:69–75.
45. Grundy SM. Small LDL, atherogenic dyslipidemia and the metabolic syndrome [Editorial]. Circulation 1997; 95:1–4.
46. Austin MA, King M-C, Vranizen KM, et al. Atherogenic lipoprotein phenotype: A proposed genetic marker for coronary heart disease risk. Circulation 1990; 82:495–506.
47. Reaven GM, Chen YD, Jeppesen J, et al. Insulin resistance and hyper-insulinemia in individuals with small, dense LDL particles. J Clin Invest 1993; 92:141–146.
48. Zambon A, Brown BG, Hokanson JE, et al. Hepatic lipase changes predict coronary artery disease progression/regression in the Familial Atherosclerosis Treatment Study (FATS) [Abstract]. Circulation 1996; 94(suppl I):I-539.
49. Blankenhorn DH, Alaupovic P, Wickham E, et al. Prediction of angiographic change in native human coronary arteries and aortocornary bypass grafts: Lipid and non-lipid factors. Circulation 1990; 81:470–476.
50. Maher VMG, Brown BG, Marcovina SM, et al. Effects of elevated LDL cholesterol on the cardiovascular risk of lipoprotein (a). JAMA 1995; 274:1771–1774.
51. Kane JP, Malloy MJ, Ports TA, et al. Regression of coronary atherosclerosis during treatment of familial hypercholesterolemia with combined drug regimens. JAMA 1990; 264:3007.
52. Gould KL, Ornish D, Scherwitz L, et al. Changes in myocardial perfusion abnormalities by positron emission tomography after long-term, intense risk factor modification. JAMA 1995; 274:894–901.
53. Schuler G, Harnbrecht R, Schlierf G, et al. Myocardial perfusion and regression of coronary artery disease in patients on a regimen of intensive physical exercise and low fat diet. J Am Coll Cardiol 1992; 19:34–42.
54. Kjekshus J, Pedersen TR, Pyorala K, et al. Effect of simvastatin on ischemic signs and symptoms in the 4S [Abstract]. J Am Coll Cardiol 1997; 29:75A.
55. Andrews TC, Raby K, Barry J, et al. Effect of cholesterol reduction on myocardial ischemia in patients with coronary disease. Circulation 1997; 95:324–328.
56. Coronary Drug Project Research Group. Clofibrate and niacin in coronary heart disease. JAMA 1975; 231:360–381.
57. Canner PL, Berge KG, Wenger NK, et al. Fifteen-year mortality in Coronary Drug Project Patients: Long-term benefit with niacin. J Am Coll Cardiol 1986; 8:1245–1255.
58. Buchwald H. Lowering of cholesterol absorption and blood levels by ileal exclusion: Experimental basis and preliminary clinical report. Circulation 1964; 29:713–720.
59. Buchwald H, Matts JP, Fitch L, et al. Changes in sequential coronary arteriograms and subsequent coronary events. JAMA 1992; 268:1429–1433.
60. Waters D, Craven TE, Lesperance J. Prognostic significance of progression of coronary atherosclerosis. Circulation 1993; 87:1067–1075.
61. 4S Investigators. Randomized trial of cholesterol lowering in 4,444 patients with coronary heart disease: The Scandinavian Simvastatin Survival Study (4S). Lancet 1994; 344:1383–1389.
62. Pedersen TR, Kjekshus J, Berg K, et al. Cholesterol-lowering and the use of health care resources: Results of the Scandinavian Simvastatin Survival Study (4S). Circulation 1996; 93:1796–1802.
63. Sacks FM, Pfeffer MA, Moye LA, et al. The effect of pravastatin on coronary events after myocardial infarction in patients with average cholesterol levels. N Engl J Med 1996; 335:1001–1009.
64. Shepherd J, Cobbe SM, Ford I, et al. Prevention of coronary heart disease with pravastatin in men with hypercholesterolemia. N Engl J Med 1995; 333:1301–1307.
65. LIPID Study Group. Design features of the LIPID Study: A randomized trial in patients with previous acute myocardial infarction and/or unstable angina pectoris. Am J Cardiol 1995; 76:474–479.
66. Downs JR, Beere PA, Whitney E, et al. Design and rationale of the Air Force/Texas Coronary Atherosclerosis Prevention Study (AFCAPS/TexCAPS). Am J Cardiol 1997; 80:287–293.
67. Brown BG, Zhao X-Q, Maher VMG, et al. HDL cholesterol as a therapeutic target in coronary disease: Current concepts and future directions. Developments Cardiovasc Med 1995; 174:29–42.
68. Furchgott RF, Zawadski JV. The obligatory role of endothelial cells in the relaxation of arterial smooth muscle by acetylcholine. Nature 1980; 299:373–376.
69. Moncada S, Palmer RM, Higgs EA. Nitric oxide physiology,

pathophysiology, and pharmacology. Pharmacol Rev 1991; 43:109–142.
70. Yokoyama I, Ohtake T, Mormomura S-I, et al. Reduced coronary flow reserve in hypercholesterolemic patients without overt coronary stenosis. Circulation 1996; 94:3232–3238.
71. Clarkson P, Celermajer DS, Donald AE, et al. Impaired vascular reactivity in insulin-dependent diabetes mellitus is related to disease duration and LDL cholesterol levels. J Am Coll Cardiol 1996; 28:573–579.
72. Lieberman EH, Gerhard MD, Uchata A, et al. Estrogen improves endothelium-dependent, flow-mediated vasodilation in post-menopausal women. Ann Intern Med 1994; 121:936–941.
73. Zeiher AM, Schchinger V, Hohnloser SH, et al. Coronary atherosclerotic wall thickening and vascular reactivity in humans: Elevated high-density lipoprotein levels ameliorate abnormal vasoconstriction in early atherosclerosis. Circulation 1994; 89:2525–2532.
74. Sorensen KE, Celermajer DS, Geogakopoulos D, et al. Impairment of endothelium-dependent dilation is an early event in children with familial hypercholesterolemia and is related to the lipoprotein (a) level. J Clin Invest 1994; 93:50–55.
75. Dyce MC, Anderson TJ, Yeung AC, et al. Indices of LDL particle size closely relate to endothelial function. Circulation 1993; 88(suppl I):I-466–I-471.
76. Panza JA, Quyzumi AA, Brush JE, et al. Abnormal endothelium-dependent vascular relaxation in patients with essential hypertension. N Engl J Med 1990; 323:22–27.
77. Brown BG, Lee AB, Bolson EL, et al. Reflex constriction of significant coronary stenosis as a mechanism contributing to ischemic ventricular dysfunction during isometric exercise. Circulation 1984; 70:18–24.
78. Hess OM, Bortone A, Eid K, et al. Coronary vasomotor tone during static and dynamic exercise. Eur Heart J 1989; 10(suppl F):105–110.
79. Harrison DG, Armstrong ML, Freeman PC, et al. Restoration of endothelium-dependent relaxation by dietary treatment of atherosclerosis. J Clin Invest 1987; 80:808–811.
80. Liao JK, Shin WS, Lee WY, et al. Oxidized low-density lipoprotein decreases the expression of endothelial nitric oxide syntheses. J Biol Chem 1995; 270:319–324.
81. Muegge A, Edwell JH, Peterson TE, et al. Chronic treatment with polyethylene-glycolated superoxide dismutase partially restores endothelium-dependent vascular relaxations in cholesterol-fed rabbits. Circ Res 1991; 69:1293–1300.
82. Leung WH, Lau CP, Wong CK. Beneficial effect of cholesterol-lowering therapy on coronary endothelium-dependent relaxation in hypercholesterolemic patients. Lancet 1993; 341:1496–1500.
83. Egoshira K, Hirooka Y, Kai H, et al. Reduction in serum cholesterol with pravastatin improved endothelium-dependent coronary vasomotion in patients with hypercholesterolemia. Circulation 1994; 89:2519–2524.
84. Treasure CB, Kleis JL, Weintroub WS, et al. Beneficial effects of cholesterol-lowering therapy on the coronary endothelium in patients with coronary artery disease. N Engl J Med 1995; 332:481–487.
85. Anderson TJ, Meredith IT, Yeung AC, et al. The effect of cholesterol-lowering and antioxidant therapy on endothelium-dependent coronary vasomotion. N Engl J Med 1995; 332:488–493.
86. Jamori O, Matsuoka H, Itabe H, et al. Single LDL apheresis improves endothelium-dependent vasodilation in hypercholesterolemic humans. Circulation 1997; 95:76–82.
87. Stroes ES, Koomons HA, de Bruin TW, et al. Vascular function in the forearm of hypercholesterolemic patients off and on lipid-lowering medication. Lancet 1995; 346:467–471.
88. Ridker PM, Vaughn DE, Stampfer MJ, et al. A cross sectional study of endogenous tissue plasminogen activator, total cholesterol, HDL cholesterol, and apolipoproteins A-I, A-II, B-100. Arterioscler Thromb Vasc Biol 1993; 13:1587–1592.
89. Ridker PM, Vaughn DE, Stampfer MJ, et al. Endogenous tissue-type plasminogen activator and risk of myocardial infarction. Lancet 1993; 341:1165–1168.
90. Linjen HR, Collen D. Impaired fibrinolysis and the risk for coronary heart disease [Editorial]. Circulation 1996; 94:2052–2054.
91. Benderly M, Graff E, Reicher-Reiss H, et al. Fibrinogen is a predictor of mortality in coronary heart disease patients. Arterioscler Thromb Vasc Biol 1996; 16:351–356.
92. Carvalho ACA, Colman RW, Less RS. Platelet formation in hypercholesterolemia. N Engl J Med 1974; 290:434–438.
93. Ichiki K, Hisao I, Haramaki N, et al. Long-term smoking impairs platelet-derived nitric oxide release. Circulation 1996; 94:3109–3114.
94. McLean JW, Tomlinson JE, Kuang WJ, et al. CDNA sequence of human apolipoprotein (a) is homologous to plasminogen. Nature 1987; 330:132–137.
95. Maher VMG, Brown BG. Lipoprotein (a) and coronary heart disease. Curr Opin Lipidol 1995; 6:229–235.
96. Jaijar KA, Gavish D, Breslow JL, et al. Lipoprotein (a) modulation of endothelial cell surface fibrinolysis and its potential role in atherosclerosis. Nature 1989; 339:303–305.
97. Haider AW, Andreotti F, Thompson GR, et al. Serum lipoprotein (a) level is related to thrombin generation and spontaneous intermittent coronary occlusion in patients with acute myocardial infarction. Circulation 1996; 94:2072–2076.
98. Moreno P, Bernardi V, Lopez-Cuellar J, et al. Macrophages, smooth muscle cells, and tissue factor in unstable angina: Implications for cell-mediated thrombogenicity in acute coronary syndromes. Circulation 1996; 94:3090–3097.
99. Gerrity RG. The role of monocyte in atherogenesis: I. Transition of blood-borne monocytes into foam cells in fatty lesions. Am J Pathol 1981; 103:181–190.
100. Ross R. The pathogenesis of atherosclerosis—an update. N Engl J Med 1986; 314:488–500.
101. Steinberg D, Parthasarathy S, Carew TE, et al. Beyond cholesterol: Modifications of low-density lipoprotein that increase its atherogenicity. N Engl J Med 1989; 320:915–924.
102. Berliner JA, Territo MC, Sevanian A, et al. Minimally modified LDL stimulates monocyte endothelial interactions. J Clin Invest 1990; 85:1260–1266.
103. Yamaguchi J, Hoff MF. Apolipoprotein B accumulation and development of foam cell lesions in coronary arteries of hypercholesterolemic swine. Lab Invest 1984; 51:325–332.
104. Krempler F, Kostner GM, Roscher A, et al. The interaction of human apoB containing lipoproteins with mouse peritoneal macrophages: A comparison of Lp(a) with LDL. J Lipid Res 1984; 25:283–287.
105. Stary HC. Changes in the cells of atherosclerotic lesions as advanced lesions evolve in coronary arteries of children and young adults. *In* Glagov S, Newman WP, Schaffer SA (eds): Pathobiology of the Human Atherosclerotic Plaque. New York, Springer-Verlag, 1990, pp 93–106.
106. Guyton JR, Klemp KF. The lipid-rich core region of human atherosclerotic fibrous plaques. Am J Pathol 1989; 134:705–717.
107. Fry DL. Mass transport, atherogenesis, and risk. Arteriosclerosis 1987; 7:88–100.
108. Guyton JR, Bocan TMA. Human aortic fibrolipid lesions: Progenitor lesions for fibrous plaques, exhibiting early formation of the cholesterol-rich core. Am J Pathol 1985; 120:193–206.
109. Smith EB, Evans PH, Pownham MD. Lipid in the aortic intima: The correlation of morphological and chemical characteristics. J Atheroscler Res 1967; 7:171–186.
110. Guyton JR, Bocan TM, Schifani TA. Quantitative ultrastructural analysis of perifibrous lipid and its association with elastin in nonatherosclerotic human aorta. Arteriosclerosis 1985; 5:644–652.
111. Kragel AH, Reddy SG, Wittes JT, et al. Morphometric analysis of the composition of atherosclerotic plaques in the four major epicardial coronary arteries in acute myocardial infarction and in sudden coronary death. Circulation 1989; 80:1747–1756.
112. Dollar AL, Kragel AH, Fernicola DJ, et al. Composition of atherosclerotic plaques in coronary arteries in women less than 40 years of age with fatal coronary artery disease and implications for plaque reversibility. Am J Cardiol 1991; 67:1223–1227.
113. Gertz SD, Malezadah S, Dollar AL, et al. Composition of atherosclerotic plaques in the four major epicardial coronary arteries in patients greater than or equal to 90 years of age. Am J Cardiol 1991; 67:1228–1233.

114. Kragel AH, Roberts WC. Composition of atherosclerotic plaques in the coronary arteries in homozygous familial hypercholesterolemia. Am Heart J 1991; 121:210–211.
115. Ambrose JA, Tannenbaum MA, Alexopoulos D, et al. Angiographic progression of coronary artery disease and the development of myocardial infarction. J Am Coll Cardiol 1988; 12:56–62.
116. Little WC, Constantinescu M, Applegate RM, et al. Can coronary angiography predict the site of a subsequent myocardial infarction in patients with mild-to-moderate coronary artery disease? Circulation 1988; 78:1157–1166.
117. Little WC. Angiographic assessment of the culprit coronary artery lesion before acute myocardial infarction. Am J Cardiol 1990; 66:44G–47G.
118. Brown BG, Lin J-T, Kelsey S, et al. Progression of coronary atherosclerosis in patients with probable familial hypercholesterolemia: Quantitative arteriographic assessment of patients in NHLBI Type II Study. Arteriosclerosis 1989; 9(suppl I):I-81–I-90.
119. Webster MWI, Chesebro JH, Smith HC, et al. Myocardial infarction and coronary artery occlusion: A prospective 5-year angiographic study [Abstract]. J Am Coll Cardiol 1990; 15(suppl A):218A.
120. Fishbein MC, Seigel RJ. How big are coronary atherosclerotic plaques that rupture. Circulation 1996; 94:2662–2666.
121. Constantinides P. Plaque hemorrhages, their genesis and their role in supra-plaque thrombosis and atherogenesis. *In* Glagov S, Newman WP, Schaffer SA (eds): Pathobiology of the Human Atherosclerotic Plaque. New York, Springer-Verlag, 1990, pp 393–411.
122. Tracey RE, Devaney K, Kissling G. Characteristics of the plaque under a coronary thrombus. Virchows Arch Pathol Anat 1985; 405:411–427.
123. Davies MJ, Krikler DM, Katz D. Atherosclerosis: Inhibition or regression as therapeutic possibilities. Br Heart J 1991; 65:302–310.
124. Lendon CL, Davies MJ, Born GVR, et al. Atherosclerotic plaque caps are locally weakened when macrophage density is increased. Atherosclerosis 1991; 87:87–90.
125. Richardson PD, Davies MJ, Born GVR. Influence of plaque configuration and stress distribution on fissuring of coronary atherosclerotic plaques. Lancet 1989; 2:941–944.
126. Loree HM, Kamm RD, Strongfellow RG, et al. Effects of fibrous cap thickness on peak circumferential stress in model atherosclerotic vessels. Circ Res 1992; 71:850–858.
127. Davies MJ. Stability and instability: Two faces of coronary atherosclerosis. The Paul Dudley White Lecture 1995. Circulation 1996; 94:2013–2020.
128. Van der Wal AC, Becker AE, Van der Loos CM, et al. Site of intimal rupture or erosion of thrombosed coronary atherosclerotic plaques is characterized by an inflammatory process irrespective of the dominant plaque morphology. Circulation 1994; 89:36–44.
129. Moreno PR, Falk E, Palacios IF, et al. Macrophage infiltration in acute coronary syndromes: Implications for plaque rupture. Circulation 1994; 90:775–778.
130. Shah PK, Falk E, Badimon JJ, et al. Human monocyte-derived macrophages express collagenase and induce collagen breakdown in atherosclerotic fibrous caps: Implication for plaque rupture [Abstract]. Circulation 1993; 88(suppl I):I-254.
131. Henney AM, Wakeley PR, Davies MJ, et al. Location of stromelysin gene in atherosclerotic plaques using in-site hybridization. Proc Natl Acad Sci U S A 1991; 88:8154–8158.
132. Davies MJ, Richardson PD, Woolf N, et al. Risk of thrombosis in human atherosclerotic plaques: Role of extracellular lipid, macrophages, and smooth muscle cell content. Br Heart J 1993; 69:377–381.
133. Hessler JR, Morel DW, Lewis LJ, et al. Lipoprotein oxidation and lipoprotein-induced cytotoxicity. Arteriosclerosis 1983; 3:215–222.
134. Yla-Herttuala S, Palinski W, Rosenfeld ME, et al. Evidence for the presence of oxidatively modified low density lipoprotein in atherosclerotic lesions of rabbit and man. J Clin Invest 1989; 84:1086–1095.
135. Galis Z, Sukhova G, Lark M, et al. Increased expression of matrix metalloproteinases and matrix degrading activity in vulnerable regions of human atherosclerotic plaques. J Clin Invest 1994; 94:2493–2503.
136. Libby P. Molecular bases of the acute coronary syndromes. Circulation 1995; 91:2844–2850.

18 Antiarrhythmic Drug Therapy

▶ William G. Stevenson
▶ Peter L. Friedman

Sudden death or cardiac arrest occurs in 2% to 4% of patients during the first or second year following an acute myocardial infarction.[1–4] Many of these deaths are due to ventricular tachycardia or ventricular fibrillation provoked either by acute ischemia or reentry in the infarct scar.[5] Reentry in the infarct may also present as sustained ventricular tachycardia without cardiac arrest. Depressed left ventricular ejection fraction, frequent ventricular ectopy, nonsustained ventricular tachycardia, depressed heart rate variability, an abnormal signal-averaged electrocardiogram, and inducible sustained ventricular tachycardia at electrophysiologic study are markers of increased risk.[1–10] Thrombolytic therapy reduces the prevalence of these markers and improves survival after myocardial infarction.[11–15] Chronic therapy with beta-adrenergic blockers and angiotensin-converting enzyme inhibitors also improves survival and reduces sudden death.[16–18] The improving survival rate of myocardial infarction survivors has had an important impact on several trials attempting to address antiarrhythmic therapies. Trials that anticipated higher mortality rates, similar to those observed in the late 1970s and early 1980s, were generally underpowered to detect survival differences in more recent populations.

Because the overall risk of fatal arrhythmias after myocardial infarction is relatively low, therapy with antiarrhythmic drugs or implantable defibrillators has only limited potential to reduce sudden cardiac death in that circumstance. Furthermore, toxicities or risks of therapy can potentially offset any benefit. Competing risks (i.e., the risk of an arrhythmia vs. the risk of therapy) are particularly important when a large portion of the population who receive treatment is at low risk for a fatal arrhythmia.[4] The patients who are not at risk for cardiac arrest have no opportunity to benefit from the therapy but are still exposed to the risks of therapy. The benefit of preventing sudden death in the patients at risk is also offset by the chance of treatment-related fatal toxicities. The benefit-risk ratio can be improved by selecting a population of patients at particularly high risk. This can potentially be accomplished by screening for arrhythmia risk using tests such as the ambulatory electrocardiogram, signal-averaged electrocardiogram, or programmed electrical stimulation. As the specificity of the tests or combinations of tests selected for screening increase, a subpopulation with progressively greater risk of sudden death is identified that is more likely to benefit from antiarrhythmic therapy. This subpopulation is composed of a progressively smaller fraction of the entire infarct population. The selection criteria for "high risk" and the toxicities of therapy are particularly important considerations for the interpretation of antiarrhythmic therapy trials in the post–myocardial infarction population.

CARDIAC ARRHYTHMIA SUPPRESSION TRIAL

Since the publication of its preliminary results in 1989, the Cardiac Arrhythmia Suppression Trial (CAST) has become widely regarded as the most seminal clinical trial in the field of arrhythmia management. Prior to the inception of the CAST, a large body of evidence had demonstrated that the presence of ventricular arrhythmias after myocardial infarction was a strong independent predictor of subsequent all-cause and sudden-death mortality, even after adjusting for ventricular dysfunction and other clinical variables known to affect outcome.[19, 20] This finding had led to the hypothesis that ventricular ectopic activity provided a triggering mechanism that, under the proper circumstances, initiated sustained ventricular tachycardia or ventricular fibrillation and, thus, sudden death in patients at risk. The corollary to this hypothesis was that abolition of ventricular ectopic activity, including nonsustained ventricular tachycardia, by an antiarrhythmic drug would improve outcome by eliminating the trigger for sustained arrhythmia. Although prior clinical trials of arrhythmia suppression using various antiarrhythmic drugs had failed to demonstrate any survival benefit of antiarrhythmic drug therapy, the results of these trials had been viewed with suspicion because of perceived flaws in their design, sample size, or the target population enrolled.[21–23] When recruitment of patients for the CAST first began, it was accompanied by great anticipation that at last a properly designed trial with sufficient power to demonstrate the benefit of antiarrhythmic drug therapy was underway.

The CAST was designed to test the hypothesis that suppression of asymptomatic or minimally symptomatic ventricular arrhythmias after myocardial infarction would reduce the arrhythmic death rate. In a pilot study (the Cardiac Arrhythmia Pilot Study [CAPS]) conducted as a prelude to CAST, encainide, flecainide, and moricizine were identified as three antiarrhythmic drugs that were suitable for use in the main trial based on their efficacy for suppression of spontaneous ventricular arrhythmia, their tolerability during long-term therapy, and their apparent low risk of causing ventricular proarrhythmia.[24] The intention in the CAST was to enroll those patients at increased risk for arrhythmic death after myocardial infarction who would be most likely to benefit from antiarrhythmic drug therapy.[25] Thus, patients with a recent myocardial infarction (qualifying Holter monitor recorded within 90 days of infarction) were eligible if their left ventricular ejection fraction was less than or equal to 55%, whereas patients with a more remote infarction (qualifying Holter monitor recorded 90 days to 2 years after infarction) were eligible only if their ejection fraction was less than or equal to 40%. The qualifying Holter monitor had to demonstrate an average of six or more ventricular premature depolarizations per hour. Patients with ventricular arrhythmias that caused syncope or presyncope were excluded, as were patients whose Holter monitor showed nonsustained ventricular tachycardia, defined as 15 or more consecutive beats at a rate greater than or equal to 120 beats/min.[25]

The design of the CAST included an initial period of open-label drug titration to identify those people who were intolerant of the antiarrhythmic drugs, had inadequate suppression of their qualifying arrhythmias, or exhibited evidence of ventricular proarrhythmia; such individuals were excluded from further participation in the trial.[25] Patients who tolerated drug therapy and who had adequate suppression of their arrhythmia were then randomly assigned to long-term treatment with one of the three antiarrhythmic drugs or matching placebo in a double-blind fashion. The primary endpoint of the CAST was a composite of arrhythmic death and cardiac arrest. The estimate of the arrhythmic death rate in the placebo group over an average of 3 years of follow-up was 11%. The CAST was originally intended to assess whether antiarrhythmic drug therapy in this population would improve outcome or have no effect. There was never any intention to investigate whether such therapy might be harmful. Thus, a one-tailed test of significance was planned. Sample size calculations suggested that recruitment of 4400 patients would result in approximately 85% power to detect a 30% treatment effect in the antiarrhythmic arm.[25]

Recruitment of patients began in June 1987. Two years later, after only 1455 patients had been randomized and had been followed for an average of only 10 months, an independent Data and Safety Monitoring Board recommended that encainide and flecainide treatment in the trial be halted because of clear evidence that these agents increased the arrhythmic death rate (Fig. 18–1).[25, 26] Death from arrhythmia occurred in 4.5% of patients treated with encainide or flecainide compared with 1.2% in placebo-assigned patients (relative risk [RR], 3.6; 95% confidence interval [CI], 1.7 to 8.5). Total mortality rates in patients treated with encainide or flecainide were also higher than in the placebo group (7.7% vs. 3.0%; RR, 2.5; 95% CI, 1.6 to 4.5). This adverse treatment effect could not be accounted for by imbalances in the randomization of patients to the different treatment groups and was a consistent finding in all major subgroups examined. One of the most surprising findings in the CAST was the exceptionally low arrhythmic death rate in the placebo group in spite of an effort when the trial was designed to recruit patients believed to be at greatest risk.[25, 26] Indeed, in the face of such a low placebo group mortality, it is difficult to imagine how one could demonstrate benefit of any intervention within the bounds of a trial with this sample size.

Although encainide and flecainide treatment was discontinued in the CAST, the Data and Safety Moni-

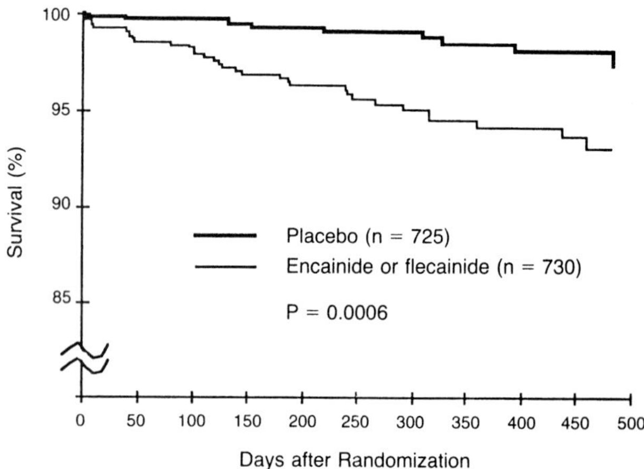

Figure 18–1 Survival curves by treatment group for the composite endpoint of arrhythmic death or cardiac arrest in the CAST. (Reprinted by permission of *The New England Journal of Medicine* from Cardiac Arrhythmia Suppression Trial [CAST] Investigators. Preliminary report: Effect of encainide and flecainide on mortality in a randomized trial of arrhythmia suppression after myocardial infarction. N Engl J Med 1989; 321:406–412. Copyright 1989, Massachusetts Medical Society.)

toring Board recommended that the trial be continued with moricizine. Because of the unexpectedly low arrhythmic death rate and all-cause mortality rate in the placebo group, several design changes were incorporated into the continuation of the trial (referred to as CAST II) to recruit a higher-risk population who would be expected to derive the maximum benefit from moricizine. In CAST II only patients with a left ventricular ejection fraction equal to or less than 0.40 and a recent (≤90 days) myocardial infarction were eligible to participate.[27] In addition, patients with nonsustained ventricular tachycardia, redefined as consecutive ventricular beats at rates greater than or equal to 120 beats/min but lasting less than 30 seconds, were now eligible for the trial, provided that the nonsustained ventricular tachycardia was not associated with syncope or presyncope.[27] CAST II was divided into two blinded, placebo-controlled phases. In the first phase patients were treated in hospital with either placebo or low-dose moricizine for 2 weeks. The primary endpoint of this short-term study was a composite of death or cardiac arrest. Patients who completed the short-term study and who had suppression of their arrhythmia with moricizine and no evidence for ventricular proarrhythmia could then undergo a dose-titration phase with higher-dose moricizine. If adequate suppression of their qualifying arrhythmia with moricizine could be achieved, these patients were then randomly allocated to outpatient long-term treatment with either moricizine or matching placebo. The primary endpoint for this phase of CAST II was a composite of arrhythmic death or cardiac arrest due to arrhythmia requiring resuscitation.[27]

In spite of the changes in trial design, CAST II was also halted prematurely because of evidence of harm in the patients assigned to moricizine treatment.[27] Moricizine had an adverse impact on mortality that was particularly evident during the short-term period of in-hospital treatment with low-dose moricizine (Fig. 18–2*A*). During this phase of the trial, 17 of 655 moricizine-assigned patients and only 3 of 660 placebo-assigned patients died or had a cardiac arrest, yielding crude death rates of 2.6% and 0.45% in the two groups, respectively (RR, 5.6; 95% CI, 1.7 to 19.1). During the outpatient long-term phase of the trial, outcomes in the moricizine-assigned and placebo-assigned patients were similar (Fig. 18–2*B*). This observation stood in sharp contrast to the results seen in CAST I with encainide and flecainide, where there was evidence of cumulative and continuing harm throughout the period of exposure to the drugs, as evidenced by divergence of the survival curves over the entire duration of the trial (see Fig. 18–1). Nonetheless, CAST II was halted because of the clear increase in early mortality in the active treatment arm and the extremely low likelihood of ever being able to demonstrate benefit during long-term outpatient therapy.[27]

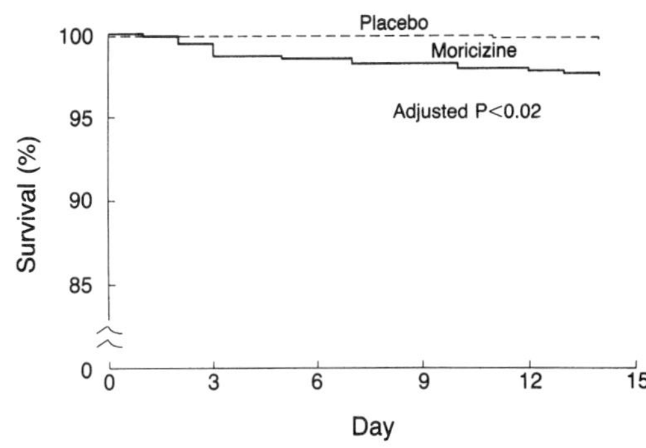

No. at risk (% surviving)

A				
	Placebo	660 (100)	659 (99.9)	658 (99.7)
	Moricizine	665 (100)	655 (98.5)	608 (97.7)

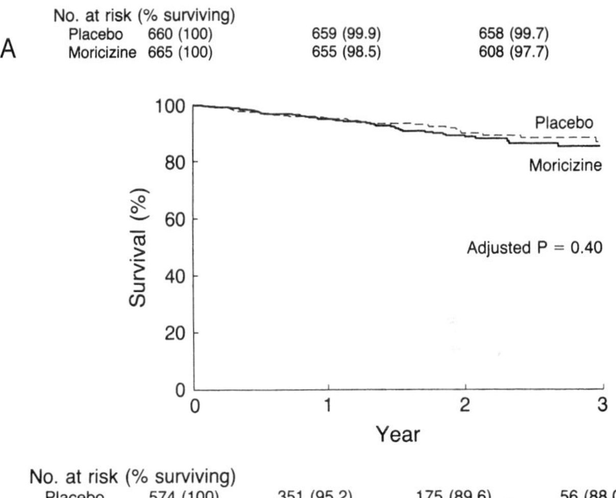

No. at risk (% surviving)

B					
	Placebo	574 (100)	351 (95.2)	175 (89.6)	56 (88.0)
	Moricizine	581 (100)	350 (94.9)	181 (88.8)	56 (85.0)

Figure 18–2 *A*, Survival curves by treatment group for the composite endpoint of death or nonfatal cardiac arrest from any cause during the inhospital phase of drug testing in CAST II. *B*, Survival curves by treatment group for the composite endpoint of death on nonfatal cardiac arrest owing to arrhythmias during the long-term treatment phase of CAST II. (*A* and *B* reprinted by permission of *The New England Journal of Medicine* from Cardiac Arrhythmia Suppression Trial II Investigators. Effect of the antiarrhythmic agent moricizine on survival after myocardial infarction. N Engl J Med 1992; 327:227–233. Copyright 1992, Massachusetts Medical Society.)

The results of CAST were met with widespread surprise and dismay in the medical community, not to mention the considerable attention accorded the trial in the lay press. The demonstration by the CAST that antiarrhythmic drug therapy after myocardial infarction not only failed to improve outcome but actually increased mortality caused an immediate reexamination of earlier, much smaller clinical trials that had either been neutral or had suggested harm but that had originally been viewed with skepticism. The principal flaw in earlier trials had been that they lacked sufficient power to enable one to draw firm conclusions about the effects of antiarrhythmic drug treatment. Using meta-analytic techniques in an attempt to overcome this flaw, Teo and associates examined the results of 51 randomized trials of class I antiarrhythmic drugs in more than 23,000 patients after myocardial infarction.[28] When all class I antiarrhythmic drugs were considered together, there were 660 deaths among 11,712 patients assigned to active therapy compared with 571 deaths among 11,517 placebo-assigned patients, yielding an odds ratio of 1.14 and a 95% CI of 1.01 to 1.28 ($P = 0.03$).[28] When results were analyzed according to individual drug subclass, there was a trend toward higher mortality among patients receiving active treatment, regardless of whether a class IA, IB, or IC agent was used.[28]

All class I antiarrhythmic drugs act predominantly by blockade of the sodium channel, reducing the rate of rise of phase 0 of the action potential and, thereby, slowing conduction velocity. The various drugs differ from one another in terms of their effects on other ion channels, particularly those responsible for repolarization. The results with three different class I agents in the CAST and the results of meta-analysis of all other trials of class I agents after myocardial infarction suggest that the adverse impact on survival owing to these drugs is related principally to their sodium channel–blocking properties. The mechanism of this adverse effect is not clear. In the CAST the observation that encainide-, flecainide-, and moricizine-treated patients had an excess of arrhythmic deaths suggests that these agents were proarrhythmic. If this assumption is correct, it challenges many previously held concepts regarding drug-induced proarrhythmia. Such proarrhythmia is usually heralded by an increase in spontaneous arrhythmia or the appearance of a new ventricular arrhythmia and yet, in the CAST, it occurred in face of demonstrable suppression of spontaneous ventricular arrhythmia.[25–27] Drug-induced proarrhythmia is believed typically to become evident early during exposure to the offending agent and yet, for encainide and flecainide in the CAST, the harmful effects of the drugs were evident continuously throughout exposure to the drugs.[25, 26] The extremely low incidence of documented nonfatal serious arrhythmic events in patients assigned to active treatment in the CAST is also difficult to reconcile with a proarrhythmic mechanism. Patients with non–Q wave infarction assigned to active therapy in CAST were at particular risk of arrhythmic death and, conversely, concomitant therapy with beta blockers was partially protective.[29, 30] This finding suggests that an interaction between ischemia and the sodium channel–blocking action of these drugs may create an increased susceptibility of treated patients to ventricular fibrillation during periods of myocardial ischemia. Whatever the mechanism, the cumulative evidence from clinical trials of class I antiarrhythmic drugs in patients with prior myocardial infarction is that such agents are harmful. These studies have dealt a serious, if not fatal, blow to the hypothesis that suppression of spontaneous ventricular arrhythmias is beneficial in this particular population.

d-SOTALOL AND *d,l*-SOTALOL TRIALS

The CAST demonstrated that class I antiarrhythmic drugs, which slow conduction velocity by blockade of the sodium channel, are associated with an increase in mortality when used to suppress spontaneous nonsustained ventricular arrhythmias in patients with a prior myocardial infarction.[25–27] This unexpected finding focused attention on class III antiarrhythmic drugs, which block potassium channels responsible for repolarization and which have little effect on conduction velocity, as agents that might be beneficial in patients at risk for sudden cardiac death after myocardial infarction. The compound *d*-sotalol, the dextrorotatory isomer of the racemate *d,l*-sotalol, blocks the rapid component of the delayed rectifier current, IKr. However, unlike *d,l*-sotalol, *d*-sotalol is practically devoid of beta-blocking activity and, thus, should be well tolerated in patients with even the most severe left ventricular dysfunction. Since *d*-sotalol is not a beta blocker and, therefore, does not appreciably slow the heart rate, it is less likely than *d,l*-sotalol to cause pause-dependent torsades de pointes ventricular tachycardia associated with QT prolongation, the major manifestation of proarrhythmia with potassium channel–blocking agents. For these reasons *d*-sotalol was selected for use in the Survival with Oral *d*-Sotalol (SWORD) trial, a multinational, multicenter, randomized, double-blind, placebo-controlled trial to test the hypothesis that a pure potassium channel blocker such as *d*-sotalol can reduce all-cause mortality in patients with a previous myocardial infarction and residual left ventricular dysfunction.[31] The SWORD trial was a postinfarction secondary prevention trial, not an arrhythmia suppression trial such as the CAST. The primary endpoint for the trial was all-cause mortality; secondary endpoints included cardiac mortality and presumed arrhythmic death.[31]

In the SWORD trial patients with left ventricular ejection fraction less than 40% and either a recent myocardial infarction (6 to 42 days) or symptomatic heart failure (New York Heart Association [NYHA] class II or III) after a remote myocardial infarction (>42 days) were randomly allocated to treatment with *d*-sotalol 100 or 200 mg per day or matching placebo. The trial was originally designed to enroll recent and remote infarction patients in a 2:1 ratio. It was estimated that the placebo group would have a 1-year all-cause mortality of 7.9% and that 6400 patients would be required to yield 90% power to detect a 20% treatment effect, using a two-tailed test.[31] Although it was originally planned to enroll 6400 patients in the trial, recruitment was halted prematurely after only 3121 patients because the advisory statistical boundary for harm was exceeded (RR, 1.65; 95% CI, 1.15 to 2.36; $P = 0.006$).[14] The majority of the excess mortality in the *d*-sotalol–treated patients was presumed arrhythmic death (RR, 1.77; 95% CI, 1.15 to 2.74; $P = 0.008$).[32]

In the SWORD trial the *d*-sotalol–associated mortality was not evenly distributed in all patients (Fig. 18–3). *d*-Sotalol–associated mortality was greater in patients with left ventricular ejection fraction of 31% to 40% as compared with those with ejection fractions less than 30% (RR, 4.0 vs. 1.2; $P = 0.007$) and was greatest in patients with remote myocardial infarction and ejection fraction of 31% to 40% (RR, 7.9; 95% CI, 2.4 to 26.2).[33] Concomitant therapy with beta blockers did not alter the adverse effect of *d*-sotalol; nor were indirect markers of residual ischemia such as nitrate use, need for revascularization, or non–Q wave infarction, associated with an enhanced risk of *d*-sotalol therapy.[33]

One of the findings in the CAST that had frequently been cited critically was the unexpected low placebo mortality. In the SWORD trial the annualized 1-year all-cause mortality was 7.8% in the placebo group, very close to the 7.9% that had been predicted during sample size calculations.[32] However, the predicted placebo group mortality had been based on the assumption that two patients with recent infarction would be enrolled for every one patient with remote infarction and that there would be a higher all-cause mortality in patients with remote infarction, who were required to have symptomatic heart failure, than in patients with recent infarction. In fact, the ratio for enrolled patients was the reverse (recent to remote = 1:2.4). Thus, reminiscent of the CAST, the placebo group mortality proved to be much lower than had been predicted. This unexpectedly low placebo group mortality can be largely attributed to the extremely low mortality in patients with remote infarction and left ventricular ejection fraction of 31% to 40%.[33]

The mechanism of the *d*-sotalol–associated mortality risk is uncertain. The trial was designed with several features to reduce the risk of torsades de pointes ventricular tachycardia, including strict exclusion criteria based on QT and QTc intervals, heart rate, serum electrolyte levels, and creatinine clearance (sotalol is excreted by the kidney) at baseline and careful attention to these variables and mandated dose adjustment during therapy. Indeed, the incidence of documented nonfatal torsades de pointes ventricular tachycardia was only 0.13%.[32] *d*-Sotalol–associated mortality was not related to drug dose, QTc at baseline, QTc after 2 weeks of therapy, duration of drug treatment, serum potassium concentration, or baseline heart rate.[33] On the other hand, women, who are more susceptible to torsade de pointes, tended to have a greater adverse *d*-sotalol–associated treatment effect (RR, 4.7; 95% CI, 2.4 to 16.5) compared with men (RR, 1.4; 95% CI, 1.0 to 2.1; $P = 0.07$ for treatment, gender interaction).[33] In addition, the presence of nonsustained ventricular tachycardia during a

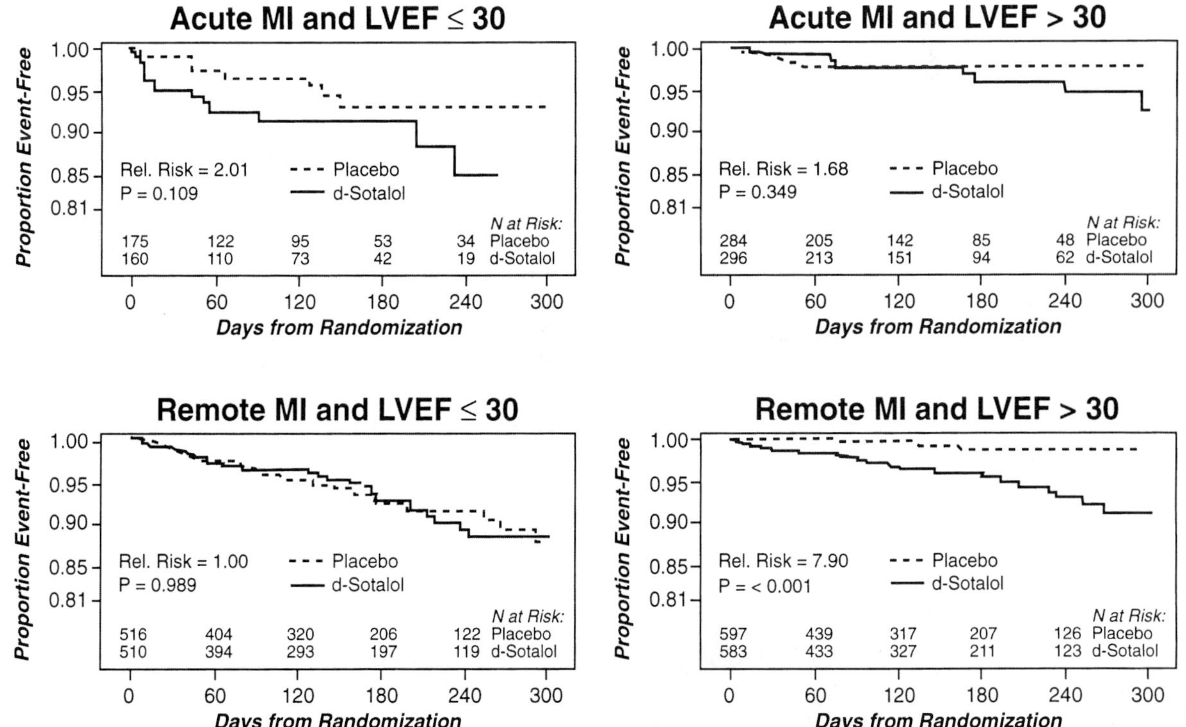

Figure 18–3 Survival curves by treatment group for all-cause mortality in various subgroups of patients in the SWORD trial. MI, myocardial infarction; LVEF, left ventricular ejection fraction (%). Acute = 6 to 42 days after MI. Remote = >42 days after MI. Patients with remote MI and LVEF >30% treated with *d*-sotalol had the greatest relative risk.

baseline Holter monitor was associated with an increased risk of *d*-sotalol–associated mortality.[33] If the excess mortality in patients treated with *d*-sotalol was due to torsades de pointes ventricular tachycardia, many widely held notions about predictors of this proarrhythmic mechanism would be challenged.

The finding in the SWORD trial that patients with relatively well-preserved ventricular function were at greatest risk of mortality during treatment with *d*-sotalol can best be explained by the concept of competing risks (Fig. 18–4). In patients with the poorest ventricular function and the greatest intrinsic risk of developing ventricular fibrillation, the drug may actually have had a beneficial antifibrillatory effect, but one that was counterbalanced by its lethal proarrhythmic effect. The overall effect of treatment in this group was neither benefit nor harm. Patients with better ventricular function, on the other hand, may have had a lower intrinsic risk of ventricular fibrillation to begin with. The antifibrillatory effect of *d*-sotalol in this group may have been masked by a proportionally greater proarrhythmic effect of the drug. The overall results of the trial appear to have been influenced largely by a subgroup that had a good prognosis to begin with, namely patients with remote myocardial infarction, clinical heart failure, and left ventricular ejection fraction of 31% to 40%.

In retrospect, the surprising finding of an adverse effect of *d*-sotalol on survival among patients with a previous myocardial infarction might have been anticipated based on the results of a clinical trial with *d,l*-sotalol that was conducted more than 20 years ago in Great Britain.[34] In this double-blind, placebo-controlled trial, 1456 patients with a recent myocardial infarction who were not being treated with a beta blocker at the time of trial entry and who had no clinical evidence of heart failure were randomly allocated to treatment with *d,l*-sotalol 320 mg per day or matching placebo. Patients were then followed prospectively for 1 year. The risk of reinfarction was significantly lower in patients assigned to treatment with *d,l*-sotalol as compared with placebo, an observation that has repeatedly been made in other clinical trials with various other beta blockers. However, cumulative mortality in patients treated with *d,l*-sotalol was not significantly different compared with placebo-assigned patients.[34] This latter finding stands in sharp contrast with other post–myocardial infarction beta-blocker trials, which have consistently demonstrated reduction in all-cause mortality by beta-blocker therapy.[35] In retrospect, this curious combination of findings in patients treated with *d,l*-sotalol could have resulted from the interplay of two disparate drug effects, namely beta blockade, which was responsible for reduction of the reinfarction rate and which should have also reduced mortality but which was counterbalanced by a lethal proarrhythmic effect of the drug, possibly related to its effects on repolarization.

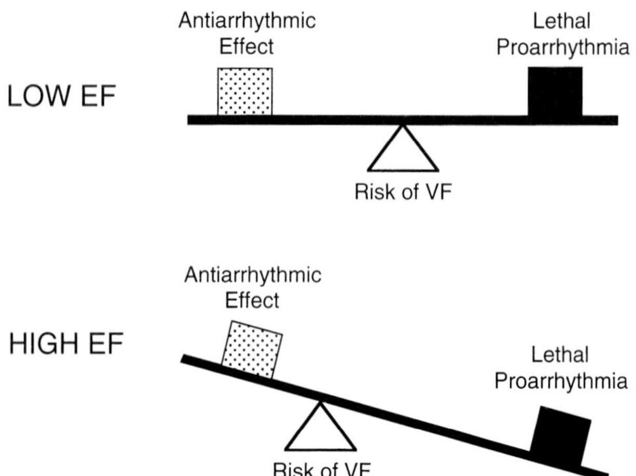

Figure 18–4 The effect of "competing risks" in antiarrhythmic drug trials. The overall effect of an antiarrhythmic drug depends on a balance between its antiarrhythmic and proarrhythmic effects as well as the intrinsic risk of arrhythmic death in the population being treated. EF, ejection fraction; VF, ventricular fibrillation.

AMIODARONE

Amiodarone is a complex drug that has a variety of actions of potential benefit to myocardial infarction survivors.[36] It is effective against a variety of supraventricular and ventricular arrhythmias; reduces the risk of ventricular fibrillation in animal models; and has antiadrenergic, vasodilating, and anti-ischemic effects. It also possesses the ability to aggravate bradyarrhythmias and to cause significant long-term toxicities, which include potentially fatal pulmonary or hepatic toxicity, and less severe neurologic and thyroid toxicities. Pulmonary toxicity occurs in up to 6% of patients but is rare at chronic maintenance doses of less than 300 mg daily.[37, 38] Hence, there is the possibility of either beneficial or adverse effects. It has been evaluated in myocardial infarction survivors believed to be at increased risk of sudden death.

In the Basel Antiarrhythmic Study of Infarct Size (BASIS), Burkart and coworkers tested the hypothesis that therapy with amiodarone or with individualized therapy of other antiarrhythmic drugs adjusted to suppress ventricular ectopy would reduce total mortality and arrhythmic events (sudden death and sustained ventricular tachycardia or ventricular fibrillation) in myocardial infarction survivors with complex ventricular ectopic activity early after myocardial infarction.[39] A desired sample size of 108 patients per group was estimated assuming a 1-year mortality of 20% and a 50% reduction in mortality by therapy ($\alpha = 0.05$; power = 80%, one tailed). Entry criteria were inhospital survival of acute myocardial infarction, age less than 71 years, and asymptomatic complex ventricular ectopic activity (multiform or repetitive ventricular ectopic beats) present in more than 2 hours of a 24-hour electrocardiographic recording prior to hospital discharge. Cardiac surgery or a symptomatic arrhythmia during the hospitalization was an exclusion. From 1981 to 1987 a total of 1220 consecutive patients admitted to one of three hospitals with acute myocardial infarction were screened for entry, 28% of these had qualifying arrhythmias, and 312 patients were randomized to one of three groups: (1) therapy with amiodarone 1000 mg daily for 5 days followed by 200 mg daily (98 patients); (2) individualized antiarrhythmic drug therapy with quinidine, mexiletine, propafenone, flecainide, sotalol, disopyramide, prajmaline, or a combination of these drugs administered to reduce total ventricular premature beats by more than 50% and abolish repetitive forms by more than 90% (100 patients); and (3) a control group who did not receive antiarrhythmic therapy (114 patients). The three groups were well balanced with respect to age (mean of 61 years), gender (86% male), peak creatine kinase enzyme (1305 IU/L), infarct location (40% anterior), and left ventricular ejection fraction (mean of 43%). At 3 months of follow-up 25% of patients were receiving beta-blocking drugs and 52% of patients were receiving antithrombotic therapy (presumably antiplatelet therapy or warfarin). Use of thrombolytic agents, angiotensin-converting enzyme inhibitors, and lipid-lowering agents was not reported. During the 1-year follow-up period 30 (9.6%) patients died; 22 (73%) deaths were sudden. By Kaplan-Meier analysis 1-year mortality was 13% in the control group, 10% in the individualized drug group, and 5% in the amiodarone group ($P < 0.05$ for amiodarone vs. control). Differences of the individualized drug group with control or amiodarone groups did not reach statistical significance. These results were the same in a Cox proportional Hazard model used to adjust for age, prior myocardial infarction, and left ventricular ejection fraction between the groups. Arrhythmic events occurred in 13%, 10%, and 5% of control, individualized therapy, and amiodarone groups, respectively; the difference between the amiodarone-treated group and the control group was significant ($P < 0.01$). In the subgroup of 126 patients with left ventricular ejection fraction less than 40% there was no benefit of amiodarone, but the number of patients and events was small.[40]

Amiodarone therapy was discontinued after 1 year of therapy. Long-term follow-up (mean 72 months, ranging from 55 to 125 months) of the amiodarone and control groups was subsequently reported.[41] Total mortality remained lower throughout the follow-up period in the amiodarone group (30% vs. 45%; $P = 0.03$). This improvement in survival was due entirely to the effect observed during the first year of therapy, while the patient was receiving active therapy, because survival after the first year was the same in both groups.

The BASIS study was not blinded, and analysis was by intention to treat. Protocol deviations or crossovers occurred in 29%; 11 control patients received antiarrhythmic therapy for symptomatic arrhythmias, 9 individually treated patients received amiodarone, and 2 patients initially randomized to receive amiodarone received sotalol because of amiodarone side effects. In addition 22% of patients (32 individualized-therapy patients and 27 amiodarone-treated patients) discontinued study medication owing to side effects or noncompliance.

Amiodarone possesses antiadrenergic effects that could be responsible in part for its benefit.[36] Thus, a greater benefit may be anticipated in infarct survivors who are not treated chronically with beta-adrenergic blocking agents, which are beneficial in infarct survivors. Ceremuzynski and coworkers conducted a feasibility study aimed at assessing the safety of low-dose amiodarone in patients who had a contraindication to therapy with beta-adrenergic blockers after surviving the acute phase of myocardial infarction.[42] No formal sample size was calculated; funding was available for a 4-year enrollment period with 1 year of follow-up. Entry criteria were a confirmed diagnosis of acute myocardial infarction and age less than 75 years. Ventricular ectopic activity was not required. Exclusions were atrial fibrillation and need for an antiarrhythmic agent or lack of contraindication to beta blockers (heart failure, asthma, treated diabetes, or claudication). Between 1986 and 1989 a total of 4212 infarct survivors at eight university hospitals were screened for entry. Of these, 3599 were excluded owing predominantly to no beta-blocker contraindication (1441) or a contraindication to amiodarone (bradycardia, 239; atrioventricular block, 393; bundle branch block, 482; prolonged QT interval, 40). A total of 613 patients were randomized 5 to 7 days after acute myocardial infarction to amiodarone (305 patients) or placebo (308 patients) in a double-blind fashion. Amiodarone was administered at a dose of 800 mg daily for 1 week, then 400 mg 6 days a week for 1 year. The dose was reduced to 100 to 200 mg daily for heart rate less than 55 beats/min or QT interval greater than 0.48 s. Compliance assessed by tablet consumption was 96%. The two groups were well balanced with respect to age (mean of 59 years), gender (70% male), infarct location (51% anterior), and left ventricular ejection fraction (<40% in 33% of patients). Therapy with thrombolytic agents, angiotensin-converting enzyme inhibitors, aspirin, and lipid-lowering agents was not reported. During the 1-year follow-up period 54 (9%) patients died; 30 (55%) of the deaths were sudden. There were 33 (10.7%) deaths in the placebo group and 21 (6.9%) in the amiodarone group (odds ratio, 0.62; 95% CI, 0.35 to 1.08; $P = 0.095$). In the placebo group all deaths were due to cardiac causes, whereas 19 of the 21 deaths in the amiodarone group were due to cardiac causes. The difference in cardiac death between the two groups reached statistical significance ($P = 0.048$; odds ratio, 0.55; 95% CI, 0.32 to 0.99). There were 10 (3.3%) sudden deaths in the amiodarone group compared with 20 (6.5%) in the control group ($P = 0.07$). Amioarone also reduced the incidence of Lown grade 4 arrhythmias during follow-up 24-hour Holter electrocardiogram recordings (7.5% compared with 19.5% in the control group; $P < 0.001$). Adverse reactions causing withdrawal of medication occurred in 10.3% of patients in the placebo group and 30.1% of amiodarone-treated patients; most commonly, bradyarrhythmias, but also hyperthyroidism and one case of pulmonary toxicity were observed. Thus, reductions in cardiac death and sudden death were observed, but they were of borderline statistical significance.

Amiodarone was compared with therapy with the beta-adrenergic blocker metoprolol and a control group in myocardial infarction survivors in the Spanish Study on Sudden Death (SSSD).[43] Assuming a 2-year mortality of at least 20%, a sample size of 600 to 700 patients was planned to detect a 30% difference in mortality with α of 0.05, two-tailed, and 80% power. Endpoints were death or resuscitation from cardiac arrest. Entry criteria were acute myocardial infarction, age less than 75 years, left ventricular ejection fraction between 20% and 45%, and an average of three or more ventricular ectopic beats per hour, or couplets or runs of ventricular tachycardia in at least one of the two 24-hour electrocardiogram recordings. Exclusions were ventricular tachycardia more than 15 beats in duration, symptomatic bradycardia, first-degree (PR > 0.24 s) or greater atrioventricular block, contraindication to therapy with a beta blocker, and severe renal or liver disease. Patients were randomized to receive amiodarone (115 patients), metoprolol (130 patients), or were left untreated (123 patients). Therapy was not placebo controlled or blinded. Amiodarone was administered as 600 mg daily for 1 week, then 400 mg daily for the second week, then 200 mg daily. Metoprolol was administered as 50 or 100 mg twice daily. Between 1987 and 1991 a total of 1342 infarct survivors at eight university hospitals were screened for entry and 368 patients were enrolled for a median of 37 days after acute myocardial infarction. After 1 year of follow-up the event rate in the control group was substantially lower than anticipated; recruitment was terminated and the follow-up period was extended to 3 years. The two groups were well balanced with respect to age (mean of 59 years), gender (90% male), infarct location (28% anterior), and left ventricular ejection fraction (mean of 34%). Thrombolytic therapy had been administered to 19% of patients. At randomization 38% of patients were receiving aspirin and 7% of patients were receiving captopril. Therapy with lipid-lowering agents was not reported. After a median follow-up of 33.4 months, 30 (8%) patients died; 17 (56%) of the deaths were sudden. By Kaplan-Meier method with two-sided log rank test, the difference in mortality between the amiodarone-treated group (3.5 ± 2%) and the control group (7.7 ± 2.5%) did not reach statistical significance ($P = 0.19$). Surprisingly, the mortality in the metoprolol-treated group (15.4 ± 3.5%) was greater than in the amiodarone-treated ($P < 0.006$) and control groups, although the latter difference did not reach statistical significance ($P = 0.14$). Sudden death occurred in 3%, 4%, and 7% of the amiodarone, control, and metoprolol groups, respectively. Amiodarone reduced the frequency of ventricular ectopic beats and repetitive ventricular ectopic beats at 1, 6, and 12 months. Adverse reactions causing withdrawal of medication occurred in six amiodarone-treated and five metoprolol-treated patients. At the end of the study, 82% and 89% of amiodarone- and metoprolol-treated patients, respectively, were still receiving the study medication. The high mortality in the beta-blocker group is surprising. In larger trials, beta-blocker therapy has consistently reduced mortality, with the greatest benefit observed in patients at increased risk owing to depressed ventricular function. Thus, the high mortality rate in the metoprolol group is likely the result of chance in this relatively small study.

Zarembski and coworkers performed a meta-analysis including 1140 patients in the three trials discussed earlier and a pilot study of 77 patients from the Canadian Amiodarone Myocardial Infarction Trial (CAMIAT) discussed in the following section (Fig. 18–5).[44] They concluded that amiodarone was associated with reductions in total mortality to 6.1% from 11.2%, and in sudden death to 3.1% from 6.9% ($P < 0.01$) but no reduction in cardiac mortality (excluding sudden deaths), which was 2.6% compared with 3.7% ($P = 0.26$).

Canadian and European Amiodarone Trials

To clarify further the effect of amiodarone on survival in patients believed to be at increased risk of sudden death after myocardial infarction, the CAMIAT and the European Myocardial Infarction Amiodarone Trial (EMIAT) were initiated. The CAMIAT was a randomized, double-blind, placebo-controlled trial in 1202 patients with a recent myocardial infarction (6 to 45 days prior to entry into the trial) and frequent spontaneous ventricular arrhythmias, defined as 10 or more ventricular premature depolarizations per hour, or

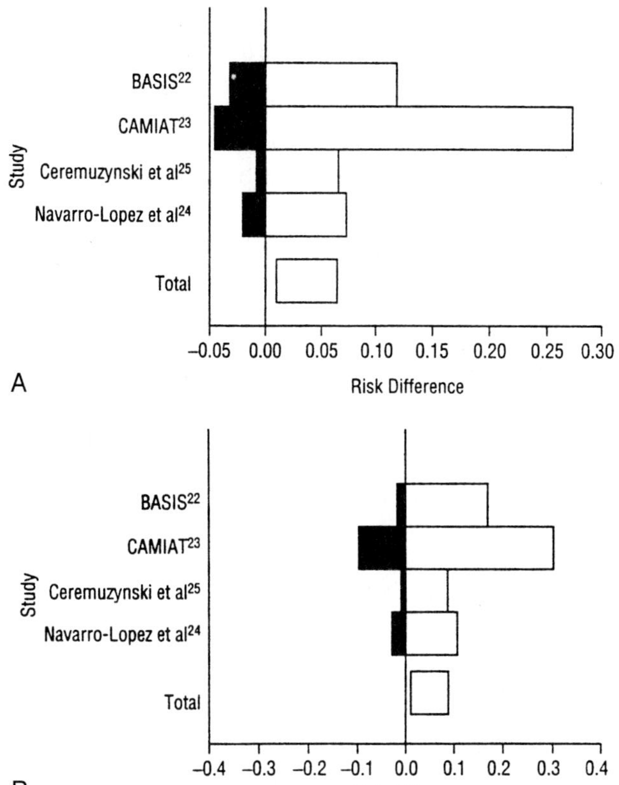

Figure 18–5 Ninety-five percent confidence intervals for risk differences describing the effects of amiodarone on sudden death *(A)* and total mortality *(B)* in BASIS, the CAMIAT pilot study; trials by Ceremuzynski et al and Navarro-Lopez et al; and the combined trials (total) are shown. For the complete citation of the references, see the original source. (From Zarembski DG, Nolan PE Jr, Slack MK, et al. Empiric long-term amiodarone prophylaxis following myocardial infarction. Arch Intern Med 1993; 153:2661–2667. Copyright 1993, American Medical Association.)

any nonsustained ventricular tachycardia.[45] Left ventricular dysfunction was not a requirement for eligibility. The trial was designed to detect among the patients receiving amiodarone a 50% reduction in the primary endpoint, which was a composite of arrhythmic death and resuscitated ventricular fibrillation. It was anticipated that this would translate into a 25% reduction in all-cause mortality but that this effect would not achieve statistical significance because of the relatively small sample size. Amiodarone was administered as a loading dose of 10 mg/kg daily for 2 weeks, followed by 200 to 400 mg daily, depending on the patient's age, body weight, and ability to tolerate the medication.[45]

In the CAMIAT the primary endpoint of arrhythmic death or resuscitated ventricular fibrillation at 2 years was reduced from 6.9% in the placebo group to 4.5% in the amiodarone-assigned patients when the data were analyzed on an intention-to-treat basis.[46] This translated into a 38.2% relative risk reduction (P = 0.029). Thirty-six percent of the amiodarone-treated patients discontinued study medication because of intolerable side effects as compared with only 25.5% in the placebo group. Study medication was stopped because of a pulmonary side effect in 3.8% of patients treated with amiodarone compared with only 1.2% in the placebo-assigned patients. Because of this extremely high discontinuation rate of amiodarone, the data were also examined according to an efficacy analysis, focused only on those patients who remained on their assigned therapy throughout the trial.[46] According to this efficacy analysis, arrhythmic death and resuscitated ventricular fibrillation was reduced from 6% in the placebo group to 3.3% in the amiodarone-treated patients, a 48.5% RR (P = 0.016). The annual all-cause mortality rate was reduced from 6.4% to 5.2% in the intention-to-treat analysis and from 5.4% to 4.4% in the efficacy analysis. As expected, these differences were not statistically significant.

The EMIAT was a randomized, double-blind, placebo-controlled trial in 1486 patients with a recent myocardial infarction (mean time of 15 ± 3.9 days prior to enrollment) and left ventricular ejection fraction less than or equal to 40%.[47] Although a baseline Holter monitor was obtained in all patients, the presence of spontaneous ventricular arrhythmia was not a requirement for study eligibility. Patients assigned to amiodarone treatment received 800 mg daily for 2 weeks, followed by 400 mg daily for 3 months and then 200 mg per day as a maintenance dose. In the design phase of the EMIAT it was estimated that the placebo group would have a 2-year all-cause mortality rate of 15% and that amiodarone would reduce total mortality by 35%. The primary endpoint of the trial was to be all-cause mortality: intention to treat was to be the primary method of analysis, although an efficacy analysis was also planned.

In the EMIAT there were 102 deaths in the placebo group and 103 deaths in amiodarone-assigned patients (risk ratio, 0.99; P = NS) during an average follow-up period of 21 months.[47] Arrhythmic deaths occurred in 50 placebo patients and 33 amiodarone patients, yielding a 35% risk reduction (P = 0.052). Three patients treated with amiodarone died of pulmonary fibrosis compared with one case of nonfatal pulmonary fibrosis in the placebo group. Twice as many patients (six versus three) treated with amiodarone developed pulmonary infiltrates as in the placebo group. Of interest, in spite of the randomized nature of the trial and the relatively large sample size, two possibly important imbalances between the two groups emerged. The amiodarone-assigned patients had a higher prevalence of remote myocardial infarction prior to the qualifying infarction (32% compared with only 26% in the placebo-assigned patients) and a more advanced degree of heart failure (NYHA class I heart failure in 45% of amiodarone-treated patients compared with 50% in the placebo patients). When adjustments were made for these variables, there was a trend toward a reduction in all-cause mortality in patients treated with amiodarone, although the difference between the two groups still did not reach statistical significance.[47]

Although neither the EMIAT nor the CAMIAT demonstrated a survival benefit from amiodarone in patients with a recent myocardial infarction, when the results of these trials are considered together, amiodarone did seem to reduce arrhythmic death significantly. This should translate into a survival benefit, although demonstration of such a survival benefit may require a larger trial targeting a population of patients at greater risk of dying from ventricular fibrillation. Nonetheless, the results of the EMIAT and the CAMIAT do stand in sharp contrast to the CAST and the SWORD trial in the sense that amiodarone at least did not increase mortality. Unlike the class I antiarrhythmic drugs and potassium channel–blocking agents like *d*-sotalol, the risk-benefit ratio for amiodarone appears to be favorable in patients with ischemic heart disease. This may reflect a lower risk of serious ventricular proarrhythmia with amiodarone. However, the relatively high incidence of adverse effects with amiodarone, including the potential for fatal pulmonary toxicity, underscores the need for development of new antiarrhythmic agents with the efficacy of amiodarone but not its toxicity.

Amiodarone in Heart Failure

The Survival Trial of Antiarrhythmic Therapy in Congestive Heart Failure (CHF-STAT) sheds further light on the use of amiodarone in patients with depressed ventricular function and asymptomatic ventricular ectopy who have not had a recent, acute infarction.[48, 49] This trial tested the hypothesis that amiodarone prolongs survival in patients with heart failure and asymptomatic but frequent and complex arrhythmias. It was conducted in U.S. Veterans Affairs Medical Centers and included patients with heart failure of a variety of causes, but the randomization was stratified for presence of coronary artery disease, present in 71% of the study population. Patients with a recent myocardial infarction, within the previous 3 months, were excluded. To detect an improvement in 2-year survival to 80% from 70% ($\alpha = 0.05$, two tailed, and power of 0.90), a desired sample size of 674 patients was estimated assuming substantial (25%) dropouts owing to drug intolerance or side effects. Entry criteria were at least 10 premature ventricular beats per hour; symptomatic congestive heart failure, with dyspnea on exertion or paroxysmal nocturnal dyspnea; left ventricular internal dimension greater than 5.5 cm or cardiothoracic ratio exceeding 0.5 on chest radiograph, and left ventricular ejection fraction of 40% or less. All patients were treated with vasodilators (angiotensin-converting enzyme inhibitors in 78%). In addition to coronary artery disease, randomization was stratified for left ventricular ejection fraction (<30%) and the participating hospital at which they were receiving care. Over the 3.5-year period of enrollment, 1303 patients seen at 24 hospitals were screened for entry, 674 were randomized to placebo or to therapy with amiodarone 800 mg daily for 2 weeks, then 400 mg daily for 50 weeks, then 300 mg daily to the end of the study. The treatment and placebo groups were well balanced with respect to age (mean of 65 and 66 years); gender (99% male); left ventricular ejection fraction less than 30% (67% and 66%); functional class; left ventricular dimension; resting heart rate (80 beats/min in both groups); and therapy with vasodilators, digitalis, and beta-adrenergic blockers (3.9% and 4.7%, respectively). Therapy with lipid-lowering agents was not reported. Analysis of survival was by intention to treat for the duration of the study, which was the 3.5-year enrollment period plus 1 year after enrollment ended (median follow-up of 45 months). There were 274 deaths during the study, 131 (39%) in the amiodarone group and 143 (42%) in the placebo group. Actuarial survival at 2 years was 69.4% in the amiodarone group and 70.8% in the placebo group. In the amiodarone group 49% of deaths were sudden as compared with 52% of the deaths in the placebo group. There was no difference between the amiodarone and the placebo groups in overall mortality or sudden death. In the 481 patients with ischemic heart disease, there was similarly no difference in overall mortality. A trend for better survival with amiodarone was present in the smaller subgroup of 193 patients without ischemic heart disease ($P = 0.07$). As in the CAST trial, suppression of ventricular arrhythmias was achieved but was not a marker for better survival. Amiodarone was associated with an improvement in left ventricular ejection fraction, which increased from 24.9% at baseline to 33.7% at 6 months, compared with an improvement from 25.7% to 29% in the placebo group ($P < 0.001$).

This study was double blinded and analyzed by intention to treat. Although pulmonary toxicity was observed in 1.2%, hepatic toxicity in 1.2%, and bradyarrhythmias in 1.7% of the amiodarone group, study medication was discontinued in 27% of the amiodarone group and 23% of the placebo group owing to real or perceived side effects. An additional 11.5% of patients withdrew or were lost to follow-up.

In summary, trials of amiodarone in various populations of patients with coronary artery disease have shown that, in contrast with flecainide, moricizine, encainide, and *d*-sotalol, amiodarone is a safe antiarrhythmic drug in patients with prior myocardial infarction and depressed ventricular function. Its effect on overall mortality is neutral, although a small beneficial effect cannot be excluded. Arrhythmic deaths are reduced. This finding suggests that the beneficial effect may be offset by some adverse competing risks that have yet to be defined, such as bradyarrhythmias, elevation of blood lipids,[50, 51] or noncardiac toxicities, or that a high enough risk population has not been studied.

IMPLANTABLE DEFIBRILLATORS

The Multicenter Automatic Defibrillator Implantation Trial (MADIT) tested the hypothesis that an implantable defibrillator would improve survival as compared with antiarrhythmic drugs in a high-risk group of myocardial infarct survivors.[52, 53] Entry criteria were a myocardial infarction 3 weeks or more prior to entry, left ventricular ejection fraction less than or equal to 35%, age 25 to 80 years, asymptomatic nonsustained ventricular tachycardia of three or more beats on 24-hour electrocardiographic recording, and inducible ventricular tachycardia at electrophysiologic testing (discussed later). Exclusion criteria were a history of sustained ventricular tachycardia, prior cardiac arrest unrelated to acute myocardial infarction, recent myocardial infarction (within 3 weeks), coronary artery bypass surgery within 2 months, coronary angioplasty within 3 months, NYHA class IV symptoms, or significant, active, myocardial ischemia. Patients meeting the initial screening criteria underwent electrophysiology study. Those who had inducible sustained ventricular tachycardia then received procainamide administered intravenously. If ventricular tachycardia remained inducible, they continued in the study and were randomized to receive either an implantable defibrillator or what was defined at the beginning of the trial as "conventional therapy," in which the choice of antiarrhythmic drug therapy was left to the patient's attending physician. In general, conventional therapy consisted of antiarrhythmic drug therapy guided by electrophysiologic testing to identify a drug that suppressed inducible ventricular tachycardia. If this could not be achieved, amiodarone was often selected. At 1 month of follow-up, 80% of patients in the drug treatment group were receiving amiodarone, 11% were receiving class I antiarrhythmic drugs, and 8% were receiving sotalol. The trial was structured as a sequential design with all-cause mortality as the primary endpoint. After the first 10 deaths, mortality was assessed weekly with the intent of stopping the trial when the log-rank statistic crossed one of the prespecified termination boundaries for either benefit, harm, or no possibility of proving either. Primary analysis used the hazard ratio (risk of death per unit time) according to intention to treat (crossovers were not excluded). An 85% power for detecting a 46% reduction in mortality was anticipated for a sample size of 140 patients per group.

Patient recruitment began in December 1990, and the boundary for mortality reduction was reached in March 1996 after 196 patients had been randomized (95 patients to implantable cardioverter-defibrillator [ICD] and 101 to antiarrhythmic drug therapy). During a mean follow-up period of 27 months, there were 15 deaths in the ICD group and 39 deaths in the drug therapy group. The hazard ratio for risk of death in the ICD group was 0.46 (95% CI, 0.26 to 0.82; $P = 0.009$). Survival at 2 years was 68% in the drug therapy group.

The long recruitment phase introduced several potential problems, that, in the end, did not appear to introduce significant bias. During the initial phase of the trial, the defibrillators were implanted with epicardial lead systems, requiring thoracotomy. Transvenous lead systems became available later in the trial, and approximately half of the ICD group received these systems. There was no operative mortality, however, with either defibrillator system, and surgical infections occurred in only two patients. ICD lead problems occurred in seven patients.

There was no control group of untreated patients. The natural history of this group of patients is not known. Of infarct survivors subjected to electrophysiologic study approximately 1 month after myocardial infarction, fewer than 20% of those who have inducible ventricular tachycardia actually went on to suffer a spontaneous episode of sustained ventricular tachycardia.[10] The risk has not been defined for patients studied later after myocardial infarction; in prior studies patients with inducible ventricular tachycardia were often treated with class I antiarrhythmic drugs. Similarly, at the beginning of MADIT class I antiarrhythmic drugs were still commonly accepted therapy. The enthusiasm for this approach waned in the wake of CAST (see earlier), which showed that these drugs increase mortality in myocardial infarction survivors. This raises the question of whether the better survival in the ICD group could be due to adverse effects of antiarrhythmic drugs in the drug-treated group. Amiodarone, which does not increase mortality in the myocardial infarction survivor (see earlier), was the therapy in 80% of antiarrhythmic drug–treated patients at 1 month. However, only 40% of the patients were still taking amiodarone at the time of last follow-up. Furthermore, many patients received class I drugs prior to amiodarone. The early mortality, potentially due to these drugs, has not yet been reported. The greatest difference in survival occurred during the first year (20% difference), and the survival curves were virtually parallel thereafter. In multivariate analysis, however, there was no effect of amiodarone on the results. There were more than twice as many deaths from nonarrhythmic and unknown causes in the drug-treated group as compared with the ICD group. It is possible that drug toxicities also contributed to these deaths. Although 60% of the ICD-tested patients received a shock within 2 years, it cannot be determined what proportion of these were for ventricular tachycardia that would have been fatal had it not been terminated, rather than a run of supraventricular tachycardia or a self-terminating ventricular tachycardia.

There were minor differences in the ICD and drug-treated groups. Patients in the drug group had slightly lower left ventricular ejection fractions, and only 9% were receiving beta-adrenergic blocking drugs at 1 month as compared with 28% of the ICD group patients. Beta-adrenergic blockers are known to improve survival and reduce sudden death in myocardial infarction survivors. Thus, the benefit of an ICD as compared with beta-adrenergic blocking drug alone in this group is not established by this trial. On the other hand, many patients with heart failure after myocardial infarction do not tolerate therapy with β-adrenergic blocking agents.

In summary, MADIT showed that an ICD improves survival as compared with antiarrhythmic drug therapy in myocardial infarction survivors who have depressed ventricular function, nonsustained ventricular tachycardia, and inducible sustained ventricular tachycardia that cannot be suppressed by procainamide. The U.S. Food and Drug Administration has approved ICD therapy for patients who fit this profile exactly. However, one should exercise caution in extrapolating these results to patients whose ventricular tachycardia *can* be suppressed by procainamide or patients who are noninducible at the outset. Outcomes in such patients were not reported in the MADIT. Equally uncertain is whether ICD therapy is better than a beta-adrenergic blocker alone for this population.

SAMPLE SIZE CONSIDERATIONS FOR FUTURE TRIALS

Although sudden cardiac death is still an important unsolved problem after myocardial infarction, the absolute risk is diminishing. This is particularly evident from analysis of placebo group survival in trials where all myocardial infarction survivors were screened for participation in the trial. For example, CAST and EMIAT screened myocardial infarction survivors for markers of increased risk and randomized only the "high-risk" patients to therapy or placebo. In the original CAST, death from arrhythmia occurred in 1.2% of the placebo group over a follow-up period of 10 months.[26] In EMIAT only 7.1% of patients in the placebo group suffered arrhythmic deaths over an average follow-up period of 22 months. The relative mortality risk from arrhythmias in the present era has important implications for future trials of arrhythmia therapy. A recent analysis estimated samples sizes (90% power, $\alpha = 0.5$) that would be required to demonstrate a favorable impact on mortality of therapies that reduced arrhythmia related death by 50% to 75% in patient populations with an approximately 3% per year risk of sudden death followed for 3 years.[4] Randomization of 1200 to 1600 patients would be required, likely representing 25% of myocardial infarction survivors screened for enrollment. The sample size could be reduced by applying further testing, such as Holter electrocardiogram recording or invasive electrophysiologic testing, to select potential populations with arrhythmic death risks of up to 30%, reducing the number of patients randomized to 200 to 500. However, to obtain this select high-risk population, the testing procedure would have to be applied to 1400 to 3500 patients, obtained from 5600 to 14,000 total infarct survivors initially screened. Trials directed at routine screening of myocardial infarction survivors require almost prohibitively large patient populations.

Trials in myocardial infarction survivors who are referred to centers participating in arrhythmia trials, such as MADIT, are likely to be composed of higher-risk groups, more likely to benefit from therapy. However, the referral process introduces a factor that makes the study population more difficult to characterize. Referring physicians probably select patients for participation in randomized trials they perceive to be either low risk or high risk, based on a variety of factors that may not have been uniformly tested in the eligible patient population. Thus, the applicability of the study results is intrinsically limited. A number of other trials of this nature are in progress evaluating various arrhythmia management strategies in patients with nonsustained ventricular tachycardia, patients with heart failure, and survivors of cardiac arrest or sustained ventricular tachycardia. Careful characterization of the patient population with attention to how patients came to participate in the study will be important to determine how the results of these studies should influence patient management.

REFERENCES

1. Statters DJ, Malik M, Redwood S, et al. Use of ventricular premature complexes for risk stratification after acute myocardial infarction in the thrombolytic era. Am J Cardiol 1996; 77:133–138.
2. Myerburg RJ, Kessler KM, Castellanos A. Sudden cardiac death: Structure, function, and time-dependence of risk. Circulation 1992; 85(1 Suppl):I2–10.
3. Pfisterer M, Salamin P-A, Schwendener R, et al. Clinical risk assessment after first myocardial infarction—is additional noninvasive testing necessary? Chest 1992; 102:1499–1506.
4. Stevenson WG, Ridker PM. Should survivors of myocardial infarction with low ejection fraction be routinely referred to arrhythmia specialists? JAMA 1996; 276:481–485.
5. Weiss JN, Nademanee K, Stevenson WG, et al. Ventricular

arrhythmias in ischemic heart disease. Ann Intern Med 1991; 114:784–797.
6. Richards DAB, Byth K, Ross DL, et al. What is the best predictor of spontaneous ventricular tachycardia and sudden death after myocardial infarction? Circulation 1991; 83:756–763.
7. Pedretti R, Etro MD, Laporta A, et al. Prediction of late arrhythmic events after acute myocardial infarction from combined use of noninvasive prognostic variables and inducibility of sustained monomorphic ventricular tachycardia. Am J Cardiol 1993; 71:1131–1141.
8. McClements BM, Adgey AAJ. Value of signal-averaged electrocardiography, radionuclide ventriculography, Holter monitoring, and clinical variables for prediction of arrhythmic events in survivors of acute myocardial infarction in the thrombolytic era. J Am Coll Cardiol 1993; 21:1419–1427.
9. Maggioni AP, Zuanetti G, Franzosi MG, et al, on behalf of GISSI-2 Investigators. Prevalence and prognostic significance of ventricular arrhythmias after acute myocardial infarction in the fibrinolytic era: GISSI-2 results. Circulation 1993; 87:312–322.
10. Bourke JP, Richards DAB, Ross DL, et al. Routine programmed electrical stimulation in survivors of acute myocardial infarction for prediction of spontaneous ventricular tachyarrhythmias during follow-up: Results, optimal stimulation protocol, and cost-effective screening. J Am Coll Cardiol 1991; 18:780–788.
11. Sager PT, Perlmutter RA, Rosenfeld LE, et al. Electrophysiologic effects of thrombolytic therapy in patients with a transmural anterior myocardial infarction complicated by left ventricular aneurysm formation. J Am Coll Cardiol 1988; 12:19–24.
12. de Chillou C, Sadoul N, Briancon S, et al. Factors determining the occurrence of late potentials on the signal-averaged electrocardiogram after a first myocardial infarction: A multivariate analysis. J Am Coll Cardiol 1991; 18:1638–1642.
13. Gang ES, Lew AS, Hong M, et al. Decreased incidence of ventricular late potentials after successful thrombolytic therapy for acute myocardial infarction. N Engl J Med 1989; 321:712–716.
14. Kersschot IE, Brugada P, Ramentol M, et al. Effects of early reperfusion in acute myocardial infarction on arrhythmias induced by programmed stimulation: A prospective, randomized study. J Am Coll Cardiol 1986; 7:1234–1242.
15. Odemuyiwa O, Jordan P, Malik M, et al. Autonomic correlates of late infarct artery patency after first myocardial infarction. Am Heart J 1993; 125:1597–1600.
16. Pfeffer MA, Braunwald E, Moye LA, et al, on behalf of the SAVE Investigators. Effect of captopril on mortality and morbidity in patients with left ventricular dysfunction after myocardial infarction. N Engl J Med 1992; 327:669–677.
17. Kober L, Torp-Penersen C, Charlsen JE, et al. A clinical trial of the angiotensin-converting enzyme inhibitor trandolapril in patients with left ventricular dysfunction after myocardial infarction. N Engl J Med 1995; 333:1670–1676.
18. Rouleau JL, Talajic M, Sussex B, et al. Myocardial infarction patients in the 1990s—their risk factors, stratification, and survival in Canada: The Canadian Assessment of Myocardial Infarction (CAMI) study. J Am Coll Cardiol 1996; 27:1119–1127.
19. Moss AJ, Davis HT, DeCamilla J, et al. Ventricular ectopic beats and their relation to sudden and nonsudden cardiac death after myocardial infarction. Circulation 1979; 60:998.
20. Bigger JT Jr, Weld FM, Rolnitzky LM. Prevalence, characteristics, and significance of ventricular tachycardia (three or more complexes) detected with ambulatory electrocardiographic recording in the late hospital phase of acute myocardial infarction. Am J Cardiol 1981; 48:814.
21. Furberg CD. Effect of antiarrhythmic drugs on mortality after myocardial infarction. Am J Cardiol 1983; 52:32C.
22. Yusuf S, Wittes J, Friedman L. Overview of results of randomized clinical trials in heart disease: I. Treatments following myocardial infarction. JAMA 1988; 260:2088.
23. IMPACT Research Group. International mexiletine and placebo antiarrhythmic coronary trial: I. Report on arrhythmia and other findings. J Am Coll Cardiol 1984; 4:1148.
24. Cardiac Arrhythmia Pilot Study (CAPS) Investigators. Effects of encainide, flecainide, imipramine, and moricizine on ventricular arrhythmias during the year after acute myocardial infarction: The CAPS. Am J Cardiol 1988; 61:501–509.
25. Cardiac Arrhythmia Suppression Trial (CAST) Investigators. Preliminary report: Effect of encainide and flecainide on mortality in a randomized trial of arrhythmia suppression after myocardial infarction. N Engl J Med 1989; 321:406–412.
26. Echt DS, Liebson PR, Mitchell LB, et al, and the CAST Investigators. Mortality and morbidity in patients receiving encainide, flecainide, or placebo: The Cardiac Arrhythmia Suppression Trial. N Engl J Med 1991; 324:781–788.
27. Cardiac Arrhythmia Suppression Trial II Investigators. Effect of the antiarrhythmic agent moricizine on survival after myocardial infarction. N Engl J Med 1992; 327:227–233.
28. Teo KK, Yusuf S, Furberg CD. Effects of prophylactic antiarrhythmic drug therapy in acute myocardial infarction. JAMA 1993; 270:1589–1595.
29. Pratt CM, Moye LA. The Cardiac Arrhythmia Suppression Trial: Background, interim results, and implications. Am J Cardiol 1990; 65:20B–29B.
30. Bigger JT Jr. Implications of the Cardiac Arrhythmia Suppression Trial for antiarrhythmic drug treatment. Am J Cardiol 1990; 65:3D–10D.
31. Waldo AL, Camm AJ, deRuyter H, et al. The SWORD trial: Survival with oral *d*-sotalol in patients with left ventricular dysfunction after myocardial infarction: Rationale, design, and methods. Am J Cardiol 1995; 75:1023–1027.
32. Waldo AL, Camm AJ, deRuyter H, et al. Effect of *d*-sotalol on mortality in patients with left ventricular dysfunction after recent and remote myocardial infarction. Lancet 1996; 348:7–12.
33. Pratt CM, Camm AJ, Cooper W, et al, for the SWORD Investigators. Mortality in the Survival with Oral *d*-Sotalol (SWORD) trial: Why did patients die? Am J Cardiol 1998; 81:869–876.
34. Julian DG, Prescott RJ, Jackson FS, et al. Controlled trial of sotalol for one year after myocardial infarction. Lancet 1982; 1(8282):1142–1147.
35. Yusuf S, Peto R, Lewis J, et al. Beta blockade during and after myocardial infarction: An overview of the randomized trials. Prog Cardiovasc Dis 1985; 27:335–371.
36. Nademanee K, Singh BN, Stevenson WG, et al. Amiodarone and post-MI patients. Circulation 1993; 88(2):764–774.
37. Wilson JS, Podrid PJ. Side effects from amiodarone. Am Heart J 1991; 121:158–171.
38. Dusman RE, Stanton MS, Miles WM, et al. Clinical features of amiodarone-induced pulmonary toxicity. Circulation 1990; 82:51–59.
39. Burkart F, Pfisterer M, Kiowski W, et al. Effect of antiarrhythmic therapy on mortality in survivors of myocardial infarction with asymptomatic complex ventricular arrhythmias: Basel Antiarrhythmic Study of Infarct (BASIS). J Am Coll Cardiol 1990; 16:1711–1718.
40. Pfisterer M, Kiowski W, Burckhardt D, et al. Beneficial effect of amiodarone on cardiac mortality in patients with asymptomatic complex ventricular arrhythmias after acute myocardial infarction and preserved but not impaired left ventricular function. Am J Cardiol 1992; 69(17):1399–1402.
41. Pfisterer M, Kiowski W, Brunner H, et al. Long-term benefit of one-year amiodarone treatment for persistent complex ventricular arrhythmias after myocardial infarction. Circulation 1993; 87:309–311.
42. Ceremuzynski L, Kleczer E, Krzeminska-Pakula M, et al. Effect of amiodarone on mortality after myocardial infarction: A double-blind, placebo-controlled pilot study. J Am Coll Cardiol 1992; 20:1056–1062.
43. Navarro-López F, Cosin J, Marrugat J, et al. Comparison of the effects of amiodarone versus metoprolol on the frequency of ventricular arrhythmias and on mortality after acute myocardial infarction. Am J Cardiol 1993; 72:1243–1248.
44. Zarembski DG, Nolan PE Jr, Slack MK, et al. Empiric long-term amiodarone prophylaxis following myocardial infarction. Arch Intern Med 1993; 153:2661–2667.
45. Cairns JA, Connolly SJ, Gent M, et al. Post–myocardial infarction mortality in patients with ventricular premature depolarization: Canadian Amiodarone Myocardial Infarction Arrhythmia Trial pilot study. Circulation 1991; 84:550–557.
46. Cairns JA, Connolly SJ, Roberts R, Gent M. Randomized trial of outcome after myocardial infarction in patients with frequent

or repetitive ventricular premature depolarisations: Canadian Amiodarone Myocardial Infarction Arrhythmia Trial (CAMIAT). Lancet 1997; 349:675–682.

47. Julian DG, Camm AJ, Frangin G, et al. Randomised trial of effect of amiodarone on mortality in patients with left ventricular dysfunction after recent myocardial infarction: European Myocardial Infarct Amiodarone Trial (EMIAT). Lancet 1997; 349:667–674.
48. Singh SN, Fletcher RD, Fisher SG, et al. Amiodarone in patients with congestive heart failure and asymptomatic ventricular arrhythmia. N Engl J Med 1995; 333:77–82.
49. Singh SN, Fletcher RD, Fisher S, et al. Veterans Affairs Congestive Heart Failure Antiarrhythmic Trial. Am J Cardiol 1993; 72:99F–102F.
50. Scandinavian Simvastatin Survival Group. Randomized trial of cholesterol lowering in 4,444 patients with coronary heart disease: The Scandinavian Simvastatin Survival Study. Lancet 1994; 344:1383–1389.
51. Wiersinga WM, Trip MD, van Berren MH, et al. An increase in plasma cholesterol independent of thyroid function during long-term amiodarone therapy: A dose-dependent relationship. Ann Intern Med 1991; 114(2):128–132.
52. MADIT Executive Committee: Multicenter Automatic Defibrillator Implantation Trial (MADIT) design and clinical protocol. Pacing Clin Electrophysiol 1991; 14(5 pt 2):920–927.
53. Moss AJ, Hall WJ, Cannom DS, et al, for the Multicenter Automatic Defibrillator Implantation Trial Investigators. Improved survival with an implanted defibrillator in patients with coronary disease at high risk for ventricular arrhythmia. N Engl J Med 1996; 335:1993–1940.

19 Antiarrhythmic Drug Therapy in Supraventricular Tachycardia

▶ Sharon C. Reimold

Clinical trials investigating the efficacy of antiarrhythmic therapy in supraventricular tachycardias are numerous. Compared with other investigative disciplines within cardiology, however, most of the randomized trials are small, single-center studies with short duration of follow-up. These studies are difficult to compare and contrast because of variability in enrollment criteria and study endpoints (Table 19–1). Many investigators have enrolled patients with various forms of supraventricular tachycardia including atrioventricular nodal reentrant tachycardia, atrioventricular reentrant tachycardia (Wolff-Parkinson-White syndrome), and atrial fibrillation in a single study. The response of a given supraventricular arrhythmia to pharmacologic therapy may be variable; therefore, combining data for arrhythmias of multiple mechanisms may be inappropriate when evaluating overall efficacy. Clinical trials designed to investigate acute termination of supraventricular arrhythmias frequently use dissimilar dosing regimens and examine the likelihood of success at intervals ranging from 1 to 8 hours after antiarrhythmic drug administration. The definition of successful therapy may extend from complete suppression of an arrhythmia to a reduction in the frequency and duration of paroxysms of an arrhythmia. For long-term suppression of these arrhythmias, the duration of follow-up is generally on the order of 3 to 12 months, a small duration given the natural history of these disorders.

TABLE 19–1 • Limitations in Comparing and Contrasting Clinical Studies of Pharmacologic Therapy in Supraventricular Tachycardia

- Small number of patients
- Combining patients with arrhythmias of varying mechanisms
  - Atrioventricular nodal reentrant tachycardia
  - Atrioventricular reentrant tachycardia
  - Atrial fibrillation/flutter
- Dose-finding/titration period
- Variable follow-up time for acute and long-term studies
- Variable dosing regimens for the same agent
- Sporadic nature of paroxysmal arrhythmias
- Different definitions of successful therapy (i.e., complete suppression of arrhythmia vs. reduction in the frequency and duration of arrhythmia)
- Multiple ways of assessing efficacy
  - Patient self-reporting
  - Electrocardiogram
  - Transtelephonic monitoring
  - Holter monitoring
- Presence of adjunctive atrioventricular nodal blocking agents
- Uneven distribution of underlying cardiac diseases
- Variable severity of underlying cardiac disorders

Trials examining suppression of paroxysmal arrhythmias most frequently employ the randomized crossover design. The duration of the crossover is variable, ranging from 1 to 3 months. These studies often incorporate a dose-finding or dose-titration phase in which patients are placed on increasing doses of a pharmacologic agent in an attempt to assess the optimal dose for a given patient. Patients who develop significant side effects or who develop worsening arrhythmia during the dose-finding phase are generally excluded from participation in the randomized component of each trial. Thus, the reported efficacy is often based on a selected subset of patients (i.e., patients who are more likely to tolerate a given medication).

Some investigators have chosen to study the impact of antiarrhythmic agents on inducible as opposed to spontaneous arrhythmias. In some supraventricular as well as ventricular arrhythmia trials, there is evidence that termination or suppression of inducible arrhythmia is predictive of the ambient response to a pharmacologic agent. Although the response of a spontaneous arrhythmia to a pharmacologic agent is the ideal endpoint to evaluate, there are some situations in which it is technically difficult to accrue sufficient patients with spontaneous arrhythmias to study effectively the likelihood of acute termination of that arrhythmia. This difficulty may be related to the duration of spontaneous rhythm disturbance as well as the likelihood of the patient being in a hospital environment at the time of arrhythmia onset.

Despite these limitations, it is useful to examine the available trials of antiarrhythmic therapy in supraventricular arrhythmias. As radiofrequency ablation gains acceptance for the long-term treatment of atrioventricular nodal reentrant and atrioventricular reentrant tachycardias on a worldwide basis, many of these clinical trials will primarily be of historical importance. This chapter focuses on the use of pharmacologic agents for (1) acute termination or heart rate control of supraventricular tachycardias, (2) long-term suppression of supraventricular tachycardias, (3) acute termination of paroxysmal atrial fibrillation, (4) long-term suppression of paroxysmal atrial fibrillation, (5) suppression of recurrent chronic atrial fibrillation, (6) prevention of supraventricular arrhythmias after cardiac surgery, and (7) control of the ventricular heart rate response in atrial fibrillation.

ACUTE TERMINATION AND HEART RATE CONTROL OF SUPRAVENTRICULAR TACHYCARDIAS

Conventional atrioventricular nodal blocking agents have been used as well as types I and III antiarrhythmic agents for the acute termination of supraventricular tachycardias. These studies have focused on acute conversion rates, the duration of time from drug administration to conversion, and adverse effects. Results from patients with atrioventricular nodal reentrant tachycardia, atrioventricular reentrant tachycardia, atrial fibrillation or flutter, and automatic atrial tachycardia have been pooled in some studies.

Heart Rate Control in Acute Arrhythmias

Esmolol has been compared with placebo in 71 patients with supraventricular arrhythmias (heart rate > 120 beats/min) lasting for at least 30 minutes.[1] This study included patients primarily with atrial fibrillation or atrial flutter but also included patients with supraventricular arrhythmias such as automatic atrial tachycardia (n = 6). Patients were randomized to esmolol (50 to 300 μg/kg per minute) or placebo and treated for up to 30 minutes. Efficacy endpoints included conversion to sinus rhythm, decrease in heart rate to less than 100 beats/min, or a 20% decrease in heart rate. Patients not responding to the initial regimen were allowed to cross over to the other regimen. Of the 32 patients randomized to esmolol, 23 patients responded to therapy, whereas only 2 of 31 patients responded to placebo therapy. Crossovers to esmolol also had a higher likelihood of response (16 of 29) as compared with placebo (1 of 8). Only two patients converted to sinus rhythm. Increasing the esmolol infusion beyond 150 μg/kg per minute did not result in any additional increase in therapeutic efficacy. Major side effects included hypotension (n = 8) and diaphoresis (n = 7) in patients treated with esmolol. There was one episode of symptomatic hypotension in a placebo-treated patient.

The Esmolol Multicenter Study Research Group compared the efficacy of esmolol and propranolol for the control of heart rate in supraventricular tachyarrhythmias.[2] Esmolol dosing, inclusion criteria, and endpoints were the same as discussed previously.[1] Atrial fibrillation or flutter was present in 95% of 127 study subjects. Esmolol and propranolol were equally effective in decreasing heart rate or converting the patient to sinus rhythm (66% for esmolol vs. 65% for propranolol). Approximately 75% of patients achieved heart rate control during the 4-hour maintenance infusion or injections for both agents. Hypotension developed in 23 of 64 patients receiving esmolol. Hypotension developed in four patients receiving propranolol. Four patients receiving propranolol also developed nausea.

Acute Termination of Supraventricular Tachyarrhythmias

Intravenous verapamil has been used extensively to terminate supraventricular arrhythmias. Supraventricular arrhythmias (atrioventricular nodal reentry [n = 9], sinus node reentry [n = 2], and atrioventricular reentry [n = 9]) were induced in 20 patients undergoing programmed electrical stimulation.[3] Fifteen of 19 patients converted to sinus rhythm with verapamil (0.075 mg/kg), whereas only 1 of 16 patients converted to sinus rhythm after receiving placebo.

Verapamil has been compared with adenosine in a larger randomized trial using a sequential dose-ranging protocol.[4] Patients had both spontaneous and induced arrhythmias. Pre-excitation was present in 22% of patients. In the first portion of this trial, adenosine was given in sequential doses of 3, 6, 9, and 12 mg (n = 137) or matching placebo was administered (n = 64). Adenosine was significantly more effective than placebo, and its efficacy increased with dose (Fig. 19–1). In the second phase of the study, patients were randomized between adenosine (n = 77, 6 mg followed by 12 mg intravenously) or verapamil (n = 81, 5 mg followed by 7.5 mg intravenously if no response). Efficacy was similar between the two agents if both doses are included (93.4% for adenosine and 90.6% for verapamil). Concomitant digoxin use, evidence of preexcitation in sinus rhythm, and mechanism of arrhythmia initiation did not influence efficacy. Facial flushing, chest pain, and dyspnea were common with adenosine (approximately 40% of patients) but were transient, generally resolving within 2 minutes. Side effects with verapamil were less com-

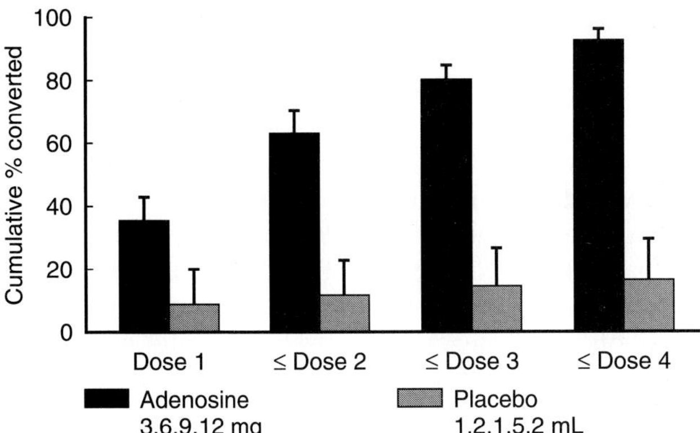

Figure 19–1 Cumulative efficacy of adenosine. The bars represent the cumulative percentage (with 95% confidence interval) of eligible patients converting to sinus rhythm after adenosine and placebo. Data on both patients initially assigned to adenosine and those who crossed over to adenosine after four placebo injections are included. Each bar represents the percent converting after completion of that dose and the preceding dose or doses with each agent. Intravenous doses of adenosine were 3, 6, 9, and 12 mg; corresponding volumes of saline injected were 1, 2, 1.5, and 2 mL. Significant differences ($P < 0.001$) were seen at each dose level. (From DiMarco JP, Miles W, Akhtar M, et al. Adenosine for paroxysmal supraventricular tachycardia: Dose ranging and comparison with verapamil—assessment in placebo-controlled, multicenter trials. Ann Intern Med 1990; 113:104–110.)

mon (12.4%) but occasionally lasted longer (hypotension in one patient lasting 20 minutes and facial flushing in one patient lasting 20 minutes).

The central intravenous administration of adenosine has been evaluated in 30 patients (atrioventricular reentrant tachycardia in 18, atrioventricular nodal reentrant tachycardia in 12) undergoing programmed electrical stimulation.[5] Sequential adenosine doses of 3, 6, 9, and 12 mg were administered by the peripheral and central routes. The dose required for central conversion was less (3.8 ± 1.6 mg) than for peripheral conversion (6.3 ± 3.3 mg). The time from drug administration to conversion was also less with central injections (12.7 ± 5.1 seconds vs. 19.2 ± 7.9 seconds). Side effects did not differ between the two arms. This time difference should not influence the clinician's decision regarding route of drug administration. Adenosine triphosphate has been compared with adenosine.[6] Efficacy rates (93% with adenosine and 88% with adenosine triphosphate) and time to conversion were similar between the two agents.

Intravenous diltiazem has been studied by two groups for the termination of paroxysmal supraventricular tachycardias.[7, 8] Dougherty and colleagues[7] found that conversion to sinus rhythm was dose dependent. Patients receiving 0.05 mg/kg of diltiazem were much less likely to convert to sinus rhythm than those patients receiving 0.15 mg/kg of diltiazem or higher. Overall efficacy for conversion was 75% (47 of 63) for all doses of diltiazem and 25% (6 of 24) for the control group. Hypotension was the most common side effect, occurring in seven (12%) patients receiving diltiazem. In another study, 34 patients with atrioventricular reentrant tachycardia and 20 patients with atrioventricular nodal reentrant tachycardia were treated with intravenous diltiazem after arrhythmia induction.[8] Diltiazem was effective in 24 of 28 (86%) patients, whereas only 5 of 26 (19%) of placebo-treated patients converted to sinus rhythm. The median time to conversion was 2 minutes after beginning the diltiazem infusion. Propafenone, sotalol, and flecainide have also been used for acute termination of supraventricular arrhythmias. In a group of 20 patients, 15 of 20 patients receiving propafenone (2 mg/kg intravenously) converted to sinus rhythm, but 0 of 11 patients receiving placebo converted to sinus rhythm.[9] Sotalol appears to be equally efficacious (conversion in 30 minutes in 83% of sotalol-treated patients and 16% of placebo-treated patients; n = 43).[10] In another study, sotalol was effective in 67% of patients compared with 14% of control patients.[11]

β-adrenergic blocking agents (esmolol and propranolol) have been shown to reduce the heart rate of patients with supraventricular tachycardias. Acute termination of atrioventricular nodal reentrant tachycardias may be achieved in almost all patients with adenosine or verapamil. Efficacy increases with dosage. The side-effect profiles vary slightly between adenosine and verapamil and may form the basis for choosing one agent versus the other. Intravenous diltiazem as well as type I or III antiarrhythmic agents are effective in terminating supraventricular arrhythmias. In many centers, these agents are not first-line therapy because of cost and concerns regarding side effects.

LONG-TERM SUPPRESSION OF SUPRAVENTRICULAR TACHYCARDIAS

Few randomized trials exist studying pharmacologic therapy for the long-term suppression of supraventricular tachycardias. Those trials that do exist frequently pool patients with atrioventricular nodal reentrant tachycardia and atrioventricular reentrant tachycardia (Wolff-Parkinson-White syndrome) into one group. Because the mechanisms of the arrhythmias are different, this pooling may ultimately influence the results obtained.

The efficacy of verapamil in suppressing supraventricular tachycardias was investigated in a small trial of 12 patients (atrioventricular nodal reentrant tachycardia [n = 7], concealed bypass tract [n = 3], Wolff-Parkinson-White syndrome [n = 2]).[12] Each patient was required to have at least two episodes of arrhythmia per month on no suppressive therapy. After a dose-finding phase, patients entered a 4-month blinded protocol of alternating verapamil and placebo therapy in a randomized fashion. Efficacy was judged by the number of episodes of arrhythmia as well as the duration of arrhythmia by patient report and weekly Holter monitor. Patients had 0.7 ± 0.7 episodes per day on placebo by Holter versus 0.3 ± 0.5 episodes per day on verapamil ($P < 0.05$). The average duration of arrhythmia fell dramatically on treatment (67 ± 111 minutes per day on placebo vs. 1 ± 2 minutes per day on verapamil [$P < 0.05$]). These results suggest a beneficial effect of verapamil on the suppression of these arrhythmias over a relatively short period.

Winniford and colleagues[13] then studied 11 patients with documented supraventricular arrhythmia occurring at least two times per month in the absence of therapy and no evidence of ventricular preexcitation. Patients received digoxin, propranolol, or verapamil for 1 month followed by a 1-week washout period. Efficacy was judged by patient diary as well as weekly Holter monitors. According to the patient diaries, the number of weekly episodes of tachycardia did not vary between agents (digoxin, 2.3 ± 3.1 episodes; propranolol, 1.5 ± 2.3 episodes; verapamil, 2.9 ± 5.7 episodes). The authors did not include a placebo arm in this small study to allow the absolute effect of these atrioventricular nodal blocking agents to be determined.

Clair and associates[14] have studied the influence of oral diltiazem on the prevention of supraventricular tachycardia in 17 patients without bypass tracts who experienced arrhythmias at least three times in 6 months. After a dose-ranging study to select the optimal dose of diltiazem (60 to 90 mg every 6 hours), patients entered a 2-month randomized phase followed by crossover to the other arm. Each randomized phase lasted for 60 days or until the first recurrence of arrhythmia. Endpoints included the duration of time until first recurrence and heart rate during tachycardia. Diltiazem did not significantly prolong the time until first recurrence but did decrease the heart rate during active therapy (average 208 beats/min without therapy to 189 beats/min on diltiazem; $P < 0.01$). This study was too small to detect anything but a large difference between diltiazem and placebo.

The type IC agents, flecainide and propafenone, have been studied in the suppression of supraventricular tachycardia. The Flecainide Supraventricular Tachycardia Study Group enrolled 34 patients with a history of at least one episode of arrhythmia in the month before drug initiation.[15] A dose-ranging trial of flecainide was performed for 3 weeks to determine the maximal tolerated drug dosage for each patient (up to 200 mg twice a day). The next phase consisted of an 8-week randomized, placebo-controlled, crossover study. Patients could cross over after the documentation of four episodes of supraventricular tachycardia. Although 51 patients qualified for the study, only 34 were available for the randomized phase. Three of these patients had adverse cardiac effects, including myocardial infarction ($n = 1$), ventricular fibrillation during programmed electrophysiologic stimulation ($n = 1$), and incessant supraventricular tachycardia after intravenous flecainide ($n = 1$). Of the patients randomized, the cumulative proportion of patients free of tachycardia at 8 weeks was 0.79 for flecainide and 0.15 for placebo. Twenty-nine of 34 patients had a least one paroxysm while on placebo as compared with 8 of 34 with at least one event on flecainide. Pritchett and colleagues[16] studied propafenone in a similar protocol in 16 patients with paroxysmal supraventricular tachycardia. The time to first recurrence was prolonged in patients receiving propafenone in this trial; data from patients with atrial fibrillation were pooled with those who had supraventricular tachycardia.

The UK Propafenone Paroxysmal Supraventricular Tachycardia (PSVT) Study Group has studied the influence of propafenone versus placebo in 52 patients with paroxysmal supraventricular tachycardia.[17] The study design included two crossover phases of propafenone 300 mg twice a day versus placebo and propafenone 300 mg three times a day versus placebo. Recurrent arrhythmia was documented by diary and transtelephonic monitor. Twenty-nine of 45 patients completing the first phase of the study were free of arrhythmia and adverse effects while on propafenone, whereas 11 of 45 were free of events while on placebo. Propafenone was even more effective at the higher dose (31 of 34 patients), but adverse events were more frequent (7 of 34 patients).

Thus, few trials are available investigating the efficacy of pharmacologic therapy in the suppression of paroxysmal supraventricular tachycardia. Trials that exist suggest that both atrioventricular nodal blocking agents and type IC antiarrhythmic agents may be effective in reducing the frequency, duration, or heart rate of episodes. Trials investigating calcium channel blockers are small and have shown equivocal results. Most of these studies are of short duration. Prescription of a given agent may depend not only on effectiveness, but also on the side-effect profiles and cost. It is unlikely that large-scale trials of these agents will be performed because no long-term suppressive therapy may be needed for the patient with rare episodes, and radiofrequency ablation may be recommended as the most effective therapy to many patients with frequent paroxysms.

ACUTE TERMINATION OF PAROXYSMAL ATRIAL FIBRILLATION

Paroxysmal atrial fibrillation is a difficult clinical entity because the acute episodes may lead to palpitations, dyspnea, lightheadedness, or chest discomfort as well as a variety of other symptoms. Patients with brief episodes may not present for acute medical attention, but patients with more severe symptoms frequently present emergently. Effective, prompt therapy is ideal for alleviating patient symptoms. A summary of the efficacy of these trials is given in Table 19–2.

Digoxin is the primary therapy that has been available to clinicians for several decades. Because of its vagally mediated effects, however, digoxin has the potential for having little effect or a negative effect on the acute termination of atrial fibrillation. One randomized trial investigating digoxin in the conversion of recent-onset atrial fibrillation has been performed.[18] Falk and colleagues[18] enrolled 36 patients with atrial fibrillation (≤7 days duration) and randomized them to treatment with digoxin or placebo (0.6, 0.4, 0.2, and 0.2 mg at 0, 4, 8, and 14 hours). Patients were monitored for 18 hours for the return of sinus rhythm. Eight of 18 patients receiving placebo and 9 of 18 patients receiving digoxin converted to sinus rhythm within the observation period. The average time to conversion was 5.1 hours with digoxin and 3.3 hours with placebo (P = NS). Thus, in this small trial, there were no significant differences between digoxin and placebo in the conversion of atrial fibrillation to sinus rhythm.

Pirmenol is a type I agent that has been investigated for the acute conversion of atrial fibrillation. In a randomized intravenous protocol, patients receiving pirmenol were more likely to convert to sinus rhythm (12 of 20) in 1 hour than those receiving placebo (3 of 20).[19] No controlled trials exist comparing other type IA agents with placebo.

Flecainide, a type IC agent, has been studied by several groups and compared with other agents as well as to placebo. In comparison to procainamide, patients receiving flecainide were more likely to convert to sinus rhythm within 1 hour of infusion (37 of 40 vs. 25 of 40).[20] The time to conversion was not different between the agents. Oral treatment has also been found to be effective for conversion to sinus rhythm, but the time to conversion is longer (104 minutes vs. 14 minutes in a group of 27 patients).[21] In another trial, flecainide (2 mg/kg) was administered concurrently with digoxin and compared with digoxin monotherapy.[22] Six hours after therapy was initiated, 34 of 51 patients receiving flecainide plus digoxin and 18 of 51 patients receiving digoxin monotherapy were in sinus rhythm.[22] Transient significant hypotension was more common in patients receiving flecainide than in the control group. In comparison to verapamil, flecainide is more effective in terminating atrial fibrillation (14 of 20 vs. 1 of 20).[23]

Oral loading of flecainide has been compared with amiodarone and placebo therapy. Flecainide was associated with a higher rate of conversion (20 of 22 vs. 10 of 21 in the placebo group) with mean conversion times of 190 ± 147 minutes.[24] Amiodarone was associated with a lower rate of conversion (7 of 19) than flecainide in the first day of therapy. In another trial with similar design but a higher dose of amiodarone (7 mg/kg), flecainide was more effective in the first 2 hours after drug administration, but this superiority was inapparent 8 hours after drug administration (flecainide 68%, amiodarone 59%, placebo 56%).[25] Amiodarone, however, was more effective in acutely controlling the ventricular rate response.

Propafenone is another type IC agent used for the treatment of atrial fibrillation. In two trials comparing propafenone with flecainide, flecainide was more effective (pooled results 28 of 40 converted to normal sinus rhythm with flecainide and 16 of 40 converted to normal sinus rhythm with propafenone).[26, 27] Hypo-

TABLE 19–2 • Effectiveness of Antiarrhythmic Agents in Terminating Acute Atrial Fibrillation

Drug 1	Drug 2	Duration of Trial (h)	Proportion in Normal Sinus Rhythm: *Drug 1*	*Drug 2*	Value	Reference
Digoxin	Placebo	18	9/18	8/18	NS	18
Pirmenol	Placebo	1	12/20	3/20	< 0.01	19
Flecainide	Procainamide	1	37/40	25/40	< 0.001	20
Flecainide plus digoxin	Digoxin	1	29/51	7/51	< 0.001	21
Flecainide	Verapamil	1	14/20	1/20	< 0.001	22
Flecainide	Amiodarone	8	20/22	17/19	NS	23
Flecainide	Amiodarone	2	20/34	11/32	NS	24
Flecainide	Propafenone	1	10/20	5/20	< 0.05	25
Flecainide	Propafenone	1	18/20	11/20	< 0.02	26
Propafenone	Placebo	24	89/98	27/84	< 0.001	27
Propafenone	Digoxin plus quinidine	24	25/29	23/29	NS	28
Sotalol	Digoxin plus quinidine	12	17/33	24/28	< 0.001	30
Amiodarone	Digoxin plus quinidine	24	31/33	27/29	NS	31
Amiodarone	Digoxin	24	24/26	17/24	NS	32

tension may be associated with either therapy. In comparison to placebo, propafenone (2 mg/kg followed by a 10 mg/kg per 24-hour infusion) was more likely to result in sinus rhythm (89 of 98 vs. 27 of 84).[28] Termination of arrhythmia was quicker in patients treated with propafenone (2.5 ± 2.8 hours vs. 17.2 ± 7.8 hours for placebo). The efficacy of oral propafenone has been contrasted with digoxin plus quinidine combination therapy and placebo in a group of 87 patients.[29] Although the 12-hour conversion rates were higher in the propafenone group as compared with the other treatment arms, the 48-hour conversion to sinus rhythm was 76% in the placebo group, which was similar to the propafenone group at this time point. Intravenous propafenone and amiodarone have been administered at home for acute conversion of atrial fibrillation.[30] The median time of conversion was shorter for propafenone (10 minutes) than for amiodarone (60 minutes). Termination of the arrhythmia was also more frequent in patients receiving propafenone (88%) than amiodarone (40%).

Acute conversion to sinus rhythm with sotalol (17 of 33) was less effective than digoxin plus quinidine (24 of 28) in an oral loading trial.[31] Asymptomatic ventricular tachycardia was observed in several patients in both arms of the trial; hypotension or bradycardia developed in nearly half of the patients receiving sotalol (80 mg at 0, 2, 6, and 10 hours).[31]

Intravenous amiodarone is also effective for the acute conversion of atrial fibrillation. Amiodarone was as effective as quinidine (31 of 33 vs. 27 of 29) over a 24-hour period.[32] Twenty-four of 26 patients receiving amiodarone achieved sinus rhythm versus 17 of 24 patients randomized to digoxin monotherapy in another trial.[33]

Although many classes of pharmacologic therapy are useful for the acute termination of arrhythmias, the primary result of antiarrhythmic administration appears to be decreasing the duration of a paroxysm. Depending on the nature of the underlying heart disease and patient symptoms, terminating an episode more quickly may help the patient feel better and decrease the use of medical resources.

ANTIARRHYTHMIC THERAPY FOR THE PREVENTION OF PAROXYSMS OF ATRIAL FIBRILLATION

Episodes of paroxysmal atrial fibrillation occur at varying frequencies but are believed to occur according to a Poisson distribution. Trials investigating the role of antiarrhythmic therapy in the prevention of recurrent paroxysms focus on endpoints such as time to first recurrence of arrhythmia, the frequency of arrhythmia recurrence, or the likelihood of total suppression of the arrhythmia. These trials are difficult to perform and interpret when the frequency of events is uncommon or rare. As a result, most trials focus on patients with frequent symptomatic atrial arrhythmias.

Van Wijk and colleagues[34] studied 49 patients with weekly episodes of paroxysmal atrial fibrillation. These patients were randomized to flecainide 100 mg twice a day or quinidine 500 mg twice a day. Drug dosages were adjusted upward for symptomatic recurrences (flecainide 150 mg twice a day or quinidine 500 mg three times a day), and patients were treated for 3 months followed by a 3-month crossover to the other drug regimen. Recurrences were documented by self-report, electrocardiogram, and monthly 24-hour Holter monitoring. At the maximal dose prescribed during this 3-month period, flecainide totally suppressed atrial fibrillation by Holter in 50% of patients, and quinidine was effective in 32% (P = NS). Twenty percent of patients discontinued quinidine because of undesirable side effects, including one patient with prolonged QT. One patient receiving flecainide developed hemodynamically well-tolerated ventricular tachycardia necessitating drug withdrawal. One patient receiving flecainide died; this death was deemed unrelated to drug therapy by the authors.

A comparison of flecainide and quinidine for this purpose was also performed by Lau and coworkers,[35] who randomized 19 patients without structural heart disease to these agents. Trial design included blinded therapy for 8 weeks followed by a crossover phase. Thirteen patients also completed a placebo phase. Transtelephonic monitoring was used to record recurrences in addition to monthly Holter monitors. All patients experienced symptoms during the placebo phase, whereas flecainide resulted in suppression of symptoms in 4 of 19 patients, and quinidine resulted in control of symptoms in 2 of 11 patients. Alternate ways of expressing the efficacy of therapy include a prolongation of the time to first recurrence of arrhythmia (placebo, 2 days; flecainide, 21 days; quinidine 15 days [$P < 0.01$]), symptomatic duration of arrhythmia (placebo, 1619 ± 616 minutes; flecainide, 975 ± 424 minutes; quinidine, 865 ± 306 minutes), and frequency of arrhythmia (placebo, 25 ± 9 episodes per 8 weeks; flecainide, 14 ± 8 episodes; quinidine, 24 ± 10 episodes). Although both quinidine and flecainide appeared to decrease the duration of therapy and the time to first recurrence, quinidine did not alter the frequency of arrhythmia.

The Flecainide Multicenter Atrial Fibrillation Study Group studied flecainide (n = 122) versus quinidine (n = 117) in patients with symptomatic paroxysmal atrial fibrillation.[36] Patients with significant ventricular arrhythmias, conduction defects, or left ventricular dysfunction were excluded from participating in the study as well as those with significant noncardiac diseases. Patients kept a diary to record characteristics and frequency of attacks on medication. Antiarrhythmic agents were discontinued for development of significant conduction defects, QT prolongation, or drug-related toxicity. These patients had frequent paroxysms of arrhythmia (13.4 per month in the flecainide group and 10.7 per month in the quinidine group). The majority of patients had been treated with antiarrhythmics previously. Approximately 10% of patients in each group (9.8% flecainide and 12.0% quinidine) discontinued therapy because of an unacceptable response. Approximately one fifth of patients (23.8% flecainide and 20.5% quinidine) had total suppression of arrhythmia during a 9-month period. In approximately three quarters of all patient months, there were no symptomatic arrhythmias with both agents. Side effects resulted in discontinuation of therapy in 29.9% of quinidine-treated patients and 18.0% of flecainide-treated patients. There were no deaths in this trial. Thus, both quinidine and flecainide effectively reduced the frequency of paroxysms of atrial fibrillation. Quinidine was more likely to be associated with adverse effects.

The Danish-Norwegian Flecainide Multicenter Study Group administered flecainide (150 mg twice a day) or placebo to 43 patients with paroxysmal atrial fibrillation for 3 months with a crossover period.[37] Entry criteria included a minimum of three symptomatic paroxysms over a 3-month interval on 3 different days lasting less than 72 hours. Flecainide decreased the mean paroxysms per week (0.2 ± 0.4) in comparison to placebo (1.9 ± 12.1) in individuals completing both treatment periods. Complete response was seen in 12 of 24 flecainide-treated patients with no response in 8 patients. Of note, two patients died during the flecainide treatment period, one with pulmonary carcinoma and one while swimming in the North Sea.

Propafenone is another type IC antiarrhythmic agent studied in the treatment of paroxysmal atrial fibrillation. Connolly and Hoffert[38] studied 18 patients with monthly symptomatic episodes of atrial fibrillation. These patients entered a randomized trial with four monthly treatment periods alternating between propafenone and placebo. Early crossovers were permitted on patient request for perceived inefficacy. Patient diaries and transtelephonic monitors were used to document arrhythmia recurrences. Only 12 of 18 patients participated in the crossover study. The other six withdrew because of side effects or inefficacy during the dose-ranging study ($n = 5$) or because of noncompliance ($n = 1$). Efficacy was judged by reduction in episodes of atrial fibrillation. During the placebo phase, patients experienced fibrillation on 51 ± 34% of days. This was reduced to 27 ± 34% of days on propafenone. Patients were more likely to cross over prematurely on placebo (45%) than on propafenone (14%). One patient receiving placebo experienced sudden death during the trial.

Pritchett and colleagues[16] investigated propafenone in 17 patients with paroxysmal atrial fibrillation. Atfer a dose-finding phase, patients were randomly assigned to placebo or propafenone for up to 60 days. The observation period began 3 days after the beginning of therapy and continued until the recurrence of arrhythmia or 60 days, the maximal length of the study period. Patients were then treated with the second agent in a similar fashion. Patients were allowed to continue digoxin therapy. Only 9 of 17 patients with paroxysmal atrial fibrillation entered the randomized phase of the study. In these nine patients, the time to first recurrence of arrhythmia was prolonged with propafenone. Data pooled from patients with supraventricular tachycardia as well as atrial fibrillation suggest that the rate of recurrent arrhythmia is approximately 21% that of placebo therapy. Cardiac adverse events included one episode of atrial flutter with a rate of 263 beats/min in one patient and the development of chest discomfort, presyncope, and dyspnea in another patient, both of whom were receiving propafenone in an open-label fashion after completion of the randomized phase.

The Flecainide AF French Study Group enrolled 97 patients with paroxysmal atrial fibrillation into a study of flecainide versus placebo.[39] Patients with heart failure, significant conduction disturbances, or recent amiodarone usage were excluded from participation. Hypertension and lone atrial fibrillation were the most common causes of underlying disease. Twenty-three percent of flecainide-treated patients and 24% of propafenone-treated patients discontinued therapy because of an inadequate response. At 1 year of therapy, the probability of successful treatment on flecainide treatment was 62% and on propafenone was 47%. One patient with hypertension receiving propafenone died during the study.

Reimold and colleagues[40] have studied propafenone and sotalol in patients with paroxysmal atrial fibrillation ($n = 47$). In their study, the randomization was stratified according to arrhythmia pattern and left atrial size. The likelihood of any recurrence of atrial fibrillation at 6 months was similar between those patients treated with propafenone (42 ± 10) and sotalol (48 ± 12) (P = NS). Thirty patients with paroxysmal atrial fibrillation received propafenone or placebo in the UK Propafenone PSVT Study Group, a 3-month double-blind, double-crossover study.[17] Patients were less likely to have adverse effects or recurrent atrial fibrillation on propafenone 300 mg twice a day (17 of 30) versus placebo (8 of 30). As the dose of propafenone increased to 300 mg three times a day, the incidence of adverse events increased to 40%.

Propafenone has been compared with hydroquinidine in a larger study of 200 patients with a minimum of three recurrences of atrial fibrillation in 6 months.[41] At 6 months after drug initiation, survival of sinus rhythm was 60% for propafenone and 56% for quinidine, suggesting similar efficacy rates.

Thus, these randomized trials investigating antiarrhythmic therapy in the prevention of episodes of paroxysmal atrial fibrillation demonstrate drug efficacy when examining parameters such as frequency of recurrence, time to first recurrence, and duration of episodes. Total suppression of arrhythmia over a long period of time seems less likely. Because the authors of these studies chose different endpoints and enrolled a heterogeneous group of patients in terms of underlying heart disease, they are difficult to compare. Most trials lasted a brief period of time relative to the duration of this chronic disease process. Extrapolating from these data to long-term efficacy is extremely difficult because the underlying disease process may not remain stable over time.

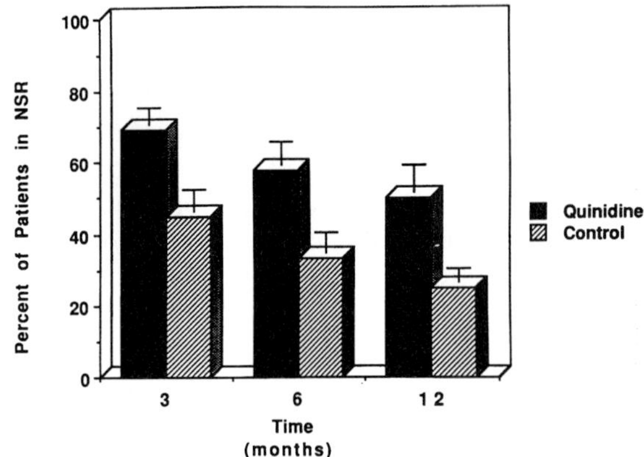

Figure 19–2 Proportion of patients remaining in normal sinus rhythm (NSR) at 3, 6, and 12 months after cardioversion was greater at all time intervals in quinidine-treated group as compared with control group ($P < 0.001$). (From Coplen SE, Antman EM, Berlin JA, et al. Efficacy and safety of quinidine therapy for maintenance of sinus rhythm after cardioversion: A meta-analysis of randomized control trials. Circulation 1990; 82:1106–1116.)

SUPPRESSION OF CHRONIC ATRIAL FIBRILLATION

Quinidine is a type IA agent that has been available for decades for the maintenance of sinus rhythm. With the advent of direct current cardioversion in the early 1960s, reestablishment of sinus rhythm became possible in a large proportion of patients with sinus rhythm, and the influence of quinidine on the maintenance of sinus rhythm over time could be observed. Coplen and coworkers[42] examined six randomized, controlled trials of quinidine in the maintenance of sinus rhythm. These six trials together enrolled 808 patients. The efficacy of quinidine in maintaining sinus rhythm was evident at 3, 6, and 12 months after cardioversion (Fig. 19–2) with an absolute difference of 24.4% (14.0, 34.8) between quinidine and placebo therapy 12 months after cardioversion. This meta-analysis raised the issue of increased mortality in patients treated with quinidine (1.8%) versus placebo (0.3%).[40] A smaller study ($n = 53$) evaluated the efficacy of verapamil versus quinidine in the conversion and maintenance of sinus rhythm.[43] There was a higher conversion to sinus rhythm with quinidine; long-term maintenance of sinus rhythm was similar between these agents at 12 and 24 months.

Disopyramide has been compared with placebo in several studies.[44, 45] The overall efficacy of disopyramide is similar to quinidine in these studies. Karlson and associates[45] studied 90 patients who were randomized to disopyramide or placebo. At 1 year after cardioversion, 54% of disopyramide and 30% of placebo patients remained in sinus rhythm.[45]

A contemporary comparison between quinidine and sotalol, a type III antiarrhythmic agent, was made by Juul-Moller and colleagues.[46] They studied 183 patients with chronic atrial fibrillation who were cardioverted to normal sinus rhythm. Two hours after conversion, patients were randomized to quinidine ($n = 85$) or sotalol ($n = 98$). At 6 months of follow-up, 52% of sotalol-treated patients and 48% of quinidine-treated patients remained in sinus rhythm (P = NS). Relapses to atrial fibrillation occurred in 34% of sotalol-treated patients and in 22% of quinidine-treated patients. Adverse effects were more likely in quinidine-treated (50%) than in sotalol-treated (28%) patients. Two patients died during the study, one receiving sotalol (posterolateral myocardial infarction) and one receiving quinidine (cerebral embolism). Ventricular tachycardia and ventricular fibrillation occurred in an additional two patients receiving quinidine; both these episodes occurred during hospital monitoring and had successful outcomes. Propafenone and sotalol were compared by Reimold and colleagues[40] in 53 patients with chronic atrial fibrillation. These agents were equally effective at maintaining sinus rhythm 6 months after starting therapy.

The efficacy of flecainide versus placebo for the maintenance of sinus rhythm was tested by Van Gelder and coworkers[47] in 81 patients with chronic atrial fibrillation. Patients without congestive heart failure or significant angina pectoris were excluded as well as those patients with myocardial infarction within 2 years of enrollment, major conduction defects, or severe systemic disease. Sinus rhythm was maintained in 49% of flecainide-treated patients versus 36% of untreated patients 12 months after initiation of therapy. This difference was nonsignificant given the small number of patients in this study. New York Heart Association (NYHA) class and flecainide treatment were predictive of outcome, whereas left atrial size and duration of atrial fibrillation were not predictive of rhythm outcome. Adverse cardiac events related to flecainide included syncope, sinus arrest, high-grade atrioventricular block, rate-related left bundle branch block, and proarrhythmic ventricular premature beats.

Although amiodarone has been shown to have improved maintenance of sinus rhythm in patients with chronic atrial fibrillation, there are no randomized trials comparing this agent with placebo. One nonrandomized trial found the 3-year likelihood of staying in sinus rhythm in patients who had failed other therapy to be 53%.[48] Another trial studying a similar group of patients ($n = 100$) found the actuarial rate of sinus rhythm survival at 3 years to be 70%, a rate far better than results with conventional therapy.[49]

Type IA and IC antiarrhythmic agents and sotalol have been shown to be effective in preventing recurrences of chronic atrial fibrillation in randomized clinical trials. This effectiveness extends over a period ranging from 6 months to 2 years in most patients. Amiodarone may be more effective than these agents, but there are no randomized controlled trials investigating its efficacy. The decision to use any agent to maintain sinus rhythm must be weighed against the potential side effects of each individual agent, especially because many of these side effects could be serious.

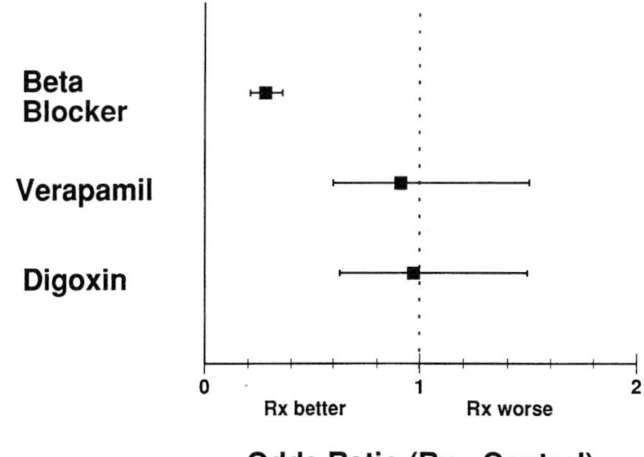

Figure 19–3 Summary odds ratio for the development of supraventricular arrhythmias as estimated by the Mantel-Haenszel method for treatment (Rx) with digoxin, verapamil, or beta blockers. The width of the horizontal lines indicates the 95% confidence intervals for the estimates of the odds ratios shown. (From Andrews TC, Reimold SC, Berlin JA, Antman EM. Prevention of supraventricular arrhythmias after coronary artery bypass surgery: A meta-analysis of randomized control trials. Circulation 1991; 84(Suppl 3):III-236–III-244.)

PREVENTION OF SUPRAVENTRICULAR ARRHYTHMIAS AFTER CARDIAC SURGERY

Supraventricular arrhythmias, most frequently atrial fibrillation, are common complications of coronary artery bypass surgery. Several randomized trials have been performed investigating the role of digoxin, β-adrenergic blocking agents, and calcium channel blocking agents in the prevention of these arrhythmias. Trial design has been variable in terms of the time of initiation of therapy (preoperatively or postoperatively), dosage and choice of agent, and duration and type of monitoring postoperatively as well as the duration of arrhythmias needed for reaching the study endpoint. Trials have also varied according to arrhythmia type included (e.g., supraventricular tachycardia, atrial fibrillation, atrial flutter). Twenty-four randomized trials published before 1990 were included in a meta-analysis published in 1991.[50] Three of these trials evaluated the efficacy of verapamil, 5 evaluated the efficacy of digoxin, and 16 examined various β-adrenergic blocking agents. Verapamil and digoxin were not associated with a reduction in supraventricular arrhythmias (Fig. 19–3). β-adrenergic blocking agents, however, were associated with a profound reduction in the development of these arrhythmias (pooled odds ratio, 0.28 [0.21 to 0.36]; $P < 0.0001$). This marked reduction in supraventricular arrhythmias was noted regardless of time of drug initiation, exact agent used, and dosage selected (for propranolol). Verapamil, digoxin, and β-adrenergic blocking agents were all associated with a reduction in the ventricular rate during supraventricular arrhythmias. Limitations in interpreting these four studies relate to the type of patient enrolled. Most patients were male, had preserved left ventricular systolic function, and had been taking β-adrenergic blocking agents preoperatively. Patients enrolled in these studies underwent coronary artery bypass grafting but did not have valvular surgery.

Other studies have focused on the use of type IA, type IC, and type III agents on the incidence of atrial fibrillation after cardiac surgery. Intravenous procainamide has been administered for the prevention of postoperative atrial fibrillation. In one series of 46 patients, procainamide reduced the number of tachycardia episodes (5 episodes per 129 patient days at risk vs. 17 episodes in 161 patient days at risk in the control group).[51] The use of procainamide to convert atrial fibrillation to sinus rhythm has been compared with digoxin in 30 patients; conversion to sinus rhythm occurred in 87% of procainamide-treated patients as opposed to 60% of digoxin-treated patients.[52] Conversion to sinus rhythm occurred sooner after the start of treatment with procainamide (40 minutes) than with digoxin (540 minutes).[52] Sotalol, a type III agent, has been used by several investigators to treat postoperative atrial fibrillation. Campbell and colleagues[53] randomized patients to sotalol (n = 22) versus disopyramide plus digoxin (n = 20). Seventeen patients in each group reverted to sinus rhythm within 12 hours. Patients on disopyramide plus digoxin were more likely to develop recurrent atrial fibrillation than those given sotalol. The efficacy of sotalol versus conventional β-adrenergic blocking agents was studied by Nystrom and colleagues[54] in 101 patients. Postoperative atrial fibrillation was more common in those patients on conventional β-adrenergic blocking agents (29%) than in those treated with sotalol (10%) (P = 0.028). In a larger series, Suttorp and coworkers[55] studied 300 patients after coronary artery bypass grafting who had been given sotalol versus placebo. Supraventricular tachycardia was seen in 24 (16%) of sotalol-treated patients and in 49 (33%) of placebo-treated patients ($P < 0.005$) consistent with a major benefit of sotalol for the prevention of post–coronary artery bypass surgery atrial arrhythmias.

Propafenone (300 mg twice daily), a type IC agent, was compared with atenolol (50 mg per day) in 207 patients undergoing bypass surgery (n = 198) or valve replacement (n = 9) for arrhythmia prophylaxis.[56] Supraventricular arrhythmias developed in 13 of 105 patients receiving propafenone and 11 of 102 receiving atenolol (P = NS). Propafenone was compared with amiodarone in the acute conversion of atrial fibrillation or flutter.[57] There was a greater likelihood of converting to sinus rhythm 1 hour after treatment initiation in those patients treated with propafenone (45%) than with amiodarone (20%). By 24 hours after the onset of therapy, there was no significant difference in the proportion of patients in sinus rhythm receiving propafenone (68%) than in those receiving amiodarone (83%).

In a population of 80 patients undergoing coronary artery bypass surgery or valve replacement who developed atrial fibrillation, oral quinidine was more effective in converting to sinus rhythm than intravenous amiodarone (64% vs. 41%) during the 16-hour study period.[58] Predictors of drug failure during this time period included preoperative atrial fibrillation, longer time from arrhythmia recognition to treatment, mitral valve operations, and concomitant propranolol therapy. This is one of the few studies including a moderate number of patients undergoing valve operations (40 patients). In comparison to placebo, intravenous amiodarone reduced the incidence of atrial fibrillation (5% vs. 21%).

Thus, a variety of antiarrhythmic agents are efficacious in decreasing supraventricular arrhythmias after coronary artery bypass grafting. Of all agents, however, β-adrenergic blocking agents are the most efficacious in decreasing the occurrence and frequency of supraventricular arrhythmias in this setting and should be considered in patients undergoing this operation.

CONTROL OF THE VENTRICULAR RESPONSE IN ATRIAL FIBRILLATION

An important use of atrioventricular nodal blocking agents is to control the ventricular response to atrial fibrillation. Many studies have been performed investigating the relative efficacies of β-adrenergic blocking agents, calcium channel blockers, digoxin, and combinations of these agents on resting and exercise heart rate control as well as exercise tolerance with these agents. Most of these trials do not use a treatment-free arm. The control arm generally consists of patients treated with digoxin. Similarly, most of the treatment arms use combination as opposed to monotherapy; combination therapy generally includes digoxin plus another agent. The combination of nadolol and digoxin therapy has been compared with digoxin in 20 patients with chronic atrial fibrillation whose baseline average heart rates were greater than 80 beats/min.[59] After a nadolol dose titration period, patients taking digoxin underwent a double-blind crossover of nadolol versus placebo. The resting heart rate decreased from 92 ± 19 beats/min to 73 ± 16 beats/min on nadolol (87 mg per day). Maximal exercise heart rate was diminished by nadolol (126 ± 25 beats/min vs. 175 ± 24 beats/min on placebo) as was maximal exercise time (380 ± 143 seconds vs. 466 ± 143 seconds). Nadolol/digoxin combination therapy and digoxin monotherapy were also compared by another group of investigators in 32 patients.[60] Using a similar trial design, the average heart rate dropped from 78 ± 4 beats/min to 63 ± 3 beats/min on combination therapy with an average daily nadolol dose of 59 ± 16 mg per day. Exercise duration was not different between the two arms of this study, but exercise-related average heart rate dropped from 154 to 120 beats/min.

The rate-controlling effects of labetalol were studied in 10 patients with chronic atrial fibrillation who underwent four phases of treatment with a randomized crossover design (placebo, digoxin, digoxin with half-dose labetalol, and full-dose labetalol).[61] Exercise duration was not reduced with labetalol. Maximal exercise heart rate was reduced with labetalol therapy (156 ± 4 beats/min vs. 177 ± 2 beats/min on placebo). The resting and exercise rate pressure products were decreased in patients receiving labetalol. Digoxin had no effect on peak exercise heart rate compared with placebo.

Pindolol, a β-adrenergic blocking agent with intrinsic sympathomimetic activity, has been combined with digoxin for controlling the heart rate in atrial fibrillation.[62] Twelve patients were treated with pindolol plus digoxin versus digoxin treatment alone or digoxin plus verapamil. The addition of pindolol therapy was useful in decreasing maximal heart rate as well as heart rate variability. The addition of verapamil therapy to digoxin resulted in a minor decrease in heart rate.

Sotalol (80 to 160 mg per day) has been combined with digoxin as therapy for the control of ventricular response in atrial fibrillation.[63] Twenty patients were randomized to placebo, DL-sotalol 80 mg per day, or DL-sotalol 160 mg per day after a dose-finding period. Digoxin was continued in the sotalol arms. Efficacy was assessed by determining the heart rate at rest as well as the exercise heart rate. Resting heart rate was significantly reduced in patients receiving sotalol (95 ± 4 beats/min at baseline to 79 ± 3 beats/min for sotalol 80 mg per day and 97 ± 4 beats/min to 79 ± 3 beats/min for sotalol 160 mg per day). The maximal heart rate during exercise was not influenced by digoxin therapy but was significantly decreased with both doses of sotalol.

The influence of verapamil, a calcium channel blocker, has been studied by several groups. In 27 patients, the resting heart rate was lower in patients treated with verapamil and digoxin (69 ± 13 beats/min) compared with digoxin alone (87 ± 20 beats/min).[64] The heart rate at the conclusion of 3 minutes of exercise was also decreased in those receiving verapamil (104 ± 14 beats/min vs. 136 ± 23 beats/min). Doses of 240 to 480 mg per day of verapamil were used to achieve this heart rate control. Lewis and colleagues[65] studied the influence of verapamil on 12 patients. Patients entered a double-blind crossover study with a placebo arm (no verapamil) versus verapamil 40 mg three times a day, 80 mg three times a day, or 120 mg three times a day. The resting heart rate was not significantly influenced by the addition of verapamil. The exercise heart rate decreased, especially with the higher doses of verapamil (postexercise digoxin, 147 ± 23 beats/min; verapamil 80 mg three times a day, 127 ± 15 beats/min; verapamil 120 mg three times day, 132 ± 30 beats/min). Exercise duration did not significantly vary between the treatment arms in this study. In another trial, 20 patients were given verapamil/digoxin combination or digoxin.[66] In these patients, exercise capacity and resting and peak exercise heart rates were decreased by verapamil therapy. In these patients, who were either in NYHA functional class II or III, exercise duration increased from 219 ± 77 seconds to 292 ± 71 seconds in those receiving verapamil. Intravenous verapamil (0.075 mg/kg) has also been found to reduce the average ventricular rate from 151 to 118 beats/min as compared to a small change from 144 to 138 beats/min.[67]

Diltiazem, another calcium channel blocker with atrioventricular nodal blocking characteristics, has been compared with propranolol. Twenty-two patients entered a study with three arms: (1) digoxin plus propranolol (20 mg three times a day), (2) digoxin plus oral diltiazem (60 mg three times a day), or (3) digoxin plus diltiazem and propranolol.[68] Resting heart rate and maximal heart rate were more dramatically influenced by the combination of digoxin, diltiazem, and propranolol. Exercise duration was not influenced by these agents. In a trial of 13 patients, Vitale and colleagues[69] noted that diltiazem reduced resting heart rate from 107 ± 19 beats/min to 85 ± 12 beats/min. Maximal exercise heart rate was also blunted by diltiazem (142 ± 13 beats/min vs. 160 ± 14 beats/min during digoxin plus placebo treatment). Diltiazem was associated with a decrease in exercise rate-pressure product but an improvement in exercise capacity.

Intravenous diltiazem has been investigated as an agent to decrease heart rate in hospitalized patients with atrial fibrillation. These trials have enrolled a moderate number of patients. Salerno and coworkers[70] reported on the results of the Diltiazem-Atrial Fibrillation/Flutter Study Group. Patients with atrial fibrillation or flutter at an average heart rate ± 120 beats/min were randomized to placebo or diltiazem (0.25 mg/kg as a 2-minute infusion) followed by a repeat injection of placebo or diltiazem (0.35 mg/kg) 15 minutes later if efficacy had not been achieved. Efficacy was defined as a decrease in the ventricular rate to less than 100 beats/min or a 20% reduction in heart rate from baseline. Nonresponders randomized to placebo were given the option to receive open-label diltiazem after the randomized phase. Patients were evenly randomized to placebo and diltiazem (113 total patients). At the low dose, 7% of placebo-treated patients and 75% of diltiazem-treated patients responded to therapy. After administration of the higher dose, 12% of the placebo-treated patients and 93% of diltiazem-treated patients reached the efficacy endpoint. The effect of diltiazem on heart rate was evident as early as 2 minutes after the initiation of intravenous therapy. Systolic blood pressure dropped by 8% in patients receiving diltiazem.

The efficacy of intravenous diltiazem in patients with moderate to severe congestive heart failure has been investigated by Goldenberg and associates,[71] who studied 37 patients in a protocol similar to Salerno. Ninety-five percent of the patients responded to either the low or high dose of diltiazem, whereas no patient responded to placebo. All placebo-treated patients ultimately received open-label diltiazem with all patients reaching a therapeutic endpoint. The only significant side effect associated with the diltiazem infusion was hypotension (4 of 37 patients).

An alternative therapy for rate control is clonidine, a centrally acting α_2-agonist that may block sympathetic outflow. This agent was compared with placebo in 20 patients presenting to the emergency department for evaluation of atrial fibrillation.[72] The clonidine was administered as a 0.075-mg dose and repeated 2 hours later if the heart rate had not decreased by 20%. In the clonidine group, the average heart rate dropped from 135 ± 26 beats/min to 82 ± 10 beats/min. There was a small decrease in heart rate in patients receiving placebo (132 ± 25 beats/min to 117 ± 31 beats/min). Six patients receiving clonidine converted to normal rhythm, whereas only one patient receiving placebo converted to sinus rhythm.

Heart rate control in atrial fibrillation may be achieved with a variety of antiarrhythmic agents. β-adrenergic blocking agents are better than digoxin therapy for blunting the exercise-related increase in heart rate. Calcium channel blockers and β-adrenergic blockers may be effective in the emergent control of heart rate. The choice of agent and route of administration depend on the urgency and nature of the clinical situation.

SUMMARY

Supraventricular tachyarrhythmias continue to be a clinical problem for many patients. The criteria for initiating pharmacologic therapy or considering radiofrequency ablation depend on clinical judgment and patient preference in most instances. Future areas of investigation include the long-term assessment of safety and efficacy of radiofrequency ablation as well as the development of newer, more effective pharmacologic agents for the treatment of these arrhythmias.

REFERENCES

1. Anderson S, Blanski L, Byrd RC, et al. Comparison of the efficacy and safety of esmolol, a short-acting beta blocker, with placebo in the treatment of supraventricular tachyarrhythmia. The Esmolol Versus Placebo Multicenter Study Group. Am Heart J 1986; 111:42–48.
2. Abrams J, Allen J, Allin D, et al. Efficacy and safety of esmolol versus propranolol in the treatment of supraventricular tachyarrhythmias: A multicenter double-blind clinical trial. The Esmolol Multicenter Study Research Group. Am Heart J 1985; 110:913–922.
3. Sung RJ, Elser B, McAllister RG Jr. Intravenous verapamil for termination of re-entrant supraventricular tachycardias: Intracardiac studies correlated with plasma verapamil concentrations. Ann Intern Med 1980; 93:682–689.
4. DiMarco JP, Miles W, Akhtar M, et al. Adenosine for paroxysmal supraventricular tachycardia: Dose ranging and comparison with verapamil: Assessment in placebo-controlled, multicenter trials. The Adenosine for PSVT Study Group. Ann Intern Med 1990; 113:104–110.
5. McIntosh-Yellin NL, Drew BJ, Scheinman MM. Safety and efficacy of central intravenous bolus administration of adenosine for termination of supraventricular tachycardia. J Am Coll Cardiol 1993; 22:741–745.
6. Rankin AC, Oldroyd KG, Chong E, et al. Adenosine or adenosine triphosphate for supraventricular tachycardias? Comparative double-blind randomized study in patients with spontaneous or inducible arrhythmias. Am Heart J 1990; 119(2 Pt 1):316–323.
7. Dougherty AH, Jackman WM, Naccarelli GV, et al. Acute conversion of paroxysmal supraventricular tachycardia with intravenous diltiazem. IV Diltiazem Study Group. Am J Cardiol 1992; 70:587–592.
8. Huycke EC, Sung RJ, Dias VC, et al, and the Multicenter Diltiazem PSVT Study Group. Intravenous diltiazem for termination of reentrant supraventricular tachycardia: A placebo-controlled, randomized, double-blind, multicenter study. J Am Coll Cardiol 1989; 13:538–544.
9. Shen EN, Keung E, Huycke E, et al. Intravenous propafenone for termination of re-entrant supraventricular tachycardia: A placebo-controlled, randomized, double-blind, crossover study. Ann Intern Med 1986; 105:655–661.
10. Jordaens L, Gorgels A, Stroobanmdt R, et al. Efficacy and safety of intravenous sotalol for termination of paroxysmal supraventricular tachycardia. The Sotalol Versus Placebo Multicenter Study Group. Am J Cardiol 1991; 68:35–40.
11. Sung RJ, Tan HL, Karagounis L, et al, and the Multicenter Study Group. Intravenous sotalol for the termination of supraventricular tachycardia and atrial fibrillation and flutter: A multicenter, randomized, double-blind, placebo-controlled study. Am Heart J 1995; 129:739–748.
12. Mauritson DR, Winniford MD, Walker WS, et al. Oral verapamil for paroxysmal supraventricular tachycardia: A long-term, double-blind randomized trial. Ann Intern Med 1982; 96:409–412.
13. Winniford MD, Fulton KL, Hillis LD. Long-term therapy of paroxysmal supraventricular tachycardia: A randomized, double-blind comparison of digoxin, propranolol and verapamil. Am J Cardiol 1984; 54:1138–1139.
14. Clair WK, Wilkinson WE, McCarthy EA, et al. Treatment of paroxysmal supraventricular tachycardia with oral diltiazem. Clin Pharmacol Ther 1992; 51:562–565.
15. Henthorn RW, Waldo AL, Anderson JL, et al. Flecainide acetate prevents recurrence of symptomatic paroxysmal supraventricular tachycardia. Circulation 1991; 83:119–125.
16. Pritchett ELC, McCarthy EA, Wilkinson WE. Propafenone treatment of symptomatic paroxysmal supraventricular arrhythmias. Ann Intern Med 1991; 114:539–544.
17. UK Propafenone PSVT Study Group. A randomized, placebo-controlled trial of propafenone in the prophylaxis of paroxysmal supraventricular tachycardia and paroxysmal atrial fibrillation. Circulation 1995; 91:2550–2557.
18. Falk RH, Knowlton AA, Bernard SA, et al. Digoxin for converting recent-onset atrial fibrillation to sinus rhythm: A randomized, double-blinded trial. Ann Intern Med 1987; 106:503–506.
19. Toivonen LK, Nieminen MS, Manninen V, et al. Conversion of paroxysmal atrial fibrillation to sinus rhythm by intravenous pirmenol: A placebo controlled study. Br Heart J 1986; 55:176–180.
20. Madrid AH, Marin-Huerta E, Novo ML, et al. Comparison of flecainide and procainamide in cardioversion of atrial fibrillation. Eur Heart J 1993; 14:1127–1131.
21. Crijns HJGM, van Wijk M, van Gilst WH, et al. Acute conversion of atrial fibrillation to sinus rhythm: Clinical efficacy of flecainide acetate: Comparison of two regimens. Eur Heart J 1988; 9:634–638.
22. Donovan KD, Dobb GJ, Coombs LJ, et al. Efficacy of flecainide for the reversion of acute onset atrial fibrillation. Am J Cardiol 1992; 70:50A–55A.
23. Suttorp MJ, Kingma JH, Lie-A-Huen L, et al. Intravenous flecainide versus verapamil for acute conversion of paroxysmal atrial fibrillation or flutter to sinus rhythm. Am J Cardiol 1989; 63:693–696.
24. Capucci A, Lenzi T, Boriani G, et al. Effectiveness of loading oral flecainide for converting recent onset atrial fibrillation to sinus rhythm in patients without organic heart disease or with only systemic hypertension. Am J Cardiol 1992; 70:69–72.
25. Donovan KD, Power BM, Hockings BEF, et al. Intravenous

flecainide versus amiodarone for recent-onset atrial fibrillation. Am J Cardiol 1995; 75:693–697.
26. Kondili A, Kastrati A, Popa Y. Comparative evaluation of verapamil, flecainide and propafenone for the acute conversion of atrial fibrillation to sinus rhythm. Wien Klin Wochenschr 1990; 102:510–513.
27. Suttorp MJ, Kingma JH, Jessurun ER, et al. The value of class IC antiarrhythmic drugs for acute conversion of paroxysmal atrial fibrillation or flutter to sinus rhythm. J Am Coll Cardiol 1990; 16:1722–1727.
28. Bellandi F, Cantini F, Pedone T, et al. Effectiveness of intravenous propafenone for conversion of recent-onset atrial fibrillation: A placebo-controlled study. Clin Cardiol 1995; 18:631–634.
29. Capucci A, Boriani G, Rubino I, et al. A controlled study on oral propafenone versus digoxin plus quinidine in converting recent onset atrial fibrillation to sinus rhytym. Int J Cardiol 1994; 43:305–313.
30. Bertini G, Conti A, Fradella G, et al. Propafenone versus amiodarone in field treatment of primary atrial tachydysrhythmias. J Emerg Med 1990; 8:15–20.
31. Halinen MO, Huttunen M, Paakkinen S, et al. Comparison of sotalol with digoxin-quinidine for conversion of acute atrial fibrillation to sinus rhythm (The Sotalol Digoxin-Quinidine Trial). Am J Cardiol 1995; 76:495–498.
32. Negrini M, Gibelli G, De Ponti C. Confronto tra amiodarone e chinidina nella conversione a ritmo sinusale della fibrillazione atriale di recente insorgenza. G Ital Cardiol 1990; 20:207–214.
33. Hou ZY, Chang MS, Chen CY, et al. Acute treatment of recent-onset atrial fibrillation and flutter with a tailored dosing regimen of intravenous amiodarone: A randomized, digoxin-controlled study. Eur Heart J 1995; 16:521–528.
34. Van Wijk LM, den Heijer P, Crijns HJ, et al. Flecainide versus quinidine in the prevention of paroxysms of atrial fibrillation. J Cardiovasc Pharmacol 1989; 13:32–36.
35. Lau CP, Leung, WH, Wong CK. A randomized double-blind crossover study comparing the efficacy and tolerability of flecainide and quinidine in the control of patients with symptomatic paroxysmal atrial fibrillation. Am Heart J 1992; 124:645–650.
36. Naccarelli GV, Dorian P, Hohnloser SH, et al. Prospective comparison of flecainide versus quinidine for the treatment of paroxysmal atrial fibrillation/flutter. Am J Cardiol 1996; 77:53A–59A.
37. Pietersen AH, Helleman H. Usefulness of flecainide for prevention of paroxysmal atrial fibrillation and flutter. Danish-Norwegian Flecainide Multicenter Study Group. Am J Cardiol 1991; 67:713–717.
38. Connolly SJ, Hoffert DL. Usefulness of propafenone for recurrent paroxysmal atrial fibrillation. Am J Cardiol 1989; 63:817–819.
39. Aliot E, Denjoy I. Comparison of the safety and efficacy of flecainide versus propafenone in hospital out-patients with symptomatic paroxysmal atrial fibrillation/flutter. Am J Cardiol 1996; 77:66A–71A.
40. Reimold SC, Cantillon CO, Friedman PL, et al. Propafenone versus sotalol for suppression of recurrent symptomatic atrial fibrillation. Am J Cardiol 1993; 71:558–563.
41. Richiardi E, Gaita F, Greco C, et al. Propafenone versus idrochinidina nella profilassi farmacologica a lungo termine della fibrillazione atriale. Cardiologia 1992; 37:123–127.
42. Coplen SE, Antman EM, Berlin JA, et al. Efficacy and safety of quinidine therapy for maintenance of sinus rhythm after cardioversion: A meta-analysis of randomized control trials. Circulation 1990; 82:1106–1116.
43. Rasmussen K, Wang H, Fausa D. Comparative efficiency of quinidine and verapamil in the maintenance of sinus rhythm after DC conversion of atrial fibrillation: A controlled clinical trial. Acta Med Scand Suppl 1981; 645:23–28.
44. Lloyd EA, Gersh BJ, Forman R. The efficacy of quinidine and disopyramide in the maintenance of sinus rhythm after electroconversion from atrial fibrillation. S Afr Med J 1984; 65:367–369.
45. Karlson BW, Torstensson I, Abjorn C, et al. Disopyramide in the maintenance of sinus rhythm after electroconversion of atrial fibrillation: A placebo-controlled one-year follow-up study. Eur Heart J 1988; 9:284–290.
46. Juul-Moller S, Edvardsson N, Rehnqvist-Ahlberg N. Sotalol versus quinidine for the maintenance of sinus rhythm after direct current conversion of atrial fibrillation. Circulation 1990; 82:1932–1939.
47. Van Gelder IC, Crijns HJ, Van Gilst WH, et al. Efficacy and safety of flecainide acetate in the maintenance of sinus rhythm after electrical cardioversion of chronic atrial fibrillation or atrial flutter. Am J Cardiol 1989; 64:1317–1321.
48. Gosselink AT, Crijns HJ, Van Gelder IC, et al. Low-dose amiodarone for maintenance of sinus rhythm after cardioversion of atrial fibrillation or flutter. JAMA 1992; 267:3289–3293.
49. Chun SH, Sager PT, Stevenson WG, et al. Long-term efficacy of amiodarone for the maintenance of normal sinus rhythm in patients with refractory atrial fibrillation or flutter. Am J Cardiol 1995; 76:47–50.
50. Andrews TC, Reimold SC, Berlin JA, et al. Prevention of supraventricular arrhythmias after coronary artery bypass surgery: A meta-analysis of randomized control trials. Circulation 1991; 84(suppl III):III-236–III-244.
51. Laub GW, Janeira L, Muralidharan S, et al. Prophylactic procainamide for prevention of atrial fibrillation after coronary artery bypass grafting: A prospective, double-blind, randomized, placabo-controlled pilot study. Crit Care Med 1993; 21:1471–1478.
52. Hjelms E. Procainamide conversion of acute atrial fibrillation after open-heart surgery compared with digoxin treatment. Scand J Thorac Cardiovasc Surg 1992; 26:193–196.
53. Campbell TJ, Gavaghan TP, Morgan JJ. Intravenous sotalol for the treatment of atrial fibrillation and flutter after cardiopulmonary bypass: Comparison with disopyramide and digoxin in a randomized trial. Br Heart J 1985; 54:86–90.
54. Nystrom U, Edvardsson N, Berggren H, et al. Oral sotalol reduces the incidence of atrial fibrillation after coronary artery bypass surgery. Thorac Cardiovasc Surg 1993; 41:34–37.
55. Suttorp MJ, Kingma JH, Peels HO, et al. Effectiveness of sotalol in preventing supraventricular tachyarrhythmias shortly after coronary artery bypass grafting. Am J Cardiol 1991; 68:1163–1169.
56. Merrick AF, Odom NJ, Keenan DJM, et al. Comparison of propafenone to atenolol for the prophylaxis of postcardiotomy supraventricular tachyarrhythmias: A prospective trial. Eur J Cardiothorac Surg 1995; 9:146–149.
57. Di Biasi P, Scrofani R, Paje A, et al. Intravenous amiodarone vs propafenone for atrial fibrillation and flutter after cardiac operation. Eur J Cardiothorac Surg 1995; 9:587–591.
58. McAlister HF, Luke RA, Whitlock RM, et al. Intravenous amiodarone bolus versus oral quinidine for atrial flutter and fibrillation after cardiac operations. J Thorac Cardiovasc Surg 1990; 99:911–918.
59. DiBianco R, Morganroth J, Freitag JA, et al. Effects of nadolol on the spontaneous and exercise-provoked heart rate of patients with chronic atrial fibrillation receiving stable dosages of digoxin. Am Heart J 1984; 108(4 Pt 2):1121–1127.
60. Zoble RG, Brewington J, Olukotun AY, et al. Comparative effects of nadolol-digoxin combination therapy and digoxin monotherapy for chronic atrial fibrillation. Am J Cardiol 1987; 60:39D–45D.
61. Wong CK, Lau CP, Leung WH, et al. Usefulness of labetalol in chronic atrial fibrillation. Am J Cardiol 1990; 66:1212–1215.
62. James MA, Channer KS, Papouchado M, et al. Improved control of atrial fibrillation with combined pindolol and digoxin therapy. Eur Heart J 1989; 10:83–90.
63. Brodsky M, Saini R, Bellinger R, et al. Comparative effects of the combination of digoxin and DL-sotalol therapy versus digoxin monotherapy for control of ventricular response in chronic atrial fibrillation. DL-Sotalol Atrial Fibrillation Study Group. Am Heart J 1994; 127:572–577.
64. Panidis IP, Morganroth J, Baessler C. Effectiveness and safety of oral verapamil to control exercise-induced tachycardia in patients with atrial fibrillation receiving digitalis. Am J Cardiol 1983; 52:1197–1201.
65. Lewis R, Lakhani M, Moreland TA, et al. A comparison of verapamil and digoxin in the treatment of atrial fibrillation. Eur Heart J 1987; 8:148–153.
66. Lang R, Klein HO, Di Segni E, et al. Verapamil improves exercise capacity in chronic atrial fibrillation: Double-blind crossover study. Am Heart J 1983; 105:820–825.
67. Waxman HL, Myerburg RJ, Appel R, et al. Verapamil for con-

trol of ventricular rate in paroxysmal supraventricular tachycardia and atrial fibrillation or flutter: A double-blind randomized cross-over study. Ann Intern Med 1981; 94:1–6.
68. Dahlstrom CG, Edvardsson N, Nasheng C, et al. Effects of diltiazem, propranolol, and their combination in the control of atrial fibrillation. Clin Cardiol 1992; 15:280–284.
69. Vitale P, Auricchio A, De Stefano R, et al. Efficacia del Diltiazem nel controllare la risposta ventricolare e migliorare la capacita di esercizio nella fibrillazione atriale cronica: Studio in doppio cieco, cross-over. Cardiologia 1989; 34:73–81.
70. Salerno DM, Dias VC, Kleiger RE, et al. Efficacy and safety of intravenous diltiazem for treatment of atrial fibrillation and atrial flutter. The Diltiazem-Atrial Fibrillation/Flutter Study Group. Am J Cardiol 1989; 63:1046–1051.
71. Goldenberg IF, Lewis WR, Dias VC, et al. Intravenous diltiazem for the treatment of patients with atrial fibrillation or flutter and moderate to severe congestive heart failure. Am J Cardiol 1994; 74:884–889.
72. Roth A, Kaluski E, Felner S, et al. Clonidine for patients with rapid atrial fibrillation. Ann Intern Med 1992; 116:388–390.

20 Antithrombotic and Anticoagulant Therapy

▶ David M. Kerins
▶ Paul M. Ridker

Patients with acute myocardial infarction (MI) are at increased risk for recurrent cardiovascular events, including reinfarction and stroke. Over the past 50 years, a series of clinical trials has addressed the benefit-risk ratio of antithrombotic and anticoagulant therapies in the secondary prevention of these events, focusing primarily on the endpoints of all-cause mortality, cardiac mortality, sudden death, nonfatal reinfarction, and stroke. In this chapter, those trials evaluating antiplatelet agents alone or in combination with warfarin are reviewed, as is the pathophysiologic basis for the use of these therapies following acute ischemia.

PLATELET FUNCTION, THROMBOSIS, AND MYOCARDIAL INFARCTION

Acute thrombosis and subsequent occlusion of flow in a coronary artery are the proximate cause of infarction in more 90% of patients with MI.[1] This observation provided a pathologic basis for the administration of thrombolytic therapy, initially via the intracoronary route and subsequently via peripheral infusion.[2] However, plaque disruption and platelet activation are also important processes in acute infarction.[3] For example, studies employing continuous electrocardiographic monitoring and serial angiography indicate that intermittent occlusion is common during the infarction process and that such intermittent disruption of coronary flow may be the result of platelet activation.[4] Further, morphologic changes in platelet shape indicative of activation have been demonstrated in electron microscopy studies performed among patients with acute MI.[5]

Biochemical evidence of increased thromboxane formation, the major vasoconstricting and platelet-aggregating eicosanoid derived from the platelet, and other markers of platelet activation have also been described during acute ischemia.[6,7] For example, in a study of acute infarction patients undergoing therapy with tissue-plasminogen activator (t-PA), a single oral aspirin (325 mg) was found sufficient to prevent increased platelet activation as assessed by urinary excretion of 2,3-dinor-thromboxane B_2.[8] Similar data have been presented for patients treated with intravenous aspirin (250 mg) in the setting of thrombolysis.[9] Finally, plasma concentrations of β thromboglobulin, a substance released from platelet α granules on activation, have been shown to increase threefold during acute infarction.[10]

Platelet aggregation studies also support a fundamental role for platelets in acute thrombosis. In retrospective data from the Caerphilly Cooperative Heart Disease Study, increased platelet aggregation in response to adenosine diphosphate was associated with a twofold increase in risk of prior MI.[11] The extent of platelet aggregation may also be of value in predicting future coronary events. In this regard, platelet hyperactivity as assessed by spontaneous platelet aggregation has been reported to significantly increase the risk of subsequent coronary events among survivors of MI.[12] An increased aggregation response to thrombin has also been reported to increase the likelihood of coronary artery disease progression.[13] This observation is of particular interest because expression of the thrombin receptor is increased in atherosclerotic as compared to normal arteries.[14]

In contrast with the role of platelet activation in the acute coronary syndromes, a major role for platelet activation in the setting of chronic stable angina has not been widely accepted. However, clinical trial data support the use of aspirin among patients with chronic, stable angina. For example, in a subgroup of 333 participants in the Physicians' Health Study who gave a history of angina, randomized assignment to 325 mg of aspirin on alternate days resulted in an 87% reduction in risk of first-ever MI ($P < 0.001$).[15] However, the use of aspirin in this trial had no effect on atherosclerotic progression[16] or on the clinical severity of events.[17] Similar data derive from the Swedish Angina Pectoris Aspirin Trial, a randomized, placebo-controlled trial of aspirin (75 mg daily) among 2035 men with chronic stable angina being treated with sotalol.[18] In that trial, aspirin use was associated with a 34% decrease in first MI or sudden death ($P = 0.003$), and a 39% reduction in nonfatal MI ($P = 0.006$).

Clinical data also support a role for antiplatelet and anticoagulant therapies as a means to potentially modify novel markers of cardiovascular risk, including intrinsic fibrinolytic function and inflammation. For example, prospective data indicate that fibrinolytic capacity as measured by baseline antigen levels of plasminogen activator inhibitor, t-PA, and D-dimer are associated with increased risks of first or recurrent MI.[19-22] However, aspirin appears to attenuate this effect, at least when fibrinolytic capacity is assessed by t-PA antigen.[20] Recent work has also demonstrated that aspirin may modify the risk of MI associated with elevated levels of C-reactive protein, a marker of inflammation that appears to be an independent risk factor for MI, stroke, and peripheral vascular disease.[23, 24] With regard to anticoagulant therapy, warfarin has been shown to reduce plasma concentrations of coagulation factor VII, an intriguing observation, because some studies suggest that factor VII activity is itself a risk factor for arterial occlusion.[25, 26] Such data, however, have not always been consistent,[27] and it remains uncertain what role these novel pathways have in the atherothrombotic process.

RANDOMIZED TRIALS OF ANTIPLATELET AGENTS IN SECONDARY PREVENTION

While the pathophysiologic basis for antiplatelet agents in the secondary prevention of MI is well-established, the initial randomized, controlled trials designed to evaluate the clinical efficacy of this approach were inconclusive. For example, the first completed trial of antiplatelet therapy among patients with prior MI randomized 1239 men in the Cardiff region of Wales to 300 mg of aspirin daily or placebo. Patients assigned to aspirin experienced a 25% mortality reduction compared with those assigned placebo (8.3% vs. 10.9%), but this did not achieve statistical significance.[28]

A second trial in Cardiff randomized 1682 post-MI patients (1434 men and 248 women) to 300 mg aspirin, three times daily, or placebo.[29, 30] In the Cardiff-II trial, aspirin treatment after 1 year was associated with a 17% mortality reduction but, as in Cardiff-I, the decrease was not statistically significant. Although the follow-up data on nonfatal events were not complete, there was a statistically significant 34% decrease in reinfarction among the aspirin group (7.1% vs. 10.9%).

The Coronary Drug Project, which conducted several trials of promising agents for the secondary prevention of MI, carried out a trial of aspirin therapy among 1529 male post-MI patients. Participants were randomly allocated to 324 mg of aspirin, three times daily, or placebo.[31] Patients assigned to active treatment experienced a 30% decreased risk of mortality and a 21% decreased risk of a combined outcome of nonfatal reinfarction plus coronary death, but neither reduction was statistically significant.

The largest single trial of aspirin in post-MI patients was the Aspirin Myocardial Infarction Study (AMIS), a multicenter trial directed by the U.S. National Heart, Lung, and Blood Institute. AMIS enrolled a total of 4524 men and women, 30 to 69 years of age, with prior MI and randomly allocated them to 1000 mg of aspirin daily or placebo.[32] After an average of 38.2 months of treatment and follow-up, aspirin-allocated patients actually had slightly higher mortality than the placebo group (10.8% vs. 9.7%; Cox adjusted Z score, 0.02), but they experienced reductions of 22% in reinfarction (6.3% vs. 8.1%; Z value, −2.34) and 40% in stroke (1.2% vs. 2.0%; Z value, −2.26). The high dose of aspirin was associated with a doubling of gastrointestinal side effects (23.7% vs. 14.9%; $P < 0.05$).

The Persantine-Aspirin ReInfarction Study (PARIS-I) randomized 2026 patients (1759 men and 267 women), 30 to 74 years of age, 8 weeks to 5 years following an acute MI. This multicenter trial enlisted clinical sites in the United States and the United Kingdom and randomized patients to 324 mg aspirin plus 75 mg Persantine (dipyridamole), each three times daily, 324 mg aspirin alone, three times daily, or to placebo.[33] After an average treatment and follow-up of 41 months, there were nonsignificant decreases in total mortality of 16% in the combined drug group and 18% in the aspirin-only group compared with placebo. There were similar nonsignificant decreases of 24% and 21% for coronary mortality and 25% and 24% for the outcome of nonfatal MI plus fatal coronary disease in the combined therapy and aspirin groups, respectively.

Post hoc analyses of PARIS-I results demonstrated that the greatest reductions in total and coronary mortality associated with the active treatments occurred among those enrolled within 6 months of their index infarction. Based on these findings, a second PARIS study was initiated, which restricted enrollment to patients who were within 4 weeks to 4 months of a qualifying MI. Although in the initial PARIS study there was little difference between the aspirin and aspirin plus Persantine groups in total and coronary death among those randomized within 6 months of infarction, the PARIS-II investigators elected not to include an aspirin-only arm, allocating patients instead to either a capsule containing 330 mg aspirin and 75 mg dipyridamole, three times daily, or placebo. A total of 3128 post-MI patients were randomized, and the average length of follow-up was 23.4 months. There was a statistically significant 24% reduction in coronary incidence (nonfatal MI plus coronary death) among those allocated to active treatment (Z value, −2.57), but no significant difference between groups in the occurrence of total and coronary mortality, the two other prespecified primary endpoints.

The German-Austrian Myocardial Infarction Study (GAMIS) randomized 946 male and female MI patients, 45 to 70 years of age, to 1.5 g of aspirin daily, phenprocoumon (target thrombotest value 5% to 12%), or placebo.[34] Patients were eligible if they were within 30 to 42 days of their index infarction. After 2 years, there were nonsignificant mortality reductions of 17% for aspirin versus placebo, and 26% for aspirin versus phenprocoumon. There were reductions that approached borderline significance in coronary death among those assigned aspirin versus phenprocoumon (46.3% reduction; $P < 0.07$), and in coronary events (nonfatal reinfarction plus coronary death) among those assigned aspirin versus placebo (36.6% reduction; $P < 0.06$).

Sulfinpyrazone, a reversible cyclooxygenase inhibitor of poor biochemical selectivity, has also been evaluated in secondary prevention trials following MI. The first of these, the Anturane Reinfarction Trial (ART), tested sulfinpyrazone (Anturane), 200 mg four times daily, versus placebo in 1558 men and women who were within 25 to 35 days of their MI. Following an average treatment and follow-up of 16 months, there was a trend toward a reduced risk of cardiac mortality in the sulfinpyrazone group (32% reduction; $P = 0.058$), and a significant 43% reduction in sudden death ($P = 0.041$). Virtually all of this apparent benefit occurred in the first 6 months after randomization, such that the authors reported that there was a significant 74% reduction ($P = 0.003$) in sudden death associated with sulfinpyrazone when considering only this early period.[35, 36] Analysis of this early postinfarct period, however, had not been prespecified, and sudden deaths constituted only a portion of all cardiac deaths, the primary prespecified study outcome. Results of the ART were thus controversial.[37] In addition, in a follow-up analysis based on a new, independent review of the study records, the reductions in cardiac and sudden death previously reported for the whole trial period were attenuated and the reduction for sudden death was no longer statistically significant.[38]

A second trial of sulfinpyrazone, the Anturane Italian Reinfarction Trial, randomized 727 patients, 15 to 25 days after infarction, to 400 mg of sulfinpyrazone, twice daily, or placebo. After a mean treatment and follow-up of 19.2 months, there was no difference in total mortality, but sulfinpyrazone treatment was associated with a significant 56% reduction in total reinfarction ($P < 0.01$) and a 66% reduction in all fatal and nonfatal events judged to be thromboembolic ($P < 0.001$).[39]

Summary and Overview of Antiplatelet Trials

Thus, the available evidence from randomized trials of antiplatelet therapy, mainly with aspirin, following MI is certainly suggestive of net clinical benefits of this treatment. However, a number of the completed trials failed individually to provide convincing proof of this. This situation is principally the result of the small sample size of many of the trials, which left them with inadequate statistical power to provide conclusive tests of the agents under study. In such a situation, one means of evaluating the available data is to perform an overview, or meta-analysis. In an overview, the results of several trials are considered in aggregate, with statistical weight given to each trial according to the number of outcome events it contributes to the analysis. By including larger numbers of subjects, an overview can diminish the play of chance in results and provide a more statistically stable estimate of a treatment effect.

In 1988, with the worldwide collaboration of investigators who had conducted randomized trials of antiplatelet therapy, an overview was published of the 25 then-completed trials of antiplatelet therapy in secondary prevention of cardiovascular disease. The overview included the results of the 10 completed trials of approximately 18,000 post-MI patients as well as 13 completed trials among approximately 9000 patients with prior cerebrovascular disease (stroke or transient ischemic attack [TIA]) and two trials among approximately 2000 patients with unstable angina.[40]

For the 10 post-MI trials, the overview demonstrated statistically significant reductions from antiplatelet treatment of 31% in nonfatal reinfarction (SD 5%), 42% in nonfatal stroke (SD 11%), 13% in total vascular mortality (SD 5%), and 25% (SD 4%) in important vascular events, a composite outcome that comprised nonfatal MI, nonfatal stroke, and vascular mortality.

With all 25 secondary prevention trials considered together, the overview demonstrated similar, conclusive benefits of antiplatelet therapy, with patients allocated to active treatment experiencing statistically significant reductions of 32% in nonfatal MI (SD 5%), 27% in nonfatal stroke (SD 6%), 15% in total vascular mortality (SD 4%), and 25% (SD 3%) in important vascular events. There was no apparent effect of antiplatelet treatment on nonvascular death, so the significant ($P = 0.0003$) benefit observed on total mortality is largely explained by the definite reduction in vascular death. Considered separately, the 13 trials of patients with cerebrovascular disease (stroke or TIA) demonstrated statistically significant reductions of 35% for MI, 22% for subsequent nonfatal stroke, 15% for vascular death, and 22% for important vascular events. Finally, for the two trials of unstable angina patients, there were statistically significant decreases of 35% in nonfatal MI, 37% in vascular death, and 36% in any vascular event. There were too few strokes in these trials to provide meaningful data.

In regard to the different antiplatelet agents tested, there was no clear evidence that aspirin plus dipyridamole was any more effective than aspirin alone, because the indirect comparison between the two risk reductions was not significant, and the overview of the direct comparisons indicated no difference whatsoever. There was also no evidence that sulfinpyrazone was superior to aspirin or that daily aspirin doses of 900 to 1500 mg were any more effective in reducing vascular events than 300 mg, the lowest dose tested.

Although the overview provided reliable evidence of the benefit of aspirin therapy in patients with prior MI, stroke, TIA, or unstable angina, it did not address directly whether such therapy would benefit other patient populations at increased risk for occlusive vascular disease, such as those with chronic stable angina or peripheral vascular disease or patients undergoing revascularization procedures. The report also did not address the question of aspirin's benefit in certain subgroups of high-risk patients, such as women and the elderly, or those with hypertension or diabetes.

In 1994, an expanded overview was published that included subsequently completed trials among a broader range of patients with prior manifestations of vascular disease (e.g., prior coronary revascularization, peripheral vascular disease, and atrial fibrillation).[41] In all, the updated overview included 133 trials of antiplatelet therapy among 53,000 patients with prior vascular disease, more than 18,000 acute MI patients, and more than 28,000 low-risk subjects in primary prevention trials (Fig. 20–1).

The findings among patients with prior MI were unchanged from the 1988 report and include only one

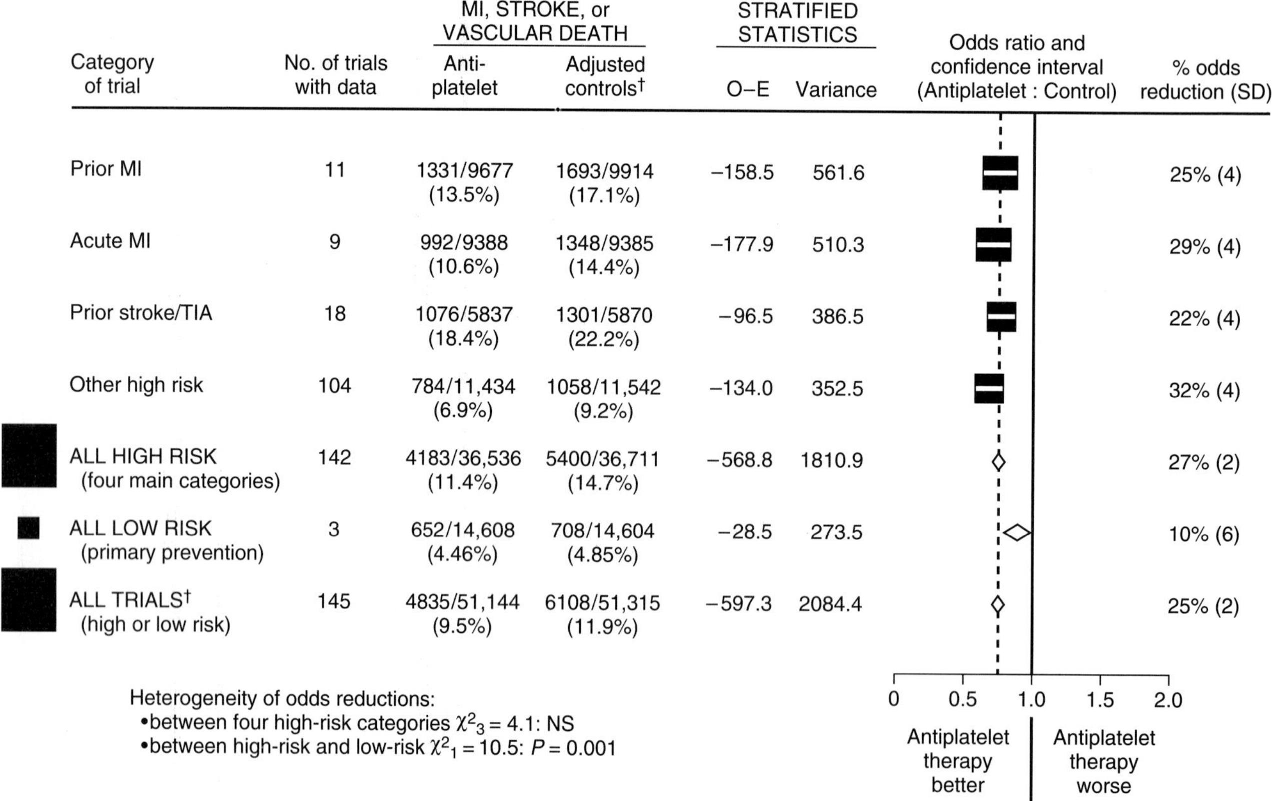

Category of trial	No. of trials with data	MI, STROKE, or VASCULAR DEATH: Anti-platelet	MI, STROKE, or VASCULAR DEATH: Adjusted controls†	STRATIFIED STATISTICS: O–E	STRATIFIED STATISTICS: Variance	% odds reduction (SD)
Prior MI	11	1331/9677 (13.5%)	1693/9914 (17.1%)	−158.5	561.6	25% (4)
Acute MI	9	992/9388 (10.6%)	1348/9385 (14.4%)	−177.9	510.3	29% (4)
Prior stroke/TIA	18	1076/5837 (18.4%)	1301/5870 (22.2%)	−96.5	386.5	22% (4)
Other high risk	104	784/11,434 (6.9%)	1058/11,542 (9.2%)	−134.0	352.5	32% (4)
ALL HIGH RISK (four main categories)	142	4183/36,536 (11.4%)	5400/36,711 (14.7%)	−568.8	1810.9	27% (2)
ALL LOW RISK (primary prevention)	3	652/14,608 (4.46%)	708/14,604 (4.85%)	−28.5	273.5	10% (6)
ALL TRIALS† (high or low risk)	145	4835/51,144 (9.5%)	6108/51,315 (11.9%)	−597.3	2084.4	25% (2)

Figure 20–1 Proportional effects of antiplatelet therapy on vascular events (myocardial infarction [MI], stroke, or vascular death) in four high-risk categories of trial and in low risk (primary prevention). O − E, Observed minus expected. Stratified ratio of odds of an event in treatment groups to that in control groups is plotted for each group of trials (black square: area proportional to amount of statistical information contributed by trial) along with its 99% confidence interval (horizontal line). Overviews of results for certain subtotals (and 95% confidence intervals) are represented by diamonds. Odds reductions observed in particular groups of trials are given to right of solid vertical line. (From Antiplatelet Trialists' Collaboration. Collaborative overview of randomized trials of antiplatelet treatment: I. Prevention of vascular death, myocardial infarction, and stroke by prolonged antiplatelet therapy in different categories of patients. BMJ 1994; 308:81–106.)

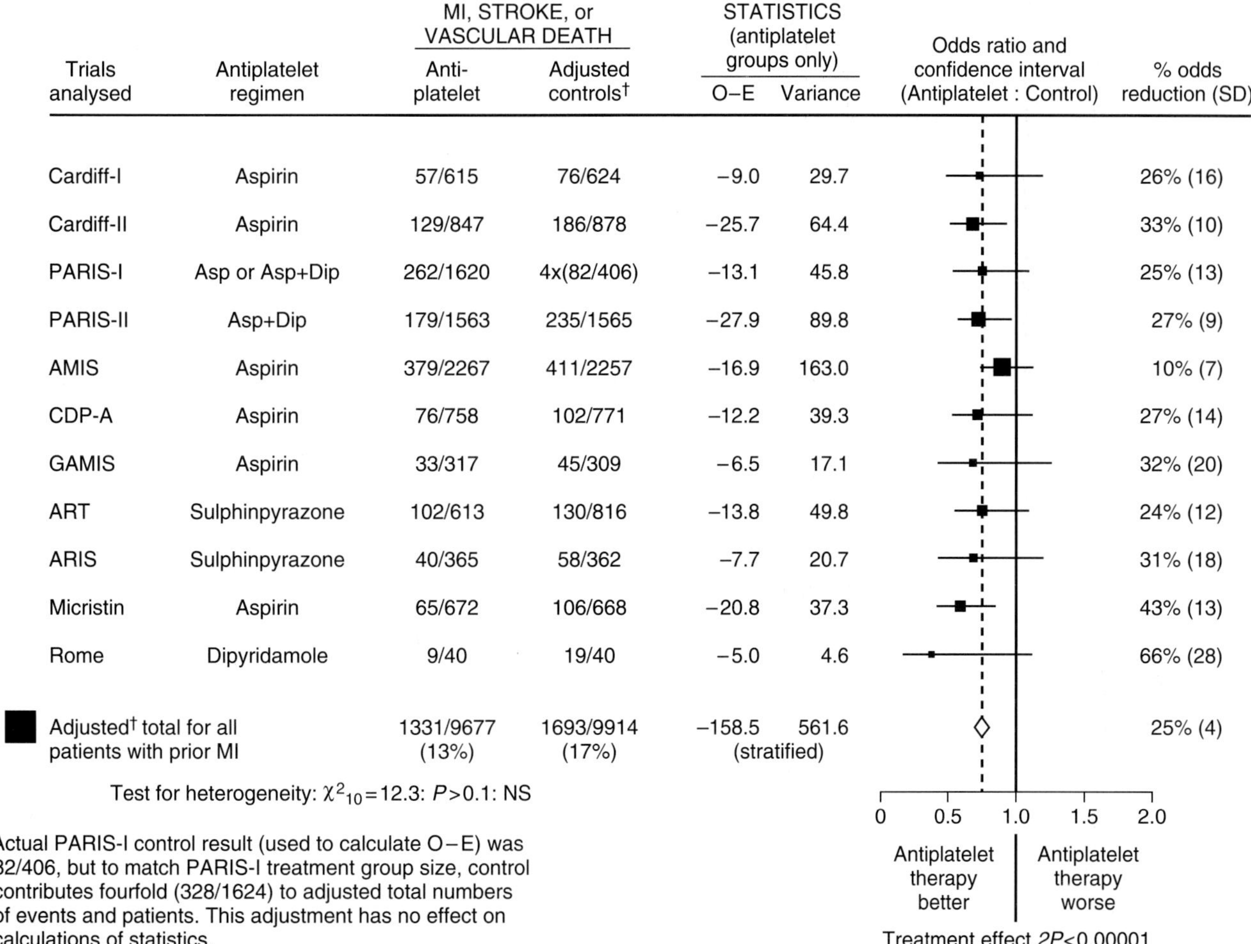

Trials analysed	Antiplatelet regimen	MI, STROKE, or VASCULAR DEATH: Anti-platelet	Adjusted controls†	STATISTICS (antiplatelet groups only): O–E	Variance	% odds reduction (SD)
Cardiff-I	Aspirin	57/615	76/624	−9.0	29.7	26% (16)
Cardiff-II	Aspirin	129/847	186/878	−25.7	64.4	33% (10)
PARIS-I	Asp or Asp+Dip	262/1620	4x(82/406)	−13.1	45.8	25% (13)
PARIS-II	Asp+Dip	179/1563	235/1565	−27.9	89.8	27% (9)
AMIS	Aspirin	379/2267	411/2257	−16.9	163.0	10% (7)
CDP-A	Aspirin	76/758	102/771	−12.2	39.3	27% (14)
GAMIS	Aspirin	33/317	45/309	−6.5	17.1	32% (20)
ART	Sulphinpyrazone	102/613	130/816	−13.8	49.8	24% (12)
ARIS	Sulphinpyrazone	40/365	58/362	−7.7	20.7	31% (18)
Micristin	Aspirin	65/672	106/668	−20.8	37.3	43% (13)
Rome	Dipyridamole	9/40	19/40	−5.0	4.6	66% (28)
Adjusted† total for all patients with prior MI		1331/9677 (13%)	1693/9914 (17%)	−158.5	561.6 (stratified)	25% (4)

†Actual PARIS-I control result (used to calculate O−E) was 82/406, but to match PARIS-I treatment group size, control contributes fourfold (328/1624) to adjusted total numbers of events and patients. This adjustment has no effect on calculations of statistics.

Figure 20–2 Proportional effects on vascular events (myocardial infarction [MI], stroke, or vascular death) in 11 randomized trials of prolonged antiplatelet therapy (for ≥1 month) versus control in patients with prior MI. O − E, observed minus expected; Asp, aspirin; Dip, dipyridamole. (In most trials patients were allocated roughly evenly between treatment groups, but in some more were deliberately allocated to active treatment. To allow direct comparisons between percentages suffering an event in each treatment group, adjusted totals have been calculated after converting any unevenly randomized trials to even ones by counting control groups more than once. Statistical calculations are, however, based on actual numbers from individual trials.) Ratio of odds of an event in treatment group to that in control group is plotted for each trial (black square: area proportional to amount of statistical information contributed by trial) along with its 99% confidence interval (horizontal line). All black squares are to left of solid vertical line, indicating benefit (but benefit is significant at $2P < 0.01$ only where, in three trials, the entire confidence interval is to the left of the line). Stratified overview of results of all trials (and 95% confidence interval) is represented by open diamond, indicating an odds ratio of 0.75 (SD 0.04) or, equivalently, odds reduction of 25% (SD 4%). (From Antiplatelet Trialists' Collaboration. Collaborative overview of randomized trials of antiplatelet treatment: I. Prevention of vascular death, myocardial infarction, and stroke by prolonged antiplatelet therapy in different categories of patients. BMJ 1994; 308:81–106.)

additional trial of 80 patients (Fig. 20–2). With respect to new patient populations included in the updated overview, the report includes the experience of approximately 22,000 patients at high risk for occlusive vascular events due to atrial fibrillation, valve surgery, peripheral vascular disease, chronic stable angina, and coronary revascularization (either coronary artery bypass graft [CABG] or percutaneous transluminal coronary angioplasty [PTCA]). When analyzed separately according to specific patient entry criteria, most comparisons of antiplatelet therapy and control failed to achieve statistical significance because of the small numbers of patients in each category. However, when the trials of these various high-risk patients were considered in aggregate, antiplatelet therapy was associated with a statistically significant 32% decrease in important vascular events.

With respect to the absolute benefits of antiplatelet treatment, for patients with prior MI, the risk reductions demonstrated in the overview translate to avoidance of approximately 40 events per 1000 patients treated over 2 years. Among other patient categories, the risk reductions correspond to avoidance of approximately 50 vascular events per 1000 unstable angina patients treated for 6 months; 40 events per 1000 patients with prior stroke or TIAs treated for 3 years; and 20 events per 1000 patients among other high-risk patients treated for 1 year.[41]

The updated overview also provides reliable data that antiplatelet treatment in high-risk patients produces vascular event reductions of similar size in various patient subgroups. Specifically, separate data for men and women were available from 29 trials conducted among approximately 40,000 men and 10,000 women. There were comparable benefits on vascular events, with reductions per 1000 patients treated of 37 events for men (SD 4; $P < 0.00001$) and 33 events for women (SD 7; $P < 0.0001$). The data from these 29 trials also demonstrate similar reductions in vascular events for middle-aged as well as older patients; in hypertensive and normotensive groups; and in diabetic and nondiabetic groups.

The updated overview included trials testing aspirin in doses ranging from 75 mg to 1500 mg per day. As in the original overview, there was no evidence that higher doses were any more effective in reducing the risk of occlusive vascular events than were lower doses. Although 300 mg was the lowest daily dose tested in trials in the original overview, the updated analysis includes approximately 5000 patients in trials testing 75 mg of aspirin per day. When analyzed separately, the trials testing daily doses of 75 mg demonstrated a statistically significant 29% reduction in vascular events associated with aspirin ($P < 0.0001$).

It has been postulated that doses even lower than 75 mg may confer greater benefit by inhibiting platelet aggregation without blocking the synthesis of prostacyclin, an enzyme with antiplatelet and vasodilative properties. However, even low daily doses appear to depress prostacyclin biosynthesis.[42] One strategy that has been proposed to enhance the biochemical selectivity of aspirin for thromboxane A_2, while sparing prostacyclin, is the use of a controlled-release aspirin preparation. A small trial comparing a controlled-release 75 mg aspirin preparation with a conventional immediate-release 75 mg preparation has demonstrated the ability of this formulation to inhibit thromboxane A_2 production, while decreasing basal prostacyclin biosynthesis only slightly.[42] A large-scale trial comparing such a preparation with conventional aspirin will be necessary to determine the clinical value, if any, of preserving prostacyclin during antiplatelet therapy.

In addition to aspirin, dipyridamole, and sulfinpyrazone, which were tested in trials included in the original overview, the updated analysis also includes three trials that tested ticlopidine versus aspirin. The updated overview demonstrates no significant differences in the efficacy of any of these various antiplatelet agents. However, any differences between antiplatelet agents will be much smaller than that between antiplatelet treatment and no antiplatelet treatment, so the results of the overview cannot exclude the possibility of a small advantage of one type of agent.

Finally, as regards the optimal duration of treatment in secondary prevention, there is no direct evidence on this question, since no large-scale randomized trials have compared different durations of treatment. For trials of patients with prior MI, stroke, or TIA that provided individual patient data, information is available on events occurring in the first, second, and subsequent years of scheduled treatment. These trials show an apparent trend toward greater effect during the earlier years. However, there are difficulties in interpreting these data, because noncompliance with treatment tends to increase with time (i.e., some in the treatment group will have stopped antiplatelet therapy and others in the control group will have initiated such treatment), so the underestimation of the effect of actual treatment tends to increase over time. In addition, even with no further divergence in event rates after the first few years, continued aspirin therapy may be preventing survival and event rate curves from converging. For this reason, absent direct evidence otherwise from randomized comparisons of different durations of treatment, and absent the development of a contraindication to its use in individual patients, it may be advisable to continue aspirin therapy indefinitely in those patients considered to be at high risk of occlusive vascular events.

As regards side effects of aspirin, although its benefits in reducing occlusive vascular events may be approximately equal over the wide dose range tested in trials to date, the principal adverse effects of aspirin appear to be strongly dose related. The United Kingdom Transient Ischemic Attack Aspirin Trial, which tested two daily dosages of aspirin as well as placebo, provides the most informative direct comparison of the side effects of different aspirin dosages.[43] This trial among 2345 patients with a history of TIAs tested 300 mg per day and 1200 mg per day of aspirin against placebo. With respect to upper gastrointestinal (GI) symptoms and GI bleeding, the percentage of participants reporting it was lowest in the placebo group, somewhat higher in the group receiving 300 mg per day, and highest among those receiving 1200 mg daily. Rates for GI symptoms were 26%, 31%, and 41%, in the three groups, respectively, the difference between the two aspirin doses being statistically significant. For GI bleeding, the rates were 1%, 3%, and 5%. For hemorrhagic stroke, the most severe potential adverse effect of aspirin, the totality of randomized trial evidence in both secondary and primary prevention indicates a small, but significant, excess with treatment versus control, but its overall occurrence was very low (0.3% vs. 0.2%) and was substantially outweighed by the definite reduction in the far more common strokes of nonhemorrhagic etiology.[41]

Taken together, available data support the use of chronic low-dose aspirin (75 to 160 mg per day) for all post-MI patients without clear evidence of contraindications. This extremely inexpensive and relatively safe treatment has also been demonstrated to confer clear benefits on subsequent vascular disease events among a broad range of patients with prior manifestations of cardiovascular disease and should be part of the clinical management plan for most patients with a history of occlusive vascular disease.

Despite its clear benefits, aspirin remains an underutilized treatment for cardiovascular disease. In a national registry of more than 1000 larger U.S. hospitals, only 77% of acute MI patients received aspirin in 1993.[44] In data from 1992 to 1993 on a sample of acute MI patients 65 years of age and older, only 61% were receiving aspirin within 2 days of hospitalization,[45] and only 76% were discharged with instructions to take aspirin.[46]

RANDOMIZED TRIALS OF ANTICOAGULANT AGENTS IN SECONDARY PREVENTION

In contrast with the clinical trials of antiplatelet therapy in the secondary prevention of MI, which have largely been conducted over the past 25 years, trials of oral anticoagulant therapy have been carried out for more than a half century. In 1946, the board of directors of the American Heart Association established a Committee for the Evaluation of Anticoagulants in the Treatment of Coronary Thrombosis with Myocardial Infarction, and 2 years later this panel reported results from a multicenter trial involving 800 patients hospitalized with acute MI.[47] The trial, which used a nonrandomized treatment allocation scheme, reported significant benefits of 30 days of anticoagulation on rates of mortality (24% vs. 15%; $P < 0.01$) and total thromboembolic events (36% vs. 14%; $P < 0.01$). The authors concluded that "anticoagulant therapy should be used in all cases of coronary thrombosis with MI unless a definite contraindication exists."[47]

Following this early, confident assessment, a number of trials of anticoagulant therapy following acute MI were conducted during the 1950s, 1960s, and 1970s.[48–60] Their findings, however, were not consistent, and, overall, it appeared that the benefits were greatest in those trials that lacked randomized treatment assignment. Benefits were also generally more pronounced for thromboembolic events than for mortality; however, many of the studies were conducted at a time when prolonged bed rest and delayed ambulation were the standard of care for MI patients, practices that would be expected to increase the overall rate of thromboembolic events. Many of the trials also predated the introduction of the coronary care unit, tested a variety of orally active anticoagulants, and used a variety of assays with reagents of varying strengths and sources to determine the degree of anticoagulation. Thus, the applicability of many of these trials to current medical management is limited. Against this background, a 1981 review concluded that the "anticoagulant era began with high hopes but ended with a whimper."[52]

In contrast with the large number of trials performed during this early phase of the anticoagulant era, recent years have been characterized by the performance of fewer trials of overall higher quality, with greater definition of patient entry requirements and more rigorous control and reporting of the degree of anticoagulation.

In the Sixty-Plus Reinfarction Study, a multicenter trial carried out in The Netherlands, 878 patients older than 60 years of age who had been placed on anticoagulant therapy following a first transmural MI were randomly assigned to continue anticoagulant treatment ($n = 439$) or to receive placebo ($n = 439$).[61, 62] The average duration of prerandomization treatment with anticoagulants was 6 years. Patients allocated to active treatment received either acenocoumarol or phenprocoumon, with a target thrombotest of 5% to 10%, corresponding to an international normalized ratio (INR) of 2.7 to 4.5. After 2 years of treatment, anticoagulant therapy was associated with an apparent, but not statistically significant, reduction in total mortality (15.7% vs. 11.6%; $P = 0.071$). "On-treatment" analysis revealed a greater mortality difference (13.4% vs. 7.6%; $P = 0.017$). For reinfarction, there was a highly significant benefit of anticoagulation (15.2% vs. 6.9%; $P = 0.0005$). With respect to intracranial events, all but two of which (1 in treatment, 1 in control) were classified as cerebrovascular in origin, there were fewer among the treatment group than placebo (13 vs. 21), but this difference was not statistically significant ($P = 0.16$). There were apparent competing effects on such events when divided by etiology, with an excess of hemorrhagic events in the anticoagulant group (7 vs. 1) and a deficit of events classified as nonhemorrhagic (2 vs. 13). As regards major extracranial hemorrhage (i.e., events leading to protocol deviation), there were 3 events in placebo versus 27 in the anticoagulant group. Minor extracranial hemorrhage was reported for 7 patients assigned placebo compared with 57 patients assigned active treatment.

Thus, the Sixty-Plus Study demonstrated a possible mortality benefit of anticoagulation, a more definite reduction in reinfarction, and possible competing effects on cerebral thrombosis and hemorrhage, with somewhat fewer total intracranial events among treated patients than control subjects. Because all patients were exposed to an extensive period of pretrial anticoagulant treatment, however, the study actually examined the effect of maintaining versus discontinuing anticoagulation and did not, therefore, address directly the question of the benefits of initiating anticoagulation in the period just following infarction.

To address this issue directly, the Warfarin Reinfarction Study (WARIS) in Norway randomized 1214 male and female patients, 75 years of age and younger, soon after acute MI (mean interval from infarct symptoms to randomization, 27 days) to warfarin or placebo.[63] Warfarin was dosed to a target range INR of 2.8 to 4.8, which corresponds approximately to a prothrombin time ratio of 1.5 to 2.0 with a typical North American thromboplastin. The average duration of trial treatment was 37 months. With this relatively intense dosing of anticoagulant therapy, warfarin treatment was associated with statistically significant reductions of 24% in total mortality (123 vs. 94 deaths; $P = 0.027$), 34% in reinfarction (124 vs. 82 events; $P = 0.0007$), and 55% in total cerebrovascular accidents (44 vs. 20 events; $P = 0.0015$). Of the 44 strokes in the placebo group, 10 were fatal, all of these deemed nonhemorrhagic. In contrast, 4 of the 20 strokes in the warfarin group were fatal, all of these of hemorrhagic etiology.

A second post-MI trial of anticoagulants in The Netherlands, the Anticoagulants in the Secondary Prevention of Events in Coronary Thrombosis (ASPECT) study, randomized 3404 hospitalized male and female survivors of acute MI, with treatment initiated as soon as possible following hospital discharge, but not more than 6 weeks later.[64] Patients were allocated at random to anticoagulation with nicoumalone or phenprocoumon or to placebo, with a target INR of 2.8 to 4.8. Following an average treatment duration of 37 months, anticoagulant-treated patients had experienced a nonsignificant 10% decrease in mortality (hazard ratio = 0.90; 95% confidence interval [CI], 0.73 to 1.11). Anticoagulant treatment was associated with significant reductions in reinfarction (114 vs. 242; hazard ratio = 0.47 [0.38 to 0.59]) and cerebrovascular events (37 vs. 62; hazard ratio = 0.60 [0.40 to 0.90]). There was, however, an excess in cerebral hemorrhage among those allocated anticoagulant treatment (17 cases, 8 fatal) compared with those assigned placebo (2 cases, neither fatal). The numbers of fatal strokes were similar (11 in anticoagulant, 8 in placebo), so that the reduction in total cerebrovascular events associated with active treatment largely reflects a decrease in nonfatal events. There were major bleeding complications in 73 patients allocated to anticoagulants and 19 assigned placebo. In on-treatment analyses, there were 55 major bleeds in the anticoagulant group and 6 in placebo. This corresponds to a rate for anticoagulant therapy of 1.5 bleeds per 100 patient-years, a rate similar to that in earlier trials and one that supports the relative safety of long-term anticoagulation with an INR of 2.8 to 4.8.

Thus, three more recent, large-scale trials have more firmly established the benefits of anticoagulant therapy in post-MI patients, demonstrating reductions in mortality, reinfarction, and stroke using moderate-intensity anticoagulation.[61–64] As with antiplatelet therapy, the optimal duration of anticoagulation is uncertain, although the results of the Sixty-Plus Study[61] suggest that this extends beyond 1 year post-MI.

COMPARISONS OF ASPIRIN AND ANTICOAGULANT THERAPY

Although a number of large-scale randomized trials and overviews of trials have demonstrated net benefits of antiplatelet therapy with aspirin as well as anticoagulant regimens in long-term therapy of post-MI patients, these data do not address directly whether one of these forms of therapy is superior or whether a combined regimen of aspirin and anticoagulation confers any net benefit over that achieved using monotherapy with either treatment alone. Several randomized have evaluated these questions.

An early trial that compared directly antithrombotic therapy with aspirin and anticoagulant therapy was the previously described German-Austrian Reinfarction Study in the 1970s.[34] This trial randomized 946 patients, 45 to 70 years of age, 30 to 42 days following infarction, to aspirin (1.5 g daily), phenprocoumon (target thrombotest value 5% to 12%), or placebo. The trial was double blind with respect to aspirin assignment, but was open label for phenprocoumon. As reviewed earlier, after 2 years of treatment, there were nonsignificant mortality reductions for aspirin versus placebo and for aspirin versus phenprocoumon, and reductions that approached borderline significance in coronary death among those assigned aspirin versus phenprocoumon (46.3% reduction; $P < 0.07$), and in coronary events (nonfatal reinfarction plus coronary death) among those assigned aspirin versus placebo (36.6% reduction; $P < 0.06$). Thus, this early comparison of aspirin and oral anticoagulation did not yield clear results, but it did suggest a possible advantage of aspirin.

The French Enquête de Prévention Secondaire de l'Infarctus du Myocarde (EPSIM) study compared aspirin (500 mg, three times daily) with oral anticoagulation (acenocoumarol, luindione, ethylbiscoumacetate, phenindioe, or tioclomarol) in 1303 post-MI men and women.[65] Participants were 30 to 70 years of age, and the mean interval from infarction to study entry was 11 days. Following an average duration of treatment of 29 months, there were no statistically significant differences between treatment groups in mortality or reinfarction. The occurrence of at least one bleeding episode was far more common among patients assigned oral anticoagulants than aspirin (104 vs. 35 patients), while aspirin-allocated patients experienced excesses in reported gastritis (18 vs. 4) and confirmed peptic ulcer (22 vs. 6).

Whether there are differences in the relative efficacy of aspirin and anticoagulants in thrombolyzed patients was the focus of a recent multicenter, international trial. The Aspirin/Anticoagulants Following Thrombolysis with Eminase in Recurrent Infarction (AFTER) Study randomized 1036 patients who had been treated with the thrombolytic drug Eminase (anistreplase) to aspirin (150 mg daily) or anticoagulation (intravenous heparin followed by oral anticoagulation, target INR 2.0 to 2.5).[66] For the primary outcome of reinfarction plus cardiac death, there was no significant difference between treatments at 30 days (11.2% for aspirin vs. 11.0% for anticoagulation) or 3 months (12.1% for aspirin vs. 13.2% for anticoagulation). Patients assigned anticoagulation were significantly more likely to have had severe bleeding or a stroke by 3 months (3.6% vs. 1.7%; $P = 0.04$), but most of this excess occurred in the first 3 days, a period during which anticoagulant patients were still receiving heparin.

A second trial among thrombolysed patients, the Antithrombotics in the Prevention of Reocclusion In Coronary Thrombolysis (APRICOT) Study, enrolled 300 patients with patent infarct-related arteries following thrombolysis and initiation of intravenous heparin.[67] Participants were allocated to one of three treatment groups: continuation of heparin and initiation of warfarin (open label) or discontinuation of heparin and initiation of either aspirin (325 mg daily) or aspirin-placebo (double blinded). The initial warfarin dose was at the discretion of the attending physician, with dose adjustments made until the INR was between 2.8 and 4.0. The primary endpoint for the trial was patency of the infarct-related artery 3 months following hospital discharge.

A total of 300 patients were randomized, with angiographic follow-up data available for 248 subjects. Reocclusion rates were not significantly different among the three groups (25% with aspirin, 30% with warfarin, and 32% with placebo). Mortality rates also did not differ. Reinfarction occurred in 3% of patients assigned aspirin, 8% of those allocated warfarin, and 11% of those on placebo (aspirin vs. placebo; $P < 0.025$; other comparisons not significant). Similarly, revascularization was lower in the aspirin group (6%) than in warfarin (13%) and placebo (16%) (aspirin vs. placebo; $P < 0.05$; other comparisons NS). Thus, the available trial data comparing anticoagulant and aspirin regimens in post-MI patients do not provide clear evidence for the superiority of one form of antithrombotic therapy.

Combined Anticoagulant/Aspirin Therapy Versus Aspirin Monotherapy

Since the pathogenesis of thrombosis is multifactorial, it has been postulated that combined therapy with aspirin and anticoagulants might inhibit both platelet activation and thrombin generation, thereby providing greater clinical benefit than monotherapy with either regimen. Trials in unstable angina patients[68] and recipients of mechanical heart valves[69] have provided some support for use of full-dose anticoagulation plus aspirin rather than therapy with either antithrombotic regimen alone. However, the increased bleeding risks observed with this dual regimen, as well as the added clinical burden and financial costs of monitoring INR values, raised the question of whether comparable benefit might be achieved, with less bleeding and clinical monitoring, using lower, fixed doses of anticoagulants as well as lower-dose aspirin.

The recent Coumadin Aspirin Reinfarction Study (CARS) was designed to address this question. This multicenter, North American trial randomly assigned 8803 post-MI patients to daily treatment with 160 mg aspirin alone, 3 mg warfarin plus 80 mg aspirin, or 1 mg warfarin plus 80 mg aspirin.[70] INR values were assessed at weeks 1, 2, 3, 4, 6, and 12, and then at 3-month intervals, but the only dose adjustments made were reductions for patients with values of 3.5 or higher. Thus, for most patients the CARS trial represents an evaluation of "fixed-dose" rather than "targeted-dose" warfarin.

The primary study endpoint was first occurrence of reinfarction, nonfatal ischemic stroke, or cardiovascular death. The trial was terminated early, at the recommendation of the data and safety monitoring committee, based on the apparent comparable efficacy of the three treatments, and an estimate that there was less than 1% chance that a statistically significant 20% difference for any comparison would emerge with additional enrollment or follow-up. At the trial termination, after a median treatment of 14 months, the relative risk of the primary endpoint for the aspirin alone group compared with the 3-mg warfarin plus aspirin group was 0.95 (0.81 to 1.12; $P = 0.57$). For the aspirin alone group compared with the 1-mg warfarin plus aspirin group, the relative risk was 1.03 (0.87 to 1.22; $P = 0.74$). For the low- versus high-dose warfarin regimens, the relative risk was 0.93 (0.78 to 1.11; $P = 0.41$). With respect to individual outcomes, there was a reduction in ischemic stroke in the aspirin-only group compared with both of the combined regimens, and the comparison with 1-mg warfarin plus 80-mg aspirin was of borderline significance ($P = 0.05$). The authors suggest this finding may support the possibility of greater benefit in preventing stroke with the higher 160-mg dose used in the aspirin-only arm, but this finding was based on small numbers of events (21 vs. 28 ischemic strokes). Overall, however, the CARS results demonstrated no clinical benefit of low fixed doses of warfarin combined with 80 mg of aspirin over that achieved with

160 mg of aspirin alone. The investigators cited recent evidence that mechanical heart value patients benefit from combined moderate-dose anticoagulation and aspirin, with low bleeding risk,[71] to support the possible use of higher-dose anticoagulation with aspirin in post-MI patients.

One such trial, the Combined Hemotherapy and Mortality Prevention (CHAMP) Study, is currently ongoing among post-MI patients. This Veterans Affairs cooperative trial is comparing aspirin alone (162 mg per day) to warfarin (INR 1.5 to 2.5) plus aspirin (81 mg per day).

Recently, the Thrombosis Prevention Trial reported results of a 2 × 2 factorial trial of low-intensity warfarin and low-dose aspirin in men without prior events but at high risk of ischemic heart disease (IHD).[72] While this was not a trial of secondary prevention, its findings add important new data to the totality of evidence on combination versus monotherapy with anticoagulants and aspirin to prevent occlusive vascular events. The trial randomized 5085 men in the United Kingdom, 45 to 69 years of age, who were at high risk for IHD based on a risk score that considered family history, smoking history, body mass index, blood pressure, cholesterol, plasma fibrinogen, and plasma factor VII activity. Anticoagulation with warfarin was adjusted toward a target INR of 1.5; aspirin was given as 75 mg daily in a controlled-release preparation. The trial accrued a median treatment duration of 6.8 years. The mean warfarin INR and dose were 1.47 and 4.1 mg daily, respectively. The primary endpoint was total IHD, defined as nonfatal MI plus coronary death.

Warfarin-treated participants experienced a 21% reduction in IHD (95% CI, 4 to 35; $P = 0.02$), chiefly because of a statistically significant 39% reduction in fatal events. Aspirin treatment was associated with a similar 20% reduction in IHD (95% CI, 1 to 35; $P = 0.04$), but this was almost entirely because of a significant 32% reduction in nonfatal MI. Combined treatment yielded a 34% reduction in IHD (95% CI, 11 to 51; $P = 0.006$). There was an excess of hemorrhagic stroke and total fatal strokes among those assigned combined therapy, the numbers of events for hemorrhagic stroke being 7 in the combined, 1 in the warfarin alone, 2 in the aspirin alone, and 0 in the placebo groups; for fatal strokes the numbers were 12 in combined therapy, 5 in warfarin alone, 2 in aspirin alone, and 1 in placebo. Taking into account the relative incidence of IHD and stroke, the trial reported that combined therapy prevented approximately 12 times as many episodes of IHD as it caused strokes, although the strokes tended to be hemorrhagic and fatal. Thus, the trial demonstrates that there may be added benefits on vascular disease events of combined therapy with warfarin and aspirin, and it further suggests that the failure to observe such an effect in the CARS investigation may have related to its use of a fixed, low dose of warfarin.

NEW ANTIPLATELET AND ANTICOAGULANT AGENTS

The thienopyridines represent a new class of antiplatelet agents that may have an advantage over aspirin. These agents act to inhibit adenosine diphosphate–dependent activation of the platelet glycoprotein IIb/IIIa complex. In a study of patients who received Palmaz-Schatz coronary artery stents, the combination of ticlopidine and aspirin was more effective than the combination of heparin, phenprocoumon, and aspirin in the prevention of the combination of death, MI, CABG, or repeat PTCA.[73] However, ticlopidine is associated with the potentially serious complication of bone marrow depression. The results of a secondary prevention trial utilizing the thienopyridine clopidogrel have been presented by the Clopidogrel Versus Aspirin in Patients at Risk of Ischaemic Events (CAPRIE) investigators.[74] A total of 19,185 patients with atherosclerotic vascular disease were randomized to clopidogrel (75 mg daily) or to aspirin (325 mg daily). Clopidogrel was associated with an 8.7% reduction in the annual risk of the composite endpoint of vascular death, MI, or ischemic stroke (5.3 vs 5.8%; $P = 0.043$). Clopidogrel use was not associated with bone marrow depression, and the overall safety profile was comparable with that of aspirin 325 mg. These data raise the possibility that newer agents, such as the thienopyridines, may have an advantage over aspirin.

CLINICAL RECOMMENDATIONS

The large number of randomized clinical trials completed to date provides strong support for the administration of antiplatelet therapy or anticoagulation therapy to patients who have survived an MI. Of the antiplatelet agents, there is presently no clear evidence from most studies that any agent provides superior benefit to that achieved with aspirin alone. In one recent trial, clopidogrel, a new oral platelet inhibitor, was shown somewhat more effective than aspirin.[74] At this time, however, it is uncertain which patient subgroups are most likely to accrue this modest benefit. Although the ideal dose of aspirin has not been established, 75 to 160 mg daily appears to be sufficient for long-term therapy. Lower doses may also confer benefit because of their decreased toxicity and potential to preserve the biosynthesis of prostacyclin, but the latter possibility has not been clinically demonstrated. Anticoagulant therapy also confers conclusive benefits in post-MI patients, but there is no evidence of superior efficacy to aspirin.

All post-MI patients should be considered for one or the other of these therapies. Strong consideration should be given to warfarin for patients with additional risk factors for thromboembolism (e.g., atrial fibrillation, prior embolism, or extensive left ventricular dysfunction). For most post-MI patients, however, aspirin alone may provide the best benefit-risk ratio, and the lack of need for clinical dose monitoring makes its use far less costly and complex than anticoagulation. Recent findings from a primary prevention trial among high-risk subjects[72] suggest there may be a modest added benefit from combined therapy with aspirin and low-intensity oral anticoagulation. Additional trial data on combined therapy are necessary, particularly in the specific setting of post-MI. However, at present, the practical dose-monitoring considerations with anticoagulation, as well as the increased bleeding risks from this therapy, may limit the widespread use of dual therapy in clinical practice.

REFERENCES

1. DeWood MA, Spores J, Notske R, et al. Prevalence of total coronary occlusion during the early hours of transmural myocardial infarction. N Engl J Med 1980; 303:897–902.
2. Rentrop KP, Blanke H, Karsch KR, et al. Selective intracoronary thrombolysis in acute myocardial infarction and unstable angina pectoris. Circulation 1981; 63:307.
3. Falk E. Unstable angina with fatal outcome: Dynamic coronary thrombosis leading to infarction and/or sudden death—autopsy evidence of recurrent mural thrombosis with peripheral embolization culminating in total vascular occlusion. Circulation 1985; 71:699–708.
4. Hackett D, Davies G, Chierchia S, et al. Intermittent coronary occlusion in acute myocardial infarction: Value of combined thrombolytic and vasodilator therapy. N Engl J Med 1987; 317:1055–1059.
5. Schatz IJ, Riddle JM. Platelet surface activation and aggregation in myocardial infarction—electron microscopic appearances. Adv Cardiol 1970; 4:143–160.
6. Fitzgerald DJ, Roy L, Catella F, et al. Platelet activation in unstable coronary disease. N Engl J Med 1986; 315:983–989.
7. Fitzgerald DJ, Catella F, Roy L, et al. Marked platelet activation in vivo after intravenous streptokinase in patients with acute myocardial infarction. Circulation 1988; 77:142–150.
8. Kerins DM, Roy L, FitzGerald GA, et al. Platelet and vascular function during coronary thrombolysis with tissue-type plasminogen activator. Circulation 1989; 80:1718–1725.
9. Rebuzzi AG, Natale A, Bianchi C, et al. Importance of reperfusion on thromboxane A_2 metabolite excretion after thrombolysis. Am Heart J 1992; 123:560–566.
10. Salvioni A, Marenzi G, Lauri G, et al. Beta-thromboglobulin plasma levels in the first week after myocardial infarction: Influence of thrombolytic therapy. Am Heart J 1994; 128:472–476.
11. Elwood PC, Renaud S, Sharp DS, et al. Ischemic heart disease and platelet aggregation: The Caerphilly Collaborative Heart Disease Study. Circulation 1991; 83:38–44.
12. Trip MD, Cats VM, van Capelle FJL, et al. Platelet hyperreactivity and prognosis in survivors of myocardial infarction. N Engl J Med 1990; 322:1549–1554.
13. Lam JYT, Latour JG, Lesperance J, et al. Platelet aggregation, coronary artery disease progression, and future coronary events. Am J Cardiol 1994; 73:333–338.
14. Nelken NA, Soifer SJ, Vu T-KH, et al. Thrombin receptor expression in normal and atherosclerotic human arteries. J Clin Invest 1992; 90:1614–1621.
15. Ridker PM, Manson JE, Gaziano MJ, et al. Low-dose aspirin therapy for chronic stable angina: A randomized clinical trial. Ann Intern Med 1991; 114:835–839.
16. Ridker PM, Manson JE, Buring JE, et al. The effect of chronic platelet inhibition with low-dose aspirin on atherosclerotic progression and acute thrombosis: Clinical evidence from the Physicians' Health Study. Am Heart J 1991; 122:1588–1592.
17. Ridker PM, Manson JE, Buring JE, et al. Clinical characteristics of nonfatal myocardial infarction among individuals on prophylactic low-dose aspirin therapy. Circulation 1991; 84:708–711.
18. Juul-Moller S, Edvardsson N, Jahnmatz B, et al. Double-blind trial of aspirin in primary prevention of myocardial infarction in patients with stable chronic angina pectoris. Lancet 1992; 340:1421–1425.
19. Hamsten A, Walldius G, Szamosi A, et al. Plasminogen activator inhibitor in plasma: Risk factor for recurrent myocardial infarction. Lancet 1987; 2:3–9.
20. Ridker PM, Vaughan DE, Stampfer MJ, et al. Endogenous tissue-type plasminogen activator and risk of myocardial infarction. Lancet 1993; 341:1165–1168.
21. Thompson SG, Kienast J, Pyke SDM, et al, for the European Concerted Action on Thrombosis and Disabilities Angina Pectoris Study Group. Hemostatic factors and the risk of myocardial infarction or sudden death in patients with angina pectoris. N Engl J Med 1995; 332:635–641.
22. Ridker PM, Hennekens CH, Cerskus A, Stampfer MJ. Plasma concentration of cross linked fibrin degradation product (D-dimer) and the risk of future myocardial infarction among apparently healthy men. Circulation 1994; 90:2236–2240.
23. Ridker PM, Cushman M, Stampfer MJ, et al. Inflammation, aspirin, and the risk of cardiovascular disease in apparently healthy men. N Engl J Med 1997; 336:973–979.
24. Ridker PM, Cushman M, Stampfer MJ, et al. Plasma concentration of C-reactive protein and risk of developing peripheral vascular disease. Circulation 1998; 97:425–428.
25. Meade TW, North WRS, Chakrabarti R, et al. Haemostatic function and cardiovascular death: Early results of a prospective study. Lancet 1980; 1:1050–1054.
26. Meade TW, Mellow S, Brazovic M, et al. Haemostatic function and ischaemic heart disease: Principal results of the Northwick Part Heart Study. Lancet 1986; 2:533–537.
27. Heinrich J, Balleisen L, Schulte H, et al. Fibrinogen and factor VII in the prediction of coronary risk: Results from the PROCAM study in healthy men. Arterioscler Thromb 1994; 14:54–59.
28. Elwood PC, Cochrane AL, Burr ML, et al. A randomized, controlled trial of acetylsalicyclic acid in the secondary prevention of mortality from myocardial infarction. BMJ 1974; 1:436–440.
29. Elwood PC, Sweetnam PM. Aspirin and secondary mortality after myocardial infarction. Lancet 1979; 2:1313–1315.
30. Elwood PC, Sweetnam PM. Aspirin and secondary mortality after myocardial infarction. Circulation 1980; 62:53–58.
31. Coronary Drug Project Research Group. Aspirin in coronary heart disease. J Chronic Dis 1976; 29:625–642.
32. Aspirin Myocardial Infarction Study Research Group. A randomized, controlled trial of aspirin in persons recovered from myocardial infarction. JAMA 1980; 243:991–999.
33. Persantine-Aspirin Reinfarction Study Research Group. Persantine and aspirin in coronary heart disease. Circulation 1980; 62:449–461.
34. Breddin K, Loew D, Lechner K, et al. Secondary prevention of myocardial infarction: A comparison of acetylsalicylic acid, placebo, and phenprocoumon. Haemostasis 1980; 9:325–344.
35. Anturane Reinfarction Trial Research Group. Sulfinpyrazone in the prevention of cardiac death after myocardial infarction: The Anturane reinfarction trial. N Engl J Med 1978; 298:289–295.
36. Anturane Reinfarction Trial Research Group. Sulfinpyrazone in the prevention of sudden death after myocardial infarction. N Engl J Med 1980; 302:250–256.
37. Temple R, Pledger GW. The FDA's critique of the Anturane reinfarction trial. N Engl J Med 1980; 303:1488–1492.

38. Anturane Reinfarction Trial Policy Committee. The Anturane reinfarction trial: Reevaluation of outcome. N Engl J Med 1982; 306:1005–1008.
39. Anturane Reinfarction Italian Study Group. Sulphinpyrazone in post-myocardial infarction: Report from the Anturane Reinfarction Italian Study. Lancet 1982; 1:237–242.
40. Antiplatelet Trialists' Collaboration. Secondary prevention of vascular disease by prolonged antiplatelet therapy. BMJ 1988; 296:320–332.
41. Antiplatelet Trialists' Collaboration. Collaborative review of randomized trials of antiplatelet therapy: I. Prevention of death, myocardial infarction, and stroke by prolonged antiplatelet therapy in various categories of patients. BMJ 1994; 308:81–206.
42. Clarke RJ, Mayo G, Price P, FitzGerald GA. Suppression of thromboxane A_2 but not of systemic prostacyclin by controlled-release aspirin. N Eng J Med 1991; 325:1137–1141.
43. UK-TIA Study Group. United Kingdom Transient Ischaemic Attack (UK-TIA) Aspirin Trial: Final results. J Neurol Neurosurg Psychiatry 1991; 54:1044–1054.
44. Rogers WJ, Bowlby LJ, Chandra NC, et al. Treatment of myocardial infarction in the United States (1990 to 1993): Observations from the National Registry of Myocardial Infarction. Circulation 1994; 90:2103–2114.
45. Krumholz HM, Radford MJ, Ellerbeck EF, et al. Aspirin in the treatment of acute myocardial infarction in elderly Medicare beneficiaries: Patterns of use and outcomes. Circulation 1995; 92:2841–2847.
46. Krumholz HM, Radford MJ, Ellerbeck EF, et al. Aspirin for secondary prevention after myocardial infarction in the elderly: Prescribed use and outcomes. Ann Intern Med 1996; 124:292–298.
47. Wright IS, Marple CD, Beck DF. Report of the committee for the evaluation of anticoagulants in the treatment of coronary thrombosis with myocardial infarction. Am Heart J 1948; 36:801–815.
48. Tulloch JA, Gilchrist AR. Anticoagulants in treatment of coronary thrombosis. BMJ 1950; 2:965–971.
49. Wright IS. The use of anticoagulants in coronary heart disease: Progress and problems—1960. Circulation 1960; 22:608–618.
50. Wasserman AJ, Gutterman LA, Yoe KB, et al. Anticoagulants in acute myocardial infarction: The failure of anticoagulants to alter mortality in a randomized trial. Am Heart J 1966; 71:43–49.
51. Loeliger EA, Kroes AH, van Dijk LM, et al. A double-blind trial of long-term anticoagulation treatment after myocardial infarction. Acta Med Scand 1967; 182:549–566.
52. Borchgrevink CF, Bjerkelund C, Abrahamsen AM, et al. Long-term anticoagulant therapy after myocardial infarction in women. BMJ 1968; 3:571–574.
53. Drapkin A, Merskey C. Anticoagulant therapy after acute myocardial infarction: Relation of therapeutic benefit to patient's age, sex, and severity of infarction. JAMA 1972; 222:541–548.
54. Ritland S, Ritland LT. Comparison of efficacy of 3 and 12 months' anticoagulant therapy after myocardial infarction. Lancet 1969; 1:122–124.
55. Working Party on Anticoagulant Therapy in Coronary Thrombosis. Assessment of short-term anticoagulant administration after cardiac infarction. BMJ 1969; 1:335–342.
56. Ebert RV, Borden CW, Hipp HR, et al. Long-term anticoagulation therapy after myocardial infarction: Final report of the Veterans Administration Cooperative Study. JAMA 1969; 207:2263–2267.
57. Ebert RV. Anticoagulants in acute myocardial infarction. JAMA 1973; 255:724–729.
58. Seaman AJ, Griswold HE, Reaume RB, et al. Long-term anticoagulant prophylaxis after myocardial infarction: Final report. N Engl J Med 1969; 281:115–119.
59. Meuwissen OJAT, Vervoorn AC, Cohen O, et al. Double-blind trial of long-term anticoagulant treatment after myocardial infarction. Acta Med Scand 1969; 186:361–368.
60. Mitchell JRA. Anticoagulants in coronary heart disease—retrospect and prospect. Lancet 1981; 1:257–262.
61. Sixty-Plus Reinfarction Study Research Group. A double-blind trial to assess long-term oral anticoagulant therapy in elderly patients after myocardial infarction. Lancet 1980; 2:889–894.
62. Sixty-Plus Reinfarction Study Research Group. Risks of long-term oral anticoagulant therapy in elderly patients after myocardial infarction: Second report of the Sixty-Plus Reinfarction Study Group. Lancet 1982; 1:64–68.
63. Smith P, Arnesen H, Holme I. The effect of warfarin on mortality and reinfarction after myocardial infarction. N Engl J Med 1990; 323:147–152.
64. Anticoagulants in the Secondary Prevention of Events in Coronary Thrombosis (ASPECT) Research Group. Effect of long-term oral anticoagulant treatment on mortality and cardiovascular morbidity after myocardial infarction. Lancet 1994; 343:499–503.
65. The EPSIM Research Group. A controlled comparison of aspirin and oral anticoagulants in prevention of death after myocardial infarction. N Engl J Med 1982; 307:701–708.
66. Julian DG, Chamberlain DA, Pocock SJ. A comparison of aspirin and anticoagulation following thrombolysis for myocardial infarction (the AFTER study): A multicentre, unblinded, randomized clinical trial. BMJ 1996; 313:1429–1431.
67. Meijer A, Verheught FWA, Werter CJPJ, et al. Aspirin versus Coumadin in the prevention of reocclusion and recurrent ischemia after successful thrombolysis: A prospective, placebo-controlled angiographic trial—results of the APRICOT study. Circulation 1993; 87:1524–1530.
68. Cohen M, Adams PC, Parry G, et al. Combination antithrombotic therapy in unstable rest angina and non–Q wave infarction in nonprior aspirin users: Primary endpoints analysis from the ATACS trial. Circulation 1994; 89:81–88.
69. Altman R, Boullon F, Rouvier J, et al. Aspirin and prophylaxis of thromboembolic complications in patients with substitute heart valves. J Thorac Cardiovasc Surg 1976; 72:127–129.
70. Coumadin Aspirin Reinfarction Study (CARS) Investigators. Randomised, double-blind trial of fixed low-dose warfarin with aspirin after myocardial infarction. Lancet 1997; 350:389–396.
71. Altman R, Rouvier J, Gurfinkel E, et al. Comparison of two levels of anticoagulant therapy in patients with substitute heart valves. J Thorac Cardiovasc Surg 1991; 101:427–431.
72. The Medical Research Council's General Practice Research Framework. Thrombosis prevention trial: Randomised trial of low-intensity oral anticoagulation with warfarin and low-dose aspirin in the primary prevention of ischaemic heart disease in men at increased risk. Lancet 1998; 351:233–241.
73. Schomig A, Neumann F-J, Kastrati A, et al. A randomized comparison of antiplatelet and anticoagulant therapy after the placement of coronary artery stents. N Engl J Med 1996; 334:1084–1108.
74. CAPRIE Steering Committee. A randomised, blinded, trial of clopidogrel versus aspirin in patients at risk of ischaemic events (CAPRIE). Lancet 1996; 348:1329–1339.

21 Anticoagulant and Antiplatelet Drug Therapy in Atrial Fibrillation

▶ Daniel E. Singer
▶ Elaine M. Hylek

Research conducted over the past two decades has established that atrial fibrillation (AF) is a potent risk factor for ischemic stroke and that this risk is largely reversible by long-term anticoagulant therapy. This chapter reviews the randomized trials that have tested anticoagulants and antiplatelet agents to prevent stroke in AF and the relevant observational studies that have extended our understanding of stroke prevention in AF.

AF occurring in patients with rheumatic heart disease, principally mitral stenosis, has long been accepted as a major stroke risk and a strong indication for lifelong anticoagulation. AF results in the loss of coordinated atrial contraction. This loss, combined with obstruction of outflow from the left atrium in mitral stenosis, leads to relative stasis of blood and presumably promotes the formation of atrial thrombi that become a source of systemic embolism. The clinical studies supporting the efficacy of anticoagulation in preventing embolism in rheumatic AF are methodologically weak.[1] Certainly no randomized trials have been conducted in this condition. Nonetheless, the frequent occurrence of thromboembolism in young patients with mitral stenosis and AF prompted acceptance of an atrioembolic mechanism, and of anticoagulation as the appropriate intervention.

NONRHEUMATIC AF AS RISK FACTOR FOR STROKE: EPIDEMIOLOGY

There was more controversy about whether nonrheumatic AF, by far the more common category of AF, also caused embolic stroke. AF is predominantly a condition occurring in older people and in those with other cardiac illnesses.[2] Stroke in such people might simply be a result of their age or comorbid conditions. Several clinical and autopsy studies appeared to link more directly nonrheumatic AF and stroke.[3, 4] High-quality epidemiologic studies[2, 5] subsequently provided firmer evidence that nonrheumatic AF is an important cause of stroke. In particular, the Framingham Heart Study demonstrated that AF was the most common cardiac arrhythmia, affecting approximately 4% of persons older than 65 years of age and 10% of those older than age 80. Most important, the Framingham Study also demonstrated that AF increased the risk of stroke fivefold. This increased relative risk (RR) occurred across the entire span of the stroke-prone older decades, establishing AF as the most potent common risk factor for stroke. A direct consequence of the sizable prevalence of AF and the strength of its association with stroke is that about 14% of all strokes in the United States can be attributed to AF.[2, 6]

RANDOMIZED TRIALS OF ANTITHROMBOTIC THERAPY TO PREVENT STROKE IN NONRHEUMATIC AF

In response to the accumulating epidemiologic evidence implicating AF as a cause of stroke, a set of five roughly contemporaneous randomized trials were begun to test whether long-term antithrombotic therapy could prevent stroke in nonrheumatic AF.[7–11] These first five trials were all primary prevention trials enrolling patients who had not had a stroke or (rarely) who had had a stroke in the distant past. All trials tested anticoagulation. Two of these trials also tested aspirin in a randomized fashion.[7, 9] Remarkably, all five trials stopped early because of the marked efficacy of anticoagulation. (The CAFA Trial [see later] stopped because of findings of other trials; all others stopped because of their own results.) We review the individual trials and the findings of a pooled analysis of their results in the following section.

CLINICAL FEATURES OF PATIENTS ENTERED INTO THE RANDOMIZED TRIALS

A recurrent concern in the interpretation of randomized trials is the generalizability of the results. Only a small fraction of apparently eligible patients with AF participated in the trials (e.g., see discussion of the SPAF Trial). As a result, it is of interest to examine the features of the participants. Patients were predominantly elderly, with a mean age of 69 years (Table 21–1); one fourth were older than 75 years of age. Although most participants were men, a large number of women were included. Most subjects had had AF for longer than a year. Only 13% had intermittent ("paroxysmal") AF; for the remainder, AF was sustained. A large number of patients had significant cardiovascular comorbid illness. One can assume that the frailest patients with AF were not included and that most participants appeared to be reasonably safe candidates for anticoagulation. Otherwise subjects in the trials had many of the features characteristic of the general population with AF.

RESULTS OF THE INDIVIDUAL RANDOMIZED TRIALS

Atrial Fibrillation, Aspirin, Anticoagulation Trial (AFASAK)

AFASAK[7] was a three-armed trial comparing warfarin at a target international normalized ratio (INR) of 2.8 to 4.2, aspirin at 75 mg per day, and an aspirin placebo (Tables 21–2 and 21–3). AFASAK did not blind warfarin therapy. AFASAK was probably the closest to a community trial of warfarin. Patients were identified at two outpatient electrocardiography laboratories used by general practitioners in Denmark. Of 1842 eligible patients, 1007 entered the trial, a high recruitment fraction. Three hundred thirty-six subjects were assigned to placebo (i.e., aspirin-placebo), 336 to aspirin, and 335 to warfarin. Thirty-eight percent of patients assigned to warfarin withdrew from the study after an average follow-up of less than 1 year. This high percentage of withdrawals may have resulted from AFASAK's high recruitment fraction; more highly selected samples of patients may have been more compliant. AFASAK reported four outcome events in the warfarin group, 20 in the aspirin group, and 21 on placebo (90% of these outcomes were ischemic strokes). There were two major hemorrhages on warfarin, including one fatal intracerebral bleed. The marked benefit of warfarin coupled with the low rate of major hemorrhage led to the early stopping of the trial.

Two additional points about AFASAK are worth noting. First, the comparisons initially reported were not, in fact, the result of an intention-to-treat analysis. Patients who withdrew from the study, in particular the 38% of those assigned to warfarin, were not counted. A subsequent standard intention-to-treat analysis resulted in a P value of approximately 0.05,[12] meeting the usual standard for statistical significance, but certainly too large to activate an early stopping rule. Table 21–2 presents the estimated intention-to-treat results. It is of interest that only one of the patients in the warfarin arm who sustained a thromboembolic event was fully anticoagulated at the time of the event.

TABLE 21–1 • First Five Trials in Atrial Fibrillation (AF) for Primary Prevention of Stroke: Clinical Features of Subjects at Entry*

Clinical Features	Data
Mean age (yr)	69
Male (%)	73
Race, white (%)	94
Onset of AF, >1 yr (%)	68
Intermittent AF (%)	13
Diagnosis (%)	
Hypertension	46
Diabetes	15
Angina	22
Myocardial infarction	14
Congestive heart failure	20

* The first five trials include AFASAK (Atrial Fibrillation, Aspirin, Anticoagulation Study), BAATAF (Boston Area Anticoagulation Trial for Atrial Fibrillation), CAFA (Canadian Atrial Fibrillation Anticoagulation Study), SPAF (Stroke Prevention in Atrial Fibrillation Study), and SPINAF (Veterans Affairs Stroke Prevention in Nonrheumatic Atrial Fibrillation Study).

Data from Atrial Fibrillation Investigators. Atrial fibrillation: Risk factors for embolization and efficacy of antithrombotic therapy. Arch Intern Med 1994; 154:1449–1457.

Boston Area Anticoagulation Trial for Atrial Fibrillation (BAATAF)

BAATAF,[8] and subsequently SPINAF[11] (see later) and CAFA,[10] made the fortuitous decision to use a low-intensity anticoagulation target, adopting the strategy successfully applied by Hull and associates in treating deep vein thrombophlebitis.[13] BAATAF randomized 212 patients to "low-dose" warfarin (target prothrombin time ratio [PTR], 1.2 to 1.5) and 208 to control (see Table 21–2). Therapy was not blinded. Subjects in the control group could take aspirin, and approximately half did. Nearly three fourths of the patients were male. Only 10% of BAATAF patients assigned to warfarin withdrew from therapy permanently.

BAATAF observed 13 strokes in the control arm versus two in warfarin, for a preventive efficacy of 86% (see Table 21–2). There were no other embolic events. There was one presumed subdural hematoma

Table 21–2 • Overview of the Randomized Trials of Anticoagulation for Atrial Fibrillation*

Features	Trials					
	AFASAK	*BAATAF*	*SPAF*	*CAFA*	*SPINAF*	*EAFT*
Anticoagulation						
Target	INR 2.8–4.2	PTR 1.2–1.5	PTR 1.3–1.8	INR 2–3	PTR 1.2–1.5	INR 2.5–4
Subjects (*n*)	335	212	210	187	260	225
Emboli (*n*)	10	2	6	7	4	20
Annual rate (%)	2.3	0.41	2.3	3.0	0.88	3.9
Control						
Subjects (*n*)	336	208	211	191	265	214
Emboli (*n*)	22	13	18	11	19	50
Annual rate (%)	5.6	3.0	7.4	4.6	4.3	12.3
Preventive efficacy (%)	59	86	67	35	79	66
95% CI	15–81	51–96	27–85	(−64)–75	52–90	43–80

* Preventive efficacy is the relative risk reduction calculated as (1 − RR) × 100, where RR is the annual rate in the anticoagulation group divided by the annual rate in the control group. The outcome events reported for the AFASAK, BAATAF, SPAF, and CAFA Trials are ischemic stroke (including lacunar stroke) plus systemic embolism. For the AFASAK Trial all events reported after withdrawal from initial therapy are assumed to have been ischemic strokes or systemic emboli. For the SPINAF Trial the outcome events shown all are ischemic strokes, since that was the study's primary outcome event. For the EAFT Study the outcome event reported is ischemic stroke only, since the number of systemic emboli could not be unambiguously calculated from the study's main report.[18] For all studies the intention-to-treat analysis is presented; for the AFASAK Study the person-years of observation in different therapy categories needed to calculate incidence rates come from the Atrial Fibrillation Investigators' pooled database.[16] Preventive efficacy and 95% CI are reproduced from the original study report for the BAATAF, SPAF, SPINAF, and EAFT Trials. For the AFASAK and CAFA Studies, where the data presented differ from the study's original report, the preventive efficacy and 95% CI were calculated using the method of Breslow and Day.[47]

See Table 21–1 for complete titles of the AFASAK, BAATAF, SPAF, CAFA, and SPINAF Trials.

EAFT, European Atrial Fibrillation Trial. INR, international normalized ratio; PTR, prothrombin time ratio; CI, confidence interval.

that was fatal in a patient on warfarin. Otherwise, the rate of serious bleeding was essentially the same in the warfarin group as in the control group. In a secondary analysis, based on a nonrandomized comparison, there was no evidence of benefit among those in the control group who took aspirin.[14]

Stroke Prevention in Atrial Fibrillation Trial (SPAF)

SPAF[9] (or SPAF-I) randomly assigned patients to warfarin (target PTR, 1.3 to 1.8), aspirin at 325 mg per day, or aspirin-placebo (Group 1) (see Table 21–2). Warfarin therapy was not blinded. SPAF also studied patients who would not or could not take warfarin. These latter patients were separately randomized to aspirin at 325 mg per day or aspirin-placebo (Group 2). SPAF estimated that a relatively small fraction of eligible patients (7%) were actually recruited, a finding consistent with other American studies.

SPAF observed that warfarin reduced the risk of ischemic stroke and systemic embolic events by 69%. Of the six patients in the warfarin arm who had strokes, four were not taking warfarin at the time of their stroke.

SPAF provided a mixed picture of aspirin's effectiveness (see Table 21–3). It reported a statistically significant overall reduction in risk of stroke and systemic emboli of 42%. However, this effect was markedly heterogeneous in its two separately randomized

TABLE 21–3 • Overview of the Randomized Trials of Aspirin for Atrial Fibrillation*

Features	Trials			
	AFASAK	*SPAF-I, 1*	*SPAF-I, 2*	*EAFT*
Aspirin				
Dose/day (mg)	75	325	325	300
Subjects	336	206	346	404
Emboli	19	1	25	87
Annual rate (%)	4.7	0.37	5.5	10.4
Control				
Subjects (*n*)	336	211	357	378
Emboli (*n*)	22	18	28	90
Annual rate (%)	5.6	6.6	6.1	12.6
Preventive efficacy (%)	16	94	8	18
95% CI	(−54, +54)	(+58, +99)	(−54, +46)	(−9, +38)

* Outcome events reported for the AFASAK and SPAF Trials are ischemic stroke plus systemic embolism. For the AFASAK Trial all events reported after withdrawal from initial therapy are assumed to have been ischemic strokes or systemic emboli. Data for SPAF-I, 1 and SPAF-I, 2 are estimated from results presented in References 9 and 19. For the EAFT Study the outcome event reported is ischemic stroke only, since the number of systemic emboli could not be unambiguously calculated from the study's main report. For all studies the intention-to-treat analysis is presented; for the AFASAK Study the person-years of observation in different therapy categories needed to calculate incidence rates come from the Atrial Fibrillation Investigators' pooled database.[16] Preventive efficacy for the SPAF Trials are those given in Reference 19. The 95% CI for all the trials are calculated using the method of Breslow and Day,[47] since none of the study reports presented results exactly as they are presented in this table.

See Tables 21–1 and 21–2 for the complete titles of the Trials. SPAF-I, 1 and SPAF-I, 2 are the two separate trials of aspirin in the (first) SPAF Study.

studies of aspirin. In Group 1, which included warfarin as a possible therapy, there was only one outcome event observed in the aspirin group contrasted with 18 in the placebo group, for a calculated efficacy of 94%. In Group 2, where patients were assigned to either aspirin or aspirin-placebo, there were 25 events on aspirin versus 28 in placebo, for an efficacy of 8% (P = NS).

Among those treated with warfarin, one patient sustained a fatal intracerebral hemorrhage and one a subdural hematoma with full recovery. Two patients in the placebo group had subdural hematomas (with full recovery). There was no increase in major bleeding from other anatomic sites with warfarin.

Canadian Atrial Fibrillation Anticoagulation Trial (CAFA)

CAFA[10] was a double-blind, placebo-controlled trial of low-dose warfarin (target INR, 2 to 3) in AF (see Table 21–2). After the AFASAK report and a preliminary report of the SPAF Trial, the CAFA investigators decided to stop their trial to allow all patients access to warfarin. CAFA counted events using an "efficacy" analysis where events occurring more than 28 days after stopping therapy would not be counted. The CAFA Study did not include apparent lacunar stroke as an endpoint. In Table 21–2 we include the one lacunar stroke and present the intention-to-treat analysis. Regardless of approach, the CAFA Study observed too few events to achieve a statistically significant result, although their findings were consistent with a sizable benefit from warfarin. Once again, most of the events in the warfarin arm of the trial occurred among subjects who were not fully anticoagulated. Major bleeding occurred in five patients on warfarin, including one fatal intracranial hemorrhage, and in one patient on placebo.

Stroke Prevention in Nonvalvular Atrial Fibrillation (SPINAF)

The SPINAF Study[11] was the only completed trial to provide a fully blinded assessment of warfarin. As a Department of Veterans Affairs study, it entered only men. SPINAF used a 12-hour cutoff to distinguish transient ischemic attacks (TIAs) from strokes, rather than the more usual 24-hour cutoff used by the other studies. In this study, warfarin at low dose (target PTR, 1.2 to 1.5) reduced the risk of stroke by 79% (see Table 21–2). There was one nonfatal intracerebral hemorrhage in the warfarin-treated group versus none in the placebo group. There were six other major hemorrhages in the warfarin group versus four in the placebo group (all gastrointestinal hemorrhages).

POOLED ANALYSIS OF ANTICOAGULATION EFFICACY IN THE PRIMARY PREVENTION TRIALS

The first five primary prevention trials provided consistent evidence for the striking efficacy of warfarin in AF. Warfarin, at relatively low intensities of anticoagulation, removed most of the risk of stroke in AF with little increase in major bleeding. These trials also demonstrated the potential advantages of multiple studies of the same intervention.[15] Each of the individual trials had features that could have added controversy to interpretation of the trial's results (such features would include unblinded use of warfarin, use of aspirin in the control arm, enrollment solely of men, and unwarranted stopping of the trial). These potentially controversial limitations were successfully addressed by similar results in other trials that did not have the given limitation. Further, since all these trials stopped early, the number of events observed in each was small, resulting in imprecision in each trial's estimate of warfarin's efficacy (i.e., wide confidence intervals [CIs}). Precise estimates of efficacy are particularly important when deciding whether to use a risky and demanding therapy such as warfarin. The presence of five trials allowed pooling of results to provide a much tighter CI describing warfarin's efficacy.[16]

The initial analysis of the pooled data focused on the effect of warfarin in the first five primary prevention trials. In the process of pooling, some data were recategorized to provide consistent definitions across the trials, and some previously unreported data were included in the analysis. The pooled estimate of warfarin's efficacy (i.e., the RR reduction) was 68%, with a 95% CI ranging from 50% to 79%. These estimates were calculated according to initial randomization status (i.e., intention-to-treat analysis). Since 29% of all strokes counted in the warfarin group occurred among patients not actually taking warfarin at the time of the stroke, it is reasonable to assume that warfarin's true efficacy is even higher. Eighty percent of the stroke risk faced by patients with AF is attributable to AF itself (assuming an RR of 5). Nearly all of this additional risk is prevented by anticoagulation. Across the five primary prevention trials the absolute risk of stroke was reduced by 3.1% per year (4.5% vs. 1.4% per year). For cardiovascular prevention trials, this effect is sizable; for example, it is about five times more effective in preventing strokes in the elderly than in treating hypertension.[17]

The pooled analysis identified the following independent clinical risk factors for stroke with AF:

1. Prior stroke or TIA (RR = 2.5)
2. Age (RR = 1.4 per decade)

3. Hypertension (RR = 1.6)
4. Diabetes (RR = 1.7)

Coronary heart disease and congestive heart failure were univariate risk factors but did not add significantly to the prediction of stroke, once the other risk factors were included in the multivariate model. Analysis of echocardiographic features has not yet been completed. For subjects younger than 65 years of age with none of the other three clinical risk factors, the annual risk of stroke was 1%, whether or not they received warfarin. For most subjects in the trials who had at least one of the risk factors and/or were 65 years of age or older, the annual untreated risk of stroke ranged from 3.5% to 8.1%. This annual risk was reduced in all categories to approximately 1.5% with anticoagulant treatment (Table 21–4). These results indicate that only the youngest, lowest risk group of patients with AF might safely forego anticoagulation.

SECONDARY PREVENTION TRIAL OF ANTICOAGULATION IN AF

European Atrial Fibrillation Trial (EAFT)

EAFT was a trial of antithrombotic therapy for patients with AF who had sustained a recent TIA or minor stroke. Patients were recruited from 108 centers in 13 countries. The structure of the trial was similar to that of SPAF-I.[18] For patients who were considered eligible for anticoagulation, there was a three-armed design of oral anticoagulation at INR 2.5 to 4.0 versus aspirin at 300 mg per day versus aspirin-placebo. Anticoagulation was not blinded, and participating physicians chose the anticoagulant agent. Acenocoumarol was the most commonly used anticoagulant, but warfarin and phenprocoumon were also used. For those who were not candidates for anticoagulation, the comparison groups were aspirin at 300 mg per day versus placebo. The rates of stroke in the placebo groups were much higher (12% per year) than those in the primary prevention trials. In EAFT anticoagulation reduced the rate of stroke by 66%, a finding that was virtually identical to that found in the pooled results of the primary prevention trials. Aspirin had no significant effect (87 ischemic strokes in the aspirin arms vs. 90 in the control arms), although the rate of stroke in those randomized to aspirin was slightly lower than those randomized to placebo (see Tables 21–2 and 21–3).

OVERVIEW OF THE EFFICACY OF ASPIRIN

Aspirin is simpler to take than oral anticoagulants and may be safer. It would be an attractive alternative to warfarin if it were comparably effective. Aspirin was tested against placebo in three trials in AF: AFASAK, SPAF-I, and EAFT (see Table 21–3).[7, 9, 18] SPAF-I included two separately randomized groups of subjects testing aspirin at 325 mg/day. Group 1 randomized subjects to one of three arms: warfarin therapy, aspirin, or aspirin-placebo. Patients in Group 2 were not considered candidates for warfarin and were assigned only to aspirin or aspirin-placebo. Patients in Group 2 were generally older than those in Group 1 (mean age 68 vs. 65 years), since age older than 75 years was initially considered a contraindication to anticoagulation in the SPAF-I Trial.[19] Although the original report of SPAF-I pooled the results of Groups 1 and 2, we report these results separately to highlight their disparate findings. We report a single pooled

TABLE 21–4 • Pooled Analysis of First Five Atrial Fibrillation Trials: Effect of Warfarin by Risk Category*

	Control		Warfarin	
Risk Category	*No. of Strokes*	*Annual Rate (95% CI)*	*No. of Strokes*	*Annual Rate (95% CI)*
Age <65 yr				
No risk factor	3	1.0 (0.3–3.1)	3	1.0 (0.3–3.0)
≥1 risk factor	16	4.9 (3.0–8.1)	6	1.7 (0.8–3.9)
Age 65–75 yr				
No risk factor	16	4.3 (2.7–7.1)	4	1.1 (0.4–2.8)
≥1 risk factor	27	5.7 (3.9–8.3)	7	1.7 (0.9–3.4)
Age >75 yr				
No risk factor	6	3.5 (1.6–7.7)	3	1.7 (0.5–5.2)
≥1 risk factor	13	8.1 (4.7–13.9)	2	1.2 (0.3–5.0)

* Risk factors are history of hypertension, diabetes, or prior stroke or transient ischemic attack. As indicated, ischemic stroke is the only outcome event reported. See Table 21–1 for complete titles of the Atrial Fibrillation Trials. CI, confidence interval.

Data from Atrial Fibrillation Investigators. Atrial fibrillation: Risk factors for embolization and efficacy of antithrombotic therapy. Arch Intern Med 1994; 154:1449–1457.

assessment of aspirin from the EAFT, which used the same design as SPAF-I, because the EAFT investigators specifically stated that the effect of aspirin in their two component trials was shown to be uniform.[18] In AFASAK (using 75 mg/day of aspirin), EAFT (using 300 mg/day of aspirin), and SPAF-I, Group 1 (using 325 mg/day of aspirin), the RR reduction (i.e., efficacy) was found to be 16%, 18%, and 8%, respectively. These effects were not statistically significant, and the CIs ranged from large negative effects to large positive effects. SPAF-I, Group 1 observed only one event in its aspirin arm versus 18 in placebo, for a highly statistically significant efficacy of 94%. Analysis of these four trials of aspirin reveals that the effect estimates are statistically significantly heterogeneous. As a result, it is not clear that pooling SPAF-I, Group 1 with the other three estimates would be meaningful. If SPAF-I, Group 1 is excluded, the pooled estimate of aspirin's efficacy remains statistically nonsignificant with a broad CI including the null value of 0. If SPAF-I, Group 1 is included, and no adjustment is made to account for the heterogeneity, the estimated efficacy of aspirin is approximately 20%. Whether this effect is statistically significant depends on the averaging technique used. In the pooled analysis of the raw data from the trials, the lower confidence bound for the effect of aspirin is 0. This pooled analysis also failed to identify any subgroup of patients where aspirin's effect was significantly enhanced. These trials support the conclusion that aspirin's efficacy in AF is small, at most.[20]

RECENTLY COMPLETED TRIALS

Stroke Prevention in Atrial Fibrillation II (SPAF-II)

SPAF-I raised the possibility that aspirin might be comparable to warfarin in efficacy. SPAF-II was an extension of SPAF-I, Group 1 with the aspirin-placebo group removed, thereby limiting the comparison to warfarin at PTR 1.3 to 1.8 (subsequently converted to a target of INR 2 to 4.5) versus aspirin at 325 mg per day.[21] With the beginning of SPAF-II patients were separately randomized according to age: 75 or younger versus older than 75. This was motivated by the finding in SPAF-I that aspirin appeared to work only in the younger patients.

SPAF-II's results stand in contrast with the earlier studies. In particular, there was a high rate of intracranial hemorrhage among patients older than 75—nearly 2% per year. Warfarin appeared to be modestly more effective than aspirin in preventing ischemic stroke in both age groups; however, when the intracranial hemorrhages were added to the ischemic strokes, the aggregate rates of strokes with residual deficit were similar in both the aspirin and warfarin groups: about 1.5% per year in the younger group and about 4.5% per year in the older group. This latter rate of "bad" events was more than double that seen in the warfarin arms of the earlier primary prevention trials.

Problems in the design and the execution of SPAF-II appear to weaken its conclusions.[22] Inclusion of SPAF-I, Group 1's anomalous findings regarding aspirin likely resulted in an overestimate of aspirin's efficacy in SPAF-II, particularly in the patients 75 and younger (the predominant age group for SPAF-I, Group 1). Analyses removing the experience of SPAF-I, Group 1 would have shown a substantial relative benefit of warfarin versus aspirin in the younger age group. In addition, many of the events occurring in the warfarin groups occurred in patients who were not actually taking warfarin. Of 56 events occurring in patients who were actually taking an antithrombotic therapy, 39 occurred in patients taking aspirin versus 17 in patients taking warfarin. This effect was seen in both age categories: 20 events versus 9 in the younger group, and 19 versus 8 in the older group. As a result of these considerations, the findings of SPAF-II are consistent with warfarin being substantially more effective than aspirin in preventing stroke in AF.

The increased rate of intracranial bleeding among the elderly observed in SPAF-II is clearly worrisome. However, the upper bound of SPAF-II's INR target, INR 4.5, was the highest of any trial in AF, and there was a suggestion that increased anticoagulant intensity was associated with intracranial bleeding.[21] In the pooled analysis of the primary prevention trials, the rate of intracranial hemorrhage among those older than 75 was only 0.3% per year,[16] and in EAFT no intracranial hemorrhages were reported.[18] Nonetheless, SPAF-II highlights the need to carefully monitor the rate of intracranial hemorrhage, particularly because warfarin is used more frequently in elderly patients.

Stroke Prevention in Atrial Fibrillation III (SPAF-III)

SPAF-III was crafted in response to the findings of the SPAF-II Trial.[23] It included a randomized trial and an observational cohort study. Patients were classified as at high and low risk of thromboembolism based on SPAF-II. Features denoting high risk included being both female and older than 75 years, having a systolic blood pressure higher than 160 mm Hg, having left ventricular dysfunction or recent congestive heart failure, or having had a recent stroke or TIA or systemic embolism. Patients with no high-risk features were believed to be adequately treated with aspirin. An observational cohort of such low-risk patients was assembled, aspirin was recommended, and follow-up for thromboembolic events was implemented.

The randomized trial in SPAF-III enrolled high-risk patients and randomized them to either warfarin alone targeted at INR 2.0 to 3.0 monitored by INR tests at least once per month or to a very low dose of warfarin plus aspirin at 325 mg per day. In this very-low-dose arm, patients were prescribed warfarin at 0.5 to 3 mg per day targeted to achieve an INR of 1.2 to 1.5. With this latter regimen, INR testing was to be done once every 3 months. This therapeutic combination had three goals: (1) protection against thromboembolism; (2) decreased bleeding risk; and (3) reduced burden of INR testing.

The SPAF-III randomized trial was stopped well before its planned termination date. Five hundred twenty-three high-risk patients with AF were randomly allocated to the INR 2.0 to 3.0 arm ("adjusted-dose" arm), and 521 were allocated to the combination-therapy arm ("fixed-dose combination" arm). The mean INR in the adjusted dose arm was 2.4, and in the fixed-dose warfarin arm the mean INR was 1.3. There were 11 strokes in the adjusted-dose arm, for a rate of 1.9% per year. There were 43 strokes plus one systemic embolism in the combination-therapy arm for a fourfold increase in the rate of thromboembolism of 7.9% per year. After adjustment for baseline blood pressure the RR reduction, INR 2.0 to 3.0 versus fixed combination therapy, was 74% (95% CI, 50% to 87%). The rate of intracranial bleeding was 0.5% per year in the INR 2.0 to 3.0 arm, compared to 0.9% per year in the combination arm (not statistically significant). Similarly, the rate of all major hemorrhage was slightly, but not significantly, higher in the combination therapy arm (2.4% vs. 2.1% per year).

SPAF-III makes it clear that for patients with AF who have a significant annual risk of stroke, both aspirin and very-low-intensity anticoagulation are ineffective. Indeed, the RR reduction in SPAF-III, standard warfarin anticoagulation versus the combination of aspirin and low-dose warfarin, is actually slightly higher than the RR reduction of warfarin targeted at INR 2 to 3 versus no antithrombotic therapy.[16]

IDENTIFYING THE OPTIMAL RANGE OF ANTICOAGULANT INTENSITY IN AF

Numerous studies have demonstrated that higher INR levels are associated with increased risks of major hemorrhage.[24–27] To optimize therapy, physicians need to know the lowest intensity of anticoagulation that is still effective in preventing stroke in AF. The lowest target intensity of anticoagulation in the randomized trials that was still fully effective was PTR 1.2 to 1.5 (see Table 21–2), corresponding roughly to INR 2.0 to 3.0. Although there have been reports that very low intensities of anticoagulation are effective in other thrombotic conditions,[28, 29] the SPAF-III results indicate that INR values just slightly above 1.0 are not effective in AF.

It is difficult to define the lowest effective INR from the completed randomized trials. Although a large percentage of the strokes observed in the anticoagulation arms of the trials occurred in patients who had either discontinued their therapy or had very low INR values,[16, 30] the total number of events was too low to precisely describe the risk of stroke at INR levels below 2.0. Studies from clinical practice provide rich alternative sources of information.[27, 31] A recent case-control analysis assembled 74 consecutive cases of ischemic stroke in patients with AF who were taking warfarin who were admitted to one general hospital.[31] These cases were compared to 222 patients with AF who had not had a stroke while anticoagulated. These latter controls were randomly selected from among eligible patients managed by the hospital's large anticoagulant therapy unit. The relative odds for stroke increased rapidly as the INR level decreased below 2.0 (Fig. 21–1). For example, the relative odds for stroke at an INR of 1.8 was 1.5 and was 2.5 at an INR of 1.6. At an INR of 1.3 the relative odds for stroke was 6.0. These values for relative odds were estimated from a logistic regression model that adjusted for the effects of other determinants of stroke in AF, such as prior stroke.

Stroke-preventive efficacy in AF does not appear to increase with INR levels above 2.0. In contrast, the risk of intracranial hemorrhage increases rapidly

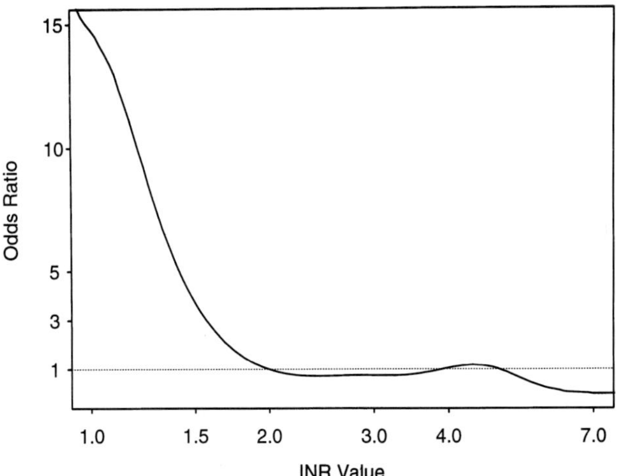

Figure 21–1 The relative odds (odds ratio) for stroke according to International Normalized Ratio (INR) value, among patients with atrial fibrillation (AF) taking warfarin. This display was generated from a case-control study comparing patients with AF who sustained a stroke while taking warfarin ("cases") with patients with AF without stroke while taking warfarin ("controls").[31] The results of the analysis that adjusted for other determinants of stroke are reported in the text.

above INR levels of 4.0 to 5.0.[26, 27] These findings indicate that the optimal INR range for AF is between 2.0 and 4.0. Published guidelines have prescribed a target INR of 2.0 to 3.0 for AF.[32] These guidelines were extrapolated from the results of the randomized trials. Thus, the target range of anticoagulation proposed by the guidelines occupies the lower end of the actual optimal INR range estimated by large observational studies.

COST EFFECTIVENESS OF ANTICOAGULATION FOR AF

In the current era of constrained resources for medical care, preventive interventions have to be justified not only on the basis of their efficacy but also on the basis of efficiency. Anticoagulation for AF appears to pass both tests. Several formal cost-effectiveness analyses indicate that strokes can be averted and quality-adjusted life years added at relatively low cost.[33, 34] Indeed, among the many patients with AF whose annual risk of stroke is above 2.6%, anticoagulation appears to be cost-saving.[33] That is, both quality-adjusted life years are added and direct medical costs are lessened by using anticoagulants. This is an extraordinary finding for preventive practices for adults. An additional attractive aspect of anticoagulation in AF is that risk of stroke is reduced immediately, providing a rapid pay-back on the investment in preventive care. Many other preventive actions take years to produce health benefits. Of course, all these calculations will be too optimistic if the management of anticoagulation in clinical practice is much worse than that in the randomized trials.

TRANSLATION OF THE FINDINGS OF THE RANDOMIZED TRIALS INTO CLINICAL PRACTICE

The results of the randomized trials of anticoagulation in AF were dramatic, demonstrating striking efficacy with low rates of complications. Nonetheless, long-term anticoagulation poses substantial burdens for both patient and physician. Patients who may be asymptomatic need to get blood tests every few weeks and need to be alert to the effects of new medications, changes in diet, or intercurrent illnesses. They also must face a new risk of hemorrhage posed by taking anticoagulants. For physicians, close monitoring of patients' INR values and the need to rapidly respond to abnormal INR levels can be burdensome. In addition, many elderly patients with AF have minor contraindications to anticoagulation (e.g., increased risk of falls), undercutting physician enthusiasm for anticoagulation. There is often slow adoption into routine care of preventive practices that have been shown to be effective in trials. One might expect adoption of anticoagulation in AF to proceed even more slowly. There is now good evidence for a clear increase in the use of anticoagulants for AF following the reports of the randomized trials.[35] Roughly 10% of patients with AF received anticoagulants before the randomized trials (Fig. 21–2). This percentage increased sharply after the first five trials to nearly 40% of patients with AF in 1993. The optimal percentage is unclear, but at least one major health maintenance organization has reported that more than 60% of their patients with AF were successfully anticoagulated.[36] One can conclude that the randomized trials have changed physician behavior but that more physician education and support (e.g., through anticoagulation clinics) will be needed to increase the numbers of patients with AF who are safely anticoagulated.

FUTURE RESEARCH

There are at least three general areas for future research in stroke prevention in AF. The first is optimizing the application of the findings of the trials in usual clinical practice. It seems clear that more widespread use of dedicated anticoagulation clinics would result in better control of INR levels—the single most important determinant of outcome among patients who are anticoagulated.[37, 38] Within the context of such clinics there should be testing of new dosing algorithms and of novel technologies such as self-testing

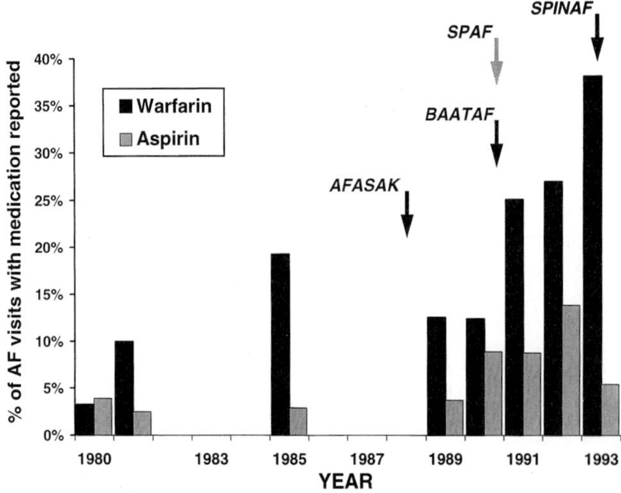

Figure 21–2 The use of anticoagulants or aspirin in patients with atrial fibrillation (AF).[35] The percentage of patients with AF is shown in which warfarin or aspirin use was reported in the National Ambulatory Medical Care Surveys. Arrows indicate the publication dates of clinical trials described in the text (see text for complete names of the trials). A shaded arrow for SPAF corresponds to this study's preliminary report.[48] The final report of the SPAF-I trial was published in 1991.[9]

apparatus.[39, 40] The goals of such research would be to define more patient-specific INR targets and monitoring schedules, to improve control of INR levels, and to achieve better patient adherence with monitoring.[39, 40, 41] Health systems should institute quality control programs to track the percentage of patients with AF who are being anticoagulated, the INR control for such patients, and the bleeding and thromboembolism rates experienced by anticoagulated patients.

A second more basic area of research should focus on new determinants of risk among patients with AF. Currently, stroke risk in AF is dictated by simple clinical features. More sophisticated hematologic measures and imaging approaches may allow physicians to discriminate better those patients who absolutely need anticoagulation from those who might safely avoid anticoagulants.[42, 43] Transesophageal echocardiography is currently being studied as such a risk marker in the context of cardioversion of AF.[44]

Finally, we should continue to search for safer and less intrusive alternatives to anticoagulation. Such alternatives would include newer antithrombotic agents,[45] as well as approaches to cardiovert AF and more successfully maintain sinus rhythm.[46]

REFERENCES

1. Szekely P. Systemic embolism and anticoagulant prophylaxis in rheumatic heart disease. BMJ 1964; 1:209–212.
2. Wolf PA, Abbott RD, Kannel WB. Atrial fibrillation: A major contributor to stroke in the elderly. Arch Intern Med 1987; 147:1561–1564.
3. Fisher CM. Reducing risks of cerebral embolism. Geriatrics 1979; 34:59–61, 65–66.
4. Hinton RC, Kistler JP, Fallon JT, et al. Influence of etiology of atrial fibrillation on incidence of systemic embolism. Am J Cardiol 1977; 40:509–513.
5. Friedman GD, Loveland DB, Ehrlich SP Jr. Relationship of stroke to other cardiovascular disease. Circulation 1968; 38:533–541.
6. Wolf PA, Abbott RD, Kannel WB. Atrial fibrillation as an independent risk factor for stroke: The Framingham Study. Stroke 1991; 22:983–988.
7. Petersen P, Godtfredsen J, Boysen G, et al. Placebo-controlled, randomised trial of warfarin and aspirin for prevention of thromboembolic complications in chronic atrial fibrillation: The Copenhagen AFASAK study. Lancet 1989; 1:175–179.
8. The Boston Area Anticoagulation Trial for Atrial Fibrillation Investigators. The effect of low-dose warfarin on the risk of stroke in patients with nonrheumatic atrial fibrillation. N Engl J Med 1990; 323:1505–1511.
9. Stroke Prevention in Atrial Fibrillation Investigators. Stroke prevention in atrial fibrillation study: Final results. Circulation 1991; 84:527–539.
10. Connolly SJ, Laupacis A, Gent M, et al. Canadian Atrial Fibrillation Anticoagulation (CAFA) study. J Am Coll Cardiol 1991; 18:349–355.
11. Ezekowitz MD, Bridgers SL, James KE, et al. Warfarin in the prevention of stroke associated with nonrheumatic atrial fibrillation. N Engl J Med 1992; 327:1406–1412.
12. Petersen P, Boysen G, Godtfredsen J, et al. Warfarin to prevent thromboembolism in chronic atrial fibrillation [Letter]. Lancet 1989; 1:670.
13. Hull R, Hirsh J, Jay R, et al. Different intensities of oral anticoagulant therapy in the treatment of proximal vein thrombosis. N Engl J Med 1982; 307:1676–1681.
14. Singer DE, Hughes RA, Gress DR, et al. The effect of aspirin on the risk of stroke in patients with non-rheumatic atrial fibrillation: The BAATAF study. Am Heart J 1992; 124:1567–1573.
15. Singer DE. Problems with stopping rules in trials of risky therapies: The case of warfarin to prevent stroke in atrial fibrillation. Clin Res 1993; 41:482–486.
16. Atrial Fibrillation Investigators. Atrial fibrillation: Risk factors for embolization and efficacy of anti-thrombotic therapy. Arch Intern Med 1994; 154:1449–1457.
17. Mulrow CD, Cornell JA, Herrera CR, et al. Hypertension in the elderly: Implications and generalizability of randomized trials. JAMA 1994; 272:1932–1938.
18. EAFT (European Atrial Fibrillation Trial) Study Group. Secondary prevention in non-rheumatic atrial fibrillation after transient ischaemic attack or minor stroke. Lancet 1993; 342:1256–1262.
19. Stroke Prevention in Atrial Fibrillation Investigators. A differential effect of aspirin on prevention of stroke in atrial fibrillation. J Stroke Cerebrovasc Dis 1993; 3:181–188.
20. Atrial Fibrillation Investigators (Laupacis A, Boysen G, Connolly S, et al). The efficacy of aspirin in patients with atrial fibrillation: Analysis of pooled data from three randomized trials. Arch Intern Med 1997; 336:243–250.
21. Stroke Prevention in Atrial Fibrillation Investigators. Warfarin versus aspirin for prevention of thromboembolism in atrial fibrillation: The Stroke Prevention in Atrial Fibrillation II Study. Lancet 1994; 343:687–691.
22. Singer DE. Anticoagulation to prevent stroke in atrial fibrillation. *In* DiMarco JP, Prystowsky EN (eds). Atrial Arrhythmias: State of the Art. Armonk, NY, Futura, 1995, pp 313–326.
23. Stroke Prevention in Atrial Fibrillation Investigators. Adjusted-dose warfarin versus low-intensity, fixed-dose warfarin plus aspirin for high-risk patients with atrial fibrillation: Stroke Prevention in Atrial Fibrillation III randomised clinical trial. Lancet 1996; 348:633–638.
24. Landefeld CS, Rosenblatt MW, Goldman L. Bleeding in outpatients treated with warfarin: Relation to the prothrombin time and important remediable lesions. Am J Med 1989; 87:153–159.
25. Fihn SD, McDonell M, Martin D, et al. Risk factors for complications of chronic anticoagulation. Ann Intern Med 1993; 118:511–520.
26. Hylek EM, Singer DE. Risk factors for intracranial hemorrhage in outpatients taking warfarin. Ann Intern Med 1994; 120:897–902.
27. Cannegieter SC, Rosendaal FR, Wintzen AR, et al. Optimal oral anticoagulant therapy in patients with mechanical heart valves. N Engl J Med 1995; 333:11–17.
28. Poller L, McKernan A, Thompson JM, et al. Fixed minidose warfarin: A new approach to prophylaxis against venous thrombosis after major surgery. BMJ 1987; 295:1309–1312.
29. Bern MM, Bothe A Jr, Bistrian B, et al. Prophylaxis against central vein thrombosis with low-dose warfarin. Surgery 1986; 99:216–220.
30. The European Atrial Fibrillation Trial Study Group. Optimal oral anticoagulant therapy in patients with nonrheumatic atrial fibrillation and recent cerebral ischemia. N Engl J Med 1995; 333:5–10.
31. Hylek EM, Skates SJ, Sheehan MA, Singer DE. An analysis of the lowest effective intensity of prophylactic anticoagulation for patients with nonrheumatic atrial fibrillation. N Engl J Med 1996; 335:540–546.
32. Laupacis A, Albers G, Dalen J, et al. Antithrombotic therapy in atrial fibrillation. Chest 1995; 108(suppl):352S–359S.
33. Gage BF, Cardinalli AB, Albers GW, Owens DK. Cost-effectiveness of warfarin and aspirin for prophylaxis of stroke in patients with nonvalvular atrial fibrillation. JAMA 1995; 274:1839–1845.
34. Gustafsson C, Asplund K, Britton M, et al. Cost effectiveness of primary stroke prevention in atrial fibrillation: Swedish national perspective. BMJ 1992; 305:1457–1460.
35. Stafford RS, Singer DE. National patterns of warfarin use in atrial fibrillation. Arch Intern Med 1996; 156:2537–2541.
36. Gottlieb LK, Salem-Schatz S. Anticoagulation in atrial fibrillation: Does efficacy in clinical trials translate into effectiveness in practice? Arch Intern Med 1994; 154:1945–1953.

37. Singer DE. Anticoagulation for atrial fibrillation: Epidemiology informing a difficult clinical decision. Proc Assoc Am Physicians 1996; 108:29–36.
38. Rosendaal FR. The Scylla and Charybdis of oral anticoagulant treatment [Editorial]. N Engl J Med 1996; 335:587–588.
39. Fihn SD, McDonell MB, Vermes D, et al. A computerized intervention to improve timing of outpatient follow-up: A multicenter randomized trial in patients treated with warfarin. National Consortium of Anticoagulation Clinics. J Gen Intern Med 1994; 9:131–139.
40. Ansell JE, Patel N, Ostrovsky D, et al. Long-term patient self-management of oral anticoagulation. Arch Intern Med 1995; 155:2185–2189.
41. Arnsten JH, Gelfand JM, Singer DE. Determinants of compliance with anticoagulation: A case-control study. Am J Med 1997; 103:11–17.
42. Bauer KA, Rosenberg RD. The pathophysiology of the prethrombotic state in humans. Blood 1987; 70:343.
43. Manning WJ, Silverman DI, Waksmonski CA, et al. Prevalence of residual left atrial thrombi among patients with acute thromboembolism and newly recognized atrial fibrillation. Arch Intern Med 1995; 155:2193–2197.
44. Black IW, Fatkin D, Sagar KB, et al. Exclusion of atrial thrombus by transesophageal echocardiography does not preclude embolism after cardioversion of atrial fibrillation: A multicenter study. Circulation 1994; 89:2509–2513.
45. Cataldo G. Warfarin versus indobufen for secondary prevention of thromboembolism in nonvalvular atrial fibrillation. The SIFA (Studio Italliano Fibrillazione Atriale) Trial [Abstract]. Circulation 1995; 92(Suppl I):485.
46. The National Heart, Lung, and Blood Institute Working Group on Atrial Fibrillation. Atrial fibrillation: Current understandings and research imperatives. J Am Coll Cardiol 1993; 22:1830–1834.
47. Breslow NE, Day NE. Statistical methods in cancer research. *In* The Analysis of Case-Control Studies, vol 1. Lyon, International Agency for Research on Cancer, 1980, p 134.
48. Stroke Prevention in Atrial Fibrillation Study Group Investigators. Preliminary report of the Stroke Prevention in Atrial Fibrillation study. N Engl J Med 1990; 322:863–868.

22 Angioplasty and Bypass Surgery

▶ Malcolm R. Bell
▶ Bernard J. Gersh

Although percutaneous transluminal coronary angioplasty (PTCA) was first introduced into clinical cardiology practice as long ago as 1977,[1] the first randomized comparison with other conventional therapy for chronic angina was not reported until 1992.[2] Prior to this time, considerable amounts of observational (primarily retrospective) data had been reported pertaining to the indications, efficacy, and safety of PTCA in patients with various coronary artery syndromes. The well-known large trials comparing coronary artery bypass graft (CABG) surgery to medical therapy had all been completed more than a decade earlier, and during this period, pleas were repeatedly made by cardiologists and cardiac surgeons alike to compare this new, but relatively established, percutaneous revascularization technique to CABG surgery, particularly among patients with chronic angina and multivessel disease. PTCA appeared to already have an established role in the treatment of single-vessel disease, although concerns existed, and were often passionately debated, that PTCA should not be offered as therapy for proximal left anterior descending (LAD) coronary artery disease. These pleas for objective, randomized trials were finally heeded, and in the late 1980s and early 1990s such trials were planned and executed in Europe and North and South America. The first publication of these trials appeared in 1993, and as of 1996 all the major trials commenced during that period have had their results published. The purpose of this chapter is to briefly summarize the most important findings of each of these recently published trials. A summary of the study populations and treatment strategies of all the trials discussed in this chapter is provided in Table 22–1.

Although all these trials compared PTCA with CABG or medical therapy, one should keep in mind that at the time these trials were performed, the understanding of the mechanisms for coronary restenosis after successful PTCA was only just evolving, and no effective prevention or therapy existed. Since then, the use of intracoronary stents has supplemented and in many centers taken over the role of PTCA as a percutaneous revascularization technique. Evidence that intracoronary stents reduce the chance of restenosis is appealing in the setting of single-vessel disease with relatively discrete lesions,[3, 4] but their efficacy in patients with multivessel disease is unknown at this stage.

Surgical revascularization techniques have also evolved since the first large trials conducted against medical therapy, particularly with the greater use of the internal thoracic artery as a bypass conduit and refinements and improvements in techniques of intraoperative myocardial protection. More recently, a less invasive surgical technique of revascularization without the need for cardiopulmonary bypass has been introduced for the treatment of single-vessel disease. Finally, effective secondary prevention treatment of patients with established coronary artery disease with lipid-lowering therapy[5] is now pursued more aggressively compared with the era in which these trials were conducted regardless of whether patients have undergone myocardial revascularization procedures. It would appear likely that aggressive lipid-lowering therapy will radically alter the natural history of medically treated disease, but a favorable effect on the long-term outcomes of both percutaneous and surgical revascularization techniques is also to be expected.

PTCA VERSUS MEDICAL THERAPY

There have been two trials comparing PTCA and medical therapy reported. The first was the Angioplasty Compared to Medicine (ACME) study,[2] and the second, with a surgical arm, was a trial examining outcomes of patients with isolated proximal LAD coronary artery disease[6] (discussed later).

ACME

The ACME study, the first randomized study comparing PTCA with conventional therapy ever to be pub-

TABLE 22–1 • Summary of Treatment Strategies and Baseline Demographic, Clinical, and Angiographic Data for Each Randomized Trial

	ACME	Lausanne	MASS	RITA	ERACI	GABI	EAST	CABRI	BARI
Patient total	212	134	214	1011	127	359	392	1054	1829
PTCA vs. CABG	No	Yes	Yes	Yes	Yes	Yes	Yes	Yes	Yes
Medical arm	Yes	No	Yes	No	No	No	No	No	No
Equivalent revascularization planned at enrollment	—	Yes	Yes	Yes	No	Yes	No	No	No
Male (%)	100	80	82	81	85	80	74	78	74
Unstable angina (%)	None	None	None	59	83	14	NP*	14	64
Single-vessel disease (%)	100	100	100	45	None	None	None	1	2
Multivessel disease (%)	None	None	None	55	100	100	100	99	98
Two (%)				43	55	82	60	57	41
Three (%)				12	44	18	40	42	57
LVEF exclusion (%)	<30	<50	<50	None	<35†	None	<25	≤35	None

* 79% of patients were classified with class III or IV angina but not whether their symptoms represented unstable angina.
† With associated three-vessel disease.
PTCA, percutaneous transluminal coronary angioplasty; CABG, coronary artery bypass graft; LVEF, left ventricular ejection fraction; NP, not provided.

lished, was reported in 1992.[2] Patients were enrolled in this study if they had a significant stenosis (70% to 90% diameter reduction) of one major coronary artery and evidence of exercise-induced myocardial ischemia and then randomized to either PTCA or medical therapy (nitrates, beta blockers, and/or calcium channel blockers). Patients were highly selected and represented only about 2% of those screened. The PTCA success rate was relatively low by contemporary standards (80%), but no deaths occurred. During follow-up, 21 of the 105 PTCA patients required additional revascularization procedures (PTCA or CABG surgery). Eleven of the 107 patients assigned to the medical arm also underwent PTCA.

The primary endpoints of this trial included a change in exercise duration at 6 months compared with baseline and frequency of anginal attacks. Exercise duration at 6 months improved by 2.1 ± 3.1 minutes in the PTCA group, significantly more than the 0.5 ± 2.2 minutes in the medical group. Time to onset of angina was also delayed in the PTCA group relative to the medical group. Among the PTCA-treated patients, 64% were angina free at 6 months compared with 46% of the medically treated patients. Approximately 91% of the PTCA patients were using some antianginal medication at 6 months, although all such medical therapy was discontinued prior to the performance of the exercise test.

Thus, the ACME trial suggests that highly selected patients with angina and single-vessel coronary disease can obtain a better functional result with PTCA compared with medical therapy. Indeed, this was also associated with greater physical and psychological improvements among PTCA-treated patients.[7] The study was not powered to examine differences in mortality or infarction rates. The most important question regarding these findings was whether or not the additional cost of performing PTCA can be justified in such patients who primarily have mild angina. However, in this trial PTCA was clearly superior therapy and could easily be justified in patients who are refractory to medical treatment. Thus, a reasonable treatment approach in patients with mild angina would be to offer medical therapy initially and later proceed with PTCA in the 50% or so who remain symptomatic.

It is not clear from the available evidence that PTCA should be the primary treatment of choice for mild, symptomatic single-vessel disease. It is of some concern that patients undergoing PTCA with single-vessel disease are likely to have such a procedure without a preceding exercise test,[8] thus supporting the notion that many physicians believe that PTCA should be universally considered in such patients. Higher PTCA success rates than seen in ACME should be anticipated in most large institutions today.

PTCA VERSUS CABG SURGERY

Single-Vessel Disease

With the exception of three trials, all the randomized revascularization trials have involved patients requiring treatment for multivessel disease. The Randomized Treatment of Angina (RITA) Trial[9] enrolled patients with single-vessel and multivessel disease, while two other trials compared the outcomes of patients treated for isolated LAD coronary disease.[6, 10]

RITA

Patients were enrolled in the British multicenter trial known as RITA if they had documented coronary artery disease and required myocardial revascularization, regardless of whether they had stable or unstable angina, although patients were not randomized if they required urgent revascularization.[9, 11] A total of

1011 patients were randomized to either PTCA or CABG surgery, 456 (45%) of whom had single-vessel disease; the remainder had multivessel disease and are discussed later in the chapter. Fifty-nine percent of patients had either class III or IV angina and 59% had symptoms of angina at rest. The assigned treatment was not performed in 95 of the 1011 patients until more than 3 months after randomization because of excessive waiting lists. PTCA was successful in 90% of patients, and 99% of patients undergoing CABG surgery had the selected vessel bypassed. Overall utilization of the internal thoracic artery was 76% for all patients undergoing surgery. Median length of hospital stay was 12 days for surgical patients and 4 days for PTCA patients.

The predefined primary endpoint of this trial was death or acute myocardial infarction, and this did not appear to depend on the number of vessels diseased at randomization. After 30 months, 40 patients had reached this endpoint with no statistical difference between the two groups (16 CABG and 24 PTCA). Further details on outcome of patients with single-vessel disease, including the need for subsequent revascularization procedures and symptomatic status, have not yet been differentiated from those patients with multivessel disease but are expected to be made available when the 5-year follow-up data are reported.

LAUSANNE TRIAL OF PROXIMAL LAD DISEASE

The outcomes of 134 patients with isolated proximal LAD disease randomized to PTCA or CABG surgery were reported from the Centre Hospitaller Universitaire Vaudois in Lausanne, Switzerland, in 1994.[10] Patients with isolated proximal (including ostial) LAD lesions with angina and documented ischemia and left ventricular ejection fractions greater than 50% were eligible for this study. Patients with unstable angina or a history of anterior Q wave myocardial infarction were excluded. Sixty-eight patients were randomized to PTCA; of the 66 patients assigned to CABG surgery, exclusively using the left internal thoracic artery as the bypass conduit, 6 actually underwent PTCA, and 1 patient received medical therapy. Patients randomized to CABG surgery all were operated on within 30 days of randomization, while PTCA patients had their procedure performed within 10 days.

There was one perioperative infarction in the CABG group. Two of the 68 PTCA patients required emergency CABG with associated non–Q wave infarctions. Two other patients had intracoronary stents placed urgently for threatened closure. There was no mortality in either group. Thus, for this initial predefined endpoint, no significant difference between the two interventions was observed.

Follow-up was reported after a median of 24 months (maximum 36 months) and focused on the remaining primary endpoint of need for repeat revascularization procedures, which occurred more frequently among the patients who had PTCA performed (17 of 68 patients) compared with patients who had undergone surgical revascularization (2 of 66 patients). There was one late cardiac-related death in the CABG group. The composite endpoint (cardiac death, myocardial infarction, or repeat revascularization) was more frequent in the PTCA group (relative risk [RR], 8.3; 95% confidence interval [CI], 4.7 to 12.0). Among secondary endpoints examined, the functional status was similar in the two groups after 1 year, although there was a slight trend toward more patients in the surgical group being asymptomatic.

Therefore, one can conclude from this study that for patients with isolated proximal LAD disease and normal left ventricular function, both PTCA and CABG were equally safe and effective in reducing patients' symptoms from angina, but at the cost of more frequent reintervention among the nonsurgically treated patients. This latter difference is almost certainly related to the expected incidence of restenosis (no patient had stents placed electively). Other differences might emerge over the next 10 years or so when graft attrition becomes more prevalent and when progression in native vessel disease develops.

MASS

The Medicine, Angioplasty, or Surgery Study (MASS) was a Brazilian trial from Sao Paulo University that enrolled 214 patients with isolated proximal LAD disease and was similar in design to the Lausanne trial except that a third randomization arm—medical therapy—was included.[6] Patients were excluded if they had unstable angina or had left ventricular dysfunction or previous infarction. A unique feature of this trial was that all 70 surgical procedures (exclusively using the internal thoracic artery) and all 72 PTCA procedures were performed by single operators, each with a vast experience in their respective fields. Additionally, the medical treatment assigned to 72 patients was supervised by a single experienced cardiologist. Success rates were high in both revascularization groups: one nonfatal perioperative myocardial infarction after CABG surgery and 96% success rate with PTCA (3 patients required emergency surgery).

The predefined endpoint of the study was the combination of cardiac death, myocardial infarction, or refractory angina requiring revascularization. Repeat PTCA in the PTCA group was not considered an endpoint. After an average of 3 years, these endpoints were reached in only 3% of surgically treated patients, significantly less than the 24% incidence among PTCA-treated patients. Seventeen percent of the medically treated patients reached these endpoints, significantly more than the surgically treated patients but also significantly less than the PTCA-treated patients. These differences were primarily related to the need for subsequent revascularization procedures because there were no significant differences in incidence of either death or infarction. Symptomatic relief and reduction in exercise-induced ischemia were achieved significantly more often in the revascularization groups compared with medically treated patients. Asymptomatic status was achieved in 98% of the surgical patients and in 82% of the PTCA patients but in only 32% of the medically treated patients.

All surviving patients agreed to have angiography performed after 2 years. Patency of the internal thoracic artery was documented in all but 1 patient. Among the surgical patients, the native LAD vessel had become occluded in 74%. This finding had occurred in 8% of the PTCA patients and 11% of the medical patients. Progression of other native vessel disease had occurred in 35% of the entire group without significant differences based on treatment received.

Similar conclusions to those from the Lausanne trial[10] can be drawn from the MASS Trial: differences in outcome in these selected patients from two relatively small trials are primarily related to the need for subsequent interventions among the PTCA-treated patients without any obvious increase in mortality or infarction. Both revascularization strategies are extremely effective in improving or abolishing angina and appear to be superior in this respect than medical therapy.

Multivessel Disease

Patients with multivessel disease represent a heterogeneous group of patients because of differences in anatomic location of coronary lesions, differences in left ventricular function, accessibility of target vessels to bypass conduits or PTCA, and extent of myocardial ischemia. In addition, differences in definitions of multivessel disease and completeness of revascularization also can potentially confuse comparisons of different studies. Two crucial issues need to be emphasized to the discerning reviewer of comparisons of outcome of treated patients with multivessel disease: distinguishing the proportions of patients with two- versus three-vessel disease and whether left ventricular function is impaired or not; the latter is particularly relevant to the outcome of patients with three-vessel disease. Finally, many patients with multivessel disease have at least one chronic (total) occlusion that may prevent any attempt at angioplasty or significantly reduce the success rate of this procedure. To date, six randomized trials have been reported comparing the use of CABG surgery with PTCA in patients with multivessel disease.

RITA

A summary of the design of the British multicenter RITA trial has been provided earlier during the discussion of single-vessel disease treatments. In addition to those with single-vessel disease, 43% (431 patients) had two-vessel disease and 12% (124 patients) had three-vessel disease. There was no absolute requirement that all diseased vessels would be revascularized, although revascularization had to be equivalent by both techniques.[11] The presence of chronic occlusions was not a reason for exclusion. Patients with significant left main coronary artery disease were excluded, but no exclusions based on left ventricular dysfunction were made. Among surgically treated patients, 97% of two-vessel disease patients and 87% of three-vessel disease patients had all selected vessels bypassed.[9] This compared with 81% and 63%, respectively, in the PTCA-treated patients. Thus, initial revascularization rates appeared to be higher in the surgical group. Success rates with angioplasty for two- and three-vessel disease patients were 84% and 77%, respectively, and 4.5% required emergency CABG surgery.

During a median of 2.5 years of follow-up, there were no significant differences in mortality or myocardial infarctions between the two revascularization strategies, regardless of the number of vessels diseased, although 5-year follow-up observations are still pending. When subsequent revascularization procedures were added to these analyses, approximately 38% of PTCA patients had experienced one of these primary events or had CABG surgery or repeat PTCA performed compared with 11% of the surgical patients. These event-free outcomes did not appear to be related to the number of diseased vessels at randomization. Regardless of time points chosen, there were greater improvements in symptoms of angina (associated with less use of antianginal medications) in the surgical compared with PTCA-treated patients (Fig. 22–1). However, 6 months or longer after randomization, no significant differences in exercise duration improvement could be discerned between the two treatment groups.

No difference among eligible patients in employment status was found,[9, 12] while quality of life measures, closely associated with persistent angina, were found to be similar between the two treatment groups after 3 years of follow-up.[12] Health service cost estimates based on data from two of the RITA sites have recently been published.[13] The initial average costs of

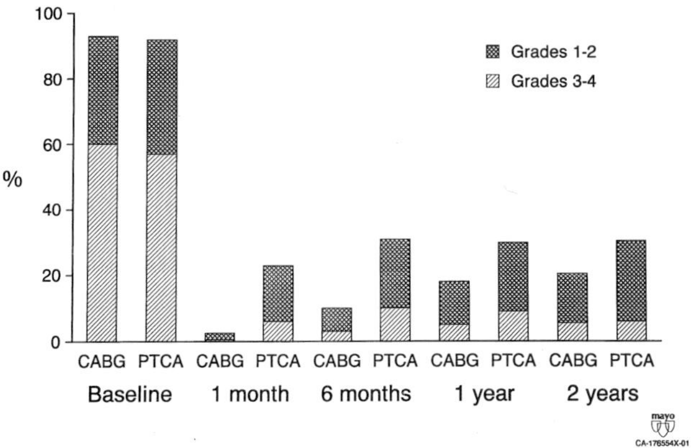

Figure 22–1 Prevalence of angina over time in the two treatment groups of the Randomized Treatment of Angina (RITA) trial, according to the Canadian Cardiovascular Society classification of angina. CABG, coronary artery bypass graft; PTCA, percutaneous transluminal coronary angioplasty. (From RITA Trial Participants. Coronary angioplasty versus coronary artery bypass surgery: The Randomized Intervention Treatment of Angina [RITA] Trial. Lancet 1993; 341:573–580. © by The Lancet Ltd. 1993.)

treating randomized patients with CABG were approximately twice those of PTCA procedures, but this difference diminished over 2 years of follow-up as more patients assigned to PTCA required additional revascularization procedures. However, after 2 years the total incremental costs were 20% higher in the CABG group, which suggests a significant cost saving in the PTCA group. Whether such a saving is cost effective or not remains to be determined, and it is unclear whether similar savings could be anticipated in other countries with differing costs and reimbursement systems.

In summary, although CABG surgery and PTCA were associated with similar initial outcomes as well as long-term risks of death or myocardial infarction, relief of angina was inferior with PTCA, and this treatment strategy was also associated with a greater need for subsequent revascularization procedures.

ERACI

The Argentine Randomized Trial of Percutaneous Transluminal Coronary Angioplasty Versus Coronary Artery Bypass Surgery in Multivessel Disease (ERACI) Trial was performed at a single hospital in Buenos Aires.[14] The trial was relatively small in comparison with the other trials of patients with multivessel disease—a total of 127 of 302 eligible patients were randomized. Patients with either stable (17%) or unstable (83%) angina were enrolled as long as multivessel disease amenable to either PTCA or surgical revascularization was present. Important exclusion criteria included those patients with dilated ischemic cardiomyopathy, left main coronary artery disease, three-vessel disease with left ventricular ejection fractions of 35% or less, or evolving myocardial infarction. Most patients in this trial had normal left ventricular ejection fractions. Approximately 55% of patients had two-vessel disease, and 45% had three-vessel disease.

Chronic occlusions were attempted by PTCA only if the target vessel supplied viable myocardium—if nonviable myocardium was present, untreated chronic occlusions were considered to represent functionally complete revascularization. Forty-four chronic occlusions were left untreated according to these guidelines. Complete revascularization (no residual stenoses >50% in severity) was achieved in 88% of the surgically treated patients compared with 51% of the PTCA-treated patients; 89% of the latter group were considered to have functionally complete revascularization.

The internal thoracic artery was used as a conduit in approximately 77% of patients who had surgery performed. Inhospital mortality was 4.6% in patients who had surgery performed compared with 1.5% who had PTCA performed. Q wave myocardial infarctions occurred in approximately 6% in each group. Stroke incidence was 3.1% and 1.5% in the surgical and PTCA patients, respectively. The overall success rate of PTCA was 92%. Success rates were 100% for type A lesions versus 64% for type C lesions, the latter of which comprised only 13% of treated lesions.

Follow-up has been reported initially at 1 year[14] and subsequently at 3 years.[15] After 1 year, there were no significant differences in survival or freedom from infarction between the two groups; however, patients treated with PTCA had a greater incidence of angina or repeat revascularization procedures than did surgically treated patients. These differences persisted at 3 years: 77% of the surgical group were alive and free of myocardial infarction, angina, and repeat revascularization compared with 47% of the PTCA-treated patients. This difference was entirely explicable on the basis of increased need for repeat revascularization procedures and more angina in the latter patients.

Thus, these findings, although from only a small group of patients, are consistent with those of the RITA Trial.

GABI

The German Angioplasty Bypass Surgery Investigation (GABI) Trial investigators at multiple sites screened almost 9000 patients and were successful in enrolling 359 patients (177 for CABG surgery and 182 for PTCA).[16] Revascularization of at least two major epicardial vessels had to be deemed feasible to ensure eligibility for the trial. Among the exclusion criteria were the presence of any chronic occlusion or a left main coronary artery stenosis of more than 30%. Also excluded were patients who had sustained a myocardial infarction within the 28 days prior to randomization. Most patients (approximately 80%) had two-vessel disease, while only 20% had three-vessel disease and only about 15% had unstable angina prior to enrollment. As witnessed in the RITA trial, there were fairly long treatment delays after randomization (median of 53 days for CABG patients and 19 for the PTCA patients). During these periods, 5 patients died and 17 refused to participate further, resulting in a total of 337 patients eventually receiving their assigned treatment.

PTCA was clinically successful in 88% of patients (1.9 ± 0.5 vessels dilated per patient), while mortality was 1.1%. An average of 2.2 vessels were bypassed in the surgical patients, but, surprisingly, only 37% received an internal thoracic artery conduit. Inhospital mortality was 2.5%, and strokes occurred in 1.2% of patients. Perioperative Q wave myocardial infarctions occurred in 8.1% of the surgical group versus 2.3% of the PTCA group. Pneumonia occurred in approximately 10% of surgical patients—a rate almost ten times higher than in the PTCA group. Median hospital stays were surprisingly long: 19 days for the surgical patients and 5 days for the PTCA patients.

After 1 year of follow-up, the risk of death or nonfatal myocardial infarction was significantly greater in the surgical group than in the PTCA group (13.6% vs. 6.0%, respectively). The primary endpoint of the GABI Trial was, however, freedom from angina (lower than class II), and this was reached by 74% of the CABG patients and 71% of the PTCA patients, although more PTCA patients were using antianginal medications. No difference in improvement in exercise workload between the two groups could be found. Finally, only 6% of the CABG group compared with 44% of the PTCA group had undergone subsequent revascularization procedures at 1 year. In a subset comprising almost two thirds of the study group, 6-month angiographic findings were reported. Among the CABG patients, 13% of all saphenous vein grafts and 7% of the internal thoracic artery grafts were occluded, while among PTCA patients, 16% of dilated vessels had either occluded or were severely narrowed.

In contrast with the other trials, the GABI trial showed significantly worse intermediate (1-year) outcome in CABG patients with respect to mortality or myocardial infarction. This difference is possibly explained by the higher inhospital complication rates observed among surgical patients and the less frequent use of the internal thoracic artery as a bypass conduit. In addition, in contrast with other studies, but probably with similar explanations, the improvement in angina status was identical in the surgical and PTCA groups. The complete exclusion of patients with chronic occlusions, probably accounting for fewer treatment failures in the PTCA group, may also explain the lack of difference in this endpoint.

EAST

The Emory Angioplasty Surgery Trial (EAST) was the first North American randomized trial of treatment in patients with multivessel disease and was conducted at Emory University Hospital in Atlanta and sponsored by the National Heart, Lung, and Blood Institute. More than 5000 patients were screened for the study, with a successful enrollment of 392.[17, 18] Patients were randomized to PTCA or CABG surgery, but equivalent revascularization was not required for eligibility. Patients with two-vessel disease constituted 60% of the study population, while the remainder had three-vessel disease. Among the exclusion criteria were chronic occlusions (>8 weeks), left main disease (≥ 30%), two or more chronic occlusions, or left ventricular ejection fraction of 25% or less. Eight percent of patients had class III or IV angina at baseline. Proximal LAD disease was present in 72% of patients, and the mean left ventricular ejection fraction was 61%.

PTCA was clinically successful in 88% of patients, while mortality was 1%; complicating Q wave infarction occurred in 3%; and CABG surgery was performed in 10.1% of patients. Among the complications experienced by surgical patients were (1) death, 1%; (2) Q wave infarction, 10.3%; and (3) stroke, 1.5%. Revascularization was considered functionally complete in 98% of surgically treated patients compared with 61% of those who underwent PTCA.

The primary endpoint of this trial was a composite of death, Q wave myocardial infarction, and large thallium defect with nuclear stress testing at 3 years. This endpoint was reached in 27.3% of the surgically treated patients compared with 28.8% of the PTCA-treated patients. Survival was virtually identical in the two groups. The major difference between the two groups after 3 years of follow-up was in the utilization of subsequent revascularization procedures: 13% of the surgical group compared with 54% of the PTCA group had undergone either CABG surgery or PTCA following their initial procedure. With respect to the surgical group, only 1% required repeat surgery, while the remainder had PTCA performed. Twenty-two percent of the PTCA group eventually had surgery performed. Persistent angina was more common in patients in the PTCA group at 3 years compared with the patients in the surgical group, as was the use of antianginal medications. Despite these differences, activity and employment levels were similar in the two groups.

Again, these findings largely confirm those of the other trials, showing that we can be reassured that survival and freedom from infarction are not influenced by choice of revascularization strategy but that with respect to symptom relief and avoidance of subsequent operations, CABG surgery is superior to

PTCA. The lack of difference in primary endpoints in this trial may be related to the overall lack of significant difference between the two procedures in achieving functionally complete revascularization.[19] A detailed cost analysis of the two procedures has revealed that although PTCA procedural costs were less expensive than those of CABG, this difference almost disappeared over the next 3 years as more PTCA patients require additional hospitalizations and procedures.[20]

CABRI

The European multinational, multicenter, randomized Coronary Angioplasty versus Bypass Revascularization Investigation (CABRI) was performed in 1054 patients after screening 23,047 patients with symptomatic multivessel coronary disease.[21] Patients were randomized to PTCA (541 patients) or CABG surgery (513 patients). Patients with overt cardiac failure, acute myocardial infarction within 10 days of randomization, or left ventricular ejection fractions of 35% or less were excluded. The upper-eligible age limit for randomization was 75 years. Patients were considered eligible if their anatomy was considered suitable for either procedure; chronic occlusions were accepted for treatment, and equivalent revascularization was not required. Most patients had class II or III angina, while only 14% had unstable symptoms. Mean left ventricular ejection fraction was 63%. Two-vessel disease was present in 57% of patients and three-vessel disease was present in 42%.

CABG surgery was performed at a median of 32 days, and PTCA was performed at a median of 19 days after randomization. Three percent of the surgically assigned patients and 1% of the PTCA-assigned patients never received their assigned treatment. Although technical success was high (94%) for PTCA procedures, the immediate clinical success rate (freedom from infarction, death, or emergency surgery) was not published. Unlike the other trials discussed earlier, in addition to conventional balloon angioplasty, the use of newer devices such as atherectomy devices and intracoronary stents was permitted in the PTCA arm, although no details have been provided regarding the number of patients so treated. Inhospital mortality was 1.9% in the surgical group and 1.3% in the PTCA group.

The primary endpoints of the trial are to be studied after 5 years of follow-up, but an initial analysis after 12 months of follow-up has been published.[21] No difference in survival was noted between the two groups after 1 year. Significant angina was present more often among PTCA-treated patients (RR, 1.54; 95% CI, 1.09 to 2.16), although this finding was only significant among women. No significant difference in the occurrence of nonfatal myocardial infarctions was noted. The use of repeat revascularization procedures, a secondary endpoint of the trial, was approximately five times more common for patients assigned PTCA than for those assigned surgery (RR, 5.23; 95% CI, 3.90 to 7.03) within the first year.

In summary, the interim analysis of the CABRI Trial suggests that survival and freedom from myocardial infarction were not associated with choice of revascularization procedure, although angina and the need for subsequent procedures were more common in the PTCA group. Further analyses over longer duration are awaited, and the relative influences of restenosis of dilated vessels and completeness of revascularization on symptomatic outcome may provide some insights into long-term functional status of patients in this trial.

BARI

The Bypass Angioplasty Revascularization Investigation (BARI) was initiated by the National Heart, Lung, and Blood Institute and recruited patients from 1988 to 1991.[22, 23] Sixteen centers in the United States and two in Canada randomized 1829 patients with multivessel disease to either PTCA (915 patients) or CABG surgery (914 patients). Thus, this is the largest of all the randomized trials reported to date that are concerned with revascularization strategies in this population of patients. A total of 25,200 patients with multivessel disease was screened; in addition to the randomized patients, a detailed registry of 2013 eligible but not randomized patients was also collected, and data from this registry should add considerable information regarding the outcome of patients selected for either PTCA or CABG. Similar registries were also maintained in the RITA and EAST Trials.

Patients were ineligible if they required emergency revascularization or had left main stenosis of 50% or greater. Patients older than 80 years of age were also excluded. PTCA or CABG had to be deemed feasible by both an interventional cardiologist and surgeon, respectively. Unstable angina was present in 64% of patients.[24] Mean left ventricular ejection fraction was 57% and was less than 50% in 21% of CABG-treated patients and 23% of PTCA-treated patients. Two-vessel disease was present in 58% of patients, three-vessel disease in 41%, and single-vessel disease in 1% (core laboratory determination). The proximal LAD coronary artery was narrowed 50% or greater in approximately one third of both CABG and PTCA patients. Assigned treatment was recommended, by protocol, to be performed within 2 weeks of randomization. This was accomplished in 91% of patients, while 99.6% had received their treatment by 8 weeks. A mean of 3.1 coronary arteries was bypassed using a mean of 2.8 grafts. The internal thoracic artery was used as a bypass conduit in 82% of patients (including 12% of patients who had both internal thoracic arteries used), although wide interinstitutional variability was evident.[25] The median hospital stay was 7 days.

PTCA was performed in multiple vessels in 70% of patients.[24] Successful dilation of at least one vessel was accomplished in 88% of patients, while in 57%, all lesions were successfully dilated. Chronic occlusions were present in 33% of patients with two-vessel disease (attempted in 46%) and present in 46% of patients with three-vessel disease (attempted in 29%).[23] Median hospital stay was 3 days.

Inhospital mortality was low (1.3% in CABG patients and 1.1% in PTCA patients). Q wave myocardial infarction was a complication in 4.6% of surgical patients and in 2.1% of PTCA patients ($P < 0.01$). Emergency CABG surgery was required in 6.3% of PTCA patients. Strokes occurred in 0.8% of surgical patients and 0.2% of PTCA patients. There was no significant difference in cumulative 5-year mortality (the primary endpoint of the study) between the two treatment groups: 89.3% versus 86.3% for patients assigned to surgery and PTCA, respectively (Fig. 22–2). Neither was there any significant difference in the incidence of Q wave myocardial infarction. Of patients assigned to CABG surgery, 8% required a subsequent revascularization procedure, predominantly PTCA, while 54% of PTCA-assigned patients required at least one additional procedure with PTCA and CABG used in equal proportions (Fig. 22–3). Most subsequent procedures in this group were performed

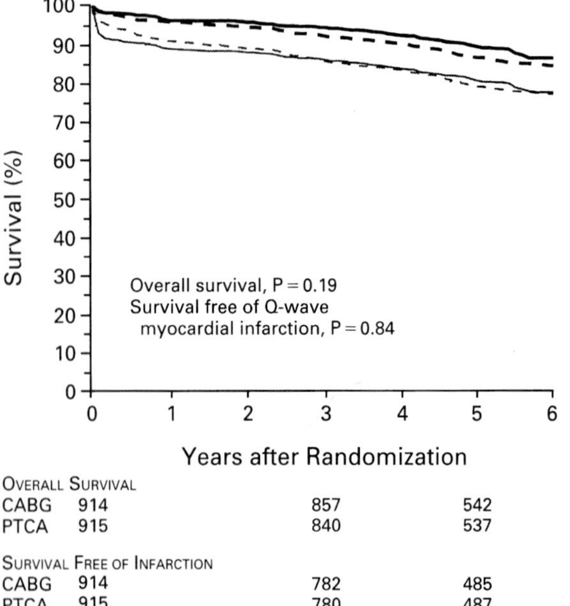

Figure 22–2 Overall survival (heavy lines) and survival free from Q wave myocardial infarction (light lines) of patients after entry into the BARI Trial. Patients who had coronary artery bypass graft (CABG) surgery are assigned the solid lines, and patients who had percutaneous transluminal coronary angioplasty (PTCA) are assigned the dashed lines. (From the BARI Trial Participants. Comparison of coronary bypass surgery with angioplasty in patients with multivessel disease. N Engl J Med 1996; 335:217–225. Copyright © 1996, Massachusetts Medical Society. All rights reserved.)

within the first 12 months of the assigned treatment, suggesting that these were used to primarily treat restenosis. Multiple revascularization procedures were performed in 19% of PTCA patients versus 3% of surgical patients and were associated with more frequent hospitalizations.

Subgroup analyses of 5-year mortality revealed no differences between the two groups with respect to the influence of the severity of angina at baseline (stable vs. unstable vs. severe ischemia), left ventricular dysfunction, two- or three-vessel disease, or lesion type. A surprising finding, but also evident in the CABRI study,[26] was that patients with treated diabetes mellitus who underwent PTCA had a mortality incidence of 15.1% greater (95% CI, 1.4 to 28.9) than those who had CABG performed. Definitive explanations for this observation have not been forthcoming, but it is not explained by higher complication rates during the initial hospitalization. Further analyses and research are required for this important group of patients focusing on whether their worse outcome with PTCA is the result of higher prevalence of three-vessel disease, especially diffuse disease, in diabetics and their worse left ventricular function or of other undefined vascular or other biologic effects of diabetes.

Therefore, the results of the BARI Trial, the largest of all the studies performed to date, indicate no survival advantages to either CABG or PTCA when compared with each other for patients with multivessel disease. Subsequent need for reintervention or surgery, as in the other trials, was common within the first year after PTCA, although this need diminished thereafter. Functional data with respect to alleviation of symptoms have yet to be released by the BARI investigators. Finally, a post hoc analysis of survival among treated diabetic patients revealed a small but significant advantage to CABG-treated patients compared with PTCA-treated patients.

CONCLUSIONS

Before drawing conclusions and making any recommendations from the trials discussed earlier, we must emphasize a few points. The patients enrolled in these studies represented only a small proportion of patients who underwent revascularization at the recruiting sites. Approximately two thirds of clinically eligible patients were excluded because of angiographic criteria and were thus never randomized. Patients who were randomized did have a preponderance of two-vessel rather than three-vessel disease, and patients generally had preserved left ventricular function. Thus, extrapolating the results from these trials to patients with severe three-vessel disease and left ventricular dysfunction must be done cautiously. Pa-

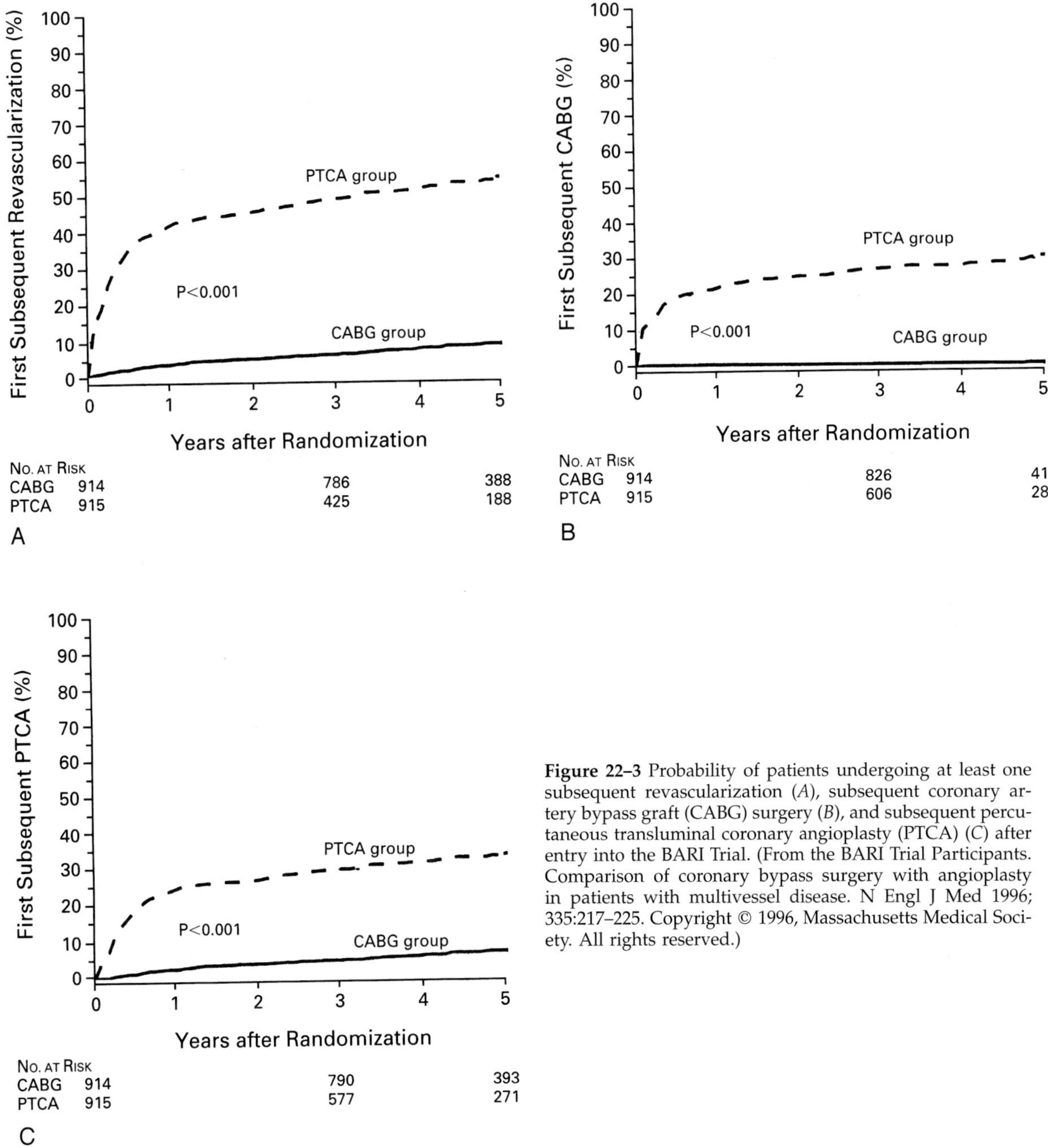

Figure 22–3 Probability of patients undergoing at least one subsequent revascularization (*A*), subsequent coronary artery bypass graft (CABG) surgery (*B*), and subsequent percutaneous transluminal coronary angioplasty (PTCA) (*C*) after entry into the BARI Trial. (From the BARI Trial Participants. Comparison of coronary bypass surgery with angioplasty in patients with multivessel disease. N Engl J Med 1996; 335:217–225. Copyright © 1996, Massachusetts Medical Society. All rights reserved.)

tients with multivessel disease and significant left ventricular function were not well represented in these trials; of the six multivessel trials, only three had no left ventricular dysfunction exclusionary criteria (see Table 22–1). In the largest of these, the BARI randomized population included only 22% with left ventricular ejection fractions less than 50%.[23] Thus, it would be wise not to generalize the overall finding of equivalency in survival following PTCA and CABG to patients with significant left ventricular dysfunction (ejection fractions <35%).

Nevertheless, there has been an overall consistency in the reported results of both the small and large randomized trials of patients with symptomatic coronary artery disease who are considered candidates for revascularization procedures. PTCA appeared to be associated with similarly low major inhospital complication rates to CABG surgery (Table 22–2). It appears that for single-vessel and multivessel disease, both PTCA and CABG are effective in alleviating symptoms of angina, although patients who have had PTCA as their initial procedure will more likely require additional revascularization procedures to achieve this. There is no evidence that one strategy is safer or associated with better survival than the other. A summary of the major outcome measures of the revascularization trials is provided in Table 22–3. The relatively high complication rates observed in the

TABLE 22–2 • Summary of PTCA Success, Utilization of the ITA During CABG, and Inhospital Outcomes for Randomized Patients from Each Trial

	ACME	Lausanne	MASS	RITA	ERACI	GABI	EAST	CABRI	BARI
PTCA clinical success (%)	80	97	96	87	92	88	88	NP	88
CABG—use of ITA (%)	NA	100	100	74	77	37	90	81	82
Inhospital mortality									
PTCA (%)	0	0		1	1.5	1.1	1	1.3	1.1
CABG (%)	—	0		1	4.6	2.5	1	1.9	1.3
Inhospital Q wave MI									
PTCA (%)	1	0		3.5*	6	2.3	3	NP	2.1
CABG (%)	—	1.5		2.4*	6	8.1	10.3	NP	4.6

* No distinction made between Q wave and non–Q wave MI.
PTCA, percutaneous transluminal coronary angioplasty; CABG, coronary artery bypass graft; ITA, internal thoracic artery; MI, myocardial infarction; NP, not provided; NA, not applicable.

GABI trial among the surgically treated patients[16] suggest the need for concentrating the performance of these procedures in high-volume centers with experienced personnel.

A meta-analysis of the randomized PTCA versus CABG trials involving 3371 patients, prior to the release of the BARI results and including unpublished data from Toulouse, France, has recently been published by Pocock and colleagues.[27] From their analysis, no differences were found between the two treatment strategies in either the risk of death or the combined endpoint of death or myocardial infarction. Almost 18% of patients who initially had PTCA underwent CABG surgery within the first year, and the rate thereafter was approximately 2% per annum. Additional revascularization (PTCA or CABG surgery) was performed in 34% of patients randomized to PTCA and 3% randomized to surgery (RR, 1.56; 95% CI, 1.30 to 1.88). This difference diminished over time, and after 3 years the RR of revascularization had fallen to 1.22 (95% CI, 0.99 to 1.54). A summary of the use of subsequent revascularization procedures among patients with multivessel disease randomized to PTCA is shown in Table 22–4.

More extended follow-up will help enable the determination of whether these observations persist as the anticipated graft attrition and progression of native vessel disease occur. Whether or not the use of intracoronary stents would substantially reduce the need for reintervention in nonsurgical patients and whether such a reduction would compare equally well to CABG surgery remain unknown at this stage. The potential impact of aggressive lipid-lowering therapy has also yet to be explored in these populations. The observations of differences in treated diabetic patients in both the BARI and CABRI Trials are important but will need further examination before PTCA should be generally discouraged in these patients. Analysis of the relative cost effectiveness of the two procedures may also provide data that will influence the choice and ultimately even the reimbursement potential of one over the other.

RECOMMENDATIONS

For selected and eligible patients with single-vessel disease who have failed medical treatment and for many patients with multivessel disease, PTCA appears to be a reasonable therapeutic option if both patient and physician are prepared for the possibility that subsequent procedures may be necessary. For patients not requiring reintervention it will clearly be the most cost-effective option. However, for patients in whom there is significant left main stenosis (generally excluded from these trials) or with three-vessel disease with left ventricular dysfunction, CABG surgery may still be the more reasonable option, particu-

TABLE 22–3 • Summary of Main Long-Term Outcomes of Patients Comparing PTCA with CABG Surgery

	Lausanne	MASS	RITA	ERACI	GABI	EAST	CABRI	BARI
Follow-up interval (yr)	2	3	2.5	3	1	3	1	5
Survival	Similar	Similar	Similar	Similar	Similar	Similar	Similar	Similar
Q wave MI	Similar	Similar	Similar*	Similar	CABG—more	Similar	NP	Similar
Relief of angina	Similar	PTCA—less	PTCA—less	PTCA—less	Similar	PTCA—less	PTCA—less	NP
Repeat revascularization	PTCA—more	PTCA—more	PTCA—more	PTCA—more	PTCA—more	PTCA—more	PTCA—more	PTCA—more

* No distinction made between Q wave and non–Q wave MI.
PTCA, percutaneous transluminal coronary angioplasty; CABG, coronary artery bypass graft; MI, myocardial infarction; NP, not provided.

TABLE 22–4 • Proportion of Patients with Multivessel Disease Who Required Repeat Revascularization Procedures After Initial Randomization to Treatment with Coronary Angioplasty

Trial	Follow-Up Duration (yr)	Repeat Revascularization	
		PTCA (%)	*CABG (%)*
RITA	2.5	18	19
ERACI	3	14	22
GABI	1	23	18
EAST	3	41	22
CABRI	1	20	15
BARI	5	23	21

PTCA, percutaneous transluminal coronary angioplasty; CABG, coronary artery bypass graft.

larly if complete revascularization is believed to be necessary.[28] Regardless of choice of strategy, revascularization of patients with multivessel disease, with or without left ventricular dysfunction, should be performed in high-volume centers with experienced teams to minimize the complication rates associated with these procedures.

REFERENCES

1. Grüntzig A. Transluminal dilatation of coronary artery stenosis [Letter]. Lancet 1978; 1:263.
2. Parisi AF, Folland ED, Hartigan P. A comparison of angioplasty with medical therapy in the treatment of single-vessel coronary artery disease: Veterans Affairs ACME Investigators. N Engl J Med 1992; 326:10–16.
3. Fischman DL, Leon MB, Baim DS, et al. A randomized comparison of coronary stent placement and balloon angioplasty in the treatment of coronary artery disease: Stent Restenosis Study. N Engl J Med 1994; 331:496–501.
4. Serruys PW, de Jaegere P, Kiemeneij F, et al. A comparison of balloon-expandable–stent implantation with balloon angioplasty in patients with coronary artery disease: Benestent Study Group. N Engl J Med 1994; 331:489–495.
5. Scandinavian Simvastatin Survival Group. Randomized trial of cholesterol lowering in 4444 patients with coronary heart disease: The Scandinavian Simvastatin Survival Study (4S). Lancet 1994; 344:1383–1389.
6. Hueb WA, Bellotti G, de Oliveira SA, et al. The Medicine, Angioplasty, or Surgery Study (MASS): A prospective, randomized trial of medical therapy, balloon angioplasty, or bypass surgery for single proximal left anterior descending artery stenoses. J Am Coll Cardiol 1995; 26:1600–1605.
7. Strauss WE, Fortin T, Hartigan P, et al. A comparison of quality of life scores in patients with angina pectoris after angioplasty compared with after medical therapy: Outcomes of a randomized clinical trial: Veterans Affairs Study of Angioplasty Compared to Medical Therapy Investigators. Circulation 1995; 92:1710–1719.
8. Topol EJ, Ellis SG, Cosgrove DM, et al. Analysis of coronary angioplasty practice in the United States with an insurance-claims data base. Circulation 1993; 87:1489–1497.
9. RITA Trial Participants. Coronary angioplasty versus coronary artery bypass surgery: The Randomized Intervention Treatment of Angina (RITA) Trial. Lancet 1993; 341:573–580.
10. Goy JJ, Eeckhout E, Burnand B, et al. Coronary angioplasty versus left internal mammary artery grafting for isolated proximal left anterior descending artery stenosis. Lancet 1994; 343:1449–1453.
11. Henderson RA. The Randomized Intervention Treatment of Angina (RITA) Trial protocol: A long-term study of coronary angioplasty and coronary artery bypass surgery in patients with angina. Br Heart J 1989; 62:411–414.
12. Pocock SJ, Henderson RA, Seed P, et al. Quality of life, employment status, and anginal symptoms after coronary angioplasty or bypass surgery: Three-year follow-up in the Randomized Intervention Treatment of Angina (RITA) Trial. Circulation 1996; 94:135–142.
13. Sculpher MJ, Seed P, Henderson RA, et al. Health service costs of coronary angioplasty and coronary artery bypass surgery: The Randomised Intervention Treatment of Angina (RITA) Trial. Lancet 1994; 344:927–930.
14. Rodriguez A, Boullon F, Perez BN, et al. Argentine Randomized Trial of Percutaneous Transluminal Coronary Angioplasty Versus Coronary Artery Bypass Surgery in Multivessel Disease (ERACI): In-hospital results and 1-year follow-up. J Am Coll Cardiol 1993; 22:1060–1067.
15. Rodriguez A, Mele E, Peyregne E, et al. Three-year follow-up of the Argentine Randomized Trial of Percutaneous Transluminal Coronary Angioplasty Versus Coronary Artery Bypass Surgery in Multivessel Disease (ERACI). J Am Coll Cardiol 1996; 27:1178–1184.
16. Hamm CW, Reimers J, Ischinger T, et al. A randomized study of coronary angioplasty compared with bypass surgery in patients with symptomatic multivessel coronary disease: German Angioplasty Bypass Surgery Investigation (GABI). N Engl J Med 1994; 331:1037–1043.
17. King SB III, Lembo NJ, Weintraub WS, et al. Emory Angioplasty Versus Surgery Trial (EAST): Design, recruitment, and baseline description of patients. Am J Cardiol 1995; 75:42C–59C.
18. King SB III, Lembo NJ, Weintraub WS, et al. A randomized trial comparing coronary angioplasty with coronary bypass surgery: Emory Angioplasty Versus Surgery Trial (EAST). N Engl J Med 1994; 331:1044–1050.
19. Zhao XQ, Brown BG, Stewart DK, et al. Effectiveness of revascularization in the Emory Angioplasty Versus Surgery Trial: A randomized comparison of coronary angioplasty with bypass surgery. Circulation 1996; 93:1954–1962.
20. Weintraub WS, Mauldin PD, Becker E, et al. A comparison of the costs of and quality of life after coronary angioplasty or coronary surgery for multivessel coronary artery disease: Results from the Emory Angioplasty Versus Surgery Trial (EAST). Circulation 1995; 92:2831–2840.
21. CABRI Trial Participants. First-year results of CABRI (Coronary Angioplasty Versus Bypass Revascularisation Investigation). Lancet 1995; 346:1179–1184.
22. Bourassa MG, Roubin GS, Detre KM, et al. Bypass Angioplasty Revascularization Investigation: Patient screening, selection, and recruitment. Am J Cardiol 1995; 75:3C–8C.
23. Rogers WJ, Alderman EL, Chaitman BR, et al. Bypass Angioplasty Revascularization Investigation (BARI): Baseline clinical and angiographic data. Am J Cardiol 1995; 75:9C–17C.
24. BARI Trial Participants. Comparison of coronary bypass surgery with angioplasty in patients with multivessel disease. N Engl J Med 1996; 335:217–225.
25. Schaff HV, Rosen AD, Shemin RJ, et al. Clinical and operative characteristics of patients randomized to coronary artery bypass surgery in the Bypass Angioplasty Revascularization Investigation (BARI). Am J Cardiol 1995; 75:18C–26C.
26. Bertrand M. Long-Term Follow-Up of European Revascularization Trials. Presented at the 68th Scientific Sessions, Plenary Session XII, American Heart Association, Anaheim, CA, November 1995.
27. Pocock SJ, Henderson RA, Rickards AF, et al. Meta-analysis of randomised trials comparing coronary angioplasty with bypass surgery. Lancet 1995; 346:1184–1189.
28. Bell MR, Gersh BJ, Schaff HV, et al. Effect of completeness of revascularization on long-term outcome of patients with three-vessel disease undergoing coronary artery bypass surgery: A report from the Coronary Artery Surgery Study (CASS) Registry. Circulation 1992; 86:446–457.

23 Exercise

▶ Barry A. Franklin
▶ Peter A. McCullough
▶ Gerald C. Timmis

Cardiac rehabilitation is characterized by comprehensive long-term services involving medical evaluation; prescribed exercise; cardiac risk factor modification; drug therapy (when appropriate); and education, counseling, and behavioral change. This *multifactorial* intervention is designed to reduce the adverse physiologic and psychological sequelae of cardiac illness, decrease the risk of fatal and nonfatal recurrent cardiac events, control cardiac symptoms, delay or reverse the atherosclerotic process, and enhance the patient's psychosocial and vocational status. The 1 million survivors of acute myocardial infarction (MI) each year and 7 million patients with stable angina pectoris are candidates for exercise-based cardiac rehabilitation, as are the nearly 700,000 patients who undergo coronary revascularization procedures annually (Fig. 23–1). An estimated 5 million patients with heart failure may also be eligible for cardiac rehabilitation, including several thousand with end-stage disease who undergo cardiac transplantation surgery. However, only 11% to 20% of patients with coronary heart disease participate in exercise-based cardiac rehabilitation programs, highlighting the vast underutilization of these services.[1]

Although the degree of left ventricular (LV) dysfunction and residual myocardial ischemia largely determines the risk of future cardiac events,[2] risk status can be influenced by numerous interventions and lifestyle changes (Fig. 23–2). Multicenter trials have confirmed that mortality from acute MI can be decreased by approximately 25% with early thrombolytic reperfusion,[3] emergent percutaneous transluminal coronary angioplasty (PTCA),[4] or both. Patients at moderate risk may experience a reduction in anginal symptoms and recurrent cardiac events from elective PTCA or coronary artery bypass graft surgery (CABGS). Aggressive risk factor interventions aimed at smoking cessation, cholesterol and blood pressure reductions, and exercise training, especially when combined with efficacious drugs, including beta blockers, aspirin, angiotensin-converting enzyme (ACE) inhibitors, and lipid-lowering agents, have produced regression or limitation of progression of the atherosclerotic process with its attendant morbidity and mortality.[5, 6] On the other hand, time (disease progression), poor patient management or compliance, and psychological dysfunction—manifested as anger, hostility, and/or social isolation—can lead to increased risk and an adverse prognosis.

The purpose of this chapter is to review the physiologic basis and rationale for exercise therapy following acute MI, with specific reference to inpatient therapy and early convalescence, exercise testing, exercise prescription, randomized trials evaluating exercise training after acute MI, pathophysiologic outcomes, safety of exercise-based cardiac rehabilitation, special patient populations, and economic considerations.

INPATIENT THERAPY AND EARLY CONVALESCENCE

Simple exposure to orthostatic or gravitational stress during the ever-decreasing bed rest stage of hospital convalescence may obviate much of the deterioration in cardiorespiratory fitness that normally follows acute MI. Attempts to prevent venous pooling during 14 days of bed rest resulted in a modest 6% decline in aerobic fitness, compared with a 15% decrease in untreated subjects (Table 23–1).[7] Thus, it appears that the deterioration in aerobic capacity ($\dot{V}O_2max$) with bed rest may be lessened simply by regular exposure to orthostatic stress, such as intermittent sitting or standing during the hospital confinement period.[8] Structured, formalized inhospital exercise programs after acute MI appear to offer little additional physiologic or behavioral (self-efficacy) benefits over routine medical care.[9, 10]

A significant increase in $\dot{V}O_2max$, corresponding to 2 to 3 metabolic equivalents (METs),* generally occurs between 3 and 11 weeks after clinically uncomplicated MI, even in patients who undergo no formal exercise

*1 MET = 3.5 mL of O_2 per kilogram per minute.

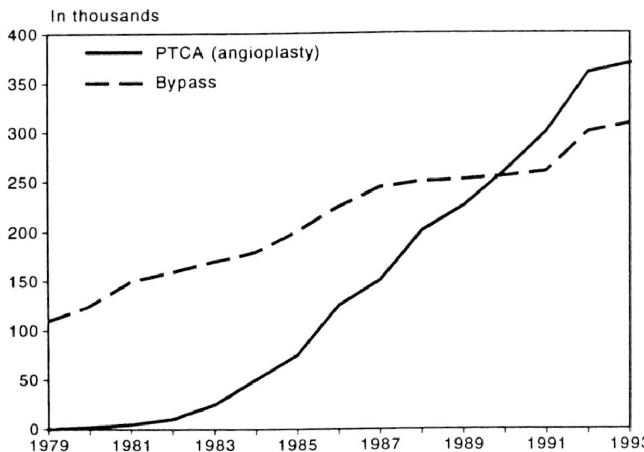

Figure 23–1 Escalating numbers of patients undergoing percutaneous transluminal coronary angioplasty (PTCA) and coronary artery bypass surgery.

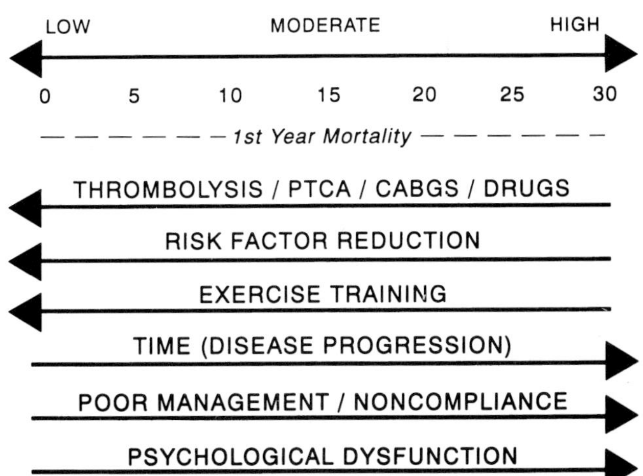

Figure 23–2 Risk stratification continuum based on the extent of myocardial ischemia and left ventricular dysfunction. Variables shown may potentially influence the patient's coronary risk status; the degree of risk is shown at the top. CABGS, coronary artery bypass graft surgery; PTCA, percutaneous transluminal coronary angioplasty.

training.[11] Similar improvements have been reported for patients who have undergone PTCA[12] or CABGS.[13] Self-care and other home activities performed by cardiac patients soon after hospital discharge frequently *evoke somatic aerobic requirements that exceed the threshold intensity for training*,[14] which may approximate 40% to 50% $\dot{V}O_2max$ in deconditioned patients.[15] These transient fluxes in cardiorespiratory activity may promote a training effect and, at least in part, account for the spontaneous improvement in aerobic capacity during the early weeks after acute MI.

EXERCISE TESTING SOON AFTER ACUTE MYOCARDIAL INFARCTION

Exercise testing of the convalescing patient after uncomplicated MI is used not only to assess functional capacity and ability to perform tasks at home and work but to evaluate the efficacy of current medications and risk for subsequent cardiac events.[16] The test also serves to promote patient self-confidence and reassurance to a spouse or employer that various physical activities can be safely undertaken.[17] Because the risk of predischarge or early exercise testing (usually within 3 months) is low,[18] it is now widely administered to many patients soon after acute MI, except those with major complications such as overt heart failure, threatening ventricular arrhythmias, or residual myocardial ischemia, manifested as significant ST-segment depression, angina pectoris, or both.[19]

Methods and Protocols

Early postinfarction exercise tests, as compared with peak or symptom-limited exercise tests, generally begin at a lower metabolic requirement (e.g., ≤2.5 METs), proceed with smaller increments of work per stage, and generally employ arbitrary submaximal endpoints. The timing of low-level exercise tests varies widely, from 3 days to 4 weeks after the acute coronary event. The protocol is designed to simulate and slightly exceed the somatic and myocardial aerobic demands of self-care and other activities that will be encountered at home during convalescence. Accordingly, these tests typically employ peak workloads of up to 5 METs, which are equivalent to stage I of the conventional Bruce[20] treadmill protocol (1.7 mph, 10% grade). However, in the absence of early adverse signs and symptoms, a test may be continued to sign- or symptom-limited workloads or volitional fatigue.[21] Symptom-limited testing is associated with an enhanced sensitivity, yielding a higher frequency of ischemic ST-segment displacement or angina pectoris than do low-level studies.[22]

The two most commonly used early postinfarction treadmill tests are the modified Bruce[23] and the Naughton[24] protocols, starting at 1.7 mph at a 0% grade, and 2.0 mph at a 0% grade, respectively. Both

TABLE 23–1 • Mean Changes in Aerobic Capacity ($\dot{V}O_2max$) Before and After Bed Rest

Remedial Treatment Mode	Bed Rest (d)	$\dot{V}O_2max$ (L/min)		
		Before	*After*	%Δ
None	14	3.9	3.3	−15
Venous pooling	14	3.3	3.1	−6

%Δ, percent change.

Data from Convertino VA, Sandler H, Webb P, et al. Induced venous pooling and cardiorespiratory responses to exercise after bed rest. J Appl Physiol 1982; 52:1343–1348.

tests employ a constant treadmill speed and increase the grade or incline every 3 minutes. A comparison of these protocols for postinfarction exercise testing revealed no significant differences in peak heart rate, rate-pressure product, or workload achieved.[25] Although the Naughton protocol resulted in a significantly longer mean maximal exercise duration (17.3 ± 5.0 vs. 14.8 ± 2.8 minutes), the protocols were equally effective in detecting ischemic responses 6 weeks after MI.

Exercise stress testing with concomitant myocardial perfusion imaging (e.g., thallium-201 or technetium 99m sestamibi) or pharmacologic stress testing using dipyridamole (Persantine IV), adenosine (Adenocard), or dobutamine (Dobutrex) with supplemental imaging may be used to assess residual myocardial ischemia in patients with uninterpretable electrocardiograms (ECGs) or those who may be unable to perform treadmill or cycle ergometer testing. Exercise echocardiography has been shown to be an effective alternative to assess residual ischemic and especially hibernating myocardium, and it has the additional advantage of being totally noninvasive with no radiation exposure.[26]

Guidelines for Terminating Low-Level Postinfarction Exercise Tests

The criteria for terminating exercise tests soon after infarction are often more conservative than those for discontinuing conventional fatigue-limited or symptom-limited exercise tests. Arbitrary "submaximal" endpoints after MI may include a predetermined relative heart rate response (70% to 75% of the age-predicted maximal heart rate [60% with beta blockade]); a peak heart rate of at least 30 beats/min above that measured at standing rest; a fixed metabolic load or aerobic requirement (usually up to 5 METs), a designated rating of perceived exertion (usually "somewhat hard" to "hard"); or adverse clinical signs or symptoms (e.g., ischemic ST-segment depression, angina pectoris, serious ventricular arrhythmias, exertional hypotension).[27]

Interpretation of Results

The responses to early postinfarction exercise tests have been shown to be useful in evaluating three clinical indicators of prognosis: (1) the degree of LV dysfunction; (2) the magnitude of residual myocardial ischemia, suggesting additional myocardium in jeopardy; and (3) the presence of threatening ventricular arrhythmias.[26] Exercise-induced ST-segment depression of 1 mm or more (horizontal or downsloping),[28] especially in the non–Q wave MI patient,[29, 30] has been shown to identify patients at increased risk for sudden cardiac death and recurrent infarction. However, other electrocardiographic (ECG) and non-ECG variables in treadmill exercise testing may also have prognostic significance (Table 23–2).[26]

A meta-analysis of 24 studies using exercise testing in the early postinfarction period with follow-up monitoring for cardiovascular events examined the following five exercise test variables as potential predictors of posthospital morbidity and/or mortality:

1. ST-segment displacement (depression or elevation)
2. Exercise-induced angina pectoris
3. Poor exercise capacity and/or an excessive heart rate response to low levels of work
4. Exertional hypotension
5. Premature ventricular contractions[31]

However, a blunted or decreasing systolic blood pressure response and low aerobic fitness were the only variables associated with a poor outcome. In the non–Q wave MI patient, exercise-induced ST-segment depression accurately identified those at increased risk.[29, 30]

EXERCISE PRESCRIPTION: AN UPDATE

Exercise training sessions should include a preliminary warm-up, a conditioning or stimulus phase, and a cool-down (Fig. 23–3). The conditioning phase should include aerobic endurance exercise and, for selected patients, upper body and resistance training.[1] Modified recreational games and related activities can be employed after the stimulus period, before the cool-down. Sustained exercise recruiting large muscle

TABLE 23–2 • ECG and Non-ECG Variables in Exercise Testing that May Have Prognostic Value in Stratifying Survivors of Acute MI

ECG Variables
ST-segment depression (≥1 mm)*
Early onset (≤3 min, Bruce protocol) of ST-segment depression
Prolonged duration (>6 min) of ST-segment depression
ST-segment elevation
Complex ventricular ectopy†
Non-ECG Variables
Angina pectoris
Chronotropic impairment (peak heart rate ≤120 beats/min)
Systolic hypotension (<140 mm Hg)
Low achieved rate-pressure product (≤15 × 10³)
Low aerobic fitness (≤7 METs, Bruce protocol)
Inability to perform exercise test

* High prognostic value in the non–Q wave MI patient.
† More likely to be associated with significant CAD and a poor prognosis in the presence of ischemic ST-segment depression.
ECG, electrocardiographic; MI, myocardial infarction; MET, metabolic equivalent.

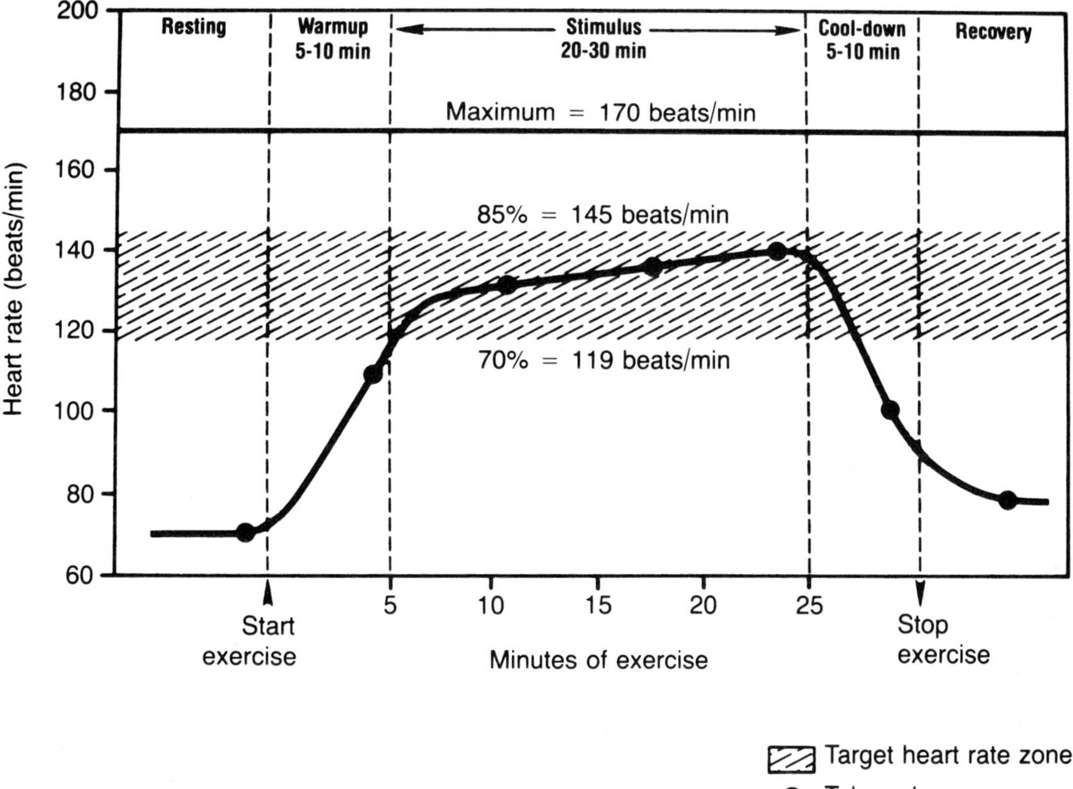

Figure 23–3 Format of a typical aerobic exercise training session, illustrating the warm-up, stimulus, and cool-down phases along with a representative heart rate response. The target heart rate zone for training corresponds to 70% to 85% of the peak heart rate achieved during symptom-limited exercise testing.

groups such as walking, jogging, stationary cycle ergometry, rowing, stepping on and off a bench, or stair climbing, is appropriate for outpatient cardiovascular conditioning. These activities, however, should be prescribed in specific terms of intensity, frequency, and duration. Using an "Exercise Prescription Form" can be helpful in this regard (Fig. 23–4).

Intensity

The prescribed exercise intensity should be above a threshold level that promotes cardiorespiratory fitness and/or health benefits, yet below the workload that evokes abnormal signs or symptoms. For most deconditioned postinfarction patients, the threshold intensity for aerobic conditioning probably lies between 40% and 60% $\dot{V}O_2max$[32]; however, considerable evidence suggests that it increases in direct proportion to the pretraining $\dot{V}O_2max$ or level of habitual physical activity. Improvement in aerobic capacity with low-to-moderate training intensities suggests that the interrelationship of the training intensity and duration may permit a decrease in the intensity to be partially or totally compensated for by increases in the exercise duration, if the total energy costs of the activities are comparable.[32]

An exercise intensity corresponding to 70% to 85% of maximal heart rate, which approximates 57% to 78% $\dot{V}O_2max$, is considered appropriate for cardiorespiratory conditioning in most cases.[32] Ratings of perceived exertion may serve as a useful and important adjunct to heart rate as an intensity guide, using either the category (6–20) or category-ratio (0–10) scales (Table 23–3*A* and *B*).[33] Ratings greater than 13 to 14 on the former scale, corresponding to "somewhat hard" exertion, or 3 to 4 on the latter scale, signifying "moderate" to "somewhat strong" exertion, suggest an exercise training intensity that is too high, regardless of the heart rate response. It should be emphasized, however, that numerous health benefits can be derived at exercise intensities that are below those generally prescribed to improve cardiorespiratory fitness or aerobic capacity.

Frequency

Although exercise is usually prescribed for 3 or 4 days per week, recent studies suggest that two exer-

TABLE 23–3*A* • The Borg RPE Scale, the 15-Grade Scale for Ratings of Perceived Exertion (RPE)

Category Scale	
6	No exertion at all
7	Extremely light
8	
9	Very light
10	
11	Light
12	
13	Somewhat hard
14	
15	Hard (heavy)
16	
17	Very hard
18	
19	Extremaly hard
20	Maximal exertion

Borg's RPE scale is constructed so that given ratings increase linearly with power and heart rate during an incremental exercise test. It is of utmost importance that the test leader administers the test in a correct way. Wrong or misleading results may otherwise be obtained. The instruction to the test leader and to the person to be tested given by Borg must be followed. See Borg (1998) as cited in the credit line below.

From Borg G. Borg's Perceived Exertion and Pain Scales. Champaign, IL, Human Kinetics, 1998, p 31. © Gunnar Borg 1970, 1985, 1994, 1998.

cise sessions per week are as effective as three per week for cardiorespiratory conditioning in early postinfarction cardiac rehabilitation.[34] In this study, subjects were randomly assigned to either a control group and restricted to "very light" physical activity (requiring ≤50% of $\dot{V}O_2max$) at home, or to one of three training groups that, in addition to very light home activity, performed moderately intense (~70% $\dot{V}O_2max$) aerobic exercise for 35 minutes either once, twice, or three times per week in a hospital-based cardiac rehabilitation program. The two- and three-session per week training regimens produced similar increases in treadmill time and aerobic capacity and decreases in submaximal heart rate (Fig. 23–5). Additional cardiorespiratory benefits of five or more training sessions per week appear to be minimal, whereas the risk of orthopedic injury increases significantly.[32]

TABLE 23–3*B* • The Old Borg CR10 Scale, a Category (C) Scale with Ratio (R) Properties for most Perceptual Continua

Category-Ratio Scale	
0	Nothing at all
0.5	Extremely weak (just noticeable)
0	Very weak
2	Weak (light)
3	Moderate
4	
5	Strong (heavy)
6	
7	Very strong
8	
9	
10	Extremely strong (Almost max)
•	Maximal

Borg's CR10 scale is constructed in a very different way than the RPE scale (Table 23–3*A*). It has different psychometric properties and a special instruction should be given. See Borg (1998) as cited in the credit line below.

From Borg G. Borg's Perceived Exertion and Pain Scales. Champaign, IL, Human Kinetics, 1998, p 41. © Gunnar Borg 1961, 1982.

Duration

The duration of exercise required to elicit a measurable training effect varies inversely with the intensity: The greater the intensity, the shorter the duration of exercise necessary to promote favorable adaptation and improvement in $\dot{V}O_2max$.[32] Although it is widely believed that aerobic benefits from exercise accrue only to *continuous* workouts of 30 minutes or longer, recent studies have shown improvements in cardiorespiratory fitness in subjects who completed three 10-minute bouts of moderate intensity exercise per

MD ________________

Name ____________ Age ____________ Starting Date ____________

Clinical Status: Normal
Arrhythmia Angina CABG CAD HTN MI PTCA VR

Note: This prescription is valid only if you remain on the same medications (type and dose), and you are in the same clinical status as on the day your exercise test was conducted.

Contraindications: Angina at rest, fever, illness
Temperature and weather extremes (below 30°F or more than 80° with high humidity)

Activities to avoid: Sudden strenuous lifting or carrying
Exertion that leads to holding your breath

Exercise Type: Aerobic types of exercise that are continuous, dynamic and repetitive in nature

Frequency: ______ times/day ______ days/week

Duration: Total duration of exercise session: ______ min

To be divided as follows:

Warm-up: (light flexibility/stretching routine) ______ min

Aerobic training activity: ______ to ______ min

Cool-down: (slow walking and stretching): ______ min

Intensity:

Target heart rate ______ to ______ beats/min

______ to ______ beats/10 sec

Perceived exertion should not exceed "somewhat hard"

Re-evaluation

Your next graded exercise test is due: ____________
Call our office to schedule an appointment. Phone: ____________

Exercise Physiologist ____________

Figure 23–4 Exercise prescription form.

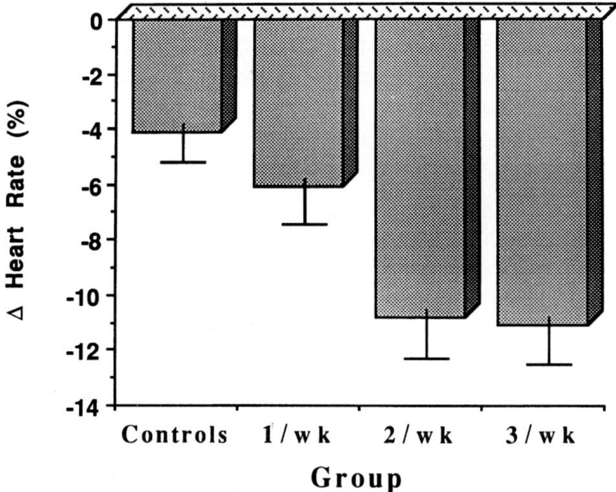

Figure 23–5 Percentage decreases (mean ± SE) in submaximal heart rate. (Adapted from Dressendorfer RH, Franklin BA, Cameron JL, et al. Exercise training frequency in early post-infarction cardiac rehabilitation: Influence on aerobic conditioning. J Cardiopulm Rehabil 1995; 15:269–276.)

day compared with those who performed one "long" exercise bout of 30 minutes, 5 days per week for 8 weeks.[35] The relative increase in measured $\dot{V}O_2$max was significantly greater in the long-bout group (13.9% vs. 7.6%); however, both groups demonstrated identical percentage increases and decreases in exercise test duration and submaximal heart rate, respectively (Table 23–4). Similarly, subjects who were randomized to one of three groups who ran the same total distance, but in one, two, or three sessions daily, demonstrated comparable improvements in aerobic fitness (measured as $\dot{V}O_2$max); moreover, high-density lipoprotein cholesterol levels increased significantly only in the group that exercised three times per day.[36] Thus, accumulation of physical activity in intermittent, short bouts is now considered an appropriate alternative to continuous exercise in achieving health and fitness goals.[37]

Arm Exercise Training

Numerous studies have investigated the physiologic adaptations of trained versus untrained muscles to chronic endurance exercise. Results have generally shown that the favorable cardiorespiratory, hemodynamic, and metabolic adaptations to exercise training are largely *specific* to the muscle groups that have been trained. For example, Clausen and associates[38] demonstrated that leg training caused a significant decrease in the heart rate response to leg exercise, but not to arm exercise. Conversely, arm training resulted in a marked reduction in the heart rate response to arm exercise, but not to leg exercise (Fig. 23–6). Similar "muscle-specific" adaptations have been shown for blood lactate[39] and pulmonary ventilation,[40] suggesting that a significant portion of the training response derives from peripheral rather than central changes, including cellular and enzymatic adaptations that increase the oxidative capacity of chronically exercised skeletal muscle.[41]

The lack of interchangeability of training benefits from one set of limbs to another appears to discredit the general practice of limiting exercise training to

TABLE 23–4 • Training Effects of Long Versus Short Bouts of Exercise in Healthy Subjects

Variable/Program	Long (30 min) (%Δ)	Short (3–10 min) (%Δ)
$\dot{V}O_2$max (mL/kg/min)	+13.9*	+7.6
Treadmill time (min)	+12	+12
Submaximal exercise heart rate (beats/min)	−6	−6

*P = 0.03 vs. short bouts; %Δ, percent change.

Reprinted from American Journal of Cardiology, vol 65: DeBusk RF, Stenestrand U, Meehan M, et al. Training effects of long versus short bouts of exercise in healthy subjects, pp 1010–1013. Copyright 1990, with permission from Excerpta Medica Inc.

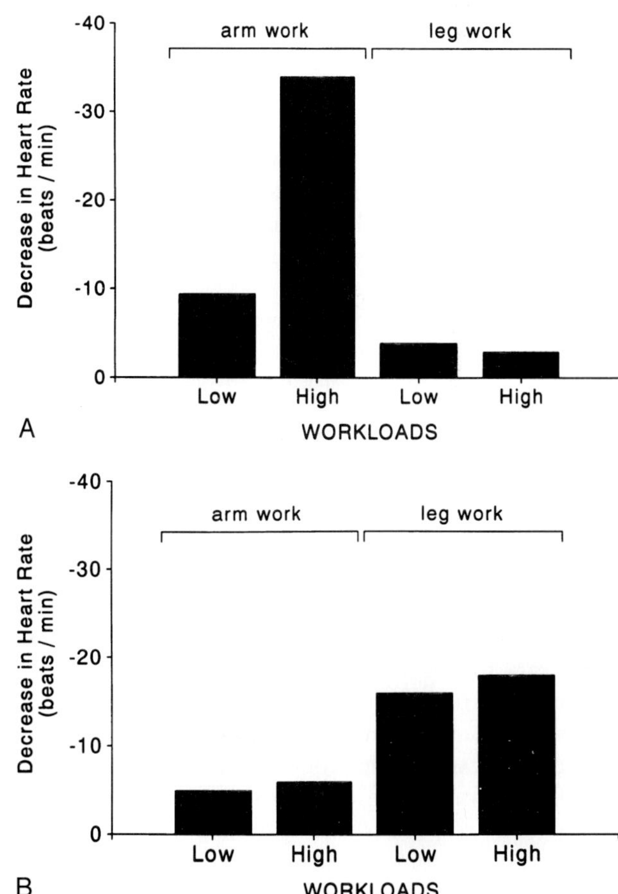

Figure 23–6 *A*, Results of *arm training* using a cycle ergometer. The heart rate response during arm exercise was markedly decreased at low and high workloads, whereas the heart rate reduction during leg work was modest. *B*, Results of *leg training* using a cycle ergometer. The heart rate response during leg work markedly decreased, whereas the heart rate reduction during arm work was minimal. (Adapted from Clausen JP, Trap-Jensen J, Lassen NA. The effects of training on the heart rate during arm and leg exercise. Scand J Clin Lab Invest 1970; 26:295–301.)

the legs alone. Many occupational and leisure-time activities require arm work to a greater extent than leg work.[42] Consequently, postinfarction survivors who rely on their upper extremities should be advised to train the arms as well as the legs, with the expectation of improved cardiorespiratory and hemodynamic responses to both forms of effort.

Although upper extremity exercise training for cardiac patients has been traditionally proscribed, at a given heart rate arm exercise elicits no greater incidence of threatening ventricular dysrhythmias, ischemic ST-segment depression, or angina pectoris than does leg exercise.[43] Moreover, recent studies suggest that the upper extremities respond to aerobic exercise conditioning in the same qualitative and quantitative manner as the lower extremities, showing comparable relative decreases in submaximal rate-pressure product and increases in peak power output and aerobic fitness for both sets of limbs when comparable exercise intensity, frequency, and duration are used for the arms and legs.[44]

ARM EXERCISE PRESCRIPTION

Guidelines for arm exercise training should include recommendations regarding three variables[45]: (1) the appropriate exercise heart rate; (2) the workrate (kilogram meters [kgm] per minute or watts [1 watt = 6 kgm/min]) that will elicit a sufficient metabolic load for training; and (3) the proper training equipment or modalities.

Arm Exercise Training Heart Rate. Although the prescribed heart rate for arm training should, ideally, be based on the results of a progressive arm ergometer test, this may not always be feasible. Research indicates that a slightly lower maximal heart rate is generally obtained during arm exercise than during leg exercise testing.[46] Consequently, an arm exercise prescription based on a maximal heart rate obtained during leg ergometry may result in an inappropriately high target heart rate for arm training. As a general guideline, we have found that the prescribed heart rate for leg training should be reduced by approximately 10 beats/min for arm training.

Workrates for Arm Training. In prescribing the appropriate workrates for arm training, it is important to emphasize that cardiorespiratory and hemodynamic responses during arm exercise are higher for any given submaximal workrate (kgm/min). Consequently, a prescribed workrate for leg training is generally too high for arm training. In our experience, workrates approximating 50% of those used for leg training are generally appropriate for arm training.[47] Thus, a patient's 300 kgm/min load for leg training would be reduced to 150 kgm/min for arm conditioning, with the expectation of comparable heart rates and perceived exertion ratings.

Arm Exercise Training Equipment/Modalities. Specially designed arm ergometers (Fig. 23–7) or combined arm/leg ergometers are commonly recommended for upper extremity training. Other equipment suitable for upper body training includes rowing machines, weight training devices, wall pulleys, light dumbbells, ladder climbing apparatuses, and cross-country skiing simulators. Pumping handheld weights while walking or jogging can also be used to facilitate training of the upper extremities,[48] as can various sport and recreational activities, including canoeing, swimming, and cross-country skiing. Specific precautions should be taken during the latter, particularly with cardiac patients, because heart rates are frequently inordinately high and do not correspond with ratings of perceived exertion.[49]

Resistance Training

New to this decade has been the demonstration that mild-to-moderate resistance training can safely and effectively improve weight-carrying tolerance and skeletal muscle strength in clinically stable coronary

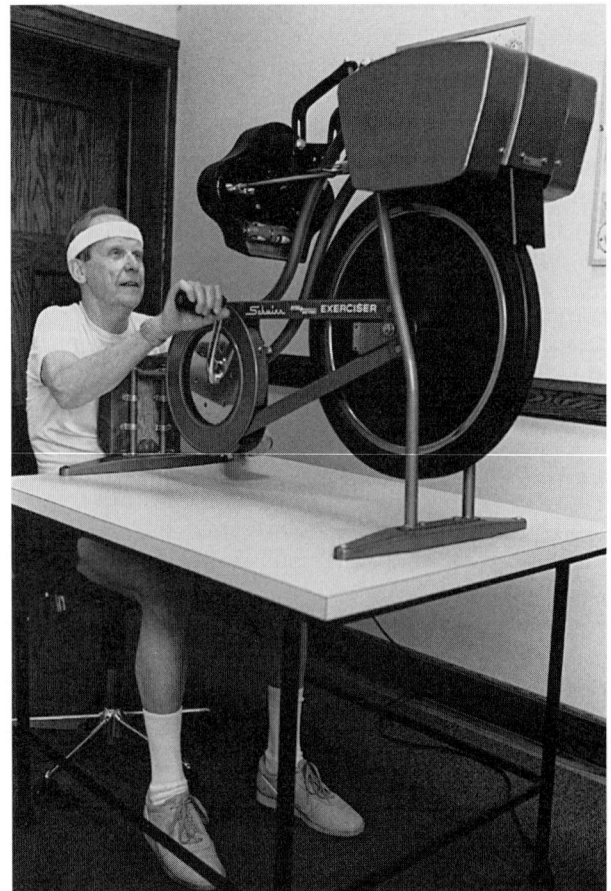

Figure 23–7 The Schwinn cycle ergometer as adapted for arm exercise. Bicycle handgrips have been fitted over the pedals, clamps secure the ergometer to a sturdy metal table, and a padded breastplate helps standardize the arm position.

patients when appropriate instruction and prescriptive guidelines are provided.[1] Moreover, signs or symptoms of myocardial ischemia, ventricular irritability, and abnormal hemodynamics occur less frequently during resistance testing than during treadmill testing to volitional fatigue. Increased subendocardial perfusion secondary to the elevated diastolic pressure that predictably accompanies resistance exercise may contribute to this response.[50] Adjunctive upper body and resistance exercise programs can also facilitate increased transfer of training benefits to occupational and recreational activities and provide greater diversity to the conditioning regimen, which may increase patient interest and adherence.

The rationale supporting resistance training as an adjunct to an exercise-based cardiac rehabilitation program stems from several lines of evidence. Sustained isometric effort is characterized by a pressor response that is proportionate to its relative intensity (percent of maximal voluntary contraction [MVC]),[51] duration, and the muscle mass involved.[52] Consequently, increased muscular strength should result in an attenuated blood pressure response to any given load, since the load now represents a lower percentage of the MVC.

Although previous studies have reported that resistance training programs offer little or no benefit to cardiovascular function,[53] these studies generally evaluated the conditioning response with dynamic treadmill or cycle ergometer testing. When comparing heart rate and blood pressure responses to a standardized lifting or isometric test before and after a strength training regimen, improvement *has* been demonstrated.[54] There are also intriguing data to suggest that strength training can increase both treadmill and cycle ergometer endurance time to fatigue without an accompanying increase in aerobic capacity (Table 23–5).[55] Progressive resistance exercise training may also have a favorable effect on resting blood pressure and lipid levels.[56]

Resistance training guidelines for selected cardiac patients are provided elsewhere, with specific reference to the appropriate number of sets and repetitions, progression, proper breathing technique, and safety concerns.[57] Interestingly, heavy resistance exercise, which may potentially increase the hemodynamic response to and risk of strength training, offers little additional benefit in actual strength gained, at least in this population.[1] Although patients are generally encouraged to perform one to three sets of each exercise, using a weight load that will allow 12 to 15 repetitions, recent studies suggest that one set of moderate-load resistance training is as effective as three sets for increasing bilateral knee extension/flexion strength and muscle size and represents a more efficient use of training time.[58]

TABLE 23–5 • Effects of Lower Extremity Strength Training on $\dot{V}O_2max$ and Endurance During Cycle Ergometer and Treadmill Exercise

	$\dot{V}O_2max$ (mL/kg/min)		Endurance (s)	
	Treadmill	*Cycle Ergometer*	*Treadmill*	*Cycle Ergometer*
Pretraining	47.8	44.0	291	278
Posttraining	48.8	44.6	325*	407*

* Pretraining vs. posttraining ($P < 0.01$).
Adapted from Hickson RC, Rosenkoetter MA, Brown MM. Strength training effects on aerobic power and short-term endurance. Med Sci Sports Exerc 1980; 12:336–339.

RANDOMIZED CLINICAL TRIALS

Numerous studies have evaluated the effects of physical training on exercise tolerance, ischemic-anginal symptoms, coronary risk profiles, and psychological well-being because these variables may potentially impact future morbidity and mortality after MI. This section reviews selected randomized, controlled trials and meta-analyses of exercise therapy conducted in patients after MI.

Major findings of nine trials over a 15-year period are summarized in Table 23–6.[59–67] Subjects were primarily men with uncomplicated MI who were not treated with reperfusion therapy. Those with recurrent or residual ischemia or LV dysfunction were, for the most part, excluded. Exercise training as the primary intervention was initiated from 2 weeks to 2 years after MI. DeBusk and colleagues,[59] in one of the largest trials to date, studied 70 post-MI patients to assess the effects of self-care and other out-of-hospital activities with or without exercise training on the $\dot{V}O_2max$. After symptom-limited treadmill exercise testing 3 weeks after infarction, 40 men were assigned to undergo 8 weeks of home (n = 12) or medically supervised gymnasium (n = 28) exercise training, whereas the remaining 30 served as control subjects, receiving no formal exercise guidelines. At 11 weeks, peak oxygen uptake increased significantly in all three groups: gymnasium training, from 6.6 to 11.0 METs (66%); home training, from 7.3 to 10.3 METs (41%); and no training, from 7.0 to 9.4 METs (34%). The investigators concluded that formal exercise training soon after clinically uncomplicated MI may not be required to restore $\dot{V}O_2max$ "to values approximating those of sedentary men of similar age without heart disease."[59]

Exercise training after MI has been shown to decrease the frequency of recurrent angina by 50% ($P <$ 0.005).[68, 69] Others have reported that patients with nonreperfused infarcts were likely to be symptom free after a period of endurance exercise training.[70]

TABLE 23–6 • Exercise Tolerance Outcomes of Cardiac Rehabilitation After Acute MI: Selected Randomized Controlled Trials

Reference/Year	Sample	Intervention	Benefit
DeBusk et al, 1979[59]	70, all men	Gym vs. home exercise vs. controls for 11 wk	All 3 groups improved; no difference between exercise groups at 11 wk; $P < 0.01$ both exercise groups vs. controls
Sivarajan et al, 1982[60]	258, 80% men	Exercise, vs. exercise + counseling, vs. controls for 3- and 6-mo follow-up	No differences among groups at 3 or 6 mo in the hemodynamic response to exercise testing
Rechnitzer et al, 1983[61]	733, all men	High-intensity vs. low-intensity exercise for 4 yr	High-intensity group had a greater reduction in exercise heart rate than the low-intensity group (10.2 vs. 4.0 beats/min; $P = 0.01$)
Stern et al, 1983[62]	91, 86% men	Exercise training, group counseling, vs. controls for 3-, 6-, and 12-mo follow-up	Improved exercise tolerance in exercise group only compared with other two groups at 3 and 6 mo ($P < 0.001$). No differences at 12 mo
Hung et al, 1984[63]	53, all men	Exercise training vs. controls, 6-mo follow-up	Exercise training group had increased peak power output (803 vs. 648 kgm/min, $P < 0.01$), but no differences on treadmill performance
DeBusk et al, 1985[64]	100, all men	Gym vs. home exercise vs. controls, 26-wk follow-up	Greater increase in exercise tolerance both exercise groups vs. controls, $P < 0.05$
Taylor et al, 1986[65]	143, all men	Gym vs. home exercise vs. controls	Exercise groups had improved fitness vs. controls ($P < 0.05$)
Giannuzzi et al, 1993[66]	103, all men	Exercise training vs. controls for 8 wk, stress testing at 6 mo	20% improved work capacity (training: 4596–5508 vs. controls: 4362–4179 kpm) at 6 mo ($P < 0.001$)
DeBusk et al, 1994[67]	585, 79% men	Home exercise and risk reduction vs. usual care, 6-mo follow-up	Exercise group had greater functional capacity than usual care (9.3 vs. 8.4 METs, $P < 0.001$) at 6 mo

MET, metabolic equivalent; kgm, kilogram meter; MI, myocardial infarction.

Reductions in myocardial oxygen demand via decreases in the submaximal rate-pressure product are largely responsible (Fig. 23–8). To date, there have been no randomized clinical trials of exercise evaluating symptom outcomes in patients after MI where reperfusion therapy has been successful.

Several trials have evaluated the efficacy of exercise training after MI to reduce coronary risk profiles and improve prognosis. Unfortunately, exercise training, with or without counseling, had little or no effect on smoking cessation rates.[68, 71] Studies evaluating alterations in lipid profiles after exercise training post-MI, where lipid-lowering drugs were not used, demonstrated a modest benefit (Table 23–7).[68, 69, 71–73] These results, however, may be confounded by diet, weight change, and concomitant drug therapy (e.g., thiazides, beta blockers) and should be interpreted with caution. A meta-analysis[74] of statistically aggregated data from 15 longitudinal studies of the effect of moderate exercise training in 490 male post-MI patients has demonstrated significant alterations in lipids and lipoproteins (Table 23–8). None of the lipid changes were significant for the control groups. However, exercise alone should not be expected to alter global coronary risk status. Rehabilitation regimens reporting the most favorable impact on coronary risk factors are multifactorial, that is, providing exercise training, dietary education and counseling, and, in some studies, pharmacologic therapy, psychological support, and behavior training.[1]

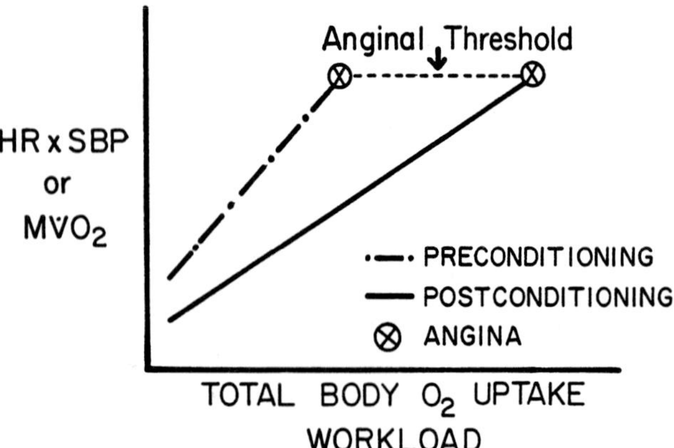

Figure 23–8 Effect of physical conditioning on the product of heart rate (HR) × systolic blood pressure (SBP) and myocardial O_2 consumption ($M\dot{V}O_2$) at submaximal and peak exercise. Peak body O_2 uptake and workload are augmented by exercise. Myocardial O_2 requirements are reduced at a given workload or O_2 uptake, but angina occurs at the same HR × SBP product.

Multiple studies have shown that exercise training after acute MI, with or without counseling, has a positive impact on health-related quality of life, including reduced anxiety, improved emotional scores, and less perceived disability.[10, 62, 65, 75, 76] Serial studies have yielded consistent findings with follow-up ranging from 3 months to 1 year, including post-MI patients with LV dysfunction.[77]

Most randomized controlled trials have shown a trend toward increased survival after MI, but one study attained borderline statistical significance.[73] Cardiac event rates (including mortality) and follow-up periods for selected randomized trials are shown in Table 23–9.[61, 63, 69, 71–73, 78–82] Because these studies

TABLE 23–7 • Effects of Exercise Training After MI on Lipid Profiles: Randomized, Controlled Trials (No Lipid-Altering Drugs Used)

Reference/Year	Sample	Intervention	Lipid Outcome
Wilhelmsen et al, 1975[72]	228 men (89% post-MI)	Supervised exercise, 1-yr follow-up	Significant decrease in C and TG for exercise and controls; no difference between groups
Kallio et al, 1979[73]	375, 80% men	Supervised exercise, 3-yr follow-up	No difference in lipid fluctuations between groups
Carson et al, 1982[71]	303 men, 8 wk post-MI	Aerobic gym exercise, 2-yr follow-up	Mean TG 182 decreased to 144 in exercise group vs. no change in controls: C unchanged in both groups
Roman et al, 1983[68]	193, 90% men	Aerobic exercise, mean follow-up 42 mo	Significant decrease in C in intervention subjects only
Vermeulen et al, 1983[69]	78 men	Exercise and risk factor modification, 5-yr follow-up	C: Intervention 271 decreased to 255 vs. 278 decreased to 276 in controls, $P < 0.005$ between groups

C, total cholesterol (mg/dL); TG, triglycerides (mg/dL); MI, myocardial infarction.

were limited by sample size, recent attempts have been made to pool data from similar randomized clinical trials. Three meta-analyses (Fig. 23–9)[83–85] have now shown that comprehensive cardiac rehabilitation provides a 20% to 24% reduction in total and cardiovascular-related mortality after acute MI (vs. 15% in exercise-only trials),[1] with no difference in the rate of nonfatal recurrent cardiac events. The influence of reperfusion therapy and improved adjunctive pharmacologic strategies (aspirin, platelet receptor inhibitors, certain antithrombin agents [e.g., Hirulog], beta blockers, and ACE inhibitors) have probably lowered the recurrent event rates to levels where mega-trials would be required to demonstrate a beneficial effect of exercise alone.

In summary, randomized trials of exercise training post-MI have demonstrated an improved functional status and lipid profile, reduced symptoms, and, importantly, an enhanced perceived quality of life by the patient. Unfortunately, these trials were hampered by small sample size and underpowered to detect significant differences in fatal and nonfatal recurrent cardiac events. Many of the best results came from multifactorial trials, making it difficult to assess the relative contribution of exercise training. Finally, most of the randomized, controlled trials of exercise-based cardiac rehabilitation were initiated and conducted prior to the application of contemporary, high-technology approaches to managing patients with cardiovascular disease. Therefore, the risk and outcomes of current-day patients may vary considerably, especially with regard to the reported reduction in coronary mortality.[83–85]

TABLE 23–8 • Effects of Exercise Training* on Serum Lipids in Post-MI Patients: A Meta-Analysis

Lipid/Lipoprotein	Pretraining	Posttraining	P
Cholesterol (mg/dL)	232	221	<0.01
LDL-cholesterol (mg/dL)	145	140	<0.01
HDL-cholesterol (mg/dL)	41	45	<0.001
Triglycerides (mg/dL)	169	149	<0.01

* Average exercise intensity was 74 ± 7% of maximal heart rate.

LDL, low-density lipoprotein; HDL, high-density lipoprotein; MI, myocardial infarction.

Data from Tran ZV, Brammell HL. Effects of exercise training on serum lipid and lipoprotein levels in post-MI patients—a meta-analysis. J Cardiopulmon Rehabil 1989; 9:250–255.

PATHOPHYSIOLOGIC OUTCOMES

Exercise training as a sole intervention does not necessarily halt the progression of coronary artery disease (CAD) or, for that matter, prevent restenosis or reinfarction, regardless of the intensity, duration, or both. However, intensive multifactorial intervention (including exercise) can result in regression or limitation of progression of angiographically documented coronary atherosclerosis.[5,6] Improvement in coronary morphology appears to depend more on the total amount of exercise accomplished or kilocalories (kcal) expended than on the specific exercise frequency, intensity, or duration. One study, which included a low-fat, low-cholesterol diet (fat <20% of energy; cholesterol <200 mg per day) showed that a minimum of 1600 kcal/week of physical activity may halt the progression of CAD, whereas regression may be achieved with an energy expenditure of 2200 kcal per week (Fig. 23–10).[86] For many patients, these goals would require walking 15 to 20 miles or more per week.

Exercise-based cardiac rehabilitation decreases myocardial ischemia assessed by exercise electrocardiography, radionuclide imaging, or both, at rate-pressure products matched before and after physical conditioning.[87] Although the mechanisms responsible for changes in the ischemic threshold remain unclear, these data suggest an increase in myocardial oxygen

TABLE 23–9 • Cardiac Event Rates, Including Mortality in Post-MI Patients Randomized to Exercise Intervention Versus Controls*

		Intervention Group		Control Group		
Reference/Year	*N*	*Event Rate (%)*	*Total Mortality (%)*	*Event Rate (%)*	*Total Mortality (%)*	**Follow-Up Duration (yr)**
Kentala, 1972[78]	152	8	7	5	14	1
Wilhelmsen et al, 1975[72]	315	16	9	18	22	4
Kallio et al, 1979[73]	325	18	22	11	30	3
Carson et al, 1982[71]	303	5	8	4	14	2
Bengtsson, 1983[79]	126	3	Not listed	6	Not listed	1
Rechnitzer et al, 1983[61]	761	10	4 cardiac	9	4 cardiac	3
Vermeulen et al, 1983[69]	98	9	4 cardiac	18	10 cardiac	5
Hung et al, 1984[63]	53	17	0	7	3	0.5
Hamalainen et al, 1989[80]	375	26	44	19	52	10
PRE Group, 1991[81]	182	12	0	16	7	Not listed
Worcester et al, 1993[82]	224	1	9	0	8	1

* All differences are $P > 0.01$.
MI, myocardial infarction.

delivery and/or decreased oxygen utilization after training. On the other hand, conventional exercise training does little to improve LV ejection fraction, regional wall motion abnormalities, resting hemodynamics, and collateral circulation. Studies describing the effects of exercise rehabilitation on ventricular arrhythmias have also produced inconsistent results.[1]

SAFETY OF EXERCISE-BASED CARDIAC REHABILITATION

Pathophysiologic evidence suggests that vigorous exercise may precipitate cardiovascular events in patients with CAD. By increasing myocardial oxygen demands and simultaneously shortening diastole, and thus coronary perfusion time, exercise may evoke a transient oxygen deficiency at the subendocardial level, which can be exacerbated by a decreased venous return resulting from an abrupt cessation of exercise. Ischemia can alter repolarization, depolarization, and conduction velocity, triggering serious ventricular arrhythmias, including ventricular tachycardia or fibrillation.[88] Intracellular sodium-potassium imbalance, catecholamine excess, and increased sympathetic outflow all may be arrhythmogenic (Fig. 23–11). Accordingly, the risk of cardiac arrest, compared with that at other times, may be more than 100-fold during or soon after vigorous physical exertion.[89] That strenuous physical exertion can trigger acute MI in habitually sedentary persons with known or occult CAD has been supported by recent studies.[90, 91] This may occur with abrupt increases in heart rate and blood pressure that disrupt vulnerable atherosclerotic plaque and lead to thrombotic occlusion of a coronary vessel.[92] An increase in platelet activation and hyperreactivity, which could contribute to (or even initiate) coronary thrombosis, has also been reported in inac-

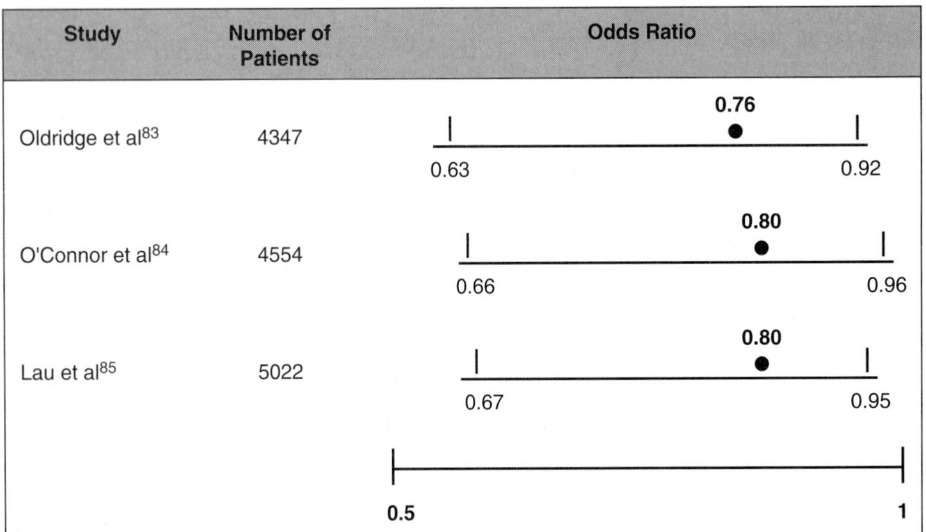

Figure 23–9 Reduced all-cause mortality in postinfarction patients who participated in exercise-based rehabilitation programs in three meta-analyses.[83–85]

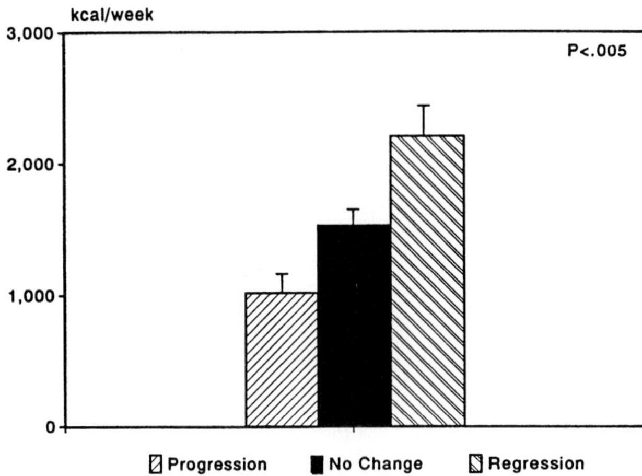

Figure 23–10 Effects of physical activity on coronary morphology in patients with coronary artery disease (CAD). The lowest activity level was noted in patients with progression of CAD (1022 ± 142 kcal/wk) compared with patients with no change (1533 ± 122 kcal/wk) or regression (2204 ± 237 kcal/wk) ($P < 0.005$). (Adapted from Hambrecht R, Niebauer J, Marburger C, et al. Various intensities of leisure time physical activity in patients with coronary artery disease: Effects of cardiorespiratory fitness and progression of coronary atherosclerotic lesions. Reprinted with permission from the American College of Cardiology [**Journal of the American College of Cardiology**, 1993, vol 22, pp 468–477.])

tive subjects who engaged in sporadic high-intensity exercise.[93] The "relative risk" of acute MI during or soon after strenuous physical exertion was two to six times greater than the risk during periods of lighter activity or rest. However, the risk varied greatly, depending on the patient's usual frequency of strenuous activity (Table 23–10).[90, 91] Regular exercise had a protective effect in decreasing the likelihood of acute MI during or soon after vigorous exertion.

Van Camp and Peterson[94] reported 29 cardiovascular complications (21 cardiac arrests and 8 MIs), including three fatal events, during 2,351,916 hours of outpatient cardiac exercise training. Accordingly, the incidence of complications was one cardiac arrest per 111,996 patient-hours, one MI per 293,990 patient-hours, and one fatality per 783,972 patient-hours of exercise. It should be emphasized, however, that this seemingly low mortality rate applies only to medically supervised programs equipped with a defibrillator and appropriate emergency drugs. Recent reports indicate that up to 90% of all patients with cardiac arrest occurring under such conditions are successfully resuscitated.

TABLE 23–10 • Relative Risk of Exertion-Related Myocardial Infarction According to the Usual Frequency of Strenuous Physical Exertion (≥6 METs)*

	Frequency of Exertion			
German Study†	<4 times/wk		≥4 times/wk	
Relative risk	6.9		1.3	
	Frequency of Exertion			
U.S. Study‡	<1	1–2	3–4	≥5
Relative risk	107	19.4	8.6	2.4

* 1 metabolic equivalent (MET) = 3.5 mL O_2/kg/min.
† Willich et al.[91]
‡ Mittleman et al.[90]

The safety of high-intensity exercise training regimens has been challenged in retrospective reports of patients with CAD who developed cardiac arrest or ventricular fibrillation during or shortly after medically supervised rehabilitation exercise.[95, 96] Patients at increased risk of untoward events were characterized by a markedly ischemic exercise ECG, an above-average exercise tolerance, or a record of poor adherence

IMMEDIATE POST-EXERCISE
ACUTE EXERCISE STRESS
Abrupt Cessation of Activity
Arterial Vasodilatation
↑Sympathetic Activity
+
↓Vagal Stimulation
Na+/K+ Imbalance
↑Catecholamines
↓Venous Return
↓Cardiac Output
↑HR, SBP
↑MVO2
↓Blood Pressure
(CHD)
↓Coronary Perfusion
↑Ischemia
↑Myocardial Irritability
Altered Depolarization/Repolarization
Altered Conduction Velocity
↑Ventricular Ectopic Activity

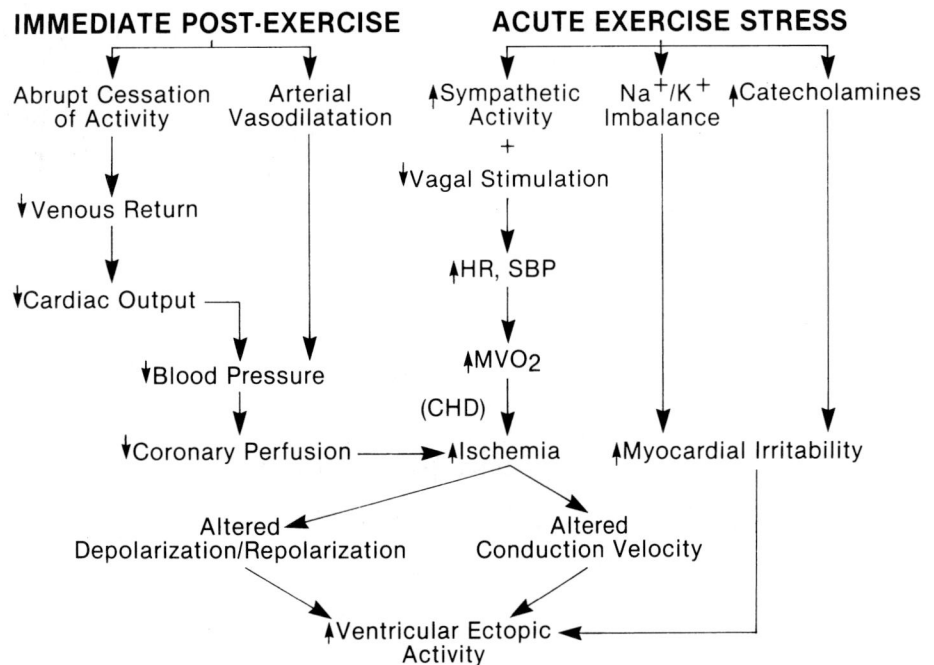

Figure 23–11 Physiologic alterations accompanying acute exercise and recovery and their possible sequelae. CHD, coronary heart disease; HR, heart rate; $M\dot{V}O_2$, myocardial oxygen uptake; Na^+/K^+, sodium/potassium ion; SBP, systolic blood pressure.

TABLE 23–11 • Patient Characteristics Associated with Exercise-Related Cardiovascular Complications

Clinical Status	Exercise Test Data
Multiple myocardial infarctions	Low or high exercise tolerance (≤4 METs or ≥10 METs)
Impaired LV function (ejection fraction <25%)	Chronotropic impairment off drugs (<120 beats/min)
Rest or unstable angina pectoris	Inotropic impairment (decrease in SBP with increasing workloads)
Serious dysrhythmias at rest	Myocardial ischemia (angina and/or ST depression ≥0.2 mV)
High-grade left anterior descending lesions and/or significant (≥75% occlusion) multivessel atherosclerosis on angiography	Complex ventricular dysrhythmias (especially in patients with significant ST depression or LV dysfunction)
Exercise Training Participation	**Other**
Disregard for appropriate warm-up and cool-down	Cigarette smoker
Consistently exceeds prescribed training heart rate (intensity violators)	Male gender

1 metabolic equivalent (MET) = 3.5 mL O_2/kg/min.
SBP, systolic blood pressure; LV, left ventricular.

to the prescribed training heart rate range (i.e., exercise intensity violators).[96] These and other recent data[97] suggest that inappropriately vigorous exercise is associated with an increased risk of cardiovascular complications in *selected* patients with CAD (Table 23–11).

SPECIFIC POPULATIONS

In the early years of cardiac rehabilitation, exercise training was considered suitable predominantly for male patients recovering from uncomplicated MI. Many categories of cardiac patients who, in prior years, were generally underserved or excluded from exercise rehabilitation now constitute an increasing percentage of the enrollees in structured exercise rehabilitation programs. These include women, elderly coronary patients, patients with heart failure, and cardiac transplant recipients.

Women

More than one half of all deaths due to CAD now occur in women, and mortality after MI is higher among women than among men.[98] Thus, the potential for cardiac rehabilitation to attenuate the progression of coronary atherosclerosis, reduce symptoms, and decrease cardiovascular-related fatal and nonfatal events in women is a critical issue. However, the effects of exercise rehabilitation in women with CAD have been less well studied than in men.[87] Indeed, only 3% of more than 4000 patients evaluated in two meta-analyses[83, 84] of randomized trials of cardiac rehabilitation after MI were women. Such a small representation makes specific conclusions regarding the efficacy of exercise-based cardiac rehabilitation in women tenuous at best.

Women are less likely to participate in formal cardiac rehabilitation programs and, when they do, their baseline physiologic and psychologic profiles may differ markedly from their male counterparts (Table 23–12).[99, 100] Moreover, women are faced with numerous gender-specific barriers to participation that may account for their lower enrollment, poorer attendance, and higher drop-out rates. For example, women are less likely to be referred to cardiac rehabilitation programs, less likely to own and drive a car, and more likely to have a dependent spouse at home and to have arthritis as a comorbid condition.[100] Nevertheless, recent studies suggest that women who participate in exercise only or intensive, multidisciplinary interventions, despite poorer compliance than men, demonstrate comparable or even greater improvements in functional capacity, lipid-lipoprotein profiles, body composition, and psychosocial well-being.[5, 6]

Elderly

Although few studies and no randomized, controlled trials have addressed the safety and effectiveness of exercise-based cardiac rehabilitation in older post-MI patients, the available studies suggest improvements similar to those of younger patients participating in these programs.[1] Two studies report that functional capacity (i.e., peak MET levels) of cardiac patients older than 65 years of age improved by 34% to 53% after 3 months of exercise training.[101, 102] Others have reported comparable improvements in cardiorespiratory fitness in elderly men and women participating in an exercise-based rehabilitation program.[100] However, referral to and participation in exercise rehabilitation are less frequent in older adults, especially women.

Heart Failure

Recent reviews have highlighted the benefits of medically supervised and home-based exercise programs

TABLE 23–12 • Characteristics of Women Versus Men Entering Outpatient Cardiac Rehabilitation Programs

Older	Higher prevalence of risk factors
Greater anxiety	More coexisting illness
Depression	Lower peak power output and $\dot{V}O_2max$
Low self-efficacy scores	More severe coronary artery disease

TABLE 23–13 • Published Studies of Exercise-Based Cardiac Rehabilitation in Patients with Congestive Heart Failure

			Peak $\dot{V}O_2$ (mL/kg/min)		
Authors	**Patients (*n*)**	**EF (%)**	***Pre-Exercise***	***Post-Exercise***	**%Δ**
Conn et al[105]	10	<27	24.5 ± 6.7	29.8 ± 10.2	22
Sullivan et al[106]	12	24 ± 10	16.8 ± 3.8	20.6 ± 4.7	23
Coats et al[107]	11	19 ± 8	14.3 ± 1.1	16.7 ± 1.3	17
Ehsani et al[108]	—	—	23 ± 1	31 ± 1	35
Davey et al[109]	22	22 ± 8	14.1 ± 2.8	15.4 ± 2.8	9
Näeveri et al[110]	15	25	21.8 ± 2.1	25.7 ± 3.2	18
Kavanagh et al[111]	17	19	15.6 ± 3.6	17.8 ± 3.3	14
Maskin et al[112]	12	21 ± 3	16.5 ± 2.1	20.4	24

EF, ejection fraction; $\dot{V}O_2$, oxygen consumption; %Δ, percent change.

in patients with moderate-to-severe LV dysfunction complicated by congestive failure.[103, 104] Exercise training increases functional capacity and exercise duration, raises the anaerobic threshold, reduces resting and submaximal exercise heart rates, decreases minute ventilation at submaximal exercise, and improves peak blood flow to exercising limbs.[87] Improvements of 9% to 35% in oxygen uptake at peak exercise have been reported (Table 23–13).[105–112] Peripheral (skeletal muscle) adaptations are primarily responsible for the increase in exercise tolerance, because cardiac output and ejection fraction are largely unchanged.[1] Moreover, symptoms are likely to resolve as the patient's quality of life improves.[107]

Cardiac Transplantation

Exercise-based rehabilitation in patients after cardiac transplantation increases exercise tolerance, raises the anaerobic threshold, and improves the ventilatory response to physical exertion.[87] Moreover, pretransplantation aerobic and resistance training may enhance operative status and recovery.[1] Detailed guidelines for the exercise rehabilitation of patients after cardiac transplantation are available elsewhere.[113]

ECONOMIC EVALUATION

Nearly a decade ago, a comprehensive cost-benefit analysis of exercise-based cardiac rehabilitation concluded that for a small investment in the early post-MI recovery period, benefits accrue over the long term and over an ensuing 5- to 10-year period may more than repay the costs of therapeutic intervention.[114] Since then, several additional studies have documented favorable economic outcomes associated with these programs and services.

In the one randomized trial of multifactorial cardiac rehabilitation initiated within 6 weeks of an acute MI encompassing a cost-benefit analysis, the best estimate of the cost/life-year gained was $21,800 (minimum $10,500 and maximum $58,200).[115] This figure can be compared with other interventions for CAD (Table 23–14). Exercise-based cardiac rehabilitation is not as cost effective as counseling for smoking cessation,[116] aspirin after acute MI,[117] simvastatin administration,[118] and β-adrenergic antagonist therapy following acute MI[119]; however, its cost/treatment benefit is comparable to that estimated for propranolol hydrochloride for diastolic hypertension[120] and lovastatin (40 mg/day) for hypercholesterolemia.[121] On the other hand, it is considerably more cost effective than is either captopril,[120] lovastatin (80 mg/day),[121] or colestipol.[122]

A nonrandomized, controlled trial in Sweden compared a comprehensive cardiac rehabilitation program with standard care (excluding the former) in 305 post-MI patients.[123] In addition to a lower rate of total cardiac events (39% vs. 53%), when hospital readmission for recurrent events was required, its duration was less (10.7 vs. 16.1 days) for the intervention group

TABLE 23–14 • Cost Effectiveness ($/Life-Year Gained) for Selected Interventions and Therapies

Interventions	**$/Life-Year Gained**
Smoking cessation advice (office visit)[116]	1,200
Aspirin for acute MI survivors[117]	3,100
β-Adrenergic antagonistic therapy[119]	5,300
Monotherapies for diastolic hypertension (>94 mm Hg)[120]	
Propranolol hydrochloride	16,000
Captopril	106,900
Hypercholesterolemia	
Simvastatin[118]	6,000–12,000
Lovastatin (40 mg/day)[121]	17,000
Lovastatin (80 mg/day)[121]	73,000
Colestipol (bulk price)[122]	104,500
Cardiac rehabilitation after MI*[115]	21,800

* 3-yr follow-up.
MI, myocardial infarction.

($P < 0.05$). Rehabilitated patients also returned to work more frequently, thereby decreasing costs owing to loss of production (sick leave). In the overall economic evaluation, rehabilitation costs were offset by lower hospital readmission rates and increased employment and work productivity, resulting in an estimated 5-year cost savings of $12,000 per patient.

A retrospective analysis of 580 postcoronary event patients (58% after CABGS, 42% after MI) in the United States, of whom 230 entered a cardiac rehabilitation program and 350 did not, revealed fewer cardiac rehospitalizations and lower costs per rehospitalization in the intervention group during 21 months of follow-up; per capita hospitalization charges for participants in cardiac rehabilitation were $739 lower than for nonparticipants, a conservative figure because physician fees were not included.[124] In particular, hospital admissions for evaluation of chest pain were 134 (38%) of 350 and 48 (21%) of 230 for nonparticipants versus rehabilitation patients, respectively ($P < 0.001$).

Another nonrandomized, controlled trial examined the effects of education, counseling, and low-level exercise training on the consumption of medical care during the first year after acute MI in patients 65 years of age or older.[125] The intervention group (n = 91) demonstrated significantly lower rates of rehospitalization ($P < 0.04$), days of rehospitalization (P = 0.05), and emergency department visits ($P = 0.005$) when compared with the control group (n = 99). Although no financial analyses were provided, these differences suggest a substantial cost savings.

Collectively, these limited data suggest that multifactorial cardiac rehabilitation after acute MI is an efficient use of medical resources and can be economically justified.[1] Nevertheless, the delivery and costs of longer-term secondary prevention services will, no doubt, require ongoing analysis in view of the challenges posed by managed care. Future secondary prevention initiatives should include broadening the armamentarium of interventions to favorably modify coronary risk, especially hyperlipidemia; restructuring and individualizing the menu of services that are currently provided; and offering alternative approaches to the delivery of cardiac rehabilitation services to increase their availability (e.g., home-based risk factor modification and exercise programs).[126]

CONCLUSION

The treatment of CAD has evolved from simple lifestyle modification in the mid-to-late 1960s, largely focused on early ambulation and exercise training, to an array of costly medical and surgical interventions that too often fail to address the underlying contributing causes—high fat and cholesterol diets, cigarette smoking, hypertension, and "hypokinetic living," all of which may be associated with insulin resistance.[127, 128] The increasing number of patients undergoing repeated PTCA and CABGS attests to the palliative nature of most coronary revascularization procedures. Moreover, acute MI frequently occurs at sites *without* a significant fixed stenosis,[129, 130] highlighting the importance of comprehensive risk reduction strategies to stabilize vulnerable coronary atherosclerotic plaques.[131] This may also explain why it has been difficult to demonstrate a reduction in nonfatal acute MI in most studies examining the effects of PTCA or CABGS.

As the millennium approaches, the importance of exercise has reemerged (Fig. 23–12) as new studies have shown that aggressive risk factor modification can result in regression or limitation of progression of angiographically documented coronary atherosclerosis.[132] Physical inactivity is now considered a *major risk factor* for cardiovascular disease,[133] which may be more amenable to "treatment" than hypercholesterolemia, cigarette smoking, and hypertension. Furthermore, a recent consensus statement on preventing heart attack and death in patients with coronary disease extolled the importance of a minimum of 30 to 60 minutes of moderate-intensity activity three or four times weekly supplemented by an increase in daily lifestyle activities; 5 to 6 hours a week was suggested for maximum cardioprotective benefits.[134] We must conclude, as the late Herman K. Hellerstein, MD, summarized in 1972,[135] that

> A planned program featuring exercise training among other measures may tangibly reduce the risk of reinfarction and greater myocardial damage.

This admonition is now time tested and has been scientifically validated.

Acknowledgment

The authors thank Brenda White for her assistance in the preparation of this manuscript.

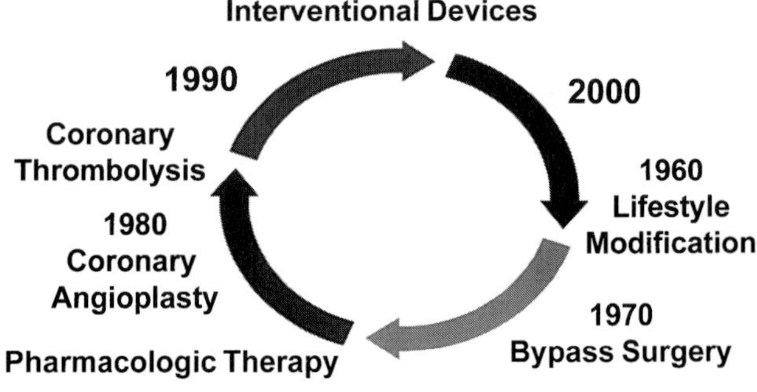

Figure 23–12 The evolution of heart disease treatment. In the 1960s, treatment of heart disease largely involved lifestyle modification, but since then, surgery, intensive pharmacotherapy, and interventional techniques have emerged. Recent studies, however, have shown that aggressive risk factor reduction, including exercise training, can stabilize and even reverse the atherosclerotic process.

REFERENCES

1. Wenger NK, Froelicher ES, Smith LK, et al. Cardiac Rehabilitation Guideline No. 17. AHCPR Publication No. 96-0672. Rockville, MD, US Department of Health and Human Services, Public Health Service, Agency for Health Care Policy and Research and the National Heart, Lung, and Blood Institute, October 1995.
2. DeBusk RF, Blomqvist CG, Kouchoukos NT, et al. Identification and treatment of low-risk patients after acute myocardial infarction and coronary artery bypass graft surgery. N Engl J Med 1986; 314:161–166.
3. Simoons ML, Serruys PW, van den Brand M, et al, for the Working Group on Therapy in Acute Myocardial Infarction of the Netherlands Interuniversity Cardiology Institute: Early thrombolysis in acute myocardial infarction: Limitation of infarct size and improved survival. J Am Coll Cardiol 1986; 7:717–772.
4. Grines CL, Browne KF, Marco J, et al, for the Primary Angioplasty in Myocardial Infarction Study Group: A comparison of immediate angioplasty with thrombolytic therapy for acute myocardial infarction. N Engl J Med 1993; 328:673–679.
5. Ornish D, Brown SE, Scherwitz LW, et al. Can lifestyle changes reverse coronary heart disease? The Lifestyle Heart Trial. Lancet 1990; 336:129–133.
6. Haskell WL, Alderman EL, Fair JM, et al. Effects of intensive multiple risk factor reduction on coronary atherosclerosis and clinical cardiac events in men and women with coronary artery disease: The Stanford Coronary Risk Intervention Project (SCRIP). Circulation 1994; 89:975–990.
7. Convertino VA, Sandler H, Webb P, et al. Induced venous pooling and cardiorespiratory responses to exercise after bedrest. J Appl Physiol 1982; 52:1343–1348.
8. Convertino VA. Effect of orthostatic stress on exercise performance after bed rest: Relation to inhospital rehabilitation. J Cardiac Rehabil 1983; 3:660–663.
9. Sivarajan ES, Bruce RA, Almes MJ, et al. In-hospital exercise after myocardial infarction does not improve treadmill performance. N Engl J Med 1981; 305:357–362.
10. Oldridge NB, Rogowski BL. Self-efficacy and in-patient cardiac rehabilitation. Am J Cardiol 1990; 66:362–365.
11. Savin WM, Haskell WL, Houston-Miller N, et al. Improvement in aerobic capacity soon after myocardial infarction. J Cardiac Rehab 1981; 1:337–342.
12. Ben-Ari E, Rothbaum DA, Linnemeir TJ, et al. Benefits of a monitored rehabilitation program versus physician care after emergency percutaneous transluminal coronary angioplasty: Follow-up of risk factors and rate of restenosis. J Cardiopulmonary Rehabil 1989; 9:281–285.
13. Weiner DA, McCabe CH, Roth RL, et al. Serial exercise testing after coronary bypass surgery. Am Heart J 1981; 101:149–154.
14. Sheldahl LM, Wilke NA, Tristani FE, et al. Heart rate responses during home activities soon after myocardial infarction. J Cardiac Rehabil 1984; 4:327–333.
15. Franklin BA, Gordon S, Timmis GC. Amount of exercise necessary for the patient with coronary artery disease. Am J Cardiol 1992; 69:1426–1432.
16. Fein SA, Klein NA, Frishman WH. Prognostic value and safety of exercise testing soon after uncomplicated myocardial infarction. Cardiovasc Clin 1983; 13:279–289.
17. Cohn PF. The role of noninvasive cardiac testing after an uncomplicated myocardial infarction. N Engl J Med 1983; 309:90–93.
18. Epstein SE, Palmeri ST, Patterson RE. Evaluation of patients after acute myocardial infarction: Indications for cardiac catheterization and surgical intervention. N Engl J Med 1982; 307:1487–1492.
19. Kozlowski JH, Ellestad MH. The exercise test as a guide to management and prognosis. Clin Sports Med 1984; 3:395–416.
20. Bruce RA, Kusumi F, Hosmer D. Maximal oxygen intake and nomographic assessment of functional aerobic impairment in cardiovascular disease. Am Heart J 1973; 85:546–562.
21. Topol EJ, Juni JE, O'Neill WW, et al. Exercise testing three days after onset of acute myocardial infarction. Am J Cardiol 1987; 60:958–962.
22. Jain A, Myers GH, Sapin PM, et al. Comparison of symptom-limited and low-level exercise tolerance tests early after myocardial infarction. J Am Coll Cardiol 1993; 22:1816–1820.
23. Bruce RA, Hornsten TR. Exercise stress testing in evaluation of patients with ischemic heart disease. Prog Cardiovasc Dis 1969; 11:371–390.
24. Naughton J, Sevelius G, Balke B. Physiological responses of normal and pathological subjects to a modified work capacity test. J Sports Med 1963; 3:201–207.
25. Handler CE, Sowton E. A comparison of the Naughton and modified Bruce treadmill exercise protocols in their ability to detect ischaemic abnormalities six weeks after myocardial infarction. Eur Hear J 1984; 5:752–755.
26. Figueredo VM. Risk stratification after acute myocardial infarction. Postgrad Med 1996; 99:207–214.
27. Weiner DA. Predischarge exercise testing after myocardial infarction: Prognostic and therapeutic features. Cardiovasc Clin North Am 1985; 15:95–104.
28. Théroux P, Waters DD, Halphen C, et al. Prognostic value of exercise testing soon after myocardial infarction. N Engl J Med 1979; 301:341–345.
29. Klein J, Froelicher V, Detrano R. Does the rest ECG after MI determine the predictive value of exercise-induced ST depression? J Am Coll Cardiol 1989; 14:305–311.
30. Krone R, Dwyer E, Greenberg H. Risk stratification in patients with first non–Q wave MI: The Multicenter Post-MI Research Group. J Am Coll Cardiol 1989; 14:31–37.
31. Froelicher V, Perdue S, Pewen W, et al. Application of meta-analysis using an electronic spreadsheet to exercise testing in patients after myocardial infarction. Am J Med 1987; 83:1045–1054.
32. American College of Sports Medicine Position Stand. The recommended quantity and quality of exercise for developing and maintaining cardiorespiratory and muscular fitness in healthy adults. Med Sci Sports Exerc 1990; 22:265–274.
33. Borg G. Psychophysical bases of perceived exertion. Med Sci Sports Exerc 1982; 14:377–381.
34. Dressendorfer RH, Franklin BA, Cameron JL, et al. Exercise training frequency in early post-infarction cardiac rehabilitation: Influence on aerobic conditioning. J Cardiopulmon Rehabil 1995; 15:269–276.
35. DeBusk RF, Stenestrand U, Sheehan M, et al. Training effects of long versus short bouts of exercise in healthy subjects. Am J Cardiol 1990; 65:1010–1013.
36. Ebisu T. Splitting the distance of endurance running on cardiovascular endurance and blood lipids. Jpn J Phys Educ 1985; 30:37–43.
37. Pate RR, Pratt M, Blair SN, et al. Physical activity and public health—a recommendation from the Centers for Disease Control and Prevention and the American College of Sports Medicine. JAMA 1995; 273:402–407.
38. Clausen JP, Trap-Jensen J, Lassen NA. The effects of training on the heart rate during arm and leg exercise. Scand J Clin Lab Invest 1970; 26:295–301.
39. Klausen K, Rasmussen B, Clausen JP, et al. Blood lactate from exercising extremities before and after arm or leg training. Am J Physiol 1974; 227:67–72.
40. Rasmussen B, Klausen K, Clausen JP, et al. Pulmonary ventilation, blood gases, and blood pH after training of the arms or the legs. J Appl Physiol 1975; 38:250–256.
41. Henriksson J, Reitman JS. Time course of changes in human skeletal muscle succinate dehydrogenase and cytochrome oxidase activities and maximal oxygen uptake with physical activity and inactivity. Acta Physiol Scand 1977; 99:91–97.
42. Franklin BA, Hellerstein HK. Realistic stress testing for activity prescription. J Cardiovasc Med 1982; 7:570–576.
43. Fardy PS, Doll NE, Reitz NL, et al. Prevalence of dysrhythmias during upper, lower, and combined upper and lower extremity exercise in cardiac patients [Abstract]. Med Sci Sports 1981; 13:137.
44. Franklin BA, Vander L, Wrisley D, et al. Trainability of arms versus legs in men with previous myocardial infarction. Chest 1994; 105:262–264.
45. Franklin BA. Exercise testing, training, and arm ergometry. Sports Med 1985; 2:100–119.
46. Franklin BA, Vander L, Wrisley D, et al. Aerobic requirements

of arm ergometry: Implications for exercise testing and training. Physician Sports Med 1983; 11:81–90.
47. Wetherbee S, Franklin BA, Hollingsworth V, et al. Relationship between arm and leg training work loads in men with heart disease: Implications for exercise prescription. Chest 1991; 99:1271–1273.
48. Makalous SL, Araujo J, Thomas TR. Energy expenditure during walking with hand weights. Physician Sports Med 1988; 16:139–148.
49. Oldridge NB, Connolly C. Oxygen uptake and heart rate during cross-country skiing and track walking after myocardial infarction. Am Heart J 1989; 117:495–497.
50. DeBusk RF, Pitts W, Haskell W, et al. Comparison of cardiovascular responses to static-dynamic and dynamic effort alone in patients with ischemic heart disease. Circulation 1979; 59:977–984.
51. Lind AR, McNichol GW. Muscular factors which determine the cardiovascular responses to sustained and rhythmic exercise. Can Med Assoc J 1967; 96:706–715.
52. Mitchell JH, Payne FC, Saltin B, et al. The role of muscle mass in the cardiovascular response to static contractions. J Physiol 1980; 309:45–54.
53. Pollock ML, Wilmore JH, Fox SM. Health and Fitness Through Physical Activity. New York, John Wiley and Sons, 1978, p 45.
54. Lewis S, Nygaard E, Sanchez J, et al. Static contraction of the quadriceps in man: Cardiovascular control and responses to one-legged strength training. Acta Physiol Scand 1984; 122:341–353.
55. Hickson RC, Rosenkoetter MA, Brown MM. Strength training effects on aerobic power and short-term endurance. Med Sci Sports Exerc 1980; 12:336–339.
56. Goldberg L, Elliot DL, Schutz RW, et al. Changes in lipid and lipoprotein levels after weight training. JAMA 1984; 252:504–506.
57. Franklin BA, Bonzheim K, Gordon S, et al. Resistance training in cardiac rehabilitation. J Cardiopulmon Rehabil 1991; 11:99–107.
58. Starkey DB, Pollock ML, Ishida Y, et al. Effect of resistance training volume on strength and muscle thickness. Med Sci Sports Exerc 1996; 28:1311–1320.
59. DeBusk RF, Houston N, Haskell W, et al. Exercise training soon after myocardial infarction. Am J Cardiol 1979; 44:1223–1229.
60. Sivarajan ES, Bruce RA, Lindskog BD, et al. Treadmill test responses to an early exercise program after myocardial infarction: A randomized study. Circulation 1982; 65:1420–1428.
61. Rechnitzer PA, Cunningham DA, Andrew GM, et al. Relation of exercise to the recurrence rate of myocardial infarction in men: Ontario Exercise-Heart Collaborative Study. Am J Cardiol 1983; 51:65–69.
62. Stern MJ, Gorman PA, Kaslow L. The group counseling versus exercise therapy study—a controlled intervention with subjects following myocardial infarction. Arch Intern Med 1983; 143:1719–1725.
63. Hung J, Gordon EP, Houston N, et al. Changes in rest and exercise myocardial perfusion and left ventricular function 3 to 26 weeks after clinically uncomplicated acute myocardial infarction: Effects of exercise training. Am J Cardiol 1984; 54:943–950.
64. DeBusk RF, Haskell WL, Miller NH, et al. Medically directed at-home rehabilitation soon after clinically uncomplicated acute myocardial infarction: A new model for patient care. Am J Cardiol 1985; 55:251–257.
65. Taylor CB, Houston-Miller N, Ahn DK, et al. The effects of exercise training programs on psychosocial improvement in uncomplicated postmyocardial infarction patients. J Psychosom Res 1986; 30:581–587.
66. Giannuzzi P, Tavazzi L, Temporelli PL, et al. Long-term physical training and left ventricular remodeling after anterior myocardial infarction: Results of the Exercise in Anterior Myocardial Infarction (EAMI) Trial: EAMI Study Group. J Am Coll Cardiol 1993; 22:1821–1829.
67. DeBusk RF, Miller NH, Superko HR, et al. A case-management system for coronary risk factor modification after acute myocardial infarction. Ann Intern Med 1994; 120:721–729.
68. Roman O, Gutierrez M, Luksic I, et al. Cardiac rehabilitation after acute myocardial infarction: Nine-year controlled follow-up study. Cardiology 1983; 70:223–231.
69. Vermeulen A, Lie KI, Durrer D. Effects of cardiac rehabilitation after myocardial infarction: Changes in coronary risk factors and long-term prognosis. Am Heart J 1983; 105:798–801.
70. Marra S, Paolillo V, Spadaccini F, et al. Long-term follow-up after a controlled randomized post-myocardial infarction rehabilitation programme: Effects on morbidity and mortality. Eur Heart J 1985; 6:656–663.
71. Carson P, Phillips R, Lloyd M, et al. Exercise after myocardial infarction: A controlled trial. J R Coll Physicians Lond 1982; 16:147–151.
72. Wilhelmsen L, Sanne H, Elmfeldt D, et al. A controlled trial of physical training after myocardial infarction: Effects on risk factors, nonfatal reinfarction, and death. Prev Med 1975; 4:491–508.
73. Kallio V, Hamalainen H, Hakkila J, et al. Reduction in sudden deaths by a multifactorial intervention programme after acute myocardial infarction. Lancet 1979; 2:1091–1094.
74. Tran ZV, Brammell HL. Effects of exercise training on serum lipid and lipoprotein levels in post-MI patients—a meta-analysis. J Cardiopulmon Rehabil 1989; 9:250–255.
75. Ott CR, Sivarajan ES, Newton KM, et al. A controlled randomized study of early cardiac rehabilitation: The Sickness Impact Profile as an assessment tool. Heart Lung 1983; 12:162–170.
76. Newton M, Mutrie N, McArthur JD. The effects of exercise in a coronary rehabilitation programme. Scott Med J 1991; 36:38–41.
77. Hertzeanu HL, Shemesh J, Aron LA, et al. Ventricular arrhythmias in rehabilitated and nonrehabilitated post-myocardial infarction patients with left ventricular dysfunction. Am J Cardiol 1993; 71:24–27.
78. Kentala E: Physical fitness and feasibility of physical rehabilitation after myocardial infarction in men of working age. Ann Clin Res 1972; 4(Suppl 9):1–84.
79. Bengtsson K: Rehabilitation after myocardial infarction—a controlled study. Scand J Rehabil Med 1983; 15:1–9.
80. Hamalainen H, Luurila OJ, Kallio V, et al. Long-term reduction in sudden deaths after a multifactorial intervention programme in patients with myocardial infarction: Ten-year results of a controlled investigation. Eur Heart J 1989; 10:55–62.
81. PRE Group: Comparison of a rehabilitation programme, a counseling programme and usual care after an acute myocardial infarction: Results of a long-term randomized trial. Eur Heart J 1991; 12:612–616.
82. Worcester MC, Hare DL, Oliver RG, et al. Early programmes of high- and low-intensity exercise and quality of life after acute myocardial infarction. BMJ 1993; 307:1244–1247.
83. Oldridge NB, Guyatt GH, Fischer ME, et al. Cardiac rehabilitation after myocardial infarction: Combined experience of randomized clinical trials. JAMA 1988; 260:945–950.
84. O'Connor GT, Buring JE, Yusuf S, et al. An overview of randomized trials of rehabilitation with exercise after myocardial infarction. Circulation 1989; 80:234–244.
85. Lau J, Antman EM, Jimenez-Silva J, et al. Cumulative meta-analysis of therapeutic trials for myocardial infarction. N Engl J Med 1992; 327:248–254.
86. Hambrecht R, Niebauer J, Marburger C, et al. Various intensities of leisure-time physical activity in patients with coronary artery disease: Effects of cardiorespiratory fitness and progression of coronary atherosclerotic lesions. J Am Coll Cardiol 1993; 22:468–477.
87. Balady GJ, Fletcher BJ, Froelicher ES, et al. Cardiac rehabilitation programs. Circulation 1994; 90:1602–1610.
88. Hoberg E, Schuler G, Kunze B, et al. Silent myocardial ischemia as a potential link between lack of premonitoring symptoms and increased risk of cardiac arrest during physical stress. Am J Cardiol 1990; 65:583–589.
89. Cobb LA, Weaver WD: Exercise—a risk for sudden death in patients with coronary heart disease. J Am Coll Cardiol 1986; 7:215–219.
90. Mittleman MA, Maclure M, Tofler GH, et al. Triggering of acute myocardial infarction by heavy physical exertion: Protection against triggering by regular exertion. N Engl J Med 1993; 329:1677–1683.

91. Willich SN, Lewis M, Löwel H, et al. Physical exertion as a trigger of acute myocardial infarction. N Engl J Med 1993; 329:1684–1690.
92. Richardson PD, Davies MJ, Born GV: Influence of plaque configuration and stress distribution on fissuring of coronary atherosclerotic plaques. Lancet 1989; 2:941–944.
93. Kestin AS, Ellis PA, Barnard MR, et al. Effect of strenuous exercise on platelet activation state and reactivity. Circulation 1993; 88:1502–1511.
94. Van Camp SP, Peterson RA. Cardiovascular complications of outpatient cardiac rehabilitation programs. JAMA 1986; 256:1160–1163.
95. Mead WF, Pyfer HR, Trombold JC, et al. Successful resuscitation of two near-simultaneous cases of cardiac arrest with a review of fifteen cases occurring during supervised exercise. Circulation 1976; 53:187–189.
96. Hossack KF, Hartwig R. Cardiac arrest associated with supervised cardiac rehabilitation. J Cardiac Rehabil 1982; 2:402–408.
97. Friedwald VE Jr, Spence DW. Sudden cardiac death associated with exercise: The risk-benefit issue. Am J Cardiol 1990; 66:183–188.
98. 1994 Heart and Stroke Facts Statistics. Dallas, American Heart Association, 1993.
99. Cannistra LB, Balady GJ, O'Malley CJ, et al. Comparison of the clinical profile and outcome of women and men in cardiac rehabilitation. Am J Cardiol 1992; 69:1274–1279.
100. Ades PA, Waldmann ML, Polk DM, et al. Referral patterns and exercise response in the rehabilitation of female coronary patients aged ≥62 years. Am J Cardiol 1992; 69:1422–1425.
101. Williams MA, Maresh CM, Esterbrooks DJ, et al. Early exercise training in patients older than age 65 years compared with that in younger patients after acute myocardial infarction or coronary artery bypass grafting. Am J Cardiol 1985; 55:263–266.
102. Lavie CJ, Milani RV, Littman AB: Benefits of cardiac rehabilitation and exercise training in secondary coronary prevention in the elderly. J Am Coll Cardiol 1993; 22:678–683.
103. Douard H, Patel P, Broustet JP. Exercise training in patients with chronic heart failure. Heart Failure 1994; April/May:80–87.
104. McKelvie RS, Teo KK, McCartney N, et al. Effects of exercise training in patients with congestive heart failure—a critical review. J Am Coll Cardiol 1995; 25:789–796.
105. Conn EH, Williams RS, Wallace AG: Exercise responses before and after physical conditioning in patients with severely depressed left ventricular function. Am J Cardiol 1982; 49:296–300.
106. Sullivan MJ, Higginbotham MB, Cobb FR: Exercise training in patients with severe left ventricular dysfunction: Hemodynamic and metabolic effects. Circulation 1988; 78:506–515.
107. Coats AJS, Adamopoulos S, Meyer T, et al. Effects of physical training in chronic heart failure. Lancet 1990; 335:63–66.
108. Ehsani AA. Adaptations to training in patients with exercise induced left ventricular dysfunction. Adv Cardiol 1986; 34:148–155.
109. Davey P, Meyer T, Coats A, et al. Ventilation in chronic heart failure: Effects of physical training. Br Heart J 1992; 68:473–477.
110. Näveri H, Kiilavuori K, Leinonen H, et al. Effect of physical training on exercise capacity and skeletal metabolism in chronic heart failure [Abstract]. Eur Heart J 1993; 14(suppl):338.
111. Kavanagh T, Myers MG, Baigrie RS, et al. Cardiac respiratory training responses to a one-year walking program in patients with chronic heart failure [Abstract]. Eur Heart J 1993; 14(suppl):415.
112. Maskin CS, Reddy HK, Gulamick M, et al. Exercise training in chronic heart failure: Improvements in cardiac performance and maximum oxygen uptake [Abstract]. Circulation 1986; 74(suppl 11):H-310.
113. Wenger NK, Haskell WL, Canter K, et al. Cardiac rehabilitation services after cardiac transplantation: Guidelines for use. American College of Cardiology policy statement. Cardiology 1991; 20:4–6.
114. Shephard RJ: Exercise in secondary and tertiary rehabilitation: Costs and benefits. J Cardiopulmon Rehabil 1989; 9:188–194.
115. Oldridge N, Furlong W, Feeny D, et al. Economic evaluation of cardiac rehabilitation soon after acute myocardial infarction. Am J Cardiol 1993; 72:154–161.
116. Cummings SR, Rubin SM, Oster G. The cost-effectiveness of counseling smokers to quit. JAMA 1988; 261:75–79.
117. Hugenholtz PG. On JUMBO and "junkie" trials: A fumbled affair, a jungle, or the ultimate solution? Int J Cardiol 1991; 33:1–4.
118. Rackley CE: Advances in the treatment of cholesterol abnormalities: The role of HMG-CoA reductase inhibitors. Postgrad Med 1996; 100:61–72.
119. Goldman L, Sai STB, Cook EF, et al. Cost-effectiveness of routine long-term beta-adrenergic antagonist therapy following acute myocardial infarction. N Engl J Med 1988; 319:152–157.
120. Edelson JT, Weinstein MC, Tosteson ANA, et al. Long-term cost-effectiveness of various initial monotherapies for mild to moderate hypertension. JAMA 1990; 263:408–413.
121. Goldman L, Weinstein MC, Goldman PA, et al. Cost-effectiveness of HMG-CoA reductase inhibition for primary and secondary prevention of heart disease. JAMA 1991; 265:1145–1151.
122. Kinosian BP, Eisenberg JM. Cutting into cholesterol: Cost-effective alternatives for treating hypercholesterolemia. JAMA 1988; 259:2249–2254.
123. Levin LA, Perk J, Hedback B. Cardiac rehabilitation—a cost analysis. J Intern Med 1991; 230:427–434.
124. Ades PA, Huang D, Weaver SO. Cardiac rehabilitation participation predicts lower hospitalization costs. Am Heart J 1992; 123:916–921.
125. Bondestam E, Breikss A, Hartford M. Effects of early rehabilitation on consumption of medial care during the first year after acute myocardial infarction in patients ≥65 years of age. Am J Cardiol 1995; 75:767–771.
126. Franklin BA, Hall L, Timmis GC. Contemporary cardiac rehabilitation services. Am J Cardiol 1997; 79:1075–1077.
127. Taegtmeyer H. Insulin resistance and atherosclerosis: Common roots for two common diseases? Circulation 1996; 93:1777–1779.
128. Reaven GM, Chen Y-DI. Insulin resistance, its consequences, and coronary heart disease: Must we choose one culprit? Circulation 1996; 93:1780–1783.
129. Little WC, Constantinescu M, Applegate RJ, et al. Can coronary angiography predict the site of a subsequent myocardial infarction in patients with mild to moderate coronary artery disease? Circulation 1988; 78:1157–1166.
130. Little WC, Gwinn NS, Burrows MT, et al. Cause of acute myocardial infarction late after successful coronary artery bypass grafting. Am J Cardiol 1990; 65:808–810.
131. Smith SC Jr. Risk-reduction therapy: The challenge to change. Circulation 1996; 93:2205–2211.
132. Franklin BA, Kahn JK. Delayed progression or regression of coronary atherosclerosis with intensive risk factor modification: Effects of diet, drugs, and exercise. Sports Med 1996; 22:306–320.
133. Fletcher GF, Balady G, Blair SN, et al. Statement on exercise: Benefits and recommendations for physical activity programs for all Americans. Circulation 1996; 94:857–862.
134. Smith SC, Blair SN, Criqui MH, et al. Preventing heart attack and death in patients with coronary disease. Circulation 1995; 92:2–4.
135. Hellerstein HK: Rehabilitation of the postinfarction patient. Hosp Pract 1972; July:45–53.

24 Congestive Heart Failure

▶ Norman Sharpe

Congestive heart failure is a major public health problem in most developed countries. Estimates of prevalence vary, but in the United States, it has been suggested that 2% of the adult population have heart failure, and about 400,000 new cases are diagnosed each year.[1] Mortality is high, with 5-year rates approximately 50%, and in the United States, about 250,000 die annually from this cause.[2]

Heart failure is also a costly condition in economic terms. In the United Kingdom, it has been estimated that annual expenditure on heart failure, which is mostly related to hospital care, was about £326 million, or about 1.5% of total health care expenditure.[3] In the United States, total national expenditure on heart failure, including hospital care, physician visits, nursing home care, and drugs, has been estimated at approximately $10 billion, with three quarters of the cost apportioned to hospital care.[4] Temporal trends indicate hospital admissions for heart failure have steadily increased in the 1970s and 1980s, despite the concurrent decline in ischemic heart disease rates and improved treatment of hypertension.[5] This increase is probably multifactorial but can be related to aging of populations and improved survival after myocardial infarction.

During the past 20 to 30 years, there have been significant advances in the management of heart failure, related to improved understanding of pathophysiology, better methods of assessment, and improved drug treatments. The aims of treatment have broadened, with increased emphasis on earlier intervention. Clinical trial activity in this area has been considerable, increasingly allowing an evidence-based approach to management. Most earlier trials of treatment were relatively short-term, small group studies with various clinical endpoints, including severity of symptoms, exercise performance, and left ventricular function assessment. Increasingly, however, a higher standard of evidence has been required, including provision of reliable, large-scale mortality trial data. This provision has been further encouraged, if not mandated, by the relatively recent appreciation that some agents may demonstrate dissociation of treatment effects, possibly dose related, with improved short-term outcomes but adverse effects on survival with prolonged treatment.[6–8]

For the clinician in practice, heart failure remains a complex condition, and lacking convenient surrogate measures is often difficult to manage.[9, 10] Barriers are recognized between presentation of clinical trial evidence and translation into practice, some of which may be removed through the use of best practice guidelines.[4]

The general principles of management of congestive heart failure encompass patient evaluation and confirmation of the diagnosis, consideration and correction of underlying remediable causes and precipitating factors, pharmacologic treatment, patient education and counseling, and planned follow-up.[4, 11] This chapter focuses primarily on the available randomized controlled clinical trial evidence related to the pharmacologic treatment of the clinical congestive heart failure syndrome. Other aspects of management, such as patient education, counseling, and planned follow-up, should be regarded as complementary to pharmacologic treatment and important to ensure compliance and optimal long-term outcomes.

CLINICAL TRIAL EVIDENCE: TRANSLATION INTO PRACTICE

Barriers to the appropriate practical application of clinical trial results exist in general, and this difficulty is well exemplified in the management of congestive heart failure. Apart from the volume and complexity of evidence, patient selection criteria for trials often differ from the typical patient group in the community. Trials based on secondary and tertiary clinical centers tend to enroll predominantly relatively younger men, who may be more amenable to the assessment procedures required. The typical patient with heart failure encountered in the community is 70 years old or older, with women more evenly represented. The aims of treatment for congestive heart failure may differ considerably with variation in age and severity and are not necessarily equated with the aims of intervention in clinical trials (Table 24–1). For

TABLE 24–1 • Aims of Treatment

Symptomatic improvement, immediate and sustained
Improved ventricular function and hemodynamics
Correction of metabolic and neurohormonal abnormalities
Prevention of progression in left ventricular dysfunction
Prevention of arrhythmias
Improved quality of life
Reduced hospital readmission
Prolonged survival

example, the priority in the frail, elderly patient with severe limitation is symptomatic relief to improve comfort and mobility. In the younger patient, with less severe failure, the aims of treatment are broader and more directed toward preventing progression and improving survival.

The appreciation that the short-term clinical outcomes and mortality effects of some treatments may be dissociated has led appropriately to more stringent regulatory requirements for drug registration. This change, however, has resulted in some difficulty for clinicians in the determination of the most appropriate clinical aims in the treatment of individual patients. The international move toward evidence-based clinical practice guidelines has been useful. Such guidelines are generally broad statements allowing flexibility in application and requiring careful clinical judgment for optimal individual outcomes.[4, 11]

Various definitions of heart failure exist, based on different hemodynamic, functional, or clinical criteria. A broad spectrum of severity can be defined, based on assessment of left ventricular size and function alone. Many patients with important left ventricular dysfunction, however, may have no symptoms or signs of congestive heart failure.[12] The syndrome of clinical congestive heart failure can be defined on the basis of symptoms and signs related to reduced cardiac output and pulmonary and systemic venous congestion, with objective evidence of cardiac dysfunction.[12] An additional criterion suggested, when the diagnosis is in doubt, is a response to treatment directed toward heart failure. With these definitions agreed, it should be emphasized that clinical congestive heart failure generally represents advanced disease progression, at which stage a poor prognosis is determined and the effectiveness of intervention relatively limited. Thus, although this clinical definition of the syndrome prevails for practical reasons, a broader definition of heart failure, based on objective assessment of left ventricular function, is now generally adopted as earlier preventive approaches to treatment are instituted.

Routine echocardiographic assessment in patients with congestive heart failure allows the recognition of varying degrees of left ventricular dilation, hypertrophy, and systolic and diastolic dysfunction. Primary diastolic dysfunction with normal or near-normal left ventricular size and systolic function may be more common in the elderly and related to left ventricular hypertrophy, previous hypertension, and coronary heart disease.[13–15] This condition requires a different emphasis in treatment and indicates the difficulty that may be encountered in extrapolating clinical trial results to the management of a more elderly patient group.

CLINICAL TRIAL ASSESSMENT AND ENDPOINTS

There are three broad categories of assessment employed in larger clinical trials, which can be related to the aims of treatment of congestive heart failure (Table 24–2)[16]: (1) symptom assessment using a variety of symptom scales or classifications, often supplemented by exercise testing, maximal or submaximal, and quality-of-life questionnaires; (2) measurement of cardiac function, either direct hemodynamic measurements or indirect measurements of ventricular size and function, as with radionuclide ventriculography or echocardiography; and (3) assessment of morbidity in terms of worsening heart failure, cardiovascular events, or hospital readmission and mortality often categorized as due to progressive heart failure or sudden death. These various outcomes may be influenced, and the aims of treatment achieved, through different mechanisms that may not necessarily be associated (Table 24–3). For example, improvement in congestive symptoms is achieved primarily through hemodynamic improvement and reduction of ele-

TABLE 24–2 • Clinical Trial Assessment

Symptom status
NYHA functional class
Patient self-assessment
Exercise testing
Maximal
Submaximal
Ventricular size and function
Direct hemodynamic measurements
Radionuclide ventriculography
Echocardiography
Neurohormone measurements
Holter monitoring
Arrhythmias
Heart rate variability
Quality-of-life questionnaires
Morbidity
Cardiovascular events
Worsening heart failure
Hospital readmission
Mortality
Progressive heart failure
Sudden death

NYHA, New York Heart Association.

TABLE 24–3 • Possible Dissociation of Treatment Aims and Mechanisms of Improvement

	Left Ventricular Function	Symptoms/ Exercise	Survival
Diuretics	↑↓	↑	?
Digitalis	↑	↑	↑↓
ACE inhibitors	↑	↑	↑
Beta blockers	↑	—	↑
Inotropes	↑	↑	↓

ACE, angiotensin-converting enzyme.

vated filling pressures. Hemodynamic improvement may also allow improved exercise performance, but longer-term peripheral circulatory improvement and muscular conditioning may be more important determinants of such change. Reduction in morbidity and mortality may also result from improvement in left ventricular function, but neurohormonal blockade is the most important mechanism by which survival improvement can be achieved. Different drug treatments have different effects on these various mechanisms and outcomes. Short-term clinical outcomes may not be correlated with, or reliable surrogates for, mortality.

Consideration of these aspects indicates the difficulty in combining endpoints in trials, an approach that is often adopted to increase power and seek a significant outcome with a smaller sample size. Clearly, such a design may or may not be appropriate, depending on the mechanisms of action of the agent under study and the combination of endpoints chosen. Interpretation of combined endpoint data may be difficult, however, and ideally endpoints should be targeted separately.

PHARMACOLOGIC TREATMENT

Diuretics

Diuretic drugs are generally accepted as first-line treatment for symptomatic congestive heart failure. They are effective in relieving symptoms of fluid retention, pulmonary congestion, and peripheral edema. Their adverse metabolic effects are well recognized, electrolyte depletion being a primary concern. Although it is accepted that diuretics can predictably improve symptoms and quality of life with short-term treatment, their effects with long-term treatment are poorly understood, and effects on mortality are unknown. Excessive diuresis may further compromise cardiac output, and diuretic-induced activation of the renin-angiotensin-aldosterone system could potentially confer long-term disadvantage.[17, 18] The combination of diuretic treatment with angiotensin-converting enzyme (ACE) inhibition is rational, combining hemodynamic and symptomatic benefits while offsetting adverse metabolic effects, particularly hypokalemia and neurohormonal activation. There have been no controlled clinical trials assessing the mortality effect of diuretic treatment, and such trials are unlikely given the importance of relief of congestive symptoms as a primary aim of therapy. Studies that have compared diuretics and ACE inhibitors as initial therapy in heart failure are few but consistent in suggesting that ACE inhibitors alone are generally insufficient for the relief of significant fluid retention.[19–22] Thus, diuretics have a long established role as essential treatment for symptomatic heart failure based on clinical observation rather than controlled trial data. In general, all other treatments subject to trial have been assessed against a background of diuretic treatment. Again, although the short-term symptomatic benefit from such treatment is undoubted, long-term effects have not been well studied, and mortality effects remain unknown.

Angiotensin-Converting Enzyme Inhibitors

ACE inhibitors were introduced initially into cardiovascular therapeutics as antihypertensive agents but during the 1980s and continuing to the present have been extensively studied in the context of congestive heart failure. As a class, they are now established as standard initial and maintenance treatment for congestive heart failure in combination with diuretics. Their application has been extended to the treatment of asymptomatic left ventricular dysfunction after myocardial infarction as well as diabetic nephropathy. Possible antiatherosclerotic effects are the subject of ongoing research at present.

No class of agent for heart failure treatment has been subject to such rigorous assessment as the ACE inhibitors. Interest in this treatment approach has also fostered a much clearer understanding of cardiovascular physiology. Although various other vasodilator agents can produce favorable acute hemodynamic responses, these effects have generally not been maintained with long-term use because of the occurrence of tolerance.[23, 24] In contrast, the large amount of clinical trial data now available with ACE inhibitors is consistent in demonstrating sustained hemodynamic and symptomatic improvement in a majority of patients and significant improvement in survival. The potent vasodilating effects of ACE inhibitors are well maintained in most patients, and tolerance appears less likely than with alternative vasodilating drugs because effective neurohormonal blockade is maintained.

CLINICAL TRIALS

Effects on Left Ventricular Function, Symptoms, and Exercise Performance

Numerous studies have demonstrated the beneficial hemodynamic, symptomatic, and exercise response to treatment with ACE inhibition, which appears to be maintained over several weeks or months.[25–31] Hemodynamic tolerance is less likely than with other vasodilators because of withdrawal of sympathetic tone rather than further activation. Sustained hemodynamic improvement with longer-term treatment is associated with improvement in symptoms and exercise performance, the latter improving gradually over several months after peripheral adaptation (Fig. 24–1).[28–31]

The Captopril Multicentre trial[32] was the first major multicenter trial of an ACE inhibitor in congestive heart failure. Ninety-two patients with New York Heart Association (NYHA) class II or III heart failure on digoxin and diuretic treatment were randomized to double-blind treatment with captopril or placebo for 12 weeks. Captopril was begun in a dosage of 25 mg three times daily, increasing to 100 mg three times

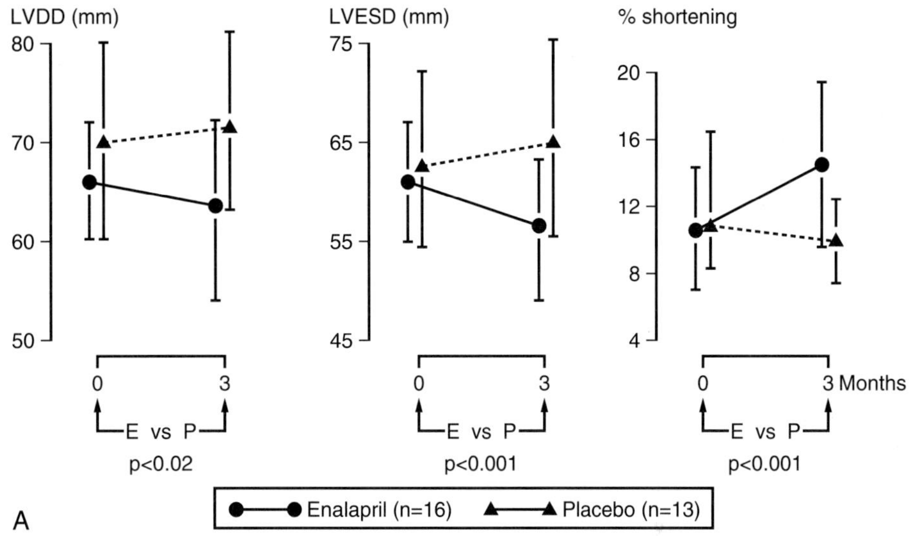

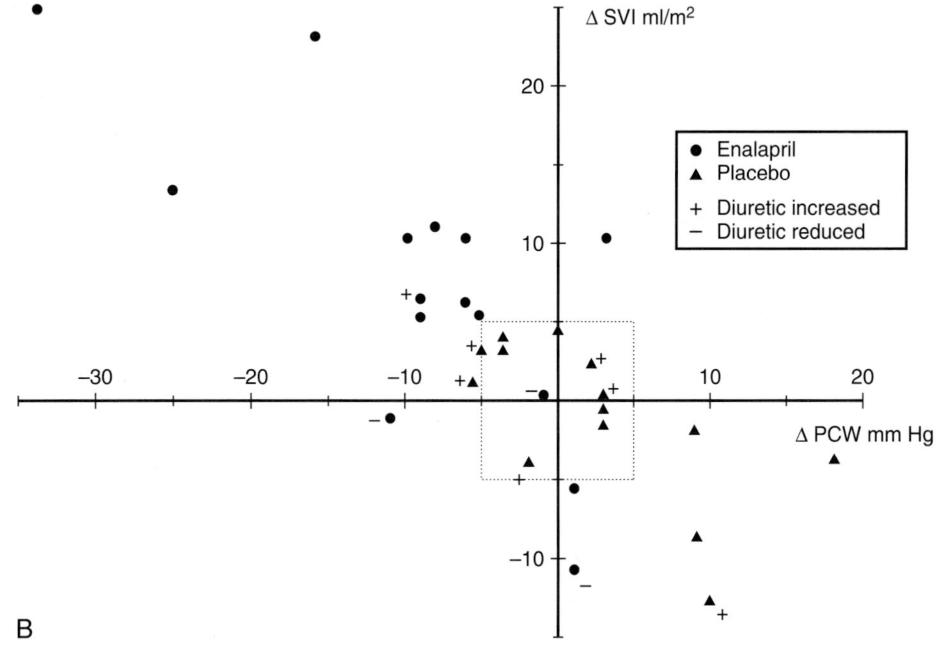

Figure 24–1 *A*, Enalapril in chronic heart failure. Echocardiographic evaluation at baseline and 3 months. Left ventricular end-diastolic dimension (LVDD) and LV end-systolic dimension (LVESD) were significantly reduced, and LV fractional shortening (% shortening) significantly increased in the enalapril group compared with the placebo group. *B*, Hemodynamic changes from baseline to 3 months for individual patients with respect to stroke volume index (SVI) and mean pulmonary capillary wedge pressure (PCW). The majority in the enalapril group showed hemodynamic improvement compared with the placebo group, which showed no change or a deterioration. (*A* and *B* From Sharpe DN, Murphy J, Coxon R, et al. Enalapril in patients with chronic heart failure: A placebo-controlled, randomized, double-blind study. Circulation 1984; 70:271–278.)

daily if tolerated. Mean exercise duration in the captopril group increased 24% from the baseline of 494 seconds to 614 seconds after 12 weeks ($P < 0.001$), whereas the placebo group did not change (Fig. 24–2). Symptoms assessed by both patients and physicians also improved in the captopril group but were unchanged in the placebo group. Captopril was generally well tolerated, and withdrawals because of death or worsening heart failure were greater in the placebo group.

The Captopril-Digoxin Multicentre study[33] was designed to compare the effects of captopril or digoxin with placebo in 300 patients with congestive heart failure, predominantly NYHA class II. Patients were randomized to double-blind treatment after stabilization on diuretics alone or no treatment, and many patients were withdrawn from previous digoxin treatment before randomization. Captopril treatment was begun at 25 mg three times daily and increased to 50 mg three times daily if tolerated. The mean change in exercise time after 6 months of treatment was significantly different in the captopril group, compared with the placebo group (82 vs. 35 seconds, $P < 0.05$) but not significantly different in the digitalis group. The mean change in left ventricular ejection fraction in the digitalis group was 4.4%, significantly different from the placebo group ($P < 0.01$) and the captopril group ($P < 0.05$). Increased requirements for diuretic treatment and hospitalization were significantly more frequent in placebo-treated patients than in either of the other groups.

An analysis of 35 published randomized, double-blind, placebo-controlled trials involving a total of 3411 patients has demonstrated the high concordance between changes in symptoms and exercise capacity with ACE inhibitor treatment.[34] Symptoms improved in 25 of the 33 trials in which this was assessed, and exercise capacity improved in 23 of the 35 trials. In 27 of the 35 trials (82%), there was concordance between the effects on symptoms and exercise capacity. Twenty-one showed improvement in both, six showed no improvement in either, and six showed discrepant results. Study size, duration of follow-up, and method of exercise testing were major factors affecting outcome. All nine trials with study size greater than 50, follow-up 3 to 6 months, and using treadmill exercise testing showed improved exercise capacity and symptoms.

Effects on Survival

The Cooperative North Scandinavian Enalapril Survival Study–1 (CONSENSUS-1) trial[35] was the first to demonstrate the survival benefit of ACE inhibition in patients with severe heart failure. In this study, 253 patients with NYHA class IV heart failure on digoxin, diuretic, and possible vasodilator treatment were randomized to double-blind treatment with enalapril 5 mg twice daily or placebo and the dosage increased to 10 mg twice daily if tolerated. At 6 and 12 months, mortality rates were 44% and 52% in the placebo group, compared with 26% and 36% in the enalapril group ($P < 0.003$), the difference being due to a reduction in deaths from progressive heart failure

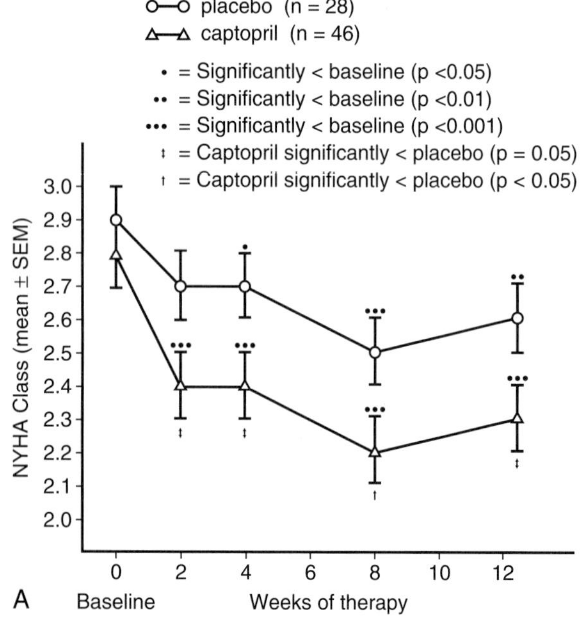

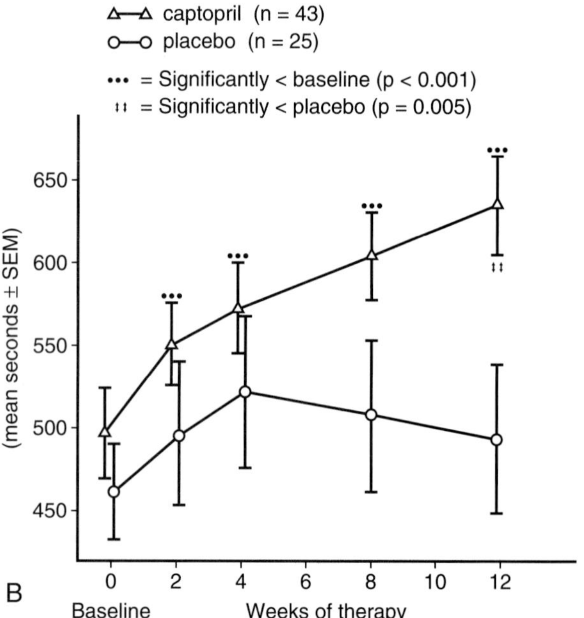

Figure 24–2 *A*, Captopril Multicenter Trial. Comparison of New York Heart Association (NYHA) functional class ratings for cohorts of patients (mean ± standard error of the mean). *B*, Comparison of exercise tolerance times for cohorts of patients (mean ± standard error of the mean). (*A* and *B* From Captopril Multicenter Research Group. A placebo-controlled trial of captopril in refractory chronic congestive heart failure. Reprinted with permission from the American College of Cardiology [Journal of the American College of Cardiology, 1983, vol 2, pp 755–763.])

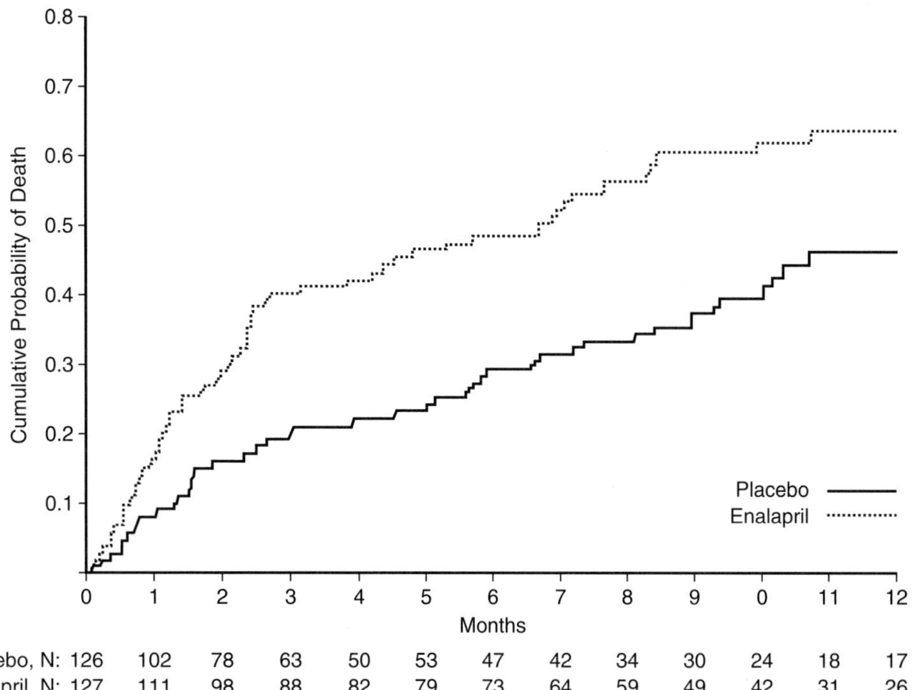

Figure 24–3 CONSENSUS-1. Cumulative probability of death in the placebo and enalapril groups. (From CONSENSUS Trial Group. Effects of enalapril on mortality in severe congestive heart failure: Results of the Cooperative North Scandinavian Enalapril Survival Study [CONSENSUS]. N Engl J Med 1987; 316:1429–1435. Copyright 1987, Massachusetts Medical Society. All rights reserved.)

(Fig. 24–3). The reduction in mortality was associated with general clinical improvement, reduction in hospital admissions, and fewer days spent in the hospital. Symptomatic hypotension was observed in 17% of the enalapril group but in none of the placebo group, although withdrawal rates were similar in both groups.

The Studies of Left Ventricular Dysfunction (SOLVD) Treatment trial[36] was conducted in patients with NYHA class II or III heart failure and left ventricular ejection fraction (LVEF) less than 35% and paralleled by a preventive trial in patients with left ventricular dysfunction (LVEF <35%) but no symptoms of heart failure. In the treatment trial, 2569 patients were randomized to double-blind treatment with enalapril or placebo in addition to standard treatment in an initial dose of 2.5 mg twice daily, increasing to 10 mg twice daily if tolerated. The mean follow-up period was 3 to 4 years, during which time enalapril treatment reduced mortality from 39.7% to 35.2% ($P = 0.0036$), principally as a result of a reduction in deaths attributed to progressive heart failure. Hospitalizations for worsening heart failure were also significantly reduced with enalapril treatment. The benefit from enalapril appeared most marked during the first 2 years of treatment.

The Veterans Administration Cooperative Heart Failure (V-HeFT)-2 trial[37] followed the first trial (V-HeFT-1),[38] in which a combination of hydralazine and isosorbide dinitrate produced a significant reduction in mortality compared with placebo and prasozin in patients with NYHA class II and III heart failure. In V-HeFT-2, the combination of hydralazine and isosorbide dinitrate was compared with enalapril in 804 patients with NYHA class II and III heart failure and evidence of left ventricular dysfunction.[37] Enalapril was begun in an initial dose of 5 mg twice daily and increased to 10 mg twice daily if tolerated. After 2 years, mortality was significantly lower in the enalapril group than in the combination treatment group (18% vs. 25%, $P = 0.016$), attributed to a reduction in the incidence of sudden death. Greatest relative benefit occurred in patients with primary cardiomyopathy and those with milder heart failure, in contrast to the placebo-controlled SOLVD treatment trial, in which most benefit was seen in patients with ischemic heart disease and class III heart failure.

An analysis of data pooled from all completed published or unpublished randomized placebo-controlled trials of ACE inhibitors in patients with heart failure indicates the consistency of benefit from this treatment in a broad range of patients.[39] From an overview of 32 randomized controlled trials in 7105 patients, there was a significant reduction in total mortality (odds ratio [OR], 0.77; 95% confidence interval [CI], 0.67 to 0.88; $P < 0.001$) and in the combined endpoint of mortality or hospitalization for congestive heart failure (OR, 0.65; 95% CI, 0.57 to 0.74; $P < 0.001$) (Table 24–4). Similar benefits were observed for several different ACE inhibitors, and reductions in total mortality and the combined endpoint were similar for various subgroups (age, sex, cause, and NYHA class). Greatest benefit was evident for patients with the lowest ejection fraction (LVEF <25%) and during the first 3 months of treatment. Mortality reduction was due primarily to fewer deaths from progressive

Table 24–4 • Overview of Angiotensin-Converting Enzyme Inhibitors in Heart Failure

	Odds Ratio	95% Confidence Interval
Total mortality	0.77	0.67–0.88
Mortality or hospitalization	0.65	0.57–0.74
Progressive heart failure	0.69	0.58–0.83
Sudden death	0.91	0.73–1.12
Fatal myocardial infarction	0.82	0.60–1.11
Total mortality		
Class 1	0.75	0.46–1.23
Class 2	0.83	0.68–1.01
Class 3	0.76	0.60–0.96
Class 4	0.55	0.36–0.84
EF >0.25	0.98	0.78–1.23
EF ≤0.25	0.69	0.57–0.85

EF, ejection fraction.
From Garg R, Yusuf S. Overview of randomized trials of angiotensin-converting enzyme inhibitors on mortality and morbidity in patients with heart failure. JAMA 1995; 273:1450. Copyright 1995, American Medical Association.

heart failure. The point estimates for effects on sudden or presumed arrhythmic deaths and fatal myocardial infarction were less than 1 but not significant.

The clinical trial data for ACE inhibitors demonstrate consistent hemodynamic and symptomatic improvement for a majority of patients with clinical congestive heart failure and concordant mortality reduction, providing the basis for recommending these agents as standard treatment. In most clinical trials, patients with hypotension (systolic blood pressure <90 to 100 mm Hg), important valvular stenosis, significant renal impairment, or primary diastolic dysfunction were excluded, and thus these conditions remain important relative contraindications to ACE inhibitor use.

Effects in Patients with Left Ventricular Dysfunction and Heart Failure After Acute Myocardial Infarction

After trials that demonstrated improved ventricular function with ACE inhibitor treatment in patients with asymptomatic left ventricular dysfunction after myocardial infarction (Fig. 24–4),[40, 41] several large-scale mortality studies were performed. In the Survival and Ventricular Enlargement (SAVE) trial,[42] 2231 patients with LVEF less than 40% but without overt heart failure were randomized to double-blind treatment 3 to 16 days after myocardial infarction with captopril 12.5 mg three times daily or placebo, increasing to 50 mg three times daily if tolerated. During an average follow-up period of 42 months, all-cause mortality was reduced significantly from 24.6% in the placebo group to 20.4% in the captopril group (relative risk reduction 19%, $P = 0.019$) (Fig. 24–5). The proportion of patients requiring hospitalization for congestive heart failure and the risk of fatal or nonfatal myocardial infarction were significantly reduced with captopril treatment.

The SOLVD Prevention trial[43] evaluated 4228 patients with LVEF less than 35% without clinical heart failure, most of whom had had previous myocardial infarction more than 1 month before entry. Patients were randomized to double-blind enalapril 2.5 mg twice daily, increasing to 10 mg twice daily, or placebo, for an average follow-up of about 3 years. During this time, mortality was 15.8% in the placebo group and 14.8% in the enalapril group (relative risk reduction 8%, $P = 0.30$). Enalapril significantly reduced the number of hospitalizations for heart failure and the incidence of heart failure, and fewer patients were observed to develop recurrent myocardial infarction.

In the Trandolapril in Patients with Reduced Left Ventricular Function After AMI (TRACE) trial,[44] 1749 patients with left ventricular dysfunction (echocardiographic wall motion index ≤1.2) were randomized to double-blind treatment 3 to 7 days after myocardial infarction with 1 mg daily of trandolapril, increasing to 4 mg daily, or placebo. Patients were followed for a minimum of 2 years. Mortality was 34.7% in the trandolapril group compared with 42.3% in the placebo group (relative risk reduction 18%, $P < 0.001$).

The Acute Infarction Ramipril Efficacy (AIRE) study[45] investigated the efficacy of therapy with ramipril in a select high-risk group of patients with clinical heart failure after acute myocardial infarction. Patients with definite myocardial infarction and clinical or radiographic evidence of left ventricular failure were randomized between day 3 and day 10 after myocardial infarction to double-blind treatment with 2.5 mg twice daily of ramipril, increasing to 5 mg twice daily, or placebo. A total of 2006 patients were randomized to treatment for a minimum of 6 months and an average of 15 months. Mortality was reduced from 23% in the placebo group to 17% in the ramipril group (relative risk reduction 27%, $P = 0.002$) (Fig. 24–6).

A number of studies have evaluated the effect of ACE inhibition with a nonselective approach to treatment begun within 24 hours of acute myocardial infarction. These studies, including the CONSENSUS-2 trial,[46] International Study of Infarct Study-4 (ISIS-4),[47] Gruppo Italiano per lo Studio della Sopravvivenza nell'Infarto Miocardico-3 (GISSI-3),[48] and the Chinese Cardiac Study-1 (CCS-1),[49] together with a number of other small trials, have been pooled together to provide an overview of the early treatment benefit derived from this generalized approach. More than 100,000 patients were randomized to ACE inhibitor treatment or placebo in these trials,[50] with follow-up from 1 to 6 months. Overall, early mortality was reduced from 7.73% to 7.27% ($P = 0.006$).

Finally, the efficacy of treatment with ACE inhibi-

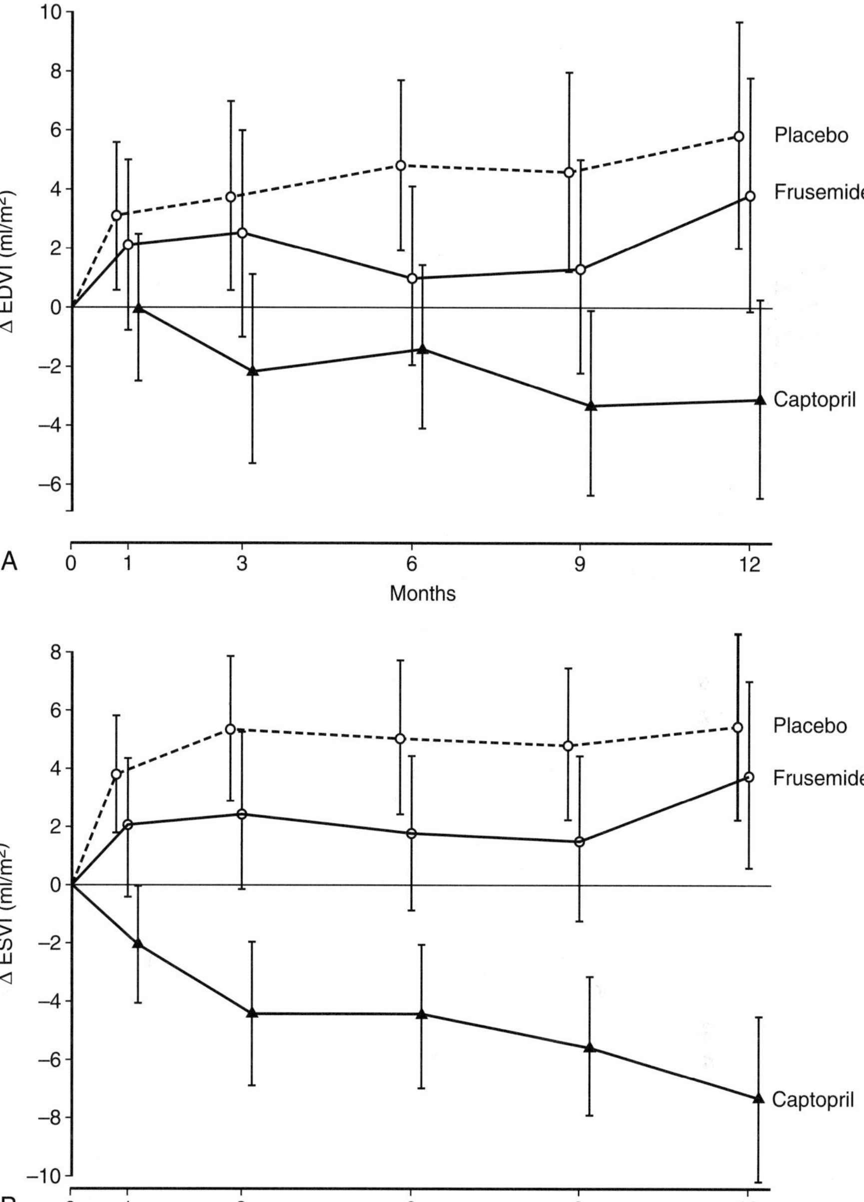

Figure 24–4 Captopril and left ventricular (LV) dysfunction after myocardial infarction: effect on LV volumes. Adjusted mean differences from baseline at 1, 3, 6, 9, and 12 months for the three treatment groups for *(A)* LV end-diastolic volume index (LVEDVI) and *(B)* LV end-systolic volume index (LVESVI). Values are least squares means with least significant difference intervals ($P < 0.05$). (*A* and *B* From Sharpe N, Murphy J, Smith H, et al. Treatment of patients with symptomless left ventricular dysfunction after myocardial infarction. Lancet 1988; 1:255–259. © by The Lancet Ltd., 1988.)

tion initiated selectively in patients with anterior myocardial infarction within 24 hours has been evaluated. In the Survival of Myocardial Infarction Long-Term Evaluation (SMILE) study,[51] zofenopril treatment in patients with acute anterior myocardial infarction not eligible for thrombolysis significantly reduced the combined endpoint of death or severe heart failure during 6 weeks of treatment.

Overall, these data allow a clear recommendation for ACE inhibitor treatment in patients with left ventricular dysfunction or heart failure after acute myocardial infarction. In general, a selective high-risk approach is favored. Treatment should be considered in patients with Q wave infarction, particularly anterior infarction, and those with left ventricular dysfunction or heart failure who are clinically stable within the first 24 to 48 hours, avoiding undue delay. Initiation of such treatment may be limited by low blood pressure, particularly if concomitant beta blocker treatment is administered. No trials have compared ACE inhibitor with beta blocker treatment, or a combination of both, after myocardial infarction. It is likely, however, that combination treatment, if tolerated, may provide complementary benefit through different mechanisms.

Digitalis

Digitalis has been applied in the treatment of heart failure for centuries and was first scientifically investi-

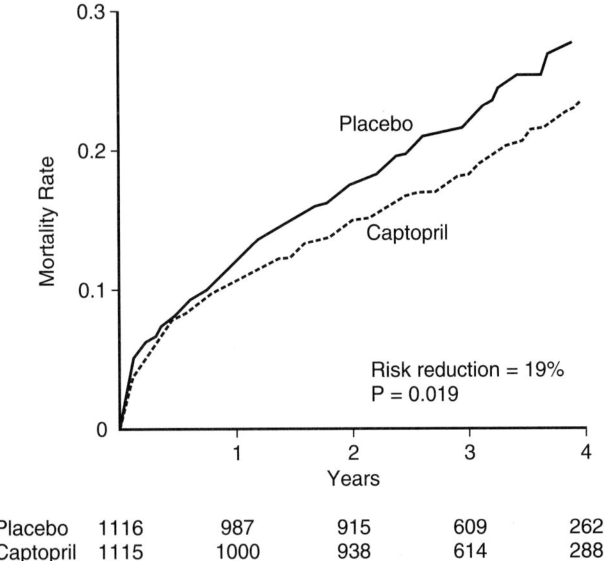

Figure 24–5 SAVE Trial: cumulative mortality from all causes in the study groups. (From Pfeffer MA, Braunwald E, Moyé LA, et al, for the SAVE Investigators. Effect of captopril on mortality and morbidity in patients with left ventricular dysfunction after myocardial infarction: Results of the Survival and Ventricular Enlargement [SAVE] trial. N Engl J Med 1992; 327:669–677. Copyright 1992, Massachusetts Medical Society. All rights reserved.)

gated more than 200 years ago.[52] Its value in the management of patients with heart failure and atrial fibrillation for heart rate control is generally accepted, but the role of digoxin in patients with heart failure in sinus rhythm has been uncertain and controversial until recently. Early studies demonstrated hemodynamic improvement after digoxin treatment in patients with chronic heart failure in sinus rhythm, but long-term efficacy remained unclear.

A number of small, single-center, randomized, controlled trials were carried out during the 1980s.[53–60]

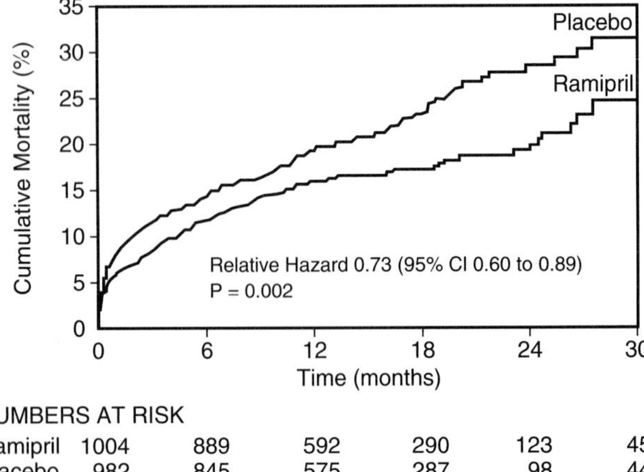

Figure 24–6 AIRE Trial: Mortality curves illustrating the primary endpoint of all-cause mortality analyzed by intention to treat. (From Acute Infarction Ramipril Efficacy (AIRE) Study Investigators. Effect of ramipril on mortality and morbidity of survivors of acute myocardial infarction with clinical evidence of heart failure. Lancet 1993; 342:821–828. © by The Lancet Ltd., 1993.)

In most of these trials, many patients had received previous digoxin treatment, and treatment withdrawal was carried out before randomization. This aspect as well as various other methodologic difficulties associated with the studies has made interpretation difficult. Overall the hemodynamic and symptomatic results from the studies were variable, although six of the seven studies that assessed left ventricular contractile function showed improvement, and four of the eight studies demonstrated a significant reduction in worsening heart failure with digoxin treatment.[53–60] From the late 1980s to the present, a further series of larger, multicenter, randomized, controlled trials has been reported, including some active controlled comparative studies, two similar withdrawal trials, and finally the recently reported definitive Digitalis Investigation Group (DIG) mortality study.[67]

The Captopril-Digoxin trial[33] (previously outlined in the ACE inhibitor section) compared captopril, digoxin, and placebo in 196 patients, 84% of whom were on diuretics and 65% of whom had previously been on digoxin. Digoxin significantly improved LVEF by 4.4%, but captopril did not produce a significant change. Captopril significantly prolonged exercise time by 14%, compared with a 6% increase in the placebo group, the intermediate 10% increase in the digoxin group being not significantly different from captopril or placebo. Worsening heart failure was significantly reduced from 29% in the placebo group to 15% in the digoxin group ($P < 0.05$), and captopril was similarly effective.

In the German and Austrian Xamoterol trial,[61] 433 patients with mild to moderate symptoms of heart failure but with no documentation of left ventricular systolic dysfunction were randomized to digoxin, xamoterol, or placebo. After 3 months, patients on digoxin therapy demonstrated some improvement in symptoms and signs of heart failure, but there was no effect on exercise capacity.

In the Milrinone Multicenter trial,[62] 230 patients with an average LVEF of 25% were stabilized on digoxin and diuretic treatment for 4 to 8 weeks then randomized to digoxin, milrinone, a combination of both, or placebo, with diuretic continuing in all groups. In the digoxin continuation group, the LVEF and exercise capacity increased significantly during the 12-week follow-up period, whereas exercise capacity was unchanged in the placebo group, in which treatment failures were greatest.

The Captopril and Digoxin study[63] evaluated the effect of captopril, 25 mg twice daily; digoxin, 0.25 mg daily; and placebo in 222 patients with mild heart failure (NYHA class II) and preserved LVEF. After 1 year of treatment, NYHA class had improved in 45% of the digoxin group, compared with 25% in the placebo group. Symptoms and quality of life improved significantly with digoxin as compared with placebo, but exercise tolerance did not change in either group.

Finally, the Dutch Ibopamine Multicenter trial[64] evaluated 161 patients with mild to moderate heart failure, treated with diuretics alone and randomized to digoxin; ibopamine, a dopamine agonist; or placebo. After 6 months of treatment, exercise capacity was significantly improved in the digoxin group compared with placebo, but there was no difference in the incidence of worsening heart failure between these groups.

Overall, this group of larger studies, despite considerable limitations in terms of study design characteristics and methodology, suggested significant long-term clinical benefit from digoxin treatment. Modest hemodynamic improvement was evident in the two studies in which this was assessed[33, 62] and a reduction in worsening heart failure in two of the five trials.[33, 62]

The Prospective Randomized Study of Ventricular Function and Efficacy of Digoxin (PROVED)[65] and Randomized Assessment of Digoxin and Inhibitors of Angiotensin-Converting Enzyme (RADIANCE)[66] trials had a similar design, the former testing the effects of digoxin withdrawal in patients receiving background treatment with diuretics, the latter testing the effects of digoxin withdrawal in patients receiving treatment with both diuretics and ACE inhibitors. Both were randomized, placebo-controlled withdrawal studies in patients with chronic heart failure and significant exercise limitation (NYHA class II or III) in sinus rhythm and with documented left ventricular systolic dysfunction (LVEF <35%, echocardiographic left ventricular end-diastolic dimension >60 mm). After dose adjustment and stabilization, patients were randomized to continue digoxin or discontinue (placebo group) for a 12-week treatment period. In the PROVED trial,[65] in which a total of 88 patients were randomized, the primary endpoints of treadmill exercise time, incidence of treatment failure, and time to treatment failure all favored the digoxin group, with no difference between groups in the 6-minute walk distance. There was a significant reduction in LVEF and increase in heart rate in the placebo group but no difference in other secondary endpoints between the groups. The results of the RADIANCE trial,[66] which included 178 patients, were similar for the primary endpoints, although the incidence of treatment failure was less in both groups than in the PROVED trial, possibly because of the effect of background ACE inhibitor treatment (Fig. 24–7). Secondary endpoints in the RADIANCE trial more consistently favored the digoxin group than occurred in the PROVED trial, probably because of a larger sample size increasing study power. The trials together clearly indicate the risk of digoxin withdrawal in such a group of patients with chronic heart failure who are stable on maintenance therapy including digoxin.

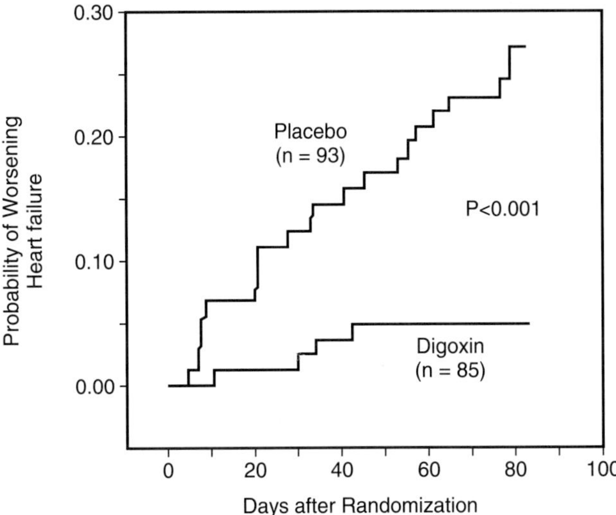

Figure 24–7 RADIANCE Trial: cumulative probability of worsening heart failure in the patients continuing to receive digoxin and those switched to placebo. (From Packer M, Gheorghiade M, Young JB, et al, for the RADIANCE Study. Withdrawal of digoxin from patients with chronic heart failure treated with angiotensin-converting enzyme inhibitors. N Engl J Med 1993; 329:1–7. Copyright 1993, Massachusetts Medical Society. All rights reserved.)

Such withdrawal studies, however, obviously include only patients in whom digoxin introduction has been tolerated and who have survived initial treatment. The question of whether initiation of digoxin is generally beneficial cannot be answered from these studies.

The DIG trial[67] was the first study to provide a reliable assessment of the mortality effect of digoxin treatment in patients with clinical heart failure and left ventricular systolic dysfunction in sinus rhythm. In 301 centers, a total of 7788 patients were randomized to digoxin or placebo and followed for an average of 3 years. Digoxin withdrawal before study entry was required in 43% of the patients, 82% were on diuretic, and 94% were on ACE inhibitor treatment. Cause of heart failure was ischemic heart disease in 69%, and average LVEF was 32%. The primary endpoint of total mortality was not different between the digoxin and placebo groups (1274 and 1263 deaths; OR, 1.0). Heart failure deaths, however, were significantly reduced in the digoxin group (401 vs. 463 deaths; OR, 0.86; $P = 0.03$), this benefit being offset by an adverse trend toward an increase in deaths because of presumed arrhythmia or myocardial infarction in the digoxin group. Hospital admissions because of heart failure were significantly reduced in the digoxin group (975 vs. 1266; OR, 0.72; $P < 0.001$).

A clear perspective on digoxin has now been provided from all these clinical trial data after many years of controversy. Digoxin has a narrow therapeutic-to-toxic ratio, does have significant long-term inotropic effects, and appears to provide modest symptomatic and clinical benefit in the majority of patients. The neutral mortality effect evident in the DIG trial[67] apparently represents the summation of a beneficial effect on heart failure progression, offset by other adverse effects. Patterns of digoxin use vary in different parts of the world, but in general it can now be justifiably recommended as a second-line treatment addition in patients in whom symptoms and signs of heart failure persist, despite optimal diuretic and ACE inhibitor combination treatment.

Alternative Inotropic Agents

Numerous inotropic agents have been assessed for heart failure treatment and can be classified in various ways. Inotropes affect myocardial contractility by increasing the availability of intracellular free calcium through several potential sites of action, and many have other associated effects, including vasodilator, diuretic, and neurohormonal modulating effects. Although beneficial short-term hemodynamic and symptomatic effects can be demonstrated with inotropic agents in general, long-term results of treatment have been disappointing because of adverse effects and, in some cases, increased mortality.

A study in severe heart failure with xamoterol, a β_1-selective partial agonist, was stopped early because a marked increase in mortality within 100 days of randomization of 9.1% was observed in the xamoterol group, compared with 3.7% in the placebo group.[68] Similarly a multicenter trial of intermittent (48 hours per week) dobutamine infusion therapy was terminated because of increased mortality with active therapy.[69]

Most extensive investigation of inotropic agents has been directed toward the phosphodiesterase inhibitors. Although these agents consistently produce short-term hemodynamic and symptomatic improvement,[70–75] tolerance can occur with long-term use,[76, 77] and mortality experience has been unfavorable. Increased mortality has been demonstrated with enoximone[6, 78] and with milrinone[7] in studies prematurely terminated.

Vesnarinone is another agent with phosphodiesterase-inhibiting properties as well as multiple effects on ion channels that has been evaluated in patients with heart failure. In a study that initially aimed at comparing 60 mg or 120 mg of vesnarinone daily with placebo, a significantly higher mortality in the patients receiving 120 mg daily was observed.[8] The study design was then altered, with exclusion of the 120-mg dosage and 60 mg of vesnarinone daily only compared with placebo, showing a significant reduction in mortality with active treatment. These findings led to the conduct of the Vesnarinone Evaluation of Survival Trial (VEST), which compared 30 or 60 mg of vesnarinone daily with placebo. Preliminary analyses reported higher mortality in both active treatment groups compared with placebo.[78a] A similar agent, pimobendan, which also produces hemodynamic and symptomatic improvement,[79, 80] is currently being assessed in a large-scale mortality trial.

Experience with flosequinan, an agent with primary vasodilator properties but with phosphodiesterase-inhibiting activity and positive inotropism at higher dosage,[81, 82] provides further support for the concept of dose-related dissociation of short-term clinical and longer-term mortality effects. This agent has been withdrawn by the manufacturers following the demonstration of increased mortality at higher dosage.[83]

In a meta-analysis of 13 randomized, placebo-controlled trials of phosphodiesterase inhibitors in heart failure, a nonsignificant trend toward an increase in mortality was demonstrated.[84] Analysis of the studies involving agents other than vesnarinone, however, suggested a significantly increased mortality (OR, 1.41) with other phosphodiesterase inhibitors and a reduction with vesnarinone (OR, 0.3). The vesnarinone data are not sufficient to allow any clear recommendation on treatment with this agent, and further clinical trials are required for a reliable estimation of treatment effects.

The clinical trial experience with alternative inotropic agents generally has been disappointing and exemplifies the possibility of both benefit and harm, perhaps dose related, from agents with multiple actions. At present, none of these agents can be recommended for use in heart failure treatment except as short-term or bridging therapy in selected cases.

Beta Blockers

Traditionally, beta blockers have been considered contraindicated in heart failure because of their acute negative inotropic effect. The first report of their application in heart failure described a small group of patients with severe idiopathic dilated cardiomyopathy who appeared to have a favorable clinical response to beta blockade with metoprolol.[85] The same workers later reported a further 24 patients (with 13 control subjects) who showed clinical improvement during beta blockade.[86] It was suggested that, in comparison with historical controls, survival was prolonged with the beta blocker treatment. A further report of patients with idiopathic dilated cardiomyopathy indicated improvement in hemodynamics and symptoms[87] with beta blockade and significant hemodynamic deterioration on withdrawal.[88]

The initial observations suggestive of benefit were all derived from nonrandomized studies, but these observations have since been followed by a number of randomized, placebo-controlled trials of beta blockers in patients with heart failure of different types (Table 24–5).[89] Earlier trials predominantly included

Table 24–5 • Randomized, Controlled Trials of Beta Blockers in Congestive Heart Failure

Trial	Year	No.	Beta Blocker	Follow-up (mo)	DEF (%)*	Exercise
Ikram	1981	17	Acebutolol	1	NA	Decrease
Currie	1984	10	Metoprolol	1	+3.0%	No change
Anderson	1985	50	Metoprolol	19	NA	No change
Engelmeier	1985	25	Metoprolol	12	+2.0%	Increase
Sano	1989	22	Metoprolol	12	NA	NA
Leung	1990	12	Labetalol	2	NA	Increase
Pollock	1990	20	Bucindolol	3	0.0%	Increase
Gilbert	1990	23	Bucindolol	3	+8.0%	No change
Woodley	1991	50	Bucindolol	3	+0.5%	No change
Paolisso	1992	10	Metoprolol	3	NA	Increase
MDC Trial	1992	383	Metoprolol	12–18	+6.0%	No change
Krum	1993	49	Carvedilol	3.5	+5.5%	NA
Olsen	1993	60	Carvedilol	4	+10.0%	NA
Wisenbaugh	1993	29	Nebivolol	3	+8.0%	No change
Fisher	1994	50	Metoprolol	6	+5.0%	NA
Bristow	1994	139	Bucindolol	3	+4.1%	Decrease
Eichhorn	1994	25	Metoprolol	3	+8.0%	NA
CIBIS	1994	641	Bisoprolol	23	NA	NA
Metra	1994	40	Carvedilol	6	+11.0%	No change
ANZ Trial	1995	415	Carvedilol	18–24	+5.2%	No change
Totals		2047			+5.7%	

*DEF = mean difference in ejection fraction % (calculated as mean change during active treatment − mean change during control, and adjusted for number of patients).

From Sharpe N. Beta blockers in heart failure. Heart Failure Rev 1996; 1:5.

patients with idiopathic dilated cardiomyopathy, although more recently more patients with ischemic cardiomyopathy have been studied. Most, but not all, have reported an improvement in symptoms and a reduction in NYHA functional class with longer-term treatment. Studies that did not report improvement generally had a short treatment period and relatively small numbers of patients.

HEMODYNAMIC EFFECTS OF BETA BLOCKADE IN HEART FAILURE

In patients with heart failure principally caused by idiopathic dilated cardiomyopathy, long-term beta blockade has been shown to result in significant hemodynamic improvement with increased left ventricular stroke work index, LVEF, and decreased pulmonary capillary wedge pressure. In the studies that measured ejection fraction, the mean increase in the beta blocker group relative to control was 5.7% (see Table 24–5).[89] The mechanisms of hemodynamic improvement with long-term beta blockade in heart failure are unclear. Acute intravenous beta blockade has been demonstrated to affect left ventricular systolic function adversely.[90] Long-term oral therapy is well tolerated, however, and can result in significant improvement. Most studies investigating the possible mechanisms of improvement have been uncontrolled and have involved small numbers of patients, and the data are conflicting.

Improved contractility after long-term beta blockade has been demonstrated in a placebo-controlled study of nebivolol, a β_1-selective antagonist with vasodilating properties, in patients with dilated cardiomyopathy.[91] This study demonstrated no significant change in wall stress, suggesting that the significant increase in ejection fraction observed was due to improved contractility rather than ventricular unloading. In addition to improvements in resting hemodynamics after beta blockade, improvements have also been demonstrated in cardiac index, stroke volume index, stroke work index, and pulmonary capillary wedge pressure with exercise.[92, 93] In association with these improvements, there was no increase in myocardial oxygen consumption, suggesting increased myocardial workload without higher metabolic costs.

EFFECTS OF BETA BLOCKADE ON EXERCISE TOLERANCE IN HEART FAILURE

The findings related to exercise capacity in these studies have been conflicting. Although some studies have reported statistically significant improvements in total exercise duration with beta blockade, others have not (see Table 24–5).[89] Long-term beta blockade can attenuate maximal oxygen consumption,[94] and, consequently, maximal exercise tolerance testing may not be the appropriate method for assessing an improvement in functional capacity. In a randomized trial of the effects of the vasodilating beta blocker carvedilol, submaximal exercise time (determined by stressing patients at a workload fixed at 85% of their baseline maximal oxygen consumption) was significantly increased in the beta blocker group compared with placebo, whereas maximal exercise time was not changed.[95] A similar study has shown a significant increase in the distance traversed during a 6-minute walk test in the beta blocker–treated group compared with the placebo group.[91] This method of assessing submaximal performance is often preferred by patients and may reflect an improvement in their regular daily physical activity that is better than maximal exercise testing might show.

EFFECTS OF BETA BLOCKADE ON SURVIVAL IN HEART FAILURE

Several larger studies have provided more reliable data on the clinical and mortality effects of beta blockers in heart failure. In these studies, the agents metoprolol, bisoprolol, and carvedilol have been used in patients on standard therapy including ACE inhibitors.

In the Metoprolol in Dilated Cardiomyopathy (MDC) study,[96] 383 patients with heart failure caused by idiopathic cardiomyopathy on standard treatment were randomized to receive either metoprolol or placebo and were followed for 12 to 18 months. There were significant improvements in hemodynamics and symptoms as well as fewer hospital readmissions in the beta blocker–treated group. There was no significant effect on total mortality, but fewer metoprolol-treated patients were placed on the transplant list.

In the Cardiac Insufficiency Bisoprolol Study (CIBIS),[97] 641 patients with heart failure of various causes on standard treatment were randomized to bisoprolol or placebo for a mean period of 1.9 years. Significantly fewer patients in the beta blocker group required hospitalization, and significantly more showed improvement in functional class. There was no significant difference between the groups in mortality.

In the Australia–New Zealand study,[98] 415 patients with chronic stable heart failure of ischemic origin were randomized to carvedilol or placebo for an average follow-up period of 20 months. After 12 months, LVEF had increased by 5.3% ($2P < 0.001$) with left ventricular dimensions significantly decreased (Fig. 24–8). No significant changes occurred in treadmill exercise duration, 6-minute walk distance, or symptom assessment. After 20 months, the rate of death or hospital admission was 50% in the carvedilol group, compared with 63% in the placebo group (relative risk reduction, 26%; $2P = 0.02$).

In a U.S. clinical trial program,[99] the effects of carvedilol were assessed in 1094 patients with chronic heart failure enrolled in a stratified program in which patients were assigned to one of four treatment protocols on the basis of their exercise capacity. Within

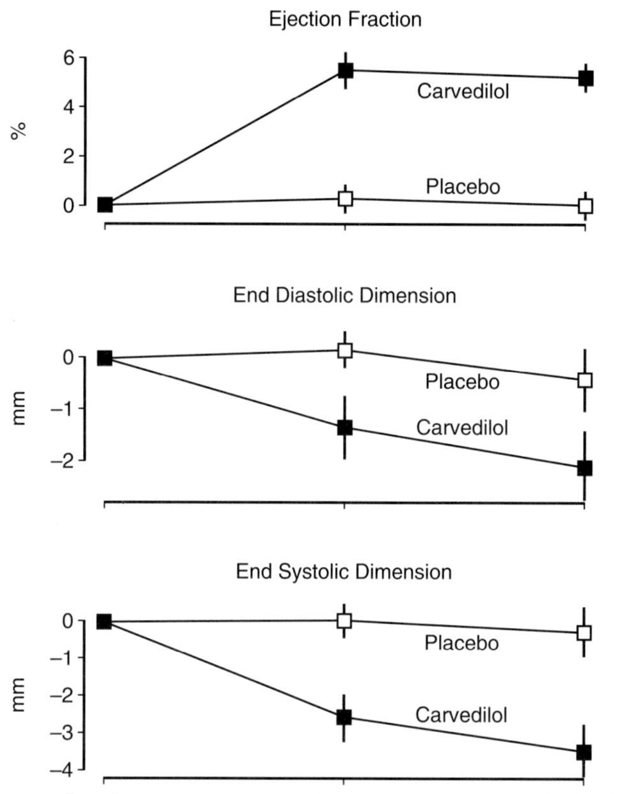

Figure 24–8 Carvedilol in congestive heart failure: effect on left ventricular (LV) function and size. Changes in radionuclide LV ejection fraction and M-mode echocardiographic LV dimensions in carvedilol and placebo groups after 6 and 12 months of follow-up. Values represent mean change from baseline ± SE. (From Randomised, placebo-controlled trial of carvedilol in patients with congestive heart failure due to ischaemic heart disease. Australia/New Zealand Heart Failure Research Collaborative Group. Lancet 1997; 349:375–380. © by The Lancet Ltd., 1997.)

each protocol, patients were randomized to carvedilol (696 patients) or placebo (398 patients). During an average follow-up period of 6.5 months that extended to a maximum of 15 months, the overall mortality rate was 7.8% in the placebo group and 3.2% in the carvedilol group (relative risk reduction, 65%; 95% CI, 39% to 80%; $P < 0.001$). This finding led the Data and Safety Monitoring Board to recommend early termination of the study. In addition, carvedilol therapy reduced the risk of hospitalization from cardiovascular causes from 19.6% to 14.1% ($P = 0.036$) and the combined risk of hospitalization or death from 24.6% to 15.8% ($P < 0.001$). The large mortality reduction with carvedilol remained significant when allowance for early prerandomization deaths during treatment run-in was made. The total number of deaths, however, was similar to that observed in the Australia–New Zealand study, in which the mortality reduction was not significant. A mortality reduction of approximately 30% to 50%, the range in which the CIs from these two studies overlap, may be more plausible as an estimate of true treatment effect.

In an overview of all 24 randomized, controlled trials of beta blocker therapy in heart failure, data involving 3141 patients, a total of 297 deaths and an average follow-up of 13 months have been analyzed.[100] Overall, there was a 31% reduction in the odds of death among patients assigned a beta blocker (95% CI, 11% to 46%; $2P = 0.0035$), representing an absolute reduction in mean annual mortality from 9.7% to 7.5% (Fig. 24–9). The effects on mortality of vasodilating beta blockers (47% reduction; standard deviation [SD] 15), principally carvedilol, were nonsignificantly greater ($2P = 0.09$) than those of standard agents (18% reduction; SD, 15), principally metoprolol. Data for carvedilol alone from 1658 patients, including a total of 105 deaths, showed a similar 49% reduction.

It appears that the most significant benefit of beta blocker treatment in heart failure is improved longevity when added to standard treatment including ACE inhibitors. Although symptoms may be improved in patients with severe heart failure, symptoms may not change in those with more stable heart failure. A cautious, closely monitored dose titration approach is required to achieve optimal outcomes and minimize possible adverse effects. Large-scale studies presently in progress will provide further data and better perspective on the role of beta blockers in future therapy.

Calcium Channel Blockers

Calcium channel blockers have generally been considered contraindicated in patients with left ventricular dysfunction or heart failure. Agents such as verapamil,[101] diltiazem,[102] nifedipine,[103, 104] nisoldipine,[105] and felodipine[106] have all been shown to produce clinical deterioration and adverse effects in such patients. Calcium channel blockers vary widely in their pharmacologic properties, however, and those with primary vasodilator action and gradual onset of action have been thought likely to be better tolerated in patients with heart failure when used primarily for the treatment of angina or hypertension.

In the Prospective Randomized Amlodipine Sur-

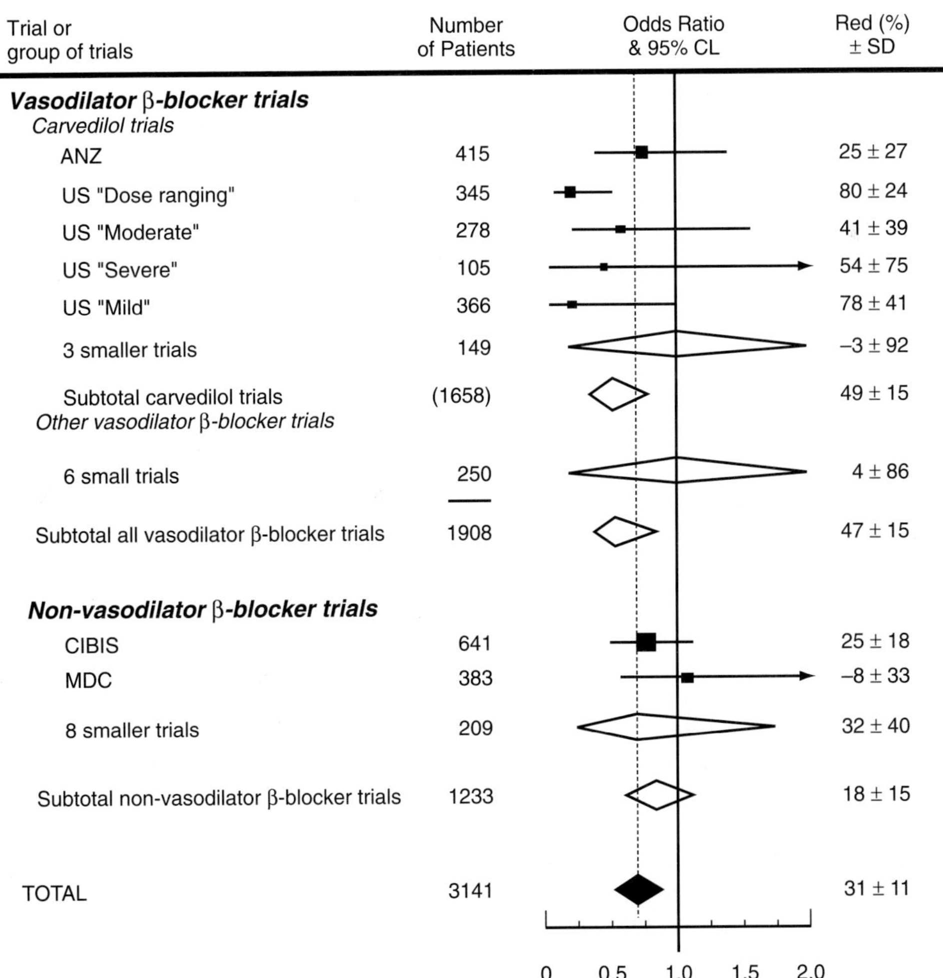

Trial or group of trials
Number of Patients
Odds Ratio & 95% CL
Red (%) ± SD
Vasodilator β-blocker trials
Carvedilol trials
ANZ 415 25 ± 27
US "Dose ranging" 345 80 ± 24
US "Moderate" 278 41 ± 39
US "Severe" 105 54 ± 75
US "Mild" 366 78 ± 41
3 smaller trials 149 –3 ± 92
Subtotal carvedilol trials (1658) 49 ± 15
Other vasodilator β-blocker trials
6 small trials 250 4 ± 86
Subtotal all vasodilator β-blocker trials 1908 47 ± 15
Non-vasodilator β-blocker trials
CIBIS 641 25 ± 18
MDC 383 –8 ± 33
8 smaller trials 209 32 ± 40
Subtotal non-vasodilator β-blocker trials 1233 18 ± 15
TOTAL 3141 31 ± 11
0 0.5 1.0 1.5 2.0

Figure 24–9 Beta blockers in heart failure: overview of mortality effect. (From Doughty RN, Rodgers A, Sharpe N, et al. Effects of beta blocker therapy on mortality in patients with heart failure: A systematic overview of randomized controlled trials. Eur Heart J 1997; 18:560–565.)

vival Evaluation (PRAISE) study,[107] the long-acting dihydropyridine agent amlodipine was assessed in a randomized, double-blind, placebo-controlled study in 1153 patients with severe chronic heart failure (LVEF $< 30\%$) and ischemic or nonischemic cause. After a minimum of 6 months' follow-up (median, 13.8 months), there was no significant difference between groups in the primary endpoint of death or hospitalization for major cardiovascular events. Mortality in the amlodipine group was 33% compared with 38% in the placebo group, a 16% relative risk reduction ($P = 0.07$). There was no difference between treatment groups among patients with ischemic heart disease for either endpoint, whereas in patients with nonischemic cause, amlodipine significantly reduced the combined risk of fatal and nonfatal events as well as the risk of death. This trial established the safety of amlodipine for the treatment of angina or hypertension in patients with heart failure. Possible mortality benefit in patients with nonischemic cardiomyopathy is now being investigated in a further trial.

Amiodarone

Many patients with heart failure die suddenly, about 25% to 50% of deaths in patients with heart failure being attributable to arrhythmias. Thus, effective antiarrhythmic treatment has the potential to reduce mortality other than that due to progressive heart failure alone. The survival benefit of beta blocker treatment may be due, in part, to antiarrhythmic action, but no other agents have been shown to be clearly beneficial.

Two studies have evaluated the role of amiodarone in patients with heart failure. This agent has vasodilator action and relatively low risk of proarrhythmia and appears well tolerated in heart failure. The Study Group on Survival of Heart Failure in Argentina (GESICA) trial from South America randomized 516 patients with heart failure to amiodarone or placebo.[108] Amiodarone dosage was relatively low at 600 mg daily for 14 days, followed by 300 mg daily. The mean follow-up period was 13 months, during which mortality was 33.5% in the amiodarone group and 41.4% in the placebo group, a risk reduction of 28% ($P = 0.024$). Hospital admissions for worsening heart failure were also significantly reduced. Five percent of patients stopped amiodarone because of side effects.

The Survival Trial of Antiarrhythmia Therapy in Congestive Heart Failure (CHF-STAT) randomized 674 patients with heart failure to amiodarone or placebo.[109] Amiodarone dosage was higher in this trial at 800 mg daily for 14 days, followed by 400 mg daily for 50 weeks, then 300 mg daily. The mean follow-up period was 45 months, with 2-year actuarial survival similar in both groups—69.4% in the amiodarone group and 70.8% in the placebo group. There was a trend toward reduced mortality among patients with nonischemic cardiomyopathy. Twenty-seven percent of patients stopped amiodarone because of side effects.

There are no obvious reasons for these disparate results, although in the GESICA trial the majority of patients had nonischemic causes, whereas in the CHF-STAT trial, nearly three quarters had ischemic heart disease. The CHF-STAT trial did show a trend toward mortality reduction among patients with nonischemic causes as was found in the GESICA trial. These studies have demonstrated the safety of amiodarone in heart failure with a possible beneficial effect in patients with nonischemic heart disease. Amiodarone is the preferred antiarrhythmic drug in patients with heart failure who require treatment for supraventricular arrhythmias or symptomatic ventricular arrhythmias. Its general use in patients with ischemic heart disease and heart failure with asymptomatic ventricular arrhythmias is not recommended.

d-Sotalol

Following studies with amiodarone, which prolongs action potential duration by potassium channel blockade, it was considered that other potassium channel blockers lacking the toxicity of amiodarone might be beneficial. Thus, *d*-sotalol, a pure potassium channel blocker with no clinically significant beta-blocking effect, was assessed in patients with an LVEF of 40% or less after myocardial infarction.[110] Patients were randomized to 100 mg of *d*-sotalol increasing to 200 mg twice daily if tolerated or placebo. The trial was stopped when approximately half the planned 6400 patients had been recruited when a significant excess mortality in the patients treated with *d*-sotalol was observed. Among 3121 patients with a mean follow-up of 148 days, there was a mortality of 5.0% in *d*-sotalol-treated patients compared with 3.1% in the placebo group (relative risk increase, 65%; $P = 0.006$). Presumed arrhythmic deaths accounted for this increase, and the effect was greater in patients with an LVEF 31% to 40% than in those with lower ejection fractions. As in other studies, this finding emphasizes the importance of mortality data rather than surrogate endpoints to define treatment effects.

New Treatments

Angiotensin II receptor antagonists offer the possibility of an alternative means of potentially more complete blockade of the renin-angiotensin-aldosterone system without the adverse effects associated with ACE inhibition. The AT_1 receptor antagonist losartan is now being applied in hypertension treatment, and its hemodynamic effects in heart failure appear similar to ACE inhibition.[111, 112] Early experience with AT_1 receptor antagonists suggests freedom from the adverse effects of cough and angioneurotic edema that can occur with ACE inhibitors. As yet, no large-scale study data are available with angiotensin II receptor antagonists in heart failure, and their role in heart failure treatment remains to be defined.

Inhibition of the neutral endopeptidase enzyme responsible for natriuretic peptide degradation increases natriuretic peptide levels, producing natriuresis, diuresis, and vasodilation without the disadvantage of renin-angiotensin-aldosterone system stimulation induced by loop diuretics. Candoxatril, an orally active prodrug metabolized to candoxatrilat, a specific inhibitor of neutral endopeptidase, produces natriuresis and reduction in pulmonary artery wedge pressure.[113] Clearance of angiotensin II may be diminished,[114] however, and thus the combination of a neutral endopeptidase inhibitor with an ACE inhibitor is currently undergoing clinical trials.[115] Such a combination would have advantages over the current standard treatment combination of a loop diuretic and ACE inhibitor.

CONCLUSIONS

The clinical trials reviewed in this chapter have defined important advances in the treatment of congestive heart failure during the past 20 to 30 years. Management can now be directed effectively toward prevention or slowing progression in early disease and symptomatic relief with improved survival in more advanced cases. Despite these advances, the prognosis for heart failure patients still remains poor, with considerable potential for improvement. There remains a need for a more comprehensive approach to heart failure management generally, including clinical assessment, treatment planning, patient education and counseling to ensure compliance, and planned follow-up. Further substantial gains can be realized with such an approach, with more general application of treatments of proven benefit currently available as well as continuing clinical research endeavors.

REFERENCES

1. Schocken DD, Arrieta MI, Leaverton PE, et al. Prevalence and mortality rate of congestive heart failure in the United States. J Am Coll Cardiol 1992; 20:301–306.
2. Yusuf S, Thom T, Abbott RD. Changes in hypertension treatment and in congestive heart failure mortality in the United States. Hypertension 1989; 13(suppl I):I74–I79.
3. McMurray J, Hart W. The economic impact of heart failure on the National Health Service. Br Heart J 1993; 69(suppl):19 (abstract).
4. U.S. Department of Health and Human Services. Clinical Practice Guideline Number 11—Heart Failure: Evaluation and care of patients with left ventricular systolic dysfunction. AHCPR Publication No. 94–0612. 1994. Washington, DC, US Government Printing Office.
5. Ghali JK, Cooper R, Ford E. Trends in hospitalisation rates for heart failure in the United States, 1973–1986. Arch Intern Med 1990; 150:769–773.
6. Cowley AJ, Skene AM. Treatment of severe heart failure: Quantity or quality of life? A trial of enoximone. Br Heart J 1994; 72:226–230.
7. Packer M, Carver JR, Rodeheffer RJ, et al. Effect of oral milrinone on mortality in severe chronic heart failure. N Engl J Med 1991; 325:1468–1475.
8. Feldman AM, Bristow MR, Parmley WW, et al. Effects of vesnarinone on morbidity and mortality in patients with heart failure. N Engl J Med 1993; 329:149–155.
9. Lipicki RJ, Packer M. Role of surrogate endpoints in the evaluation of drugs for heart failure. J Am Coll Cardiol 1993; 22(suppl A):179A–184A.
10. Cohn J. Who should treat heart failure? J Cardiac Failure 1995; 1:97–99.
11. ACC/AHA Task Force. Committee on Evaluation and Management of Heart Failure: Guidelines for the evaluation and management of heart failure. J Am Coll Cardiol 1995; 26:1376–1398.
12. Task Force on Heart Failure of the ESC. Guidelines for the diagnosis of heart failure. Eur Heart J 1995; 16:741–751.
13. Wong WF, Gold S, Fukuyama O, et al. Diastolic dysfunction in elderly patients with congestive heart failure. Am J Cardiol 1989; 63:1526–1528.
14. Bonow RO, Udelsen JE. Left ventricular diastolic dysfunction as a cause of congestive cardiac failure: Mechanisms and management. Ann Intern Med 1992; 117:502–510.
15. Brutsaert DL, Sys SU, Gillebert TC. Diastolic heart failure: Pathophysiology and therapeutic implications. J Am Coll Cardiol 1993; 22:318–325.
16. Poole-Wilson PA. What are we trying to achieve when we treat heart failure? *In* McMurray JJV, Cleland JGF (eds). Heart Failure in Clinical Practice. London, Martin Dunitz Ltd, 1996
17. Bayliss J, Norell M, Canepa-Anson R, et al. Untreated heart failure: Clinical and neuroendocrine effects of introducing diuretics. Br Heart J 1987; 57:17–22.
18. Ikram H, Chan W, Espiner EA, et al. Haemodynamic and humoral response to acute and chronic furosemide therapy in congestive heart failure. Clin Sci 1980; 59:443–449.
19. Richardson A, Bayliss J, Scriven AJ, et al. Double-blind comparison of captopril alone against furosemide plus amiloride in mild heart failure. Lancet 1987; 2:709–711.
20. Cowley AJ, Stainer K, Wynne, et al. Symptomatic assessment of patients with heart failure: Double-blind comparison of increasing doses of diuretics and captopril in moderate heart failure. Lancet 1986; 2:770–772.
21. Dzau VJ, Hollenberg NK. Renal response to captopril in severe heart failure: Role of furosemide in natriuresis and reversal of hyponatremia. Ann Intern Med 1984; 100:777–782.
22. Anand IS, Kalka KS, Ferrari R, et al. Enalapril as sole treatment in severe chronic heart failure with sodium retention. Int J Cardiol 1990; 28:341–346.
23. Arnold SB, Williams RL, Ports TH, et al. Attenuation of prazosin effect on cardiac output in chronic heart failure. Ann Intern Med 1979; 91:345–349.
24. Flaherty JT. Nitrate tolerance—a review of the evidence. Drugs 1989; 37:523–550.
25. David R, Ribner HS, Keung E, et al. Treatment of chronic congestive heart failure with captopril, an oral inhibitor of angiotensin converting enzyme. N Engl J Med 1979; 301:117–121.
26. Ader R, Chatterjee K, Ports T, et al. Immediate and sustained hemodynamic and clinical improvement in chronic heart failure by angiotensin-converting enzyme inhibitors. Circulation 1980; 61:931–937.
27. Levine TB, Franciosa JA, Cohn JN. Acute and long-term response to an oral converting enzyme inhibitor, captopril, in congestive heart failure. Circulation 1980; 62:35–41.
28. Creager MA, Massie BM, Faxon DP, et al. Acute and long-

term effects of enalapril on the cardiovascular response to exercise and exercise tolerance in patients with congestive heart failure. J Am Coll Cardiol 1985; 6:163–170.
29. Kramer BL, Massie BM, Topic N. Controlled trial of captopril in chronic heart failure: A rest and exercise hemodynamic study. Circulation 1983; 67:807–816.
30. Sharpe DN, Murphy J, Coxon R, et al. Enalapril in patients with chronic heart failure: A placebo-controlled, randomized, double-blind study. Circulation 1984; 70:271–278.
31. Cleland JGF, Dargie HJ, Hodsman GP, et al. Captopril in heart failure: A double-blind controlled trial. Br Heart J 1984; 52:530–535.
32. Captopril Multicentre Research Group. A placebo-controlled trial of captopril in refractory chronic congestive heart failure. J Am Coll Cardiol 1983; 2:755–763.
33. Captopril-Digoxin Multicentre Research Group. Comparative effects of therapy with captopril and digoxin in patients with mild to moderate heart failure. JAMA 1988; 259:539–544.
34. Narang R, Swedberg K, Cleland JGF. What is the ideal study design for evaluation of treatment for heart failure? Insights from trials assessing the effect of ACE inhibitors on exercise capacity. Eur Heart J 1996; 17:120–134.
35. CONSENSUS Trial Group. Effects of enalapril on mortality in severe congestive heart failure: Results of the Cooperative North Scandanavian Enalapril Survival Study (CONSENSUS). N Engl J Med 1987; 316:1429–1435.
36. SOLVD Investigators. Effect of enalapril on survival in patients with reduced left ventricular ejection fractions and congestive heart failure. N Engl J Med 1991; 325:293–302.
37. Cohn JN, Johnson G, Ziesche S, et al. A comparison of enalapril with hydralazine-isosorbide dinitrate in the treatment of chronic congestive heart failure. N Engl J Med 1991; 325:303–310.
38. Cohn JN, Archibald DG, Ziesche S, et al. Effect of vasodilator therapy on mortality in chronic congestive heart failure. N Engl J Med 1986; 314:1547–1552.
39. Garg R, Yusuf S. Overview of randomized trials of angiotensin-converting enzyme inhibitors on mortality and morbidity in patients with heart failure. JAMA 1995; 273:1450–1456.
40. Sharpe N, Murphy J, Smith H, et al. Treatment of patients with symptomless left ventricular dysfunction after myocardial infarction. Lancet 1988; 1:255–259.
41. Pfeffer MA, Lamas GA, Vaughan DE, et al. Effect of captopril on progressive ventricular dilatation after anterior myocardial infarction. N Engl J Med 1988; 319:80–86.
42. Pfeffer MA, Braunwald E, Moyé LA, et al, for the SAVE Investigators. Effect of captopril on mortality and morbidity in patients with left ventricular dysfunction after myocardial infarction: Results of the Survival and Ventricular Enlargement (SAVE) trial. N Engl J Med 1992; 327:669–677.
43. SOLVD Investigators. Effect of enalapril on mortality and the development of heart failure in asymptomatic patients with reduced left ventricular ejection fractions. N Engl J Med 1992; 327:685–691.
44. Kober L, Torp-Pedersen C, Carlsen JE, et al. A clinical trial of the angiotensin-converting-enzyme inhibitor trandolapril in patients with left ventricular dysfunction after myocardial infarction. N Engl J Med 1995; 333:1670–1676.
45. Acute Infarction Ramipril Efficacy (AIRE) Study Investigators. Effect of ramipril on mortality and morbidity of survivors of acute myocardial infarction with clinical evidence of heart failure. Lancet 1993; 342:821–828.
46. Swedberg K, Held P, Kjekshus J, et al, for the CONSENSUS II Study Group. Effects of the early administration of enalapril on mortality in patients with acute myocardial infarction. N Engl J Med 1992; 327:678–684.
47. ISIS-4 Collaborative Group. ISIS-4: A randomized factorial trial assessing early oral captopril, oral mononitrate and intravenous magnesium sulphate in 58,050 patients with suspected acute myocardial infarction. Lancet 1995; 345:669–685.
48. Gruppo Italiano per lo Studio della Sopravvivenza nell'Infarto Miocardico. GISSI-3: Effects of lisinopril and transdermal glyceryl trinitrate singly and together on 6-week mortality and ventricular function after acute myocardial infarction. Lancet 1994; 343:1115–1122.
49. Chinese Cardiac Study Collaborative Group. Oral captopril versus placebo among 13,634 patients with suspected acute myocardial infarction: Interim report from the Chinese Cardiac Study (CCS-1). Lancet 1995; 345:686–687.
50. Latini R, Maggioni AP, Flather M, et al. ACE inhibitor use in patients with myocardial infarction. Circulation 1995; 92:3132–3137.
51. Ambrosioni E, Borghi C, Magnani B, for the Survival of Myocardial Infarction Long-term Evaluation (SMILE) Study Investigators. The effect of the angiotensin-converting-enzyme inhibitor zofenopril on mortality and morbidity after anterior myocardial infarction. N Engl J Med 1995; 332:80–85.
52. Withering W. An Account of the Foxglove and Some of Its Medical Uses: With Practical Remarks on Dropsy and Other Diseases. London, M Swinney, 1785.
53. Dobbs S, Kenyon W, Dobbs R. Maintenance digoxin after an episode of heart failure: Placebo controlled trial in outpatients. BMJ 1977; 1:749–752.
54. Lee D, Johnson R, Bingham J, et al. Heart failure in outpatients: A randomized trial of digoxin versus placebo. N Engl J Med 1982; 306:699–705.
55. Fleg L, Gottlieb S, Lakalta E. Is digoxin really important in compensated heart failure? Am J Med 1982; 73:244–250.
56. Taggart A, Johnston G, McDevitt D. Digoxin withdrawal after cardiac failure in patients with sinus rhythm. J Cardiovasc Pharmacol 1983; 5:229–234.
57. Guyatt G, Sullivan M, Fallen E, et al. A controlled trial of digoxin in congestive heart failure. Am J Cardiol 1988; 61:371–375.
58. Pugh S, White N, Aronson J, et al. Clinical, hemodynamic and pharmacological effects of withdrawal and reintroduction of digoxin in patients with heart failure in sinus rhythm after long-term treatment. Br Heart J 1989; 61:529–539.
59. Fleg J, Rothfeld B, Gottlieb S. Effect of maintenance digoxin therapy on aerobic performance and exercise left ventricular function in mild to moderate heart failure due to coronary artery disease: A randomise placebo-controlled crossover trial. J Am Coll Cardiol 1991; 17:743–751.
60. Haerer W, Bauer U, Hetzel M, et al. Long-term effects of digoxin and diuretics in congestive heart failure: Results of a placebo-controlled randomized double-blind study. Circulation 1988; 78:53.
61. German and Austrian Xamoterol Study Group. Double-blind placebo-controlled comparison of digoxin and xamoterol in chronic heart failure. Lancet 1988; 1:489–493.
62. DiBianco R, Shabetai R, Kostuk W, et al, for the Milrinone Multicenter Trial Group. A comparison of oral milrinone, digoxin and their combination in the treatment of patients with chronic heart failure. N Engl J Med 1989; 320:677–683.
63. Just H, Drexler H, Taylor SH, et al. Captopril versus digoxin in patients with coronary artery disease and mild heart failure: A prospective, double-blind, placebo-controlled multicenter study. The CADS Study Group. Herz 1993; 18(suppl 1):436–443.
64. van Veldhuisen DJ, Man in't Veld AJ, Dunselman PH, et al. Double-blind placebo-controlled study of ibopamine and digoxin in patients with mild to moderate heart failure: Results of the Dutch Ibopamine Multicenter Trial (DIMT). J Am Coll Cardiol 1993; 22:1564–1573.
65. Uretsky BF, Young JB, Shahidi FE, et al. Randomised study assessing the effect of digoxin withdrawal in patients with mild to moderate congestive heart failure: Results of the PROVED trial. PROVED Investigative Group. J Am Coll Cardiol 1993; 22:955–962.
66. Packer M, Gheorghiade M, Young JB, et al, for the RADIANCE Study. Withdrawal of digoxin from patients with chronic heart failure treated with angiotensin-converting enzyme inhibitors. N Engl J Med 1993; 329:1–7.
67. Digitalis Investigation Group. The effect of digoxin on mortality and morbidity in patients with heart failure. N Engl J Med 1997; 336:525–533.
68. Xamoterol in Severe Heart Failure Study Group. Xamoterol in severe heart failure. Lancet 1990; 336:1–6.
69. Dies F, Knell MJ, Whitlow P, et al. Intermittent dobutamine in ambulatory outpatients with chronic cardiac failure. Circulation 1984; 74(suppl II):II-39.
70. Maskin CS, Forman R, Klein NA, et al. Long term amrinone

therapy in patients with severe heart failure: Drug dependent hemodynamic benefits despite progression of the disease. Am J Med 1982; 72:113–118.
71. Baim DS, McDowell AD, Cherniles J, et al. Evaluation of a new bipyridine inotropic agent—milrinone—in patients with severe congestive heart failure. N Engl J Med 1983; 309:748–756.
72. Petein M, Levine TB, Cohn JN. Persistent hemodynamic effects without long term clinical benefits in response to oral piroximone (MDL 19205) in patients with congestive heart failure. Circulation 1986; 73(suppl III):III-230.
73. Hermann HC, Ruddy TD, Dec GW, et al. Inotropic effect of enoximone in patients with severe heart failure: Demonstration by left ventricular end systolic pressure volume analysis. J Am Coll Cardiol 1987; 9:1117–1123.
74. Packer M, Narahara KA, Elkayam U, et al. Double-blind, placebo-controlled study of the efficacy of flosequinan in patients with chronic heart failure. J Am Coll Cardiol 1993; 22:65–72.
75. Asanoi H, Sassayama S, Kameyama T, et al. Sustained inotropic effects of a new cardiotonic agent OPC-8212 in patients with chronic heart failure. Clin Cardiol 1989; 12:133–138.
76. Packer M, Medina N, Yushak M. Haemodynamic and clinical limitations of long-term inotropic therapy with amrinone in patients with severe chronic heart failure. Circulation 1984; 70:1038–1047.
77. Shah PK, Amin DK, Hilse S, et al. Inotropic therapy for refractory congestive heart failure with oral fenoximone (MDL 17,043): Poor long term results despite early hemodynamic and clinical improvement. Circulation 1985; 71:326–331.
78. Uretsky BF, Jessup M, Konstam MA, et al. Multicenter trial of oral enoximone in patients with mderate to moderately severe congestive heart failure: Lack of benefit compared with placebo. Circulation 1990; 82:774–780.
78a. Feldman AM, Young J, Bourge R, et al. Mechanism of increased mortality from vesnarinone in the severe heart failure trial (VEST). J Am Coll Cardiol 1997; 29(2 Suppl A):64A.
79. Hasenfuss G, Holubarsch C, Heiss HW, et al. Influence of the calcium sensitiser UDCG-115 on haemodynamics and myocardial energetics in patients with idiopathic dilated cardiomyopathy: Comparison with nitroprusside. *In* Just HJ, Holubarsch CH, Scholz H (eds). Inotropic Stimulation and Myocardial Energetics. New York, Springer, 1989, pp 225–233.
80. Kubo SH, Gollub S, Bourge R, et al. Beneficial effects of pimobendan on exercise tolerance and quality of life in patients with heart failure: Results of a multicenter trial. Circulation 1992; 85:942–949.
81. Weishaar RE, Kirker ML, Wallace AM, et al. Relationship between inotropic activity and phosphodiesterase activity inhibition for flosequinan and milrinone. Eur J Pharmacol 1993; 236:363–366.
82. Kelso EJ, McDermott BJ, Silke B. Actions of the novel vasodilator, flosequinan, in isolated ventricular cardiomyocytes. J Cardiovasc Pharmacol 1995; 25:376–386.
83. Boots Company. Warning on flosequinan. Lancet 1993; 341:1146.
84. Nony P, Boissel JP, Leizorovic A, et al. Evaluation of the effect of phosphodiesterase inhibitors in mortality on chronic heart failure patients. Eur J Clin Pharmacol 1994; 46:191–196.
85. Waagstein F, Hjalmarson A, Varnauskas E, et al. Effect of chronic beta-adrenergic receptor blockade in congestive cardiomyopathy. Br Heart J 1975; 37:1022–1036.
86. Swedberg K, Hjalmarson A, Waagstein F, et al. Prolongation of survival in congestive cardiomyopathy by beta-receptor blockade. Lancet 1979; 1:1374–1377.
87. Swedberg K, Hjalmarson A, Waagstein F, et al. Beneficial effects of long term beta blockade in congestive cardiomyopathy. Br Heart J 1980; 44:117–133.
88. Swedberg K, Hjalmarson A, Waagstein F, et al. Adverse effects of beta blockade withdrawal in patients with congestive cardiomyopathy. Br Heart J 1980; 44:134–142.
89. Sharpe N. Beta blockers in heart failure. Heart Failure Reviews 1996; 1:5–13.
90. Haber HL, Gimple LW, Simek CI, et al. Why do patients with congestive heart failure tolerate the initiation of beta blocker therapy? Circulation 1992; 86(suppl I):17 (abstract).
91. Wisenbaugh T, Katz I, Davis J, et al. Long term (3 month) effects of a new beta blocker (nebivolol) on cardiac performance in dilated cardiomyopathy. J Am Coll Cardiol 1993; 21:1094–1100.
92. Anderson FL, Port JD, Reid BB, et al. Myocardial catecholamine and neuropeptide Y depletion in failing ventricles of patients with idopathic dilated cardiomyopathy: Correlation with beta-adrenergic receptor down regulation. Circulation 1992; 85:46–53.
93. Nemanich JW, Veith RC, Abrass IB, et al. Effects of metoprolol on rest and exercise cardiac function and plasma catecholomines in chronic congestive heart failure secondary to ischemic or idiopathic cardiomyopathy. Am J Cardiol 1990; 66:843–848.
94. Sweeney ME, Fletcher BJ, Fletcher GF. Exercise testing and training with beta-adrenergic blockade: Role of drug washout period in "unmasking" a training effect. Am Heart J 1989; 118:941–946.
95. Olsen SL, Yanowitz FG, Gilbert EM, et al. Beta blocker related improvement in submaximal exercise tolerance in heart failure from idiopathic dilated cardiomyopathy. J Am Coll Cardiol 1992; 19(suppl A):146A (abstract).
96. Waagstein F, Bristow MR, Swedberg K, et al, for the Metoprolol in Dilated Cardiomyopathy (MDC) Trial Study Group. Beneficial effects of metoprolol in idiopathic dilated cardiomyopathy. Lancet 1993; 342:1441–1446.
97. CIBIS Investigators. A randomized trial of beta blockade in heart failure. The Cardiac Insufficiency Bisoprolol Study. Circulation 1994; 90:1765–1773.
98. Australia–New Zealand Heart Failure Research Collaborative Group. Randomised, placebo-controlled trial of carvedilol in patients with congestive heart failure due to ischemic heart disease. Lancet 1997; 349:375–380.
99. Packer M, Bristow MR, Cohn JN, et al, for the U.S. Carvedilol Heart Failure Study Group. The effect of carvedilol on morbidity and mortality in patients with chronic heart failure. N Engl J Med 1996; 334:1349–1355.
100. Doughty RN, Rodgers A, Sharpe N, et al. Effects of beta blocker therapy on mortality in patients with heart failure: A systematic overview of randomized controlled trials. Eur Heart J 1997; 18:560–565.
101. Mohindra SK, Udeani GO. Long acting verapamil and heart failure. JAMA 1989; 261:994.
102. Goldstein RE, Boccuzzi SJ, Cruess D, et al. Diltiazem increases late inset congestive heart failure in postinfarction patients with early reduction in ejection fraction. Circulation 1991; 83:52–60.
103. Packer M, Lee WH, Medina N, et al. Prognostic importance of the immediate hemodynamic response to nifedipine in patients with severe left ventricular dysfunction. J Am Coll Cardiol 1987; 10:1303–1311.
104. Elayam U, Weber L, McKay C, et al. Spectrum of acute hemodynamic effects of nifedipine in severe congestive heart failure. Am J Cardiol 1985; 56:560–566.
105. Barjon JN, Rouleau JL, Bichet D, et al. Chronic renal and neurohormonal effects of the calcium entry blocker nisoldipine in patients with congestive heart failure. J Am Coll Cardiol 1987; 9:622–630.
106. Littler WA, Sheridan DJ. Placebo controlled trial of felodipine in patients with mild to moderate heart failure: UK Study Group. Br Heart J 1995; 73:428–433.
107. Packer M, O'Connor CM, Ghali JK, et al, for the PRAISE Study Group. Effect of amlodipine on morbidity and mortality in severe chronic heart failure. N Engl J Med 1996; 335:1107–1114.
108. Doval HC, Nul DR, Grancelli HO, et al. Randomised trial of low dose amiodarone in severe congestive heart failure. Lancet 1994; 344:493–498.
109. Singh SN, Fletcher RD, Fisher SG, et al. Amiodarone in patients with congestive heart failure and asymptomatic ventricular arrhythmia. N Engl J Med 1995; 333:77–82.
110. Waldo AL, Camm AJ, de Ruyter H, et al. Effect of d-sotalol on mortality in patients with left ventricular dysfunction after recent and remote myocardial infarction. Lancet 1996; 348:7–12.
111. Gottlieb SS, Dickstein K, Fleck E, et al. Haemodynamic and

neurohormonal effects of the angiotensin II antagonist losartan in patients with congestive heart failure. Circulation 1993; 88:1602–1609.

112. Crozier I, Ikram H, Awan N, et al. Losartan in heart failure: Haemodynamic effects and tolerability. Circulation 1995; 91:691–697.

113. Northridge DB, Jackson NC, Metcalfe MJ, et al. Effects of candoxatril, a novel endopeptidase inhibitor compared to frusemide in mild chronic heart failure. Br J Clin Pharm 1991; 32:645.

114. Richards AM, Wittert GA, Espiner EA, et al. Effect of inhibition of neutral endopeptidase 24.11 on responses to angiotensin II in normal volunteers. Circ Res 1992; 71:1501–1507.

115. Asaad MM, Cheung HS, Brittain R, et al. Inhibitory Selectivity of BMS-186716 and BMS-189921. Princeton, Bristol Myers Squibb Cardiovascular Biochem Report, 1995.

25 Psychosocial Factors*

▶ Robert Allan
▶ Stephen Scheidt

A number of noteworthy clinical trials have demonstrated that psychosocial intervention, generally using group psychotherapy, can improve prognosis for patients with coronary heart disease (CHD). These trials are supported by a rapidly accumulating epidemiologic and laboratory database that links psychosocial factors, such as depression, social isolation, type A behavior, hostility, and vital exhaustion, with poor outcome from CHD. A new specialty, *cardiac psychology*, has emerged from what is now a fairly substantial empiric literature.[1] Within the most recent past, however, one large clinical trial has reported null findings with a psychological intervention[2] and another, using home visits by nurses,[3] found that psychosocial intervention *increased* mortality for women. Thus, the field, with a longstanding history of controversy since the introduction of the type A behavior pattern (TABP) in the late 1950s, continues to be highly provocative.

Important recent developments in clinical cardiology suggest that lifestyle intervention programs *should* be helpful for patients with CHD. First, observations made during repeat cardiac catheterization show that subclinical atherosclerotic lesions can progress rapidly, within only 6 months to a year, to become culprit lesions, triggering cardiac events such as myocardial infarction (MI) and sudden cardiac death (SCD).[4–6] Indeed, Little and associates[7] reported that more than half of MIs occur at sites without a significant visible stenosis on a previous angiogram. Additionally, patients suffering from unstable angina, even if medically stabilized, may be particularly vulnerable to rapid progression of atherosclerosis, particularly at sites of complex lesions.[8, 9] Clearly, it is important that CHD patients slow or halt the progression of atherosclerosis to avoid future morbid events.

Second, a number of clinical trials have demonstrated that it is possible to stabilize and even reverse atherosclerotic plaques[4, 5, 10–12] and improve myocardial perfusion.[13] Although the degree of regression has been small (generally only 1% to 2% of coronary artery diameter over short-term follow-up periods, often 1 to 5 years), angina has been reduced dramatically and cardiac events such as unstable angina and MI have been reduced substantially.[14]

Third, in a conclusion reached by a recent consensus panel of distinguished cardiologists[15] and endorsed by the Board of Trustees of the American College of Cardiology,

> Compelling scientific evidence, including data from recent studies in patients with coronary artery disease, demonstrates that comprehensive risk factor interventions: extend overall survival, improve quality of life, decrease need for interventional procedures such as angioplasty and bypass grafting, and reduce the incidence of subsequent myocardial infarction.

However, the panel also noted that

> Studies have demonstrated that only approximately one third of eligible patients continue risk factor interventions over the long term.

Why are so many cardiac patients unable to *maintain* heart-healthy lifestyle changes? We often hear earnest resolutions to reduce coronary-prone behavior from patients in the coronary care units of our hospitals. Such "foxhole resolutions" and "death-bed promises" have typically waned with the passage of time. Perhaps this lessened motivation to change is, in part, a result of reduced fear after patients leave the alien hospital atmosphere and return to their former environments, and cues that in the past have been stimuli for smoking cigarettes, eating high-fat, high-cholesterol foods, maintaining a sedentary lifestyle, and suffering from maladaptive psychosocial behavior patterns, such as easily aroused hostility, social isolation, depression, and vital exhaustion, that have

*Supported in part by the Horace W. Goldsmith Foundation, the Pinewood Foundation, the Nathaniel and Josephine Sokolski Foundation, and the Terner Foundation.

been linked with poor prognosis from CHD. Typically, once patients are past the life-and-death crisis and reinstalled in comfortable surroundings, the powerful forces of "cardiac denial" take hold as many people minimize their status as a "cardiac patient" and return to a "normal life." As one observant patient put it, "you don't notice that the roof leaks until it starts to rain." Apparently, once the sun shines again, psychological defenses insulate many against the unsettling awareness that they are indeed cardiac patients, suffering from the progressive disease that is the leading cause of death and disability in the United States.

Table 25–1 presents the lifestyle changes requested by a typical cardiologist after a patient is diagnosed with CHD. An important question is whether these changes can be managed most effectively by patients independently or with formal intervention. Further, a number of psychosocial factors have been implicated in the development of CHD, such as anger and hostility, type A behavior, psychological stress, "vital exhaustion" (a debilitated emotional and physical condition), anxiety, job strain, and social isolation. Some psychosocial factors, such as depression,[16] social isolation,[17–19] vital exhaustion,[20–23] type D (distressed) personality,[23a] and anger[23] negatively impact prognosis after diagnosis of CHD. Additionally, strenuous exertion,[24] particularly for those who are sedentary (one might wonder about the psychological factors at play when a sedentary person chooses to engage in strenuous exertion), and episodes of anger[25] have been shown to trigger the onset of MI.

A number of studies have demonstrated that modification of psychosocial factors has improved prognosis after diagnosis of CHD.[10, 11, 13, 26, 27] Quality of life is another important consideration, and many CHD patients, particularly those who have had coronary artery bypass graft (CABG) surgery, suffer new-onset depression and/or do not return to work.[28] Psychosocial intervention with such patients may help ameliorate these conditions as well.

TABLE 25–1 • Lifestyle and Behavior Changes Commonly Demanded by Cardiologists at the Time of CHD Diagnosis (Especially Acute MI)

1. Immediate cessation of smoking
2. Major dietary change (prudent diet)
3. Weight loss
4. Various mood- and physiology-altering drugs, especially beta blockers
5. Short-term major decrease in physical, mental, sexual activity
6. (often) Long-term increase in physical activity for fitness
7. (sometimes) Major changes in work responsibilities, including retirement
8. (not infrequently) Body invasion: cardiac catheterization, PTCA, CABG

See text for abbreviations.

CLINICAL TRIALS USING LIFESTYLE INTERVENTION

The literature on psychosocial intervention programs for managing CHD is not large. However, two meta-analyses have examined the interventions that have been tested. In 1987, Nunes and associates[29] reviewed 18 controlled studies for psychological treatment of TABP. Of these, only two provided sufficient information to be included in an analysis of "hard" cardiac endpoints. Nonetheless, these two interventions, a 1979 study by Rahe and colleagues[30] and the 1986 Friedman and associates' Recurrent Coronary Prevention Project (RCPP),[26] reduced recurrent and fatal MI by approximately 50% over 3 years. A 1996 meta-analysis of psychosocial intervention by Linden and associates[31] examined 23 randomized clinical trials, with a total of 2024 patients and 1156 controls. Several of the same studies were included in both meta-analyses. The more recent meta-analysis[31] concluded that the addition of a psychosocial component to standard cardiac rehabilitation protocols reduces cardiac morbidity and mortality, psychological distress, and some biologic risk factors, with benefits clearly evident within the first 2 years, although less marked afterward. Improvements occurred irrespective of the theoretical orientation of the intervention, suggesting that a wide range of psychological theories may be useful in helping CHD patients change lifestyle. Control subjects generally showed a worsening of risk factors and disease.

Table 25–2 describes the studies included in the Linden and associates'[31] meta-analysis. Many of these trials used small numbers of patients and a variety of health care providers and educators, and some studies were completed more than 20 years ago. All interventions took place in groups, a highly cost-effective treatment, particularly when compared with costs for hospitalization and invasive cardiology procedures. Only 14 of the 23 studies reported subsequent mortality or recurrent MI outcomes, endpoints likely considered most important by cardiologists.

Highlights from the Clinical Trial Literature

Clinical trials are the gold standard for scientific validation in both medicine and psychology. One of the strongest arguments for increased attention to cardiac psychology is the reduced morbidity and mortality achieved in a few noteworthy trials. Following are highlights from the most important ones.

Most recently, Blumenthal and associates[32] studied a group of 107 patients with coronary artery disease who demonstrated myocardial ischemia during men-

TABLE 25–2 • Psychosocial Interventions

Source, Year	Ref	Total *N*	Type of Intervention*	Therapists	Available Clinical Endpoints *Anx*	*Dep*	*BP*	*HR*	*Lip*	*Mort*	*Rec*
Adsett and Bruhn, 1968	33	12	Group psychotherapy	MD, PhD	x	x	x	x	x	x	x
Bohachick, 1984	34	37	Relaxation (b)	Unknown	x	x	—	—	—	—	—
Burell, 1996	27	49	Type A behavior reduction, SMT (a)	MD, PhD	—	—	x	x	x	x	x
Burgess et al, 1987	35	180	Individual cognitive therapy	Nurse	x	x	—	—	—	x	—
Clark et al, 1992	36	155	Group education	Health educator	x	—	—	—	—	—	—
Fielding, 1979	40	55	Group counseling, SMT, relaxation training	Unknown	—	x	—	—	—	—	x
Frasure-Smith and Prince, 1989	41	461	As needed psychological support	Nurse	—	—	—	—	—	x	x
Friedman et al, 1986	26	1013	Type A behavior reduction	MD, PhD	—	—	—	—	x	x	x
Gruen, 1975	42	75	Individual counseling	PhD	x	—	—	—	—	x	—
Guzetta, 1989	43	80	Relaxation therapy, music therapy	Nurse	—	—	—	x	—	—	x
Horlick et al, 1984	44	116	Group education and support with spouse	PhD, nurse	x	x	—	—	—	x	—
Munro et al, 1988	45	57	Relaxation therapy with spouse (b)	Nurse	—	—	x	x	—	—	—
Pozen et al, 1977	46	112	Group SMT, education; individual counseling	Nurse	x	—	—	—	—	—	—
Rahe et al, 1975	47	57	Group psychotherapy	MD	—	—	—	—	—	x	x
Rahe et al, 1979	30	44	Group psychotherapy	MD	—	—	—	—	—	x	x
Schulte et al, 1986	48	45	Group psychotherapy	MD, layperson	x	x	—	—	—	—	—
Stern et al, 1983	49	106	Group counseling + relaxation training	MD, nurse, social worker	—	x	—	—	—	x	x
Thompson, 1989	50	60	Group education + individual counseling with spouse	Nurse	x	x	—	—	—	—	—
Thompson and Meddis, 1990	51	60	Individual counseling, education	Nurse	x	x	—	—	—	x	—
Turner et al, 1995	52	24	SMT (b)	Nurse	—	—	x	x	—	—	—
Van Dixhoorn et al, 1987	37	90	Individual therapy, breathing therapy (b)	MD, PhD, PT	—	—	—	—	—	x	x
Van Dixhoorn et al, 1989, 1990	38 39	156	Individual therapy, breathing therapy (b)	MD, PhD, PT	x	—	x	x	—	—	—

*Intervention compared with usual care unless otherwise specified: (a) vs. drugs and group education; (b) vs. drugs and exercise.
Anx, anxiety; Dep, depression; BP, blood pressure; HR, heart rate; Lip, lipids; Mort, mortality; Rec, recurrence; SMT, stress management training; PT, physiotherapist.
Adapted from Linden W, Stossel C, Maurice J. Psychosocial interventions for patients with coronary artery disease. Arch Intern Med 1996; 156:745–752. Copyright 1996, American Medical Association.

tal stress testing or ambulatory electrocardiographic monitoring. Patients were randomly assigned to a 4-month program of "stress management" or exercise training and followed up for a mean of 38 ± 17 (SD) months. The stress management program consisted of 16 1½-hour group sessions and was based on a cognitive-social learning model of behavior. Initial sessions were largely educational and provided information about coronary disease, the structure and function of the heart, risk factors, and psychological stress. Later sessions focused on person-environment interactions and provided techniques for reducing the affective, behavioral, cognitive, and physiologic bases of stress. Patients were also taught progressive muscle relaxation and had at least 2 sessions of electromyographic biofeedback training.

Exercise patients received aerobic group training three times per week, much akin to standard cardiac rehabilitation protocols. A "comparison group" of patients, who lived too far from Duke University Medical Center for regular participation in a follow-up program, served as a nonrandom control.

Compared with controls, stress management patients had a lower relative risk (RR) of a cardiac event (death, nonfatal MI, CABG, or percutaneous transluminal coronary angioplasty [PTCA]), after controlling for ejection fraction, previous MI, and age (RR, 0.26; 95% confidence interval [CI], 0.07 to 0.93; P = 0.04). While the RR of a cardic event was lower for the exercise group than for control subjects, results were not statistically significant.

Additionally, patients in the stress management

group reported less distress ($P < 0.001$) on the General Health Questionnaire (GHQ) and had lower hostility scale scores ($P < 0.05$) than usual-care controls. Patients who experienced more frequent episodes of myocardial ischemia at baseline demonstrated a significant reduction in the number of episodes with both exercise ($P = 0.008$) and stress management ($P = 0.001$), compared with usual-care controls. This study has demonstrated improved cardiac morbidity and quality of life with stress management.

The Lifestyle Heart Trial,[10, 11, 13] by Ornish and associates, demonstrated angiographic evidence for *reversal* of coronary atherosclerosis with lifestyle modification, without drugs or surgery. In addition, positron emission tomography has shown increased perfusion in myocardium that was previously considered necrotic.[13] In this prospective trial, 48 CHD patients were randomized to either a lifestyle intervention program or routine medical care. The program began with a week-long retreat and became a major focus in participants' lives: twice-weekly group sessions included exercise, stress management, yoga and meditation, a communal meal, and group support psychotherapy. A spouse or significant other was encouraged to attend these 4-hour evening meetings. Patients ate a very-low-fat (<7% of calories derived from fat) vegetarian diet. The program required daily yoga practice, including stretching and meditation for 1 hour as well as moderate exercise on days when there were no group sessions. Patients underwent coronary arteriograms before entering the study and again at the end of 1 and 4 years, with coronary artery lesions analyzed by quantitative angiography. After 1 year, 82% of experimental subjects showed regression in atherosclerotic lesions compared with only 42% of controls.[10] After 4 years, average stenosis diameter decreased from 43.6% to 39.7% in experimental patients but progressed from 41.6% to 51.4% in the control group.[11] Patients in the experimental group reported dramatic reductions in the frequency, duration, and severity of angina compared with increases in the control group. Regression of lesions was associated with overall adherence to the program in a dose-response relationship. Quite provocatively, yoga practice was more strongly related to reductions in low-density lipoprotein (LDL) cholesterol levels and regression of coronary lesions than either diet or exercise.[53] Favorable changes in myocardial perfusion, assessed by positron emission tomography, were reported recently, after 5 years of intervention.[13]

One important question raised by the Ornish and colleagues' studies is whether such a radical lifestyle is necessary to delay progression of atherosclerosis. Schuler and associates[12] studied a group of 18 patients with stable angina pectoris "with no more than average motivation and discipline" and found regression of CHD with a more modest lifestyle change program that included a low-fat (<20% of calories), low-cholesterol (<200 mg per day) diet, and at least 3 hours of exercise per week. Patients and their spouses participated in four group discussions during the year and were provided opportunities to talk about personal problems after exercise sessions. At the end of 1 year, 105 stenoses were evaluated by digital angiography, which revealed regression of atherosclerotic lesions in 7 of 18 patients in the treatment group but in only 1 of the 12 patients receiving usual care. Progression of atherosclerosis also occurred at a significantly slower rate in treated patients than controls.

The RCPP[26] was a large ($N = 1012$) TABP modification program for prevention of CHD events after MI. This study demonstrated a 44% reduction in second MI for patients who received 4.5 years of group counseling for TABP and traditional cardiac risk factors compared with controls who received counseling only about traditional cardiac risk factors. The control group was subsequently offered type A counseling and showed a similar reduction in MI recurrence rates over an additional year.[54] The RCPP also determined that type A counseling was most protective against cardiac death for patients with less severe MI,[55] suggesting that psychosocial intervention is most effective when people are still relatively healthy but less beneficial when disease is advanced and physiologic processes predominate. Further, there was a significant reduction in sudden, but not nonsudden, cardiac death for people manifesting type A behavior during a standardized videotaped clinical examination at entry into the study,[56] providing support for the hypothesis that behavioral factors may precipitate lethal arrhythmias.

In a modified replication of the RCPP in Sweden, Burell[27] randomized 268 nonsmoking post-CABG patients to a group program for modification of TABP and cardiac risk factor education or a control group that received routine care by their own physicians. During the first year, intervention patients met for 17 3-hour group sessions with five or six "booster sessions" in years 2 and 3. The behavioral treatment was modeled after the RCPP, with patients encouraged to reduce anger, impatience, annoyance, and irritation in daily life. "Homework assignments," "drills," and relaxation techniques were provided to facilitate self-observation and reduce type A behavior. At follow-up 4.5 years after surgery, there was a significant difference in total (7 vs. 16; $P = 0.02$) and cardiovascular (5 vs. 8; NS) deaths between treatment and control patients, respectively. There were 14 fatal and nonfatal cardiovascular events (reinfarction, reoperation, or PTCA in the intervention group versus 19 in the control group ($P = 0.04$).

Friedman and colleagues[57] were also able to demonstrate reduced myocardial ischemia with psychosocial intervention. In this small study, type A counseling was provided to 10 post-MI volunteers who manifested *silent* ischemia (SI) (>1 mm ST-segment depression on 48-hour Holter monitoring). These studies suggest that SI patients, a sizable segment of the CHD population, might benefit from stress management. SI patients may place themselves in jeopardy because they do not consciously experience anginal pain and are thus unaware of their myocardial ischemia. This may be a particularly fertile population for future research. Both of these interventions were modeled after the treatment provided in the RCPP,[26] described below.

In a creative and practical approach, Frasure-Smith and Prince[41, 58] assessed 461 post-MI male patients' stress levels from the GHQ administered prior to discharge from the hospital and in monthly telephone interviews. Whenever symptoms exceeded a threshold score, nurses made home visits and attempted to resolve whatever problems were causing the patient's distress. An average of five home visits was made during 1 year of intervention. Patients with high inhospital stress scores ($N = 61$) had a nearly threefold risk of cardiac mortality over the next 5 years compared with those with low scores on the initial GHQ ($N = 168$). However, highly stressed patients who were randomized to the home visit intervention did not suffer increased cardiac mortality or recurrent MI compared with controls who had similar high stress scores but did not receive the special intervention. Thus, intervention provided little benefit for patients who had low inhospital stress scores but considerable benefit for patients who were distressed while in the hospital. Although this was an encouraging study, an unexpectedly high proportion of lower-socioeconomic subjects in the control group limited generalizability to the population at large.[59]

A much larger replication using a similar protocol with men *and* women, the Montreal Heart Attack Readjustment Trial (M-HART), was recently reported by Frasure-Smith and coworkers.[3] In this study, 1376 post-MI patients (473 women) were randomized to 1 year of special treatment or usual care. Treated patients received monthly telephone calls to assess stress levels. Over the year, 75% of patients had elevated stress scores on at least one occasion, and they received an average of six 1-hour home visits by nurses with cardiac experience who were under the supervision of psychiatrists. Individually tailored treatment consisted of education, support, and referral to other health resources. There was no overall treatment impact on mortality and no impact on men. Surprisingly, women who received special treatment were marginally more likely to die than those in usual care (hazards ratio, 1.94; CI, 0.89 to 3.80; $P = 0.055$). Frasure-Smith (personal communication, April 17, 1997) speculated that increased mortality may have occurred because home visits interfered with the women's usual coping mechanisms, *elevating* their stress levels. In many cases death was arrhythmogenic in women with low ejection fractions, who may have been physiologically vulnerable to stress. The nurses who made home visits had no special training in mental health but were rather trained in cardiac care and perhaps exacerbated, rather than alleviated, patients' stress.

One recent large study attempted to assess the effectiveness of psychological intervention independent of modification of standard risk factors. Jones and West[2] randomized 2328 post-MI patients in Wales to either seven 2-hour psychological interventions, which included education about CHD and stress, relaxation training, stress management, and individual and group counseling, or routine cardiac care. Although there were reductions in angina and cardiac mortality at 6 months, after 1 year there were no significant differences in psychological factors, which included anxiety and depression, or cardiac endpoints, including utilization of medical services, angina, and mortality.

This study is noteworthy for at least two important reasons. First, the large number of subjects is two thirds as large as all of the interventions combined in the Linden and coworkers' meta-analysis.[31] Second, it shows that seven 2-hour psychotherapy sessions are not sufficient for bringing about behavioral change profound enough to affect either psychological or physiologic variables in the long term. The study was designed according to available financial resources and the "wisdom of the time." However, both data and our clinical experience suggest that it is unlikely that such brief intervention would achieve positive results. The RCPP[26] provided 28 90-minute sessions in the first year before beginning to achieve a reduction in recurrent MI; Project New Life[27] provided 15 or 16 3-hour sessions in the first year followed by "booster sessions" in years 2 and 3 and demonstrated reduced morbidity and mortality; and the Ornish Lifestyle Heart Trial[10, 11, 13] required 14 hours per week to achieve its results, which included improved myocardial perfusion and angiographic evidence of regression of coronary atherosclerosis. In our experience it has been quite difficult for most cardiac patients to change lifelong health habits, and when successful, intervention requires a sustained period of treatment. Jones and West note that their patients rated the program highly but wished that it was more extensive.

The results of this trial and M-HART[3] are disappointing and troubling. Results from M-HART suggest extreme caution in the design of future trials for women. Some have speculated that psychosocial intervention is, at worst, harmless, the greatest downside risk being wasted words and time. We now know that even a well-designed and carefully implemented replication of a promising design can cause harm and must be exceedingly cautious about future trials.

Other noteworthy trials done some time in the past offer more encouraging results. In Finland, Hamalainen and associates[60] studied a group of 375 acute MI patients (74 women) younger than 65 years of age at entry into the study who were provided a comprehensive rehabilitation program that included optimal medical care, exercise, smoking cessation, dietary advice, and discussion of psychological problems. Intervention was most intensive during the first 3 months post MI, but there was close contact with the health care team for 3 years. Patients have been followed for 15 years, with a significantly lower incidence of sudden death (16.5% vs. 28.9%; $P = 0.006$) and coronary mortality (47.9% vs. 58.5%; $P = 0.04$) in the intervention compared with the control group. Total mortality, however, was similar between groups, with death from cancer a "competitive" cause for this aging population. Quite dramatically, the protective effects of the comprehensive cardiac rehabilitation program were significant 12 years after all intervention had ceased.

Some behavioral interventions have focused on psychosocial rather than medical outcomes. In a "wait list control study" performed in England, Trzcieniecka-Green and Steptoe[60a] randomized 50 post-MI and 50 CABG patients to a 10-week relaxation-based stress management program or usual care. After the initial treatment, control subjects were offered the stress management program. Significantly greater improvements were noted for both MI and CABG patients on the Hospital Anxiety and Depression Scale ($P < 0.005$), the Psychological General Well-being Index ($P < 0.001$), activities of daily living, satisfaction with health, and disruption due to chest pain. Relatives also reported better emotional states for treatment patients compared with control subjects. When controls underwent treatment, they too showed reductions in anxiety and depression, but no changes in social or functional status, suggesting that psychosocial intervention is most beneficial in close proximity to a cardic event. "Hard" endpoints, such as recurrent MI or cardiac death, were not assessed.

Outcomes have been attempted at a number of different stages in recovery from MI. Thompson and Meddis[51] reported reduced anxiety and depression for 30 first-time MI patients who received inhospital counseling compared with 30 routine-care control subjects, with benefits sustained for 6 months after discharge. A companion intervention[61] showed lowered anxiety levels for spouses who received counseling compared with routine-care control subjects, both at discharge and 6 months later. Spouses often suffer profound emotional distress around their significant other's cardiac illness and are typically neglected by modern medicine's focus on treating the acute event. This intervention demonstrated the value of including the spouse in treatment, which typically requires major long-term adjustments in living for the entire family.

In a nonrandomized design, Dracup and coworkers[62] compared the results of a 3-month multidimensional rehabilitation program for 41 post-MI and post-CABG patients with 100 routine medical care control subjects. The intervention group received stress management, risk factor counseling, and education that emphasized patient responsibility for health outcome, in addition to three monitored exercise sessions a week for 12 weeks. At 6-month follow-up, patients who attended the comprehensive program were less anxious and depressed and showed better adjustment and marital satisfaction than nonparticipants.

The cited studies are highlights from the clinical trial literature of psychosocial intervention with cardiac patients. Results appear encouraging for future trials using a variety of interventional theories and styles. In the following section we present some of the issues that nearly every cardiac patient is forced to confront. We believe from the available data and more than a decade of clinical experience that risk factor modification will be shown to be far more effective when supported by comprehensive programs led by teams of dedicated health care professionals than if patients are left to make and maintain such changes independently. Changing lifelong habits is difficult, particularly when they are deeply ingrained, as in mid-life, as evidenced by the two thirds of CHD patients who do not maintain heart-healthy habits.[13]

UNIVERSAL ISSUES IN PSYCHOLOGICAL ADJUSTMENT TO CHD

Acceptance of the Diagnosis

Many patients have difficulty truly accepting a diagnosis of CHD: "They tell me I had a heart attack, but I can't believe it" is often heard. Minimization and denial can lead to avoidance of necessary lifestyle change. At least one study found favorable short-term, but unfavorable long-term, effects with denial. Levine and coworkers[63] reported that MI patients scoring high on a denial scale spent fewer days in the coronary care unit than those who scored low; however, 1 year later, high deniers had a greater number of recurrent coronary events and more time in the hospital than those who did not engage in as much denial. These results suggest that health practitioners should wait until after the acute phase of a patient's recovery from MI, when denial may be beneficial, before attempting to overcome this powerful defense mechanism.

Acceptance of the Need for Lifestyle Change

We believe that the optimum time for beginning the rehabilitation process is once the patient is out of life-threatening danger, in the step-down coronary care unit. Coronary risk reduction classes have been widely appreciated by patients at our hospital because they have come to realize that while they have overcome their acute medical crisis, important lifestyle factors may well have contributed to their illness, particularly if they are young and have often indulged in health-damaging behaviors. CHD patients appear highly motivated while still in the hospital, and this is a good time to enroll them in an outpatient program.

The Denial-Overprotectiveness Syndrome

The effect of CHD on the spouse or significant other and members of the patient's family is also an important consideration. Initially, family members often regard the patient as fragile, as if any little stress might trigger another heart attack. This can occur at the expense of the patient's self-image as a strong and capable adult.

Once healing from MI or CABG is nearly complete, one ubiquitous problem is how to deal with the patient when he or she fails to follow important medical or lifestyle recommendations. How *should* a caring family member (or friend) respond when a patient is making a poor health choice? Is there an *appropriate and effective response* to the patient who resumes smoking cigarettes, returns to a high-fat diet, stops exercising, and is chronically angry and exhausted? Often, a caring family member "fills in the void" of the patient's missing motivation, sometimes with nagging and even anger. We have termed this pattern the *denial-overprotectiveness syndrome*: when the patient minimizes or denies the significance of risk behaviors, a caring spouse is seemingly *forced* to supply the missing motivation. Sometimes this pattern is made more complex by the spouse's guilt, such as "what am I doing wrong that he [or she] won't change?" which can lead to an even more relentless effort to "change the patient." Too often, we have seen patients resume unhealthful behaviors in spite of the best efforts of family, friends, and medical personnel. From our experience, *gentle* though *consistent* reminders are most successful for helping patients overcome this enormous problem.

Another variation on regression may occur if the significant other continues to engage in coronary risk behaviors, "tempting" the patient by smoking cigarettes and/or eating high-fat, high-cholesterol foods. Thus, effective treatment of CHD risk factors is often a family affair, suggesting that programs should be designed to include spouses and perhaps other family members.

Others' Reactions to the Cardiac Patient

An important issue for many is how others respond to their CHD. An MI can be seen as a "badge of honor," in the popular mind a sign of working, and perhaps playing, too hard over many years. However, employers sometimes regard the post-MI or post-CABG patient as "damaged goods," and there is often a deep-seated fear among patients that their careers are in jeopardy. Further, it is questionable whether such patients should allow themselves to frequently become exhausted for the sake of their jobs. Indeed, a recent study reported that post-PTCA patients were more likely to suffer increased cardiac morbidity, invasive procedures, and hospitalization if they were "vitally exhausted" 2 weeks after PTCA.[23] These data, along with other studies on vital exhaustion,[20–22] suggest that PTCA patients, and likely post-MI patients, should avoid exhaustion.

Dealing with Ongoing Controversies in Cardiology

Many patients feel that they cannot keep pace with the rapid advances in clinical cardiology. This is a field that is often in the news, and to some patients, it appears that what is true one day is not true the next. Although there is a theoretical consistency in what has been considered a heart-healthy diet, there have been many changes in recommendations by health experts over recent years. Reductions in levels of dietary cholesterol and fat intake have characterized standards provided by the American Heart Association (AHA) over past decades. Many CHD patients who believed that they had been following a prudent diet have discovered to their dismay that newer recommendations are more stringent. There is also ongoing debate over whether the diet commonly recommended for those with or at high risk of CHD (the AHA "Type I" prudent diet) is a sufficient reduction in total and saturated fat for high-risk patients.

Following are a number of other ongoing controversies within the cardiology community that directly affect patients' lifestyle choices. Addressing these issues in coronary risk reduction programs has been beneficial to our patients in that it provides *choices* for patients to make themselves, in light of a lack of consensus within the medical community.

1. Should cardiac patients become vegetarian?
2. Should cardiac patients (and others) take dietary supplements, such as antioxidant vitamins?
3. Should CHD patients, and those at risk owing to family history, take aspirin? If so, at what dose?
4. How much exercise is optimal? How soon after PTCA, MI, or CABG? Should exercise be electrocardiographically monitored? If so, for how long before the patient can exercise on his or her own?
5. Should alcohol be encouraged?

CONCLUSION

Lifestyle intervention programs have demonstrated encouraging results for managing CHD, although there have been some recent null and even negative findings. Although the database is small, this is clearly an area that merits further clinical trials. There has been considerable research, and great controversy, over the importance of psychosocial factors for CHD over the past 4 decades. Because CHD is the leading cause of death and disability in the United States and industrialized western world, reducing the risk factors that have been associated with development of the disease should be a high priority. Given the promising results from most of the clinical trials that have been attempted, cardiac psychology deserves increased attention.

A major focus of future research should be how to increase the motivation, and overcome the resistance to long-term change, of the two thirds of cardiac patients who do not sustain lifestyle changes. We suggest that small groups with an empathic leader well trained in both psychotherapy and cardiology are likely to be accepted by patients and highly cost effective in solving this problem. A caveat from recent negative findings is that treatment must be sufficiently intensive and extensive to attain psychologic and cardiac benefits.

From our experience as a psychologist-cardiologist team over more than a decade, psychosocial intervention has clearly improved the quality of life of many cardiac patients.

REFERENCES

1. Allan R, Scheidt S (eds). Heart and Mind: The Practice of Cardiac Psychology. Washington, DC, American Psychological Association, 1996.
2. Jones DA, West RR. Psychological rehabilitation after myocardial infarction: Multicentre randomised controlled trial. BMJ 1996; 313:1517–1521.
3. Frasure-Smith N, Lesperance F, Prince R, et al. Randomized trial of home-based psychosocial nursing intervention for patients recovering from myocardial infarction. Lancet 1997; 350:473–479.
4. Brown GM, Albers JJ, Fisher LD, et al. Regression of coronary artery disease as a result of intensive lipid-lowering therapy in men with high levels of apolipoprotein B. N Engl J Med 1990; 323:1289–1298.
5. Watts GF, Lewis B, Brunt JN, et al. Effects on coronary artery disease of lipid-lowering diet, or diet plus cholestyramine in the St. Thomas Atherosclerosis Regression Study (STARS). Lancet 1992; 339:563–569.
6. Kaski JC, Chester MR, Chen L, Katritis D. Rapid angiographic progression of coronary artery disease in patients with angina pectoris: The role of complex stenosis morphology. Circulation 1995; 92:2058–2065.
7. Little WC, Gwinn NS, Burrows MT, et al. Cause of myocardial infarction late after successful coronary artery bypass grafting. Am J Cardiol 1990; 65:808–810.
8. Ambrose JA, Winters SL, Arora RR, et al. Angiographic evolution of coronary artery morphology in unstable angina. J Am Coll Cardiol 1986; 7:472–478.
9. Chen L, Chester MR, Redwood S, et al. Angiographic stenosis progression and coronary events in patients with "stabilized" unstable angina pectoris. Circulation 1995; 91:2319–2324.
10. Ornish D, Brown SE, Scherwitz LW, et al. Can lifestyle changes reverse coronary heart disease? Lancet 1990; 336:129–133.
11. Ornish D, Brown SE, Billings JH, et al. Can lifestyle changes reverse coronary atherosclerosis? Four-year results of the Lifestyle Heart Trial [Abstract]. Circulation 1993; 88:I-385.
12. Schuler G, Hambrecht R, Schlier G, et al. Myocardial perfusion and regression of coronary artery disease in patients on a regimen of intensive physical exercise and low-fat diet. J Am Coll Cardiol 1992; 19:34–42.
13. Gould KL, Ornish D, Scherwitz L, et al. Changes in myocardial perfusion abnormalities by positron emission tomography after long-term, intense risk factor modification. JAMA 1995; 274:894–901.
14. Deedwania PC. Clinical perspectives on primary and secondary prevention of coronary atherosclerosis. Med Clin North Am 1995; 79:973–998.
15. Smith SC, Blair SN, Criqui MH, et al. The Secondary Prevention Panel: Preventing heart attack and death in patients with coronary disease. Circulation 1995; 92:2–4.
16. Frasure-Smith N, Lesperance F, Talajic M. Depression following myocardial infarction. JAMA 1993; 270:1819–1825.
17. Case RB, Moss AJ, Case N, et al. Living alone after myocardial infarction: Impact on prognosis. JAMA 1992; 267:515–519.
18. Williams RB, Barefoot JC, Califf RM. Prognostic importance of social and economic resources among medically treated patients with angiographically documented coronary artery disease. JAMA 1992; 267:520–524.
19. Berkman LF, Leo-Summers L, Horwitz RI. Emotional support and survival after myocardial infarction. Ann Intern Med 1992; 117:1003–1009.
20. Appels A. Mental precursors of myocardial infarction. Br J Psychiatry 1990; 156:465–471.
21. Appels A, Mulder P. Fatigue and heart disease: The association between "vital exhaustion" and past, present, and future coronary heart disease. J Psychosom Res 1989; 33:727–738.
22. Appels A, Schouten E. Waking up exhausted as risk indicator of myocardial infarction. Am J Cardiol 1991; 68:395–398.
23. Mendes de Leon CF, Kop WJ, de Swart HB, et al. Psychosocial characteristics and recurrent events after percutaneous transluminal coronary angioplasty. Am J Cardiology 1996; 77:252–255.

23a. Denollet J, Brutsaert DL. Personality, disease severity, and the risk of long-term cardiac events in patients with a decreased ejection fraction after myocardial infarction. Circulation 1998; 97:167–173.

24. Mittleman MA, Maclure M, Tofler GH, et al. Triggering of acute myocardial infarction by heavy physical exertion. N Engl J Med 1993; 329:1677–1683.
25. Mittleman MA, Maclure M, Sherwood JB, et al for the Determinants of Myocardial Infarction Onset Study Investigators. Triggering of acute myocardial infarction onset by episodes of anger. Circulation 1995; 92:1720–1725.
26. Friedman M, Thoresen CE, Gill JJ, et al. Alteration of type A behavior and its effect on cardiac recurrences in post–myocardial infarction patients: Summary results of the Recurrent Coronary Prevention Project. Am Heart J 1986; 112:653–665.

27. Burell G. Group psychotherapy in Project New Life: Treatment of coronary-prone behavior for post–coronary artery bypass patients. *In* Allan R, Scheidt S (eds). Heart and Mind: The Practice of Cardiac Psychology. Washington, DC, American Psychological Association, 1996.
28. Gold J. Psychological issues and coronary artery bypass graft surgery. *In* Allan R, Scheidt S (eds). Heart and Mind: The Practice of Cardiac Psychology. Washington, DC, American Psychological Association, 1996.
29. Nunes EV, Frank KA, Kornfeld DS. Psychologic treatment for the type A behavior pattern and for coronary heart disease: A meta-analysis of the literature. Psychosom Med 1987; 48:159–173.
30. Rahe RH, Ward HW, Hayes V. Brief group therapy in myocardial infarction rehabilitation: Three- to four-year follow-up of a controlled trial. Psychosom Med 1979; 41:229–242.
31. Linden W, Stossel C, Maurice J. Psychosocial interventions for patients with coronary artery disease. Arch Intern Med 1996; 156:745–752.
32. Blumenthal JA, Jiang W, Babyak MA, et al. Stress management and exercise training in cardiac patients with myocardial ischemia. Arch Intern Med 1997; 157:2213–2223.
33. Adsett CA, Bruhn JG. Short-term group psychotherapy for post–myocardial patients and their wives. Can Med Assoc J 1968; 99:577–584.
34. Bohachick P. Progressive relaxation training in cardiac rehabilitation: Effect on psychologic variables. Nurs Res 1984; 33:283–287.
35. Burgess AW, Lerner DJ, D'Agostino RB, et al. A randomized, controlled trial of cardiac rehabilitation. Soc Sci Med 1987; 24:359–370.
36. Clark NM, Janz NK, Becker MH, et al. Impact of self-management education on the functional health status of older adults with heart disease. Gerontologist 1992; 32:438–443.
37. Van Dixhoorn J, Duivenvoorden HJ, Staal HA, et al. Cardiac events after myocardial infarction: Possible effects of relaxation therapy. Eur Heart J 1987; 8:1210–1214.
38. Van Dixhoorn J, Duivenvoorden HJ, Staal HA, Pool J. Physical training and relaxation therapy in cardiac rehabilitation assessed through a composite criterion for training outcome. Am Heart J 1989; 118:545–552.
39. Van Dixhoorn J, Duivenvoorden HJ, Pool J, Verhage F. Psychic effects of physical training and relaxation therapy after myocardial infarction. J Psychosom Res 1990; 34:327–337.
40. Fielding R. A note on behavioral treatment in the rehabilitation of myocardial infarction patients. Br J Soc Clin Psychol 1979; 19:157–161.
41. Frasure-Smith N, Prince R. Long-term follow-up of the Ischemic Heart Disease Life Stress Monitoring Program. Psychosom Med 1989; 51:485–513.
42. Gruen W. Effects of brief psychotherapy during the hospitalization period on the recovery process in heart attacks. J Consult Clin Psychol 1975; 43:223–232.
43. Guzetta CE. Effects of relaxation and music therapy on patients in a coronary care unit with presumptive acute myocardial infarction. Heart Lung 1989; 18:609–616.
44. Horlick L, Cameron R, Firor W, et al. The effects of education and group discussion in the post–myocardial infarction patient. J Psychosom Res 1984; 28:485–492.
45. Munro BH, Creamer AM, Haggerty MR, Cooper FS. Effect of relaxation therapy on post–myocardial infarction patients' rehabilitation. Nurs Res 1988; 37:231–235.
46. Pozen MW, Stechmiller JA, Harris W, et al. A nurse rehabilitator's impact on patients with myocardial infarction. Med Care 1977; 15:830–837.
47. Rahe RH, O'Neil T, Hagan A, Arthur RJ. Brief group therapy following myocardial infarction: Eighteen-month follow-up of a controlled trial. Int J Psychiatry Med 1975; 6:349–358.
48. Schulte MB, Pluym B, Van Schendel G. Reintegration with duos: A self-care program following myocardial infarction. Patient Educ Counsel 1986; 8:233–244.
49. Stern MJ, Gorman PA, Kaslow L. The group counseling versus exercise therapy study: A controlled intervention with subjects following myocardial infarction. Arch Intern Med 1983; 143:1719–1725.
50. Thompson DR. A randomized controlled trial of in-hospital nursing support for first-time myocardial infarction patients and their partners: Effects on anxiety and depression. J Adv Nurs 1989; 14:291–297.
51. Thompson DR, Meddis R. A prospective evaluation of in-hospital counseling for first-time myocardial infarction men. J Pychosom Res 1990; 34:237–248.
52. Turner L, Linden W, VanderWal R, Schamberger W. Stress management for patients with cardiac disease: A pilot study. Heart Lung 1995; 24:145–153.
53. Scherwitz L, Ornish DM, Billings JH, Merritt TA. Yoga and lifestyle change in the Lifestyle Heart Trial. Paper presented at the Fourth International Congress of Behavioral Medicine, Washington, DC, March 16, 1996.
54. Friedman M, Powell LH, Thoresen CE, et al. Effect of discontinuance of type A behavioral counseling on type A behavior and cardiac recurrence rate of post–myocardial infarction patients. Am Heart J 1987; 114:483–490.
55. Powell LH, Thoresen CE. Effects of type A behavioral counseling and severity of prior acute myocardial infarction on survival. Am J Cardiol 1988; 62:1159–1163.
56. Brackett CD, Powell LH. Psychosocial and physiological predictors of sudden cardiac death after healing of acute myocardial infarction. Am J Cardiol 1988; 61:979–983.
57. Friedman M, Breall WS, Goodwin ML, et al. Effect of type A behavioral counseling on frequency of episodes of silent myocardial ischemia in coronary patients. Am Heart J 1996; 132:933–937.
58. Frasure-Smith N. In-hospital symptoms of psychological stress as predictors of long-term outcome after acute myocardial infarction in men. Am J Cardiol 1991; 67:121–127.
59. Powell LH. Unanswered questions in the ischemic heart disease life stress monitoring program. Psychosom Med 1989; 51:479–484.
60. Hamalainen H, Luurila OJ, Kallio V, Knuts L-R. Reduction in sudden deaths and coronary mortality in myocardial infarction patients after rehabilitation: Fifteen-year follow-up study. Eur Heart J 1995; 16:1839–1844.

60a. Trzcieniecka-Green A, Steptoe A. The effects of stress management on the quality of life of patients following acute myocardial infarction or coronary bypass surgery. Eur Heart J 1996; 17:1663–1670.

61. Thompson DR, Meddis R. Wives' responses to counseling early after myocardial infarction. J Psychosom Res 1990; 34:249–258.
62. Dracup K, Moser DK, Marsden C, et al. Effects of a multidimensional cardiopulmonary rehabilitation program on psychosocial function. Am J Cardiol 1991; 68:31–34.
63. Levine J, Warrenburg S, Kerns R, et al. The role of denial in recovery from coronary heart disease. Psychosom Med 1987; 49:109–117.

Section Editor

▶ **JoAnn E. Manson**

SECTION

III PREVENTION TRIALS

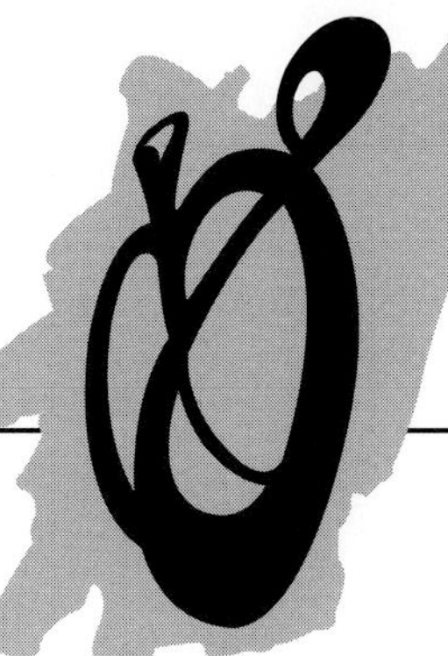

26 Cholesterol Reduction

▶ J. Michael Gaziano
▶ William P. Castelli

The stimulus to intervene in lipoprotein abnormalities came from animal, case-control clinical, and prospective epidemiologic studies that demonstrated an association between levels of the various blood lipids, including total cholesterol, triglyceride, low-density lipoprotein (LDL) cholesterol, high-density lipoprotein (HDL) cholesterol, and very-low-density lipoprotein (VLDL) cholesterol and coronary heart disease (CHD). These associations were present in young and old, men and women. Guidelines for the screening and intervention for hyperlipidemia in primary prevention of atherosclerotic disease are based largely on the results of large-scale primary prevention randomized trials as well as extrapolation from secondary prevention trials.

In this chapter we discuss a number of issues related to cholesterol screening and treatment among those without known cardiovascular disease. Lipid-lowering therapy in secondary prevention is covered in elsewhere in this textbook (see Chapter 17). We begin with discussion of the clear benefits of intervention in terms of CHD followed by a discussion of the controversies over the role of lipid-lowering therapy in stroke prevention. Consideration of any intervention in a lower-risk population must include all potential risks. For this reason we present issues of nonvascular and total mortality in detail. The cost efficacy of lipid-lowering therapy is also discussed. Finally, we summarize issues related to cholesterol reduction among the elderly and women.

CORONARY HEART DISEASE

Observational Epidemiology

Based on human observational evidence, there is little doubt that elevated cholesterol levels increase the risk of CHD.[1] Observational research indicates a linear relationship, with a 20% increase in risk of CHD for each 10% increase in serum cholesterol.[2] This dose-response effect occurs at any level of cholesterol[3] and is apparent in both men and women and blacks and whites.

These estimates from prospective data may underestimate the true risk associated with lipoprotein abnormalities because the relationship is generally based on a single measure of total cholesterol.[2] The underestimation results from two forms of bias. First, regression dilution bias, which results from random fluctuation of cholesterol levels over time in any subject and inaccuracies in the assays, would introduce random misclassification that would tend to underestimate the size of the true association. Second, surrogate dilution bias results from the less-than-perfect correlation between LDL cholesterol and total cholesterol levels. Since LDL cholesterol tends to be a stronger predictor of CHD than total cholesterol, this value would also tend to underestimate the association. Correction for these two forms of bias involves using repeated measures of LDL cholesterol and yields an approximate 27% increase in risk of CHD for each increase of 10% in serum cholesterol.[4]

Randomized Trials

Findings from randomized trials are consistent with human observational evidence. Data from individual randomized trials have consistently shown a reduction in risk of both fatal and nonfatal CHD in both primary and secondary prevention. Several multifactorial primary prevention trials included a dietary component to lower cholesterol[5–8] (Table 26–1). Although these trials tended to show lower rates of CHD among those in the intervention arm, the magnitude of the benefit cannot be ascribed fully to the cholesterol reduction component alone, given the simultaneous modification of other risk factors.

There are seven large-scale primary prevention trials of cholesterol-lowering alone, including one dietary[9] and six pharmacologic trials (Table 26–2).[10–18] Trials of dietary treatment of coronary risk or disease grew out of knowledge of what foods influence the levels, initially of cholesterol alone, but eventually of most of the major categories of lipoproteins. The earliest trial was the Los Angeles Veterans Affairs Cooper-

TABLE 26–1 • Randomized Trials of Cholesterol Lowering in the Primary Prevention of Cardiovascular Disease

Study	Year of Publication	Intervention
Multiple-Intervention Studies		
Oslo Study Group[8]	1981	Diet
MRFIT[6]	1982	Diet
Miettinen, et al.[7]	1985	Diet/Clofibrate
Goteburg[5]	1986	Diet
Single-Intervention Studies		
LA VA[9]	1969	Diet
Colestipol Trial, Door[10]	1978	Colestipol
World Health Organization Clofibrate[11–13]	1984	Clofibrate
Helsinki Heart Study[14]	1987	Gemfibrozil
Lipid Research Clinics Coronary Primary Prevention Trial[15]	1984	Cholestyramine
West of Scotland Coronary Prevention Study[16]	1995	Pravastatin
Air Force/Texas Coronary Atherosclerosis Prevention Study (AFCAPS/Tex CAPS)[17]	1998	Lovastatin

ative Study (LA VA), which randomized 846 subjects to either a low-fat diet or no dietary change.[9] Mean cholesterol reduction was 12.7% among those in the diet-modification arm. After a mean follow-up of 7 years, there was a reduction in risk of fatal and nonfatal CHD events.

The first large-scale primary prevention trial of a pharmacologic agent used the resin colestipol.[10] Investigators randomized 2278 subjects to colestipol or placebo. Mean cholesterol level was reduced by 9.8% among those in the active treatment group compared with those on placebo. After a mean follow-up of only 2 years, the treatment group showed reductions in CHD events and deaths and a trend toward a lower total mortality rate.

The World Health Organization clofibrate trial investigators randomized 10,621 subjects to clofibrate or placebo and followed them for an average of 5.3 years.[11–13] Active treatment with clofibrate was associated with an 8.5% reduction in total cholesterol. There was a 25% reduction in the risk of nonfatal MI; however, there was no reduction in CHD mortality. There tended to be higher rates of non-CHD, as well as total, death among those assigned to clofibrate compared with those assigned to placebo.

The Helsinki Heart Study randomized 4081 subjects to either gemfibrozil or placebo and followed subjects for an average of 5 years.[14] The mean reduction in total cholesterol of 9.9% resulted in a clear reduction in nonfatal MI (34%) and incident CHD (37%) rates among those allocated to gemfibrozil.

The Lipid Research Clinics Coronary Primary Prevention Trial (LRC-CPPT) investigators randomized 3806 subjects to either cholestyramine or placebo, with a 9% reduction in total cholesterol among those assigned active drug.[15] After a mean follow-up period of 7.4 years, those receiving cholestyramine, compared with those receiving placebo, experienced a 19% reduction in risk of a definite CHD event and a 24% reduction in fatal CHD as well as 20% to 25% reductions in risk of a positive stress test, angina, or bypass surgery. The risk of total death was only slightly (7%) and nonsignificantly reduced.

In all these early primary prevention trials the mean reduction in total cholesterol was modest and the overall event rates were low. Thus, these studies were not generally powered to detect differences in total or CHD mortality. The newest class of cholesterol-lowering drug, 3-hydroxy-3-methylglutaryl coenzyme A (HMG-CoA) reductase inhibitors, or statins, produce much larger reductions in cholesterol than do earlier agents. There are two large-scale primary prevention trials of cholesterol reduction using statins.[16, 17]

TABLE 26–2 • Summary of Single Intervention Large-Scale Primary Prevention Trials of Cholesterol Lowering

Study	Study Population	Number Randomized	Major Findings Associated with Active Treatment
LA VA[9]	Middle-aged men	846	Reduced risks of fatal and nonfatal CHD events
Colestipol Trial[10]	Middle-aged men and women	2278	Reduced risks of fatal and nonfatal CHD events. Trend toward lower rates of total death
World Health Organization Clofibrate[11–13]	Middle-aged men	10,621	Reduced risk of nonfatal MI. No reduction in fatal CHD. Trend toward increased risk from non CHD and total deaths
Lipid Research Clinic Coronary Primary Prevention Trial[15]	Middle-aged men	3806	Reduced risks of CHD events and fatal CHD. Trend toward lower total deaths
Helsinki Heart Study[14]	Middle-aged men	4081	Reduced risks of nonfatal MI and incident CHD
West of Scotland Coronary Prevention Study[16]	Middle-aged men and women	6595	Reduced risks of total CHD events, revascularization, CHD death, and fatal CHD
Air Force/Texas Coronary Atherosclerosis Prevention Study (AFCAPS/TexCAPS)[17]	Middle-aged men and women	6595	Reduced risks of MI, unstable angina, coronary revascularization, total coronary events, and total cardiovascular events

CHD, coronary heart disease; MI, myocardial infarction.

In the West of Scotland Coronary Prevention Study, 6595 hyperlipidemic subjects were randomized to either pravastatin or its placebo. Compared with those assigned to the placebo group, mean total cholesterol reduction among those receiving active treatment was approximately twice that of the previous primary prevention trials (20%). After 4.9 years of follow-up there were clear reductions in CHD events (31%) and revascularization procedures (37%) as well CHD death. There was also a borderline significant 22% reduction in total mortality in the pravastatin group.

Recently, data were presented from the Air Force and Texas Coronary Atherosclerosis Prevention Study (AFCAPS/TexCAPS),[17] a large-scale primary prevention trial among those with only modest elevations in LDL cholesterol. Lovastatin reduced LDL cholesterol by 25%. Compared with those assigned placebo, those given lovastatin had clear reductions in risk of myocardial infarction (relative risk [RR], 0.60), unstable angina (RR, 0.68), coronary revascularization procedures (RR, 0.67), total coronary events (RR, 0.75), and total cardiovascular events (RR, 0.75).

Meta-Analyses of Randomized Trials

Most primary prevention trials are underpowered to fully assess the balance of benefits and any potential risks. A number of meta-analyses provide valuable insight on the role of lipid lowering in primary as well as secondary prevention.[18–26] A comprehensive overview by Law and coworkers[24, 25] of 28 trials of cholesterol reduction in the prestatin era, including six multiple intervention trials with a cholesterol-lowering arm, indicate that a 10% reduction in serum cholesterol results in highly significant reductions of 10% for CHD death and 18% for coronary events. When the duration of treatment is 5 years or more, the event rate reductions reported from this meta-analysis of randomized trials are consistent with what would be expected based on observational data. Specifically, a 10% reduction in cholesterol was associated with a 25% reduction in coronary events (95% confidence interval [CI], 15% to 35%) among those treated for more than 5 years.[24]

Recent overviews of statin trials reveal similar findings in terms of CHD, with greater reductions in cholesterol associated with greater reductions in CHD event rates and deaths. In a recent meta-analysis, which included all trials that used a single pharmacologic intervention, including statins, the additional information provided by the recent statin trials did not alter the regression line predicting the amount of benefit in terms of cardiovascular events or total mortality for primary or secondary prevention, in relation to the amount of lipid lowering.[27] An earlier analysis by these authors[26] predicted the magnitude of the effect that would result from the greater lipid-lowering effects of statin drugs. This analysis suggests the primary effect of statins in reducing CHD rates is due to the reduction in cholesterol rather than some other statin-specific mechanism.

The strength and consistency of the cholesterol-CHD association as well as dose-response and duration effects provide strong support for a judgment of cause and effect. The available observational evidence clearly indicates that higher cholesterol levels increase the risk of CHD, and available randomized trial data demonstrate that cholesterol lowering results in comparable reductions in CHD risks in primary as well as secondary prevention.

STROKE

Although cholesterol level is a clear risk factor for CHD, its role as a precursor to stroke is much less certain.[28] Some observational studies suggest that cholesterol level is positively associated with the risk of stroke, and ischemic stroke in particular,[29] but others have failed to find this association.[30, 31] A recently published overview of 45 prospective observational cohorts including 450,000 individuals and 13,000 strokes, however, demonstrated an independent association between baseline blood cholesterol and stroke risk.[32]

One difficulty in assessing the association of cholesterol level with risk of stroke is that the relationship may differ by the cause of cerebrovascular events. The Multiple Risk Factor Intervention Trial screening data showed a positive association between cholesterol level and ischemic stroke but an inverse relationship for hemorrhagic stroke.[29] These findings are compatible with other observational studies of populations with low blood cholesterol levels.[33, 34] They are also compatible with studies of Japanese populations that have adopted Western eating habits, either in Japan as a result of secular lifestyle changes or on migration to the United States.[34–37] The Japanese typically consume less animal fat and have lower blood cholesterol levels than do their U.S. counterparts. They also have a higher incidence of stroke, which is primarily hemorrhagic rather than ischemic, but a lower incidence of CHD. With the adoption of Western eating habits, their blood cholesterol levels rise and the incidence of CHD increases, while the proportion of stroke attributable to hemorrhage decreases. These findings raise the possibility that detecting any benefits of cholesterol lowering on risks of stroke from randomized trials would require far larger samples as well as reliable classification by ischemic or hemorrhagic cause.

Randomized trials have clearly demonstrated that cholesterol lowering decreases risk of coronary heart disease in both primary as well as secondary prevention,[18–27] but whether it decreases risk of stroke remains unclear. Overviews of all randomized trials that provided data on stroke outcomes prior to the large-scale statin trials revealed no reduction in stroke among those treated with cholesterol-lowering agents compared with placebo.[38, 39] These overviews included trials among those with and without known coronary artery disease. None was designed to include those with prior stroke. In one overview of more than 36,000 individuals,[38] the mean reduction in cholesterol level in the treated group as compared with the control subjects ranged from 6% to 23% (Table 26–3). Those assigned to treatment experienced no significant reduction in all (fatal plus nonfatal) stroke (RR, 1.0; 95% CI, 0.8 to 1.2) or fatal strokes (RR 1.1; CI 0.8 to 1.6). There were no clear differences between primary and secondary prevention trials. Insufficient cholesterol lowering and inadequate sample size are plausible explanations for the inability to detect reductions in stroke in earlier individual trials and their overviews.

With the recent publication of several large trials using statins, which produce larger reductions of cholesterol than previous lipid-lowering drugs,[16, 17, 40–43] additional evidence on the role of cholesterol reduction in the prevention of stroke is emerging. Several of these trials reported lower stroke rates among those treated with statins. In a subsequent overview of randomized trials that used statins, there was a substantial reduction in risk of ischemic stroke.[44] A total of 16 individual trials including approximately 29,000 subjects treated and followed up an average of 3.3 years were included in the overview. The average reductions in total and LDL cholesterol were large—22% and 30%, respectively (see Table 26–3). A total of 454 strokes (fatal plus nonfatal) occurred during follow-up. Those assigned to statin drugs experienced a significant reduction in risk of total stroke of 29% (95% CI, 14% to 41%) but no apparent reduction in risk of fatal stroke. This overview of all published randomized trials of statin drugs demonstrates large reductions in cholesterol and evidence of benefit on stroke.

TABLE 26–3 • Results from Overviews of Cholesterol-Lowering Trials with Data on Stroke Events

Endpoint	Overview of Prestatin Studies[38]	Overview of Statin Studies[44]
Total death	—	0.78 (0.69–0.88)
CVD death	—	0.72 (0.63–0.84)
Non-CVD death	—	0.93 (0.75–1.14)
Total stroke	1.0 (0.8–1.2)	0.71 (0.59–0.86)
Primary prevention trials	1.0 (0.8–1.3)	0.80 (0.54–1.16)
Secondary prevention trials	1.0 (0.7–1.3)	0.68 (0.55–0.85)
Stroke death	1.1 (0.8–1.6)	1.17 (0.69–1.97)
Primary prevention trials	1.5 (0.9–2.6)	0.86 (0.29–2.56)
Secondary prevention trials	0.9 (0.6–1.4)	1.28 (0.71–2.32)

There are several possible explanations for the discrepancy between the reduced stroke rates observed in statin trials and earlier randomized trials as well as observational studies that do not support a role of cholesterol reduction in stroke prevention. Large reductions in cholesterol level may be necessary to provide a large enough reduction in ischemic strokes to be detected. Another explanation may relate to the fact that much of the statin data are from secondary prevention trials among those with CHD. The statins may prevent stroke secondary to reducing risk of myocardial infarction (MI). Stroke risk following an MI is increased and may be attributable to the formation of mural thrombi that can produce embolic strokes. The greater reductions in coronary disease achieved with the statins may, therefore, result in prevention of stroke. Though less likely, it remains possible that statins reduce stroke by a mechanism unrelated to the lipid-lowering effect. Additional randomized trial data will be required to clarify the role of lipid-lowering agents in stroke prevention.

NONVASCULAR MORTALITY

Although there is little doubt that cholesterol reduction results in reduced risks of CHD and possibly stroke, questions have been raised regarding the increased risk of nonvascular deaths observed in some trials.[45, 46] This is of particular importance in primary prevention, in which benefits could be offset by any potential risks of nonvascular mortality because of lower baseline risks of cardiovascular disease. The hypothesis that there is a potential hazard associated with lowering cholesterol is based primarily on two observations: (1) observational data have raised the possibility of an association between low serum cholesterol and increased risk of nonvascular mortality, and (2) there has been no benefit from cholesterol reduction on total mortality in early randomized trials despite a clear reduction in risks of CHD. For several reasons, as outlined below, the currently available evidence does not support the hypothesis that cholesterol reduction increases nonvascular mortality overall or mortality due to any specific cause.[47]

First, unlike the association between cholesterol and risk of CHD, randomized trial data do not reinforce concerns raised by observational data. The observational studies suggest that those with the lowest cholesterol levels in a given population are at increased risk of nonvascular death. These low levels of cholesterol have never been achieved in randomized trials. It has been postulated that rapid reductions in blood cholesterol observed in randomized trials may lead to nonvascular events[48]; however, it is highly unlikely that those in observational studies with the lowest cholesterol achieved these levels by a rapid fall. Thus, data from observational studies and randomized trials support two causally distinct hypotheses.

Second, although individuals with very low cholesterol levels have higher rates of nonvascular mortality,[2] it is unclear whether low cholesterol is a marker for or a cause of these increased nonvascular mortality rates. The association from observational studies of an increase in nonvascular deaths at lower cholesterol levels may be the result of confounding by the existence of subclinical disease. This is suggested by the attenuation of the relationship if deaths within the first 5 years are excluded.[2]

Given the long latency period for some nonvascular causes of death, such as liver disease and lung cancer, even exclusion of events in the first 5 years of follow-up may not eliminate all residual confounding. Indirect support for this comes from the observation that the association of lower cholesterol and increased non-CHD mortality from prospective cohort studies varies, depending on whether the study populations were employment- or community-based.[4] In employment-based cohorts, there was no evidence of increased non-CHD mortality among those with low cholesterol, which was defined as levels less than 5.0 mmol/L (193 mg/dL) (RR, 1.00; 95% CI, 0.94 to 1.06). In addition to the point estimate indicating a null result, the upper bound of the CI (1.06) excludes any substantial increased risk. In contrast, there was an apparent increased risk of non-CHD deaths among those in community-based cohorts (RR, 1.20; 95% CI, 1.15 to 1.24).

If low cholesterol levels increase non-CHD mortality rates, these discrepant results are difficult to explain. An alternative explanation is that in contrast to employee-based cohorts, among community-based populations there may be higher prevalence of premorbid disease, such as cancer, liver disease, and depression, all of which result in low cholesterol levels. The association of low cholesterol level with cause-specific mortality also varies, depending on whether the populations studied were employment or community based. In employment-based cohorts, among those with the lowest cholesterol levels there was no increased risk of death from non-CHD vascular disease (RR, 0.92; 95% CI, 0.80 to 1.05), cancer (RR, 1.00; 95% CI, 0.91 to 1.10), trauma deaths (which includes deaths due to accidents or suicide) (RR, 0.95; 95% CI, 0.70 to 1.30), or other causes (RR, 0.97; 95% CI, 0.97 to 1.21). This is in contrast with studies of community-based cohorts, in which those with the lowest cholesterol levels are at increased risk of death from cancer (RR, 1.23; 95% CI, 1.17 to 1.30), trauma (RR, 1.29; 95% CI, 1.13 to 1.47), or other causes (RR, 1.26; 95% CI, 1.15 to 1.24). Thus, any relationship of low cholesterol with non-CHD death seems more likely to be due to confounding factors rather than a causal relationship.

Third, in contrast with the cholesterol-heart disease relationship, evidence for a dose-response relationship between low cholesterol and nonvascular mortality is quite limited. The lack of a dose-response relationship raises the possibility of a threshold effect. However, when comparing studies cross-culturally, it is the relative rather than the absolute level of cholesterol that is associated with increased risk of nonvascular mortality.[18] For example, the mean cholesterol among the lowest quartile of adults in Finland, where levels tend to be high, corresponds to average values in the United States, whereas average levels in Japan would be considered low in the United States. This argues against a causal relationship between an absolute level of low cholesterol and nonvascular disease. A plausible explanation for these cross-cultural differences is that chronic diseases that lead to death lower cholesterol levels, regardless of the absolute values, which vary from population to population.

This lack of dose response is apparent in randomized trials as well. In a recent meta-analysis, Gordon[48a] analyzed data by the extent of cholesterol reduction (11 studies with cholesterol reduction of 12% or more compared with 11 with less than 12% reductions). As expected, greater cholesterol reduction resulted in greater reduction in CHD incidence (31% vs. 11%) and mortality (27% vs. 2%). In contrast, greater reduction in cholesterol was associated with less of an increase in rates of nonvascular mortality (11% vs. 30%). These results are further confirmed by the recent data from the Scandinavian Simvastatin Survival Study (4S),[40] where drug therapy resulted in a 25% reduction in total cholesterol (larger than the reduction in any previous trial), yet there was no increase in nonvascular deaths (49 in placebo vs. 46 in the treatment group). Similarly, there were no increases in nonvascular mortality in other individual large-scale statin trials[16, 17, 40–43] or in a recent overview of all completed statin trials[44] (RR, 0.93; 95% CI, 0.75 to 1.14).

Fourth, there is no consistent association with any specific cause of death,[23, 24] and apparent increases in cause-specific mortality are confined to relatively few studies. The trend for cancer is primarily accounted for by one relatively large drug trial, the World Health Organization (WHO) Clofibrate Trial,[11–13] and one large dietary trial, the LA VA Study,[9] in which cholesterol reductions were 9% and 13%, respectively (Table 26–4). In both cases, the differences in mortality from cancer in the intervention and control groups, which, if real, might have been expected to persist or even become more accentuated owing to the long latency period of cancer, were in fact diminished with extended follow-up. In addition, the recent overview of

TABLE 26–4 • Cancer Deaths by Type of Cholesterol-Lowering Intervention in the Cholesterol-Lowering Trialists' Overview[23]

Trial/Type of Intervention	Deaths		
	Treated vs. Control	*O-E*	*Z*
WHO Clofibrate Trial	74 vs. 2	+10.8	1.9 (NS)
All other clofibrate trials	16 vs. 20	−0.6	0.2 (NS)
Los Angeles Diet (LA VA)	33 vs. 20	+6.4	1.8 (NS)
All other diet trials	26 vs. 30	−2.2	0.6 (NS)
All other trials	49 vs. 55*	−0.8	0.1 (NS)
Total	**198 vs. 177**	**+13.1**	**1.4 (NS)†**

*Half CDP control deaths in each group.
†The results are unchanged by giving proportionally more weight to trials of longer duration and trials with larger cholesterol reductions.
CDP, Coronary Drug Project; O-E, observed-expected.

completed large-scale statin trials demonstrated no increase in cancer risk (RR, 1.03; CI 0.90 to 1.17). The apparent excess in trauma deaths among those treated was most apparent in the Helsinki trial of gemfibrozil (15 vs. 4 trauma deaths)[14] and the Lipid Research Clinics trial of cholestyramine (11 vs. 4),[15] in which the net cholesterol reductions were 9% and 10%, respectively (Table 26–5). This raises the possibility that increases in cancer or trauma mortality may be intervention specific and not related to cholesterol reduction in itself or, equally plausibly, simply the result of the play of chance.

Until recently, data from individual randomized trials have been insufficient to address the issue of cholesterol lowering and nonvascular mortality. The lack of a statistically significant benefit on overall mortality, particularly in the early primary prevention trials, has led some to speculate that this is evidence of an offsetting of the reduction in cardiovascular disease risk by an increase in nonvascular mortality.

However, the recently completed large-scale primary and secondary prevention trials of statins provide reassuring data supporting the conclusion that cholesterol reduction does not increase the risk of nonvascular mortality. Randomized trials with the statins result in greater cholesterol reductions than those achieved with earlier agents, and there is no apparent increase in nonvascular mortality in the individual statin trials or recent meta-analyses of their findings.[16, 17, 40–43]

In summary, the potential for confounding by the presence of subclinical disease, the lack of a dose-response or threshold effect, the lack of a consistent effect for any specific cause of death, the appearance of adverse effects in just a few trials, along with the lack of evidence from basic research all argue against a causal relationship between lower cholesterol and nonvascular causes of death.

TOTAL MORTALITY

Most randomized cholesterol-lowering trials in primary prevention do not show a lower total mortality; however, it is important to distinguish between the finding of no effect and the inability to detect an effect. Specifically, randomized trials of cholesterol lowering conducted to date were designed to test specifically for differences in the incidence of fatal plus nonfatal CHD events. In fact, no completed primary prevention trial was designed to test for the effects of cholesterol lowering on either total or nonvascular mortality, much less cause-specific nonvascular mortality.

TABLE 26–5 • Trauma Deaths by Type of Cholesterol-Lowering Intervention in the Cholesterol Trialists' Overview[23]

Trial/Type of Intervention	Deaths		
	Treated vs. Control	*O-E*	*Z*
Helsinki gemfibrozil trial	10 vs. 4	+3.0	1.6 (NS)
All other fibric acid trials	31 vs. 32*	−0.3	0.7 (NS)
LRC cholestyramine	11 vs. 4	+3.5	1.8 (NS)
All other bile acid sequestrants	2 vs. 1	+0.5	0.6 (NS)
Minnesota diet trial	33 vs. 28*	+2.3	0.6 (NS)
All other trials	11 vs. 8*	+3.1	1.3 (NS)
Total	**98 vs. 77**	**+12.0**	**1.8 (NS)**

*Half CDP control deaths in each group.
CDP, Coronary Drug Project; LRC, Lipid Research Clinics; O-E, observed-expected.

Mean cholesterol reduction in the early trials was relatively modest (6 to 10 mg/dL), and the early trials were underpowered to detect a benefit on total mortality. Overviews of these early trials were consistent with a modest trend toward lower mortality in the range of what would be anticipated, given the modest reduction in CHD mortality. Most overviews of the randomized trials of lipid lowering, whether they include primary prevention trials, secondary prevention trials, or both, have reported a small statistically nonsignificant reduction in total mortality.[18–21] In the two recent comprehensive overviews[23, 24] the observed reduction in total mortality from all randomized trials was 4% (95% CI, 10% reduction to 2% increase). Although statistically inconclusive, such data are compatible with the expected 6% overall decline in mortality anticipated with 9% to 10% decline in CHD death, assuming no excess risk of nonvascular death.

Based on the state of knowledge on the relationship of cholesterol lowering and total mortality prior to the large-scale statin trials, there was no clear evidence of benefit, but there was also no clear evidence of lack of benefit. Data were simply insufficient to address this issue definitively, either in individual trials or in an overview. Recently, however, the West of Scotland trial demonstrated a 22% reduction in total mortality among those without known coronary artery disease[16] and recent overviews of statin trials suggest clear reductions in total mortality.

Even if reductions in total mortality are only modest in primary prevention, the public health benefits of cholesterol lowering in reducing nonfatal CHD events are still likely to far outweigh the risks. This is illustrated by data from the LRC trial.[15] Although there was no clear benefit in terms of total mortality (68 deaths among treated subjects compared with 71 among nontreated subjects—a nonsignificant reduction of 4.3%, which is consistent with the 4% estimate from overviews[23, 24]) there were 206 fewer nonfatal CHD events among those treated (906 vs. 1112). The reduction in morbidity is likely to have substantial public health benefit in terms of quality of life and productivity.

CHOLESTEROL REDUCTION IN THE ELDERLY

Although most trials have demonstrated clear benefits of cholesterol reduction, they have not included subjects older than 65 years of age in sufficient numbers to determine whether there are qualitative differences in benefits or risks in the elderly compared with younger individuals. This lack of trial data among those older than 65 years of age, along with the controversy over the predictive value of total cholesterol among the elderly, have led to divergent opinions on the role of screening and treatment among those older than 65. The National Cholesterol Education Program (NCEP)[49, 50] recommends screening for all adults older than 20 years of age, whereas the guidelines set forth by the American College of Physicians (ACP)[51, 52] do not recommend screening for anyone older than 75 years of age, and no recommendations are provided for or against screening among those aged 65 to 75 years.

Recent large-scale statin trials have included larger numbers of older people (Table 26–6). Among the approximately 2300 participants aged 60 years or older enrolled in 4S, those assigned to receive simvastatin were 29% (95% CI, 14% to 40%) less likely to have a major coronary event than those assigned to receive placebo. Among those younger than age 60, there was a 39% (95% CI, 27% to 49%) risk reduction.[40] In the Cholesterol and Recurrent Events (CARE) Trial, a secondary prevention trial among those with prior MI, more than half of the 4159 participants, who ranged from 21 to 75 years of age, were 60 years old or older.[43] Compared with those assigned placebo, those randomized to receive pravastatin and who were aged 60 years or older had a 27% (95% CI, 9% to 36%) reduction in the risk of a major coronary event, compared with a 20% (95% CI, 4% to 33%) risk reduction for those younger than 60. In the West of Scotland Coronary Prevention Study, the first large-scale primary prevention trial of a statin, no subjects aged 65 or older were enrolled.[16] There was an apparently larger reduction in risk for those younger than 55 years of age than in those aged 55 years or older (40% [95% CI, 16% to 56%] vs. 27% [95% CI, 8% to 43%]).

These data suggest that people older than 55 to 60 years of age may benefit from lipid-lowering therapy. Although these findings must be interpreted cautiously because they rely on relatively small subgroups (based on the number of endpoints), as illustrated by the wide confidence intervals around each estimate, they strongly suggest that there are no qualitative differences in the benefits of lipid-lowering therapy for older individuals. This is in contrast with the observational evidence on the predictive value of total cholesterol in the elderly. No single trial has enrolled sufficient numbers of people older than 70 years of age to assess fully the effects of lipid lowering in the elderly in either primary or secondary prevention. Several additional ongoing trials will provide further data on those older than age 60, but information on those older than 75 will remain limited.

Although many trials have provided some age-specific data, more of such data, particularly from the recent large-scale statin trials, is needed. Age-specific analyses are reportedly under way on the recent

TABLE 26–6 • Events and Relative Risks of Major Coronary Events in Large-Scale Primary and Secondary Prevention Statin Trials by Age and Gender

Trials	*Total Randomized*	Events: *Placebo*	Events: *Active Agent*	Relative Risk (95% Confidence Interval)
PRIMARY PREVENTION TRIALS				
West of Scotland Coronary Prevention Study[16]				
Men	—	—	—	—
Women	—	—	—	—
<60 y	3225	96	57	0.60 (0.44 to 0.84)
≥60 y	3370	152	117	0.73 (0.57 to 0.92)
Air Force/Texas Coronary Atherosclerosis Prevention Study (AFCAPS/TexCAPS)[17]				
Men	5608	170	109	0.64 (0.51 to 0.81)*
Women	997	13	7	0.54 (0.22 to 1.34)*
At median or below	3425	71	58	0.54 (0.36 to 0.80)*
Above median	3180	112	78	0.67 (0.53 to 0.86)*
SECONDARY PREVENTION TRIALS				
Scandinavian Simvastatin Survival Study (4S)[40]				
Men	3917	91	59	0.65 (0.47 to 0.91)
Women	827	531	372	0.66 (0.58 to 0.76)
<60 y	2162	303	188	0.61 (0.51 to 0.73)
≥60 y	2282	319	243	0.71 (0.60 to 0.86)
CARE[43]				
Men	3583	469	384	0.80 (0.70 to 0.92)
Women	576	80	46	0.64 (0.38 to 0.78)
<60 y	2030	258	217	0.80 (0.67 to 0.96)
≥60 y	2179	291	213	0.73 (0.62 to 0.88)

*Estimate based on number of events in each group assuming equivalent follow-up time by treatment assignment.

large-scale statin trials. Additional data from ongoing trials, including the Gruppo Italiano per lo Studio Della Streptochinasi nell'Infarto Miocardio (GISSI) Prevention Study (recently stopped prematurely on ethical grounds after the publication of the CARE study results), Long-Term Intervention with Pravastatin in Ischaemic Heart Disease, the Heart Protection Study, and the Veterans Administration Cooperative HDL Intervention Trial will be available in the next few years. Long-Term Intervention with Pravastatin in Ischaemic Heart Disease enrolled 3600 participants aged 65 years and older. Pooled data from randomized trials will provide better estimates of the balance of the benefits and risks of lipid lowering among the elderly than could be derived from any single completed or ongoing trial and are also likely to greatly enhance cost-effectiveness models.

CHOLESTEROL REDUCTION IN WOMEN

Observational data suggest that cholesterol represents a potent risk factor for heart disease in men and women. The magnitude of the relative risk appears to be similar by gender. However, when addressing cholesterol lowering in primary prevention among women, the absolute risk of CHD must be considered. At every age women are at lower absolute risk of CHD than men. This has two main effects on the overall assessment of cholesterol reduction in primary prevention. First, since absolute benefits are less than in men, even modest risks may have an important impact in offsetting modest absolute benefits. Second, with lower levels of absolute risk, the cost effectiveness of any intervention will be affected.

Although observational data clearly indicate the relative importance of cholesterol determinations in men and women, randomized data on women, particularly in primary prevention, are limited because trials have generally included far fewer women than men. Recent large-scale trials of statins have begun to include larger numbers of women,[16, 17, 40–43] and these studies generally indicate that the qualitative risk reductions among women are comparable to those in men (see Table 26–6). Unfortunately, no single trial is powered to determine whether or not there are small quantitative differences in risk reduction by gender. Until more data from individual large-scale trials and meta-analyses are available, based on available data it is reasonable to assume that relative risk reductions among men and women are comparable.

Even if one assumes comparable risk reductions among women, the cost efficacy will vary, given differences in absolute rates of CHD among those without cardiovascular disease. To save one life from CHD, one would have to treat more women than

TABLE 26–7 • Cost Effectiveness of Cholesterol Reduction in Secondary Prevention

A. Estimated Cost per Year of Life Saved for Lovastatin in Secondary Prevention*

	Age (y)				
Lovastatin Dose	35–44	45–54	55–64	65–74	75–84
20 mg/d					
Men	Savings	Savings	$1,600	$10,000	$19,000
Women	$4,500	$3,500	$8,100	$12,000	$15,000
40 mg/d					
Men	$14,000	$8,600	$17,000	$27,000	$38,000
Women	$49,000	$30,000	$29,000	$30,000	$29,000

*Based on the coronary heart disease policy model.
Adapted from Goldman, L, Weinstein MC, Goldman PA, et al. Cost effectiveness of HMG-CoA reductase inhibition for primary and secondary prevention of coronary heart disease. JAMA 1991; 265:1145–1151. Copyright 1991, American Medical Association.

B. Estimated Cost per Year of Life Saved for Simvastatin in Secondary Prevention†

	Age (y)		
Cholesterol Level	35	59	70
213 mg/dL			
Men	$11,400	$7,000	$6,200
Women	$27,000	$16,400	$13,300
261 mg/dL			
Men	$8,800	$5,500	$4,700
Women	$18,800	$16,400	$8,500
309 mg/dL			
Men	$6,700	$4,200	$3,800
Women	$13,200	$7,100	$6,200

†Based on the 4S Trial.
Adapted with permission from Johannesson M, Jonssan B, Kjekshus J, et al. Cost effectiveness of simvastatin treatment to lower cholesterol levels in patients with coronary heart disease. N Engl J Med 1997; 336:332–336. Copyright 1997, Massachusetts Medical Society. All rights reserved.

similarly aged men if all other risk factors are equivalent. This increases the cost per life saved among women. This has been illustrated in several cost-benefit analyses (see following discussion). Tables 26–7 and 26–8 illustrate clear and dramatic differences in the cost per year of life saved between men and women at all ages and both primary and secondary prevention.

TABLE 26–8 • Estimated Cost Per Year of Life Saved for Lovastatin in Primary Prevention*

	Age (y)				
Cholesterol Level	*35–44*	*45–54*	*55–64*	*65–74*	*75–84*
LOW RISK†					
>300 mg/dL					
Men	$330,000	$110,000	$58,000	$58,000	$150,000
Women	$1,500,000	$320,000	$86,000	$68,000	$111,000
>250 mg/dL					
Men	$690,000	$220,000	$93,000	$85,000	$210,000
HIGH RISK‡					
>300 mg/dL					
Men	$24,000	$13,000	$15,000	$23,000	$66,000
Women	$195,000	$62,000	$34,000	$39,000	$67,000
>250 mg/dL					
Men	$70,000	$36,000	$27,000	$33,000	$89,000

*Based on coronary heart disease policy model.
†No major cardiovascular risk factors.
‡Hypertension, cigarette smoking, and obesity (130% of ideal body weight).
Adapted from Goldman L, Weinstein MC, Goldman PA, et al. Cost effectiveness of HMG-CoA reductase inhibition for primary and secondary prevention of coronary heart disease. JAMA 1991; 265:1145–1151. Copyright 1991, American Medical Association.

The differences in the costs per year of life saved among men and women, particularly in primary prevention in younger adults, has prompted the ACP to adopt different cutpoints for initiation of screening among men and women.[51] Specifically, their guidelines recommend against screening for younger women (<45 years of age) and men younger than 35 years of age. The NCEP, in contrast, recommends screening for all adults older than 20 years of age, regardless of gender. More data from large-scale trials are needed to further clarify this issue.

COSTS OF CHOLESTEROL REDUCTION

The cost effectiveness of interventions to prevent heart disease is of particular concern due to the prevalence of CHD and the high cost of treating it with technologically advanced interventions. Several issues in the interpretation of cost analyses must be considered. Analyses of preventive measures have a long time horizon, and thus models are necessarily complex. The consequences of initial assumptions for the prevention of chronic diseases can be much more significant than those of interventions with a short time horizon, such as treatment of acute MI (with a 30-day primary outcome). The estimates used for some of the major assumptions are often based on limited data.

Cost-effectiveness estimates are calculated as the ratio of net costs to the gain in life expectancy and are usually presented as the cost per quality-adjusted life-year. Interventions with an incremental cost-effectiveness ratio of less than $40,000 per quality-adjusted life-year are comparable to other chronic interventions, such as hypertension management and hemodialysis. Those less than $20,000 are very favorable. On the other hand, the costs per year of life saved considerably above $40,000 tend to be higher than is generally accepted by most providers.

The cost effectiveness of screening and treatment of high cholesterol has been explored with several models and using various baseline assumptions. One well-known model is the Coronary Heart Disease Policy Model.[53] This model, developed at the Harvard School of Public Health, has been used extensively for the estimation of the cost effectiveness of various preventive interventions, including cholesterol reduction. All model projections are based on the assumption that data from observational cohort studies and randomized trials can be applied broadly to estimate the risk of coronary events and that the incidence of these events will influence mortality.

Although other models use a similar methodology, the source of information for baseline assumptions varies widely. Accordingly, the results of cost-effectiveness analyses of cholesterol reduction vary widely, depending on the baseline assumptions used for the model and the underlying risk of the individual being studied.

Secondary Prevention

Individuals with known CHD are at a considerably higher risk of subsequent events and death than are those without underlying CHD and thus they tend to have more favorable costs per year of life saved than those without disease. Studies of the cost effectiveness of cholesterol reduction were recently reviewed by Kupersmith and associates.[54] The early cost-effectiveness analyses of cholesterol reduction for secondary prevention (which used early trial data on cholestyramine) resulted in very costly interventions, largely because the drugs were relatively ineffective compared with the more effective statin drugs.[55, 56] Estimates for secondary prevention were generally greater than $40,000 per year of life saved.

The first comprehensive statin analysis used the coronary heart disease policy model, estimated costs for both primary and secondary prevention.[57] For secondary prevention, cost-effectiveness ratios were generally favorable (less than $40,000) for lovastatin at doses of 20 and 40 mg (see Table 26–7*A*) for those with cholesterol levels greater than 250 mg/dL. The relationship between cost per year and age was U shaped; in other words, the costs tended to be highest for younger and older individuals and lowest for the middle aged. For those with lower cholesterol levels, ratios were generally favorable at a dose of 20 mg/dL. The costs per year were even more favorable when estimated using the 40% reduction in drug costs that is expected when lovastatin comes off patent in 2001.

The cost per life-year gained was recently estimated for simvastatin, using data from the 4S[58] (see Table 26–7*B*). The investigators modified a Markov model with data from that study. Although there are many similarities to the Goldman estimates for secondary prevention, there are also notable differences in the two sets of estimates. These estimates are based on actual experience in a randomized trial of simvastatin rather than on extrapolation of possible effects from observational data. The probabilities of transition from one of the predefined states to another state were based on the hazard functions for the placebo group. Four functions were used to estimate the probability of four transitions, depending on the baseline presence of a prior event and the nature of the subsequent event. Costs of events were provided by the Swedish Institute for Health Services and ranged from $653 for chest pain admission to $80,178 for cardiac transplantation. The direct cost of simvastatin was estimated at $604 per year of treatment.

The direct cost per life-year saved was $5400 for men and $10,500 for women. As expected, costs decreased as the baseline cholesterol level increased. For example, the direct cost per life saved was $11,400 for a man with a baseline total cholesterol of 213 mg/dL and $6700 for a man with a cholesterol level of 309 mg/dL (see Table 26–7*B*). In contrast with the Goldman estimates, there was not a U-shaped relationship with age. In fact, direct costs tended to be lower with increasing age. This is a key difference between the two models and may reflect the base assumptions in each model.

In the 4S, the estimated indirect costs included estimates for lost productivity.[58] Estimates of productivity were based on work status collected every 6 months during the study. The indirect cost per life-year saved was $1600 for men and $5100 for women. The indirect costs were higher for older than for younger individuals, because older individuals tended to work at a much lower frequency. The use of lost productivity in the analysis tends to value working individuals more than those not working and has not been considered in most models for that reason. The overall, incremental costs of treatment in all groups analyzed were attractive by most standards; direct costs were well below $20,000, except for 35-year-old women with a cholesterol level of 213 mg/dL ($27,400).

Primary Prevention

The cost-effectiveness data on primary prevention are limited. Weinstein and Stason,[55] using data from the LRC-CPPT of cholestyramine, estimated a cost of $237,400 per year of life saved. Oster and Epstein[56] estimated the cost effectiveness of this same intervention, presenting a range of costs from $99,500 to $1.7 million, depending on age and other risk factors; the greatest cost-effectiveness ratio was found for older individuals with fewer risk factors. The CHD policy model made estimates for lovastatin,[57] finding that favorable costs per life-year were largely confined to middle-aged men with multiple coronary risk factors (see Table 26–8). Again, there was a U-shaped relationship, with costs increasing among the elderly compared with the young. Costs were generally prohibitive among women and among those with lower cholesterol levels. Although there are as yet no data from a trial of primary prevention estimating cost effectiveness, analyses are under way and should be available shortly. If direct costs decrease with age for primary prevention, as they did for the 4S analysis of secondary prevention, then cost-effectiveness estimates for the elderly would be more favorable for primary prevention in the elderly than for the middle aged.

GUIDELINES

To reduce the prevalence of elevated cholesterol levels in the United States, the NCEP issued its first Adult Treatment Panel (ATP) report in 1988[48] and a second report in 1993.[50] The NCEP recommends lowering levels of total and LDL cholesterol to decrease risks of CHD. These guidelines recommend nonpharmacologic interventions for approximately 30% of American adults and cholesterol-lowering drugs for about 7%.

The goals of intervention are based on the level of CHD risk for an individual (Table 26–9). The NCEP recommends a goal of LDL cholesterol lower than 160 mg/dL for people over that level with only one other risk factor and no disease. For people without disease but with two other risk factors (family history under age 55 years, hypertension, cigarette smoking, HDL cholesterol less than 35 mg/dL), the goal is an LDL cholesterol lower than 130 mg/dL. For people with prior cardiovascular disease, the goal is an LDL cholesterol lower than 100 mg/dL. Those with diabetes are considered at highest risk, and the LDL goal is lower than 100 mg/dL.

For primary prevention the NCEP recommends a Step 1 diet to lower fat intake to 30% of total calories.

TABLE 26–9 • National Cholesterol Education Program Adult Treatment Panel Guidelines

	LDL Goal (mg/dL)	Initial Diet Therapy (mg/dL)	Initial Drug (mg/dL)
With CHD or diabetes	<100	100	≥130
Without CHD but with ≥2 risk factors*	≥130	130	≥160
Without CHD but with <2 risk factors	≥160	160	≥190

*Risk factors include age and gender (male ≥ 45 years, female ≥ 55 years), family history of heart disease, cigarette smoking, hypertension, diabetes mellitus, and low high-density lipoprotein level (<35 mg/dL).

CHD, coronary heart disease, LDL, low-density lipoprotein.

From Expert Panel on Detection, Evaluation, and Treatment of High Blood Cholesterol in Adults: Summary of the second report of the National Cholesterol Education Program (NCEP) Expert Panel on detection, evaluation, and treatment of high blood cholesterol in adults (Adult Treatment Panel II). JAMA 1993; 269:3015–3023.

Of this, saturated fat should be less than 10% with polyunsaturated and monounsaturated fat each less than 10%. Carbohydrates are 55% and protein 15% of calories. Cholesterol intake is no more than 300 mg/day. If after 3 months the goals of therapy are not met or the patient already has vascular disease of some kind, the Step 2 diet is recommended, consisting of less than 7% of calories from saturated fat and 10% from polyunsaturated fat with the remained in monounsaturated fat (13%). Cholesterol intake is limited to 200 mg/day. For patients who find it difficult to understand amounts based on a percentage of calories, it may be helpful to translate these guidelines into grams of fat, protein, and other dietary constituents, the reporting of which is now mandated on labels of all foods sold in the United States. In addition, professional dietetic counseling with food records may be helpful.

If targets are not met after diet to lower the LDL cholesterol to target, drug therapy is started. The fundamental principle of drug therapy is to use the lowest dose of drugs to reach the goals. This means starting with the lowest dose of a drug, waiting a month to assess its effects, and then adding the next dose.

SUMMARY

The totality of evidence supports the judgment of a causal relationship of elevated serum cholesterol and risk of CHD. Specifically, a 10% increase in serum cholesterol is associated with a 20% to 30% increase in risk of CHD, and elevations earlier in life seem to be associated with even higher increases in risk. Randomized trials have demonstrated that treatment to lower cholesterol levels by 10% will reduce risks of CHD death by 10% and events by 18%, and treatment for more than 5 years yields a 25% reduction in CHD events. Recent statin trials raise the possibility that these potent lipid-lowering agents also may reduce the risk of stroke, though additional randomized trial data will be helpful in better clarifying this effect.

Existing data do not support a causal role of cholesterol lowering in increasing nonvascular mortality or any specific nonvascular cause of death. Results from recent overviews of randomized trials are most consistent with a reduction in total mortality associated with cholesterol reduction in primary prevention as well as secondary prevention. The ongoing large-scale mortality trials with their anticipated larger cholesterol reductions will provide more reliable data on total, nonvascular, and cause-specific nonvascular mortality. These trials will add greatly to our understanding of treatment for hyperlipidemia.

At present, recommendations for cholesterol reduction as outlined by the NCEP weigh the clear benefits in terms of CHD against any possible, but as yet unproved, risks in terms of nonvascular morbidity and mortality.[50] In secondary prevention the benefits of cholesterol lowering on CHD and total mortality, and the cost effectiveness of this therapy, have been clearly demonstrated. For those who have not had a CHD event, the following three strategies have been outlined to reduce risks of CHD by cholesterol reduction:

1. Public health measures aimed at reducing the mean population cholesterol level
2. Primary prevention measures that stress nonpharmacologic interventions among those at higher than average risk
3. Aggressive cholesterol reduction, including pharmacologic intervention, among those at highest risk (those with diabetes) or with underlying atherosclerotic disease.

Mean age-adjusted cholesterol levels have fallen in the United States since the mid-1960s.[59] It has been estimated that approximately 30% of the decline in CHD mortality in the 1970s and early 1980s in the United States could be attributed to cholesterol reduction.[60] Therefore, public health measures to further reduce the mean cholesterol of the population represent safe, effective, and inexpensive means of CHD prevention that clearly appear warranted. For the 30% of the adult U.S. population recommended for nonpharmacologic intervention, lifestyle modification avoids costs and any potential risks associated with drug therapy. Recommendations for drug therapy have focused on those at highest risk for CHD events, and approximately 7% of the adult population meet ATP II guidelines for pharmacologic intervention. Pending the outcome of the ongoing trials, current NCEP ATP II recommendations seem both justified and warranted.

REFERENCES

1. Consensus Conference. Lowering blood cholesterol to prevent heart disease. JAMA 1985; 253:2080–2086.
2. LaRosa JC, Hunninhake D, Bush D, et al. The cholesterol facts: A summary of the evidence relating dietary fats, serum cholesterol, and coronary heart disease: A joint statement by the American Heart Association and the National Heart, Lung, and Blood Institute. AHA Medical/Scientific Statement, AHA and NHLBI, 1990, pp 1721–1733.
3. Chen Z, Peto R, Collins R, et al. Serum cholesterol concentration and coronary heart disease in population with low cholesterol concentrations. BMJ 1991; 303:276–282.
4. Law MR, Wald NJ, Wu T, et al. Systematic underestimation of association between serum cholesterol concentration and ischaemic heart disease in observational studies: Data from the BUPA study. BMJ 1994; 308:363–366.
5. Wilhelmsen L, Berglund G, Elmfeldt D, et al. The multifactor primary prevention trial in Goteborg, Sweden. Eur Heart J 1986; 7:279–288.
6. Multiple Risk Factor Intervention Trial Research Group. Multi-

ple Risk Factor Intervention Trial: Risk factor changes and mortality results. JAMA 1982; 248:1465–1477.
7. Miettinen TA, Huttunen JK, Naukkarinen V. Multifactorial primary prevention of cardiovascular diseases in middle-aged men: Risk factor changes, incidence, and mortality. JAMA 1985; 254:2097–2102.
8. Hjerman I, Byre KV, Holme I, Leren P. Effect of diet and smoking on the incidence of coronary heart disease: Report from the Oslo Study Group of a randomized trial of healthy men. Lancet 1981; 2:1303–1310.
9. Dayton S, Pearce ML, Hashimoto S, et al. A controlled clinical trial of a diet high in unsaturated fat in preventing complications of atherosclerosis. Circulation 1969; 39, 40 (suppl 2):1–63.
10. Dorr AE, Gunderson K, Schneider JC, et al. Colestipol hydrochloride in hypercholesterolemic patients: Effect on serum cholesterol and mortality. J Chronic Dis 1978; 31:5–14.
11. Committee of Principal Investigators, World Health Organization Clofibrate Trial. A cooperative trial in the primary prevention of ischemic heart disease using clofibrate. Br Heart J 1978; 40:1069–1118.
12. Committee of Principal Investigators. World Health Organization cooperative trial on primary prevention of ischaemic heart disease with clofibrate to lower serum cholesterol: Final mortality follow-up. Lancet 1984; 2:600–604.
13. Heady JN, Morris JN, Oliver MF. WHO clofibrate/cholesterol trial clarifications (letter). Lancet 1992; 340:1405–1406.
14. Frick MH, Elo O, Haapa K, et al. Helsinki Heart Study: Primary prevention trial with gemfibrozil in middle-aged men with dyslipidemia: Safety of treatment, changes in risk factors, and incidence of coronary heart disease. N Engl J Med 1987; 317:1237–1245.
15. Lipid Research Clinics Program. The Lipid Research Clinics Coronary Primary Prevention Trial results: I. Reduction in the incidence of coronary heart disease. JAMA 1984; 251:351–364.
16. Shepherd J, Cobbe SM, Ford I, et al. Prevention of coronary heart disease with pravastatin in men with hypercholesterolemia. N Engl J Med 1995; 333:1301–1307.
17. Downs JR, Clearfield M, Weis S, et al. Primary prevention of acute coronary events with lovastatin in men and women with average cholesterol levels. JAMA 1998; 279:1615–1622.
18. Muldoon MF, Manuck SB, Matthew KA. Lowering cholesterol concentrations and mortality: A quantitative review of primary prevention trials. BMJ 1990; 301:309–314.
19. Rossouw JE, Lewis B, Rifkind BM. The value of lowering cholesterol after myocardial infarction. N Engl J Med 1990; 323:1112–1119.
20. Holme I. An analysis of randomized trials evaluating the effects of cholesterol reduction on total mortality and coronary heart disease incidence. Circulation 1990; 82:1916–1924.
21. Ravnskov U. Cholesterol-lowering trials in coronary heart disease: Frequency of citation and outcome. BMJ 1992; 305:15–19.
22. Collins R, Keech A, Peto R, et al. Cholesterol and total mortality: Need for larger trials. BMJ 1992; 304:1689.
23. Peto R, Yusuf S, Collins R. Cholesterol-lowering trials: Results in their epidemiologic context (abstract). Circulation 1985; 72:111–451.
24. Law MR, Wald NJ, Thompson SG. By how much and how quickly does reduction in serum cholesterol concentration lower risk of ischaemic heart disease? BMJ 1994; 308:367–372.
25. Law MR, Thompson SG, Wald NJ. Assessing possible hazards of reducing serum cholesterol. BMJ 1994; 308:373–379.
26. Gould LA, Rossouw JE, Santanello NC, et al. Cholesterol reduction yields clinical benefit: A new look at old data. Circulation 1995; 91:2274–2282.
27. Gould AL, Rossouw JE, Santanello NC, et al. Cholesterol reduction yields clinical benefit: Impact of statin trials. Circulation 1998; 97:946–952.
28. Wolf PA, Kannel WB, Verter J. Current status of risk factors for stroke. Neurol Clin 1983; 1:317–343.
29. Iso H, Jacobs DR Jr, Wentworth D, et al. Serum cholesterol levels and six-year mortality from stroke in 350,977 men screened for the Multiple Risk Factor Intervention Trial. N Engl J Med 1989; 320:904–910.
30. Smith GD, Shipley MJ, Mermot MG, Rose G. Plasma cholesterol concentration and mortality: The White Hall Study. JAMA 1992; 267:70–76.
31. Chen ZM, Collins R, Peto R, Li XY. No association between serum cholesterol and stroke rates in a Chinese population. N Engl J Med 1989; 321:1339–1340.
32. Prospective Studies Collaboration. Cholesterol, diastolic blood pressure, and stroke: 13,000 strokes in 450,000 people in 45 prospective cohorts. Lancet 195; 346:1647–1653.
33. Tanaka H, Ueda Y, Hayashi M, et al. Risk factors for cerebral hemorrhage and cerebral infarction in a Japanese rural community. Stroke 1982; 13:62–73.
34. Kaga A, Popper JS, Rhoads GG. Factors related to stroke incidence in Hawaiian Japanese men: The Honolulu Heart Study. Stroke 1980; 11:14–21.
35. Blackburn H, Jacobs DR. The ongoing natural experiment of cardiovascular diseases in Japan. Circulation 1989; 79:718–720.
36. Shimamotot T, Komachi Y, Inada H, et al. Trends for coronary heart disease and stroke and their risk factors in Japan. Circulation 1989; 79:503–515.
37. Robertson TL, Kato H, Rhoads GG, et al. Epidemiologic studies of coronary heart disease and stroke in Japanese men living in Japan, Hawaii, and California. Am J Cardiol 1977; 39:239–243.
38. Hebert PR, Gaziano JM, Hennekens CH. An overview of trials of cholesterol lowering and risk of stroke. Arch Intern Med 1995; 155:50–55.
39. Atkins D, Psaty BM, Koepsell TD, et al. Cholesterol reduction and the risk of stroke in men. Ann Intern Med 1993; 119:136–145.
40. Scandinavian Simvastatin Survival Study Group. Randomised trial of cholesterol lowering in 4444 patients with coronary heart disease: The Scandinavian Simvastatin Survival Study (4S). Lancet 1994; 344:1383–1389.
41. Scandinavian Simvastatin Survival Study Group. Baseline serum cholesterol and treatment effect in the Scandinavian Simvastatin Survival Study (4S). Lancet 1995; 345:1274–1275.
42. The West of Scotland Coronary Prevention Study Group. A coronary primary prevention study of Scottish men aged 45–64 years: Trial design. J Clin Epidemiol 1992; 45:489–860.
43. Sacks FM, Pfeffer MA, Moye LA, et al. The effect of pravastatin on coronary events after myocardial infarction in patients with average cholesterol levels. N Engl J Med 1996; 335:1001–1009.
44. Hebert PR, Gaziano JM, Chan KS, Hennekens CH. Cholesterol lowering with statin drugs, risk of stroke, and total mortality: An overview of randomized trials. JAMA 1997; 278:313–321.
45. Davey Smith GD, Pekkanen J. Should there be a moratorium on the use of cholesterol lowering drugs? BMJ 1992; 304:431–434.
46. Oliver MF. Might treatment of hypercholesterolaemia increase non-cardiac mortality? Lancet 1991; 337:1529–1531.
47. Gaziano JM, Hebert PR, Hennekens CH. Cholesterol reduction: Weighing the benefits and risks. Ann Intern Med 1996; 124:914–918.
48. Engelberg H. Low serum cholesterol and suicide. Lancet 1992; 339:727–729.
48a. Gordon DJ. Cholesterol lowering and total mortality. *In* Rifkind B (ed). Lowering Cholesterol in High-Risk Individuals and Populations. New York, Marcel Dekker, 1995, pp 33–48.
49. The Expert Panel. Report of the National Cholesterol Education Program Expert Panel on detection, evaluation, and treatment of high blood pressure in adults. Arch Intern Med 1988; 148:36–69.
50. Expert Panel on Detection, Evaluation, and Treatment of High Blood Cholesterol in Adults: Summary of the second report of the National Cholesterol Education program (NCEP) Expert Panel on detection, evaluation, and treatment of high blood cholesterol in adults (Adult Treatment Panel II). JAMA 1993; 269:3015–3023.
51. American College of Physicians. Clinical Guideline, Part 1. Guidelines for using serum cholesterol, high-density lipoprotein cholesterol, and triglyceride levels as screening tests for preventing coronary heart disease in adults. Ann Intern Med 1996; 124:515–517.
52. Garber AM, Browner WS, Hulley SB. Clinical Guideline, Part 2. Cholesterol Screening in asymptomatic adults, revisited. Ann Intern Med 1996; 124:518–531.
53. Weinstein MC, Coxson PG, Williams LW, et al. Forecasting coronary heart disease incidence, mortality, and cost: The Coronary Heart Disease Policy Model. Am J Public Health 1987; 77:1417–1426.

54. Kupersmith J, Holmes-Rovner M, Hogan A, et al. Cost-effectiveness analysis in heart disease, Part II: Preventive therapies. Progr Cardiovasc Dis 1995; 37:243–271.
55. Weinstein MC, Stason WB. Cost-effectiveness of interventions to prevent or treat coronary heart disease. Annu Rev Publ Health 1985; 6:41–63.
56. Oster G, Epstein AM. Cost-effectiveness of antihyperlipidemic therapy in the prevention of coronary heart disease: The case of cholestyramine. JAMA 1987; 258:2381–2387.
57. Goldman L, Weinstein MC, Goldman PA, Williams LW. Cost-effectiveness of HMG-CoA reductase inhibition for primary and secondary prevention of coronary heart disease. JAMA 1991; 265:1145–1151.
58. Johannesson M, Jonsson B, Kjekshus J, et al. Cost-effectiveness of simvastatin treatment to lower cholesterol levels in patients with coronary heart disease. N Engl J Med 1997; 336:332–336.
59. National Center for Health Statistics—National Heart, Lung, and Blood Institute Collaborative Lipid Group. Trends in serum cholesterol levels among U.S. adults aged 20 to 74 years: Data from the National Health and Nutrition Examination Surveys, 1960 to 1980. JAMA 1987; 257(7):937–942.
60. Goldman L, Cook EF. The decline in ischemic heart disease mortality rates: An analysis of the comparative effects of medical interventions and changes in lifestyle. Ann Intern Med 1984; 101:825–836.

27 Blood Pressure Reduction

▶ Paul K. Whelton
▶ Jiang He

Estimates of the prevalence of high blood pressure (BP) as well as the awareness, treatment, and control of hypertension are available for many countries and ethnic groups.[1, 2] The prevalence of hypertension varies substantially depending on geographic setting, characteristics of the survey sample, criteria for diagnosis, and BP measurement methods. Studies have consistently identified a high prevalence of hypertension in economically developed countries, and high BP is being noted with increasing frequency in the economically developing world. In contrast, surveys of isolated populations have consistently identified a low average level of BP and little, if any, hypertension. Recognizing this, studies in both isolated and economically developed populations have identified a similar pattern for relationships between BP and environmental factors such as diet and exercise. In addition, migration studies have demonstrated that persons from low BP populations are prone to experience a progressively higher BP and increased risk of developing hypertension as they move from their natural environment to a setting where environmental exposures favor a high prevalence of hypertension.[3, 4] In aggregate, these studies indicate that hypertension is not an inevitable consequence of life. Most humans, however, have a strong genetic predisposition to develop hypertension when exposed to the unfavorable environment found in economically developed societies.

PREVALENCE OF HYPERTENSION

Results from the most recent U.S. national survey indicate that 24% of the adult, noninstitutionalized population of the United States, representing 43,186,000 persons, meet the criteria for diagnosis of hypertension proposed by the Fifth Joint National Committee for Detection, Evaluation, and Treatment of Hypertension (average systolic BP ≥ 140 mm Hg, or average diastolic BP ≥ 90 mm Hg, or treatment with antihypertensive medication).[5] An additional 7.1%, representing 12,744,000 persons, who did not meet the criteria for diagnosis at the time of the survey had been told by a "doctor or other health care professional" that they had hypertension. The prevalence of hypertension rose progressively with increasing age, from the teens to the 70s. As a consequence, hypertension was noted in less than 10% of those 18 to 29 years old but in approximately 60% to 70% of their counterparts in their 60s and 70s. During the second half of life, much of the age-related increase in prevalence of hypertension was due to a progressive rise in systolic BP. Diastolic BP rose until about the 40s but declined in succeeding years. As a result, much of the hypertension in later years was attributable to an isolated elevation of systolic BP. In addition to age, prevalence varied by race and gender. The age-adjusted prevalence of hypertension in non-Hispanic blacks was almost 50% higher than the corresponding prevalence in non-Hispanic whites and Mexican-Americans. Men had a higher prevalence of hypertension during the first half of life, but the reverse was true after the 60s. For those aged 60 years and older, the prevalence of isolated systolic hypertension (systolic BP > 140 mm Hg and diastolic BP < 90 mm Hg) was slightly higher for women (66%) compared with men (63%).[6] The magnitude of the gender-associated differences in prevalence was, however, much smaller than the previously described associations for age and race. Overall, approximately two thirds of those with hypertension were aware of their diagnosis (69%), 53% were being treated with antihypertensive medications, and 24% had a systolic BP less than 140 mm Hg and a diastolic BP less than 90 mm Hg while being treated with antihypertensive medications.

BLOOD PRESSURE–ASSOCIATED RISK OF CARDIOVASCULAR AND RENAL DISEASE

Epidemiologic studies have repeatedly demonstrated that high BP is an important, independent predictor of cardiovascular disease risk.[7] MacMahon and colleagues[8] conducted a pooled analysis of nine prospective cohort studies in which 418,343 adults, aged 25 to 84 years, were followed for an average of 10 years to study the relationship between baseline BP and subsequent occurrence of coronary heart disease (CHD) and stroke. At the outset, none of the study participants had clinical evidence of CHD or stroke. The authors' findings were corrected for the regression dilution bias, which occurs when studying variables that can be measured only in an imprecise manner. The difference between the highest (105 mm Hg) and lowest (76 mm Hg) category of mean usual diastolic BP at entry was only about 30 mm Hg. Even so, the risk of CHD and stroke was about fivefold and tenfold higher for those at the higher compared with the lower end of this BP range. A 5 to 6 mm Hg difference in diastolic BP at entry was associated with a 20% to 25% difference in the corresponding risk of CHD and a 35% to 40% difference in the risk of stroke. The relationship between BP and renal disease in observational studies has been equally impressive.[9] In a 16-year follow-up of 332,544 men who were screened for possible participation in the Multiple Risk Factor Intervention Trial (MRFIT), hypertension appeared to be the underlying cause in almost half (49%) of the 814 instances in which end-stage renal disease (ESRD) occurred during follow-up.[10] Among those who survived the first 10 years of follow-up without suffering from ESRD, the relative risk of eventually developing ESRD was 2.8 times higher for those who had stage 1 hypertension (systolic BP 140 to 159 mm Hg or diastolic BP 90 to 99 mm Hg) at baseline compared with their counterparts who did not have hypertension. The corresponding relative risks were 5.0 for those with stage 2 hypertension (systolic BP 160 to 179 mm Hg or diastolic BP 100 to 109 mm Hg), 8.4 for those with stage 3 hypertension (systolic BP 180 to 209 mm Hg or diastolic BP 110 to 119 mm Hg), and 12.4 for those with stage 4 hypertension (systolic BP ≥ 210 mm Hg or diastolic BP ≥ 120 mm Hg). The risk of ESRD was highest for those with both a high level of systolic and diastolic BP at baseline, but much of the risk was due to the effects of a high systolic BP.

Taking both prevalence and corresponding risk into account, the approximately 5% of the population with stages 2 to 4 hypertension (systolic BP ≥ 160 mm Hg or diastolic BP ≥ 100 mm Hg) account for about a quarter of the excess BP-related CHD risk; the approximately 20% with stage 1 hypertension (systolic BP 140 to 159 mm Hg or diastolic BP 90 to 99 mm Hg) account for more than 40% of the population excess risk; and much of the remaining BP-related excess in risk (≥20%) occurs in the approximately 25% who have a high normal BP (systolic BP 130 to 139 mm Hg or diastolic BP 80 to 89 mm Hg).[6] Although stroke and ESRD are somewhat more BP-dependent diseases, the overall pattern for BP-related population excess risk for these two complications appears to be quite similar.

In aggregate, the previously mentioned epidemiologic data provide a strong scientific basis for interest in detection, treatment, and control of hypertension, both in the individual patient and in the community as a whole. The data also underscore the potential for risk reduction after application of effective treatment in those with less severe hypertension. Not only is the risk of serious outcomes such as CHD, stroke, and ESRD twofold to threefold higher in those with stage 1 hypertension compared with their counterparts with an optimal level of BP (<120 mm Hg systolic and <80 mm Hg diastolic), but also stage 1 hypertensives account for nearly half of the BP-related excess in risk of these outcomes in the general population. Finally, the data indicate the importance of concurrent efforts aimed at prevention of hypertension.[11] Although not the focus of this chapter, primary prevention of hypertension complements and extends the risk reduction goals of treating established hypertension. Furthermore, it provides a potential means to interrupt and reduce the need for the continuing costly and only modestly successful cycle of detecting and treating hypertensive patients.

ANTIHYPERTENSIVE DRUG TREATMENT TRIALS

Over the past four decades, numerous antihypertensive drug treatment trials have been conducted to determine whether BP reduction decreases the risk of cardiovascular disease. During the 1950s and early 1960s, several nonrandomized, historically controlled trials were conducted in patients with malignant hypertension.[12–14] Although the antihypertensive drugs used in these trials were crude by current standards, their effect on all-cause mortality was so impressive that the value of treatment in this context was rapidly and widely accepted by the medical community. Over the next decade, the value of antihypertensive drug therapy was documented in patients with severe (stages 3 to 4) but nonmalignant hypertension.[15–17] In each of these trials, treatment benefits were apparent within months of initiating antihypertensive drug therapy and were primarily due to a substantial reduction in the frequency of hypertensive complications, such as hemorrhagic stroke, congestive heart failure, and uremia.

Despite their value, the trials of the 1950s and 1960s contributed little to knowledge of the effect of antihypertensive drug therapy on CHD, ischemic stroke, and other BP-related atherosclerotic complications. Such information has come from the larger, more prolonged trials that were subsequently conducted in patients with less severe hypertension.[18–35] Most of these trials have demonstrated a statistically significant and impressive reduction in the incidence of fatal and nonfatal stroke. The impact of antihypertensive drug therapy on CHD has been less striking, however, and, with a few exceptions,[25, 26, 33] the risk reduction in individual trials has not been statistically significant. These nonsignificant findings for CHD reduction have led to uncertainty regarding the effects of antihypertensive drug treatment on CHD. In large part, however, this lack of statistical significance may simply reflect a lack of sufficient statistical power to detect moderate reductions in CHD event rates in the individual trials. To overcome this problem, several authors have pooled results from individual drug treatment trials to obtain a more reliable estimate of the effect of antihypertensive treatment on clinical outcomes.[36–39]

Characteristics of Participants in 17 Blood Pressure Reduction Trials

Using standard methods,[37] the authors pooled the results from 17 major randomized, controlled trials in which the effects of antihypertensive drug therapy on clinical outcomes have been evaluated.[16–35] Characteristics of the 47,653 trial participants who were enrolled in these trials as well as important elements of the study design employed in each trial are summarized in Table 27–1. The number of participants enrolled in individual trials ranged from fewer than 100 to more than 17,000, with a median sample size of 840 participants per trial. An elevated diastolic BP was the primary inclusion criterion in most studies, but in some trials participants were required to have both a high systolic and a high diastolic BP at entry.[21, 31, 32, 34, 35] One trial enrolled only patients with isolated systolic hypertension.[33] In five trials, participation was restricted to participants with a diastolic BP less than 110 mm Hg,[23, 24, 27–30, 33] and in four more enrollment was confined to those with a diastolic BP 115 mm Hg or less.[18, 21, 22, 35] In the Hypertension Detection and Follow-up Program (HDFP), trial results were reported separately for participants within three strata of diastolic BP at entry (diastolic BP < 110 mm Hg, diastolic BP 110 to 115 mm Hg, and diastolic BP > 115 mm Hg).[25, 26]

The mean age (weighted by sample size) of the participants in the 17 trials was 56 years, but the average age in individual trials varied from 38 to 76 years. Five trials with 12,483 participants were conducted exclusively in individuals who were over 60 years of age at entry.[31–35] Men and women were represented in approximately equal numbers. In most trials, the participants were followed for 4 to 5 years. In the U.S. Public Health Service Hospitals Cooperative Group (USPHS) trial and Medical Research Council (MRC) trial in older adults, a longer period of follow-up was employed, however, and in five trials the participants were followed for less than 3 years.[16, 17, 20, 21, 23, 24] Treatment was double-blind in nine of the trials, single-blind in four, and open in the remaining four. Diuretics were used as first-step drug therapy in 12 of the 17 trials. Exceptions to this rule were the Wolff and Lindeman trial,[16] in which reserpine was the active therapy; the two MRC trials,[30, 35] in which the participants were randomly assigned to active treatment with either a beta blocker or a diuretic; the Swedish Trial in Old Patients with Hypertension (STOP-Hypertension) trial,[34] in which either a diuretic (hydrochlorothiazide plus the potassium sparing agent amiloride) or a beta blocker (atenolol or pindolol) could be used as first-step therapy; and the general practice trial conducted by Coope and Warrender,[32] in which atenolol was compared with no treatment. In most of the trials, the goal in the active treatment group was to achieve and maintain a diastolic BP 90 mm Hg or less. With the exception of the HDFP trial, in which the control group was assigned to receive usual care, antihypertensive drug therapy was not recommended as a routine treatment for participants in the control group. About one quarter of the participants randomized to control therapy received antihypertensive drug therapy at some stage during their follow-up, however.

The mean reduction in BP during follow-up for those assigned to active treatment compared with their counterparts in the corresponding control group varied by trial. Specifically the mean net reduction in diastolic BP for those assigned to active treatment compared with control ranged from 4 to 27 mm Hg, with an overall average net reduction of 6.5 mm Hg (weighted by sample size). The true overall net reduction in BP may have been somewhat smaller, however, because BP measurements were obtained only in those who continued to participate in the follow-up examinations. Information on systolic BP during follow-up was available for 9 of the 17 trials. In these studies, the overall weighted average net reduction in systolic BP was 16 mm Hg. For both systolic and diastolic BP, the observed reduction was greater in trials in which the participants had a higher level of BP at entry.

Effects of Blood Pressure Reduction on Coronary Heart Disease and Stroke

Overall, 934 CHD events occurred in the participants who were assigned to active treatment, and 1104 CHD events occurred in those who were allocated to con-

TABLE 27–1 • Characteristics of Participants and Study Design for 17 Randomized Trials of Antihypertensive Drug Therapy

Trial and Year	Sample Size	Entry DBP (mm Hg)	Entry SBP (mm Hg)	Mean Age (y)	Men (%)	Mean Follow-up (y)	Blinding	Main Drug Type(s)	Mean DBP Reduction (mm Hg)*	Mean SBP Reduction (mm Hg)*
Wolff and Lindeman, 1966[16]	87	100–130	—	49	32	1.4	Double	A	20	—
Veterans Administration, 1967[17]	143	115–129	—	51	100	1.5	Double	D + A + V	27	43
Veterans Administration, 1970[18]	380	90–114	—	51	100	3.3	Double	D + A + V	19	31
Carter, 1970[19]	97	≥110	—	—	57	4	Open	D	—	—
Barraclough et al, 1973[20]	116	100–120	—	56	43	2	Single	D/M	13	—
Hypertension-Stroke Study, 1974[21]	452	90–115	140–220	59	41	2.3	Double	D	12	25
USPHS Study, 1977[22]	389	90–114	—	44	80	7	Double	D + A	10	18
VA-NHLBI Study, 1977[23, 24]	1012	85–105	—	38	81	1.5	Double	D	7	—
HDFP, 1979[25, 26]	10,940	≥90	—	51	55	5	Open	D	6	—
Oslo Study, 1980[27]	785	90–109	—	45	100	5.5	Open	D	10	—
Australian National Study, 1980[29]	3427	95–109	<200	50	63	4	Single	D	6	—
MRC Study (younger), 1985[30]	17,354	90–109	<200	52	52	5	Single	BB/D	6	—
EWPHE Study, 1985[31]	840	90–119	160–239	72	30	4.7	Double	D	8	20
Coope and Warrender, 1986[32]	884	105–120	<280	69	31	4.4	Open	BB	11	18
SHEP Study, 1991[33]	4736	<90	160–219	72	43	4.5	Double	D + BB	4	12
STOP-Hypertension Study, 1991[34]	1627	90–120	180–230	76	37	2.1	Double	BB/D	8	20
MRC Study (older), 1992[35]	4396	<115	160–209	70	42	5.8	Single	BB/D	7	14
Mean or total	47,653	—	—	56	52	4.7	—	—	6.5	16

* The difference in mean blood pressure was based on data from those who attended follow-up for blood pressure measurement.
DBP, diastolic blood pressure; SBP, systolic blood pressure; A, alkaloid; D, diuretic; V, vasodilator; M, methyldopa; BB, beta blocker.

TABLE 27–2 • Reduction in Risk for Coronary Heart Disease, Stroke, Cardiovascular Disease, and All-Cause Mortality: Results from 17 Randomized Trials with 23,847 Active Treatment and 23,806 Control Participants

	No. of Events			
	Active	*Control*	% Risk Reduction (95% CI)*	*P* Value
Total coronary heart disease	934	1104	16 (8–23)	<0.001
Fatal coronary heart disease	470	560	16 (5–26)	0.006
Total stroke	525	835	38 (31–45)	<0.001
Fatal stroke	140	234	40 (26–51)	<0.001
Cardiovascular disease deaths	768	964	21 (13–28)	<0.001
All-cause deaths	1435	1634	13 (6–19)	<0.001

* Risk reduction = 1 − odds ratio.
CI, confidence interval.

trol (Table 27–2). When results from the 17 trials were pooled, a highly significant reduction in the odds of total CHD ($P < 0.001$) and fatal CHD ($P = 0.006$) was observed among the participants allocated to active treatment. The reduction in total CHD was 16% (95% confidence interval [CI], 8% to 23%) as was the reduction in fatal CHD (95% CI, 5% to 26%). As shown in Figure 27–1, antihypertensive drug treatment was associated with a reduction in total CHD in 13 of the 17 trials. The reduction was statistically significant in only two of the trials, however.[25, 26, 33] In the HDFP trial, total CHD was reduced by 21% (95% CI, 7% to 33%),[25, 26] and in the Systolic Hypertension in the Elderly Program (SHEP) trial, total CHD was reduced by 28% (95% CI, 6% to 44%).[33]

Overall, 525 strokes occurred in participants who were allocated to active treatment, and 768 occurred in those who were assigned to control (see Table 27–2). Compared with control, those in active treatment experienced a 38% reduction in the odds of total stroke (95% CI, 31% to 45%; $P < 0.001$) and a 40% reduction in the odds of fatal stroke (95% CI, 26% to 51%; $P < 0.001$). In 14 of the 17 trials, the odds ratio for total stroke was reduced in those assigned to active compared with control treatment, and in 9 of the trials, the reduction was statistically significant (Fig. 27–2).

Although the proportional reduction in CHD was less than half that noted for stroke, the absolute reduction in CHD and stroke was less discrepant, given the greater frequency of CHD. Specifically the absolute reductions in total and fatal CHD were 7 and 4 events per 1000 persons, whereas the corresponding absolute reductions in total and fatal stroke were 13 and 4 events per 1000 persons.

Temporal trends from the 17 trials indicated that most of the reduction in stroke risk was achieved within the first year of initiating antihypertensive drug treatment. In contrast, the reduction in CHD risk after institution of antihypertensive or lipid-lowering drug therapy is not usually manifest for 2 to 3 years. The results of the authors' meta-analysis and others indicate, however, that only about two thirds of the expected reduction in CHD has been achieved in the trials conducted to date. This shortfall in risk reduction may simply reflect the effect of random variation. In the authors' meta-analysis, the upper band of the 95% CI for reduction in the risk of total (fatal) CHD was 23% (26%). Alternatively, it may indicate that a

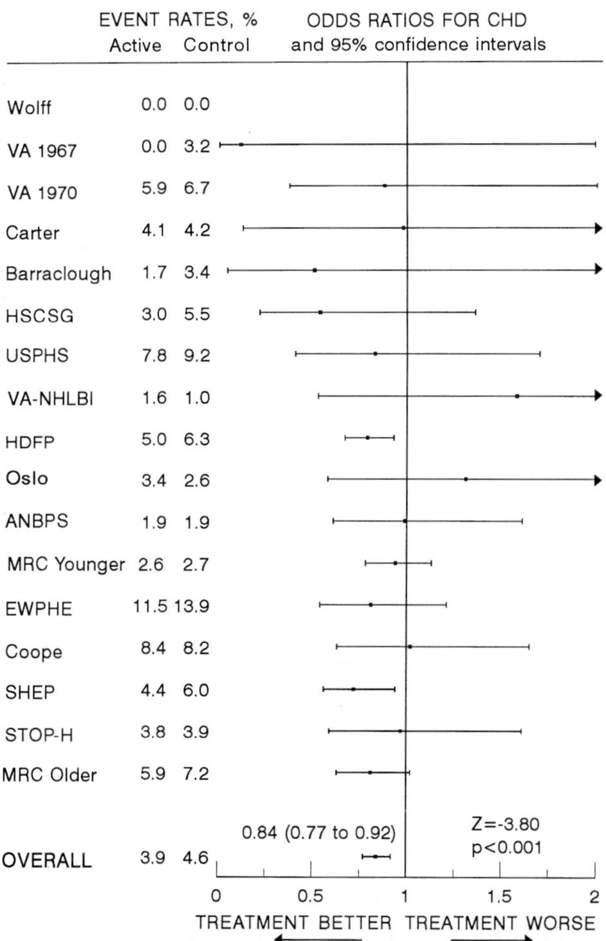

Figure 27–1 Odds ratios and 95% confidence intervals for total (fatal and nonfatal) coronary heart disease (CHD) related to antihypertensive drug treatment. Results from 17 individual randomized, controlled trials and a pooled estimate of their findings.

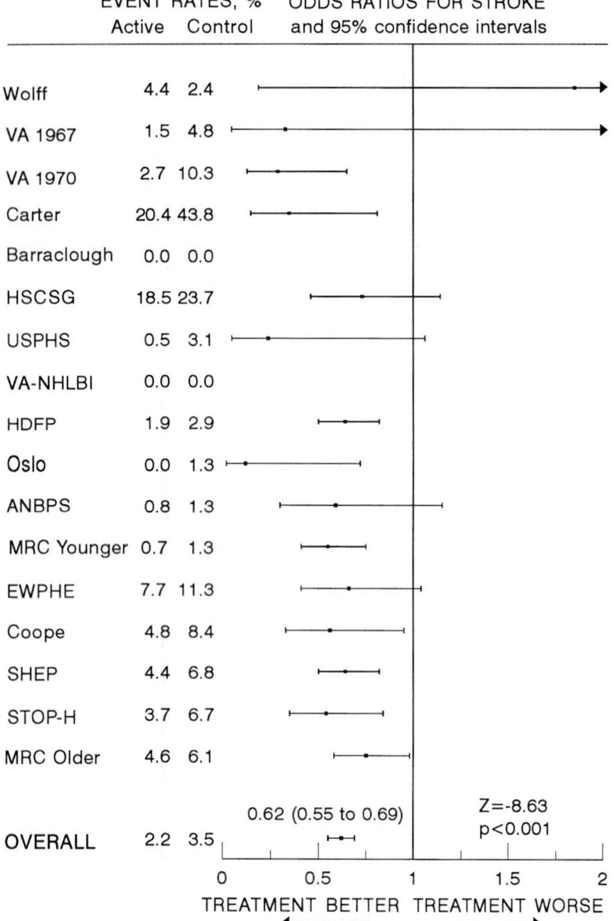

Figure 27–2 Odds ratios and 95% confidence intervals for total (fatal and nonfatal) stroke related to antihypertensive drug treatment. Results from 17 individual randomized, controlled trials and a pooled estimate of their findings. See Table 27–1 for studies listed.

longer period of treatment is necessary to reverse completely the atherosclerotic changes induced by a prolonged elevation of BP.[40–42] A third possibility is that some of the antihypertensive drug treatments used in the trials conducted to date may have produced cardiotoxic side effects that diminished but did not eliminate the beneficial effects of reducing BP. Diuretics were the principal form of drug therapy prescribed in most of the 17 trials, and in several instances they were administered at doses that are now considered to be relatively high. Diuretics can adversely affect a patient's level of serum potassium, total and low-density lipoprotein cholesterol, and glucose. The relevance of this third possibility is currently being evaluated in a number of trials, which are described later in this chapter.

Effects of Blood Pressure Reduction on Total Cardiovascular Disease and All-Cause Mortality

Overall, 768 deaths from cardiovascular disease occurred in the participants who were allocated to active treatment, and 964 deaths occurred in their counterparts who were allocated to a control group (see Table 27–2). The overall reduction in cardiovascular disease mortality for active treatment compared with control was 21% (95% CI, 12% to 28%; $P < 0.001$). In 6 of the 17 trials, the reduction in cardiovascular disease mortality was statistically significant (Fig. 27–3). Non–cardiovascular disease mortality was evenly distributed between the treatment and control groups (667 vs. 670). All-cause mortality was reduced by 13% (95% CI, 6% to 19%; $P < 0.001$) in those allocated to active compared with control treatment (see Table 27–2; Fig. 27–4).

Reduction in Coronary Heart Disease and Stroke by Level of Blood Pressure

Reduction in CHD and stroke risk by baseline level of diastolic BP is presented in Table 27–3. The reduc-

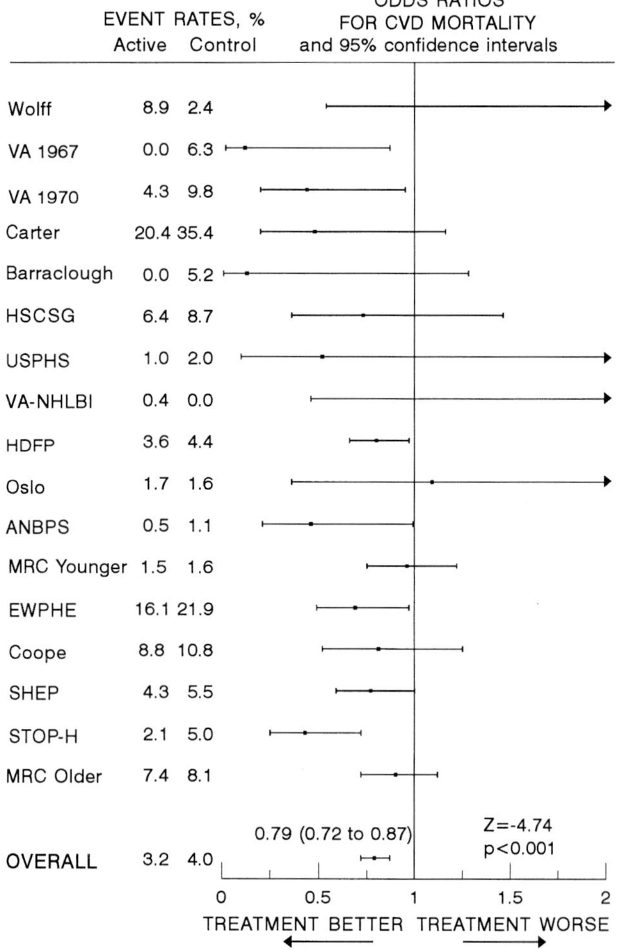

Figure 27–3 Odds ratios and 95% confidence intervals for cardiovascular disease (CVD) mortality related to antihypertensive drug treatment. Results from 17 individual randomized, controlled trials and a pooled estimate of their findings. See Table 27–1 for studies listed.

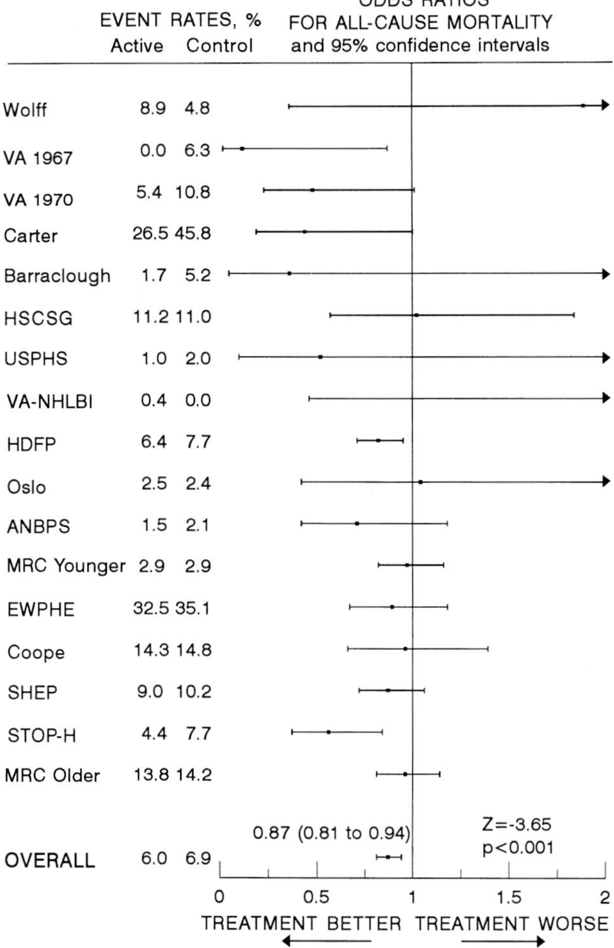

Figure 27–4 Odds ratios and 95% confidence intervals for all-cause mortality related to antihypertensive drug treatment. Results from 17 individual randomized, controlled trials and a pooled estimate of their findings. See Table 27–1 for studies listed.

tion in risk for CHD was greater in those with a higher level of BP at entry, although the differences among the three BP strata were not statistically significant. The proportional reductions in risk for participants with an entry diastolic BP less than 110 mm Hg, 110 to 115 mm Hg, and greater than 115 mm Hg were 14% (95% CI, 4% to 23%), 17% (95% CI, 1% to 31%), and 21% (95% CI, 1% to 37%). The absolute reduction in risk was even greater in participants with a higher level of BP at entry because of the higher event rate in this group. For example, the absolute reduction in risk for total CHD was 5, 12, and 15 events per 1000 persons for participants with an entry diastolic BP less than 110 mm Hg, 110 to 115 mm Hg, and greater than 115 mm Hg. The proportional reduction in risk for stroke did not differ significantly by level of diastolic BP at entry. There was an impressive relationship between absolute reduction in risk and BP at entry, however, because of the higher stroke event rate in those with a higher level of BP. The absolute reduction in risk was 9, 19, and 35 events per 1000 persons in participants with an entry diastolic BP less than 110 mm Hg, 110 to 115 mm Hg, and greater than 115 mm Hg.

Reduction in Coronary Heart Disease and Stroke by Age and Gender

Comparison of the results from 5 trials that were conducted exclusively in older participants[31–35] with the corresponding findings from the remaining 12 trials identified a similar reduction in relative risk but a greater reduction in absolute risk in the trials that were conducted in older participants (Table 27–4). For CHD (fatal and nonfatal), the relative reduction in risk was 19% (95% CI, 7% to 30%) for the trials that were conducted exclusively in older participants and 14% (95% CI, 4% to 23%) for the remaining 12 trials. The corresponding reductions in absolute risk were 13 and 5 events per 1000 persons. For fatal and nonfatal stroke, the proportional reduction in risk was 34% (95% CI, 24% to 44%) for the 5 trials conducted in older participants and 42% (95% CI, 32% to 51%) for the remaining 12 trials. The corresponding absolute reductions in risk were 23 and 9 events per 1000 persons.

Only two trials reported risk reduction by gender.[30, 35] In these two trials, there was no evidence of a gender-related difference in risk reduction.

Reduction in Coronary Heart Disease and Stroke by Trial Duration

Six trials had an intervention duration that was as long or longer than the overall weighted mean duration of 4.7 years.[22, 25, 27, 30, 31, 35] The treatment-related reduction in risk for CHD and stroke was slightly but nonsignificantly lower in this group of trials compared with the remaining 11 trials with a longer duration of follow-up (Table 27–5). For CHD (fatal and nonfatal), the reduction in the odds ratio was 16% (95% CI, 6% to 24%) for the group of trials with a longer duration compared with 17% (95% CI, 1% to 30%) for the group with a shorter duration. For stroke (fatal and nonfatal), the reduction in the odds ratio was 36% (95% CI, 26% to 45%) for the 6 trials with a longer duration compared with 41% (95% CI, 30% to 50%) for the 11 trials with a shorter duration. This discrepancy in risk reduction may simply reflect the difference in mean BP at baseline.

Comparison of Risk Reduction During Diuretic and Beta Blocker Treatment

The effects of first-step therapy with a diuretic compared with a beta-receptor blocker have been ex-

TABLE 27–3 • Risk Reduction in Coronary Heart Disease and Stroke, by Blood Pressure at Trial Entry

Participants' Entry Diastolic Blood Pressure* (mm Hg) (no. of trials)	Active Treatment			Control Treatment			% Risk Reduction (95% CI)		*P* Value	
	No. of Fatal Events	*Total No. of Events*	*No. of Participants*	*No. of Fatal Events*	*Total No. of Events*	*No. of Participants*	*Fatal Events*	*Total Events*	*Fatal Events*	*Total Events*
CORONARY HEART DISEASE										
All <110 ($n = 6$)	264	572	17,603	291	660	17,536	10 (−7–24)	14 (4–23)	0.2	0.01
Some ≥110, all ≤115 ($n = 5$)	124	222	3843	152	265	3826	19 (−3–36)	17 (1–31)	0.09	0.04
Some or all >115 ($n = 8$)	82	140	2401	117	179	2444	29 (5–46)	21 (1–37)	0.02	0.04
STROKE										
All <110 ($n = 6$)	50	237	17,603	83	386	17,536	39 (15–57)	39 (28–48)	0.004	<0.001
Some ≥110, all ≤115 ($n = 5$)	52	175	3843	71	248	3826	27 (−4–49)	32 (17–44)	0.08	<0.001
Some or all >115 ($n = 8$)	38	113	2401	80	201	2444	52 (30–67)	45 (30–56)	<0.001	<0.001

* Hypertension Detection and Follow-up Program had three entry diastolic blood pressure strata.
CI, confidence interval.

TABLE 27–4 • Risk Reduction in Coronary Heart Disease and Stroke, by Age

Participants' Age (no. of trials)	Active Treatment			Control Treatment			% Risk Reduction (95% CI)		*P* Value	
	No. of Fatal Events	*Total No. of Events*	*No. of Participants*	*No. of Fatal Events*	*Total No. of Events*	*No. of Participants*	*Fatal Events*	*Total Events*	*Fatal Events*	*Total Events*
					CORONARY HEART DISEASE					
Some or all <60 years (n = 12)	262	588	17,652	281	674	17,518	7 (−10–22)	14 (4–23)	0.3	0.01
All ≥60 years (n = 5)	208	346	6195	279	430	6288	25 (10–37)	19 (7–30)	0.002	0.004
					STROKE					
Some or all <60 years (n = 12)	62	237	17,652	114	397	17,518	46 (27–60)	42 (32–51)	<0.001	<0.001
All ≥60 years (n = 5)	78	288	6195	120	438	6288	34 (12–50)	34 (24–44)	0.004	<0.001

CI, confidence interval.

TABLE 27–5 • Risk Reduction in Coronary Heart Disease and Stroke, by Trial Duration

Duration of Intervention (no. of trials)	Active Treatment			Control Treatment			% Risk Reduction (95% CI)		P Value	
	No. of Fatal Events	*Total No. of Events*	*No. of Participants*	*No. of Fatal Events*	*Total No. of Events*	*No. of Participants*	*Fatal Events*	*Total Events*	*Fatal Events*	*Total Events*
Coronary Heart Disease										
<4.7 y (n = 11)	111	232	6464	152	281	6485	26 (5–42)	17 (1–30)	0.02	0.04
≥4.7 y (n = 6)	359	702	17,383	408	823	17,321	12 (−1–24)	16 (6–24)	0.08	0.001
Stroke										
<4.7 y (n = 11)	35	229	6464	80	375	6485	55 (35–69)	41 (30–50)	<0.001	<0.001
≥4.7 y (n = 6)	105	296	17,383	154	460	17,321	32 (13–47)	36 (26–45)	0.002	<0.001

plored in four randomized, controlled trials.[30, 35, 43, 44] In the first MRC trial, diuretic treatment yielded a statistically significant 54% (95% CI, 24% to 72%) reduction in the odds of stroke (fatal and nonfatal) compared with treatment with a beta blocker.[30] There was a similar, albeit nonsignificant trend in the second MRC trial conducted in the elderly. In a pooled estimate of the results from all four trials, however, diuretics were associated with only a nonsignificant 13% (95% CI, –8% to 30%) reduction in stroke risk compared with treatment with beta blockers (Fig. 27–5). The MRC trial in older adults identified a statistically significant 40% (95% CI, 14% to 58%) reduction in the odds of CHD for diuretic compared with beta blocker treatment.[35] Again, however, the pooled estimate identified a nonsignificant difference of 4% (95% CI, −11% to 17%) between the treatment effect with diuretics and beta blockers.

Newer classes of antihypertensive drugs, such as angiotensin-converting enzyme (ACE) inhibitors, calcium channel blockers (CCB), and α_1-receptor blockers, are well tolerated and are especially valuable for treatment of patients with specific comorbidities, such as congestive heart failure (ACE inhibitors), angina pectoris (CCB), diabetic nephropathy (ACE inhibitors), and prostatic hypertrophy (α_1-receptor blockers). Whether these newer agents are more effective than diuretics or beta blockers in reducing the risk of CHD and stroke in most patients, however, is unknown. In a meta-analysis of randomized trials comparing short-acting nifedipine with placebo in patients with CHD, CCB treatment was associated with a statistically significant 16% excess in all-cause mortality.[45] Likewise, in a case-control study of hypertensive patients, treatment with short-acting CCBs was associated with an increased risk of myocardial infarction.[46] Compared with those who were treated with diuretics alone, the adjusted risk ratio of myocardial infarction among CCB users, with or without diuretics, was increased by about 60% (risk ratio, 1.62; 95% CI, 1.11 to 2.34; $P = 0.01$). The Multicenter Isradipine Diuretic Atherosclerosis Study (MIDAS) trial showed a trend toward an increased risk of major vascular events in those randomized to a short-acting CCB (isradipine) group compared with their counterparts who were treated with diuretics.[47] The total number of cardiovascular disease events was small ($n = 39$), however, and the difference did not reach statistical significance. In contrast to the findings in MIDAS, treatment with a short-acting formulation of nifedipine was associated with a 57% reduction (95% CI, 23% to 76%) in the risk of stroke compared with placebo in the Shanghai Trial of Nifedipine in the Elderly (STONE) trial.[48] The risk of myocardial infarction was no different in the nifedipine treatment group compared with placebo (relative risk, 0.94; 95% CI, 0.13 to 6.66), but only four cases of myocardial infarction were reported in this trial. The findings in the STONE trial must be tempered by the knowledge that the investigation was single-blind and employed a nonrandomized treatment allocation schedule.

This overview provides strong evidence for a bene-

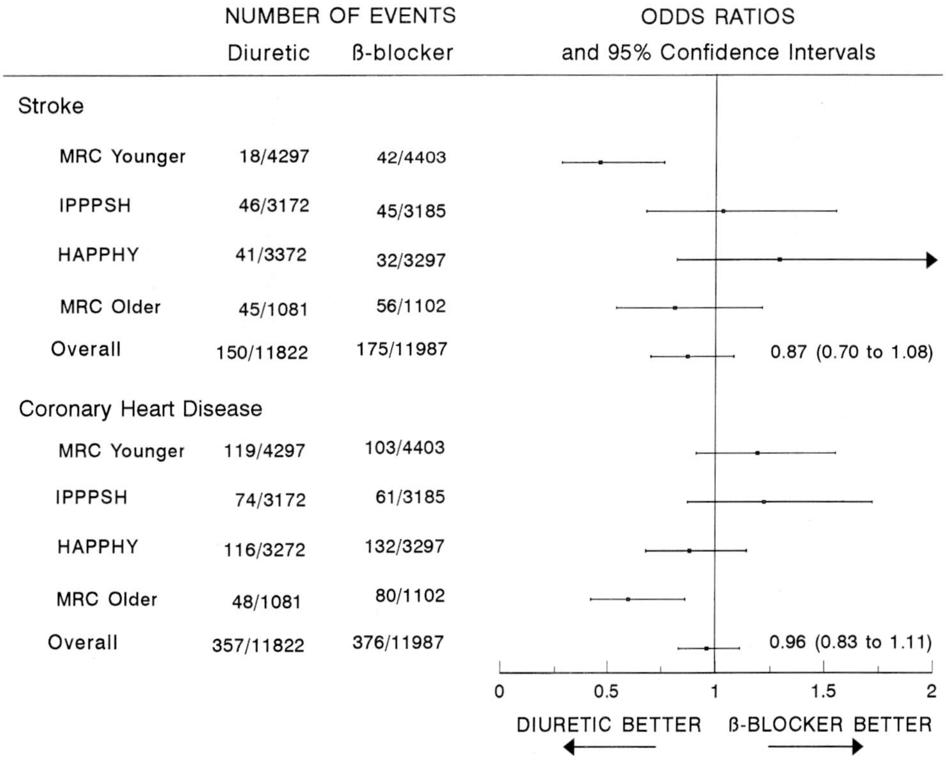

	NUMBER OF EVENTS Diuretic	ß-blocker	ODDS RATIOS and 95% Confidence Intervals
Stroke			
MRC Younger	18/4297	42/4403	
IPPPSH	46/3172	45/3185	
HAPPHY	41/3372	32/3297	
MRC Older	45/1081	56/1102	
Overall	150/11822	175/11987	0.87 (0.70 to 1.08)
Coronary Heart Disease			
MRC Younger	119/4297	103/4403	
IPPPSH	74/3172	61/3185	
HAPPHY	116/3272	132/3297	
MRC Older	48/1081	80/1102	
Overall	357/11822	376/11987	0.96 (0.83 to 1.11)

0 0.5 1 1.5 2

DIURETIC BETTER ß-BLOCKER BETTER

Figure 27–5 Odds ratios and 95% confidence intervals for stroke and coronary heart disease in four randomized, controlled trials comparing predominantly diuretic with predominantly beta blocker as the first step therapy of hypertension. HAPPHY, Heart Attack Primary Prevention in Hypertension; IPPPSH, International Prospective Primary Prevention Study in Hypertension; MRC, Medical Research Council.

ficial effect of antihypertensive drug treatment on the risk of CHD, stroke, total cardiovascular disease, and all-cause mortality in hypertensive patients. Furthermore, the data indicate that absolute reduction in risk is greater in those who are older compared with those who are younger and in those with a higher compared with a lower level of diastolic BP at the outset.

ONGOING TRIALS

Newer Classes of Antihypertensive Medications

A number of unpublished trials will help strengthen the base of knowledge regarding selection of patients for treatment with antihypertensive medications and questions related to the optimal goals for reduction of BP in different clinical settings. The names, study design, and participant characteristics for 32 such randomized controlled trials are presented in Tables 27–6, 27–7, and 27–8.[49–72] In some instances, it was a challenge to obtain or confirm relevant details for Tables 27–7 and 27–8. This was particularly the case for trials in which a separate rationale and design publication from the investigators could not be found. As such, the information presented should be considered as a general guide rather than as a definitive presentation of study design characteristics. The 32 trials have been designed to address two principal treatment questions. The first is whether choice of first-step antihypertensive medication influences treatment outcome, and the second is whether the outcome is affected by intensity of BP control.

Ongoing Trials Comparing Different First-Step Antihypertensive Drug Therapies

The effect of treatment regimens with different first-step antihypertensive drugs is being evaluated in 31 of the 32 trials.[49–59, 61–72] All major classes of antihypertensive drug therapy, including representative agents from each of the three CCB subgroups, are being evaluated (see Table 27–7). In most of the trials, the primary focus is on comparison of first-step therapy with a traditional agent, such as a diuretic or a beta blocker, with one or more first-step representatives of the newer classes of antihypertensive drug therapy. Diastolic hypertension is a requirement for enrollment in a majority of the trials, but some include normotensives,[51, 67] and a few are limited to study of isolated systolic hypertension[69, 71, 72] or are predominantly focused on hypertension in older persons (see Table 27–8).[52–54, 56, 59–62, 64, 66, 70] The trial participants encompass a wide range of ages and a broad array of comorbidities. Both diabetes and renal insufficiency are well represented. The 32 trials are also addressing a heterogeneous group of outcomes. These include clinical events, such as CHD, stroke, and all-cause mortality, as well as major morbidity, such as renal insufficiency, and surrogate outcomes, such as left ventricular hypertrophy and vessel wall thickness. Several of the trials that will provide information on clinical events are concurrently focusing interest on intermediate outcomes related to cardiac, cerebral,

TABLE 27–6 • Names and Acronyms of 32 Unpublished Randomized, Controlled Trials Evaluating the Effect of Antihypertensive Drugs

Trial Name	Acronym
African-American Study of Kidney Disease and Hypertension	AASK
Appropriate Blood Pressure Control in Diabetes	ABCD
Antihypertensive Therapy and Lipid Lowering to Prevent Heart Attack Trial	ALLHAT
Australian National Blood Pressure Study 2	ANBP-2
Anglo-Scandinavian Cardiac Outcomes Trial	ASCOT
Bergamo Nephrology Diabetes Complication Trial	BENEDICT
Captopril Prevention Project	CAPP
Controlled Onset Verapamil Investigation for Cardiovascular Endpoints	CONVINCE
Collaborative Study Group Trial on Effect of Irbesartan	CSGTEI
Diabetes Hypertension Cardiovascular Morbidity-Mortality and Ramipril	DIABHYCAR
European Lacidipine Study of Atherosclerosis	ELSA
Hypertension in Diabetes Study	HDS
Heart Outcomes Prevention Evaluation Study	HOPE
Hypertension Optimal Treatment Trial	HOT
Hypertension in the Very Elderly Trial	HYVET
International Nifedipine GITS Study Intervention as a Goal for Hypertension Therapy	INSIGHT
Losartan Intervention for Endpoint Reduction in Hypertension	LIFE
National Intervention Cooperative Study in Elderly Hypertensives	NICS-EH
Nordic Diltiazem Study	NORDIL
Prevention of Atherosclerosis with Ramipril	PART-2
Plaque Hypertension Lipid Lowering Italian Study	PHYLLIS
Prospective Randomized Enalapril Study Evaluating Regression of Ventricular Enlargement	PRESERVE
Prospective Randomized Evaluation of Vascular Effects of Norvasc	PREVENT
Perindopril Protection Against Recurrent Stroke Study	PROGRESS
Perindopril Regression of Vascular Thickning European Community Trial	PROTECT
Quinapril Ischaemia Event Trial	QUIET
Randomized Evaluation of NIDDM with the All Antagonist Losartan	RENAAL
Study of Cognition and Prognosis in Patients with Hypertension	SCOPE
Systolic Hypertension in the Elderly Lacidipine Long-Term Study	SHELL
Swedish Trial in Old Patients with Hypertension	STOP-2
SYST-EUR Multicentre Trial on the Treatment of Isolated Systolic Hypertension in the Elderly	Syst-Eur
Verapamil in Hypertension Atherosclerosis Study	VHAS

TABLE 27–7 • First-Step Medications Employed in 32 Unpublished Randomized, Controlled Trials Evaluating Effects of Antihypertensive Drug Therapy

Trial Acronym	Calcium Channel Blocker*		Angiotensin-Converting Enzyme Inhibitor/ Angiotensin II Antagonist		Diuretic		Beta-Receptor Blocker	α_1-Receptor Blocker	Other
AASK[49]	Amlodipine		Ramipril				Metoprolol		
ABCD[50, 51]	Nisoldipine		Enalapril						
ALLHAT[52, 53]	Amlodipine		Lisinopril		Chlorthalidone			Doxazosin	
ANBP-2[54]			ACE inhibitor		Thiazide				
ASCOT[55]	Amlodipine	*with or without*	ACE inhibitor		Thiazide	*with or without*	Beta blocker		
BENEDICT	CCB		ACE inhibitor						Placebo
CAPP[56]			Captopril		Diuretic	*or*	Beta blocker		
CONVINCE[57]	Verapamil				Hydrochlorothiazide	*or*	Atenolol		
CSGTEI[57]	Amlodipine		Angiotensin II antagonist (Irbesartan)						Placebo
DIABHYCAR[55]			Ramipril						Placebo
ELSA[58]	Lacidipine						Atenolol		
HDS[59]			Captopril				Atenolol		No treatment
HOPE[60]			Ramipril						Placebo
HOT[61]	Felodipine								
HYVET[62]			Lisinopril		Bendrofluazide				No treatment
INSIGHT[63]	Nifedipine				Hydrochlorothiazide/amiloride				
LIFE[54, 57, 64]			Angiotensin II antagonist (Losartan)				Atenolol		
NICS-EH	Nicardipine				Trichlormethiazide				
NORDIL[65]	Diltiazem				Diuretic	*or*	Beta blocker		
PART-2			Ramipril						Placebo
PHYLLIS[66]			Fosinopril		Hydrochlorothiazide				
PRESERVE[67]	Nifedipine		Enalapril						
PREVENT	Amlodipine								Placebo
PROGRESS[68]			Perindopril	*with or without*	Indapamide				Placebo
PROTECT[69]			Perindopril		Hydrochlorothiazide				
QUIET			Quinapril						Placebo
RENAAL			Angiotensin II antagonist (Losartan)						Placebo
SCOPE			ACE inhibitor						Placebo
SHELL[70]	Lacidipine				Chlorthalidone				
STOP-2[71]	Felodipine or isradipine		Enalapril or lisinopril		Moduretic	*or*	Beta blocker		
Syst-Eur[72]	Nitrendipine								Placebo
VHAS[66]	Verapamil				Chlorthalidone				

*All long acting.
ACE, angiotensin-converting enzyme; CCB, calcium channel blocker.

TABLE 27–8 • Characteristics of Participants and Study Design in 32 Unpublished Randomized, Controlled Trials Evaluating Effects of Antihypertensive Drug Therapy

Trial Acronym	Participant Characteristics	Age for Eligibility (y)	Study Design	Primary Outcome	No. of Participants	Duration of Follow-up (y)	Expected Year of Termination	Location of Clinical Centers
AASK[49]	HT + GFR 20–65 mL/min/1.73 m^2	18–70	Double-blind	Change in GFR	1200	4	2000	U.S.
ABCD[50, 51]	NIDDM −HT and NT strata	40–74	Double-blind	Change in creatinine clearance	950	5	1997	U.S.
ALLHAT[52, 53]	HT + 1 other major CVD risk factor	≥55	Double-blind	CHD	40,000	6	2002	U.S. & Canada
ANBP-2[54]	HT	65–84	Open (blinded endpoint)	CVD morbidity and mortality	6000	5	—	Australia
ASCOT[55]	HT	40–80	Open (blinded endpoint)	Nonfatal myocardial infarction and fatal CHD	18,000	5	2003	United Kingdom & Scandinavia
BENEDICT	NIDDM + HT	≥40	Double-blind	(a) Microalbuminuria (b) Proteinuria	2400	3	2001	Italy
CAPP[56]	HT	25–66	Open (blinded endpoint)	CVD mortality	10,800	5	1999	Sweden & Finland
CONVINCE[57]	HT + 1 other major CVD risk factor	≥55	Double-blind	CVD mortality and incident nonfatal CHD and stroke	15,000	6	2002	Worldwide
CSGTEI[57]	SBP ≥135 or DBP ≥85 mm Hg + NIDDM nephropathy	30–70	Double-blind	Doubling or serum creatinine or ESRD	1650	3	2000	Worldwide
DIABHYCAR[55]	NIDDM + albuminuria	>50	Double-blind	Fatal and nonfatal CVD	4000	3	—	France
ELSA[58]	HT	45–75	Double-blind	Vessel wall thickness	2251	4	2000	Europe (7 countries)
HDS[59]	HT + NIDDM	25–65	Open	CVD/renal and other morbidity and mortality	1060	9.4	1998	U.K.
HOPE[60]	High CVD risk	≥55	Double-blind	MI, stroke, and CVD mortality	9541	4.7	1999	U.S., Europe, & South America
HOT[61]	HT	50–80	Open (blinded endpoint)	CVD morbidity and mortality	19,000	2.5	1998	Worldwide (26 countries)
HYVET[62]	HT	>80	Open (blinded endpoint)	Stroke	2100	5	2000	Europe (esp. U.K.)
INSIGHT[63]	HT + 1 other major CVD risk factor	55–80	Double-blind	CVD morbidity and mortality	5274	3	1999	Europe & Israel (6 countries)

LIFE[54, 57, 64]	HT + LVH	55–80	Double-blind	CVD morbidity and mortality	8300	4	2001	Southern Europe & U.S.
NICS-EH	HT	≥60	Double-blind	Stroke	1000	5	1995	Japan
NORDIL[65]	HT	50–69	Open (blinded endpoint)	Fatal CVD	12,000	5	1999	Sweden & Norway
PART-2	CHD, TIA, or PVD	18–75	Double-blind	Coronary artery wall thickness	617	4	1998	New Zealand
PHYLLIS[66]	HT + high LDL cholesterol + ≥1 carotid plaque	—	Double-blind	Change in wall thickness	800	3	—	Italy
PRESERVE[67]	HT + increased LV mass	≥50	Double-blind	Reduction in LV mass	480	1	1998	China, Hong Kong, Europe, Israel, New Zealand, & U.S.
PREVENT	MI, stroke, or angina	30–80	Double-blind	Progression of coronary and carotid atherosclerosis	825	3	1997	U.S.
PROGRESS[68]	Stroke survivors	None	Double-blind	Stroke	6000	4	2000	Australia/New Zealand, China, Japan, & Europe
PROTECT[69]	HT + intima/media vessel wall thickness ≥0.8 mm	35–65	Double-blind	Change in wall thickness	800	2	—	Europe (7 countries)
QUIET	PTCA or laser/mechanical atherectomy	<75	Double-blind	Ischemic events or progression of atherosclerosis	1750	3	1996	North America and Europe
RENAAL	NIDDM + proteinuria	31–70	Double-blind	Doubling of serum creatinine, ESRD, or death	1520	4	2002	U.S.
SCOPE	HT	70–89	Double-blind	CHD/stroke	4000	2.5	2003	—
SHELL[70]	ISH	≥60	Open (blinded endpoint)	Total CVD/stroke	4800	5	1999	Italy
STOP-2[71]	HT	70–84	Open (blinded endpoint)	Fatal CVD	6600	4	1998	Sweden
Syst-Eur[72]	ISH	≥60	Double-blind	Stroke	4695	2	1998	Europe
VHAS[66]	HT	40–65	Double-blind	Carotid atherosclerosis	1500	4	1996	Europe

HT, hypertension; GFR, glomerular filtration rate; NIDDM, non–insulin-dependent diabetes mellitus; CVD, cardiovascular disease; ISH, isolated systolic hypertension; SBP, systolic blood pressure; DBP, diastolic blood pressure; CHD, coronary heart disease; ESRD, end-stage renal disease; MI, myocardial infarction; LVH, left ventricular hypertrophy; TIA, transient ischemic attack; LDL, low-density lipoprotein; LV, left ventricle; PTCA, percutaneous transluminal coronary angioplasty; PVD, peripheral vascular disease; NT, normotension.

and renal function. Twenty-three of the 32 trials are employing a double-blind design, and 8 of the remaining 9 trials are using the Prospective Randomized, Open, Blinded End-point Evaluation (PROBE) design.[73] As the name suggests, trials that use this design are conducted in a context in which participants and therapists are aware of the individual's treatment assignment. Compared with the double-blind gold standard design, the PROBE design reduces cost and provides the potential for recruitment of a more representative sample of study participants. A shortcoming of the PROBE design, however, is its associated potential for observer and cotreatment bias. The former shortcoming is especially a problem when the outcome is subjective in nature. Sample size varies considerably across the 32 trials from less than 500 to 40,000. Most of the trials are based on a 4- to 6-year period of follow-up, but the expected duration of study is somewhat shorter in a few instances and much longer in one trial.[59] In large part, the variation in sample size and length of follow-up reflects the diversity of risk for the participants being studied and the heterogeneity of the outcomes of interest. Trial participants are being enrolled in many countries, including the United States, Europe, Australia, New Zealand, and China. This diversity in geographic location provides an excellent opportunity to explore the effect of treatment in different ethnic groups as well as varying socioeconomic and cultural settings. Several of the trials employ a factorial design or separate randomization in subgroups to address other treatment questions.[49–53, 58] Given its size and the fact that it compares four first-step therapies, the Antihypertensive and Lipid Lowering Treatment to Prevent Heart Attack Trial (ALLHAT) study deserves special mention. This trial is primarily being conducted in primary care practices and is powered to detect a 20% or greater difference in fatal CHD and nonfatal myocardial infarction with any of the newer treatments (ACE inhibitors, CCB, or α_1-receptor blocker) compared with diuretic.[52, 53] As such, ALLHAT provides the single best opportunity to establish whether the newer agents are more cardioprotective than traditional therapy and to resolve the current controversy surrounding the potential for serious adverse effects during CCB therapy.[74]

One trial that was not included in Tables 27–6 through 27–8 deserves special mention. The Syst-China trial on the treatment of isolated systolic hypertension in the elderly uses the same design and protocol as the Syst-Eur trial except that treatment has been allocated by placing alternative participants on nitrendipine or placebo rather than by use of a random assignment method.[75] In addition, the number of participants enrolled in the Syst-China trial (n = 2379) is about half as many as are participating in the Syst-Eur trial.

Ongoing Trials of Optimal Goals for Blood Pressure Reduction

Observational epidemiologic studies have typically demonstrated a direct relationship between level of BP and risk of subsequent cardiovascular or renal disease.[6–10] A J-shaped relationship between BP and cardiovascular disease has been noted, however, in nonconcurrent prospective analyses of some cohorts who have been treated with antihypertensive drug therapy.[76] Several groups of investigators have demonstrated that treated hypertensives have a higher risk of cardiovascular disease compared with suitably matched normotensives.[77–80] One explanation for this finding is insufficient lowering of BP, whereas an alternative possibility is that excessive lowering of BP triggers ischemia and infarction in the coronary and cerebral circulations. Clinical trials in which participants are randomly assigned to different intensities of BP lowering provide the best opportunity to determine which of these two possibilities is most likely to explain the findings. One such trial has been conducted, but it had insufficient statistical power to answer the question.[81] Four ongoing trials have been designed to shed additional light on the question.[49–51, 59, 61] Of these, the largest is the Hypertension Optimal Treatment (HOT) trial.[61] The main goal of the HOT trial is to compare fatal and nonfatal cardiovascular disease clinical event rates in slightly more than 19,000 hypertensive patients who have been randomly allocated to three different levels of goal diastolic BP (≤90 mm Hg, ≤85 mm Hg, and ≤80 mm Hg). The study is being conducted in 26 countries in Europe and North America, and the participants are being followed for 2.5 years. The study, which is also evaluating the effects of low-dose (75 mg) aspirin, will soon be over, and the main results should be available shortly thereafter. The other three studies are considerably smaller, but they are being conducted in high-risk groups and are addressing surrogate endpoints rather than clinical events.[49–51, 59] The African-American Study of Kidney Disease and Hypertension (AASK) is investigating whether treatment to a mean arterial BP (MAP) of 92 mm Hg or less will reduce the rate of decline in renal function compared with achievement of a more traditional MAP goal of 102 to 107 mm Hg in approximately 1200 African-American adults with BP-related renal insufficiency.[49] The AASK investigators are employing a factorial study design, which will also yield information on the comparative value of three first-step approaches to antihypertensive drug therapy. The Appropriate Blood Pressure Control in Diabetes (ABCD) trial is testing the effect of two levels of blood pressure control (usual control and about 10 mm Hg lower than usual) and two antihypertensive regimens (primary treatment with an ACE inhibitor or a CCB) in almost

1000 type II diabetics in two strata of blood pressure (hypertension present or absent).[50, 51] The Hypertension in Diabetes Study (HDS) is being conducted in 1060 hypertensive participants enrolled in the UK Prospective Diabetes Study (UKPDS).[59] Approximately two thirds of the HDS participants were randomly assigned to receive active treatment aimed at achieving a systolic BP of 150 mm Hg or less and a diastolic BP of 85 mm Hg or less, whereas BP in the remaining one third was largely untreated unless the participant's systolic BP was 200 mm Hg or greater or the diastolic BP was 105 mm Hg or greater. Those assigned to active therapy were randomly assigned to receive either an ACE inhibitor (captopril) or a beta blocker (atenolol). Given their sample size and length of follow-up, the ABCD and HDS trial results will be of special value in determining the goal for BP reduction in type II diabetics with high BP. Likewise, their comparison of the effects of different antihypertensive agents on intermediate endpoints will complement the experience with clinical outcomes in larger studies, such as ALLHAT, which include a substantial minority of type II diabetics.

SUMMARY

A substantial body of experience supports the importance of high BP as a risk factor for vascular damage to the heart, brain, kidney, and other organs. Likewise, clinical trials have repeatedly demonstrated the clear net benefits of antihypertensive drug therapy in patients with hypertension. Pooling of information from trials that have already published their results indicates that approximately 5 years of first-step therapy with a diuretic or a beta blocker virtually eliminates the BP-related risk of stroke and substantially reduces the corresponding BP-related risk of CHD. A large number of ongoing trials will complement and expand this existing base of knowledge by clarifying the "whom to treat" and "how to treat" questions that face practitioners and their patients on a daily basis. The ongoing trials will help clarify the effects of antihypertensive drug therapy on a variety of outcomes, including CHD, stroke, renal insufficiency, left ventricular hypertrophy, and vessel wall thickness. More than this, they will provide comparative information regarding the relative capacity of treatment with different first-step therapies to prevent complications in patients with high BP, the appropriateness of starting treatment at lower than usual levels of BP in patients who are at particularly high risk for BP-related vascular complications, and the optimal goal for reduction of BP when treating hypertension. Within the next decade, practitioners will have an unprecedented body of BP-reduction clinical trial information to guide therapeutic decisions. This will not only be a great advantage compared with what was available to their colleagues who faced similar treatment questions in previous years but is a testament to the unique value of clinical trials in detecting small to moderate treatment effects and strengthening the scientific base for clinical decision making.

REFERENCES

1. Whelton PK, He J, Klag MJ. Blood pressure in Westernized populations. *In* Swales JD (ed): Textbook of Hypertension. Oxford, Blackwell Scientific Publications, 1994, pp 11–21.
2. Poulter NR, Sever PS. Low blood pressure populations and the impact of rural-urban migration. *In* Swales JD (ed): Textbook of Hypertension. Oxford, Blackwell Scientific Publications, 1994, pp 22–36.
3. He J, Klag MJ, Whelton PK, et al. Migration, blood pressure pattern, and hypertension. Am J Epidemiol 1991; 134:1085–1101.
4. Poulter NR, Khaw KT, Hopwood BEC, et al. The Kenyan Luo migration study: Observations on the initiation of a rise in blood pressure. BMJ 1990; 300:967–972.
5. Burt V, Whelton PK, Roccella E, et al. Prevalence of hypertension in the US adult population: Results from the Third National Health and Nutrition Examination Survey, 1988–91. Hypertension 1995; 25:305–313.
6. National High Blood Pressure Education Program Working Group. National High Blood Pressure Education Program Working Group report on hypertension in the elderly. Hypertension 1994; 23:275–285.
7. Whelton PK. Epidemiology of hypertension. Lancet 1994; 344:101–106.
8. MacMahon S, Peto R, Cutler J, et al. Blood pressure, stroke, and coronary heart disease: Part 1. Prolonged differences in blood pressure. Prospective observational studies corrected for the regression dilution bias. Lancet 1990; 335:765–774.
9. Whelton PK, Perneger TV, He J, et al. The role of blood pressure as a risk factor for renal disease: A review of the epidemiologic evidence. J Hum Hypertens 1996; 10:683–689.
10. Klag MJ, Whelton PK, Randall BL, et al. A prospective study of blood pressure and incidence of end-stage renal disease in 332,544 men. N Engl J Med 1996; 334:13–18.
11. Working Group on Primary Prevention of Hypertension. Report of the National High Blood Pressure Education Program Working Group on Primary Prevention of Hypertension. Arch Intern Med 1993; 153:186–208.
12. Harrington M, Kincaid-Smith P, McMichael J. Results of treatment of malignant hypertension. BMJ 1959; 2:969–989.
13. Mohler ER, Freis ED. Five-year survival of patients with malignant hypertension treated with antihypertensive agents. Am Heart J 1960; 60:329–335.
14. Bjork S, Sannerstedt R, Falkheden T, et al. The effect of active drug treatment in severe antihypertensive disease. Acta Med Scand 1961; 169:673–689.
15. Hamilton M, Thompson EW, Wisniewski TKM. The role of blood pressure control in preventing complications of hypertension. Lancet 1964; 1:235–238.
16. Wolff FW, Lindeman RD. Effects of treatment in hypertension: Results of a controlled study. J Chron Dis 1966; 19:227–240.
17. Veterans Administration Cooperative Study Group on Antihypertensive Agents. Effects of treatment on morbidity in hypertension: Results in patients with diastolic blood pressure averaging 115 through 129 mmHg. JAMA 1967; 202:1028–1034.
18. Veterans Administration Cooperative Study Group on Antihypertensive Agents. Effects of treatment on morbidity in hypertension: II. Results in patients with diastolic blood pressure averaging 90 through 114 mmHg. JAMA 1970; 213:1143–1152.
19. Carter AB. Hypotensive therapy in stroke survivors. Lancet 1970; 1:485–489.
20. Barraclough M, Bainton D, Joy MD, et al. Control of moderately raised blood pressure: Report of a co-operative randomized controlled trial. BMJ 1973; 3:434–436.

21. Hypertension-Stroke Cooperative Study Group. Effect of antihypertensive treatment on stroke recurrence. JAMA 1974; 229:409–418.
22. U.S. Public Health Service Hospitals Cooperative Study Group. Treatment of mild hypertension: Results of a ten-year intervention trial. Circ Res 1977; 40:I-98–I-105.
23. Veterans Administration–National Heart, Lung, and Blood Institute Study Group for Cooperative Studies on Antihypertensive Therapy. Mild Hypertension (Perry HM): Treatment of mild hypertension: Preliminary results of a two-year feasibility trial. Circ Res 1977; 40(suppl 1):180–187.
24. Veterans Administration–National Heart, Lung, and Blood Institute Study Group for Evaluating Treatment in Mild Hypertension. Evaluation of drug treatment in mild hypertension: VA-NHLBI Feasibility Trial. Ann N Y Acad Sci 1978; 304:267–288.
25. Hypertension Detection and Follow-up Program Cooperative Group. Five-year findings of the hypertension detection and follow-up program: I. Reduction in mortality of persons with high blood pressure, including mild hypertension. JAMA 1979; 242:2562–2571.
26. Hypertension Detection and Follow-up Program Cooperative Group. Five-year findings of the hypertension detection and follow-up program: II. Mortality by race, sex and age. JAMA 1979; 242:2572–2577.
27. Helgeland A. Treatment of mild hypertension: A five-year controlled drug trial. The Oslo Study. Am J Med 1980; 69:725–732.
28. Leren P, Helgeland A. Oslo Hypertension Study. Drugs 1986; 31(suppl 1):41–45.
29. Australian National Blood Pressure Study Management Committee. The Australian therapeutic trial in mild hypertension. Lancet 1980; 1:1261–1267.
30. Medical Research Council Working Party. MRC trial of treatment of mild hypertension: Principal results. BMJ 1985; 291:97–104.
31. Amery A, Birkenhager W, Brixko P, et al. Mortality and morbidity results from the European working party on high blood pressure in the elderly trial. Lancet 1985; 1:1349–1354.
32. Coope J, Warrender TS. Randomized trial of treatment of hypertension in elderly patients in primary care. BMJ 1986; 293:1145–1151.
33. SHEP Cooperative Research Group. Prevention of stroke by antihypertensive drug treatment in older persons with isolated systolic hypertension: Final results of the Systolic Hypertension in the Elderly Program (SHEP). JAMA 1991; 265:3255–3264.
34. Dahlof B, Lindholm LH, Hansson L, et al. Morbidity and mortality in the Swedish Trial in Old Patients with Hypertension (STOP-Hypertension). Lancet 1991; 338:1281–1285.
35. MRC Working Party. Medical Research Council trial of treatment of hypertension in older adults: Principal results. BMJ 1992; 304:405–412.
36. Cutler JA, MacMahon SW, Furberg CD. Controlled clinical trials of drug treatment for hypertension: A review. Hypertension 1989; 13(suppl I):I-36–I-44.
37. Collins R, Peto R, MacMahon SW, et al. Blood pressure, stroke, and CHD: Part 2. Short-term reductions in blood pressure: Overview of randomized drug trials in their epidemiological context. Lancet 1990; 335:827–838.
38. Hebert PR, Moser M, Mayer J, et al. Recent evidence on drug therapy of mild to moderate hypertension and decreased risk of CHD. Arch Intern Med 1993; 153:578–581.
39. Collins R, MacMahon S. Blood pressure, antihypertensive drug treatment and the risks of stroke and of CHD. Br Med Bull 1994; 50:272–298.
40. Lipid Research Clinics Program. The Lipid Research Clinics Coronary Primary Prevention Trial results: I. Reduction in incidence of CHD. JAMA 1984; 251:351–364.
41. Frick MH, Elo O, Haapa K, et al. Helsinki Heart Study: Primary-prevention trial with gemfibrozil in middle-aged men with dyslipidemia: Safety of treatment, changes in risk factors, and incidence of CHD. N Engl J Med 1987; 317:1237–1245.
42. Multiple Risk Factor Intervention Trial Research Group. Mortality rates after 10.5 years for participants in the Multiple Risk Factor Intervention Trial: Findings related to a priori hypotheses of the trial. JAMA 1990; 263:1795–1801.
43. IPPPSH Collaborative Group. Cardiovascular risk and risk factors in a randomized trial of treatment based on the beta-blocker oxprenolol. The International Prospective Primary Prevention Study in Hypertension (IPPPSH). J Hypertens 1985; 3:379–392.
44. Wilhelmsen L, Berglund G, Elmfeldt D, et al. Beta-blockers versus diuretics in hypertensive men: Main results from the HAPPHY trial. J Hypertens 1987; 5:561–572.
45. Furberg CD, Psaty BM, Meyer JV. Nifedipine: Dose-related increase in mortality in patients with CHD. Circulation 1995; 92:1326–1331.
46. Psaty BM, Heckbert SR, Koepsell TD, et al. The risk of myocardial infarction associated with antihypertensive drug therapies. JAMA 1995; 274:620–625.
47. Borhani NO, Mercuri M, Borhani PA, et al. Final outcome results of the Multicenter Isradipine Diuretic Atherosclerosis Study (MIDAS): A randomized controlled trial. JAMA 1996; 276:785–791.
48. Gong LS, Zhang WZ, Zhu YJ, et al. Shanghai trial of nifedipine in the elderly (STONE). J Hypertens 1996; 14:1237–1245.
49. Wright JT, Kusek JW, Toto RD, et al, for the AASK Pilot Study investigators. Design and baseline characteristics of participants in the African American Study of Kidney Disease and Hypertension (AASK) Pilot Study. Controlled Clin Trials 1996; 16:3S–16S.
50. Savage S, Johnson Nagel N, Estacio RO, et al. The ABCD (appropriate control in diabetes) trial: Rationale and design of a trial of hypertension control (moderate or intensive) in type II diabetes. Online J Curr Trials 1993 Nov 24; 1993 (Doc No 104).
51. Schrier RW, Savage S. Appropriate Blood Pressure Control in Type II Diabetes (ABCD) trial: Implications for complications. Am J Kidney Dis 1992; 6:653–657.
52. Davis BR, Cutler JA, Gordon DJ, et al, for the ALLHAT Research Group. Rationale and design for the Antihypertensive and Lipid Lowering Treatment to Prevent Heart Attack Trial (ALLHAT). Am J Hypertens 1996; 9:342–360.
53. Whelton PK, Williamson JD, Louis GT, et al, for the ALLHAT Research Group. Experimental approaches to determining the choice of first-step therapy for patients with hypertension. Clin Exp Hypertens 1996; 18:569–579.
54. Hansson L. The benefits of lowering elevated blood pressure: A critical review of studies of cardiovascular morbidity and mortality in hypertension. J Hypertens 1996; 14:537–544.
55. Sever PS, Mackay JA. The hypertension trials. J Hypertens 1996; 14(suppl 2):S29–S34.
56. CAPP Group. The Captopril Prevention Project: A prospective intervention trial of angiotensin converting enzyme inhibition in the treatment of hypertension. J Hypertens 1990; 8:985–990.
57. Nwachuku CE, Cutler JA. The explosion of morbidity trials in hypertension. Curr Opin Nephrol Hypertens 1997; 6:230–236.
58. Bond G, Dal Palu C, Hansson L, et al, on behalf of the E.L.S.A. investigators. The E.L.S.A. Trial: Protocol of randomized trials to explore the differential effect of antihypertensive drugs on atherosclerosis in hypertension. J Cardiovasc Pharmacol 1994; 23(suppl 5):S85–S87.
59. UK Prospective Diabetes Study Group. UK Prospective Diabetes Study (UKPDS): VIII. Study design, progress and performance. Diabetologia 1991; 34:877–890.
60. Mindlen F, Nordaby R, Ruiz M, et al. The HOPE (Heart Outcomes Prevention Evaluation) Study: The design of a large, simple randomized trial of an angiotensin converting enzyme inhibitor (ramipril) and vitamin E in patients at high risk of cardiovascular events. Can J Cardiol 1996; 12:127–137.
61. HOT Study Group. The Hypertension Optimal Treatment (HOT) Study—a prospective study of the optimal therapeutic goal and the value of low-dose aspirin in antihypertensive treatment. Blood Pressure 1993; 2:113–119.
62. Bulpitt C, Fletcher AE, Amery A, et al. The hypertension in the very elderly trial (HYVET). J Hum Hypertens 1994; 8:631–632.
63. Brown MJ, Castaigne A, Roulope LM, et al. INSIGHT: International Nifedipine GITS study intervention as a goal in hypertension treatment. J Hum Hypertens 1996; 10(suppl 3):S157–S160.
64. Dahlof B. Effect of angiotensin II blockade on cardiac hypertrophy and remodeling: A review. J Hum Hypertens 1995; 9(suppl 5):S34–S37.
65. Nordil Study Group. The Nordic Diltiazem Study (NORDIL):

A prospective intervention trial of calcium antagonist therapy in hypertension. Blood Pressure 1993; 2:312–321.
66. Zanchetti A. Trials investigating the anti-atherosclerotic effects of antihypertensive drugs. J Hypertens 1996; 14(suppl 2):S77–S81.
67. Devereux RB, Dahlof B, Levy D, et al. Comparison of enalapril versus nifedipine to decrease left ventricular hypertrophy in systemic hypertension (the PRESERVE trial). Am J Cardiol 1996; 78:61–65.
68. Neal B, MacMahon S. The Progress Study: Rationale and design. J Hypertens 1995; 13:1869–1873.
69. Stumpe KO, Ludwig M, Heagerty AM, et al, for the PROTECT Study Group. Vascular wall thickness in hypertension: The perindopril regression of vascular thickening European Community trial (PROTECT). Am J Cardiol 1995; 76:50E–54E.
70. Malacco E, Gnemmi AE, Romagnoli A, et al, for the SHELL Study Group. Systolic Hypertension in the Elderly: Long term lacidipine treatment (SHELL). J Cardiovasc Pharmacol 1994; 23(suppl 5):S62–S66.
71. Dahlof B, Hansson L, Lindholm L, et al. STOP-Hypertension 2: A prospective international trial of newer versus older treatment alternatives in old patients with hypertension. Blood Pressure 1993; 2:136–141.
72. Amery A, Birkenhager W, Bulpitt CJ, et al. SYST-EUR: A multicenter trial on the treatment of isolated systolic hypertension in the elderly: Objective, protocol and organization. Aging 1991; 3:287–302.
73. Hansson L, Hedner T, Dahlof B. Prospective Randomized Open Blinded End-point (PROBE) study: A novel design for intervention trials. Blood Pressure 1992; 1:113–119.
74. Cohen JD. 1995: The year of the calcium antagonist controversy. Curr Opin Nephrol Hypertens 1996; 5:214–218.
75. Lisheng L. Effects of hypertension control on stroke incidence and fatality: Report from SYST-CHINA and post-stroke antihypertensive treatment. J Hum Hypertens 1996; 10(suppl 1):S9–S11.
76. Hansson L. The optimal blood pressure reduction. J Hypertens 1996; 14:(suppl 2):S55–S59.
77. Coresh J, Whelton PK, Mead LA, et al. Increased cardiovascular disease risk in treated hypertensive men. J Hypertens 1994; 12(suppl 3):S73.
78. Lindholm L, Ejlertsson G, Scherstein B. High risk of cerebro-cardiovascular morbidity in well treated male hypertensives: A retrospective study of 40–59-year-old hypertensives in a Swedish primary care district. Acta Med Scand 1984; 216:251–259.
79. Samuelsson O. Hypertension in middle-aged men: Management, morbidity and prognostic factors during long-term hypertensive care. Acta Med Scand 1985; 218(suppl 702):1–79.
80. Isles CG, Walker LM, Beevers DG, et al. Mortality in patients of the Glasgow Blood Pressure Clinic. J Hypertens 1986; 4:141–156.
81. Hansson L, for the BBB Study Group. The BBB study: The effect of intensified antihypertensive treatment on the level of blood pressure, side effects, morbidity and mortality in "well-treated" hypertensive patients. Blood Pressure 1994; 3:248–254.

28 Smoking Cessation

▶ Nancy A. Rigotti
▶ Richard C. Pasternak

Tobacco smoking is the leading preventable cause of death in the United States.[1–3] Of the more than 2 million U.S. deaths in 1990, 418,690, or approximately one in every five, was attributable to cigarette smoking.[4] Ischemic heart disease was the cause of nearly 25% of these smoking-related deaths, and all cardiovascular diseases accounted for an estimated 43% of these deaths. Smoking prevalence has declined dramatically since its peak in 1965, at which time 40% of adults (50% of men and 32% of women) smoked.[1, 5] Nonetheless, in 1995, 24.7% of adult Americans (27% of men and 23% of women) smoked cigarettes.[6] Nearly 90% of them began to smoke before the age of 20.[7] In the United States, smoking prevalence is highest among young adults (aged 25 to 44 years) and among individuals with less education and lower socioeconomic status.[1, 6]

This chapter summarizes epidemiologic evidence concerning the relationship between tobacco use and cardiovascular disease, particularly coronary heart disease (CHD), and reviews the evidence that smoking cessation prevents cardiovascular morbidity and mortality. The chapter begins with a summary of the pathophysiologic effects of tobacco use to establish the biologic plausibility for a relationship between smoking and heart disease.

PATHOPHYSIOLOGY

Tobacco smoking influences a vast array of physiologic and biochemical factors, which, acting together, inflict a considerable burden on the cardiovascular system and provide the biologic underpinnings to account for the observed epidemiologic associations. Substantial focused research has helped to elucidate individual effects of specific components of tobacco smoke on the cardiovascular system at several points along the pathophysiologic spectrum. These data most strongly link nicotine and carbon monoxide as the components of tobacco smoke that are involved in the development of cardiovascular disease.[8, 9] Smoking accelerates the fundamental atherosclerotic process, prematurely producing plaque in arteries of all important vascular territories.[10, 11] Smoking also triggers the clinical consequences of atherosclerosis and is associated with unstable angina, acute myocardial infarction, sudden death, stroke, and worsening of peripheral vascular disease symptoms.[8]

SYSTEMIC EFFECTS

Smoking cigarettes, both acutely and chronically, unfavorably alters the critical balance between myocardial oxygen supply and demand. The smoke of one cigarette rapidly increases blood pressure and heart rate.[10] The increase in blood pressure is directly related to the increase in plasma nicotine concentration,[12] suggesting that nicotine, a well-known adrenergic agonist that increases norepinephrine and epinephrine levels,[13] mediates an important component of this immediate hemodynamic response. Although these changes are observed in both smokers and nonsmokers, they are slightly greater in individuals not previously exposed to cigarette smoke or nicotine.[14] As a consequence of these hemodynamic changes or the nicotine-related increase in plasma catecholamines, or both, smoking increases the potential for cardiac arrhythmias and has been shown to be associated with a higher incidence of sudden cardiac arrest.[15] Other components of cigarette smoke may also have important systemic effects. Carbon monoxide, which composes 2% to 6% of cigarette smoke, binds to hemoglobin, reducing oxygen carrying capacity among smokers. A direct dose-response relationship has been demonstrated between carbon monoxide concentrations and ischemic threshold.[16]

VASCULAR EFFECTS

The acute and chronic effects of cigarette smoking on the peripheral and coronary vasculature have been well studied. In the presence of coronary and peripheral atherosclerosis, the normal vascular dilating capacity is impaired, and vasoconstrictive responses are potentiated. A decrease in distensibility in both carotid and brachial arteries has been demonstrated after exposure to cigarette smoke,[14] and the smoke of a single cigarette has been shown to increase acutely coronary vascular resistance and decrease coronary flow velocity.[17] In susceptible individuals, smoke from a single cigarette is capable of producing a sudden marked epicardial coronary vasoconstriction.[17] In a patient with a vulnerable plaque, this could expose such an individual to plaque rupture, which is one mechanism by which smoking may produce acute coronary events. Further evidence of the direct vascular effect of smoking comes from the observation that smoking directly exacerbates vasospastic angina in patients without obstructive epicardial coronary artery lesions[18] and that *silent* ischemia occurs among cigarette smokers in association with demonstrable regional myocardial perfusion abnormalities.[19] A direct effect of smoking on coronary endothelium is presumed, based on several lines of evidence. Endothelial-dependent, flow-mediated vascular forearm dilation is impaired in smokers.[20] Abnormalities in endothelium-derived relaxing factor (nitric oxide) have been detected in smokers,[21, 22] and coronary vasodilation is impaired in smokers.[23, 24]

METABOLIC EFFECTS

Smoking induces a small to moderate change in serum lipids.[25] It increases the triglyceride level by approximately 9%, decreases high-density lipoprotein (HDL) cholesterol by 6%, and increases total cholesterol by 3%. Although smoking does not alter low-density lipoprotein (LDL) cholesterol levels directly, it appears to contribute to the susceptibility of the LDL molecule to oxidative modification,[26] perhaps influencing the outcomes of clinical trials of antioxidants among smokers (see Chapter 32). Smoking cessation is associated with an increase in HDL cholesterol.[10, 27]

THROMBOSIS

Acute thrombus formation at the site of a ruptured plaque is responsible for the majority of coronary disease events, whereas chronic thrombotic activity is associated with atherosclerotic progression. Smoking appears to influence both acute and chronic aspects of the thrombotic process. The influence of smoking on the clotting system is complex and includes demonstrable changes in the fibrinolytic system, the clotting cascade, and platelet function.[10, 28, 29] Fibrinogen and factor VII levels are higher in smokers than in nonsmokers, and both gradually improve with smoking cessation.[10] The effects of smoking on platelet function have been particularly carefully studied. Smoking increases the production of platelet-derived growth factor (PDGF), an atherogenic mitogen.[30] Smoking has been shown to increase a number of proaggregatory prostanoids, an effect likely responsible for the observation that smoking as few as two cigarettes can increase platelet activation more than 100-fold.[31] The influence of smoking on clotting function has been shown to be both nicotine dependent and independent,[28] and the complexity of the clotting system itself suggests that many different components of cigarette smoke are likely to influence the pathophysiology of clotting.

Smoking influences the cardiovascular system through the interplay of a wide range of pathophysiologic and biochemical factors.[9] Some of these effects, such as elevated carbon monoxide levels, increased platelet activation, and coronary artery spasm, are likely to be rapidly reversible after smoking cessation. Other effects, such as the development of atherosclerosis, are at best likely to be only gradually reversible after smoking cessation. Hence, there is a biologic rationale for both an initial rapid decline and a later gradual fall in cardiovascular disease risk among former smokers compared with continuing smokers.

CIGARETTE SMOKING AND CARDIOVASCULAR DISEASE RISK

The epidemiologic evidence supporting a causal relationship between cigarette smoking and cardiovascular disease is overwhelming. Multiple observational epidemiologic studies conducted in many nations have demonstrated a relationship between smoking and various measures of cardiovascular disease morbidity and mortality. The evidence is consistent, the relationship is strong, a dose-response relationship has been demonstrated between CHD and the duration and intensity of smoking, a reduction in risk has been documented after smoking cessation, and the association is biologically plausible. These facts meet the epidemiologic criteria for establishing causality.[1, 5, 32, 33] The relationship was first observed among men but has since been demonstrated in women as well. In both men and women, smoking is a major cause of cardiovascular disease, including myocardial infarction, sudden death, ischemic stroke, peripheral vascular disease, and aortic aneurysm.[1, 30, 34–36] Compared with nonsmokers, current smokers have a 70% increased risk of fatal CHD and a twofold to fourfold higher risk of nonfatal CHD and sudden death.[32] Cigarette smoking is synergistic with the other two major CHD risk factors, hypertension and hyperlipidemia, to increase markedly the risk of CHD. Oral contraceptive use is also synergistic with smoking to increase substantially the risk of myocardial infarction, subarachnoid hemorrhage, and ischemic stroke in women.[32, 37] There is no safe level of tobacco use. The risk of myocardial infarction and cardiovascular mortality is increased in individuals who smoke as few as one to four cigarettes daily.[34] Smoking cigarettes with lower tar and nicotine content does not reduce the smoking-related risk of cardiovascular disease.[1]

Nonsmokers can be harmed by chronic exposure to tobacco smoke in the environment, a phenomenon known as *passive smoking*.[38] Children whose parents smoke have more serious respiratory infections during infancy and childhood, more respiratory symptoms, and a greater risk of chronic otitis media and asthma than the children of nonsmokers. Regular passive smoke exposure also increases the risk of lung cancer among nonsmokers. The evidence was summarized by the Environmental Protection Agency in 1992, when it identified passive smoke as a carcinogen responsible for approximately 3000 lung cancer deaths per year in U.S. nonsmokers.[38] A growing body of epidemiologic and laboratory evidence indicates that passive smoke exposure increases the risk of death from ischemic heart disease among nonsmokers living with smokers by approximately 30%.[39–43] An even higher risk was reported by the largest and most recent study, which included more than 30,000 women.[39] Women with regular exposure to passive smoke at home or work had a 91% greater risk of CHD, even after adjustment for cardiovascular risk factors, than women not exposed to passive smoke. The risk was 58% higher for women with only occasional exposure to passive smoke. According to one estimate, passive smoking was responsible for nearly 40,000 cardiovascular deaths per year in the United States.[41]

SMOKING CESSATION AND CARDIOVASCULAR DISEASE RISK

Randomized, controlled clinical trials provide the highest quality of evidence for demonstrating conclusively that altering a cardiac risk factor reduces cardiovascular disease morbidity or mortality. For example, the value of treating hypertension or hyperlipidemia for cardiovascular disease prevention became widely accepted only after benefits had been demonstrated in randomized clinical trials. In contrast, no randomized, controlled trial specifically designed to assess the effect of smoking cessation as a single intervention to reduce cardiovascular morbidity or mortality or overall mortality has been conducted. There have been hundreds of randomized, controlled trials to assess the efficacy of interventions for producing smoking cessation,[5] but only one of them[43a, 43b] has reported the impact of a smoking intervention on disease endpoints (morbidity or mortality) in addition to behavioral outcomes. Nonetheless, an impressive body of epidemiologic evidence has accumulated to support a strong conclusion that smoking cessation reduces cardiovascular morbidity and mortality.

The strongest evidence about the benefits of smoking cessation for the primary prevention of cardiovascular disease derives from a series of large prospective observational epidemiologic studies with a decade or more of follow-up. These have compared the frequency of cardiovascular events and mortality among cohorts of current smokers, former smokers, and nonsmokers without cardiovascular disease at study entry (Table 28–1). The largest and longest of these primary prevention studies include cohorts of British physicians (40 years' follow-up),[33] U.S. veterans (26 years' follow-up),[44] volunteers recruited by the American Cancer Society (12 years' follow-up),[45, 46] men in seven countries (10 years' follow-up),[47] British civil servants (10 years' follow-up),[48] Swedish twin pairs (10 years' follow-up),[49] and Northern California Kaiser Permanente subscribers (6 years' follow-up).[50] These cohorts consisted largely of middle-aged white men until recently, when data from substantial numbers of women became available from the Nurses' Health Study (12 years' follow-up).[35, 51] Little is known about the effects of cessation in nonwhites, although there is no a priori reason to expect that they would be different. Case-control studies comparing the smoking history of patients with and without cardiovascular disease provide further support for a cardiovascular benefit of smoking cessation (Table 28–2). A third line of evidence derives from randomized, controlled trials comparing the effect of a multiple risk factor intervention including smoking cessation with usual care. These trials have the advantage of randomized allocation of treatment, but the presence of the other interventions complicates the interpretation of the independent effect of smoking cessation on cardiovascular outcomes.

The value of smoking cessation for the secondary prevention of cardiovascular disease (e.g., the prevention of recurrent events and death among individuals with diagnosed heart disease) has been demonstrated by longitudinal observational studies of cohorts of smokers with established CHD. Outcomes are compared between smokers who stop smoking and those who continue smoking after entry into the cohort. Randomized clinical trials of therapeutic interventions (e.g., bypass surgery or angioplasty) provide additional evidence to support the benefit of smoking cessation in patients with established CHD. In these studies, the survival of smokers who quit has been

TABLE 28–1 • Cohort Studies of Coronary Heart Disease Risk Among Former and Current Smokers

			Relative Risks Compared with Never-Smokers*	
Reference	**Population**	**Follow-up**	***Former Smokers***	***Current Smokers***
Doll and Peto (1976)[83]	British physicians: 34,440 men	20 y for CHD deaths	Age 30–54: 1.3–1.9 depending on years quit Age 55–64: 1.3–1.9 depending on years quit Age ≥65: 1.0–1.3 depending on years quit	3.5 1.7 1.3
Doll et al (1980)[84]	British physicians: 6194 women	22 y for CHD deaths	0.91	1.0–2.2 depending on amount smoked
Doll et al (1994)[33]	British physicians: 34,439 men	40 y for CHD deaths	1.2	1.6
Hammond and Horn (1958)[85]	187,783 men aged 50–60	44 mo for CHD deaths	PREVIOUSLY ≥1 ppd Quit <1 y 3.00 1–10 y 2.06 >10 y 1.60	2.20
Hammond and Garfinkel (1969)[86]	ACS CPS-I: 358,534 men free of diagnosed CHD	6 y for CHD deaths	PREVIOUSLY ≥1 ppd Quit <1 y 1.61 1–4 yr 1.51 5–9 y 1.16 10–14 y 1.25 ≥15 y 1.05	2.55
Burns et al (1997)[46]	ACS CSP-I: 1,051,042 men and women aged ≥30	12 y for CHD deaths	YEARS QUIT / MEN / WOMEN 2–4 2.66 2.23 5–9 1.64 1.53 10–14 1.37 0.98 15–19 1.13 0.84 20–24 0.99 0.88 25–29 0.96 0.96	1.85 (men) 1.68 (women)
Thun et al (1997)[45]	ACS CPS-I & II men and women aged >30 CPS I: 786,387 CPS II: 711,363	6 y for CHD deaths		MEN CPS-I: 1.7 (1.6–1.8) CPS-II: 1.9 (1.8–2.0) WOMEN CPS-I: 1.4 (1.3–1.5) CPS-II: 1.8 (1.7–2.0)
Kahn (1966)[87]; Rogot and Murray (1980)[88]	U.S. veterans: 248,046 men	16 y for cardiovascular deaths	Overall 1.15 <5 y 1.40 5–9 y 1.40 10–14 y 1.30 15–19 y 1.20 ≥20 y 1.00	1.58
Hrubec and McLaughlin (1997)[44]	U.S. veterans: 248,046 men	26 y for CHD deaths	Overall 1.2 (1.2–1.2) <5 y 1.7 (1.5–1.9) 5–9 y 1.5 (1.4–1.6) 10–19 y 1.4 (1.3–1.4) 20–29 y 1.2 (1.1–1.2) 30–39 y 1.1 (1.0–1.1) ≥40 y 1.0 (1.0–1.1)	
Doyle et al (1962)[89]	Framingham and Albany cohorts of 4120 healthy men aged 30–62	10 y (Framingham) 8 y (Albany) MI and CHD deaths	1.1 (0.5–2.2)	2.0–3.0 depending on amount smoked
Rosenman et al (1975)[90]	3154 healthy California men aged 39–59	8–9 y for fatal and nonfatal CHD	Aged 39–40 1.9 Aged 50–59 1.1	2.5
Cederlof et al (1975)[91]	Sample of 51,911 Swedish men aged 18–69	10 y for deaths	Quit 1–9 y 1.5 total Quit ≥10 y 1.0 total	1.7
Fuller et al (1983)[48]	Whitehall civil servants: 18,403 men aged 40–64	10 y for CHD deaths	Normoglycemic 1.3 Glucose intolerant 0.7 Diabetics 3.8	2.5 1.5 2.9

TABLE 28–1 • Cohort Studies of Coronary Heart Disease Risk Among Former and Current Smokers *Continued*

			Relative Risks Compared with Never-Smokers*	
Reference	**Population**	**Follow-up**	***Former Smokers***	***Current Smokers***
Friedman et al (1981)[93]	25,917 Kaiser-Permanente subscribers in the San Francisco area aged 20–79	4 y for CHD deaths	0.9	1.6
Friedman et al (1997)[50]	60,838 Kaiser-Permanente subscribers in San Francisco area, aged ≥35	6.1 y for CHD deaths	YEARS QUIT / MEN / WOMEN 2–20: 1.3 / 1.4 >20: 1.0 / 1.1	CIGARETTES/D / MEN / WOMEN <20: 1.4 / 1.4 ≥20: 2.0 / 2.2
Keys (1980)[47]	7-countries study of 12,096 men free of CHD	10 y for CHD deaths	2.3 (Northern Europe) 0.8 (Italy, Greece, Yugoslavia) 0.7 (U.S.)	2.4–4.5 depending on amount 0.7–1.8 depending on amount 1.6–3.0 depending on amount
Floderus et al (1988)[95]	10,495 Swedish twins aged 36–75	21 y for CHD deaths	Men: 1.0 (0.8–1.1) Women: 0.6 (0.4–1.0)	1.4–1.8 depending on amount smoked
Netterstrom and Juel (1988)[96]	2465 Danish bus drivers	7.75 y for MI and CHD death	3.2 (0.4–25.6)	5.0 (0.7–6.0)
Kawachi et al (1993, 1997)[35, 51]	Nurses Health Study: 121,700 U.S. women aged 30–55	12 y for cardiovascular deaths	1.6 (1.2–21)	3.7 (2.9–4.9)
Tervahauta et al (1995)[58]	647 Finnish men aged 65–84 171 with CHD 476 without CHD	5 y for fatal MI	1.3 (0.4–3.9) 1.1 (0.4–2.7)	>9 cigarettes/d 6.0 (1.4–25.0) 1.6 (0.4–4.7)

*95% confidence intervals shown in parentheses when available.

CHD, coronary heart disease; ppd, packs/day; ACS CPS-I and II, American Cancer Society Prevention Studies I and II; MI, myocardial infarction.

Adapted and updated from Department of Health and Human Services. The Health Benefits of Smoking Cessation: A Report of the Surgeon General. DHHS Publication No. (CDC) 90-8416. U.S. DHHS, Public Health Service, Centers for Disease Control, Office on Smoking and Health. Washington, DC, U.S. Government Printing Office, 1990.

compared with that of continuing smokers, adjusting for the effect of the intervention tested in the trial.

The lack of strong randomized, controlled clinical trial data, the highest standard of epidemiologic evidence, should not preclude a firm conclusion that smoking cessation reduces cardiovascular disease risk. Rose,[54a] for decades one of the leading minds in prevention, defined a standard *rule of prevention*—that the benefit of a preventive therapy must exceed the risk as shown in randomized clinical trials, *unless* the intervention itself equals restoration of a biologic or evolutionary norm, a circumstance certainly true for smoking cessation. The consistency, strength, and biologic plausibility of the observational epidemiologic data collected from men and women as well as the clear dose-response relationship between reduction in risk and years of tobacco abstinence make a conclusive case for the benefits of smoking cessation for cardiovascular disease prevention.[5] Given the current consensus about the benefits of smoking cessation, a randomized trial is unlikely ever to be conducted because it would be deemed unethical.

PRIMARY PREVENTION OF CARDIOVASCULAR DISEASE

Observational Epidemiologic Evidence

The 1990 Surgeon General's Report on Smoking[5] reviewed the evidence and summarized the health benefits for smoking cessation for individuals of all ages. It concluded that overall mortality of former smokers declines gradually, approaching that of never-smokers after 10 to 15 years of abstinence or perhaps sooner.[5] In otherwise healthy individuals, smoking cessation reduces cardiovascular disease risk more rapidly than the risk of lung cancer or overall mortality. Tables 28–1 and 28–2 summarize the major cohort and case-control studies, including those reviewed in the Surgeon General's Report and several published subsequently. These tables demonstrate that despite diversity of design and geographic location, the risk of CHD incidence and mortality is consistently lower

TABLE 28–2 • Case-Control Studies of Coronary Heart Disease Risk Among Former Smokers

Reference	Population	No. of Cases	No. of Controls	No. of Cases Among Former Smokers	Relative Risk as Compared with Never-Smokers*		
					Former Smokers		*Current Smokers*
Willet et al (1981)[97]	Nurses Health Study: women aged 30–55	263	5260	29	1.0 (0.7–1.6)		3.0 (2.3–4.0)
Rosenberg et al (1985)[52]	Eastern U.S. men aged <55	1873	2775	348	1.1 (0.9–1.4)		2.9 (2.4–3.4)
Rosenberg et al (1985)[98]	Eastern U.S. women aged <50	555	1864	35	1.0 (0.7–1.6)		1.4–7.0 depending on cigarettes/d
Lavecchia et al (1987)[99]	Italian women aged <55	168	251	3	0.8 (0.2–3.8)		3.6–13.1 depending on cigarettes/d
Rosenberg et al (1990)[53]	Eastern U.S. women aged <65	910	2375	149	1.2 (1.0–1.7)		3.6 (3.0–4.4)
Dobson et al (1991)[54]	Australian men aged 35–69	895	1039	374	1.3 (0.9–1.6)		2.7 (2.1–3.5)
	Australian women aged 35–69	387	1031	86	1.5 (1.1–2.2)		4.7 (3.4–6.6)
Negri et al (1994)[94]	Italian men and women aged <75	916	1106	NR	YEARS QUIT		
					1	1.6 (0.8–3.2)	2.9 (2.2–3.9)
					2–5	1.4 (0.9–2.1)	
					6–10	1.2 (0.7–2.1)	
					>10	1.1 (0.8–1.8)	

*95% confidence interval shown in parentheses when available.
NR, not reported.
Adapted and updated from Department of Health and Human Services. The Health Benefits of Smoking Cessation: A Report of the Surgeon General. DHHS Publication No. (CDC) 90-8416. U.S. DHHS, Public Health Service, Centersfor Disease Control, Office on Smoking and Health. Washington, DC, U.S. Government Printing Office, 1990.

among former smokers compared with individuals who continue to smoke.

Less clear from these data is how much time is required for total mortality and cardiovascular mortality among former smokers to decline to the level of never-smokers. The initial benefit is rapid, with as much as half the risk reduction occurring within 1 year of smoking cessation. Excess risk continues to decline, albeit more gradually, over the following 10 to 15 years. Three case-control studies suggested that approximately half of the excess risk of nonfatal myocardial infarction is eliminated within the first year of quitting smoking, and the risk of former smokers approaches that of never-smokers within 5 years.[52–54] Cohort studies in middle-aged men also suggest that the excess risk of heart disease is halved within 1 year, but most have observed a more gradual decline in risk, reaching the level of never-smokers after 10 to 15 years of abstinence, although in a few studies a small excess risk persists for 20 years or more.[5] More recent studies in women generally confirm this finding. An analysis of the Nurses' Health Study, the largest cohort study, reported that cessation reduced one third of the excess risk of CHD over 2 years and that the excess risk disappeared over 10 to 14 years of abstinence.[51, 55]

The evidence also demonstrates that the degree to which smokers benefit from cessation depends on their total exposure to tobacco, the time since quitting, and the presence or absence of comorbid conditions. In general, the observational studies cited in Table 28–1 support a dose-response relationship among all aspects of smoking and outcomes.[5] An analysis of the Nurses' Health Study confirms both a dose and a duration effect in women. The highest mortality and cardiovascular risks were seen among women who began smoking before the age of 15.[35]

Many of the studies cited attempted to adjust for the potentially confounding effects of demographic and other risk factors that could independently influence CHD mortality and morbidity. The Surgeon General's Report analysis concludes that "in the studies of primary prevention, none of these differences could explain even a minor portion of the decreased risk among quitters."[5] Nonetheless, similar to all observational studies, these have the inherent limitation that an unknown confounding factor could theoretically contribute to the difference in outcomes between smokers and ex-smokers.

The evidence that elderly individuals benefit from smoking cessation has been less certain, although that is the conclusion of the largest study, which was conducted among 7178 men and women over age 65 in three cities.[56] Former smokers had rates of cardiovascular mortality similar to those who had never smoked, regardless of the age of cessation. Jajich and colleagues,[57] who studied 2674 Chicago residents aged 64 to 75 at study entry, reached a similar conclusion. Over 4 years' follow-up, former smokers had a relative risk of 1.1 for CHD mortality compared with 1.9 for current smokers. In contrast, late follow-up from the Finnish Cohort of the Seven Countries Study addressed the influence of classic risk factors on coronary risk and total mortality among elderly men. For those without coronary disease at the 25-year follow-up, smoking more than nine cigarettes per day was associated with higher risks of developing coronary disease events in the subsequent 5 years, but this association was not statistically significant, and the risk of relationship was less strong than that seen for elevated serum cholesterol.[58]

Randomized, Controlled Clinical Trials

Only one of the many randomized, controlled trials of smoking cessation as a single factor intervention has reported long-term health outcomes.[43b] In the early 1970s, Rose and Hamilton[43a] tested the impact of smoking cessation advice versus no advice in 1445 British male civil servants at high risk of heart disease based on a risk factor assessment. Men in the intervention group received individualized information on the health risks of smoking and strong advice to quit. Over 10 years, the self-reported daily cigarette consumption was 53% lower in the intervention group than it was in the control group, but in the next 10 years of follow-up, this difference narrowed as increasing numbers of men in the control group reduced their cigarette use. At 20-year follow-up, the intervention group, compared with controls, had a 7% lower overall mortality rate, a 13% lower CHD mortality rate, and an 11% lower lung cancer incidence rate. The differences were not statistically significant, reflecting the low power in a trial not designed to detect differences in disease rates and a smaller than expected difference in exposure to tobacco because of the intervention group's imperfect compliance with smoking cessation recommendations and the control group's reduction in smoking over time.

Several other clinical trials have evaluated the effect of simultaneously altering several cardiovascular risk factors, including smoking (Table 28–3). The Multiple Risk Factor Intervention Trial (MRFIT) is the best known of these trials.[59] Its design most clearly approaches the standard now common for randomized, controlled clinical trials. More than 12,000 high-risk men, aged 35 to 57, were randomized to a special intervention or usual care and followed for an average of 10.5 years. Participants in the special intervention group underwent intensive, consistent, and recurring instructions regarding diet and smoking and aggressive, standardized hypertension therapy. Mortality at the study's end was slightly but not significantly lower (7%) in the intervention group compared with usual care for a series of complex reasons discussed elsewhere in this text (see Chapter 34). A separate analysis of those who quit smoking during the trial suggested a powerful benefit of smoking cessation. After adjustment for the presence of other risk factors, CHD risk was 42% lower among participants who had quit at the first annual follow-up visit.[60] Persistent quitters had a 65% 3-year risk reduction compared with persistent smokers. A smaller but similar study from Oslo that enrolled normotensive men aged 40 to 49 with other cardiac risk factors demonstrated a 44% decline in coronary disease events 102 months after institution of the diet and smoking intervention.[61] It was estimated that smoking cessation was responsible for 25% of the difference between the intervention and usual care groups.

Public Health Implications

The public health impact of smoking cessation on CHD events was estimated by Tosteson and coworkers,[62] using epidemiologic data and a complex computer simulation of the U.S. male population. The analysis suggests that interventions that would reduce the prevalence of smoking by 25% would generate a significant fall in the incidence of CHD among men under the age of 65. Paradoxically the model projects a slight *increase* in the incidence of CHD among men 65 or older. This occurs because of a smoking cessation–related decrease in non–coronary disease mortality that allows more former smokers to survive to age 65. This larger cohort of older smokers is then exposed to other (nonsmoking) risk for coronary disease events. Table 28–4 displays the results of this analysis. It projects, for example, a 2% *higher* incidence of CHD among a group of men turning 75 years old, half of whom stopped smoking 25 years earlier, as compared with a group of male smokers with no prior smoking cessation. Conversely a 50-year-old group, half of whom quit, would have an 8% *lower* incidence of CHD. Despite the artifactually increased cardiovascular mortality among the elderly, this analysis confirms that smoking cessation will succeed in preventing *premature* cardiovascular disease in the U.S. population.

SECONDARY PREVENTION

Observational epidemiologic evidence demonstrates that the favorable impact of smoking cessation ex-

TABLE 28–3 • Single and Multiple Risk Factor Intervention Trials of Smoking Cessation and Coronary Heart Disease Risk

Reference	Population	Intervention	Outcome	Overall Effect of Intervention	Effect of Smoking Cessation (Nonrandomized)
SINGLE RISK FACTOR					
Rose and Colwell (1992)[43b]	1445 healthy British civil servants at high CHD risk	Antismoking advice	CHD deaths	13% reduction in intervention group at 20 years (not statistically significant)	NR
MULTIPLE RISK FACTORS					
MRFIT Research Group (1982)[59]	MRFIT: 12,866 healthy U.S. men aged 35–57 at high CHD risk	Diet, weight control, hypertension, and smoking	CHD deaths	7% decline in intervention group	44% reduction compared with persistent smokers
Ockene et al (1990)[60]	MRFIT: 6943 participant smokers at entry	Diet, weight control, hypertension, and smoking	CHD deaths	—	At 3-y follow-up, quitters had 65% reduction (37–80%) compared with persistent smokers
Hjermann et al (1981)[61]	Oslo study: 1232 healthy men aged 40–49 at high CHD risk	Diet and smoking	Fatal and nonfatal MI	44% decline in intervention group at 102 mo	Smoking cessation accounted for about 25% of the difference between groups
Kornitzer et al (1983)[110]	19,409 male Belgian factory workers, aged 40–59	Smoking and hypertension	Fatal and nonfatal MI	25% reduction in intervention group	No specific analysis for effect of smoking cessation
Rose et al (1983)[111]	12 pairs of factories in UK, 18,210 men aged 40–59	Diet, smoking, hypertension control	Nonfatal MI and CHD deaths	4% net reduction in prevalence of current smoking, virtually no difference in outcome between the two groups	No specific analysis of ex-smokers
Wilhelmsen et al (1986)[112]	10,004 random Göteborg men aged 45–55	Hypertension control, dietary, and antismoking advice	Major CHD	No difference	Intervention achieved only small differences between groups for any risk factor

CHD, coronary heart disease; MRFIT, Multiple Risk Factor Intervention Trial; MI, myocardial infarction; NR, not reported.
Adapted and updated from Department of Health and Human Services. The Health Benefits of Smoking Cessation: A Report of the Surgeon General. DHHS Publication No. (CDC) 90-8416. U.S. DHHS, Public Health Service, Centers for Disease Control, Office on Smoking and Health. Washington, DC, U.S. Government Printing Office, 1990.

tends to individuals who quit after the diagnosis of CHD. Most studies have focused on survivors of myocardial infarction and out-of-hospital cardiac arrest. It has been possible to demonstrate the benefit of smoking cessation in the secondary prevention setting with smaller sample sizes because the risk of future CHD events is as much as 10-fold higher among those with established disease compared with those free of clinical evidence of coronary artery disease. Nonetheless, the dependence on observational studies provides the same methodologic issues as applied to the primary prevention setting.

The 1990 Surgeon General's Report reviewed studies of smokers with diagnosed CHD.[5] These studies, summarized in Table 28–5, demonstrate that survivors of myocardial infarction or cardiac arrest benefit from stopping smoking, with a mortality advantage of up to 50%.[5, 15, 63] As in primary prevention, the reduction in risk is most pronounced earlier (at 6 to 12 months) with lesser risk reduction in later follow-up periods. Similar results were reported in a more recently published study of a large unselected population of myocardial infarction patients.[64] Smoking cessation after the index event was associated with 17% 5-year mortality, compared with 31% mortality among patients who continue to smoke. Much of this benefit, however, was accounted for by higher baseline risk among those who failed to quit, includ-

TABLE 28–4 • Projected Percent Changes Over Baseline Values for Absolute Coronary Heart Disease Incidence Among Men Free of Coronary Heart Disease, 25 Years After Each Level of Smoking Reduction Is Achieved

	Change in Absolute Incidence for Each Level of Smoking Reduction		
Age (y)	25%	50%	75%
35–44	−9	−16	−22
45–54	−4	−8	−11
55–64	0	−1	−1
65–74	+1	+2	+4
75–84	+1	+2	+3

Adapted from Tosteson AN, Weinstein MC, Williams LW, et al. Long-term impact of smoking cessation on the incidence of coronary heart disease. Am J Public Health 1990; 80:1481–1486.

ing history of prior myocardial infarction and congestive heart failure. This is in contrast to most other studies, which have demonstrated *higher* baseline risk among quitters compared with nonquitters.[5]

It has been suggested[5] that observational studies of patients with coronary disease are likely to underestimate the favorable effect of quitting for two reasons. First, as noted previously, smokers who quit after myocardial infarction often have a greater disease burden, which provides them with a greater motivation to quit compared with less severely ill individuals but also gives them a worse prognosis at the time of cessation. Second, most observational studies of quitting after a cardiac event have not routinely used biochemical validation of smoking cessation. The individuals classified as quitters likely include some who continue to smoke despite a self-report of cessation.[5]

Additional evidence to support the benefit of smoking cessation derives from several controlled trials of therapeutic interventions for CHD. These studies have analyzed the effect of smoking cessation on risk among former smokers, independent of the intervention being studied. In the Norwegian Timolol Post-MI Trial, smoking cessation was associated with a 33% reduction in the risk of reinfarction, at an average of 17 months follow-up.[65] At this early follow-up, however, no difference in total mortality was seen. Interestingly, follow-up from a similarly designed trial of practolol demonstrated a benefit of smoking cessation beginning at 18 months, and by 24 months a 30% risk reduction in coronary disease events was demonstrated.[66]

In a prospectively planned analysis of the Cardiac Arrhythmia Suppression Trial (CAST), a study evaluating patients with ventricular ectopic activity and left ventricular dysfunction after acute myocardial infarction, smoking cessation was associated with a marked reduction in arrhythmic death as well as total mortality.[67] This major benefit occurred in patients not receiving thrombolytic therapy or undergoing coronary revascularization. These results are consistent with earlier studies of cardiac arrest survivors whose long-term prognosis is apparently improved by smoking cessation.[15]

In the Coronary Artery Surgical Study (CASS), death rates at follow-up were compared among never-smokers, persistent smokers, and persistent quitters. At baseline, quitters had a worse prognosis than did persistent smokers. At every level of risk, however, after adjustment for baseline characteristics, 5-year survival was better for quitters compared with smokers, with a risk reduction of 40%[68] (see Table 28–3). A more recent CASS follow-up communication reported 10-year total mortality of smokers and quitters.[69] Survival was better among smokers who stopped smoking during follow-up compared with those who continued to smoke (82% vs. 77%; $P = 0.025$). The difference in survival was more pronounced for patients randomized to coronary bypass graft surgery (84% among quitters vs. 68% among nonquitters; $P = 0.018$) than among medically treated patients (75% for quitters vs. 71% for nonquitters; $P =$ NS). Most other cardiac endpoints were considerably more frequent among nonquitters in both medical and surgical groups, including hospitalizations for myocardial infarction, stroke, cardiac catheterization, and peripheral vascular surgery.

Observational studies of patients undergoing bypass surgery and coronary angioplasty provide further support for a long-term benefit of smoking cessation among patients undergoing revascularization. Smoking cessation after bypass surgery appears to reduce substantially the risk of myocardial infarction, repeat bypass surgery, and angina pectoris at 15 years.[70] Similarly an observational study of almost 5000 patients from the Mayo Clinic after coronary angioplasty demonstrated a much higher relative risk of mortality (relative risk [RR], 1.76) and of Q wave myocardial infarction (RR, 2.08) in persistent smokers compared with nonsmokers. The need for repeat revascularization, either by percutaneous transluminal coronary angioplasty or surgery, was reduced by as much as one third.[71] The effects of smoking cessation on other CHD endpoints have been less consistent. This is particularly true for restenosis after coronary angioplasty. Although one such study[72] suggested a 17% higher absolute rate of restenosis among those who continued to smoke compared with quitters, other studies have not regularly detected such a benefit for restenosis with smoking cessation. In most randomized trials of interventions to reduce restenosis, smoking has not influenced the restenosis rate.[73]

A surprising finding emerged from several studies in the thrombolytic era with respect to outcomes in smokers compared with nonsmokers. Paradoxically, smoking predicted a better prognosis after acute myo-

TABLE 28–5 • Major Studies of the Effect of Smoking Cessation on Persons with Diagnosed Coronary Heart Disease

Reference	Population	Follow-up	Cases Among Former Smokers	Reduction in Risk Compared with Persistent Smokers*
Mulcahy et al (1977)[100]	190 Dublin men aged <60 who smoked at time of first MI or unstable angina	5 y	13 deaths	50%
Daly et al (1987)[101]	373 men aged <60 who smoked at time of first MI or unstable angina and survived 2 y	Average 9.4 y; ≤16 y	NR	10% for sudden death; 40% for total mortality
Hubert et al (1982)[102]	Framingham Heart Study: subjects with angina	≤26 y	NR	10-y follow-up: <60 y: 90% ≥60 y: 60%
Salonen (1980)[103]	North Karelia, Finland: 523 men aged <65 who smoked at first MI	3 y	22 CHD deaths	40% (0–60)
Ronnevik et al (1985)[104]†	1330 participants in the Norwegian timolol trial who smoked at time of MI	17 mo	44 recurrent nonfatal MI	33% reduction 8% in quitters 12% in persistent smokers
Aberg et al (1983)[105]	983 Göteborg male smokers at time of MI	≤10.5 y	104 recurrent nonfatal MI; 80 CHD deaths	30%; difference between groups increased with time
Vlietstra et al (1986)[68]†	11,605 patients in CASS who smoked at time CHD was diagnosed by angiography	5 y	234	40% (20–50)
Hermanson et al (1988)[106]†	3045 CASS patients with CHD aged 35–54 1893 CASS patients with CHD aged ≥55	5.3 y for MI or death	35–54 y: NR 55–69 y: 239 >70 y: 29	40% (30–50) 30% (20–50) 70% (30–80)
Cavender et al (1992)[69]†	780 CASS patients	10 y for death	NR	35%
Hallstrom et al (1986)[15]	310 survivors of out-of-hospital arrest, smokers at that time	Mean 47.5 mo		35% for fatal recurrent cardiac arrest
Green (1987)[107]†	2199 men who smoked at time of MI	2 y	NR	30% for CHD
Phillips et al (1988)[108]	530 male British former smokers with non-MI CHD	Mean 7.5 y		33% for fatal or nonfatal CHD
Goldberg et al (1981)[109]	325 post-MI patients	≤10 y		SURVIVAL Quit at MI / Not Quit 1 y: 99% / 98% 5 y: 97% / 84% 10 y: 95% / 51%

*95% confidence intervals reported in parentheses where available.

†Data come from a randomized, controlled trial; however, analyses are not derived from intention-to-treat analyses. All other studies in the table are observational studies.

MI, myocardial infarction; NR, not reported; CASS, Coronary Artery Surgery Study; CHD, coronary heart disease.

Adapted and updated from Department of Health and Human Services. The Health Benefits of Smoking Cessation: A Report of the Surgeon General. DHHS Publication No. (CDC) 90-8416. U.S. DHHS, Public Health Service, Centers for Disease Control, Office on Smoking and Health. Washington, DC, U.S. Government Printing Office, 1990.

cardial infarction, particularly at early follow-up.[74–76] In some studies, even smokers not actually undergoing thrombolytic therapy appeared to have better in-hospital and 6-month prognosis.[77, 78] Interventional studies[79, 80] of acute myocardial infarction have shown better early coronary flow after thrombolytic therapy in smokers compared with nonsmokers, suggesting a greater clot burden or thrombogenicity in smokers with, perhaps, less severe underlying atherosclerosis. It has been suggested that this *smoker's paradox* could be explained by the development of myocardial infarction at younger ages with a more favorable risk factor pattern in smokers compared with nonsmokers who develop myocardial infarction.[81] This hypothesis is largely confirmed by large observational studies of myocardial infarction,[76, 78] including one from Israel in which the better prognosis of smokers disappeared after adjustment for age and baseline clinical variables, including risk factors.[82] Cohort studies in which the short-term *benefit* conferred by smoking was not abolished by adjustment for baseline characteristics have not adjusted for atherosclerotic risk factors, which are likely to reflect more accurately underlying atherosclerotic burden than do clinical characteristics (such as history of previous myocardial infarction or angina) at the time of myocardial infarction presentation. Furthermore, studies showing an *advantage* for smoking were not generally consecutive series of patients but rather studies of patients eligible for thrombolytic therapy, who are generally younger with better baseline characteristics than those not eligible for thrombolytic therapy.

CONCLUSION

Despite the absence of data from randomized, controlled clinical trials, a considerable amount of prospective observational epidemiologic data regarding the effect of smoking cessation on cardiovascular disease has been collected for more than 40 years. The evidence is diverse in design and site and includes cohort studies of both primary and secondary prevention, multiple risk factor intervention trials, and subgroup analyses of cardiovascular treatment trials. The overwhelming totality of this evidence demonstrates that smoking cessation promptly, dependably, and substantially lowers morbidity and mortality from coronary artery disease, compared with continuing to smoke, regardless of how long or how much one has smoked. The effect is present in both men and women and at all ages, but little information is available about nonwhites. The data suggest that there is a rapid initial decline in excess cardiovascular risk, up to 50% within the first 1 to 2 years after cessation, followed by a more gradual decline. The risk among former smokers approaches that of never-smokers over approximately 10 to 15 years of abstinence. The benefit of smoking cessation persists even after the diagnosis of cardiovascular disease; a risk reduction of up to 50% has been reported. This pattern is consistent with the multiple effects of smoking on the pathogenesis of cardiovascular disease, which includes both short-term and long-term effects. Given the broad consensus about the benefit of smoking cessation, the issue is not likely to be testable for ethical reasons in any future prospective, randomized clinical trial. Such data are really not necessary to guide medical and public health practice. The substantial prevalence of tobacco smoking and the epidemiologic evidence of the magnitude of the benefit of smoking cessation indicate that it is a leading modifiable risk factor for cardiovascular disease and that efforts to reduce smoking prevalence deserve a high priority.

REFERENCES

1. U.S. Department of Health and Human Services. Reducing the Health Consequences of Smoking: 25 Years of Progress. A Report of the Surgeon General. DHHS Publication No. (CDC) 89–8411. Bethesda, MD, U.S. Department of Health and Human Services, Public Health Service, Centers for Disease Control, Office on Smoking and Health, 1989.
2. McGinnis JM, Foege WH. Actual causes of death in the United States. JAMA 1993; 270:2207.
3. Bartecchi CE, MacKenzie TK, Schrier RW. The human cost of tobacco use. N Engl J Med 1994; 330:907–912, 975–980.
4. Centers for Disease Control and Prevention. Cigarette-attributable mortality and years of potential life lost—United States, 1990. MMWR 1993; 42:645–649.
5. Department of Health and Human Services. The Health Benefits of Smoking Cessation. A Report of the Surgeon General. DHHS Publication No. (CDC) 90–8416. Bethesda, MD, U.S. Department of Health and Human Services, Public Health Service, Centers for Disease Control, Office on Smoking and Health, 1990.
6. Cigarette smoking among adults—United States, 1995. MMWR 1997; 46:1217–1219.
7. U.S. Department of Health and Human Services. Preventing Tobacco Use Among Young People. A Report of the Surgeon General. Bethesda, MD, U.S. Department of Health and Human Services, Public Health Service, Centers for Disease Control, Office on Smoking and Health, 1994.
8. Benowitz NL. Pharmacologic aspects of cigarette smoking and nicotine addiction. N Engl J Med 1988; 319:1318–1330.
9. Benowitz NL, Gourlay SG. Cardiovascular toxicity of nicotine: Implications for nicotine replacement therapy. J Am Coll Cardiol 1997; 29:1422–1431.
10. McBride PE. The health consequences of smoking. Med Clin North Am 1992; 76:333–353.
11. McGill HC. The cardiovascular pathology of smoking. Am Heart J 1988; 115:250–257.
12. Kurihara S. Effect of age on blood pressure response to cigarette smoking. Cardiology 1995; 86:102–107.
13. Cryer PE, Haymond MW, Santiago JV, et al. Norepinephrine and epinephrine release and adrenergic mediation of smoking-associated hemodynamic and metabolic events. N Engl J Med 1976; 295:573–577.
14. Kool MJF, Hoeks APG, Struijker Boudier HAJ, et al. Short- and long-term effects of smoking on arterial wall properties in habitual smokers. J Am Coll Cardiol 1993; 22:1881–1886.
15. Hallstrom AP, Cobb LA, Ray R. Smoking as a risk factor for recurrence of sudden cardiac arrest. N Engl J Med 1986; 314:271–275.
16. Anderson EW, Andelman RJ, Strauch JM, et al. Effect of low-level carbon monoxide exposure on onset and duration of angina pectoris. Ann Intern Med 1973; 79:46–50.
17. Quillen JE, Rossen JD, Oskarsson HJ, et al. Acute effect of cigarette smoking on the coronary circulation: Constriction of epicardial and resistance vessels. J Am Coll Cardiol 1993; 22:642–647.
18. Sugiishi M. Cigarette smoking is a major risk factor for coronary spasm. Circulation 1993; 87:76–79.
19. Deanfield JE, Sheat MJ, Wilson RA, et al. Direct effects of smoking on the heart: Silent ischemic disturbances of coronary flow. Am J Cardiol 1986; 57:1005–1009.
20. Celermajer DS, Sorensen KE, Georgakopoulos D. Cigarette smoking is associated with dose-related and potentially reversible impairment of endothelium-dependent dilation in healthy young adults. Circulation 1993; 88:2149–2155.
21. Blann AD. The acute influence of smoking on the endothelium. Atherosclerosis 1992; 96:249–250.
22. McVeigh GE, LeMay L, Morgan DJ, et al. Cigarette smoking inhibits basal but not stimulated release of nitric oxide from the forearm vasculature. J Am Coll Cardiol 1995; 26:337A.
23. Zeiher AM, Schachinger V, Minners J. Smoking selectively impairs endothelium-mediated coronary vasodilation. Circulation 1994; 90:I-512.
24. Heitzer T, Kurz S, Munzel T. Cigarette smoking potentiates endothelial dysfunction in patients with hypercholesterolemia. Circulation 1994; 90:I-513.
25. Craig WY, Palomaki GE, Haddow JE. Cigarette smoking and serum lipid and lipoprotein concentrations: An analysis of published data. BMJ 1989; 298:784–788.
26. Harats D, BenNaim M, Dabach Y, et al. Cigarette smoking renders LDL susceptible to peroxidative modification and enhanced metabolism by macrophages. Atherosclerosis 1989; 79:245–252.
27. Stamford BA, Matter S, Fell RD, et al. Effects of smoking cessation on weight gain, metabolic rate, caloric consumption, and blood lipids. Am J Clin Nutr 1986; 43:486–494.

28. Benowitz NL, Fitzgerald GA, Wilson M, et al. Nicotine effects on eicosanoid formation and hemostatic function: Comparison of transdermal nicotine and cigarette smoking. J Am Coll Cardiol 1993; 22:1159–1167.
29. Eliasson M, Asplund K, Evrin P-E, et al. Relationship of cigarette smoking and snuff dipping to plasma fibrinogen, fibrinolytic variables and serum insulin. The Northern Sweden MONICA study. Atherosclerosis 1995; 113:41–53.
30. Shah PK, Helfant RH. Smoking and coronary artery disease. Chest 1988; 94:449–452.
31. Pittilo RM, Clarke JM, Harris D, et al. Cigarette smoking and platelet adhesion. Br J Haematol 1984; 58:627–632.
32. Jonas MA, Oates JA, Ockene JK, et al. Statement on smoking and cardiovascular disease for health care professionals. AHA Medical/Scientific Statement. Circulation 1992; 86:1664–1669.
33. Doll R, Peto R, Wheatley K, et al. Mortality in relation to smoking: 40 years' observations on male British doctors. BMJ 1994; 309:901–911.
34. Willett WC, Green A, Stampfer MJ, et al. Relative and absolute excess risks of coronary heart disease among women who smoke cigarettes. N Engl J Med 1987; 317:1303–1309.
35. Kawachi I, Colditz GA, Stampfer MJ, et al. Smoking cessation in relation to total mortality rates in women: A prospective cohort study. Ann Intern Med. 1993; 119:992–1000.
36. Kawachi I, Colditz GA, Stampfer MJ, et al. Smoking cessation and decreased risk of stroke in women. JAMA 1993; 269:232–236.
37. Layde PM, Beral V. Further analyses of mortality in oral contraceptive users. Royal College of General Practitioners' Oral Contraception Study. Lancet 1981; 1:541–546.
38. Environmental Protection Agency. Respiratory health effects of passive smoking: Lung cancer and other disorders. Washington, DC, Office of Health and Environmental Assessment, 1992.
39. Kawachi I, Coditz GA, Speizer FE, et al. A prospective study of passive smoking and coronary heart disease. Circulation 1997; 95:2374–2379.
40. Glantz SA, Parmley WW. Passive smoking and heart disease: Epidemiology, physiology, and biochemistry. Circulation 1991; 83:1–12.
41. Glantz SA, Parmley WW. Passive smoking and heart disease: Mechanisms and risk. JAMA 1995; 273:1047–1053.
42. Steenland K. Passive smoking and the risk of heart disease. JAMA 1992; 267:94–99.
43. Taylor AE, Johnson DC, Kazemi H. Environmental tobacco smoke and cardiovascular disease: A position paper from the Council on Cardiopulmonary and Critical Care, American Heart Association. Circulation 1992; 86:699–702.
43a. Rose G, Hamilton PJS. A randomised controlled trial of the effect on middle-aged men of advice to stop smoking. J Epidemiol Commun Health 1978; 32:275–281.
43b. Rose G, Colwell L. Randomised controlled trial of anti-smoking advice: Final (20 year) results. J Epidemiol Commun Health 1992; 46:75–77.
44. Hrubec Z, McLaughlin JK. Former cigarette smoking and mortality among U.S. veterans: A 26-year followup, 1954–1980. *In* Changes in Cigarette-Related Disease Risks and Their Implication for Prevention and Control: Smoking and Tobacco Control Monograph. NIH Publication No. 97-4213. National Cancer Institute. Washington, DC, U.S. Government Printing Office, 1997, pp 501–530.
45. Thun MJ, Day-Lally C, Myers DG, et al. Trends in tobacco smoking and mortality from cigarette use in Cancer Prevention Studies I (1959 through 1965) and II (1982 through 1988). *In* Changes in Cigarette-Related Disease Risks and Their Implication for Prevention and Control: Smoking and Tobacco Control Monograph. NIH Publication No. 97–4213. National Cancer Institute. Washington, DC, U.S. Government Printing Office, 1997, pp 305–382.
46. Burns DM, Shanks TG, Choi W, et al. The American Cancer Society Cancer Prevention Study: I. 12-year followup of 1 million men and women. *In* Changes in Cigarette-Related Disease Risks and Their Implication for Prevention and Control: Smoking and Tobacco Control Monograph. NIH Publication No. 97–4213. National Cancer Institute. Washington, DC, U.S. Government Printing Office, 1997, pp 113–304.
47. Keys A. Smoking habits. *In* Keys A (ed). Seven Countries: A Multivariate Analysis of Death and Coronary Heart Disease. Cambridge, MA, Harvard University Press, 1980, pp 136–160.
48. Fuller JH, Shipley MJ, Rose G, et al. Mortality from coronary heart disease and stroke in relation to degree of glycaemia: The Whitehall Study. BMJ 1983; 287:867–870.
49. Cederlof R, Friberg L, Hrubec Z, et al. The relationship of smoking and some social covariables to mortality and cancer morbidity: A ten year follow-up in a probability sample of 55,000 Swedish subjects age 18–69, Part ½. Stockholm, Karolinska Institute, Department of Environmental Hygiene, 1975.
50. Friedman GD, Tekawa I, Sadler M, et al. Smoking and mortality: The Kaiser Permanente experience. *In* Changes in Cigarette-Related Disease Risks and Their Implication for Prevention and Control: Smoking and Tobacco Control Monograph. NIH Publication No. 97–4213. National Cancer Institute. Washington, DC, U.S. Government Printing Office, 1997, pp 477–497.
51. Kawachi I, Colditz GA, Stampfer MJ, et al. Smoking cessation and decreased risks of total mortality, stroke, and coronary heart disease incidence among women: A prospective cohort study. *In* Changes in Cigarette-Related Disease Risks and Their Implication for Prevention and Control: Smoking and Tobacco Control Monograph. NIH Publication No. 97–4213. National Cancer Institute. Washington, DC, U.S. Government Printing Office, 1997, pp 531–564.
52. Rosenberg L, Kaufman DW, Helmrich SP, et al. The risk of myocardial infarction after quitting smoking in men under 55 years of age. N Engl J Med 1985; 313:1511–1514.
53. Rosenberg L, Palmer JR, Shapiro S. Decline in the risk of myocardial infarction among women who stop smoking. N Engl J Med 1990; 322:213–217.
54. Dobson AJ, Alexander HM, Heller RF, et al. How soon after quitting smoking does risk of heart attack decline? J Clin Epidemiol 1991; 44:1247–1253.
54a. Rose G. Strategy of prevention: Lessons from cardiovascular disease. Br Med J 1981; 282:1847–1851.
55. Kawachi I, Colditz GA, Stampfer MJ, et al. Smoking cessation and time course of decreased risks of coronary heart disease in middle-aged women. Arch Intern Med 1994; 154:169–175.
56. LaCroix AZ, Lang J, Scherr P, et al. Smoking and mortality among older men and women in three communities. N Engl J Med 1991; 324:1619–1625.
57. Jajich CL, Ostfeld AM, Freeman DH. Smoking and coronary heart disease mortality in the elderly. JAMA 1984; 252:2831–2834.
58. Tervahauta M, Pekkanen J, Nissinen A. Risk factors of coronary heart disease and total mortality among elderly men with and without pre-existing coronary heart disease. Finnish Cohorts of the Seven Countries Study. J Am Coll Cardiol 1995; 26:1623–1629.
59. Multiple Risk Factor Intervention Trial Research Group. Multiple Risk Factor Intervention Trial: Risk factor changes and mortality results. JAMA 1982; 248:1465–1477.
60. Ockene JK, Kuller LH, Svendsen KH, et al. The relationship of smoking cessation to coronary heart disease and lung cancer in the Multiple Risk Factor Intervention Trial (MRFIT). Am J Public Health 1990; 80:954–958.
61. Hjermann I, Holme I, Leren P. Oslo study diet and antismoking trial: Results after 102 months. Am J Med 1986; 80(suppl 2A):7–12.
62. Tosteson AN, Weinstein MC, Williams LW, et al. Long-term impact of smoking cessation on the incidence of coronary heart disease. Am J Public Health 1990; 80:1481–1486.
63. Sparrow D, Dawber TR, Colton T. The influence of cigarette smoking on prognosis after a first myocardial infarction: A report from the Framingham Study. J Chronic Dis 1978; 31:425–432.
64. Herlitz J, Bengtson A, Hjalmarson A, et al. Smoking habits in consecutive patients with acute myocardial infarction: Prognosis in relation to other risk indicators and to whether or not they quit smoking. Cardiology 1995; 86:496–502.
65. Von Der Lippe G, Lund-Johansen P. Reduction of sudden deaths after myocardial infarction by treatment with beta-blocking drugs. *In* Zanchetti A (ed): Advances in Beta-Blocker

Therapy II. Proceedings of the Second International Bayer Beta-Blocker Symposium, Venice, 1981. 1982, pp 100–105.
66. Green KG. Falsely favourable early prognosis for continuing smokers following recovery from acute myocardial infarction: Information from the multi-centre practolol trial. Br J Clin Pract 1987; 41:785–788.
67. Peters RW, Brooks MM, Todd L, et al, for the Cardiac Arrhythmia Suppression Trial (CAST) Investigators. Smoking cessation and arrhythmic death: The CAST experience. J Am Coll Cardiol 1995; 26:1287–1292.
68. Vlietstra RE, Kronmal RA, Oberman A, et al. Effect of cigarette smoking on survival of patients with angiographically documented coronary artery disease:. Report from the CASS Registry. JAMA 1986; 255:1023–1027.
69. Cavender JB, Rogers WJ, Fisher LD, et al. Effects of smoking on survival and morbidity in patients randomized to medical or surgical therapy in the coronary artery surgery study (CASS): 10-year follow-up. J Am Coll Cardiol 1992; 20:287–294.
70. Voors AA, vanBrussel BL, Plokker HWT, et al. Smoking and cardiac events after venous coronary bypass surgery: A 15-year follow-up study. Circulation 1996; 93:42–47.
71. Hasdai D, Garatt KN, Grill DE, et al. Effect of smoking status on the long-term outcome after successful percutaneous coronary revascularization. N Engl J Med 1997; 336:755–761.
72. Galan KM, Beligonul U, Kern MJ, et al. Increased frequency of restenosis in patients continuing to smoke cigarettes after percutaneous transluminal coronary angioplasty. Am J Cardiol 1988; 61:260–263.
73. Moliterno DJ, Topol EJ. Clinical evaluation of restenosis. *In* Fuster V, Ross R, Topol EJ (eds). Atherosclerosis and Coronary Artery Diseases. Philadelphia, Lippincott-Raven, 1996, pp 1505–1526.
74. Barbash GI, White HD, Modan M, et al, for the Investigators of the International Tissue Plasminogen Activator/Streptokinase Mortality Trial. Significance of smoking in patients receiving thrombolytic therapy for acute myocardial infarction. Circulation 1993; 87:53–58.
75. Lee KL, Woodlief LH, Topol EJ, et al, for the GUSTO-1 Investigators. Predictors of 30-day mortality in the area of reperfusion for acute myocardial infarction: Results from an international trial of 41,021 patients. Circulation 1995; 91:1659–1668.
76. Maggioni AP, Maeri A, Fresco C, et al, on behalf of the Gruppo Italiano per lo Studio Della Soproavivenza nell Infarto Miocardico (GISSI-2). Age-related increase in mortality among patients with first myocardial infarctions treated with thrombolysis. N Engl J Med 1993; 329:1442–1448.
77. Molstad P. First myocardial infarction in smokers. Eur Heart J 1991; 12:753–759.
78. Maynard C, Weaver WD, Litwin PE, et al, for the MITI Project Investigators. Hospital mortality in acute myocardial infarction in the era of reperfusion therapy (the Myocardial Infarction Triage and Intervention Project). Am J Cardiol 1993; 72:877–882.
79. Grines CL, Topol EJ, O Neill WW, et al. Effect of cigarette smoking on outcome after thrombolytic therapy for myocardial infarction. Circulation 1995; 91:298–303.
80. Zahger D, Cerek B, Cannon CP, et al. How do smokers differ from nonsmokers in their response to thrombolysis (the TIMI-4 trial)? Am J Cardiol 1995; 75:232–236.
81. Ockene IS, Ockene JK. Smoking after acute myocardial infarction: A good thing? Circulation 1993; 87:297–299.
82. Gottlieb S, Boyko V, Zahger D, et al, for the Israeli Thrombolytic Survey Group. Smoking and prognosis after acute myocardial infarction in the thrombolytic era (Israeli Thrombolytic National Survey). J Am Coll Cardiol 1996; 28:1506–1513.
83. Doll R, Peto R. Mortality in relation to smoking: 20 years' observations on male British doctors. BMJ 1976; 2:1525–1536.
84. Doll R, Gray R, Hafner B, et al. Mortality in relation to smoking: 22 years' observations on female British doctors. BMJ 1980; 280:967–971.
85. Hammond EC, Horn D. Smoking and death rates—report on forty-four months of follow-up of 187,783 men: I. Total mortality. JAMA 1958; 166:1159–1172, 1294–1308.
86. Hammond EC, Garfinkel L. Coronary heart disease, stroke, and aortic aneurysm: Factors in etiology. Arch Environ Health 1969; 19:167–182.
87. Kahn HA. The Dorn study of smoking and mortality among U.S. veterans: Report on eight and one-half years of observation. *In* Haenszel W (ed). Epidemiological Approaches to the Study of Cancer and other Chronic Disease. NCI Monograph No. 19. Bethesda, MD, U.S. Department of Health, Education and Welfare, U.S. Public Health Service, National Cancer Institute, 1966, pp 1–125.
88. Rogot E, Murray JL. Smoking and causes of death among U.S. veterans: 16 years of observation. Public Health Rep 1980; 95:213–222.
89. Doyle JT, Dawber TR, Kannel WB, et al. Cigarette smoking and coronary heart disease: Combined experience of the Albany and Framingham studies. N Engl J Med 1962; 266:796–801.
90. Rosenman RH, Brand RJ, Jenkins CD, et al. Coronary heart disease in the Western Collaborative Group Study: Final follow-up experience of 8.5 years. JAMA 1975; 233:872–877.
91. Cederlof R, Friberg, L, Hrubec, Z, et al. The relationship of smoking and some social covariables to mortality and cancer morbidity: A ten year follow-up in a probability sample of 55,000 Swedish subjects age 18–69, Part ½. Stockholm, Karolinska Institute, Department of Environmental Hygiene, 1975.
92. Fuller JH, Shipley MJ, Rose G, et al. Mortality from coronary heart disease and stroke in relation to degree of glycaemia: The Whitehall Study. BMJ 1983; 287:867–870.
93. Friedman GD, Petitti DB, Bawol RD, et al. Mortality in cigarette smokers and quitters: Effect of base-line differences. N Engl J Med 1981; 304:1407–1410.
94. Negri E, LaVecchia C, D'Avanzo B, et al. Acute myocardial infarction: Association with time since stopping smoking in Italy. GISSI-EFRIM Investigators. J Epidemiol Commun Health 1994; 48:129–133.
95. Floderus B, Cederlof R, Friberg L. Smoking and mortality: A 21-year follow-up based on the Swedish Twin Registry. Int J Epidemiol 1988; 17:332–340.
96. Netterstrom B, Juel K. Impact of work-related and psychosocial factors on the development of ischemic heart disease among urban bus drivers in Denmark. Scand J Work Environ Health 1988; 14:231–238.
97. Willett WC, Hennekens CH, Bain C, et al. Cigarette smoking and non-fatal myocardial infarction in women. Am J Epidemiol 1981; 113:575–582.
98. Rosenberg L, Kaufman DW, Helmrich SP, et al. The risk of myocardial infarction after quitting smoking in men under 55 years of age. N Engl J Med 1985; 313:1511–1514.
99. Lavecchia C, Franceschi S, DeCarli A, et al. Risk factors for myocardial infarction in young women. Am J Epidemiol 1987; 125:832–843.
100. Mulcahy R, Hickey N, Graham IM, et al. Factors affecting the 5 year survival rate of men following acute coronary heart disease. Am Heart J 1977; 93:556–559.
101. Daly LE, Hickey N, Graham IM, et al. Predictors of sudden death up to 18 years after a first attack of unstable angina or myocardial infarction. Br Heart J 1987; 58:567–571.
102. Hubert HB, Holford TR, Kannel WB. Clinical characteristics and cigarette smoking in relation to prognosis of angina pectoris in Framingham. Am J Epidemiol 1982; 115:231–242.
103. Salonen JT. Stopping smoking and long-term mortality after acute myocardial infarction. Br Heart J 1980; 43:463–469.
104. Ronnevik PK, Gundersen T, Abrahamsen AM. Effect of smoking habits and timolol treatment on mortality and reinfarction in patients surviving acute myocardial infarction. Br Heart J 1985; 54:134–139.
105. Aberg A, Bergstrand R, Johansson S, et al. Cessation of smoking after myocardial infarction: Effects on mortality after 10 years. Br Heart J 1983; 49:416–422.
106. Hermanson B, Omenn GS, Kronmal RA, et al. Beneficial six-year outcome of smoking cessation in older men and women with coronary artery disease: Results from the CASS registry. N Engl J Med 1988; 319:1365–1369.
107. Green KG. Falsely favourable early prognosis for continuing smokers following recovery from acute myocardial infarction: Information from the multi-centre practolol trial. Br J Clin Pract 1987; 41:785–788.
108. Phillips AN, Shaper AG, Pocock SJ, et al. The role of risk factors in heart attacks occurring in men with pre-existing ischaemic heart disease. Br Heart J 1988; 60:404–410.

109. Goldberg R, Szklo M, Chandra V. The effect of cigarette smoking on the long-term prognosis of myocardial infarction. Am J Epidemiol 1981; 114:431.
110. Kornitzer M, DeBacker G, Dramaix M, et al. Belgian Heart Disease Prevention Project: Incidence and mortality results. Lancet 1983; 1:1066–1070.
111. Rose G, Tunstall-Pedoe HD, Heller RF. UK Heart Disease Prevention Project: Incidence and mortality results. Lancet 1983; 1:1062–1065.
112. Wilhelmsen L, Berglund G, Elmfeldt D, et al. The Multifactor Primary Prevention Trial in Goteborg, Sweden. Eur Heart J 1986; 7:279–288.

29 Exercise and Weight Loss

▶ Marcia L. Stefanick

The National Institutes of Health (NIH) Consensus Development Conference on the Health Implications of Obesity recognized hypercholesterolemia, hypertension, and non–insulin-dependent diabetes mellitus (NIDDM) as adverse effects of obesity, defined as excess body fat.[1] Subsequently, severe obesity, defined as being more than 30% above ideal body weight, was identified as an independent risk factor for coronary heart disease (CHD) in the National Cholesterol Education Program (NCEP) Adult Treatment Panel Guidelines.[2] In the Expert Panel's second report, however, obesity, defined as body mass index (BMI) greater than 27 kg/m^2, was not listed as a risk factor because "it operates through other risk factors that are included," specifically hyperlipidemia, decreased high-density lipoprotein (HDL) cholesterol, hypertension, and diabetes mellitus,[3] and it was for these reasons that weight loss was encouraged in overweight patients, particularly in those with visceral obesity.[3, 4]

Physical inactivity was also absent from the NCEP list of major CHD risk factors,[2–4] despite considerable evidence from observational studies that has supported a role of physical inactivity in the etiology of CHD.[5, 6] The American Heart Association (AHA) Committee on Exercise and Cardiac Rehabilitation of the Council on Clinical Cardiology, however, concluded that physical inactivity is a risk factor for coronary artery disease,[7] and the Centers for Disease Control and Prevention (CDC) and the American College of Sports Medicine (ACSM) provided arguments supporting a causal relationship for the association between physical activity and CHD.[8] More recently, the panel of the NIH Consensus Development Conference on Physical Activity and Cardiovascular Health concluded that accumulating evidence indicates that physical inactivity is a major risk factor for cardiovascular disease.[9] Furthermore, the NIH Consensus Panel supported the recommendations from the CDC and ACSM[8] that every American adult should accumulate at least 30 minutes of moderate-intensity physical activity on most, preferably all, days of the week.[9]

Therefore, while controversy continues regarding the independent role of obesity in promoting CHD, there is growing consensus that a sedentary lifestyle promotes CHD, independent of other risk factors. *Physical activity,* defined as "bodily movements produced by skeletal muscles that require energy expenditure,"[8] includes many different types of exercise (both aerobic and anaerobic) that can be performed at different intensity levels, with a wide range of doses, that is, frequency per week (or day) and duration of exercise bouts. Different exercise regimens may have substantially different effects on CHD risk.

Different methods of losing weight also vary in their effects on CHD risk, possibly owing to differences in the proportion of fat or lean weight lost. For example, diet-induced weight loss often includes substantial lean weight loss[10] and fat weight loss is generally greater when diet is combined with exercise.[10, 11] Furthermore, caloric restriction can be achieved by a variety of changes in diet composition, which may influence CHD risk differently. For example, reduced saturated fat intake is expected to lower low-density lipoprotein (LDL) cholesterol (LDL-C), even in the absence of weight change and may bring about greater weight loss than a comparable calorie restriction that does not involve a change in diet composition.[12] On the other hand, significant reduction of dietary fat can occur without causing major weight loss, as was demonstrated in the Multiple Risk Factor Intervention Trial.[13]

Several moderate-sized, moderate-duration clinical trials, many of which are reviewed here, have addressed the role of weight loss, by various strategies, or exercise, of different types, intensities, and doses, in altering CHD risk factors, particularly the lipoprotein profile, blood pressure (BP), and glucose tolerance. Unfortunately, authors often report changes within treatment groups in these trials, rather than versus controls, and often do not define a primary outcome or make statistical adjustments for multiple primary outcome variables, or adhere to other principles of randomized, controlled clinical trials, such as analysis by intention to treat. Obviously, masking subjects from treatment assignment is virtually impossible in such studies and adherence issues extend beyond pill taking. The unique subject pool attracted to such studies may raise issues about the generalizability of the findings. Furthermore, initial training or fitness level, obesity status, and CHD risk profile may have a profound influence on how these lifestyle changes alter risk factors, and these issues are considered in the chapter. Finally, gender, ethnicity, socioeconomic status, and other cultural factors should be considered.

This review separates lifestyle studies conducted in populations that were not selected for cardiovascular risk, other than being obese or sedentary at baseline, and were defined as generally healthy (see Table 29–1) from those that included pharmaceutical weight loss approaches in healthy, but obese, people (see Table 29–2), as well as from studies of people who were recruited specifically because they had a specific elevated cardiovascular risk factor but were not known to have CHD, which may include lifestyle only and lifestyle plus pharmacologic interventions (see Table 29–3) or secondary prevention trials involving people with known cardiovascular disease (see Table 29–4).

CLINICAL TRIALS OF EXERCISE AND WEIGHT LOSS FOR CHD RISK IN HEALTHY PEOPLE

The studies reviewed in this section are summarized in Table 29–1. Although primary prevention trials of weight loss or exercise have not been conducted, the feasibility of a primary prevention trial of exercise was tested in a 2-year randomized, controlled study of 184 initially healthy subjects (79 men, 105 women), aged 60 years or older, who were assigned to long-term ($n = 80$) or short-term ($n = 42$) aerobic exercise (primarily stationary bicycle) training or control ($n = 62$) and followed for new cardiovascular diagnoses and time to onset.[14] Maximal oxygen uptake ($\dot{V}O_2max$) increased by the end of the 4-month supervised training program in both exercise groups and was maintained in the long-term, but not the short-term, group, and unchanged in controls. During the study, 8 controls had new cardiovascular diagnoses (1 myocardial infarction, 2 anginas, 2 atrial fibrillations, 2 supraventricular arrhythmias, and 1 paroxysmal atrial tachycardia), versus 2 new diagnoses (both angina) in the long-term exercise group and 1 (atrial fibrillation) in the short-term exercise group, so that 12.9% of controls experienced new conditions versus 2.4% of all exercisers ($P < 0.02$).

Among the investigations of a possible role of increased aerobic exercise in reducing CHD risk are several trials designed to determine whether a causal relationship underlies the positive association reported between physical activity and HDL cholesterol (HDL-C) in observational studies.[15] With HDL-C as the primary outcome, the Stanford Exercise Study[16] randomly assigned 81 sedentary men, aged 30 to 55, for 1 year to either (1) *control*—no major change in activity level ($N = 33$) or (2) *aerobic exercise*—approximately 45 minutes of supervised walking or jogging three times per week ($N = 48$), with no instruction on diet to either group. One-year tests were conducted on 96% of the men. Compared with controls, exercisers increased $\dot{V}O_2max$ (9.0 mL/kg per minute; $P < 0.0001$), lost significant weight (2.5 kg; $P < 0.001$), and reduced percent body fat (3.8%; $P < 0.0001$), but did not differ in changes in caloric intake or percentage of calories from any given food source (based on 3-day food records). Despite these differences, no significant differences were detected between exercisers and controls in any of the lipoprotein variables studied: HDL-C, total cholesterol (TC), LDL-C, triglycerides (TG), and apolipoproteins AI, AII, and B.

Secondary analyses[16] that separated exercisers into four "treatment-dose" groups (based on weekly mileage achieved: 0–3.9; 4–7.9; 8–12.9; and 13+ miles), however, revealed significant treatment effects for HDL-C (Spearman's rho $= 0.48$; $P < 0.001$) and LDL-C ($r = -0.31$; $P = 0.04$). In exercisers who averaged at least 8 miles (12.9 km) per week ($N = 25$), HDL-C increased by 4.4 mg/dL ($P < 0.05$) compared with controls. Further exploratory analyses, which excluded exercisers who reported active dieting, showed that the weekly mileage correlated significantly with body fat changes ($r = -0.49$; $P = 0.002$), which were significantly related to HDL-C changes ($r = -0.47$; $P = 0.004$), suggesting that weight loss could be responsible for the HDL-C increases seen with increased exercise.[17]

To address this question, the first Stanford Weight Control Project (SWCP-I)[18] randomly assigned 155 sedentary, moderately overweight (20% to 50% above ideal body weight) men, aged 35 to 59 years, to one of three groups for 1 year: *control*: no change in caloric intake, diet composition, or physical activity; *weight loss by caloric restriction*, without changing diet composition or activity level ($N = 51$); or *weight loss by increased aerobic exercise*, consisting of approximately 45 minutes of supervised walking or jogging three times per week, with no dietary changes ($N = 52$). One-year measurements were made on 81% of controls, 82% of dieters, and 90% of exercisers. Caloric reduction, assessed by 7-day food records, was sig-

TABLE 29–1 • Randomized Trials of Exercise or Weight Loss (by Diet or Exercise) for CHD Risk Factors in Healthy Individuals

Study Title or Key Feature of Study (Reference)	Intervention(s) (#: Treatment Groups)	Study Population	Length	Primary Outcome (Secondary Outcomes)	Major Results
Primary prevention, exercise, feasibility (Posner et al, 1990)	1: Exercise, long-term 2: Exercise, short-term 3: Control	79 men, 105 women Age > 60 y	2 y	New cardiovascular events (time of onset)	Fewer events in 1 + 2 vs. 3 ($P < 0.02$) (sooner, 3 vs. 1 + 2)
Stanford Exercise Study (Wood et al, 1983)	1: Exercise (aerobic) 2: Control	81 men Age: 30–55 y Sedentary	1 y	HDL-cholesterol (other CHD risk factors)	HDL-C, NS, 1 vs. 2 (no other differences)
Stanford Weight Control Project, I (Wood et al, 1988)	1: Wt loss, exercise (aerobic) 2: Wt loss, diet (calories) 3: Control	155 men Age: 35–59 y Obese, sedentary	1 y	HDL-cholesterol (other CHD risk factors)	HDL-C incr (TG decr) in 1 and 2 vs. 3 (LDL-C, NS)
Overweight, middle aged and older men (Katzel et al, 1995)	1: Wt loss, diet (low fat) 2: Exercise (aerobic) 3: Control	170 men Age: 46–80 y Obese, sedentary	9 mo	CHD risk factors: HDL-C, LDL-C, TG, BP, glucose; primary, unspecified ($\dot{V}O_2$max)	HDL incr, BP, glucose decr 1 vs. 3, not 2 vs. 3; glucose decr, 1 vs 2; LDL-C, TG decr, 1 and 2 vs. 3; 1 improved >2, overall ($\dot{V}O_2$max incr, 2 vs. 1 and 3)
Stanford-Sunnyvale Health Improvement Project (Older Adults) (King et al, 1991, 1995)	1–3: Exercise (aerobic: group- vs. home-based; high- vs. low-intensity) 4: Control	197 men, 160 women (postmenopausal) Age: 50–64 y Sedentary	1 y; 2nd y, without control	Treadmill exercise test performance, $\dot{V}O_2$max (CHD risk factors)	$\dot{V}O_2$max incr 1, 2, 3, vs. 4 (lipoproteins, BP, NS) Year 2: HDL incr from baseline in both low-intensity groups
Multiple short bouts vs. one continuous (Jakicic et al, 1995)	Wt loss, diet (calories) + 1: Exercise (20–40-min bout) 2: Exercise (2–4 10-min bouts)	56 women Age: 25–50 y Obese, sedentary	20 wk	Adherence, cardiovascular fitness (weight loss)	Adherence and fitness greater in 2 vs. 1 (Wt loss, NS 1 vs. 2)
Stanford Weight Control Project, II (Wood et al, 1991)	1: Wt loss, diet (low fat) 2: Wt loss, diet (low fat) + exercise (aerobic) 3: Control	132 men, 132 women (premenopausal) Age: 25–49 y Obese, sedentary	1 y	HDL-cholesterol (other CHD risk factors)	*Men:* HDL incr, 2 vs. 3, not 1 vs. 2 or 3 (LDL, NS) *Women:* HDL incr 2 vs. 1, not 1 or 2 vs. 3 (LDL decr 1 and 2 vs. 3)
Gender differences (Wing and Jeffery, 1995)	1–4: Different behavioral strategies 5: Control	101 men, 101 women Age: 25–45 y Obese	18 mo	CHD risk factors (weight loss)	Men incr HDL, decr wt, TG, BP vs. women (men had lower baseline HDL, higher TG, BP and lost more wt)
Aerobic + anerobic exercise + diet (Svendsen et al, 1993)	1: Wt loss, diet (calories) 2: Wt loss, diet + exercise (aerobic + anaerobic) 3: Control	121 women Age: 45–54 y Obese	12 wk	CHD risk factors (weight loss)	HDL-C, NS LDL-C, TG decr 1 and 2 vs. 3; NS 1 vs. 2 Wt decr, 1 and 2 vs. 3
Anaerobic exercise (Boyden et al, 1993)	1: Exercise (anaerobic) 2: Control	113 women Age: 28–39 y Obese	5 mo	Lipoproteins (weight loss)	HDL-C, TG (Wt), NS LDL-C decr 1 vs. 2

CHD, coronary heart disease; Wt, weight; HDL or HDL-C, high-density lipoprotein cholesterol (change); LDL or LDL-C, low-density lipoprotein cholesterol (change); TG, triglyceride (change); BP, blood pressure (change); $\dot{V}O_2$max, maximal oxygen consumption; incr (decr), increased (decreased) significantly; NS, not significant (among all groups, if not specified).

nificant ($P < 0.01$) in dieters versus controls at 7 months (about 335 kcal per day) and 1 year (about 240 kcal per day), while caloric intake did not differ between exercisers and controls at either time point. At 1 year, $\dot{V}O_2max$ had increased in exercisers, compared with controls (6.5 mL/kg per minute; $P < 0.001$) and dieters (4.1 mL/kg per minute; $P < 0.001$). Compared with controls, total and fat weight losses were significantly greater ($P < 0.001$) in both dieters (7.8 kg and 6.2 kg, respectively) and exercisers (4.6 kg and 4.4 kg). Lean mass loss was greater only in dieters (2.1 kg), who also lost more lean weight than exercisers (1.4 kg; $P < 0.01$). Fat weight loss did not differ significantly between dieters and exercisers. HDL-C was elevated ($P < 0.01$) in both dieters (4.2 mg/dL) and exercisers (4.6 mg/dL) at 1 year, compared with controls, while TG was reduced (−23.9 and −14.2 mg/dL, respectively; $P < 0.05$). These changes did not differ significantly between the two weight loss groups. LDL-C did not differ significantly across groups.

Thus, weight loss achieved by caloric restriction alone, with no change in the proportion of calories from fat, or by exercise with no dietary changes, improved HDL-C and TG levels, and there was no greater benefit of this amount of weight loss by exercise versus caloric restriction.[18] Clinic resting BP decreased similarly in all three groups; however, daytime and evening ambulatory BP decreased significantly in both dieters and exercisers, compared with controls ($P < 0.05$), but did not differ between weight loss groups.[19]

To specifically compare the effects of weight loss (achieved without a change in activity level) to aerobic exercise (not accompanied by weight loss), Katzel and colleagues[20] randomly assigned 170 sedentary, obese (120% to 160% of ideal body weight) men, aged 46 to 80 years, for 1 year to one of three groups: *control*, no weight loss or change in activity level ($N = 26$); *weight loss*, hypocaloric, reduced-fat diet, similar to the NCEP Step I diet[4] (i.e., total fat ≤ 30% of calories, saturated fat ≤ 10% of calories, and dietary cholesterol ≤ 300 mg per day) ($N = 73$); or *aerobic exercise*, consisting of 45 minutes of treadmill and cycle ergonometer workouts, three times per week ($N = 71$). Prior to baseline testing, all three groups were instructed for 3 months on an isoenergetic reduced-fat diet and men in both the aerobic exercise and control groups were encouraged to continue this diet, without losing weight, throughout the trial. One-year measurements were made on 69% of controls, 60% of men assigned to weight loss, and 69% of men assigned to exercise. Of those who completed the trial, men assigned to weight loss lost about 9.5 kg, 75% of which was fat mass, and did not change $\dot{V}O_2max$; whereas exercisers did not change average weight, although percent body fat was decreased 0.8% ($P < 0.005$), but did increase $\dot{V}O_2max$ (about 7.0 mL/kg of fat free mass per minute, i.e., 17% above baseline) compared with the other two groups ($P < 0.001$). Compared with controls, HDL-C was significantly ($P < 0.01$) increased (about 4.6 mg/dL) in the weight loss group but not in the exercise group, while TG, TC, and LDL-C were decreased ($P < 0.05$) in both the weight loss and exercise groups, with no differences between them. Systolic and diastolic blood pressures (SBPs and DBPs) were reduced in men in the weight loss group, compared with controls ($P < 0.01$) and with exercisers ($P < 0.05$), while BP changes did not differ between the exercisers and controls. There were also significant reductions in fasting plasma glucose and insulin in the weight loss group versus controls ($P < 0.01$) and the exercise group ($P < 0.05$). In summary, weight loss by a hypocaloric, reduced-fat diet resulted in significantly greater CHD risk factor reduction than was achieved by increasing physical activity without substantial weight loss.

The Stanford-Sunnyvale Health Improvement Program (SSHIP) Trial[21] provided further evidence that aerobic exercise training may not bring about significant improvements in lipid levels or BP in older men, or in postmenopausal women, in the absence of substantial weight loss or dietary change. SSHIP randomly assigned 197 men and 160 women, aged 50 to 65 years, to one of four 1-year groups: *control*, no change in activity level; *high-intensity, group-based aerobic exercise*, involving three 40-minute endurance training sessions per week at 73% to 88% of peak treadmill heart rate; *high-intensity, home-based aerobic exercise*, the same prescription, but performed by people from their home; and *low-intensity home-based aerobic exercise*, five 30-minute sessions per week at 60% to 73% of maximum heart rate. One-year assessments were completed on 85% of randomized subjects. All three exercise training conditions resulted in significant ($P < 0.03$) improvements in $\dot{V}O_2max$, averaging 5% increase, compared with controls, with no significant weight or body composition changes. Neither men nor women in any of the exercise conditions showed significant changes, versus control, in HDL-C, LDL-C, TC, TG, or resting BP.

At the end of the 1-year, controlled trial, SSHIP controls were offered an exercise program, while men and women randomized into the three exercise groups were encouraged to continue their originally assigned exercise prescriptions for a second year.[22] At the end of this year, significant HDL-C increases ($P < 0.01$) were seen within each of the two home-based groups (sexes combined), compared with their baseline values. Furthermore, these increases were especially pronounced for the lower-intensity, home-based group, despite greater exercise adherence rates in the higher-intensity, home-based group ($P < 0.003$), who also most successfully maintained their treadmill exercise test performance. The investigators suggested that the frequency of exercise bouts may be particularly important for achieving such changes. For all exercise conditions, HDL-C increases were associated with decreases in waist-to-hip ratio, in both men and women ($P < 0.04$).

The frequency, duration, and intensity of exercise, including the possibility of breaking up daily exercise into multiple short bouts rather than employing single long bouts, has become an area of increasing interest. To investigate the possible benefit of multiple short bouts for weight loss, 56 overweight women, aged 25 to 50 years, were randomly assigned to a behavioral weight loss program consisting of a calorie-restricted diet combined with 5 days per week of either *single aerobic exercise bouts per day,* starting as 20-minute bouts (weeks 1 to 4), increasing to 30-minute bouts (weeks 5 to 8) and to 40-minute bouts (weeks 9 to 20); or *multiple 10-minute bouts per day,* starting as 2 bouts per day, increasing to 3, then 4, respectively.[23] Both groups reduced calories and percentage of calories from fat significantly. Women performing multiple short bouts lost 8.9 kg in the 20-week period, whereas those exercising in single long bouts lost 6.4 kg (no significance [NS]). Because the dietary changes (caloric restriction) probably contributed the most to weight loss, it was not possible to determine the independent contribution of the exercise components; however, exercising in multiple short bouts was shown to improve adherence to exercise and to result in significantly greater improvement in aerobic capacity, as well as a trend for greater weight loss.

The effects of combining aerobic exercise (single bout) with a weight-reducing, reduced-fat diet, versus the diet only, were studied in initially sedentary, moderately overweight premenopausal women (BMI = 24 to 30 kg/m^2) and men (BMI = 28 to 34 kg/m^2), aged 25 to 49 years, in a second SWCP.[24] SWCP-II randomly assigned 132 women and 132 men for 1 year to one of three groups: *control*: no changes in diet or physical activity level; *weight loss by a hypocaloric, reduced-fat diet*: specifically reducing fat calories, to achieve an NCEP Step I diet[4] and weight loss; or *weight loss by the hypocaloric, reduced-fat diet plus aerobic exercise*: identical diet combined with approximately 45 minutes of supervised walking or jogging, three times per week. One-year measurements were completed on about 90% of men and women in each treatment group, except for diet-only women (74%; NS). Total calories, percentage of calories from total and saturated fat, and dietary cholesterol were reduced in both diet-only and diet plus exercise groups of men and women, versus control ($P < 0.001$). These reductions did not differ between diet-only and diet plus exercise women, nor did changes in saturated fat and cholesterol intake differ between diet-only and diet plus exercise men; however, diet plus exercise men reduced total fat and increased carbohydrate intake relative to diet-only men ($P < 0.05$). Aerobic capacity (mL/kg per minute) improved significantly ($P < 0.001$) in diet plus exercise men, compared with control (8.8) and diet-only (7.0) men, and in diet plus exercise women, versus control (6.4) and diet-only (5.0) women.

In SWCP-II men,[24] weight loss was significant ($P < 0.001$) in both dieters (6.8 kg) and dieting exercisers (10.4 kg), compared with controls, as was fat weight loss (5.5 kg and 9.0 kg, respectively), with greater fat loss in dieting exercisers versus dieters ($P < 0.001$). Lean mass loss was also significant ($P < 0.05$) in dieters (1.3 kg) and dieting exercisers (1.4 kg) versus control but did not differ between dieters and dieting exercisers. HDL-C was significantly increased in dieting exercisers (7.3 mg/dL; $P < 0.001$), as was apolipoprotein AI (7.2 mg/dL; $P < 0.01$), compared with controls, whereas HDL-C was not significantly increased in dieters (2.7 mg/dL). HDL-C increases in dieting exercisers were significant ($P < 0.01$) compared with diet only. Diet plus exercise men also decreased TG versus control (−58.5 mg/dL; $P < 0.001$) and diet-only (−31.9 mg/dL; $P < 0.05$) men. In contrast, LDL-C decreases were not significant in either dieters (−7.4 mg/dL) or dieting exercisers (−2.8 mg/dL) compared with controls, who decreased LDL-C by about 5% from baseline; however, apolipoprotein B was reduced ($P < 0.01$) in both dieters (−5.8 mg/dL) and dieting exercisers (−6.0 mg/dL) versus controls. On the other hand, reductions in the LDL-C to HDL-C ratio were significant in both diet-only and diet plus exercise men versus control ($P < 0.05$), with no differences between the two weight loss groups. There was also a significant reduction in the ratio of apolipoprotein B to apolipoprotein AI in dieters ($P < 0.01$) and dieting exercisers ($P < 0.001$) versus control, and this reduction was greater in the men who exercised versus those who only dieted ($P < 0.05$). Compared with controls, both dieters and dieting exercisers reduced resting SBP ($P < 0.05$) and DBP ($P < 0.001$), but there were no differences between the two weight loss groups.

In SWCP-II women,[24] weight loss was significant ($P < 0.001$) in both dieters (5.4 kg) and dieting exercisers (6.4 kg), compared with controls, as was fat weight loss (4.5 kg and 6.0 kg, respectively), with no significant differences between weight loss groups. Lean mass loss did not differ between groups. Compared with controls, women assigned to weight loss by the reduced-fat diet, without exercise, decreased HDL-C (−3.9 mg/dL; NS), HDL$_2$-C (−4.3 mg/dL; $P < 0.05$), and apolipoprotein AI (−8.8 mg/dL; $P < 0.05$), whereas diet plus exercise women increased HDL-C (2.7 mg/dL; NS) and apolipoprotein AI (1.9 mg/dL; NS) and decreased TG (−13.3 mg/dL; $P < 0.05$), so that HDL-C was significantly ($P < 0.01$) increased in diet plus exercise versus diet-only women (6.6 mg/dL). Compared with controls, both dieters and dieting exercisers reduced TC (−13.9 and −9.7 mg/dL, respectively; $P < 0.05$), LDL-C (−9.7 and −10.1 mg/dL; $P < 0.05$), and apolipoprotein B (−5.8 and −6.0 mg/dL; $P < 0.01$), and there were no differences between dieters and dieting exercisers. Compared with controls, neither the LDL-C to HDL-C nor the apolipoprotein B to AI ratios were improved in dieters, whereas both ratios were reduced in dieting exercisers ($P < 0.05$). Resting SBP ($P < 0.05$) and DBP ($P < 0.01$) were also reduced in diet and diet plus exercise women versus controls, with no differences between the two weight loss groups. Therefore, in both men and women, the addition of exercise to a reduced-fat, weight-reducing diet improved HDL-C, compared with the diet alone, and improved the lipoprotein profile compared with controls but did not produce further reductions in BP.

When results from the diet-only men in the SWCP-I[18] are compared with those from the diet-only men in SWCP-II,[24] it appears that diet composition influences the effects of diet-induced weight loss on lipoproteins. Men in SWCP-I, who reduced caloric intake by reducing portion sizes, without changing diet composition, lost only slightly more total and fat body weight (7.8 and 6.2 kg, respectively) than did men in SWCP-II (6.8 and 5.5 kg), who targeted dietary fat to reduce caloric intake; however, HDL-C was significantly increased in SWCP-I,[18] but not in SWCP-II[24] men. These results suggest an antagonistic effect of a reduction in dietary fat on the HDL-C–raising effect of weight loss, which would also explain why SWCP-II women, who were assigned to weight loss by the reduced-fat diet, did not achieve HDL-C elevations. Greater weight loss, or the addition of exercise, may be necessary to raise HDL-C with a reduced-fat diet. Thus, the significant HDL-C increases in the men who lost weight with a hypocaloric NCEP Step I diet in the study by Katzel and colleagues[20] may be explained by the fact that the men who completed that trial lost more weight (9.5 kg total) than men in the SWCP-II diet-only group (7.1 kg fat weight).

Wing and Jeffery addressed the question of a possibly greater CHD risk factor reduction from weight loss in men versus women in secondary analyses of a randomized, controlled trial of 159 men and women, aged 25 to 45 years, 13.6 to 31.8 kg above ideal body weight.[25] Participants were assigned to *control* (receiving a weight loss manual, but no treatment) or to one of four groups that received an 18-month behavioral *weight control program with various interventions* to produce adherence to weight loss. Men were shown to experience greater increases in HDL-C with weight loss and greater decreases in TG and BP than women; however, the gender difference appeared to derive from differences in CHD risk factors at baseline; that is, women started with significantly higher HDL-C and lower TG and BP than men, and differences in weight loss (i.e., men lost significantly more weight than women).

Effects on CHD risk factors of combined aerobic and anaerobic exercise, added to a weight loss diet, were studied in a trial of 121 overweight (self-reported BMI ≥ 25 kg/m^2) postmenopausal women, aged 45 to 54 years,[26] who were randomly assigned for 12 weeks to *control*: no change in diet or exercise ($N = 21$); *energy-restricted diet*: a formula diet (NUPO) within which all international recommendations for proteins, essential amino acids, vitamins, minerals, and trace elements were met, with additional energy consumption of food not to exceed a total of about 1000 kcal per day ($N = 51$); or *diet plus combined aerobic and anaerobic exercise*: the NUPO diet plus three sessions per week of 1 to 1.5 hours of aerobic exercise (bicycling, stair climbing, treadmill running) and resistance training ($N = 49$). More than 97% of women completed the trial. Total energy intake and percentage of calories from fat decreased in the two dieting groups versus controls but did not differ between diet only and diet plus exercise. Aerobic capacity (mL/kg per minute) increased in the dieting exercisers, compared with controls (5.1) and dieters (4.6). Total weight loss was significant in both diet-only (10.0 kg) and diet plus exercise (10.8 kg) women, compared with controls, and did not differ between groups; however, the dieting exercisers lost significantly ($P < 0.001$) more fat weight (1.8 kg) than diet only. The latter also lost 1.2 kg lean weight, while dieting exercisers lost none ($P < 0.05$ versus dieters). Despite considerable weight loss in the diet and diet plus exercise groups, HDL-C changes did not differ among groups; however, TG, TC, and LDL-C decreased in dieters and dieting exercisers compared with controls ($P < 0.001$), and these changes did not differ between the two weight loss groups. SBP was also reduced in both weight loss groups versus control but did not differ between dieters and dieting exercisers. Therefore, the addition of combined aerobic and anaerobic exercise to a hypocaloric, reduced-fat diet that effected substantial weight loss produced no greater CHD risk factor reduction in postmenopausal women than what was seen with the diet alone by 12 weeks.

To address whether anaerobic exercise alone may improve lipoproteins in women,[27] a randomized clinical trial was conducted in eumenorrheic, premenopausal women, aged 28 to 39 years, who were randomly assigned for 5 months to *control* ($N = 47$) or *supervised resistance exercise training* ($N = 56$). Eighty-nine percent of controls and 82% of exercisers completed the trial. Although fat free mass increased 1.2 kg in exercisers relative to controls ($P < 0.001$), there were no significant changes in total body weight,

HDL-C, or TG. Exercisers, however, reduced TC (about 9.5 mg/dL) and LDL-C (about 11.5 mg/dL) significantly versus controls ($P < 0.04$). Further clinical trials designed to investigate differences between aerobic and resistance exercise seem warranted.

CLINICAL TRIALS OF DRUG-INDUCED WEIGHT LOSS FOR CHD RISK

Following the report of significant weight loss by a calorie-restricted diet combined with dexfenfluramine (dF), 15 mg twice daily, versus placebo in a large 1-year trial involving 822 obese patients from nine European countries,[28] despite more transient side effects (tiredness, diarrhea, dry mouth, polyuria, and drowsiness) in dF patients, great interest arose in the health benefits and risks of long-term pharmacotherapy of obesity. Studies known to have measured CHD risk factors are reviewed here (Table 29–2).

To investigate the value of anorexiant medications as an adjunct to other forms of weight control therapy, Weintraub and colleagues[29] randomized 121 moderately overweight (130% to 180% of ideal body weight) people (89 women, 32 men), aged 18 to 60 years, to 34 weeks of double-blind *fenfluramine plus phentermine resin* or *placebo*, added to behavior modification, caloric restriction, and aerobic exercise (to expend 300 kcal above daily living energy output, three times per week). With 93% of subjects returning for 34-week tests, those receiving active medication (n = 58) lost an average of 14.2 kg (15.9% of initial weight), while the placebo group (n = 54) lost 4.6 kg (4.9%; $P <$ 0.001). BP decreases did not differ between groups. HDL-C was increased significantly, and similarly, in both groups (10% in the active medication group, 11% in placebo); however, TG reductions, which were also significant in both groups, were significantly greater (P = 0.025) in the fenfluramine plus phentermine group.[30]

dF treatment also improved cardiovascular risk factors in a placebo-controlled, double-blind 12-month trial of 52 obese female patients (BMI 35.1 ± 7.8 kg/m^2, age 43.3 ± 6.4 years),[30] particularly in those with upper body obesity, who had significantly greater reductions in SBP than did women with lower body obesity ($P < 0.05$). In women with upper body obesity, blood glucose, serum insulin, and TGs decreased and HDL-C increased significantly ($P < 0.05$) during fenfluramine treatment, whereas in lower body obesity, cardiovascular risk factors were in the normal range and did not change significantly during the study, despite significant weight loss.[31]

A shorter (3-month) randomized, double-blind, placebo-controlled trial of dF in 50 obese (BMI = 30 to 44 kg/m^2) women (n = 45) and men (n = 5), in which patients ate as desired and were not instructed to exercise,[32] also showed greater weight loss in the drug group, compared with placebo (3.8 vs. 1.1 kg; $P < 0.01$), as well as greater reduction in DBP (−5 vs. −1.5 mm Hg; $P < 0.05$) and improved insulin sensitivity, measured during continuous infusion of glucose with model assessment (+11% vs. 4%; $P <$ 0.03). These changes were seen after 1 week of treatment, during which time weight did not change, which the authors suggested could be a direct effect of the agent on insulin binding or result from brief calorie restriction. Whether medication has any inde-

TABLE 29–2 • Clinical Trials of Weight Loss Effects on CHD Risk with Anorexiant Medications in Healthy Individuals

Study Title or Key Feature of Study (Reference)	Intervention(s) (#: Treatment Groups)	Study Population	Length	Primary Outcome (Secondary Outcomes)	Major Results
Dexfenfluramine (Guy-Grand et al, 1989)	Wt loss, diet +: 1: Dexfenfluramine 2: Placebo	160 men, 662 women Age = 18–74 y	1 y	Weight loss (side effects [CHD risk factors not studied])	Wt decr, 1 vs. 2 (more side effects, 1 vs. 2)
Fenfluramine (Weintraub et al, 1992)	Wt loss, diet + exercise + 1: Fenfluramine + phentermine resin 2: Placebo	32 men, 89 women Age: 18–60 y Obese	34 wk	Weight loss (CHD risk factors)	Wt decr, 1 vs. 2 (HDL NS, incr in both from baseline; TG decr, 1 vs. 2; BP, NS)
Upper vs. lower body obesity (Ditschuneit, 1996)	Wt loss, diet +: 1: Dexfenfluramine 2: Placebo	52 women Mean age: 43.3 ± 6.4 y Obese	1 y	CHD risk factors	SBP decr UBO vs. LBO, overall, > CHD and improvement in UBO
Dexfenfluramine (Holdaway et al, 1995)	1: Dexfenfluramine 2: Placebo	5 men, 45 women Age = 35–59 y	3 mo	Weight loss (CHD risk factors)	Wt decr, 1 vs. 2 (DBP decr and insulin sensitivity incr, 1 vs. 2)

CHD, coronary heart disease; Wt, weight; HDL or HDL-C, high-density lipoprotein cholesterol (change); TG, triglyceride changes; BP (SBP, DBP), blood pressure (BP) (change), systolic BP, diastolic BP; UOB, LOB, upper body obesity, lower body obesity; incr (decr), increased (decreased) significantly; NS, not significant (among all groups, if not specified).

pendent effects on risk factors for obesity-related disease remains unknown.[33]

Any preceived benefit from the use of these medications, related to reductions in obesity-related cardiovascular risk factors, may be offset or overridden by an increased risk of valvulopathy, which has recently been identified by the Food and Drug Administration as a possible adverse outcome of these medications. (Dexfenfluramine and fenfluramine have now both been withdrawn from the market.)

CLINICAL TRIALS OF EXERCISE AND WEIGHT LOSS IN PEOPLE WITH CHD RISK FACTORS

Several weight loss or exercise studies have been conducted in men and women with specific CHD risk factors, as described in this section (Table 29–3). To study the impact of aerobic exercise or a reduced-fat diet or the combination thereof on CHD risk factors in middle-aged, nonobese men with slightly to moderately elevated TC,[34] 158 normoglycemic, healthy men, aged 35 to 60 years, were randomly assigned to 6 months of *control* ($n = 40$); *reduced-fat diet*: NCEP Step I goals,[4] including advice on caloric intake to reach or maintain desirable body weight ($N = 40$); *aerobic exercise*: 30 to 45 minutes of activities such as walking and jogging at 60% to 80% of maximal heart rate, two or three times per week ($n = 39$); or *diet plus exercise* ($N = 39$). Ninety-nine percent of men completed 6-month assessments. Total energy intake was reduced only in the dieting exercisers, while the percentage of calories from fat was significantly reduced in diet-only and diet plus exercise men, versus control. Exercise and diet plus exercise men reported more activity than control and diet-only men; however, aerobic capacity was not measured. Reductions in BMI (kg/m^2) were slight but significant ($P < 0.01$) versus control, in diet only (-0.6), exercise only (-0.6), and diet plus exercise (-0.9); however, there were no significant differences in lipoprotein changes between groups. BP was significantly reduced in dieters and exercisers versus controls, but not in dieting exercisers.

The Diet and Exercise for Elevated Risk (DEER) Trial[35] investigated the effects of a reduced-fat diet, aerobic exercise, and the combination thereof on the lipoprotein profile of normotensive, euglycemic men or postmenopausal women who were at elevated CHD risk by having both low HDL-C and elevated LDL-C levels. The DEER trial randomly assigned 197 men, aged 30 to 64 years, and 180 postmenopausal women, aged 45 to 64 years, who had HDL-C levels below the sex-specific mean of the population (≤ 44 mg/dL for men; ≤ 59 mg/dL for women) combined with moderately elevated LDL-C (125 to 189 mg/dL for men; 125 to 209 mg/dL for women) and were not severely overweight (BMI ≤ 34 kg/m^2 for men; BMI ≤ 32 kg/m^2 for women), for 1 year to one of four groups: *control*: no change in caloric intake or activity ($N = 47$ men; 46 women); *aerobic exercise*: 45 minutes of walking, jogging, or comparable activity, at 60% to 80% of maximum heart rate, at least three times per week ($N = 50$ men; 44 women); *NCEP Step II diet*[4] (saturated fat $\leq 7\%$ of calories, total fat $\leq 30\%$ of calories, dietary cholesterol ≤ 200 mg/day, and advice on caloric intake to reach or maintain desirable body weight) ($N = 49$ men; 47 women); or *NCEP Step II diet plus aerobic exercise* ($N = 51$ men; 43 women). Over 95% of men and women completed 1-year tests in each group. Mean dietary goals were achieved by both diet and diet plus exercise men and women, as assessed by five unannounced 24-hour recalls at baseline and 1 year, and dietary fat and cholesterol changes were significant versus control and exercise only in both sexes. Aerobic capacity (mL/kg per minute) was significantly increased, compared with controls, in exercise (2.7) and diet plus exercise (5.5) men and in exercise (3.4) and diet plus exercise (4.7) women and was similarly increased in exercisers and dieting exercisers.

DEER participants were not selected to be obese; the mean baseline BMI was 27.0 kg/m^2 in men and 26.3 kg/m^2 in women, and a large percentage of subjects assigned to the NCEP Step II were not advised to lose weight. Nonetheless, at 1 year, total and fat weight losses were significant compared with controls in dieters and dieting exercisers in both sexes but did not differ between diet-only and diet plus exercise in either sex. In men, dieters lost a mean of 3.3 kg (2.1 kg fat weight) and dieting exercisers lost 4.7 kg (3.5 kg fat weight) compared with controls, while weight loss in exercisers (1.2 kg, 1.0 kg fat weight) was not significant. Lean mass loss did not differ between dieters or dieting exercisers and control men but was significantly greater in both dieting groups compared with exercise only (1.3 kg for both). In DEER women, dieters lost a mean of 3.5 kg and dieting exercisers lost 3.9 kg compared with controls, while weight loss in exercisers (1.2 kg) was not significant. Lean mass losses were minimal and did not differ between groups.

HDL-C changes did not differ between any treatment groups, in men or women, in the DEER Trial[34]; therefore, neither the modest weight loss achieved by the NCEP Step II diet nor exercise, alone or combined with the diet, increased HDL-C in men or women who would be encouraged to adopt these lifestyle changes to improve their lipoprotein profile. Furthermore, compared with controls, LDL-C reductions were not significant in men or women who adopted the NCEP Step II diet without increasing activity level. LDL-C changes were not significant in men or

TABLE 29–3 • Randomized Trials of Exercise or Weight Loss in Individuals with CHD Risk Factors

Study Title or Key Feature of Study (Reference)	Intervention(s) (#: Treatment Groups)	Study Population	Length	Primary Outcome (Secondary Outcomes)	Major Results
Slight to moderately elevated CHD risk (Hellenius et al, 1993)	1: Diet (low fat) 2: Exercise (aerobic) 3: Diet + exercise 4: Control	158 men Age: 35–60 y Elevated total cholesterol	6 mo	CHD risk factors (weight loss)	Lipoproteins, NS BP decr 1 and 2 vs. 4, not 3 vs. 4 (Wt decr 1, 2, and 3 vs. 4)
Diet and Exercise for Elevated Risk (DEER) Trial (Stefanick et al, 1998)	1: Diet (low fat) 2: Exercise (aerobic) 3: Diet + exercise 4: Control	197 men, 180 women (postmenopausal) Age: 30–64 y, men; 45–64 y, women Low HDL + high LDL	12 mo	HDL-cholesterol (other CHD risk factors)	HDL (TG, BP) NS, either sex (LDL decr, 3 vs. 4, both sexes; not 1 vs. 4, either sex; glucose decr, 1 and 3 vs. 4, both sexes)
Campbell's Center for Nutrition & Wellness Study (McCarron et al, 1997)	1: Diet (CCNW Plan) 2: Diet (AHA Step I/II)	246 men, 314 women Age: 26–70 y CHD risk factors	10 wk	CHD risk factors (body weight)	SBP, DBP decr, 1 vs. 2; HDL, LDL, TG, NS (improved vs. baseline)
Diet and Moderate Exercise Trial, South Asian population (Singh et al, 1992)	1: Diet (AHA Step I + fruits + vegetables) + exercise 2: Diet (AHA Step I only)	419 men, 44 women Age: 25–65 y CHD risk factors	24 wk	CHD risk factors (body weight)	LDL, TG, BP, glucose decr, HDL incr, 1 vs. 2 (Wt decr 1 vs. 2)
Hypertension Prevention Trial (HPT Research Group, 1990)	[If obese, 1–4; otherwise, only 2 or 4] 1: Diet (reduced calories) 2: Low sodium 3: Diet + low sodium 4: Control	549 men, 292 women Age: 25–49 y DBP (mm Hg): 78–89	3 y	DBP; SBP (weight loss)	BP decr in all vs. baseline, most in 1 + 3 (Wt decr most in 1 + 3)
Trials of Hypertension Prevention (TOHP) (Stevens et al, 1993)	1: Wt loss, diet (calories) + exercise, behavior 2: Control	385 men, 179 women Age: 30–54 y DBP (mm Hg): 80–89, obese	18 mo	DBP; SBP (weight loss)	BP reduced more with greater weight loss (Wt decr 1 vs. 2)
Trial of Antihypertensive Interventions and Management (TAIM) (Wassertheil-Smoller, 1992)	9 Groups: 1 of **3 drugs** (chlorthalidone, atenolol, or placebo) *combined with* 1 of **3 diets:** Wt loss (calories), low sodium + incr potassium, usual	878 men and women (more than 50% men) Age: 21–65 y DBP (mm Hg): 90–100, obese	6 mo	DBP; SBP (weight loss)	BP decreased more with drugs vs. diet, more with drugs + diet vs. drugs alone, more with low-calorie vs. usual or low sodium/incr potassium diet
Treatment of Mild Hypertension Study (Neaton et al, 1993)	Lifestyle (low calorie, salt, and alcohol + exercise) + 1: Chlorthalidone 2: Acebutol 3: Doxazosin mesylate 4: Amlodipine maleate 5: Enalapril maleate 6: Placebo	557 men, 345 women Age: 45–69 y Stage 1 hypertension	4 y	DBP; SBP (other CHD risk factors)	BP decr 1–5 vs. 6; SBP, DBP decr and lipoproteins improved in all groups vs. baseline
Exercise for mild hypertension (Blumenthal et al, 1991)	1: Exercise (aerobic) 2: Strength and flexibility training 3: Control	57 men, 42 women Age: 29–59 y SBP (mm Hg): 140–180 DBP (mm Hg): 90–105	4 mo	DBP; SBP (weight loss)	SBP, DBP, (Wt), NS; SBP, DBP decr in all from baseline

CHD, coronary heart disease; HDL or HDL-C, high-density lipoprotein cholesterol (change); LDL or LDL-C, low-density lipoprotein cholesterol (change); TG, triglyceride changes; Wt, weight; BP, blood pressure (change); SBP, systolic BP; DBP, diastolic BP; incr (decr), increased (decreased) significantly; NS, not significant (among all groups, if not specified).

women who increased their exercise level without altering their diet; however, significant LDL-C reductions were seen in both men and women assigned to the diet plus aerobic exercise. (Even when analyses combined men and women, thereby increasing the number of subjects per treatment group, LDL-C decreases were not significant in the diet-only group, versus control, nor did HDL-C changes differ significantly among groups.)

Neither TGs nor BP changes differed significantly in men or women among DEER groups, whereas fasting glucose was reduced in both diet-only and diet plus exercise men and women, relative to controls ($P < 0.01$), and in men, glucose was reduced 2 hours after consumption of oral glucose in both dieters and dieting exercisers, versus controls. (This was not seen in women.) Neither fasting nor 2-hour glucose reductions differed between dieters and dieting exercisers in either sex. Therefore, in both men, aged 30 to 64 years, and postmenopausal women, aged 45 to 64 years, with high-risk lipoprotein profiles, the NCEP Step II diet, which was accompanied by modest weight loss, reduced blood glucose levels whether exercise was added to the diet or not; however, the addition of exercise to the diet improved LDL-C more than by the diet alone.

Modest, but substantial, weight loss was achieved in a multicenter, randomized trial of nutritional intervention[36] in 560 people (246 men and 314 women), aged 26 to 70 years, with one or more CHD risk factors: dyslipidemia (TC 220 to 300 mg/dL or TG levels 200 to 1000 mg/dL); hypertension (sitting SBP of 140 to 180 mm Hg and/or DBP of 90 to 105 mm Hg); or NIDDM (fasting glucose > 140 mg/dL, but not taking hypoglycemic agents). Participants were randomized to the *Campbell's Center for Nutrition and Wellness (CCNW) plan*, which is composed of prepackaged breakfast, lunch, and dinner meals provided to participants, or to a *nutritionist-guided AHA Step I and Step II diet*, in which participants self-selected foods to meet their nutrition prescription for 10 weeks. Mean weight loss with the CCNW and self-selected AHA Step I/II plans, respectively, was as follows: men, −4.5 kg and −3.5 kg; women, −4.8 and −2.8 kg, which was significant between groups when sexes were combined ($P = 0.03$). The 10-week visit was completed by 92.6% of the CCNW group and 96.8% of the self-selected diet group. Participants in both groups decreased energy intake and significantly changed intake of most nutrients, compared with baseline, with greater reduction in percentage of calories from fat in the CCNW versus self-selected AHA Step I/II group ($P < 0.001$). There was no group that did not change their diet (or weight). Compared with their baseline values, both diet groups had significant ($P < 0.01$) decreases in TC, HDL-C, LDL-C, and TG, but not LDL-C/HDL-C, and fasting glucose, insulin, glycosylated hemoglobin, hemoglobin A_{1c}, and fructosamine, but none of these changes differed between groups. Sitting SBP and DBP reductions were also significant in both diet groups, compared with their baseline, and were greater in the CCNW versus self-selected AHA Step I/II group, sexes combined. It was not clear whether risk reduction was specific to those at elevated risk for a given factor, that is, that lipoproteins were improved in those with lipid disorders or that BP was reduced in hypertensive subjects; however, this study demonstrated that diets that bring about weight loss may also reduce CHD risk factor status.

The Diet and Moderate Exercise Trial (DAMET) also focused on free-living persons with one or more CHD risk factors: BP 150/95 mm Hg or higher; diabetes mellitus by a positive glucose tolerance test; TC level higher than 250 mg/dL; TG level higher than 190 mg/dL; smoking less than 10 cigarettes per day; obesity more than 10% of normal weight for that age, sex, and height (per LIC, India); physical inactivity less than 1 km walking per day; family history of CHD; or personal history of CHD.[37, 38] DAMET randomly assigned 419 men and 44 women from a South Asian population, with stratification for each risk factor, to one of two groups for 24 weeks: *group A, AHA Step I (reduced-fat) diet plus fruits and vegetables plus exercise*: AHA Step I diet plus 400 g per day of fruits and vegetables rich in dietary fiber and antioxidants (vitamins A, C, E, carotene, copper, selenium, and magnesium), plus, after 4 weeks of diet only, moderate exercise was added, consisting of brisk walking 3 to 4 km per day or spot running 10 to 15 minutes per day ($N = 231$); or *group B, AHA Step I diet only* ($N = 232$). Data were analyzed at 4 weeks, when the two interventions differed only by the fruit-and-vegetable component of the diet, at which time no significant differences were seen between groups for changes in body weight or CHD risk factor status. At 24 weeks, after 20 weeks of exercise in addition to the dietary regimen, group A had lost 6.5 kg (9.8% reduction from baseline), while group B had lost only 0.3 kg ($P < 0.01$ vs. A). Group A showed significantly ($P < 0.01$) greater decreases in TC, LDL-C, TG, fasting blood glucose, and BPs and a greater increase in HDL-C, compared with group B. Whether these differences were due to differences in diet composition between groups, to the addition of moderate exercise in group A, or to the greater weight loss in group A is unclear.

In addition to optimal lifestyle approaches (specific diets, types of exercise) to achieving cardiovascular risk reduction, there is also growing interest in the settings in which these interventions are most effective. This is a particularly important issue for people who are identified as being at elevated risk, which generally occurs within a clinical setting, such as by a primary care physician or other clinician. The NIH recently initiated the Activity Counseling Trial (ACT), a multicenter, randomized clinical trial designed to evaluate the efficacy of two primary care, practice-based physical activity behavioral interventions compared with (recommended) standard care (i.e., with verbal encouragement to exercise), with specific recruitment targets to ensure adequate participation of men and women and minorities and to answer research questions separately in men and women. $\dot{V}O_2max$ and kilocalories expended in physical activity are the primary outcomes; however, secondary outcomes related to CHD risk factor status include plasma lipids, lipoproteins, insulin and fibrinogen, BP, body composition, and smoking. The goal is to randomize approximately 393 women and 417 men, aged 35 to 75 years (67% whites, 20% blacks, 10% Hispanics, 3% other minorities [Asians, Native Americans]) to *standard care; staff assistance* (engaging other on-site clinic staff); or *staff counseling* (including referral to off-site health educators). ACT will be completed by the year 2000.

Weight Loss Trials for Prevention of Hypertension

Prospective studies of factors that influence BP regulation have consistently identified weight or BMI as the strongest predictor of human BP; furthermore, it has been estimated that in up to 50% of the adults in the United States whose hypertension is being pharmacologically managed, the need for drug therapy could be alleviated with only modest reductions in body weight.[39] Although the association between BP decreases and increased amounts of physical activity, which generally accompany weight loss efforts, is less clear, the National Heart, Lung, and Blood Institute Joint National Committee on Detection, Evaluation, and Treatment of High Blood Pressure recommended that all hypertensive patients who are above their ideal weight be placed on individualized, monitored weight-reduction programs involving restriction of energy intake and regular physical activity.[40] Weight loss has been investigated in a number of trials focusing on prevention of hypertension. A decrease in BP with weight loss through calorie restriction was noted in five of the weight reduction, randomized, controlled trials involving hypertensives reviewed by MacMahon and colleagues.[41] Subsequent trials are reviewed here (see Table 29–3).

The Hypertension Prevention Trial (HPT)[42] randomly assigned 841 healthy adults (549 men and 292 women), aged 25 to 49 years, with diastolic BPs of 78 to 89 mm Hg, to 3-year treatment groups, depending on BMI; specifically, men with BMI less than 25 kg/m^2 and women with BMI less than 23 kg/m^2 (N = 211 total) were not assigned to calorie restriction; otherwise, people were assigned to the following groups: *control*: no dietary counseling (N = 196); *reduced calories:* to achieve desirable body weight (N = 125); *reduced sodium:* to reduce urine sodium excretion to 70 mmol or less per day (N = 196); *reduced calories and reduced sodium* (N = 129); and *reduced sodium and increased potassium*: to also increase urine potassium excretion to 100 mmol or more per day and achieve a group mean 24-hour sodium-potassium excretion ratio of 1:1 (N = 195). About 90% of subjects in each group completed the 3-year visit, and 88% of all follow-up visits were completed. The treatment groups with the largest weight changes were the two calorie restriction groups (3.4 kg vs. control for the group instructed to reduce calories only and somewhat less for those also reducing sodium). Net weight reductions attributable to calorie counseling were 3.5 kg ($P < 0.001$) at 3 years. BP, relative to baseline, decreased in all treatment groups, including control; however, the largest reduction was in the calorie-restricted group. The net effect of calorie counseling was to reduce mean DBP by 1.8 mm Hg and mean SBP by 2.4 mm Hg at 3 years ($P < 0.05$). At 6 months, the net effect of calorie counseling on DBP and SBP had been greater (2.8 and 5.1 mm Hg, respectively), as was weight loss attributable to calorie counseling (5.8 kg; $P < 0.001$). The results are consistent with a beneficial effect on BP of counseling overweight people on calorie restriction; however, they also highlight the importance of maintaining weight loss.

The Trials of Hypertension Prevention (TOHP)[43] was also a randomized, controlled clinical trial designed to determine the feasibility and efficacy of weight loss in reducing or preventing an increase in DBP. Participants, aged 30 to 54 years, who had a high-normal DBP (80 to 89 mm Hg) and were 115% to 165% of desirable body weight, were randomly assigned to an 18-month *usual-care control* condition (N = 256) or *weight loss* intervention (N = 308), consisting of counseling on nutrition and calorie restriction, increasing physical activity by increasing daily energy expenditure, starting with walking 20 minutes at least 3 days per week and increasing to 30 to 45 minutes of activity at 40% to 55% heart rate reserve, four or five times per week, and behavioral self-management techniques (n = 308). Compared with the usual-care group, the average weight losses in the intervention group at 6, 12, and 18 months of follow-up were 6.5, 5.6, and 4.7 kg, respectively, for men ($P < 0.001$) and 3.7, 2.9, and 1.8 kg, respectively, for women ($P < 0.01$). Mean changes in DBP and SBP for the weight loss group compared with controls at 18 months were −2.8 and −3.1 mm Hg for men and −1.1 and −2.0 mm Hg for women, respectively. BP reductions were greater for those who lost more weight. Sex-related differences in BP reduction were largely due to a smaller amount of weight loss by women, and sex differences in weight loss could be accounted for by higher baseline body weight in men. Therefore, the TOHP demonstrated that weight loss, achieved by a combination of caloric restriction and physical exercise, is an effective means to reduce BP in overweight adults with high-normal BP. The independent contribution of exercise, however, cannot be determined from these data.

Kumanyaka and colleagues examined race-specific weight loss results from these two trials and reported that mean weight change from baseline averaged 2.7 kg less in black women than in white women and 1.4 kg less in black versus white men during the 36-month follow-up in HPT and 2.2 kg less in black versus white women and 2.0 kg less in black versus white men during 18 months of follow-up in TOHP.[44] Such differences make it difficult to determine whether hypertension can be effectively treated by weight loss in blacks, for whom obesity is much more prevalent than in whites.[11]

The Trial of Antihypertensive Interventions and Management (TAIM)[45] was a multicenter double-blind, placebo-controlled clinical trial of drug and diet combinations for the treatment of mild hypertension among 878 participants, aged 21 to 65 years, who were 110% to 160% of ideal weight with a baseline DBP of 90 to 100 mm Hg. Individuals were randomly assigned, after stratification by center and race, to take one of three drugs for 6 months: *placebo*; diuretic, *chlorthalidone* (25 mg/day); or beta blocker, *atenolol* (50 mg/day); *combined with one of three diets*: *usual* (no change in diet); *weight reduction*; or *sodium restriction and potassium increase*. Of the 878 patients randomized, 787 (89.6%) had BP readings at both baseline and 6 months; more than half were men, about a third were black, and about two thirds had been on drug therapy at entry that was withdrawn prior to randomization. DBP fell in all nine diet/drug combination groups. Drugs outperformed diet in terms of antihypertensive effect; however, the weight loss diet was significantly better than usual diet or sodium restriction with increased potassium, and the addition of weight loss to either drug regimen resulted in a greater BP reduction, by 4 mm Hg for the diuretic and 2 mm Hg for the beta blocker. Subjects on placebo and assigned to weight reduction who lost more than 4.5 kg (and those on sodium restriction who reduced sodium to <70 mEq daily) lowered BP to a similar extent as those on either of the two drugs alone. The TAIM Investigators concluded that weight loss added to either drug provided the most beneficial regimen.

The Treatment of Mild Hypertension Study (TOMHS)[46–48] was a 4-year randomized, double-blind, placebo-controlled clinical trial in 557 men and 345 women, aged 45 to 69 years, with stage 1 hypertension (DBP < 100 mm Hg), assigned to one of six antihypertensive treatments: *placebo* (N = 234); diuretic, *chlorthalidone* (N = 136); beta blocker, *acebutolol* (N = 132); α_1-antagonist, *doxazosin mesylate* (N = 134); calcium antagonist, *amlodipine maleate* (N = 131); or angiotensin-converting enzyme inhibitor, *enalapril maleate* (N = 135), all of which were combined with sustained nutritional-hygienic advice to reduce weight, dietary sodium intake, and alcohol intake and to increase physical activity. On average, participants were obese at baseline, being 30% over desirable weight, with a mean BMI of 28.9 kg/m^2. Lifestyle intervention was identical for all groups, resulting in an average loss of 3.6 kg in participants overall, with significant decreases from baseline in reported energy intake, dietary cholesterol, and intake of fats.[47] BP reductions were sizable in all six groups but were significantly (P < 0.001) greater for participants assigned to drug treatment than placebo (SBP, −15.9 vs. −9.1 mm Hg; DBP, −12.3 vs. −8.6 mm Hg); however, the lifestyle intervention was associated with substantial reductions in SBP and DBP, so that fewer than one third of participants assigned to the placebo group were taking antihypertensive drugs after 4 years of follow-up. Mean changes in all plasma lipids were also favorable in all groups, and the degree of weight loss was significantly related to favorable lipid changes, although there were significant differences (P < 0.01) among treatment groups for average lipid changes.[47, 48] Reported leisure time physical activity increased by 86% at 1 year and remained 50% above baseline at 4 years.[48] Although the independent contribution of physical activity to weight loss and changes in BP or lipids is unclear in TOMHS, the fact that more than 50% of initial weight loss was maintained during the 4 years of the trial is consistent with the concept that adoption of exercise improves long-term maintenance of weight loss.[11, 12]

A randomized, controlled trial designed to assess the independent effects of exercise training in patients with mild, untreated hypertension (SBP, 140 to 180 mm Hg; DBP, 90 to 105 mm Hg) assigned 57 men and 42 women to 4 months of *aerobic exercise training*, consisting of three sessions per week of warm-up, 35 minutes of walking or jogging at 70% of baseline aerobic capacity (N = 39); *strength and flexibility training*, consisting of 20 minutes of flexibility exercises, followed by 30 minutes of circuit training, two or three times per week (N = 31); or a waiting list *control group*, no changes in exercise (N = 22).[49] Ninety-three percent of subjects completed the study. Aerobic exercisers increased aerobic capacity (mL/kg per minute) by 15.6% (5.1), which was significant (P < 0.01) compared with small increases in strength trainers (4.4%; 1.1) and controls (0.8%; 0.2), which did not differ from each other. There were no changes in diet or weight within or between groups. All groups showed significant (P < 0.001) decreases from baseline in SBP (−7 to −9 mm Hg) and DBP (−6 mm Hg in all); however, there were no significant differences between groups, suggesting that a program of moderate exercise without dietary changes in hypertensive patients of normal body weight and average level of fitness offers relatively little benefit to BP reduction.

In addition to the consensus that weight loss is effective for treating hypertension in people who are overweight,[39, 40] significant improvement in glucose homeostasis can usually be obtained by weight loss; therefore, weight loss is recommended for patients with NIDDM.[50] Furthermore, although the effect of regular physical exercise alone on metabolic control in NIDDM is quite variable and frequently small in magnitude, regular exercise is also recommended for patients with NIDDM,[49] partially because of its benefits in producing weight loss.[11, 12]

TRIALS OF EXERCISE AND WEIGHT LOSS IN INDIVIDUALS WITH CARDIOVASCULAR DISEASE

Several clinical trials have been designed to determine whether lifestyle changes, such as exercise and diets that may cause weight loss, can facilitate secondary prevention of CHD. Four are reviewed here and presented in Table 29–4. In the Lifestyle Heart Trial,[51] patients with angiographically documented coronary artery disease were assigned for 1 year to a *usual-care control* group ($N = 19$) or an *experimental group* ($N = 22$), involving adoption of a low-fat, vegetarian diet (about 10% calories from fat, with no animal products, including fruits, vegetables, grains, legumes, and soybean products, without calorie restriction) and moderate exercise (typically walking at 50% to 80% of maximum heart rate) as well as stopping smoking and stress management training. The experimental group lost significant weight (10.1 kg) compared with controls ($P < 0.0001$), who gained 1.4 kg, and the lifestyle change group decreased LDL-C (37.4%) versus control ($P < 0.01$); however, HDL-C, TG, and BP changes were minimal and did not differ between groups. CHD symptoms decreased markedly in the experimental group, while they increased in the usual-care group. Moreover, the average percentage diameter stenosis regressed in the experimental group but progressed in the control group. Overall, 82% of experimental group patients had an average change toward regression and adherence to the lifestyle changes was reported to be strongly related to changes in lesions in a "dose-response" manner. While the independent contribution of weight loss or exercise on CHD risk reduction cannot be determined, these data are consistent with the concept that these lifestyle changes are beneficial, even in the absence of BP reduction that would have been expected to occur

TABLE 29–4 • Randomized Trials with Exercise or Weight Loss Interventions in Individuals with Cardiovascular Disease

Study Title or Key Feature of Study (Reference)	Intervention(s) (#: Treatment Groups)	Study Population	Length	Primary Outcome (Secondary Outcomes)	Major Results
Lifestyle Heart Trial (Ornish et al, 1990)	1: Lifestyle (low-fat, vegetarian diet, stop smoking, exercise + stress reduction) 2: Usual care	36 men, 5 women Age: 35–75 y Angiographically documented CAD	12 mo	Coronary lesions; (progression, regression) (CHD risk factors)	Less progression, more regression, and reduced symptoms, 1 vs. 2 (HDL, TG, BP, NS; LDL, Wt decr, 1 vs. 2)
(Singh et al, 1992)	1: Diet (low fat) 2: Diet (low fat + fruits, vegetables, nuts)	505 people Age: unspecified Definite/possible MI	12 mo	Cardiac events, mortality (CHD risk factors)	Incidence and mortality lower, 2 vs. 1 (LDL, TG, SBP, DBP, glucose decr, HDL incr, 2 vs. 1)
(Schuller et al, 1992)	1: Exercise + diet (low-fat) 2: Usual care	113 people Age: unspecified Stable angina pectoris	12 mo	Coronary lesions (CHD risk factors)	Less progression, more regression, 1 vs. 2 (HDL, LDL, SBP, NS; Wt decr, 1 vs. 2)
Stanford Coronary Risk Intervention Project (Haskell et al, 1994)	1: Multifactorial risk reduction, including diet + exercise + smoking cessation 2: Usual care	259 men, 41 women Age: 25–65 y Angiographically documented CAD	4 y	Coronary lesions (progression, regression) (CHD risk factors)	Lower rate of narrowing and fewer hospitalizations for cardiac events, 1 vs. 2 (LDL, TG, Wt, glucose decr, HDL incr, 1 vs. 2)

CHD, coronary heart disease; CAD, coronary artery disease; MI, myocardial infarction; HDL, high-density lipoprotein cholesterol (change); LDL, low-density lipoprotein cholesterol (change); TG, triglyceride changes; Wt, weight; BP, blood pressure (change); SBP, systolic BP; DBP, diastolic BP; incr (decr), increased (decreased) significantly; NS, not significantly different.

with the major weight loss seen in the trial, or HDL-C elevation, which might be related to the extreme reduction in dietary fat.

Another randomized trial that involved increasing fruit and vegetable and reducing fat intake, without other lifestyle interventions, in patients with a definite or possible acute myocardial infarction,[52] randomly assigned 202 people to adopt a reduced-fat diet, reflecting *AHA Step I dietary recommendations*, but with usual care after initial advice, and 204 people to the *AHA Step I/II reduced-fat diet, with the addition of increased fruits, vegetables, and nuts* and regular reinforcement. Adherence to the diet was significantly higher in the group that received the more intensive counseling, and after 1 year this group had lost 6.3 kg, compared with 2.4 kg in the less-intensive group ($P < 0.01$). The intensive-diet group showed significant reductions in LDL-C, TG, fasting blood glucose, and SBP and DBP and increases in HDL-C compared with the less-intensive group; furthermore, the incidence of cardiac events was significantly lower in the intensive-diet group (50 vs. 82; $P < 0.001$), who also had lower total mortality (21 vs. 38; $P < 0.01$). The differences were attributed to the more comprehensive dietary changes and greater weight loss of the group that reduced fat and increased fruits, vegetables, and nuts.

The effects of intensive physical exercise and low-fat diet on coronary morphology and myocardial perfusion were studied in patients who were recruited after routine coronary angiography for stable angina pectoris[53] and randomized to *usual care* ($N = 57$) or *intervention* ($N = 56$), consisting of group exercise training at least two times per week and daily home exercise on a bicycle ergometer, 30 minutes a day at 75% maximum heart rate, and an AHA Phase 3 low-fat (<20% of calories), low-cholesterol (<200 mg per day) diet. Patients in the intervention group decreased total calories and decreased body weight (by 5%), which was significant versus the usual-care group ($P < 0.001$). Fat consumption and dietary cholesterol were also significantly reduced versus control, as were TC and TG. Change in body weight was significantly correlated to change in cholesterol ($P < 0.001$), as was compliance with attending group exercise sessions. HDL-C, LDL-C, and resting SBP changes did not differ between groups. Progression of coronary artery disease was reduced in patients in the diet and exercise group, while regression was greater, compared with usual care ($P < 0.001$).

The Stanford Coronary Risk Intervention Project (SCRIP) randomly assigned 259 men and 41 women with angiographically defined coronary atherosclerosis[54] to 4 years of *usual care* ($N = 155$) or *multifactorial risk reduction* ($N = 145$), which included instruction on a low-fat (<20% of calories; <6% of calories from saturated fat), low-cholesterol (<75 mg per day) diet and caloric restriction to reduce weight to 100% to 110% of ideal body weight, and a physical activity program consisting of an increase in daily activities such as walking, climbing stairs, and household chores, as well as a stop-smoking and relapse-prevention program for smokers. If LDL-C goals (110 mg/dL) were not likely to be achieved in a risk-reduction participant within the first year without drug therapy, a cholesterol-lowering drug regimen was added. Of 300 patients randomized, 274 (91.3%) had follow-up arteriograms, 28 of which could not be analyzed. The risk-reduction group significantly reduced dietary fat, including saturated fat, and cholesterol and improved exercise test performance, compared with usual care. Body weight was significantly reduced in the risk-reduction group versus usual care (3.9 kg; $P < 0.001$). Significant differences were achieved in TC, LDL-C, HDL-C, TG, and apolipoprotein B in the risk-reduction group compared with control, as well as in fasting and 1-hour postload glucose levels. The risk-reduction group showed a rate of narrowing of diseased coronary artery segments that was 47% less than that for usual care (-0.024 vs. -0.045 mm per year change in minimal diameter; $P < 0.02$), and there were fewer hospitalizations initiated by clinical cardiac events in the risk-reduction group than usual care (25 vs. 44; rate ratio, 0.61; $P = 0.05$). The independent contribution of weight loss and exercise could not be determined within this multiple-risk-factor intervention; however, the data are consistent with the concept that weight loss and exercise contribute to the secondary prevention of CHD.

Trials of Cardiac Rehabilitation Exercise Training

Cardiac rehabilitation exercise training is also generally incorporated into a multifactorial approach. The reader is referred to a recent publication by the U.S. Department of Health and Human Services for a review of randomized, controlled trials of cardiac rehabilitation exercise training.[55] Of 11 trials that reported on body weight changes, most were multifactorial; it was concluded that exercise is not recommended as a sole intervention for controlling weight in cardiac patients. Eighteen trials reported changes in lipid and lipoprotein levels (TC, LDL-C, HDL-C, TG); of 26 significant favorable changes reported, 22 resulted from multifactorial rehabilitation, that is, dietary and behavioral strategies in addition to exercise training. Likewise, of 20 lipid comparisons that showed no significant differences, 13 came from multifactorial interventions. Thus, favorable changes in lipid levels were reported to result primarily from multifactorial rehabilitation, so that exercise training was not recommended as a sole intervention for lipids. On the other hand, eight of 12 randomized, controlled trials that addressed the effect of exercise training on symptoms reported significant improvement in cardiovascular symptoms (decreased angina pectoris in patients with disease and decreases in symptoms of heart failure in patients with left ventricular systolic dysfunction) in intervention groups versus controls, and seven of these had exercise as the sole intervention.

Fifteen randomized trials pertained to cardiovascular morbidity, including 10 involving only exercise training and 5 multifactorial studies.[55] None of these reported significant differences in rates of reinfarction for rehabilitation compared with control patients; therefore, there was no evidence for reduction in cardiac morbidity, most specifically nonfatal reinfarction. The safety of moderate exercise postinfarction is well established, however, with rates of infarction and cardiovascular complications during exercise being quite low.[55] The scientific evidence pertaining to the relationship of cardiac rehabilitation exercise training with mortality included 16 randomized, controlled trials,[55] which suggested a survival benefit among patients participating in exercise training as a component of multifactorial cardiac rehabilitation. The benefit, however, could not be attributed solely to exercise.

SUMMARY AND CONCLUSION

A number of trials of exercise or weight loss have been conducted to determine the value of these lifestyle changes on risk of CHD. These studies vary considerably in design, both with respect to specific exercise interventions or weight loss strategies, and study populations, but on the whole demonstrate benefits of exercise or weight loss (for people who need to lose weight) on several specific CHD risk factors, particularly lipoproteins and BP. Nonetheless, considerably more work is needed to understand the key components of exercise and weight loss programs that affect cardiovascular risk before these lifestyle interventions may be fully endorsed by the medical community as an effective alternative or adjunct to pharmacologic and other mainstream medical approaches to improving health. For example, it is important to understand gender and age differences better, in both the health benefits of and the barriers to adopting these lifestyles. Furthermore, most of the published trials have been conducted in predominantly white populations of relatively upper socioeconomic and educational status. Major questions remain regarding the benefits of these lifestyle approaches in other segments of the population, which generally have poorer health.

There is great interest in identifying behavioral approaches and key components of interventions that can increase physical activity in the general population,[56] improve adherence to dietary regimens,[57, 58] and determine optimal methods for voluntary weight loss and control.[59] As evidence accumulates to support the importance of achieving and maintaining ideal body weight[1] and an active lifestyle for CHD risk management and other health benefits,[9, 60] it is likely that even greater emphasis will be placed on identifying minimal intervention programs that are effective in community (rather than research) settings. Hopefully, studies such as the ACT (described in the section on trials for individuals with CHD risk factors) will determine whether a primary care setting can be an effective site for such programs or demonstrate the value of referrals to community programs, so the medical community will understand how to bring about and promote the successful adoption of healthy lifestyles for CHD risk management.

Despite our need for much more information, the potential benefits of exercise and weight control seem well enough supported and the risks seem small enough to justify endorsement of these lifestyle interventions by the medical community for improving the cardiovascular health of men and women across a wide age range.

REFERENCES

1. National Institutes of Health Consensus Development Panel. Health implications of obesity: National Institutes of Health consensus development conference statement. Ann Intern Med 1985; 103:1073–1077.
2. National Cholesterol Education Program. Highlights of the Report of the Expert Panel on Detection, Evaluation, and Treatment of High Blood Cholesterol in Adults. NIH Publication No. 88–2926. Bethesda, MD, National Institutes of Health, 1987.
3. National Cholesterol Education Program Expert Panel on Detection, Evaluation, and Treatment of High Blood Cholesterol in Adults (Adult Treatment Panel II). NIH Publication No. 93–3095. Bethesda, MD, National Institutes of Health, 1993.
4. Expert Panel on Detection, Evaluation, and Treatment of High Blood Cholesterol in Adults. Summary of the second report of the National Cholesterol Education Program (NCEP) Expert Panel on Detection, Evaluation, and Treatment of High Blood Cholesterol in Adults (Adult Treatment Panel II). JAMA 1993; 269:3015.
5. Powell KE, Thompson PD, Caspersen CJ, Kendrick JS. Physical activity and the incidence of coronary heart disease. Annu Rev Public Health 1987; 8:253–287.
6. Blair SN. Physical activity, fitness, and coronary heart disease. *In* Bouchard C, Shephard RJ, Stephens T (eds). Physical Activity, Fitness, and Health: International Proceedings and Consensus Statement. Champaign, IL, Human Kinetics, 1994, pp 579–590.
7. Fletcher GF, Blair SN, Blumenthal J, et al. Statement on exercise: Benefits and recommendations for physical activity programs for all Americans: A statement for health professionals by the Committee on Exercise and Cardiac Rehabilitation of the Council on Clinical Cardiology, American Heart Association. Circulation 1992; 86:340–344.
8. Pate RR, Pratt M, Blair SN, et al. Physical activity and public health: A recommendation from the Centers for Disease Control and Prevention and the American College of Sports Medicine. JAMA 1995; 273:402–407.
9. National Institutes of Health Consensus Development Panel on Physical Activity and Cardiovascular Disease. Physical activity and cardiovascular health. JAMA 1996; 276:241–246.

10. Stefanick ML. Exercise and weight control. *In* Holloszy JO (ed). Exercise and Sport Sciences Reviews, 21. American College of Sports Medicine Series. Baltimore, Williams & Wilkins, 1993, pp 363–396
11. King AC, Tribble DL. The role of exercise in weight regulation in nonathletes. Sports Med 1991; 11:331–349.
12. Sheppard L, Kristal AT, Kushi LH. Weight loss in women participating in a randomized trial of low-fat diets. Am J Clin Nutr 1991; 54:821–828.
13. Stamler J, Briefel RR, Milas C, et al. Relation of changes in dietary lipids and weight, trial years 1–6, to changes in blood lipids in the special intervention and usual care groups in the Multiple Risk Factor Intervention Trial. Am J Clin Nutr 1997; 65(suppl):272S–288S.
14. Posner JD, Borman KM, Gitlin LN, et al. Effects of exercise training in the elderly on the occurrence and time to onset of cardiovascular diagnoses. J Am Geriatr Soc 1990; 38:205–210.
15. Stefanick ML. Exercise, lipoproteins, and cardiovascular disease. *In* Fletcher GF (ed). Cardiovascular Response to Exercise. Mount Kisco, NY, Futura, 1994, pp 325–345.
16. Wood PD, Haskell WL, Blair SN, et al. Increased exercise level and plasma lipoprotein concentrations: A one-year, randomized, controlled study in sedentary, middle-aged men. Metabolism 1983; 32:31–39.
17. Williams PT, Wood PD, Krauss RM, et al. Does weight loss cause the exercise-induced increase in plasma high density lipoproteins? Atherosclerosis 1983; 47:173–185.
18. Wood PD, Stefanick ML, Dreon DM, et al. Changes in plasma lipids and lipoproteins in overweight men during weight loss through dieting as compared with exercise. N Engl J Med 1988; 319:1173–1179.
19. Fortmann SP, Haskell WL, Wood PD. Effects of weight loss on clinic and ambulatory blood pressure in normotensive men. Am J Cardiol 1988; 62:89–93.
20. Katzel LI, Bleecker ET, Colman EB, et al. Effects of weight loss versus aerobic exercise training on risk factors for coronary disease in healthy, obese, middle-aged and older men: A randomized controlled trial. JAMA 1995; 274:1915–1921.
21. King AC, Haskell WL, Taylor CB, et al. Group- versus home-based exercise training in healthy older men and women: A community-based clinical trial. JAMA 1991; 266:1535–1542.
22. King AC, Haskell WL, Young DR, et al. Long-term effects of varying intensities and formats of physical activity on participation rates, fitness, and lipoproteins in men and women aged 50–65 years. Circulation 1995; 91:2596–2604.
23. Jakicic JM, Wing RR, Butler BA, Robertson RJ. Prescribing exercise in multiple short bouts versus one continuous bout: Effects on adherence, cardiorespiratory fitness, and weight loss in overweight women. Int J Obesity 1995; 19:893–901.
24. Wood PD, Stefanick ML, Williams PT, Haskell WL. The effects on plasma lipoproteins of a prudent weight-reducing diet, with or without exercise, in overweight men and women. N Engl J Med 1991; 325:461–466.
25. Wing RR, Jeffery RW. Effect of modest weight loss on changes in cardiovascular risk factors: Are there differences between men and women or between weight loss and maintenance? Int J Obesity 1995; 19:67–73.
26. Svendsen OL, Hassager C, Christiansen C. Effect of an energy-restrictive diet with or without exercise on lean tissue, resting metabolic rate, cardiovascular risk factors, and bone in overweight postmenopausal women. Am J Med 1993; 95:131–140.
27. Boyden TW, Pamenter RW, Going SB, et al. Resistance exercise training is associated with decreases in serum low-density lipoprotein cholesterol levels in premenopausal women. Arch Intern Med 1993; 153:97–100.
28. Guy-Grand B, Appelbaum M, Crepaldi G, et al. International trial of long-term dexfenfluramine in obesity. Lancet 1989; 1:1142–1145.
29. Weintraub M, Sundaresan PR, Madan M, et al. Long-term weight control study: I (weeks 0 to 34). The enhancement of behavior modification, caloric restriction, and exercise by fenfluramine plus phentermine versus placebo. Clin Pharmacol Ther 1992; 51:586–594.
30. Weintraub M, Sundaresan PR, Schuster B. Long-term weight control study: VII (weeks 0 to 210). Serum lipid changes. Clin Pharmacol Ther 1992; 51:634–641.
31. Ditschuneit HH, Fletchner-Mors M, Adler G. The effects of dexfenfluramine on weight loss and cardiovascular risk factors in female patients with upper and lower body obesity. J Cardiovasc Risk 1996; 3:397–403.
32. Holdaway IM, Wallace E, Westbrooke L, Gamble G. Effect of dexfenfluramine on body weight, blood pressure, insulin resistance, and serum cholesterol in obese individuals. Int J Obesity 1995; 19:749–751.
33. National Task Force on the Prevention and Treatment of Obesity. Long-term pharmacotherapy in the management of obesity. JAMA 1996; 276:1907–1915.
34. Hellenius ML, de Faire UH, Berglund BH, et al. Diet and exercise are equally effective in reducing risk for cardiovascular disease: Results of a randomized controlled study in men with slightly to moderately raised cardiovascular risk factors. Atherosclerosis 1993; 103:81–91.
35. Stefanick ML, Mackey S, Sheehan M, et al. Effects of the NCEP Step 2 diet and exercise on lipoproteins in postmenopausal women and men with low HDL-cholesterol and high LDL-cholesterol. N Engl J Med 1998; in press.
36. McCarron DA, Oparil S, Chait A, et al. Nutritional management of cardiovascular risk factors: A randomized clinical trial. Arch Intern Med 1997; 157:169–177.
37. Singh RB, Sharma VK, Gupta RK, Singh R. Nutritional modulators of lipoprotein metabolism in patients with risk factors for coronary heart disease: Diet and Moderate Exercise Trial. J Am Coll Nutr 1992; 11:391–398.
38. Singh RB, Rastogi SS, Ghosh S, et al. The Diet and Moderate Exercise Trial (DAMET): Results after 24 weeks. Acta Cardiol 1993; 48:543–557.
39. McCarron DA, Reusser ME. Body weight and blood pressure regulation. Am J Clin Nutr 1996; 63 (suppl):423S–425S.
40. Joint National Committee on Detection, Evaluation, and Treatment of High Blood Pressure. The fifth report of the Joint National Committee on Detection, Evaluation, and Treatment of High Blood Pressure (JNC-V). Arch Intern Med 1993; 153:154–183.
41. MacMahon S, Cutler J, Brittain E, Higgins M. Obesity and hypertension: Epidemiological and clinical issues. Eur Heart J 1987; 8(suppl B):57–70.
42. Hypertension Prevention Trial Research Group. The Hypertension Prevention Trial: Three-year effects of dietary changes on blood pressure. Arch Intern Med 1990; 150:153–162.
43. Stevens VJ, Corrigan SA, Obarzanek E, et al. Weight loss intervention in phase 1 of the Trials of Hypertension Prevention: The TOHP Collaborative Research Group. Arch Intern Med 1993; 153:849–858.
44. Kumanyaka SK, Obarzanek E, Stevens VJ, et al. Weight-loss experience of black and white participants in NHLBI-sponsored clinical trials. Am J Clin Nutr 1991; 53:1631S–1638S.
45. Wassertheil-Smoller S, Blaufox MD, Oberman AS, et al. The Trial of Antihypertensive Interventions and Management (TAIM) Study: Adequate weight loss, alone and combined with drug therapy in the treatment of mild hypertension. Arch Intern Med 1992; 152:131–136.
46. Neaton JD, Grimm RH, Prineas RJ, et al. Treatment of Mild Hypertension Study: Final results. JAMA 1993; 270:713–724.
47. Grimm RH, Flack JM, Grandits GA, et al. Long-term effects on plasma lipids of diet and drugs to treat hypertension: Treatment of Mild Hypertension Study (TOMHS) Research Group. JAMA 1996; 275:1549–1556.
48. Elmer PJ, Grimm R, Laing B, et al. Lifestyle intervention: Results of the Treatment of Mild Hypertension Study (TOMHS). Prev Med 1995; 24:378–388.
49. Blumenthal JA, Siegel WC, Appelbaum M. Failure of exercise to reduce blood pressure in patients with mild hypertension—results of a randomized controlled trial. JAMA 1991; 266:2098–2104.
50. Consensus Development Conference on Diet and Exercise in Non-Insulin-Dependent Diabetes Mellitus. Diabetes Care 1987; 10(5):639–643.
51. Ornish D, Brown SE, Scherwitz LW, et al. Can lifestyle changes reverse coronary heart disease? Lancet 1990; 336:129–133.
52. Singh RB, Rastogi SS, Verma R, et al. Randomized controlled trial of cardioprotective diet in patients with recent acute myo-

cardial infarction: Results of one-year follow-up. BMJ 1992; 304:1015–1019.

53. Schuller G, Hambrecht R, Schlierf G, et al. Regular physical exercise and low-fat diet—effects on progression of coronary artery disease. Circulation 1992; 86:1–11.
54. Haskell WL, Alderman EL, Fair JM, et al. Effects of intensive multiple risk factor reduction on coronary atherosclerosis and clinical cardiac effects in men and women with coronary artery disease: The Stanford Coronary Risk Intervention Project (SCRIP). Circulation 1994; 89:975–990.
55. Wenger NK, Froelicher ES, Smith LK, et al. Cardiac Rehabilitation. Clinical Practice Guideline No. 17. AHCPR Publication No. 96–0672. Rockville, MD, US Department of Health and Human Services, Public Health Service, Agency for Health Care Policy and Research and the National Heart, Lung, and Blood Institute, October 1995.
56. Dishman RK, Buckworth J. Increasing physical activity: A quantitative synthesis. Med Sci Sports Exerc 1996; 28:706–719.
57. Brownell KD, Cohen LR. Adherence to dietary regimens: I. An overview of research. Behav Med 1995; 20:149–154.
58. Brownell KD, Cohen LR. Adherence to dietary regimens: II. Components of effective interventions. Behav Med 1995; 20:155–164.
59. National Institutes of Health Technology Assessment Conference Panel. Methods for voluntary weight loss and control. Ann Intern Med 1993; 119:764–770.
60. US Department of Health and Human Services. Physical Activity and Health: A Report of the Surgeon General. Atlanta, US Department of Health and Human Services, Centers for Disease Control and Prevention, National Center for Chronic Disease Prevention and Health Promotion, 1996.

30 Aspirin

► Julie E. Buring
► Charles H. Hennekens

The history of aspirin dates to the fifth century B.C., when Hippocrates discovered that an extract of willow bark had analgesic properties. The pain-killing effect was the result of salicin, a naturally occurring chemical in willow bark, which is closely related to the synthetic aspirin available today, acetylsalicylic acid. Aspirin was synthesized in 1897 by Felix Hoffmann, a chemist working in the laboratory of Friedrich Bayer in Wuppertal, Germany. Hoffmann was motivated, in part, by humanitarian concerns to find a tolerable as well as effective pain reliever for his father, who had painful and crippling arthritis. Despite becoming the most widely used drug in the world in the twentieth century, only over the past few decades has attention focused on the potential role of aspirin in reducing the risks of occlusive vascular disease.

MECHANISM

The hypothesized mechanism for aspirin's benefit derives from its ability to decrease platelet aggregation and thereby reduce the risk of thrombotic vascular events. The disruption of platelet- and fibrin-rich atherosclerotic plaque may lead to aggressive platelet deposition and, ultimately, to the formation of a thrombus, which can precipitate an acute clinical event. Findings from basic research demonstrate that, in platelets, small amounts of aspirin (i.e., 50 to 80 mg daily) irreversibly acetylate the active site of cyclooxygenase, which is required for the production of thromboxane A_2, a powerful promoter of aggregation.[1] This effect persists for the entire life of the platelet (about 10 days) and is so pronounced that higher doses of aspirin appear to yield no additional benefit. Indeed, the basic research findings raise the possibility that less than daily frequency of administration (e.g., alternate-day dosing) might be as effective as a daily regimen, whereas very high doses might, in theory, compromise the favorable effects of aspirin, due to activation of reversible vessel wall enzymes.

TRIALS OF SECONDARY PREVENTION AND ACUTE EVOLVING MYOCARDIAL INFARCTION

The evidence on the role of aspirin in the secondary prevention or treatment of cardiovascular disease (CVD) as well as in acute evolving myocardial infarction (MI) has been discussed in detail previously in this textbook (see Chapters 7 and 20), and other publications.[2–4] In brief, long-term aspirin therapy has been shown to confer conclusive net benefits on risk of subsequent MI, stroke, and vascular death among patients with a wide range of prior manifestations of CVD.[5, 6] The 1994 Antiplatelet Trialists' Collaboration[6] overview analyzed results of randomized trials of antiplatelet therapy among more than 54,000 high-risk patients with prior MI, stroke, transient ischemic attack (TIA), unstable or stable angina, revascularization surgery, angioplasty, atrial fibrillation, vascular disease, and peripheral vascular disease. Aspirin therapy was associated with a statistically significant reduction in risk of subsequent vascular events of about 25%, regardless of age, gender, hypertensive status, and history of diabetes. Aspirin was tested in these trials in dosages ranging from 75 to 1500 mg per day. There was no evidence that higher doses were any more effective in reducing risk of occlusive vascular events than lower doses.

Aspirin therapy has also been shown to be of proven value in the treatment of acute MI. In the Second International Study of Infarct Survival (ISIS-2),[7] 162 mg of aspirin daily, given within 24 hours of onset of symptoms and continued for 30 days, conferred statistically significant reductions in risk of subsequent vascular mortality (23%), nonfatal reinfarction (49%) and nonfatal stroke (46%). In the 1980s, the U.S. Food and Drug Administration (FDA) approved professional labeling indications for aspirin in patients with prior MI and unstable angina[8] as well as for men with prior TIAs.[9] In January 1997, at a joint meeting of the FDA Nonprescription Drugs and Cardiovascular and Renal Drugs Advisory Commit-

TABLE 30–1 • Adverse Effects in the United Kingdom Transient Ischemic Attack Trial (number and percent of patients)

	Aspirin 1200 mg/day (n = 815)	Aspirin 300 mg/day (n = 806)	Placebo (n = 814)
Upper gastrointestinal symptoms*	338 (41)	253 (31)	209 (26)
Constipation	56 (7)	48 (6)	20 (2)
Gastrointestinal hemorrhage	39 (51)	25 (3)	9 (1)

*300 mg aspirin vs. 1200 mg aspirin; $p < 0.05$.

For each type of adverse effect, patients were counted only once. If a patient had more than one type of adverse effect, he or she was counted more than once.

Adapted from UK-TIA Study Group. United Kingdom transient ischaemic attack (UK-TIA) aspirin trial: Final results. J Neurol Neurosurg Psychiatry 1991; 54:1044–1054.

tees, members voted to recommend that the FDA expand the professional labeling indications to include acute MI, women as well as men with prior TIAs, and patients with prior occlusive stroke or chronic stable angina. Wider use of aspirin in these patient categories could avoid 10,000 premature deaths each year in the United States.[10]

PRIMARY PREVENTION

None of the previously summarized data, however, addresses directly the role of aspirin in the primary prevention of CVD among those at usual risk. In primary prevention, the benefit-risk ratio for aspirin must be even more carefully weighed. Any agent that inhibits platelet aggregation may pose a risk of increased bleeding. Although these risks may be deemed acceptable for those at high risk of a CVD event due to prior CVD history or an acute MI, they must be carefully weighed against the likely benefits for those at lower baseline risk of occlusive vascular events. The dose of aspirin must also be carefully considered, since the benefits on CVD may be comparable over the wide dose range tested in trials to date, but the principal side effects of the drug appear to be strongly dose related.

The United Kingdom Transient Ischemic Attack trial, which tested two daily dosages of aspirin as well as placebo, provides the most informative direct comparison of the side effects of different aspirin dosages.[11] This trial among 2345 patients with a history of TIA tested dosages of 300 mg per day and 1200 mg per day of aspirin versus placebo. For each category of symptom, including upper gastrointestinal (GI) symptoms, GI hemorrhage, and constipation, the percentage of participants reporting it was lowest in the placebo group, somewhat higher in the group receiving 300 mg per day, and highest among those receiving 1200 mg daily (Table 30–1). Thus the goal for primary prevention is to choose the lowest possible dose of aspirin that has a cardioprotective effect, while minimizing side effects.

Aspirin has been evaluated in two completed primary prevention trials among men at usual risk of CVD. The Physicians' Health Study was a randomized, double-blind, placebo-controlled trial of 325 mg of aspirin on alternate days, as well as 50 mg of β-carotene on alternate days, conducted among 22,071 U.S. male physicians, 40 to 84 years of age.[12] The trial was stopped prematurely by the external Data Monitoring Board after an average follow-up of 60.2 months, primarily because of the finding of a statistically extreme 44% reduction in risk of a first MI among those randomized to aspirin ($P < 0.00001$) (Table 30–2). The findings for stroke (Table 30–3) as well as for cardiovascular mortality (Table 30–4) were inconclusive due to inadequate numbers of events. The available data did not suggest any reduction in stroke, however, with a nonsignificant 22% increase in total stroke. There was a possible increase in hemorrhagic strokes in the aspirin group, with 23 events versus 12 in placebo ($P = 0.06$).

With respect to various subgroups, the effects of aspirin on MI risk were modified by two coronary risk factors: age and blood cholesterol level (Table 30–5). Specifically, the benefit of aspirin was apparent only among those 50 years of age or older ($P = 0.02$), whereas for cholesterol, the benefit was apparent in

TABLE 30–2 • Aspirin and Myocardial Infarction in the Physicians' Health Study

Endpoint	Aspirin Group (n = 11,037)	Placebo Group (n = 11,034)	Relative Risk	95% Confidence Interval	P Value
Myocardial infarction					
Fatal	10	26	0.34	0.15–0.75	0.007
Nonfatal	129	213	0.59	0.47–0.74	<0.00001
Total	39	239	0.56	0.45–0.70	<0.00001
Person-years of observation	54,560.0	54,355.7	—	—	—

From Steering Committee of the Physicians' Health Study Research Group. Final report on the aspirin component of the ongoing Physicians' Health Study. N Engl J Med 1989; 321:129–135.

TABLE 30–3 • Aspirin and Stroke in the Physicians' Health Study

Type of Stroke	Aspirin Group (n = 11,037)	Placebo Group (n = 11,034)	Relative Risk	95% Confidence Interval	P Value
Ischemic					
Mild	69	61	1.13	0.80–1.60	0.48
Moderate, severe or fatal	21	20	1.05	0.57–1.95	0.88
Unknown severity	1	1			
Total	**91**	**82**	**1.11**	**0.82–1.50**	**0.50**
Hemorrhagic					
Mild	10	6	1.67	0.61–4.57	0.32
Moderate, severe or fatal	13	6	2.19	0.84–5.69	0.11
Total	**23**	**12**	**2.14**	**0.96–4.77**	**0.06**
Unknown cause					
Mild	2	1	—	—	—
Moderate, severe or fatal	1	2	—	—	—
Unknown severity	2	1	—	—	—
Total	**5**	**4**	—	—	—
Total	**119**	**98**	**1.22**	**0.93–1.60**	**0.15**

Severity was defined as follows: mild, impairment not affecting functioning; moderate, functional impairment; and severe, a major change in way of life or dependence.

From Steering Committee of the Physicians' Health Study Research Group. Final report on the aspirin component of the ongoing Physicians' Health Study. N Engl J Med 1989; 321:129–135.

all strata but appeared greatest at low levels (P = 0.04). Thus, there was no apparent modification of aspirin's effects according to smoking status, diabetes, blood pressure, alcohol use, exercise habits, or body mass index.

In an analysis involving the 333 men who entered the trial with chronic stable angina and/or prior coronary revascularization, aspirin assignment was associated with a marked decrease in MI (7 vs. 20 events; relative risk = 0.30; 95% confidence interval [CI], 0.14 to 0.63; P = 0.003).[13] There was also an apparent increase in stroke among this subgroup, but this was based on a smaller number of events (11 in aspirin vs. 2 in placebo). Among the more than 21,000 participants with no history of coronary disease at baseline, aspirin appeared to provide no benefit on the development of angina pectoris during the trial.[14] Meanwhile, the benefit on MI was apparent in the early months of the trial and its magnitude did not change over the 5-year course of treatment.[15] This finding supports the view that low-dose aspirin's principal benefit relates to an acute effect on risk of thrombosis, whereas the lack of apparent benefit on the development of angina suggests that treatment with low-dose aspirin for up to 5 years does not materially slow the initiation and progression of atherosclerosis.

The other primary prevention trial was conducted among 5139 male physicians, 50 to 78 years of age, in Great Britain. The British trial tested a daily dose of 500 mg of aspirin, and the control group was asked to avoid aspirin or any aspirin-containing compounds. After 6 years of treatment and follow-up, there were no significant differences for nonfatal MI, nonfatal stroke, vascular death, or all important vascular

TABLE 30–4 • Aspirin and Mortality in the Physicians' Health Study

Cause	Aspirin Group (n = 11,037)	Placebo Group (n = 11,034)	Relative Risk	95% Confidence Interval	P Value
Total cardiovascular deaths	81	83	0.96	0.60–1.54	0.87
Acute myocardial infarction	10	28	0.31	0.14–0.68	0.004
Other ischemic heart disease	24	25	0.97	0.60–1.55	0.89
Sudden death	22	12	1.96	0.91–4.22	0.09
Stroke	10	7	1.44	0.54–3.88	0.47
Other cardiovascular	15	11	1.38	0.62–3.05	0.43
Total noncardiovascular deaths	124	133	0.93	0.72–1.20	0.59
Total deaths with confirmed cause	205	216	0.95	0.79–1.15	0.60
Total deaths	217	227	0.96	0.80–1.14	0.64
Person-years of observation	54,894.6	54,864.2	—	—	—

From Steering Committee of the Physicians' Health Study Research Group. Final report on the aspirin component of the ongoing Physicians' Health Study. N Engl J Med 1989; 321:129–135.

TABLE 30–5 • Risk of Total Myocardial Infarction (MI) Associated with Aspirin Use in the Physicians' Health Study According to Level of Coronary Risk Factors

	Aspirin Group (MI/total n) (%)	Placebo Group (MI/total n) (%)	Relative Risk	*P* Value of Trend in Relative Risk
Age (yr)				
40–49	27/4527 (0.6)	24/4524 (0.5)	1.12	
50–59	51/3725 (1.4)	87/3725 (2.3)	0.58	0.02
60–69	39/2045 (1.9)	84/2045 (4.1)	0.46	
70–84	22/740 (3.0)	44/740 (6.0)	0.49	
Cigarette smoking				
Never	55/5431 (1.0)	96/5488 (1.8)	0.58	
Past	63/4373 (1.4)	105/4301 (2.4)	0.59	0.99
Current	21/1213 (1.7)	37/1225 (3.0)	0.57	
Diabetes mellitus				
Yes	11/275 (4.0)	26/258 (10.1)	0.39	0.22
No	128/10,750 (1.2)	213/10,763 (2.0)	0.60	
Parental history of MI				
Yes	23/1420 (1.6)	39/1432 (2.7)	0.59	0.97
No	112/9505 (1.2)	192/9481 (2.0)	0.58	
Cholesterol level (mg/100 mL)*				
<159	2/382 (0.5)	9/406 (2.2)	0.23	
160–209	12/1587 (0.8)	37/1511 (2.5)	0.29	0.04
210–259	26/1435 (1.8)	43/1444 (3.0)	0.61	
≥260	14/582 (2.4)	23/570 (4.0)	0.59	
Diastolic blood pressure (mm Hg)				
≤69	2/583 (0.3)	9/562 (1.6)	0.21	
70–79	24/2999 (0.8)	40/3076 (1.3)	0.61	0.88
80–89	71/5061 (1.4)	128/5083 (2.5)	0.55	
≥90	26/1037 (2.5)	43/970 (4.4)	0.56	
Systolic blood pressure (mm Hg)				
<109	1/330 (0.3)	4/296 (1.4)	0.22	
110–129	40/5072 (0.8)	75/5129 (1.5)	0.52	0.48
130–149	63/3829 (1.7)	115/3861 (3.0)	0.55	
≥150	19/454 (4.2)	26/412 (6.3)	0.65	
Alcohol use				
Daily	26/2718 (1.0)	55/2727 (2.0)	0.45	
Weekly	70/5419 (1.3)	112/5313 (2.1)	0.61	0.26
Rarely	40/2802 (1.4)	65/2897 (2.2)	0.63	
Vigorous exercise at least once a week				
Yes	91/7910 (1.2)	140/7861 (1.8)	0.65	0.21
No	45/2997 (1.5)	92/3060 (3.0)	0.49	
Body mass index†				
<23.0126	26/2872 (0.9)	41/2807 (1.5)	0.61	
23.0127–24.4075	32/2700 (1.2)	46/2627 (1.8)	0.68	0.90
24.4076–26.3865	32/2713 (1.2)	75/2823 (2.7)	0.44	
≥26.3866	49/2750 (1.8)	76/2776 (2.7)	0.65	

*To convert cholesterol value to millimoles per liter, multiply by 0.02586.
†Body mass index is the weight (in kilograms) times the height (in meters) squared.
From Steering Committee of the Physicians' Health Study Research Group. Final report on the aspirin component of the ongoing Physicians' Health Study. N Engl J Med 1989; 321:129–135.

events.[16] It was not possible to distinguish reliably between thrombotic and hemorrhagic strokes. There was, however, an increase of borderline statistical significance ($P = 0.05$) in the aspirin group of the subgroup of strokes self-reported as "disabling." It is difficult to determine whether this reflects a real increase in such events, which might be more likely to be hemorrhagic in origin, or is the result of bias in the self-reporting of residual impairment due to the study's open design without placebo control.

There were several design differences between the two primary prevention trials. Whereas the U.S. trial tested 325 mg on alternate days, the British study used a daily dose of 500 mg. The U.S. trial was double blind and placebo controlled, whereas the British trial was single blind and not placebo controlled. The most striking difference was in sample size, with the United States trial more than four times as large.

To consider the available primary prevention trial data in aggregate, an overview was performed of the

U.S. and British trials.[2, 17] Because the U.S. study was so much larger, the overview demonstrated a highly significant 32% reduction in the risk of nonfatal MI (Table 30–6). For stroke and vascular death, even when the trials were considered together, there were too few endpoints on which to draw firm conclusions.

The recently completed Thrombosis Prevention Trial in the United Kingdom used a 2 × 2 factorial design to evaluate low-dose aspirin (75 mg daily) and warfarin (target international normalized ratio, 1.5) in men without a prior history of CVD events but at high risk of ischemic heart disease.[18] The trial randomized 5085 men, aged 45 to 69, who were judged to be at elevated risk for ischemic heart disease based on a risk score that included family history, smoking history, body mass index, blood pressure, cholesterol, plasma fibrinogen, and plasma factor VII activity. After a median treatment duration of 6.8 years, aspirin treatment was associated with a 20% reduction in the primary endpoint of total ischemic heart disease (nonfatal MI plus coronary death) (95% CI 1% to 35%; $P = 0.04$). This benefit resulted almost entirely from a statistically significant 32% reduction in nonfatal MI. In contrast, warfarin-treated participants experienced a 21% reduction in ischemic heart disease (95% CI 4% to 35%; $P = 0.02$), which was due chiefly to a significant 39% reduction in fatal events. Combined treatment was associated with a 34% reduction in ischemic heart disease (95% CI 11% to 51%; $P = 0.006$). There was an excess of hemorrhagic stroke and total fatal strokes among those assigned both agents (hemorrhagic stroke: 7 events in combined therapy vs. 1 in warfarin alone, 2 in aspirin alone, and none in placebo; fatal stroke: 12 in combined therapy vs. 5 in warfarin alone, 2 in aspirin alone, and 1 in placebo).

Additional data in primary prevention are needed for complete assessment of aspirin's benefit-risk ratio in apparently healthy persons. In addition, since only men have been studied in the trials of aspirin in primary prevention to date, there is need for direct randomized trial data in this setting in women. The only data available on aspirin use and CVD in apparently healthy women derive from observational studies. Not surprisingly, the findings are inconsistent, with two studies suggesting benefits[19, 20] one reporting no apparent effect,[21] and one suggesting an increased risk of ischemic heart disease.[22] The primary concern in extrapolating findings from trial data in men is that the benefit-risk ratio for prophylactic aspirin use in women may differ from that in men. The reason for this is that women's risk of MI, the principal outcome that aspirin may prevent, is lower at almost all ages than men's risk, while women and men have roughly comparable rates of stroke, the hemorrhagic forms of which may be increased by aspirin. To evaluate directly the benefits and risks of low-dose aspirin among apparently healthy women, a large-scale randomized trial was begun in 1992. The ongoing Women's Health Study, which has randomized approximately 40,000 U.S. female health professionals, 45 years of age and older, to low-dose aspirin (100 mg every other day) or placebo will provide direct randomized trial evidence in women as well as provide conclusive findings on aspirin's effect on stroke and total vascular mortality.[23, 24]

TABLE 30–6 • Overview of the Two Randomized Trials of Aspirin in Primary Prevention of Cardiovascular Disease

	Reduction (% ± SD) Among Those Assigned Aspirin		
Endpoint	*U.S. Physicians' Health Study*	*British Doctors' Trial*	*Overview*
Nonfatal myocardial infarction	39 ± 9	3 ± 19	32 ± 8
Nonfatal stroke	↑ 19 ± 15	↑ 13 ± 24	↑ 18 ± 13
Total vascular mortality	2 ± 15	7 ± 14	5 ± 10
Important vascular events	18 ± 7	4 ± 12	13 ± 6

↑ Nonsignificant increase among aspirin-allocated subjects.

From Hennekens CH, Buring JE, Sandercock P, et al. Aspirin and other antiplatelet agents in the secondary and primary prevention of cardiovascular disease. Circulation 1989; 80:749–756.

Pending the results of the Women's Health Study, any formal policy recommendation concerning aspirin in the primary prevention of CVD would be premature. The U.S. Preventive Services Task Force has concluded that there is insufficient evidence to recommend for or against routine aspirin prophylaxis in primary prevention and that any use should be an individual clinical judgment.[25] While awaiting definitive data on the balance of aspirin's benefits and risks, however, available data suggest that aspirin may be beneficial in primary prevention for those whose risk of MI is sufficiently high to warrant exposure to any risks of long-term administration of this drug. For example, a 60-year-old woman with a cholesterol level of 250 mg/dL and a recent diagnosis of type II diabetes would appear to be a strong candidate for prophylactic aspirin use. Similarly, aspirin may be warranted for a middle-aged man who is a current smoker and has a strong family history of premature CVD. On the other hand, aspirin would not appear to be indicated—and may even be contraindicated—in a 44-year-old premenopausal woman whose only cardiovascular risk factor is poorly controlled hypertension (average readings of 160/100 mm Hg), because she is at significantly greater risk of stroke than MI.

While these clinical scenarios suggest that aspirin may be most appropriate for those with one or more coronary risk factors, even if this intervention is proven conclusively to confer net benefits in primary prevention in both men and women, it should always be viewed as a possible adjunct, not alternative, to the control or elimination of other cardiovascular risk factors. In addition, aspirin therapy should be initiated only on the recommendation of a physician or other primary health care provider. Such a recommendation should be based on an individual clinical judgment that considers the cardiovascular risks of the patient, the adverse effects of the drug, and the documented benefits on various manifestations of CVD in different categories of patients.

SUMMARY

Aspirin therapy is of proven value in treatment of acute MI as well as long-term use in patients with a wide range of prior manifestations of CVD. For primary prevention, there is conclusive evidence of reduction associated with low-dose aspirin in the risk of a first MI in men. However, the evidence concerning stroke and vascular mortality remains inconclusive owing to inadequate numbers of endpoints in both primary prevention trials of aspirin as well as in the overview of their findings. Ongoing trials in women at usual risk as well as high-risk individuals will provide importantly relevant information to formulate policy recommendations for use of aspirin in apparently healthy people. Until then, use of aspirin in primary prevention of MI should remain an individual clinical judgment and should be viewed as an adjunct, not an alternative, to management of other coronary risk factors.

REFERENCES

1. Vane JR. Inhibition of prostaglandin synthesis as a mechanism of action for aspirin-like drugs. Nat N Biol 1971; 231:232–235.
2. Hennekens CH, Buring JE, Sandercock P, et al. Aspirin and other antiplatelet agents in the secondary and primary prevention of cardiovascular disease. Circulation 1989; 80:749–756.
3. Fuster V, Dyken ML, Vokonas PS, Hennekens CH. Aspirin as a therapeutic agent in cardiovascular disease: AHA Scientific Statement. Circulation 1993; 87:659–675.
4. Hennekens CH, Dyken ML, Fuster V. Aspirin as a therapeutic agent in cardiovascular disease: AHA Scientific Statement. Circulation 1997; 96:2751–2758.
5. Antiplatelet Trialists' Collaboration. Secondary prevention of vascular disease by prolonged antiplatelet therapy. BMJ 1988; 296:320–332.
6. Antiplatelet Trialists' Collaboration. Collaborative overview of randomized trials of antiplatelet treatment: I. Prevention of vascular death, myocardial infarction, and stroke by prolonged antiplatelet therapy in different categories of patients. BMJ 1994; 308:81–106.
7. ISIS-2 (Second International Study of Infarct Survival) Collaborative Group. Randomized trial of intravenous streptokinase, oral aspirin, both, or neither among 17,187 cases of suspected acute myocardial infarction: ISIS-2. Lancet 1988; 2:349–360.
8. Aspirin for heart patients. FDA Drug Bull 1985; 15:34–36.
9. Aspirin for TIAs. FDA Drug Bull 1980; 10:2
10. Hennekens CH, Jonas MA, Buring JE. The benefits of aspirin in acute myocardial infarction: Still a well-kept secret in the US. Arch Intern Med 1994; 154:37–39.
11. UK-TIA Study Group. United Kingdom transient ischaemic attack (UK-TIA) aspirin trial: Final results. J Neurol Neurosurg Psychiatry 1991; 54:1044–1054.
12. Steering Committee of the Physicians' Health Study Research Group. Final report on the aspirin component of the ongoing Physicians' Health Study. N Engl J Med 1989; 321:129–135.
13. Ridker PM, Manson JE, Gaziano JM, et al. Low-dose aspirin therapy for chronic stable angina. Ann Intern Med 1991; 114:835–39.
14. Manson JE, Grobbee DE, Stampfer MJ, et al. Aspirin in the primary prevention of angina pectoris in a randomized trial of US physicians. Am J Med 1990; 89:772–776.
15. Ridker PM, Manson JE, Buring JE, et al. The effect of chronic platelet inhibition with low-dose aspirin on atherosclerotic progression and acute thrombosis. Am Heart J 1991; 122:1588–1592.
16. Peto R, Gray, R, Collins R, et al. A randomised trial of the effects of prophylactic daily aspirin among male British doctors. BMJ 1988; 296:313–316.
17. Hennekens CH, Peto R, Hutchison GB, et al. An overview of the British and American aspirin studies. N Engl J Med 1988; 318:923–924.
18. The Medical Research Council's General Practice Research Framework. Thrombosis prevention trial: Randomised trial of low-intensity oral anticoagulation with warfarin and low-dose aspirin in the primary prevention of ischaemic heart disease in men at increased risk. Lancet 1998; 351:233–241.
19. Boston Collaborative Drug Surveillance Group. Regular aspirin intake and acute myocardial infarction. BMJ 1974; 1:440–443.
20. Manson JE, Stampfer MJ, Colditz GA, et al. A prospective study of aspirin use and primary prevention of cardiovascular disease in women. JAMA 1991; 266:521–527.
21. Hammond EC, Garfinkel L. Aspirin and coronary heart disease: Findings of a prospective study. BMJ 1975; 2:269–271.
22. Paganini-Hill A, Chao A, Ross RK, et al. Aspirin use and chronic diseases: A cohort of the elderly. BMJ 1989; 299:1247–1250.
23. Buring JE, Hennekens CH, for the Women's Health Study Research Group. The Women's Health Study: Summary of the study design. J Myocard Ischemia 1992; 4:27–29.
24. Buring JE, Hennekens CH, for the Women's Health Study Research Group. Women's Health Study: Rationale and background. J Myocard Ischemia 1992; 4:30–40.
25. US Preventive Services Task Force. Guide to Clinical Preventive Services, 2nd ed. Baltimore, Williams & Wilkins, 1996.

31 Postmenopausal Hormone Replacement Therapy

▶ Claudia U. Chae
▶ JoAnn E. Manson

Postmenopausal hormone replacement therapy (HRT) is a medical intervention in evolution. HRT is increasingly being considered by women and physicians largely based on favorable results from observational epidemiologic studies and studies of biologic intermediates, although there is a notable lack of randomized trial data assessing clinical outcomes or the balance of risks with benefits. Limited data exist about the effects of combined estrogen-progestin therapy and the net benefit/risk profile of long-term HRT, which are increasingly important issues in current clinical practice. Nearly 40% of women in the United States will be older than 45 years of age by the year 2000,[1] with increasing female life expectancy resulting in more than one third of life being spent in the postmenopausal state. This underscores the potential public health impact of HRT and the need for large randomized clinical trials (RCTs) to clarify its role.

Much of the potential health impact of HRT is driven by the fact that cardiovascular disease (CVD) is the leading cause of mortality in women in developed countries, causing 500,000 deaths annually among women in the United States, half of which are due to coronary heart disease (CHD).[2] Epidemiologic evidence of a cardioprotective effect of estrogen includes the low CHD risk in premenopausal women, greater CHD risk in young women with bilateral oophorectomy who are not on HRT, closing of the gender gap in CHD risk after menopause, and reduced risk of CHD and mortality with HRT in observational studies. A plausible biologic basis exists for these findings, because estrogen may influence a diverse array of mechanisms, including lipid metabolism and oxidative status, thrombosis, vascular tone, intimal hyperplasia, and insulin sensitivity, all of which are involved in the pathogenesis of atherosclerosis and acute coronary syndromes.

Several issues should be considered when the clinical trial data currently available for HRT are evaluated. These data are limited to biologic intermediates, especially lipids, as outcomes. Many of the trials are small in size and few are placebo controlled. HRT's effects are influenced by the dose, type of estrogen or progestin used, mode of administration (e.g., oral vs. transdermal), and whether progestin is administered on a cyclic or continuous basis. Variability in these factors complicates the interpretation and comparison of trial results. Many trials are also of short duration, which may not reflect a biologic steady-state or HRT's effects in the longer time frame relevant to clinical use. Evaluating HRT's net effects on dynamic, complex biologic systems (e.g., hemostasis) is also difficult. Only recently have large, placebo-controlled RCTs of HRT been established, with many of their results still pending.

In this chapter, we review existing clinical trial data regarding the possible cardioprotective effects of HRT, including the results of the Postmenopausal Estrogen/Progestin Interventions (PEPI) Trial, the first major randomized, double-blind, placebo-controlled trial of HRT. PEPI evaluated the effects of estrogen and combined estrogen-progestin HRT on CHD risk factors, including lipids, systolic blood pressure, serum insulin, and fibrinogen. We also describe the expected contributions of ongoing large-scale RCTs such as the Women's Health Initiative (WHI) and the results of the Heart and Estrogen/Progestin Replacement Study.

LIPID EFFECTS

Menopause is associated with adverse changes in the lipid profile, including higher low-density lipoprotein (LDL) levels and lower high-density lipoprotein (HDL) and HDL_2 levels.[3,4] A substantial body of clinical trial data supports the following conclusions:

1. Oral estrogen replacement therapy (ERT) significantly reduces LDL and raises HDL, both by about 10% to 15%.

2. An added progestin attenuates the HDL-raising effect of estrogen alone, in proportion to its androgenicity, but does not affect the reduction in LDL.

3. HRT is associated with a modest increase in triglycerides (TGs). HRT may lower lipoprotein(a) (Lp[a]) and inhibit LDL oxidation, but further clinical data are needed.

HDL/LDL Effects

Estrogen-Only HRT. Oral ERT consistently reduced LDL and raised HDL in small clinical trials.[5, 6] However, the observed magnitude of effect varied considerably owing to heterogeneity in type, dose, and duration of treatment, as well as small sample sizes and lack of placebo control groups. An exception is the randomized, double-blind, placebo-controlled crossover trial by Walsh and associates,[7] in which 3 months of 0.625 mg or 1.25 mg per day of conjugated equine estrogen (CEE) in 31 normolipidemic postmenopausal women resulted in significant, consistent increases in HDL (16% and 18%, respectively) and decreases in LDL (15% and 19%, respectively). Transdermal estrogen had no effect on HDL or LDL.

Recent large randomized trials of HRT have used 0.625 mg per day of CEE. As the most commonly prescribed oral estrogen, CEE is the predominant formulation in observational studies showing lower CHD risk with HRT.[8] The dosage of 0.625 mg/d is the lowest established level known to relieve menopausal symptoms and prevent osteoporosis, while minimizing adverse effects such as thrombotic complications and hypertriglyceridemia. Low-dose CEE (0.3 mg per day) has shown promise, but more clinical data are needed.

In the 3-year randomized, double-blind, placebo-controlled PEPI Trial,[8] 875 postmenopausal women aged 45 to 64 years were randomized to placebo, or 0.625 mg per day of CEE alone or combined with different progestin regimens (discussed later). With CEE alone, there was a 9% rise (+5.6 mg/dL) in HDL and a 10.3% fall (−14.5 mg/dL) in LDL compared with baseline; the placebo group had slight decreases in both HDL (−1.2 mg/dL or −2%) and LDL (−4.1 mg/dL or −2.9%) from baseline (Table 31–1). The PEPI data also showed how lipid values with HRT vary over time (Fig. 31–1); the most marked changes occur in the first 6 to 12 months and level off over the next 2 years, underscoring the caution with which one must interpret data from trials of short duration. Two other large randomized comparison trials[9, 10] of estrogen and estrogen-progestin regimens lacked placebo controls but found comparable effects of CEE-only HRT on HDL and LDL (Table 31–2).

These HDL/LDL changes depend on the first-pass hepatic effect of orally delivered estrogen.[7] Estrogen raises HDL (primarily HDL_2)[5, 7, 9, 11] by decreasing the activity of hepatic lipase, which promotes HDL uptake by hepatocytes and HDL_2 catabolism.[12] Estrogen

TABLE 31–1 • Results of the PEPI Trial*

	Placebo	CEE Only	CEE + Cyclic MPA	CEE + Contin MPA	CEE + Cyclic MP	*P* Value
n	174	175	174	174	178	
HDL (mg/dL)	−1.2 [−2.2, −0.20]	+5.6 [4.5, 6.7]	+1.6 [0.5, 2.7]	+1.2 [0.1, 2.2]	+4.1 [3.1, 5.1]	< 0.001
% change	(−2%)	(+9%)	(+2.5%)	(+1.9%)	(+6.6%)	
LDL (mg/dL)	−4.1 [−6.5, −1.8]	−14.5 [−16.8, −12.1]	−17.7 [−20.1, −15.4]	−16.5 [−18.8, −14.2]	−14.8 [−17.0, −12.5]	< 0.001
% change	(−2.9%)	(−10.3%)	(−12.9%)	(−11.6%)	(−10.9%)	
TG (mg/dL)	−3.2 [−7.2, 0.7]	+13.7 [9.3, 18.0]	+12.7 [8.5, 16.8]	+11.4 [7.0, 15.9]	+13.4 [9.1, 17.7]	< 0.001
% change	(−3.2%)	(+13.9%)	(+13.5%)	(+11.1%)	(+13.7%)	
Fibrinogen (g/L)	+0.10 [0.04, 0.16]	−0.2 [−0.08, 0.04]	+0.06 [0.0, 0.12]	+0.01 [−0.04, 0.07]	+0.01 [−0.04, 0.07]	< 0.001
% change	(+3.5%)	(−7.3%)	(+2.2%)	(+0.4%)	(+0.4%)	
OGTT						
Insulin (pmol/L)						
Fasting	+3.8 [−0.8, 8.3]	−1.7 [−5.6, 2.2]	+1.3 [−2.8, 5.5]	−3.8 [−8.0, 0.3]	−3.5 [−7.4, 0.4]	0.07
2-h	−13.7 [−45.6, 18.2]	−8.0 [−37.4, 21.4]	+13.4 [−17.8, 44.6]	+1.2 [−28.2, 30.6]	−25.1 [−54.9, 4.7]	0.29
Glucose (mg/dL)						
Fasting	−0.6 [−1.6, 06]	−2.8 [−4.0, −1.7]	−2.7 [−3.8, −1.7]	−2.1 [−2.9, −1.2]	−2.5 [−3.6, −1.4]	0.03
2-h	−0.1 [−4.0, 3.9]	+2.0 [−2.3, 6.4]	+7.5 [4.0, 11.1]	+6.9 [3.3, 10.5]	+3.0 [−0.6, 6.7]	0.01
BP (mm Hg)						
Systolic	+1.2 [−0.1, 2.6]	+0.5 [−0.7, 1.8]	+0.7 [−0.6, 2.1]	+1.8 [0.6, 3.0]	+0.1 [−1.0, 1.1]	0.83
Diastolic	0.0 [−0.9, 0.9]	−0.7 [−1.5, 0.1]	−1.0 [−1.8, −0.1]	+0.2 [−0.5, 0.9]	−0.6 [−1.3, 0.0]	0.29

*Three-year results, given as mean change from baseline [95% confidence interval]; % change denotes percent change from baseline.

HDL, high-density lipoprotein; LDL, low-density lipoprotein; TG, triglycerides; CEE, conjugated equine estrogen; MPA, medroxyprogesterone acetate; cyclic, days 1–12; contin, continuous; MP, micronized progesterone; OGTT, oral glucose tolerance test; BP, blood pressure.

Adapted from the Writing Group for the PEPI Trial. Effects of estrogen or estrogen/progestin regimens on heart disease risk factors in postmenopausal women: The Postmenopausal Estrogen/Progestin Interventions (PEPI) Trial. JAMA 1995; 273:199–208. Copyright 1995, American Medical Association.

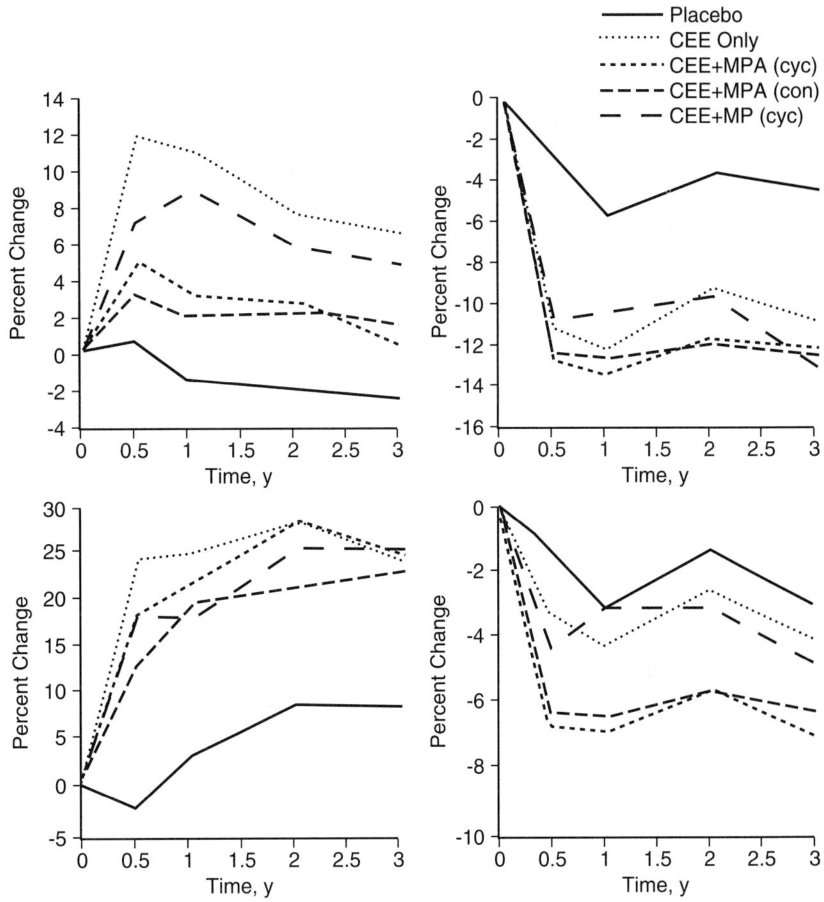

Figure 31–1 Changes in lipid fractions over time in the Postmenopausal Estrogen/Progestin Interventions (PEPI) Trial: Mean percent change from baseline by treatment arm for high-density lipoprotein cholesterol (top left), low-density lipoprotein cholesterol (top right), triglycerides (bottom left), and total cholesterol (bottom right). See Table 31–1 for an explanation of treatment groups. (From The Writing Group for the PEPI Trial. Effects of estrogen or estrogen/progestin regimens on heart disease risk factors in postmenopausal women: The Postmenopausal Estrogen/Progestin Interventions [PEPI] Trial. JAMA 1995; 273:199–208. Copyright 1995, American Medical Association.)

lowers LDL by promoting its catabolism[7] via increased LDL receptors on cell surfaces[13, 14] and greater hepatic 7α-hydroxylase activity, enhancing conversion of cholesterol to bile acids.[15] Perhaps because of the lack of the first-pass hepatic effect or lower systemic estrogen levels, transdermal ERT had no effect on HDL and LDL in one placebo-controlled trial,[7] or inconsistent and less marked effects in small non–placebo-controlled trials compared with oral ERT.[16–18]

Estrogen-Progestin HRT. Progestin is commonly added to protect against endometrial hyperplasia from unopposed estrogen but has raised concerns

TABLE 31–2 • Comparison of Selected Trials of HRT and Lipid Profiles*

	N	Age (yr)	Placebo	Duration	HRT Regimen	% HDL	% LDL	% TG
PEPI[8]	875	45–64	Yes	3 yr	CEE (0.625 mg/d)	+9§	−10.3§	+13.9§
					CEE + cyclic MPA (10 mg/d × 12 d)	+2.5§¶	−12.9§	+13.5§
					CEE + contin MPA (2.5 mg/d)	+1.9§¶	−11.6§	+11.1§
					CEE + cyclic MP (200 mg/d × 12 d)	+6.6§	−10.9§	+13.7§
Lobo et al[9]†	525	45–65	No	13 mo	CEE (0.625 mg/d)	+12§	−8§	+40§
					CEE + contin MPA (2.5 mg/d)	+3§¶	−12§	+24§¶
					CEE + contin MPA (5 mg/d)	+3§¶	−10§	+18§¶
					CEE + cyclic MP (5 mg/d × 14 d)	+3§¶	−10§	+27§¶
					CEE + cyclic MPA (10 mg/d × 14 d)	+2¶	−14§¶	+22§¶
Medical Research Council[10]‡	321	35–59	No	1 yr	CEE (0.625 mg/d)	+8.1§	−13.9§	+24§
					CEE + cyclic norgestrel (0.15 mg/d × 12 d)	−0.7¶	−12.9§	−1.3¶

*Results given as percent change from baseline.
†Data from Lobo et al approximated from bar graphs.
‡MRC trial subjects were all surgically menopausal; HDL and LDL data available on 137 and 128 subjects; data listed are from all randomized patients (116 subjects were on HRT at trial entry and were randomly reassigned; see Reference 10 for data for those not on prior HRT).
§Significant ($P < 0.05$) change from baseline.
¶Significant ($P < 0.05$) change from CEE alone.
CEE, conjugated equine estrogen; MPA, medroxyprogesterone acetate; MP, micronized progesterone; contin, continuous; HRT, hormone replacement therapy; HDL, high-density lipoprotein; LDL, low-density lipoprotein; TG, triglycerides.

about potential attenuation of estrogen's HDL effect. In contrast to estrogen, progestins induce hepatic lipase activity[12, 19] and thus lower HDL. This occurs in direct proportion to the dose and degree of androgenicity,[6, 12, 19] which declines from the 19-nortestosterones (e.g., levonorgestrel and norethindrone), to 17-hydroxyprogesterones (e.g., medroxyprogesterone acetate [MPA]), to natural "micronized" progesterone (MP) as first observed in small clinical trials.[11, 20–22]

In PEPI,[8] 875 postmenopausal women aged 45 to 64 years were randomized to (1) placebo (2) 0.625 mg per day of CEE; (3) 0.625 mg per day of CEE plus cyclic MPA, 10 mg per day for 12 days per month; (4) 0.625 mg per day of CEE plus consecutive MPA, 2.5 mg per day; or (5) 0.625 mg per day of CEE plus cyclic MP, 200 mg per day for 12 days per month. At 3 years, 37% of women assigned to CEE alone had stopped treatment (vs. 16% to 21% in other groups), largely owing to adenomatous or atypical endometrial hyperplasia. CEE alone and CEE plus cyclic MP had the greatest effects on HDL, with comparable increases from baseline of +5.6 mg/dL and +4.1 mg/dL, respectively. Cyclic MPA (+1.6 mg/dL) and continuous MPA (+1.2 mg/dL) attenuated estrogen's HDL effect, but all HRT groups had significantly higher HDL levels (+2.4 to 6.8 mg/dL) than the placebo group. All HRT groups had similar, significant reductions in LDL (−15.9 mg/dL on average) (see Table 31–1). MP's minimal effect on HDL in PEPI and in small trials[18, 23, 24] merits further study, given the desirability of retaining progestin's endometrial protection while preserving estrogen's HDL benefit.

Two large 1-year randomized double-blind trials compared CEE alone and CEE-progestin regimens, without a placebo control group (see Table 31–2). Although hampered by unreported baseline values, lack of a placebo group and dropout rates of 10% to 23%, Lobo and colleagues[9] found similar patterns of HDL and LDL effects with CEE and CEE plus MPA, as did PEPI. Significant rises in HDL_2 were greatest with CEE alone (70%) but also present with all MPA groups (30% to 40%). A comparison trial of CEE versus CEE plus norgestrel by the Medical Research Council's (MRC) general practice research framework in the United Kingdom[10] was limited by dropout rates of 30% to 36%, lack of a placebo group, nonfasting lipid measurements, and lipid data available only in a subset of subjects. One hundred sixteen women were already on HRT (90% on ERT) at trial entry and were randomly reassigned, but it is not stated if a washout period was used. HDL was unaffected by CEE plus norgestrel, which is a relatively androgenic progestin. LDL was significantly lower in both HRT groups.

In the Continuous Hormones as Replacement Therapy (CHART) Study,[25] a 2-year, double-blind, placebo-controlled, parallel group trial, 1265 postmenopausal women with intact uteri were randomized to placebo or one of eight treatment groups of ethinyl estradiol (EE_2) alone or plus norethindrone acetate (NA) (Fig. 31–2). All HRT groups had significantly lower LDLs. Although all EE_2-only groups had significantly increased HDL, the EE_2-NA groups had HDL levels below baseline due to NA's relative androgenicity. Similarly, in a 2-year placebo-controlled trial involving 113 postmenopausal women, continuous or sequential 17β-estradiol (2 mg per day) plus NA (1 mg per day) resulted in significantly lower LDLs (10% to 13%), but HDL was reduced (−14%) or unchanged, respectively.[26]

Thus, clinical trial data support significant increases in HDL and reductions in LDL with ERT, with an added progestin attenuating the HDL benefit, depending on its androgenicity. These lipoprotein effects may have important implications for CHD risk reduction. Higher HDL may be a more potent predictor of lower CHD risk in women than in men.[27, 28] No clinical trial data exist, but in observational studies, a 1 mg/dL increase in HDL is associated with a 3% lower CHD risk and 4.7% lower CVD mortality risk.[29] The rise in HDL with ERT (e.g., 4 to 5 mg/dL in PEPI) may thus markedly lower CHD risk, and even modest attenuation by progestin may affect CHD risk. ERT and combined HRT both lower LDL, although LDL is not as strong as HDL as a predictor of primary CHD risk in women.[27, 28] In secondary prevention trials,[28, 30, 31] LDL reduction has comparable, and perhaps greater,[31] benefits in women as in men.

Triglycerides. Estrogen raises TGs by increasing production of very-low-density lipoprotein (VLDL).[32] Because this VLDL undergoes hepatic breakdown and is not converted into LDL or small VLDL, it may be less atherogenic than the VLDL from impaired lipolysis in endogenous hypertriglyceridemia.[33] Progestins decrease VLDL catabolism[6] and reduced TG with short-term use in earlier small trials,[11, 20] suggesting that they may counteract estrogen's effect on TG. However, in PEPI,[8] all HRT groups had higher TG (mean +12.8 mg/dL) with no difference between ERT or combined HRT. This is in contrast to other trials[9, 10, 25] in which progestins appeared to partly or completely attenuate the rise in TG with estrogen, but the strengths of PEPI's trial design add weight to its findings. The role of TGs in CHD risk in women requires further study.

Lipoprotein(a). Lp(a) is composed of the LDL apolipoprotein B-100 linked to apolipoprotein(a), which is highly homologous with plasminogen. Lp(a) may be atherogenic via oxidative modification, foam cell formation, and antifibrinolytic effects. It is uncertain if Lp(a) is an independent CHD risk factor,[34] with conflicting data from prospective studies in men[35–37] that may be due in part to heterogeneity in Lp(a) and its assays.[38] Higher Lp(a) levels in older women may

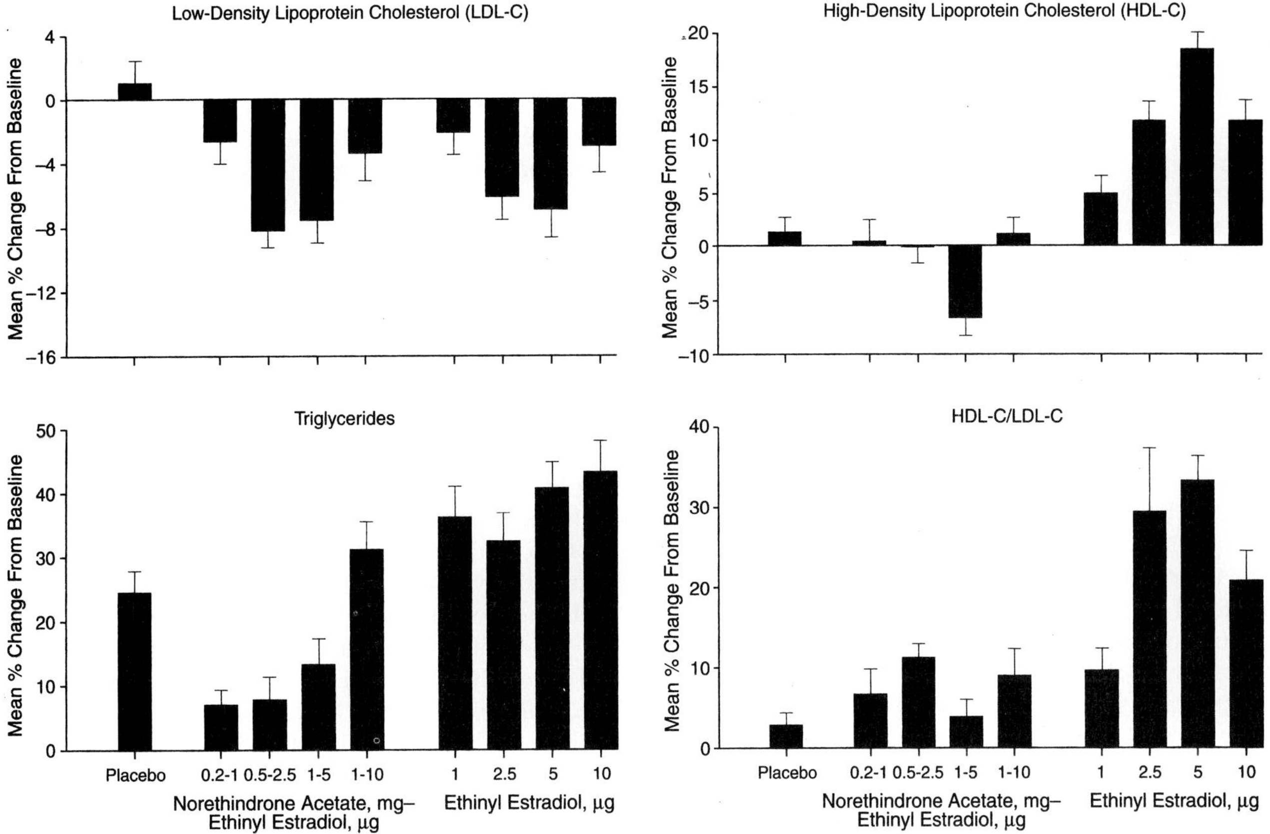

Figure 31–2 Results from the Continuous Hormones as Replacement Therapy (CHART) Study. Data reported as mean percent change (+ standard error) from baseline in lipid parameters at the end of treatment at month 24. Active treatment groups included continuous (A) 0.2 mg norethindrone acetate (NA) + 1 µg ethinyl estradiol (EE_2), (B) 0.5 mg NA + 2.5 µg EE_2, (C) 1 mg NA + 5 µg EE_2, (D) 1 mg NA + 10 µg EE_2, (E) 1 µg EE_2, (F) 2.5 µg EE_2, (G) 5 µg EE_2, and (H) 10 µg EE_2. (From Speroff L, Rowan J, Symons J, et al, for the CHART Study Group. The comparative effect on bone density, endometrium, and lipids of continuous hormones as replacement therapy [CHART Study]. JAMA 1996; 276:1397–1403. Copyright 1996, American Medical Association.)

be due to menopause[39] or age alone[40]; some data[41–43] suggest Lp(a) may be associated with CHD risk only in younger women. In the PEPI trial, Lp(a) was measured in a subset of women (N = 366) at baseline, 12 months, and 36 months. All HRT groups had a 17% to 23% reduction in Lp(a) levels compared with placebo ($P < 0.0001$), which was maintained over the course of the trial.[43a] Progestins (MPA or MP) had little effect on the impact of CEE on Lp(a). These results are generally consistent with the results of prior observational studies[44] and small, short-term clinical trials[9, 45–51] that suggested that HRT reduces Lp(a) by 10% to 50%, depending on the dose, duration, and type of estrogen. However, no clinical data exist to show that lowering Lp(a) reduces CHD risk, and the usefulness of routine screening is unclear given the current lack of effective treatments for high Lp(a).

Is estrogen's favorable impact on CHD risk and atherosclerosis due only to its lipid effects? If so, with other lipid-lowering therapy available, HRT may be less attractive in CHD prevention, given its potential risks.[52] However, HRT's HDL/LDL effects explained only 25% to 50% of the observed CHD risk reduction in earlier studies.[53–55] In the Nurses' Health Study, CHD risk was comparably reduced in current users who did not report hypercholesterolemia or other CHD risk factors.[56] In animals, reduced coronary[57–59] and aortic atherosclerosis[60–62] with ERT or combined HRT could not be explained by changes in serum lipids. Thus, estrogen may also be antiatherogenic by mechanisms unrelated to lipid lowering or by functional changes in lipids such as an antioxidant effect.

Antioxidant Action. Oxidatively modified LDL in the vessel wall promotes atherogenesis by several mechanisms, including enhanced monocyte chemotaxis, foam cell formation, and direct endothelial cytotoxicity. At supraphysiologic levels in vitro, estrogen has antioxidant properties,[63–67] but there are sparse data in humans using physiologic estrogen doses. In a trial involving 18 postmenopausal women, acute intravenous 17β-estradiol or 3 weeks of transdermal estrogen (0.1 mg per day) inhibited LDL oxidative lag time from baseline by 11% (134 to 167 minutes, P = 0.01) and 16% (132 to 178 minutes, P = 0.009), respectively.[68] Stopping the drug reversed this effect, and oxidative lag time was not correlated with post-treatment estradiol levels or lipid levels. In a non–placebo-controlled, randomized crossover trial,[51] 1 month of CEE (0.625 mg per day) alone or plus MPA (2.5 mg per day) did not affect LDL oxidation in 30 postmenopausal women. However, transdermal estradiol (0.1 mg per day) alone or plus MPA (2.5 mg per day) in 20 other subjects caused a modest increase in oxidative lag time (76 to 84 minutes, $P < 0.05$; 78 to 84 minutes, P = NS, respectively).

HEMOSTATIC EFFECTS

Thrombosis plays an integral role in atherosclerosis progression and acute coronary syndromes. Menopause may be associated with increases in fibrinogen, factor VII, and plasminogen activator inhibitor-1 (PAI-1),[69–71] a potentially hypercoagulable state that may be countered by increases in natural anticoagulants such as antithrombin III (AT-III).[72] Potential thrombotic risk factors may be modifiable by HRT, but evaluation of existing data is complicated by the complex dynamics of the coagulation system, which makes assessment of causality difficult.[73] Large randomized trials are needed to adequately control for potential confounders such as age, obesity, smoking, lipids, and alcohol use and to discern what specific effects HRT has on hemostasis.

In PEPI,[8] ERT and combined HRT reduced fibrinogen but no other hemostatic factors were measured. Limited data from observational studies and small trials suggest a host of hemostatic responses to HRT. Oral ERT may have a procoagulant effect with increased factor VII, prothrombin fragment 1 + 2 (F1+2), and fibrinopeptide A (FPA) levels, and a fibrinolytic effect via lowered fibrinogen, AT-III, and PAI-1. However, the existence and direction of causality in this relationship remain to be determined. Finally, no clinical trials of HRT have assessed clinical thrombotic events as endpoints.

Fibrinogen. Fibrinogen may influence atherogenesis and thrombosis via its role in the coagulation cascade as the substrate for thrombin, and its effects on platelet aggregation, blood viscosity, and proliferation and migration of fibroblasts and smooth muscle cells (SMCs). Fibrinogen appears to be an independent CHD risk factor in prospective cohort studies in men[74–78] and in women,[74] with a 2.3-fold increased CVD risk for those in the highest versus lowest tertiles in a meta-analysis.[79] Menopause is independently associated with higher fibrinogen levels in some[69, 80, 81] but not all[70, 82–84] cross-sectional studies.

In PEPI, fibrinogen was significantly higher in the placebo group compared with that in the active treatment groups (+0.10 g/L vs. −0.02 to 0.06 g/L) after 3 years, with no significant differences between HRT groups (see Table 31–1).[8] The maximum difference (+0.11 g/L) in fibrinogen levels may translate into a halved risk of CHD with HRT.[79]

In the Estradiol Clotting Factors Study,[85] a 1-year parallel group, placebo-controlled trial, 255 postmenopausal women were randomized to (1) cyclic transdermal estradiol (E_2) (0.05 mg per day on days 1 to 21, placebo on days 22 to 28) plus MPA (10 mg per day on days 10 to 21; placebo on other days); (2) continuous transdermal E_2 (0.05 mg per day × 28 days) plus MPA (10 mg per day on days 14 to 25, placebo on other days); or (3) placebo. Of the 188 women who completed the trial, 167 had complete hemostatic data. Continuous and cyclic transdermal E_2-MPA lowered fibrinogen (−21.5 mg/dL and −18 mg/dL, respectively), but the reduction was statistically significant only for continuous E_2-MPA. In contrast to PEPI, fibrinogen levels in the placebo group were relatively stable. No large RCTs have directly compared oral versus transdermal estrogen's effects on hemostatic variables such as fibrinogen.

Factor VII. Factor VII has a key role in tissue factor-mediated coagulation[86] and is another proposed marker of thrombotic risk. Its role as an independent CHD risk factor is uncertain based on limited prospective data in men,[75, 77] as is the relative importance of its mass or activity.[87] Menopause is independently associated with higher factor VIIc levels (which may reflect mass, activity, or both) in some[69, 70] but not all[80] observational studies. Using a recently developed assay specific for factor VII activity (FVIIa),[88] only age and menopausal status were independently associated with higher FVIIa levels in women.[71]

Oral ERT may be associated with increased factor VIIc,[10, 44, 89] a potentially procoagulant effect that may be attenuated by progestin, but clinical trial data are limited. In non–placebo-controlled trials, factor VII and factor VIIc levels were 20% higher than baseline with oral CEE (0.625 mg per day) but were unchanged with CEE-MPA[9] and CEE-norgestrel.[10] Sparse data suggest that transdermal ERT may differ from oral ERT in its effects on factor VII.[71] In the Estradiol Clotting Factors Study,[85] the continuous transdermal E_2-MPA group had significantly lower levels of factor VII (−15%), fibrinogen (−21.5%), AT-III (−6.9%), and protein S (−6.9%) versus placebo. Cyclic transdermal E_2-MPA had no effect on factor VII.

Other Coagulation Measures. Because of the complex dynamics of the clotting system, measurement of activation peptides (e.g., FPA and F1+2) and enzyme-inhibitor complexes (e.g., thrombin–AT-III complex [TAT]) may be more sensitive than changes in individual hemostatic factors in detecting the prethrombotic state.[90] In a randomized, double-blind, placebo-controlled crossover trial involving 29 postmenopausal women,[91] evidence of coagulation activation was seen after 3 months of oral CEE (0.625 mg or 1.25 mg per day), with significant dose-dependent increases in thrombin production (F1 + 2) and activity (FPA), and decreases in AT-III and protein S. In an open non–placebo-controlled crossover trial,[89] 23 women with surgical menopause were given oral CEE (0.625 mg per day) or transdermal E_2 (0.05 mg per day) for 6 weeks, then crossed over (with no washout period). Both groups had significantly higher factor VIIc, factor VIIAg, and F1 + 2 levels (but lower TAT levels). The CEE group had significant decreases in PAI-1 and AT-III. There are no clinical data for combined HRT's effects on markers of thrombin production and activity.

Fibrinolysis. Endogenous fibrinolysis is mediated by plasminogen activators (e.g., tissue-type plasminogen activator [t-PA]), and is inhibited by PAI-1. Higher PAI-1 or t-PA antigen levels, which may reflect impairment or imbalance of fibrinolysis, are linked to greater risk of CVD and mortality.[92] It is not clear if menopause is independently associated with increased PAI-1 and t-PA.[93, 94] In cross-sectional studies,[93, 94] HRT users had lower PAI-1 and t-PA antigen levels than nonusers. ERT users tended to have lower PAI-1 levels than combined HRT users.[93]

In two small non–placebo-controlled, crossover trials, PAI-1 levels were reduced approximately 50% from baseline after 1 month of oral CEE (0.625 mg per day) alone or plus MPA (2.5 mg per day),[51] or 6 weeks of oral CEE (0.625 mg per day).[89] Transdermal estrogen (0.05 mg per day or 0.10 mg per day) had no effect on PAI-1.[51, 89] Reduced PAI-1 with CEE was associated with significantly higher D-dimer levels, suggesting enhanced fibrinolysis.[51] However, little data exist regarding longer-term HRT and fibrinolysis. In a small 1-year non–placebo-controlled comparison trial (with no estrogen-only arm), PAI-1 levels fell transiently by 40% to 45% after 1 month of oral 17β-estradiol (2 mg) plus NA (0.5 mg) or megestrol acetate (2.5 mg or 5 mg), but returned to baseline levels by 12 months.[95]

Platelets/Prostacyclin. Sparse data exist concerning estrogen's effects on platelets and on prostacyclin (PGI_2), the endothelium-derived vasodilator and inhibitor of platelet aggregation. Estrogens, but not progestins, inhibit platelet aggregation in animals.[96, 97] Small trials in humans have had conflicting results regarding HRT's effects on platelet aggregation and thromboxane A_2.[98–100] Estrogen-treated atherosclerotic rabbits had greater PGI_2 synthesis and lower thromboxane B_2 levels,[101] but in vitro studies are inconsistent.[102–105]

HEMODYNAMIC AND VASCULAR EFFECTS

A growing body of literature suggests that estrogen is a vasoactive substance, with the presence of estrogen receptors (ERs) throughout the vasculature suggesting multiple target sites. Potential mechanisms include modulation of the vascular endothelium, direct effects on arterial SMCs, calcium channel antagonism, and effects on catechols and other vasoactive substances. These effects may be mediated by genomic, plasma membrane, and ion channel mechanisms and may vary with the target vessels, dose, and duration of estrogen.

Systemic/Peripheral Effects. In animal models, acute[106] and chronic[107] estrogen treatment raises cardiac output and lowers systemic vascular resistance, without affecting mean arterial pressure. In humans, peripheral vasodilation was observed with estrogen in forearm resistance vessels,[108] uterine arteries,[109] and carotid arteries.[110] In PEPI,[8] blood pressure was unchanged among treatment groups at 3 years (see Table 31–1).

Endothelial-Dependent Vasodilation. Estrogen may be cardioprotective in part owing to beneficial effects on the endothelium, which regulates vascular tone and coronary flow reserve, and has antiplatelet, antithrombotic, and fibrinolytic actions. Mediated by endothelium-derived relaxation factor/nitric oxide (NO),[111, 112] endothelial-dependent relaxation requires intact endothelium[113] and is impaired in the presence of atherosclerosis or coronary risk factors, resulting in paradoxical vasoconstriction by acetylcholine (Ach).[114]

Estrogen replacement may improve endothelial-dependent coronary vasodilation, as seen in animals ex vivo,[115] acutely,[116] and after 2 years of ERT in hyperlipidemic ovariectomized monkeys (independent of reduced plaque size).[117] In postmenopausal women, acute intravenous EE_2[118] or intracoronary 17β-estradiol[119, 120] reversed Ach-induced vasoconstriction of atherosclerotic coronary arteries and potentiated the vasodilator response of the microvasculature to Ach.[119, 120] This reaction occurred in the absence of systemic hemodynamic changes and cannot be due to changes in lipid levels or plaque size, given the acute administration of estrogen. Physiologic doses of intracoronary estrogen alone did not affect basal coronary diameter or blood flow[119, 120]; the epicardial coronary dilation seen by Reis and coworkers[118] may be due to the supraphysiologic estrogen dose, which has direct smooth muscle relaxant effects.[121] Enhanced endothelium-dependent vasodilation was also observed in the brachial artery with physiologic doses of acute intra-arterial 17β-estradiol.[122] Little data exist as to longer-term estrogen's effects on endothelial-dependent vasodilation in humans. In a double-blind, placebo-controlled crossover trial involving 13 postmenopausal women, 9 weeks of oral estradiol (1 mg or 2 mg per day) caused significantly improved endothelium-dependent, flow-mediated vasodilation in the brachial artery.[123]

Several mechanisms may explain these findings.

First, NO release[124] and synthesis[125–127] may be estrogen dependent, as seen in animal models. Roselli and associates[128] randomized 26 postmenopausal women to 2 years of transdermal estrogen (0.05 mg per day) plus cyclic NA (1 mg per day, days 1 to 12) or no HRT, and found evidence of significantly greater NO synthetase (NOS) activity in the HRT group. Second, estrogen may inhibit LDL oxidation, which contributes to endothelial dysfunction. In hyperlipidemic ovariectomized animals treated with estrogen, the degrees of LDL oxidative inhibition and endothelial-dependent vasodilation were highly correlated with plasma estrogen levels and were unrelated to lipid levels.[129] Third, estrogen may inhibit endothelium-derived vasoconstrictors like endothelin-1.[130, 131] In a 30-day, placebo-controlled trial involving 18 hypertensive or hyperlipidemic postmenopausal women, oral estrone sulfate (0.625 mg per day) or transdermal E_2 (0.05 mg per day) resulted in significantly lower endothelin-1 levels.[132]

Improved endothelial vasoreactivity[120] and reduced atherosclerosis[61] with estrogen appear to be gender-specific and thus may be mediated via ERs. ERs are ubiquitous in the vasculature and were recently identified in female human coronary artery SMCs, inversely to the degree of atherosclerosis.[133] ERs may be fewer in males (although ER immunostaining is equally intense in male and female endothelial cells),[134] or less responsive and capable of upregulation.[127, 135] In animals, longer-term estrogen therapy resulted in increased NOS messenger RNA,[127] suggesting the classic hormone/receptor interaction influencing transcriptional mechanisms. However, the acute,[116, 118–120] gender-specific[120] endothelial vasomotor response suggests the existence of other mechanisms, such as (1) a novel ER interaction leading to nontranscriptional signaling events[136]; (2) acute binding of estrogen to cell surface receptors, which are distinct from the classic ER, resulting in activation of intracellular second messenger pathways[137]; or (3) ER-independent mechanisms such as free radical scavenging[129, 136] (although this would seem less likely to be a sex-specific effect).

Sparse data exist regarding the influence of progestin on endothelial-dependent vasoreactivity. In female canine coronary arteries, estrogen's effect on endothelial vasoreactivity was inhibited by progestin.[138] In nonvascular animal tissue, progestin had no effect on NOS activity.[127] However, in humans, the increase in NOS activity with estrogen was not seen during the progestin period of cyclic combined HRT.[128]

Endothelium-Independent Vasodilation. Supraphysiologic estrogen doses cause endothelial-independent vasodilation in isolated animal coronary arteries,[121, 130, 139, 140] possibly via calcium channel inhibition. Physiologic estrogen doses, however, do not directly affect human SMCs[116] or cause acute coronary vasodilation.[119, 120] Estrogen also causes vasodilation by activating large-conductance, calcium- and voltage-activated potassium (K^+) channels, the primary K^+ channel in coronary smooth muscle, via cyclic guanosine monophosphate–dependent phosphorylation.[141]

Other Effects. Estrogen appears to be a calcium channel blocker[142] as seen ex vivo in animal coronary arteries[121, 130, 139] and in isolated ventricular cardiac myocytes.[143] Estrogen reduces SMC proliferation[61, 144, 145] and decreases myointimal hyperplasia in rabbit aortic allografts[146] and in hyperlipidemic animals.[59] After balloon injury of rat carotid arteries, reduced myointimal proliferation and *c-myc* expression was estrogen dependent and sex specific,[147] and estradiol accelerated re-endothelization and endothelial recovery, as reflected by greater NO production.[148] Estrogen may promote angiogenesis[149] and reduces collagen and elastin synthesis.[150, 151] In a canine model of ischemia/reperfusion injury, myocardial dysfunction and reperfusion arrhythmias were prevented by 17β-estradiol, in association with decreased release of free radicals and increased NO production.[152] Small trials reported a reduction in the frequency of angina with ERT in postmenopausal women with syndrome X[153] and lower serum homocysteine levels with combined HRT,[154] but further data are needed.

HRT and Myocardial Ischemia. Two small placebo-controlled clinical trials have examined estrogen's effect on myocardial ischemia in postmenopausal women with CHD, in whom antianginal medications were withdrawn. In one trial,[155] 11 women given sublingual 17β-estradiol (1 mg) or placebo 40 minutes before exercise treadmill testing had increased time to 1-mm ST segment depression (456 vs. 579 seconds, respectively; $P < 0.004$) and total exercise time (569 vs. 658 seconds, $P < 0.01$). Possible mechanisms include direct coronary vasodilation or reduced peripheral resistance (resting blood pressure tended to be lower after 17β-estradiol). In another trial ($n = 16$), no differences in hemodynamics or treadmill performance were observed after 24 hours of physiologic HRT (transdermal estradiol, 0.050 mg per day).[156] Differences in study populations (as reflected in markedly different baseline treadmill performance) and estrogen dose may have contributed to the contrasting results. Long-term HRT's effects on treadmill performance or other functional measures of myocardial ischemia are not known.

Insulin. Hyperinsulinemia appears to be an independent risk factor for CHD[157] that may be modifiable by HRT. In PEPI,[8] all groups had lower postchallenge insulin levels; however, the HRT groups had significant decreases in fasting glucose and nonsignificant reductions in fasting insulin levels, which may be a better marker for insulin resistance than postchallenge insulin levels (see Table 31–1).

EPIDEMIOLOGIC OVERVIEW

Estrogen-Only HRT. The weight of epidemiologic evidence supports a lower risk of CHD with postmenopausal ERT,[158] with significant risk reductions seen in prospective cohort studies, population or community-based case-control studies, and cross-sectional angiographic studies (Table 31–3). Combining all study types, the relative risk (RR) of CHD of ever-users versus never-users was 0.64 (95% confidence interval [CI], 0.59 to 0.68); the RR for current users versus nonusers was 0.50 (95% CI, 0.45 to 0.59).[158] Risk reduction was not seen only in hospital-based case-control studies, which are most susceptible to selection bias. A meta-analysis by Grady and colleagues[159] reported a similar RR of 0.65 (95% CI, 0.59 to 0.71) of CHD in ever-users versus nonusers. In a recent updated report from the Nurses' Health Study, a prospective cohort study of 59,337 women followed for 16 years, ERT users had an adjusted RR of CHD of 0.60 (95% CI, 0.43 to 0.83) versus never-users.[160]

Combined HRT. Data are limited but in observational studies,[161–163] combined HRT was associated with a reduced risk of myocardial infarction (MI) similar to that with ERT, with an RR of CHD of 0.65 to 0.80 in a meta-analysis.[159] In the Nurses' Health Study, CHD risk was comparably reduced in users of combined HRT (adjusted RR, 0.39; 95% CI, 0.19 to 0.78) and ERT (adjusted RR, 0.60; 95% CI, 0.43 to 0.83) versus never-users.[160] In some[57–60] but not all[61] animal models, reduced atherosclerosis with estrogen was unaffected by an added progestin.

Secondary Prevention. Limited data suggest that HRT is at least as effective in women with pre-existing CHD as in those free of CHD. ERT was an independent predictor of 10-year survival in postmenopausal women with CHD on angiography, with an RR of 0.16 (95% CI, 0.04 to 0.66).[164] Bush and associates[54] found that in women with CVD, the death rate in estrogen users was 13.8/10,000 versus 66.3/10,000 in nonusers (compared with death rates of 12.8/10,000 vs. 30.2/10,000, respectively, in women without CVD). In other studies, subgroups of women with prior MI[53] or MI or angina[165] had similar risk reductions with HRT as did women without CHD. In a meta-analysis, the largest gains in life expectancy with HRT were in women with CHD (+2.1 years with ERT, and +0.9 to +2.2 years with combined HRT).[159] The Heart and Estrogen/progestin Replacement Study addresses HRT's role in secondary prevention of CHD (see later).

TABLE 31–3 • Observational Studies of Coronary Heart Disease and Postmenopausal Estrogen Replacement Therapy: Comparison of Women Who Have Ever Used Estrogen (Ever-Use) with Never-Users

Type of Study	*N*	Summary RR	95% CI
Prospective cohort	16	0.50	[0.63, 0.77]
Population/community-based case control	9	0.76	[0.66, 0.88]
Cross-sectional angiographic studies*	4	0.39	[0.33, 0.47]
Hospital-based case control	6	1.33	[0.93, 1.31]
All studies combined	**35**	**0.64**	**[0.59, 0.68]**

*Comparing women with coronary stenoses to those without.
RR, relative risk; CI, confidence interval.
Adapted from Grodstein F, Stampfer M. The epidemiology of coronary heart disease and estrogen replacement in postmenopausal women. Prog Cardiovasc Dis 1995; 38:199–210.

Stroke. There are sparse data regarding HRT and stroke risk. In a meta-analysis, estrogen users had a pooled RR of stroke of 0.96 (95% CI, 0.82 to 1.13).[159] In the Nurses' Health Study,[160] ERT (adjusted RR, 1.27; 95% CI, 0.95 to 1.69) or combined HRT (adjusted RR, 1.09; 95% CI, 0.66 to 1.80) was not associated with stroke, although there were trends of increased stroke risk with higher estrogen doses and a higher risk of ischemic stroke in current users. Stroke mortality, however, may be lower in HRT users.[159, 166] In the Nurses' Health Study, which had a small number of deaths owing to stroke, current HRT users had an RR of stroke mortality of 0.68 (95% CI, 0.39 to 1.16).[167]

Venous Thromboembolism. In large case-control studies, current HRT users had an odds ratio (OR) of 3.5 (95% CI, 1.8 to 7.0)[168] and 3.6 (95% CI, 1.6 to 7.8)[169] of deep venous thrombosis or pulmonary embolism (PE) versus nonusers. In the Nurses' Health Study,[170] current users had an RR of PE of 2.1 (95% CI, 1.2 to 3.8). There were no apparent differences in risk between oral and transdermal estrogen or between ERT and combined HRT, but data are limited.[168] While these results support an increased risk of venous thromboembolic events with HRT, the incidence rates of these outcomes are low.

Benefits/Risks. The value of HRT lies in the net balance between its potential benefits (CHD, osteoporosis, menopausal symptoms) and potential risks (endometrial cancer, breast cancer, gallstones, venous thromboembolism). Adding progestin protects the endometrium but less is known about its effects on other clinical endpoints. In evaluating HRT's benefit/risk ratio, it is essential to distinguish relative risks from absolute risks. In white women, the cumulative absolute risk of cause-specific death from ages 50 to 94 years is 31% from CHD, 2.8% from breast cancer, 2.8% from hip fractures, and 0.7% from endometrial cancer.[171] Whether HRT increases breast cancer risk remains controversial.[172–174] Although not a uniform finding, some studies suggest a moderate risk may exist especially with longer therapy, that is, 30% to 100% after 10 to 15 years of use.[167, 173, 175] Progestin does not appear to alter the effect of estrogen on breast cancer risk.[175, 176]

Because CVD is responsible for such a large propor-

TABLE 31–4 • Relative Risk of Selected Conditions for a 50-Year-Old White Woman Treated with Long-Term Hormone Replacement

	Relative Risk (%)*	
Condition	*Estrogen Therapy*	*Estrogen plus Progestin*
Coronary heart disease	0.65	0.65 to 0.80
Stroke	0.96	0.96
Hip fracture	0.75	0.75
Breast cancer	1.25	1.25 to 2.00
Endometrial cancer	8.22	1.00

*"Best" estimates of the relative risk for developing each condition in long-term hormone users compared with nonusers. These estimates were used in our model of the risks and benefits of hormone therapy. The same relative-risk estimate was used for dying of each condition in long-term users compared with nonusers except for endometrial cancer, where a relative risk of 3.0 was used.

From Grady D, Rubin SM, Pettiti DB, et al. Hormone therapy to prevent disease and prolong life in postmenopausal women. Ann Intern Med 1992; 117:1016–1037.

tion of morbidity and mortality in women, HRT's impact on CVD risk will heavily weight the net direction of benefit/risk analyses. Grady and associates[159] reported a net benefit with HRT (Table 31–4), which is modified by baseline risk factor status and by progestin's potential influence on CHD risk (Table 31–5). The greatest gains in life expectancy with HRT are in women at risk for CHD or with known CHD, and the least benefit is in women at high risk for breast cancer, especially if at low risk for CHD. In a decision analysis,[177] the risk of CHD versus breast cancer also determined the net benefit of HRT for an individual woman. Women with at least one CHD risk factor, regardless of breast cancer risk, had a gain in life expectancy with HRT. Those without any risk factors for CHD or hip fracture but with two first-degree relatives with breast cancer would not benefit from HRT (Fig. 31–3).

TABLE 31–5 • Net Change in Life Expectancy for a 50-Year-Old White Woman Treated with Long-Term Hormone Replacement

		Net Change in Life Expectancy		
	Life Expectancy	*Estrogen*	*E + P**	*E + P†*
Variable	←	y		→
White-woman, 50 years old				
No risk factors	82.8	+0.9	+1.0	+0.1
With hysterectomy	82.8	+1.1		
With history of coronary heart disease	76.0	+2.1	+2.2	+0.9
At risk for coronary heart disease	79.6	+1.5	+1.6	+0.6
At risk for breast cancer	82.3	+0.7	+0.8	−0.5
At risk for hip fracture	82.4	+1.0	+1.1	+0.2

*Assuming that the addition of a progestin to the estrogen regimen does not alter any of the relative risks for disease seen with estrogen therapy, except to prevent the increased risk due to endometrial cancer (relative risk for endometrial cancer estimated to be 1.0).

†Assuming that the addition of a progestin to the estrogen regimen provides only two thirds of the coronary heart disease risk reduction afforded by estrogen therapy (relative risk for coronary heart disease estimated to be 0.8) and relative risk for breast cancer in treated women is 2.0.

E + P, estrogen plus progestin.

From Grady D, Rubin SM, Pettiti DB, et al. Hormone therapy to prevent disease and prolong life in postmenopausal women. Ann Intern Med 1992; 117:1016–1037.

These analyses are of particular interest in light of recent data from the Nurses' Health Study[167] examining HRT's effect on mortality. Current HRT users had a lower risk of death (adjusted RR, 0.63; 95% CI, 0.56 to 0.70) than never-users. This risk reduction was partly attenuated after more than 10 years of use (RR, 0.80; 95% CI, 0.67 to 0.96) owing to an increase in breast cancer mortality. The largest risk reduction was in current HRT users with at least one CHD risk factor (RR, 0.51; 95% CI, 0.45 to 0.57). No clear benefit was observed in those with no cardiac risk factors (RR, 0.89; 95% CI, 0.62 to 1.28).

Limitations of Observational Epidemiologic Studies. Observational epidemiologic studies support a reduced risk of CHD with postmenopausal HRT, but for small effects, the amount of selection bias and uncontrolled confounding may be as large as the possible benefits. Estrogen users have fewer cardiac risk factors, healthier lifestyles, and greater medical compliance and access to medical care than nonusers.[178–180] Despite statistical control for many of these variables, residual confounding by these factors may contribute

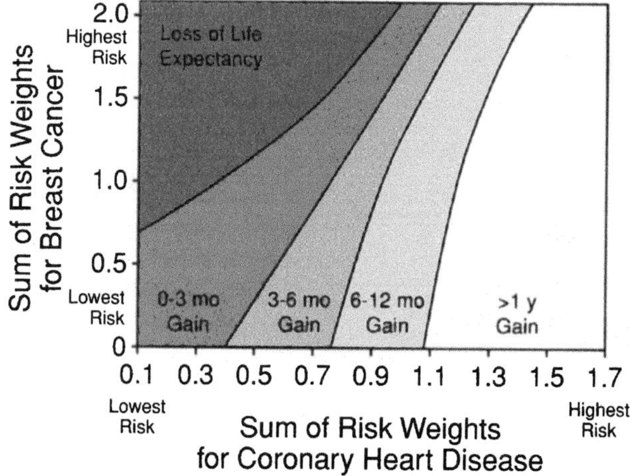

Figure 31–3 Magnitude of gains from hormone replacement therapy associated with different risks for developing coronary heart disease and breast cancer. Each axis represents the sum of risk weights for coronary heart disease and breast cancer, respectively, among women whose risk score for hip fracture is 0 (corresponding to average hip fracture risk among American women). See also Table 1 in Reference 177 to calculate an individual's sum of risk weights. (From Col NF, Eckman MH, Karas RH, et al. Patient-specific decisions about hormone replacement therapy in postmenopausal women. JAMA 1997; 277:1140–1147. Copyright 1997, American Medical Association.)

to the risk reduction observed in these studies. Thus, large RCTs are needed to confirm or refute these findings.

Ongoing Clinical Trials. The National Institutes of Health–sponsored WHI is a double-blind, placebo-controlled, randomized primary prevention trial involving more than 27,000 women in the HRT component. WHI will assess the effects of HRT (0.625 mg per day of oral CEE plus 2.5 mg per day MPA in women with an intact uterus, or 0.625 mg per day of oral CEE for women who have had a hysterectomy) on CHD risk, breast cancer, osteoporosis, and Alzheimer's disease. With its planned 9-year follow-up, WHI will add critical information as to the benefit/risk ratio of long-term HRT.

Heart and Estrogen/progestin Replacement Study (HERS). This trial addressed the role of HRT in secondary prevention of CHD.[183] A total of 2763 postmenopausal women (mean age 66.7 years) with intact uteri and pre-existing CHD (defined by history of MI [17%], ≥ 50% stenosis in at least one coronary artery on angiography, coronary artery bypass grafting [42%], or percutaneous transluminal coronary angioplasty [45%]) were randomized to 0.625 mg of oral CEE plus 2.5 mg of progesterone daily, or placebo. Over 4.1 years of mean follow-up, 348 women reached the primary combined endpoint of nonfatal MI or CHD death, with no observed difference in overall risk between the two randomized comparison groups (RR, 0.99; 95% CI, 0.80 to 1.22). A time-trend analysis of the data suggested a possible increase in risk of CHD events in the first year with a decrease in risk in subsequent years, which the authors speculated may be due to chance, or to an early risk with HRT (e.g., due to prothrombotic effects) that is later outweighed by benefits on atherosclerosis or other disease mechanisms. The study was not adequately powered to detect differences in other endpoints such as cancer and total mortality.

There are several possible explanations for the discrepancy between the null results of the HERS trial and the apparent benefit of HRT in secondary prevention suggested in prior observational studies, albeit with relatively limited data. Observational studies are subject to selection bias and uncontrolled confounding, which may at least partially explain the apparent benefit associated with HRT use. Study populations in observational studies tended to be younger, with a higher prevalence of estrogen-only HRT. The HERS trial tested only combined HRT with estrogen and continuous oral medroxyprogesterone acetate, which may attenuate estrogen's beneficial effects on HDL,[8] atherosclerosis, and endothelial-dependent vasodilation.[138] It is also plausible that a beneficial effect of HRT in secondary prevention may become evident with longer duration of follow-up, especially if its major mechanisms of benefit are antiatherogenic. The time-trend analysis must be interpreted with caution but raises the possibility of a later benefit of treatment. Furthermore, the HERS trial may have been underpowered to detect the most plausible small-to-moderate benefit of HRT, because CHD event rates were lower than anticipated. Although HERS contributes important information, more data are needed about the role of HRT in secondary prevention, particularly over longer duration of follow-up, and addressing possible differences between estrogen-only HRT and combined estrogen-progestin regimens.

Trials of Selective Estrogen Receptor Modulators (SERMs). Because raloxifene appears to function as an antiestrogen in breast and uterine tissue but as an estrogen agonist in bone and lipid metabolism,[184] the SERMs have provoked great interest as "designer estrogens" that may favorably alter the benefit/risk ratio of HRT. The tissue-specific actions of raloxifene may be mediated in part by a novel pathway for estrogen receptor–mediated gene activation.[185] In a 24-month placebo-controlled, randomized clinical trial involving 601 postmenopausal women, raloxifene significantly reduced LDL (median change from baseline −6.2 ± 0.8%; −10.1 ± 1.4%, and −14.1 ± 1.6% for 30, 60, or 150 mg daily of raloxifene, respectively) but had no effect on HDL or triglycerides; increased bone mass density; and had no adverse uterine effects.[186] In a 6-month placebo-controlled trial involving 390 postmenopausal women,[187] the effects of raloxifene (60 mg/d or 120 mg/d) and combined HRT (CEE 0.625 mg/d plus MPA 2.5 mg/d) on lipids and coagulation parameters were compared. No differences were observed between raloxifene dosages. Raloxifene and HRT reduced LDL to a similar degree (−12% and −14%, respectively; both $P < 0.001$ vs. placebo). Raloxifene had no effect on HDL (vs. 11% increase with HRT), and increased HDL_2 by 15% to 17% ($P < 0.05$) compared with 33% by HRT ($P < 0.001$ vs. placebo). Triglycerides were unaffected by raloxifene but increased 20% with HRT ($P < 0.001$ vs. placebo). Raloxifene lowered Lp(a) to a lesser degree than did HRT (7% to 8% vs. 19%, both $P < 0.001$ vs. placebo). Raloxifene lowered fibrinogen by 12% to 14% ($P < 0.001$), whereas HRT had no effect, in contrast with the PEPI data.[8] PAI-1 was unaffected by raloxifene but increased 29% with HRT ($P < 0.001$); however, no changes in FPA or F_{1+2} were observed with either therapy. Interpretation of this trial is somewhat limited by the lack of an estrogen-only arm.

SERMs are potentially promising new therapies in HRT, but more data are clearly needed. Most important, the cardioprotective effect of estrogen itself has yet to be proven. Whether or not this is borne out in trials such as WHI, clinical trials have already been launched to determine if raloxifene is cardioprotective and to what degree. Compared with estrogen, raloxifene has a less impressive overall effect on lipids (and bone mass density), particularly because raloxifene does not increase HDL. In animal models, raloxifene reduces atherosclerosis to a lesser degree than estrogen.[188, 189] It remains to be seen if the potential reduction in risk of breast and uterine cancer with raloxifene is offset by lesser cardioprotective effects, or if raloxifene will prove to be an equal or better alternative to traditional HRT for some or all women.

CONCLUSION

ERT is likely to decrease the risk of CHD, as strongly suggested by observational epidemiologic data as well as accumulating data regarding plausible biologic mechanisms by which estrogen may inhibit atherosclerosis, decrease plaque vulnerability, reduce thrombus formation, and improve vascular responsiveness. These data primarily derive from observational studies, animal or in vitro studies, and evaluation of biologic intermediates such as lipids. It remains to be seen whether these effects will translate into improved clinical outcomes.[182] Additional data are also needed regarding the effect of an added progestin; the optimal dose, type, and duration of hormone used; whether HRT's benefits are universal or confined primarily to subgroups of women (e.g., by age or risk of CHD); whether HRT is more beneficial than other interventions, such as lipid-lowering agents; effects on quality of life; and the benefit/risk balance of long-term HRT. Novel estrogen-like compounds such as raloxifene represent intriguing new areas for research. HRT is a promising and exciting intervention in maintaining health in postmenopausal women, but data from large RCTs are urgently needed to address the many questions remaining about HRT.

REFERENCES

1. US Senate Special Committee on Aging. Aging America: Trends and Projections. Washington DC, US Department of Health and Human Services, 1988.
2. Heart and Stroke Facts. Dallas, TX, American Heart Association, 1992.
3. Matthews KA, Meilahn E, Kuller LH, et al. Menopause and risk factors for coronary artery disease. N Engl J Med 1989; 321:641–646.
4. Stevenson JC, Crook D, Godsland IF. Influence of age and menopause on serum lipids and lipoproteins in healthy women. Atherosclerosis 1993; 98:83–90.
5. Bush TL, Miller VT. Effects of pharmacologic agents used during menopause: Impact on lipids and lipoproteins. *In* Mishell DR (ed). Menopause: Physiology and Pharmacology. Chicago, Year Book, 1987, pp 187–208.
6. Sacks FM, Walsh BW. The effects of reproductive hormones on serum lipoproteins: Unresolved issues in biology and clinical practice. Ann NY Acad Sci 1990; 592:272–285.
7. Walsh BW, Schiff I, Rosner B, et al. Effects of postmenopausal estrogen replacement on the concentrations and metabolism of plasma lipoproteins. N Engl J Med 1991; 325:1196–1204.
8. The Writing Group for the PEPI Trial. Effects of estrogen or estrogen/progestin regimens on heart disease risk factors in postmenopausal women: The Postmenopausal Estrogen/Progestin Interventions (PEPI) Trial. JAMA 1995; 273:199–208.
9. Lobo RA, Pickar JH, Wild RA, et al, for the Menopause Study Group. Metabolic impact of adding medroxyprogesterone acetate to conjugated estrogen therapy in postmenopausal women. Obstet Gynecol 1994; 84:987–995.
10. Medical Research Council's General Practice Research Framework. Randomized comparison of oestrogen versus oestrogen plus progestogen hormone replacement therapy in women with hysterectomy. BMJ 1996; 312:473–478.
11. Rijpkema AHM, van der Sanden AA, Ruijs AHC. Effects of post-menopausal oestrogen-progestogen replacement therapy on serum lipids and lipoproteins: A review. Maturitas 1990; 12:259–285.
12. Tikkanen MJ, Nikkilä EA, Kuusi T, Sipinen S. High-density lipoprotein-2 and hepatic lipase: Reciprocal changes produced by estrogen and norgestrel. J Clin Endocrinol Metab 1982; 54:1113–1117.
13. Windler EET, Kovanen PT, Chao Y-S, et al. The estradiol-stimulated lipoprotein receptor of rat liver. J Biol Chem 1980; 255:10464–10471.
14. Veldhuis JD, Gwynne JT. Estrogen regulates low-density lipoprotein metabolism by cultured swine granulosa cells. Endocrinology 1985; 117:1321–1327.
15. Kushwaha RS, Born KM. Effect of estrogen and progesterone on the hepatic cholesterol 7-alpha-hydoxylase activity in ovariectomized baboons. Biochim et Biophys Acta 1991; 1084:300–302.
16. Chetkowski RJ, Meldrum DR, Steingold KA, et al. Biologic effects of transdermal estradiol. N Engl J Med 314:1615–1620.
17. Stanczyk FZ, Shoupe D, Nunez V, et al. A randomized comparison of nonoral estradiol delivery in postmenopausal women. Am J Obstet Gynecol 1988; 159:1540–1546.
18. Moorjani S, Dupont A, Labrie F, et al. Changes in lipoprotein and apolipoprotein composition in relation to oral versus percutaneous administration of estrogen alone or in cyclic association with utrogestan in menopausal women. J Clin Endocrinol Metab 1991; 73:373–379.
19. Tikkanen MJ, Nikkilä EA, Kuusi T, Sipinen S. Different effects of two progestins on plasma high-density lipoprotein (HDL_2) and postheparin plasma hepatic lipase activity. Atherosclerosis 1981; 40:365–369.
20. Tikkanen MJ, Kuusi T, Nikkilä EA, Sipinen S. Postmenopausal hormone replacement therapy: Effects of progestogens on serum lipids and lipoproteins—a review. Maturitas 1986; 8:7–17.
21. Silfverstolpe G, Gustafson A, Samsioe G, Svanborg A. Lipid metabolic studies in oophorectomised women: Effects on serum lipids and lipoproteins of three synthetic progestogens. Maturitas 1982; 4:103–111.
22. Miller VT, Muesing RA, LaRosa JC, et al. Effects of conjugated equine estrogen with and without three different progestogens on lipoproteins, high-density lipoprotein subfractions, and apolipoprotein A-1. Obstet Gynecol 1991; 77:235–240.
23. Ottoson UB, Johansson BG, von Schoultz B. Subfractions of high-density lipoprotein cholesterol: A comparison between progestogens and natural progesterone. Am J Obstet Gynecol 1985; 151:746–750.
24. Fahraeus L, Larsson-Cohn U, Wallentin L. L-norgestrel and progesterone have different influences on plasma lipoproteins. Eur J Clin Invest 1983; 13:447–453.
25. Speroff L, Rowan J, Symons J, et al, for the CHART Study Group. The comparative effect on bone density, endometrium, and lipids of continuous hormones as replacement therapy (CHART Study). JAMA 1996; 276:1397–1403.
26. Munk-Jensen N, Ulrich LG, Obel EB, et al. Continuous combined and sequential estradiol and norethindrone acetate treatment of postmenopausal women: Effect on plasma lipoproteins in a two-year placebo-controlled trial. Am J Obstet Gynecol 1994; 171:132–138.
27. Bass KM, Newschaffer CJ, Klag MJ, Bush TL. Plasma lipoprotein levels as predictors of cardiovascular death in women. Arch Intern Med 1993; 153:2209–2216.
28. Walsh JME, Grady D. Treatment of hyperlipidemia in women. JAMA 1995; 274:1152–1158.

29. Gordon DJ, Probstfield JL, Garrison RJ, et al. High-density lipoprotein cholesterol and cardiovascular disease: Four prospective American studies. Circulation 1989; 79:8–15.
30. Scandinavian Simvastatin Survival Study Group. Randomized trial of cholesterol lowering in 4444 patients with coronary heart disease: The Scandinavian Simvastatin Survival Study (4S). Lancet 1994; 344:1383–1389.
31. Sacks FM, Pfeffer MA, Moye LA, et al, for the Cholesterol and Recurrent Events Trial Investigators. The effect of pravastatin on coronary events after myocardial infarction in patients with average cholesterol levels. N Engl J Med 1996; 335:1001–1009.
32. Schaefer EJ, Foster DM, Zech LA, et al. The effects of estrogen administration on plasma lipoprotein metabolism in premenopausal females. J Clin Endocrinol Metab 1983; 57:262–267.
33. Walsh BW, Sacks FM. Effects of low-dose oral contraceptives on very-low-density and low-density lipoprotein metabolism. J Clin Invest 1993; 91:2126–2132.
34. Ridker PM. An epidemiologic reassessment of lipoprotein(a) and atherothrombotic risk. Trends Cardiovasc Med 1995; 5:225–229.
35. Schaefer EJ, Lamon-Fava S, Jenner JL, et al. Lipoprotein(a) levels and risk of coronary heart disease in men: The Lipid Research Clinics Coronary Primary Prevention Trial. JAMA 1994; 271:999–1003.
36. Bostom AG, Cupples LA, Jenner JL, et al. Elevated plasma lipoprotein(a) and coronary heart disease in men aged 55 years and younger: A prospective study. JAMA 1996; 276:544–548.
37. Ridker PM, Hennekens CH, Stampfer MJ. A prospective study of lipoprotein(a) and the risk of myocardial infarction. JAMA 1993; 270:2195–2199.
38. Fortmann SP, Marcovina SM. Lipoprotein(a), a clinically elusive lipoprotein particle. Circulation 1997; 95:295–296.
39. Brown SA, Hutchinson R, Morrisett J, et al, for the ARIC Study Group. Plasma lipid, lipoprotein cholesterol, and apoprotein distribution in selected US communities: The Atherosclerosis Risk in Communities (ARIC) Study. Arterioscler Thromb 1993; 13:1139–1158.
40. Jenner JL, Ordovas JM, Lamon-Fava S, et al. Effects of age, sex, and menopausal status on plasma lipoprotein(a) levels: The Framingham Offspring Study. Circulation 1993; 87:1135–1141.
41. Bostom AG, Gagnon DR, Cupples LA, et al. A prospective investigation of elevated lipoprotein(a) detected by electrophoresis and cardiovascular disease in women: The Framingham Heart Study. Circulation 1994; 90:1688–1695.
42. Orth-Gomér K, Mittleman MA, Schenck-Gustafsson K, et al. Lipoprotein(a) as a determinant of coronary heart disease in young women. Circulation 1997; 95:329–334.
43. Sunayama S, Daida H, Mokuno H, et al. Lack of increased coronary atherosclerotic risk due to elevated lipoprotein(a) in women $\geq$ 55 years of age. Circulation 1996; 94:1263–1268.
43a. Espeland MA, Marcovina SM, Miller V, et al, for the PEPI Investigators. Effect of postmenopausal hormone therapy on lipoprotein(a) concentration. Circulation 1998; 97:979–986.
44. Nabulsi AA, Folsom AR, White A, et al, for the Atherosclerosis Risk in Communities Study Investigators. Association of hormone-replacement therapy with various cardiovascular risk factors in postmenopausal women. N Engl J Med 1993; 328:1069–1075.
45. Soma MR, Osnago-Gadda I, Paoletti R, et al. The lowering of lipoprotein(a) induced by estrogen plus progesterone replacement therapy in postmenopausal women. Arch Intern Med 1993; 153:1462–1468.
46. Sacks FM, McPherson R, Walsh BW. Effect of postmenopausal estrogen replacement on plasma Lp(a) lipoprotein concentrations. Arch Intern Med 1994; 154:1106–1110.
47. Shewmon DA, Stock JL, Rosen CJ, et al. Tamoxifen and estrogen lower circulating lipoprotein(a) concentrations in healthy postmenopausal women. Arterioscler Thromb 1994; 14:1586–1593.
48. Kim CJ, Jang HC, Cho DH, Min YK. Effects of hormone replacement therapy on lipoprotein(a) and lipids in postmenopausal women. Arterioscler Thromb 1994; 14:275–281.
49. Haines C, Chung T, Chang A, et al. Effect of oral estradiol on Lp(a) and other lipoproteins in postmenopausal women: A randomized, double-blind, placebo-controlled crossover study. Arch Intern Med 1996; 156:866–872.
50. Taskinen M-R, Puolakka J, Pyorala T, et al. Hormone replacement therapy lowers plasma Lp(a) concentrations: Comparison of cyclic transdermal and continuous estrogen-progestin regimens. Atheroscler Thromb Vasc Biol 1996; 16:1215–1221.
51. Koh KK, Minemoyer R, Bui MN, et al. Effects of hormone replacement therapy on fibrinolysis in postmenopausal women. N Engl J Med 1997; 336:683–690.
52. Guetta V, Cannon RO. Cardiovascular effects of estrogen and lipid-lowering therapies in postmenopausal women. Circulation 1996; 93:1928–1937.
53. Gruchow HW, Anderson AJ, Barboriak JJ, Sobocinski KA. Postmenopausal use of estrogen and occlusion of coronary arteries. Am Heart J 1988; 115:954–963.
54. Bush TL, Barrett-Connor E, Cowan LD, et al. Cardiovascular mortality and noncontraceptive use of estrogens in women: Results from the Lipid Research Clinics Program Follow-up Study. Circulation 1987; 75:1102–1109.
55. Barrett-Connor E, Bush TL. Estrogen and coronary heart disease in women. JAMA 1991; 265:1861–1867.
56. Stampfer MJ, Colditz GA, Willett WC, et al. Postmenopausal estrogen therapy and cardiovascular disease: Ten-year follow-up from the Nurses' Health Study. N Engl J Med 1991; 325:756–762.
57. Adams MR, Kaplan JR, Manuck SB, et al. Inhibition of coronary artery atherosclerosis by 17-beta estradiol in ovariectomized monkeys: Lack of an effect of added progesterone. Arteriosclerosis 1990; 10:1051–1057.
58. Wagner JD, Clarkson TB, St Clair RW, et al. Estrogen and progesterone replacement therapy reduces low-density lipoprotein accumulation in the coronary arteries of surgically postmenopausal cynomolgus monkeys. J Clin Invest 1991; 88:1995–2002.
59. Clarkson TB, Shively CA, Morgan TM, et al. Oral contraceptives and coronary artery atherosclerosis of cynomolgus monkeys. Obstet Gynecol 1990; 75:217–222.
60. Haarbo J, Leth-Espensen P, Stender S, Christiansen C. Estrogen monotherapy and combined estrogen-progestogen replacement therapy attenuate aortic accumulation of cholesterol in ovariectomized cholesterol-fed rabbits. J Clin Invest 1991; 87:1274–1279.
61. Hanke H, Hanke S, Finking G, et al. Different effects of estrogen and progesterone on experimental atherosclerosis in female versus male rabbits: Quantification of cellular proliferation by bromodeoxyuridine. Circulation 1996; 94:175–181.
62. Hough JL, Zilversmit DB. Effect of 17-beta estradiol on aortic cholesterol content and metabolism in cholesterol-fed rabbits. Arteriosclerosis 1986; 6:57–63.
63. Sugioka K, Shimosegawa Y, Nakano M. Estrogens as natural antioxidants of membrane phospholipid peroxidation. FEBS Lett 1987; 210:37–39.
64. Yagi K, Komura S. Inhibitory effect of female hormones on lipid peroxidation. Biochem Int 1986; 13:1051–1055.
65. Huber LA, Scheffler E, Poll T, et al. 17β-estradiol inhibits LDL oxidation and cholesteryl ester formation in cultured macrophages. Free Radic Res Commun 1990; 8:167–173.
66. Mazière C, Auclair M, Ronveaux M-F, et al. Estrogens inhibit copper and cell-mediated modification of low-density lipoprotein. Atherosclerosis 1991; 89:175–182.
67. Nègre-Salvayre A, Pieraggi M-T, Mabile L, et al. Protective effect of 17β-estradiol against the cytotoxicity of minimally oxidized LDL to cultured bovine aortic endothelial cells. Atherosclerosis 1993; 99:207–217.
68. Sack MN, Rader DJ, Cannon RO. Oestrogen and inhibition of oxidation of low-density lipoproteins in postmenopausal women. Lancet 1994; 343:269–270.
69. Meade TW, Haines AP, Imeson JD, et al. Menopausal status and haemostatic variables. Lancet 1983; 1:22–24.
70. Scarabin P-Y, Plu-Bureau G, Bara L, et al. Haemostatic variables and menopausal status: Influence of hormone replacement therapy. Thromb Haemostas 1993; 70:584–587.
71. Scarabin P-Y, Vissac A-M, Kirzin J-M, et al. Population correlates of coagulation factor VII: Importance of age, sex, and menopausal status as determinants of activated factor VII. Arterioscler Thromb Vasc Biol 1996; 16:1170–1176.

72. Meade TW, Dyer S, Howarth DJ, et al. Antithrombin III and procoagulant activity: Sex differences and effects of the menopause. Br J Haematol 1990; 74:77–81.
73. Chae CU, Ridker PM, Manson JE. Postmenopausal hormone replacement therapy and cardiovascular disease. Thromb Haemost 1997; 78:770–780.
74. Kannel WB, D'Agostino RB, Belanger AJ. Update on fibrinogen as a cardiovascular risk factor. Ann Epidemiol 1992; 2:457–466.
75. Meade TW, Mellows S, Brozovic M, et al. Haemostatic function and ischaemic heart disease: Principal results of the Northwick Park Heart Study. Lancet 1986; 2:533–537.
76. Wilhelmsen L, Svärdsudd K, Korsan-Bengtsen K, et al. Fibrinogen as a risk factor for stroke and myocardial infarction. N Engl J Med 1984; 311:501–505.
77. Heinrich J, Balleisen L, Schulte H, et al. Fibrinogen and factor VII in the prediction of coronary risk: Results from the PROCAM Study in healthy men. Arterioscler Thromb 1994; 14:54–59.
78. Yarnell JWG, Baker IA, Sweetnam PM, et al. Fibrinogen, viscosity, and white blood cell count are major risk factors for ischemic heart disease: The Caerphilly and Speedwell Collaborative Heart Disease Studies. Circulation 1991; 83:836–844.
79. Ernst E, Resch KL. Fibrinogen as a cardiovascular risk factor: A meta-analysis and review of the literature. Ann Intern Med 1993; 118:956–963.
80. Folsom AR, Wu KK, Davis CE, et al. Population correlates of plasma fibrinogen and factor VII—putative cardiac risk factors. Atherosclerosis 1991; 91:191–205.
81. Lee AJ, Lowe GOD, Smith WCS, Turnstall-Pedoe H. Plasma fibrinogen in women: Relationships with oral contraception, the menopause, and hormone replacement therapy. Br J Haematol 1993; 83:616–621.
82. Balleisen L, Bailey J, Epping P-H, et al. Epidemiological study on factor VII, factor VIII, and fibrinogen in an industrial population: I. Baseline data on the relation to age, gender, body weight, smoking, alcohol, pill-using, and menopause. Thromb Haemost 1985; 54:475–479.
83. Bonithon-Kopp C, Scarabin P-Y, Darne B, et al. Menopause-related changes in lipoproteins and some other cardiovascular risk factors. Int J Epidemiol 1990; 19:42–48.
84. Meilahn EN, Kuller LH, Matthews KA, Kiss JE. Hemostatic factors according to menopausal status and use of hormone replacement therapy. Ann Epidemiol 1992; 2:445–455.
85. The Writing Group for the Estradiol Clotting Factors Study. Effects on haemostasis of hormone replacement therapy with transdermal estradiol and oral sequential medroxyprogesterone acetate: A 1-year, double-blind, placebo-controlled study. Thromb Haemost 1996; 75:476–480.
86. Morrissey JH. Tissue factor interactions with factor VII: Measurement and clinical significance of factor VIIa in plasma. Blood Coag Fibrinol 1995; 6:S14–S19.
87. Hayes TE, Pike J, Tracy RP. Factor VII assays. Arch Pathol Lab Med 1993; 117:52–57.
88. Morrissey JH, Macik BG, Neuenschwander PF, Comp PC. Quantitation of activated factor VII levels in plasma using a tissue factor mutant selectively deficient in promoting factor VII activation. Blood 1993; 81:734–744.
89. Kroon U-B, Silfverstolpe G, Tengborn L. The effects of transdermal estradiol and oral conjugated estrogens on haemostasis variables. Thromb Haemost 1994; 71:420–423.
90. Mannucci PM, Giangrande PLF. Detection of the prethrombotic state due to procoagulant imbalance. Eur J Haematol 1992; 48:65–69.
91. Caine YG, Bauer KA, Barzegar S, et al. Coagulation activation following estrogen administration to postmenopausal women. Thromb Haemost 1992; 68:392–395.
92. Ridker PM. Fibrinolytic and inflammatory markers for arterial occlusion: The evolving epidemiology of thrombosis and haemostasis. Thromb Haemost 1997; 78:53–59.
93. Gebara OCE, Mittleman MA, Sutherland P, et al. Association between increased estrogen status and increased fibrinolytic potential in the Framingham Offspring Study. Circulation 1995; 91:1952–1958.
94. Shahar E, Folsom AR, Salomaa VV, et al, for the Atherosclerosis Risk in Communities (ARIC) Study Investigators. Relation of hormone-replacement therapy to measures of plasma fibrinolytic activity. Circulation 1996; 93:1970–1975.
95. Sporrong T, Mattsson L-ÅA, Samsioe G, et al. Haemostatic changes during continuous oestradiol-progestogen treatment of postmenopausal women. Br J Obstet Gynaecol 1990; 97:939–944.
96. Mitchell HC. Effect of estrogen and a progestogen on platelet adhesiveness and aggregation in rabbits. J Lab Clin Med 1974; 83:79–89.
97. Johnson M, Ramey E, Ramwell PW. Androgen-mediated sensitivity in platelet aggregation. Am J Physiol 1977; 232:H381–H385.
98. Aune B, Øian P, Omsjø I, Østerud B. Hormone replacement therapy reduces the reactivity of monocytes and platelets in whole blood—A beneficial effect on atherogenesis and thrombus formation? Am J Obstet Gynecol 1995; 173:1816–1820.
99. Bar J, Tepper R, Fuchs J, et al. The effect of estrogen replacement therapy on platelet aggregation and adenosine triphosphate release in postmenopausal women. Obstet Gynecol 1993; 81:261–264.
100. Viinikka L, Orpana A, Puolakka J, et al. Different effects of oral and transdermal hormonal replacement on prostacyclin and thromboxane A_2. Obstet Gynecol 1997; 89:104–107.
101. Fogelberg M, Vesterqvist O, Diczfalusy U, Henriksson P. Experimental atherosclerosis: Effects of oestrogen and atherosclerosis on thromboxane and prostacyclin formation. Eur J Clin Invest 1990; 20:105–110.
102. Chang W-C, Nakao J, Orimo H, Murota S-I. Stimulation of prostaglandin cyclooxygenase and prostacyclin synthetase activities by estradiol in rat aortic smooth muscle cells. Biochim Biophys Acta 1980; 620:472–482.
103. Seillan C, Ody C, Russo-Marie F, Duval D. Differential effects of sex steroids on prostaglandin secretion by male and female cultured piglet endothelial cells. Prostaglandins 1983; 26:3–12.
104. David M, Griesmacher A, Müller MM. 17-alpha-ethinylestradiol decreases production and release of prostacyclin in cultured human umbilical vein endothelial cells. Prostaglandins 1989; 38:431–438.
105. Redmond EM, Cherian MN, Wetzel RC. 17β-estradiol inhibits flow- and acute hypoxia–induced prostacyclin release from perfused endocardial endothelial cells. Circulation 1994; 90:2519–2524.
106. Magness RR, Rosenfeld CR. Local and systemic estradiol-17β: Effects on uterine and systemic vasodilation. Am J Physiol 1989:256:E536–E542.
107. Magness RR, Oarker CR, Rosenfeld CR. Systemic and uterine responses to chronic infusion of estradiol-17β. Am J Physiol 1993; 265:E690–E698.
108. Volterrani M, Rosano G, Coats A, et al. Estrogen acutely increases peripheral blood flow in postmenopausal women. Am J Med 1995; 99:119–122.
109. Bourne T, Hillard TC, Whitehead MI, et al. Oestrogens, arterial status, and postmenopausal women. Lancet 1990; 335:1470–1471.
110. Gangar KF, Vyas S, Whitehead M, et al. Pulsatility index in internal carotid artery in relation to transdermal estradiol and time since menopause. Lancet 1991; 338:839–842.
111. Griffith TM, Edwards DH, Lewis MJ, et al. The nature of endothelium-derived vascular relaxant factor. Nature 1984; 308:645–647.
112. Palmer RMJ, Ferrige AG, Moncada S. Nitric oxide release accounts for the biological activity of endothelium-derived relaxing factor. Nature 1987; 327:524–526.
113. Furchgott RF, Zawadzki JV. The obligatory role of endothelial cells in the relaxation of arterial smooth muscle by acetylcholine. Nature 1980; 288:373–376.
114. Ludmer PL, Selwyn AP, Shook TL, et al. Paradoxical vasoconstriction induced by acetylcholine in atherosclerotic coronary arteries. N Engl J Med 1986; 315:1046–1051.
115. Gisclard V, Miller VM, Vanhoutte PM. Effect of 17β-estradiol on endothelium-dependent responses in the rabbit. J Pharmacol Exp Ther 1988; 244:19–22.
116. Williams JK, Adams MR, Herrington DM, Clarkson TB. Short-term administration of estrogen and vascular responses of atherosclerotic coronary arteries. J Am Coll Cardiol 1992; 20:452–457.

117. Williams JK, Adams MR, Klopfenstein HS. Estrogen modulates responses of atherosclerotic coronary arteries. Circulation 1990; 81:1680–1687.
118. Reis SE, Gloth ST, Blumenthal RS, et al. Ethinyl estradiol acutely attenuates abnormal coronary vasomotor responses to acetylcholine in postmenopausal women. Circulation 1994; 89:52–60.
119. Gilligan DM, Quyyumi AA, Cannon RO. Effects of physiological levels of estrogen on coronary vasomotor function in postmenopausal women. Circulation 1994; 89:2545–2551.
120. Collins P, Rosano GMC, Sarrel PM, et al. 17β-estradiol attenuates acetylcholine-induced coronary arterial constriction in women but not men with coronary heart disease. Circulation 1995; 92:24–30.
121. Jiang C, Sarrel PM, Lindsay DC, et al. Endothelium-independent relaxation of rabbit coronary artery by 17β-estradiol *in vitro*. Br J Pharmacol 1991; 104:1033–1037.
122. Gilligan DM, Badar DM, Panza JA, et al. Acute vascular effects of estrogen in postmenopausal women. Circulation 1994; 90:786–791.
123. Lieberman EH, Gerhard MD, Uehata A, et al. Estrogen improves endothelium-dependent, flow-mediated vasodilation in postmenopausal women. Ann Intern Med 1994; 121:936–941.
124. Hayashi T, Fukuto JM, Ignarro LJ, Chaudhuri G. Basal release of nitric oxide from aortic rings is greater in female rabbits than in male rabbits: Implications for atherosclerosis. Proc Natl Acad Sci USA 1992; 89:11259–11263.
125. Collins P, Shay J, Jiang C, Moss J. Nitric oxide accounts for dose-dependent estrogen-mediated coronary relaxation following acute estrogen withdrawal. Circulation 1994; 90:1964–1968.
126. Van Buren GA, Yang D, Clark KE. Estrogen-induced uterine vasodilation is antagonized by L-nitroarginine methyl ester, an inhibitor of nitric oxide synthesis. Am J Obstet Gynecol 1992; 167:828–833.
127. Weiner CP, Lizasoain I, Baylis SA, et al. Induction of calcium-dependent nitric oxide synthases by sex hormones. Proc Natl Acad Sci USA 1994; 91:5212–5216.
128. Roselli M, Imthurn B, Keller PJ, et al. Circulating nitric oxide (nitrite/nitrate) levels in postmenopausal women substituted with 17β-estradiol and norethisterone acetate: A two-year follow-up study. Hypertension 1995; 25(part 2):848–853.
129. Keaney JF, Shwaery GT, Xu A, et al. 17β-estradiol preserves endothelial vasodilator function and limits low-density lipoprotein oxidation in hypercholesterolemic swine. Circulation 1994; 89:2251–2259.
130. Jiang C, Sarrel PM, Poole-Wilson PA, Collins P. Acute effect of 17β-estradiol on rabbit coronary artery contractile responses to endothelin-1. Am J Physiol 1992; 263:H271–H275.
131. Polderman KH, Stehouwer CDA, van Kamp GJ, et al. Influence of sex hormones on plasma endothelin levels. Ann Intern Med 1993; 118:429–432.
132. Wilcox JG, Hatch IE, Gentzschein E, et al. Endothelin-1 levels decrease after oral and nonoral estrogen in postmenopausal women with increased cardiovascular risk factors. Fertil Steril 1997; 67:273–277.
133. Losordo DW, Kearney M, Kim EA, et al. Variable expression of the estrogen receptor in normal and atherosclerotic coronary arteries of premenopausal women. Circulation 1994; 89:1501–1510.
134. Kim-Schulze S, McGowan KA, Hubchak SC, et al. Expression of an estrogen receptor by human coronary artery and umbilical vein endothelial cells. Circulation 1996; 94:1402–1407.
135. Rosser M, Chorich L, Howard E, et al. Changes in rat uterine estrogen receptor messenger ribonucleic acid levels during estrogen- and progesterone-induced estrogen receptor depletion and subsequent replenishment. Biol Reprod 1993; 48:89–98.
136. Gerhard M, Ganz P. How do we explain the clinical benefits of estrogen? From bedside to bench. Circulation 1995; 92:5–8.
137. Hardy SP, Valverde MA. Novel plasma membrane action of estrogen and antiestrogens revealed by their regulation of a large conductance chloride channel. FASEB J 1994; 8:760–765.
138. Miller VM, Vanhoutte PM. Progesterone and modulation of endothelium-dependent responses in canine coronary arteries. Am J Physiol 1992; 261:R1022–R1027.
139. Han S-Z, Karaki H, Ouchi Y, et al. 17β-estradiol inhibits Ca^{++} influx and Ca^{++} release induced by thromboxane A_2 in porcine coronary artery. Circulation 1995; 91:2619–2626.
140. Sudhir K, Chou TM, Mullen WL, et al. Mechanisms of estrogen-induced vasodilation: In vivo studies in canine coronary conductance and resistance arteries. J Am Coll Cardiol 1995; 26:807–814.
141. White RE, Darkow DJ, Falvo-Lang JL. Estrogen relaxes coronary arteries by opening BK_{Ca} channels through a cGMP-dependent mechanism. Circ Res 1995; 77:936–942.
142. Collins P, Rosano GMC, Jiang C, et al. Cardiovascular protection by oestrogen—a calcium antagonist effect? Lancet 1993; 341:1264–1265.
143. Jiang C, Poole-Wilson PA, Sarrel PM, et al. Effect of 17β-oestradiol on contraction, Ca^{++} current and intracellular free Ca^{++} in guinea pig isolated cardiac myocytes. Br J Pharmacol 1992; 106:739–745.
144. Vargas R, Wroblewska B, Rego A, et al. Oestradiol inhibits smooth muscle cell proliferation of pig coronary artery. Br J Pharmacol 1993; 109:612–617.
145. Fischer-Dzoga K, Wissler RW, Vesselinovitch D. The effect of estradiol on the proliferation of rabbit aortic medial tissue culture cells induced by hyperlipemic serum. Exp Mol Pathol 1983; 39:355–363.
146. Cheng LP, Kuwahara M, Jacobsson J, Foegh ML. Inhibition of myointimal hyperplasia and macrophage infiltration by estradiol in aorta allografts. Transplantation 1991; 52:967–972.
147. Chen S-J, Li H, Durand J, et al. Estrogen reduces myointimal proliferation after balloon injury of rat carotid artery. Circulation 1996; 93:577–584.
148. Krasinski K, Spyridopoulos I, Asahara T, et al. Estradiol accelerates functional endothelial recovery after arterial injury. Circulation 1997; 95:1768–1772.
149. Morales DE, McGowan KA, Grant DS, et al. Estrogen promotes angiogenic activity in human umbilical vein endothelial cells in vitro and in a murine model. Circulation 1995; 91:755–763.
150. Fischer GM, Cherian K, Swain ML. Increased synthesis of aortic collagen and elastin in experimental atherosclerosis. Atherosclerosis 1981; 39:463–467.
151. Fischer GM, Swain ML. Effects of estradiol and progesterone on the increased synthesis of collagen in atherosclerotic rabbit aortas. Atherosclerosis 1985; 54:1770–1785.
152. Kim YD, Chen B, Beauregard J, et al. 17β-estradiol prevents dysfunction of canine coronary endothelium and myocardium and reperfusion arrhythmias after brief ischemia/reperfusion. Circulation 1996; 94:2901–2908.
153. Rosano GMC, Peters NS, Lefroy D, et al. 17-beta-estradiol therapy lessens angina in postmenopausal women with syndrome X. J Am Coll Cardiol 1996; 28:1500–1505.
154. van der Mooren MJ, Wouters MGAJ, Blom HJ, et al. Hormone replacement therapy may reduce high serum homocysteine in postmenopausal women. Eur J Clin Invest 1994; 24:733–736.
155. Rosano GMC, Sarrel PM, Poole-Wilson PA, Collins P. Beneficial effect of oestrogen on exercise-induced myocardial ischaemia in women with coronary artery disease. Lancet 1993; 342:133–136.
156. Holdright DR, Sullivan AK, Wright CA, et al. Acute effect of oestrogen replacement on treadmill performance in postmenopausal women with coronary artery disease. Eur Heart J 1995; 16:1566–1570.
157. Despres J-P, Lamarche B, Mauriege P, et al. Hyperinsulinemia as an independent risk factor for ischemic heart disease. N Engl J Med 1996; 334:952–957.
158. Grodstein F, Stampfer M. The epidemiology of coronary heart disease and estrogen replacement in postmenopausal women. Prog Cardiovasc Dis 1995; 38:199–210.
159. Grady D, Rubin SM, Pettiti DB, et al. Hormone therapy to prevent disease and prolong life in postmenopausal women. Ann Intern Med 1992; 117:1016–1037.
160. Grodstein F, Stampfer MJ, Manson JE, et al. Postmenopausal estrogen and progestin use and the risk of cardiovascular disease. N Engl J Med 1996; 335:453–461.
161. Falkeborn M, Persson I, Adami H-O, et al. The risk of acute

myocardial infarction after oestrogen and oestrogen-progestogen replacement. Br J Obstet Gynaecol 1992; 99:821–828.
162. Hunt K, Vessey M, McPherson K, Coleman M. Long-term surveillance of mortality and cancer incidence in women receiving hormone replacement therapy. Br J Obstet Gynaecol 1987; 94:620–635.
163. Psaty BM, Heckbert SR, Atkins D, et al. The risk of myocardial infarction associated with the combined use of estrogens and progestins in postmenopausal women. Arch Intern Med 1994; 154:1333–1339.
164. Sullivan JM, Vander Zwaag R, Hughes JP, et al. Estrogen replacement and coronary artery disease: Effect on survival in postmenopausal women. Arch Intern Med 1990; 150:2557–2562.
165. Henderson BE, Paganini-Hill A, Ross RK. Decreased mortality in users of estrogen replacement therapy. Arch Intern Med 1991; 151:75–78.
166. Paganini-Hill A. Estrogen replacement therapy and stroke. Prog Cardiovasc Dis 1995; 38:223–242.
167. Grodstein F, Stampfer MJ, Colditz GA, et al. Postmenopausal hormone therapy and mortality. N Engl J Med 1997; 336:1769–1775.
168. Daly E, Vessey MP, Hawkins MM, et al. Risk of venous thromboembolism in users of hormone replacement therapy. Lancet 1996; 348:977–980.
169. Jick H, Derby LE, Myers MW, et al. Risk of hospital admission for idiopathic venous thromboembolism among users of postmenopausal oestrogens. Lancet 1996; 348:981–983.
170. Grodstein F, Stampfer MJ, Goldhaber SZ, et al. Prospective study of exogenous hormones and risk of pulmonary embolism in women. Lancet 1996; 348:983–987.
171. Cummings SR, Black DM, Rubin SM. Lifetime risks of hip, Colles', or vertebral fracture and coronary heart disease among white postmenopausal women. Arch Intern Med 1989; 149:2445–2448.
172. Brinton LA, Schairer C. Estrogen replacement therapy and breast cancer risk. Epidemiol Rev 1993; 15:66–79.
173. Adami H-O, Persson I. Hormone replacement and breast cancer: A remaining controversy? JAMA 1995; 274:178–179.
174. Speroff L. Postmenopausal hormone therapy and breast cancer. Obstet Gynecol 1996; 87(Suppl):44S–54S.
175. Colditz GA, Hankinson SE, Hunter DJ, et al. The use of estrogens and progestins and the risk of breast cancer in postmenopausal women. N Engl J Med 1995; 332:1589–1593.
176. Stanford JL, Thomas DB. Exogenous progestins and breast cancer. Epidemiol Rev 1993; 15:98–107.
177. Col NF, Eckman MH, Karas RH, et al. Patient-specific decisions about hormone replacement therapy in postmenopausal women. JAMA 1997; 277:1140–1147.
178. Barrett-Connor E. Postmenopausal estrogen use and prevention bias. Ann Intern Med 1991; 115:455–456.
179. Matthews KA, Kuller LH, Wing RR, et al. Prior to use of estrogen replacement therapy, are users healthier than nonusers? Am J Epidemiol 1996; 143:971–978.
180. Grodstein F. Can selection bias explain the cardiovascular benefits of estrogen replacement therapy? Am J Epidemiol 1996; 143:979–982.
181. Schrott HG, Bittner V, Vittinghoff E, et al, for the HERS Research Group. Adherence to National Cholesterol Education Program Treatment Goals in Postmenopausal women with heart disease: The Heart and Estrogen/progestin Replacement Study (HERS). JAMA 1997; 277:1281–1286.
182. Rossouw JE. Estrogens for the prevention of coronary heart disease: Putting the brakes on the bandwagon. Circulation 1996; 94:2982–2985.
183. Hulley S, Grady D, Bush T, et al, for the Heart and Estrogen/progestin Replacement Study (HERS) Research Group. Randomized trial of estrogen plus progestin for secondary prevention of coronary heart disease in postmenopausal women. JAMA 1998; 280:605–613.
184. Fuchs-Young R, Glasebrook AL, Short LL, et al. Raloxifene is a tissue-selective agonist/antagonist that functions through the estrogen receptor. Ann NY Acad Sci 1995; 761:355–360.
185. Yang NN, Venugopalan M, Hardikar S, Glasebrook A. Identification of an estrogen response element activated by metabolites of 17β-estradiol and raloxifene. Science 1996; 273:1222–1225.
186. Delmas PD, Bjarnason NH, Mitlak BH, et al. Effects of raloxifene on bone mineral density, serum cholesterol concentrations, and uterine endometrium in postmenopausal women. N Engl J Med 1997; 337:1641–1647.
187. Walsh BW, Kuller LH, Wild RA, et al. Effects of raloxifene on serum lipids and coagulation factors in healthy postmenopausal women. JAMA 1998; 279:1445–1451.
188. Bjarnason NH, Haarbo J, Byrjalsen I, et al. Raloxifene inhibits aortic accumulation of cholesterol in ovariectomized, cholesterol-fed rabbits. Circulation 1997; 96:1964–1969.
189. Clarkson TB, Anthony MS, Jerome CP. Lack of effect of raloxifene on coronary artery atherosclerosis of postmenopausal monkeys. J Clin Endocrinol Metab 1998; 83:721–726.

32 Antioxidant Vitamins

▶ J. Michael Gaziano
▶ JoAnn E. Manson

One of the most consistent findings in dietary research is that those who consume higher amounts of fruits and vegetables have lower rates of heart disease and stroke as well as cancer. The precise mechanisms for these apparent protective effects are not entirely clear. Possible explanations include the association between higher fruit and vegetable intake and higher dietary fiber intake or the replacement of fats and cholesterol. Alternative hypotheses focus on the micronutrient content of fruits and vegetables. Recently a great deal of attention has centered on the notion that micronutrients with antioxidant properties might be responsible for the associated lower rates of chronic diseases.

Basic research provides a plausible mechanism by which antioxidants might reduce the risk of atherosclerosis through inhibition of oxidative damage. A large number of descriptive, case-control, and cohort studies provide data suggesting that consumption of antioxidant vitamins is associated with reduced risks of cardiovascular disease. These data raise the question of a possible role of antioxidants, such as vitamins C and E and β-carotene, in the primary prevention of cardiovascular disease but do not provide a definitive answer. Results from several large-scale, randomized trials of antioxidant supplements are now available, but they are not entirely consistent. In this chapter, the rationale for conducting large-scale trials of natural antioxidants is discussed, followed by a summary of available trial data and ongoing trials.

BASIC RESEARCH

Basic research findings suggest that oxidative damage plays a role in the pathogenesis of many chronic diseases, including atherosclerosis, cancer, arthritis, eye disease, and reperfusion injury during myocardial infarction. Data from in vitro and in vivo studies suggest that oxidative damage to low-density lipoprotein (LDL) promotes several steps in atherogenesis,[1] including endothelial cell damage,[2, 3] foam cell accumulation,[4–6] and growth[7, 8] and synthesis of autoantibodies.[9] In addition, animal studies suggest that free radicals may directly damage arterial endothelium,[10] promote thrombosis,[11] and interfere with normal vasomotor regulation.[12] Therefore, oxidative damage may enhance atherogenesis by a cascade of reactions.

Elaborate systems have evolved in aerobic organisms to minimize the damaging effects of uncontrolled oxidation (Table 32–1). First, there are several mechanisms to prevent the formation of unintended free radicals. Oxidative metabolism is carefully compartmentalized, and molecular oxygen and its highly reactive species are tightly bound to enzymes involved in that process. Biologic systems take great care to safely bind heavy metal ions such as copper and iron to storage or transport proteins to prevent the catalytic reactions with oxygen species that could result in the formation of free radicals. Second, enzymatic (e.g., superoxide dismutase, catalase, glutathione peroxidase) and nonenzymatic (e.g., vitamins E and C, urate) antioxidants scavenge free radicals, thereby minimizing the damage they can cause once they have been formed. Finally, there are mechanisms for repairing the damage from unintended oxidative reactions.

Antioxidant vitamins represent one of the many

TABLE 32–1 • Natural Defense Mechanisms Against Oxidative Damage

Compartmentalization of oxidative metabolism
Binding of molecular oxygen and reactive species to proteins to prevent random oxidative reactions
Binding of transition metals (e.g., iron and copper) to transport and storage proteins to prevent involvement in free radical reactions
Enzymatic antioxidants (e.g., superoxide dismutase, catalase, and glutathione peroxidase)
Nonenzymatic antioxidants (e.g., vitamin C, vitamin E, β-carotene, urate, bilirubin, and ubiquinols)
Mechanisms to repair or dispose of damaged DNA, proteins, lipids, and carbohydrates

nonenzymatic antioxidant defense mechanisms. Ascorbic acid (vitamin C), α-tocopherol (a major component of vitamin E), and β-carotene (a provitamin A) are among the most abundant and most widely studied natural antioxidants. However, there are hundreds or thousands of other dietary compounds that may function as antioxidants. In vitro data have demonstrated the possible role of these antioxidants in preventing or retarding various steps in atherogenesis by inhibiting oxidation of LDL or other free radical reactions. These antioxidants have also been shown to prevent experimental atherogenesis in many but not all animal models of atherosclerosis.

HUMAN OBSERVATIONAL EPIDEMIOLOGY

Although basic research provides a plausible mechanism for a reduction in risk of cardiovascular disease by antioxidant vitamins, the efficacy of any intervention must rely on data from human studies. The hypothesis that antioxidant vitamins might reduce cardiovascular disease risk has been explored in a number of human observational epidemiologic studies. These descriptive, case-control, and cohort studies provide data suggesting that consumption of foods rich in antioxidant vitamins reduces the risks of developing heart disease and stroke.[13]

The data from both dietary intake and blood-based studies are compatible with a possible benefit of antioxidants; however, the available observational data are not all consistent. Additional observational data would certainly be a valuable contribution to the body of evidence concerning antioxidants and cardiovascular disease. Regardless of the number or sample size of such studies, or the consistency of their findings, these observational investigations are limited in their ability to provide reliable data on the most plausible small-to-moderate benefits of factors such as antioxidants. Observational studies can control for the effects of known potential confounding variables, but they cannot take into account unknown or unmeasured confounding factors. For example, greater dietary intake of antioxidants, measured by blood levels or a diet assessment questionnaire, may be only a marker for some other dietary practice or even nondietary lifestyle variable that is truly protective. It is, in fact, plausible that intake of antioxidant-rich foods is indeed protective; however, the benefit results not from their antioxidant properties but some other component these foods have in common. In addition, the intake of individual dietary antioxidants is often highly correlated, making it difficult to determine the specific benefit of any one antioxidant.

RATIONALE FOR RANDOMIZED TRIALS

Based on published reports of the basic and human observational data, there has been a rapid increase in the consumption of supplements with these micronutrients. However, available evidence raises the question of a possible role of antioxidants, such as vitamins C and E and β-carotene, in the prevention of cardiovascular disease as well as cancer but does not provide a definitive answer. For most hypotheses randomized trials are neither necessary nor desirable[14]; however, when searching for small-to-moderate effects, the amount of uncontrolled confounding inherent in observational studies may be as large as the likely risk reduction. For these reasons, reliable data on the relationship of antioxidants and cardiovascular disease can emerge only from large-scale randomized trials of adequate dose and duration, in which investigators allocate subjects at random to either active treatment or placebo. When the sample size is sufficient, randomized trials can avoid some limitations of observational studies by distributing the known and unknown confounding variables among treatment groups. For these reasons, the U.S. National Heart, Lung, and Blood Institute's conference, "Antioxidants in the Prevention of Human Atherosclerosis," concluded that data from large-scale randomized trials are required to test the hypothesis that dietary antioxidants reduce the risk of cardiovascular disease and recommended randomized trials examining the role of vitamins C and E and β-carotene in the primary and secondary prevention of cardiovascular disease.[15] Well-designed, well-conducted large-scale randomized trials are necessary to provide a definitive positive or negative result on which public policy can be based.

Further, a distinction must be made between interventions and therapies that are restricted (e.g., by the U.S. Food and Drug Administration) and those interventions that are readily available over the counter. Despite the fact that the health benefits as well as risks of supplementation with antioxidant vitamins are largely unknown, antioxidant vitamins are among the most widely consumed individual nutritional supplements, and their use is rapidly increasing. In the United States, the supplemental vitamin industry reports annual sales of $3 billion to $4 billion. With increasing consumption rates, it is essential to evaluate risks and benefits clearly to establish prudent recommendations for clinical decision making and public health policy. If the trend toward increasing use of vitamins E and C continues, it may be difficult to conduct randomized trials with sufficient numbers of participants willing to be randomized to placebo. Given the high rates of supplemental vitamin consumption, an informative null would be of value;

therefore, there is urgency to conduct randomized trials to assess the long-term benefits of antioxidant vitamins. Even null results from randomized trials that are truly informative would provide more reliable data on which the public can base decisions regarding antioxidant supplementation and permit the rechanneling of already limited resources to other areas of research.

PRIMARY PREVENTION TRIALS

In the 1980s several large-scale, randomized trials of antioxidants were designed to test the hypothesis that various antioxidant vitamin supplements (alone or in combination) reduce the risk of epithelial cancers (Table 32–2). Most, but not all, of these trials were conducted among subjects at higher than usual risk for various epithelial cancers.[16–18] Only one trial was conducted among those at usual risk.[19] With the emergence of the hypothesis that antioxidants might prevent or retard atherogenesis, these early large-scale trials provided the first opportunity to assess the role of several antioxidants in the primary prevention of cardiovascular disease.

Chinese Cancer Prevention Trial

The first large-scale, randomized primary prevention trial of vitamin supplements in the prevention of cancer was conducted among a poorly nourished population in Linxian, China, who were at high risk of upper gastrointestinal cancers.[16] A total of 29,584 men and women were randomized to one of eight treatment arms comprised of various combinations of nine vitamins and minerals. There was a significant reduction in the overall mortality rate among those assigned a cocktail of β-carotene (15 mg daily), α-tocopherol (30 mg daily), and selenium (50 μg daily). The mortality reduction was largely accounted for by a reduction in stomach cancer mortality. Results for cardiovascular mortality were also assessed; however, heart disease rates were relatively low. Even though the mortality rate from ischemic heart disease was less than 9% of the total deaths, the cerebrovascular mortality rate comprised 26% of the total. There was an apparent, though nonsignificant, reduction in the risk of cerebrovascular disease mortality (relative risk [RR], 0.90; 95% confidence interval [CI], 0.76 to 1.07). In this population most strokes were likely to have been hemorrhagic rather than thromboembolic. The latter type is generally due to atherosclerotic disease; however, this is not the case for the former. Therefore, the relevance of these findings in terms of atherosclerotic disease prevention is not yet clear.

α-Tocopherol, β-Carotene Cancer Prevention Trial

The α-Tocopherol, β-Carotene (ATBC) Cancer Prevention Trial was the first large-scale, randomized trial of antioxidant vitamins in a well-nourished population at high risk for lung cancer due to cigarette smoking. This 2 × 2 factorial trial tested the effect of synthetic α-tocopherol (50 mg daily) and synthetic β-carotene (20 mg daily) in the prevention of lung cancer among 29,133 Finnish male smokers.[17] After adjustment for testing multiple hypotheses, there were no increases or decreases in the risk of cause-specific morbidity or mortality that could not be explained plausibly by chance. Nevertheless, some findings were unexpected. For α-tocopherol, there was no reduction in

TABLE 32–2 • Completed Large-Scale Trials of Antioxidants

Trial	Study Population	Agents Tested	Cardiovascular Findings
Primary Prevention			
Chinese Cancer Prevention Trial	29,584 men and women	*Combination:* β-carotene, vitamin E, and selenium	Apparent reduction in risk of stroke
Finnish α-Tocopherol, β-Carotene Cancer Prevention Trial	29,133 men smokers	2 × 2 *Factorial:* β-carotene and vitamin E	*β-Carotene:* no benefit on CHD *Vitamin E:* no benefit on CHD; apparent increase in hemorrhagic stroke
U.S. Physicians' Health Study (PHS)	22,071 men physicians	β-Carotene	No benefit on CHD
β-Carotene and Retinol Efficacy Trial (CARET)	18,314 men smokers and asbestos workers	*Combination:* β-carotene and retinol	No benefit on CHD
Skin Cancer Prevention Study	1805 men and women with skin cancer	β-Carotene	No benefit on CHD
Secondary Prevention			
Cambridge Heart Antioxidant Study (CHAOS)	2002 men and women with coronary artery disease	Vitamin E	Significant decrease in risk of myocardial infarction; apparent increase in cardiovascular death

CHD, cardiovascular heart disease.

the rate of lung cancer, the primary endpoint. Further, there was no clear reduction in risk of ischemic heart disease (RR, 0.95; 95% CI, 0.85 to 1.05) or ischemic stroke mortality (RR, 0.84; 95% CI, 0.59 to 1.19) among those assigned to vitamin E. In a subsequent report the risk of developing angina was slightly lower among those assigned vitamin E (RR, 0.91; 95% CI, 0.83 to 0.99).[20] The vitamin E dose was not much higher than the U.S. recommended daily allowance. Some observational research suggests that supplementation at higher doses may be required to reduce the risk of heart disease. The apparent benefits among those who took vitamin E supplements in the Nurses' Health Study[21] and the Health Professionals' Follow-Up Study[22] were largely confined to those who used an average daily dose of 100 IU or more per day, which is higher than the dosage of 50 mg used in this trial.

There was an apparent increase in the risk of hemorrhagic stroke in the α-tocopherol treatment group compared with those assigned to placebo (RR, 1.50; 95% CI, 1.03 to 2.20), a finding not compatible with the lower stroke rates among those assigned antioxidant vitamins in the Linxian, China, trial. Hemorrhagic stroke was not a prespecified endpoint, and although this finding is compatible with an antiplatelet effect of vitamin E, it remains plausible that it could have been the result of chance.

With respect to β-carotene, there were unexpected excess lung cancers among those assigned active treatment. There was no apparent protective effect of supplementation with respect to deaths from ischemic heart disease and stroke; in fact, there were slightly more ischemic heart disease deaths (RR, 1.12; 95% CI, 1.00 to 1.25) among those assigned to β-carotene. There was no reduction in risk of angina among the β-carotene group (RR, 1.06; 95% CI, 0.97 to 1.16).[18]

The Physicians' Health Study

The Physicians' Health Study (PHS) is a randomized, double-blind, placebo-controlled trial of β-carotene (50 mg on alternate days) among 22,071 U.S. male physicians, aged 40 to 84 years, of whom 11% were current and 39% past smokers at baseline in 1982.[19] By December 31, 1995, the scheduled end of the trial, fewer than 1% were lost to morbidity and mortality follow-up and compliance with active pills was 78%. After more than 12 years of treatment and follow-up, among 11,036 participants randomized to β-carotene and 11,035 to placebo, there were virtually no early or late differences for cardiovascular disease deaths (RR, 1.09; 95% CI, 0.93 to 1.27); myocardial infarction (RR, 0.96; 95% CI, 0.84 to 1.09); stroke (RR, 0.96; 95% CI, 0.83 to 1.11); or a composite of the previous three endpoints (RR, 1.00; 95% CI, 0.91 to 1.09) between treatment groups. There was also no significant benefit or harm for total malignant neoplasms (RR, 0.98; 95% CI, 0.91 to 1.06), cancer mortality (RR, 1.02; 95% CI, 0.89 to 1.18), or lung cancer. Among current or past smokers, there were likewise no significant early or late effects of β-carotene on any of these endpoints. This large-scale, randomized trial among apparently healthy, well-nourished men provides substantial evidence that 12 years of β-carotene supplementation causes neither benefit nor harm in relation to cardiovascular disease mortality or malignant neoplasms.

The β-Carotene and Retinol Efficacy Trial

The β-Carotene and Retinol Efficacy Trial (CARET) among 18,314 men and women at high risk of lung cancer owing to a history of cigarette smoking and/or occupational exposure to asbestos evaluated a combined treatment of β-carotene (30 mg daily) and retinol (25,000 IU daily).[18] The primary aim of the study was to test whether β-carotene in combination with retinol would reduce the risk of lung cancer. Data were collected at annual clinic visits. The study was stopped prematurely because of an inability to detect a benefit over the projected funding period and a trend toward increased lung cancer in the treatment group. After 4 years of treatment and follow-up, there was an excess of total deaths (RR, 1.17; 95% CI, 1.03 to 1.33) and a trend toward excess cardiovascular deaths (RR, 1.26; 95% CI, 0.99 to 1.61) as well as excess cases of lung cancer among those assigned β-carotene and vitamin A. Data on other specific cardiovascular outcomes, including nonfatal events, are not yet available.

Skin Cancer Prevention Study

Investigators in the Skin Cancer Prevention Study, a multicenter, double-blind, placebo-controlled trial, randomized 1805 men and women with a history of skin cancer to 50 mg of β-carotene daily or placebo.[23] More than 80% of participants reported taking more than 50% of their study pills after a median follow-up of 8.2 years. Follow-up was by questionnaire and by visits to a dermatologist. Death certificates were obtained for all deaths that occurred during the follow-up period, and cause of death was coded by a trained nosologist. There was no significant risk reduction in terms of total deaths (RR, 1.05; 95% CI, 0.83 to 1.32) or cardiovascular deaths (RR, 1.15; 95% CI, 0.81 to 1.63).

SECONDARY PREVENTION TRIALS

Beginning in the 1950s, several small-scale trials tested the effects of antioxidants among people with various forms of atherosclerotic disease, including claudication and angina, as well as following angioplasty. Benefits of supplemental vitamin E were observed in each of three studies among patients with claudication.[24–26] However, the usefulness of these data is limited by small sample sizes, high dropout rates, and lack of blinding.

Two more recent trials tested the effect of vitamin E in the treatment of angina pectoris with equivocal results. There was a nonsignificant trend toward improved angina pain score in a 9-week placebo-controlled trial among stable angina patients consuming 3200 IU of vitamin E daily compared with placebo.[27] Gillian and associates[28] tested 1600 IU of vitamin E daily for 6 months in a double-blind, crossover trial of 52 angina pectoris patients, reporting no apparent benefit of vitamin E treatment as measured by exercise tolerance, symptoms of angina pectoris, or left ventricular function. These studies provide no clear evidence of benefit of short-term treatment of angina with vitamin E; however, both the small sample size and the short duration of treatment may have limited the ability of these studies to detect small-to-moderate benefits.

One small-scale trial tested the effect of vitamin E supplementation on subsequent restenosis rates among 100 subjects following percutaneous transluminal coronary angioplasty.[29] Restenosis is likely the result of an accelerated form of the atherosclerotic process. Subjects were treated with 400 IU of vitamin E daily following angioplasty. There was an apparent, though not statistically significant, 30% reduction in the risk of restenosis as measured by subsequent catheterization or exercise test.

A subgroup analysis within the PHS was conducted among 333 participants who had no prior history of myocardial infarction or stroke but who did have a history of chronic stable angina or who had a prior coronary revascularization procedure.[30] Among subjects who received β-carotene, there was a suggestion of reduced cardiovascular events after 5 years of follow-up, but the effect sizes were attenuated after additional follow-up. There were apparent, but not significant, reductions in the risk of major cardiovascular events after an average of 12 years of treatment. Specifically, compared with placebo those assigned β-carotene had apparent but nonsignificant reductions in risk of nonfatal myocardial infarction (RR, 0.76; 95% CI, 0.36 to 1.60), nonfatal stroke (RR, 0.66; 95% CI, 0.28 to 1.58), and subsequent revascularizations (RR, 0.66; 95% CI, 0.34 to 1.30) but an apparent but nonsignificant increase in cardiovascular death (RR, 1.42; 95% CI, 0.72 to 2.80) after multivariate adjustment. These findings must be cautiously interpreted because they are the result of a small subgroup analysis that was not prespecified and therefore merit further evaluation in other large-scale trials.

In a subgroup analysis from the ATBC Cancer Prevention Trial, investigators analyzed the frequency of major coronary events in men with previous myocardial infarction.[31] Participation in this cancer prevention trial was limited to those with no prior proven malignant disease. In addition those with severe angina were excluded. However, 1862 subjects with a report of prior myocardial infarction were included in this cohort. After a median follow-up of 5.3 years there were 424 major coronary events (nonfatal myocardial infarction and fatal coronary heart disease). There were no significant differences in the risk of total major coronary events by treatment group compared with placebo. There was a suggestion of reduced risk of nonfatal myocardial infarction among those assigned α-tocopherol (RR, 0.62; 95% CI, 0.41 to 0.96), β-carotene (RR, 0.67; 95% CI, 0.44 to 1.02), and combined treatment with α-tocopherol and β-carotene (RR, 0.86; 95% CI, 0.58 to 1.26) compared with placebo after multivariate adjustment for available coronary risk factors. However, there were apparent increases in risk of fatal coronary heart disease events among those assigned α-tocopherol (RR, 1.33; 95% CI, 0.86 to 2.05); β-carotene (RR, 1.58; 95% CI, 1.05 to 2.40), and combined treatment with α-tocopherol and β-carotene (RR, 1.75; 95% CI, 1.16 to 2.64) compared with placebo. No results for stroke were provided. These findings also must be interpreted cautiously because they derive from a small subgroup that was not prespecified.

Cambridge Heart Antioxidant Study

In the Cambridge Heart Antioxidant Study (CHAOS), a randomized, double-blind, placebo-controlled trial, 2002 patients with angiographically proven coronary artery disease were assigned to supplemental vitamin E (n = 1035 [546 patients treated with 800 IU and the remainder with 400 IU daily after a protocol change]) or placebo (n = 967).[32] Median follow-up was 510 days. Compared with those receiving placebo, those assigned to vitamin E had a significantly lower risk of subsequent nonfatal myocardial infarction (RR, 0.23; 95% CI, 0.11 to 0.47) and a combined endpoint of nonfatal myocardial infarction and cardiovascular death (RR, 0.53; 95% CI, 0.34 to 0.83). However, there was a nonsignificant excess of cardiovascular deaths (RR, 1.18; 95% CI, 0.62 to 2.27). Because of the relatively small sample size, there were imbalances in various baseline characteristics between the two treatment groups, including trends toward fewer women, lower cholesterol levels, and lower systolic blood pressure levels in the placebo group.

ONGOING LARGE-SCALE TRIALS

More reliable data should be forthcoming soon that will further define the role of antioxidants in the prevention and treatment of atherosclerotic disease. Currently, several large-scale, randomized trials of dietary antioxidants are testing the role of these agents in both primary and secondary prevention of cardiovascular disease and cancer (Table 32–3). Three large-scale trials are testing antioxidant supplements among those without known atherosclerotic disease. The Women's Health Study (WHS) is testing vitamin E (600 IU of natural vitamin E on alternate days) and low-dose aspirin in the primary prevention of cardiovascular disease and cancer in 40,000 healthy U.S. women health professionals. The Heart Protection Study is testing a daily cocktail of vitamin E (600 IU), β-carotene (20 mg), and vitamin C (250 mg) in a factorial design with a cholesterol-lowering medicine among 20,000 higher-risk people with coronary risk factors but no known cardiovascular disease. The PHS, a randomized trial of more than 22,000 healthy U.S. male physicians, will continue treatment with β-carotene (50 mg on alternate days) for an additional 5 years among willing participants. In addition, vitamin E (400 IU on alternate days), vitamin C (500 mg daily), and a multivitamin will be added in a factorial design.

Three large-scale secondary prevention trials are currently underway. The Women's Antioxidant Cardiovascular Study (WACS) is a secondary prevention trial of vitamin C (500 mg daily), natural vitamin E (600 IU on alternate days), and β-carotene (50 mg on alternate days) in a factorial design that has randomized approximately 8000 women health professionals with reported cardiovascular disease or with several coronary risk factors. The Heart Outcomes Prevention Evaluation (HOPE) study is testing vitamin E (400 IU daily) among 9000 men and women with prior myocardial infarction or stroke or known peripheral vascular disease. The Gruppo Italiano per lo Studio della Sopravvivenza nell'Infarto Miocardico (GISSI) is conducting an unblinded trial of vitamin E (400 IU daily) among 12,000 men and women with a recent myocardial infarction. In addition, there are several small-scale angiographic trials testing antioxidant supplements alone or in various combinations among those with coronary artery disease or endothelial dysfunction.

CONCLUSIONS

Available basic research findings strongly suggest that oxidative stress may play an important role in the development of atherosclerotic disease and that antioxidant vitamins may delay or prevent various steps in atherogenesis. Human observational data are compatible with the possibility that antioxidant intake either from foods or supplements may reduce the risk of cardiovascular disease. However, neither basic nor human observational research has provided conclusive evidence. The available basic and human observational data, together with the increasingly widespread use of antioxidant supplements despite lack of documented benefit, strongly support the urgent need for large-scale trials of antioxidant supplements.

The available randomized trial data are not yet sufficient to fully assess the role of antioxidants in the primary or secondary prevention of atherosclerotic disease. Most trials have been relatively short, particularly with respect to primary prevention. In addition, studies vary greatly in the dose and form of antioxidant vitamins.

TABLE 32–3 • Ongoing Large-Scale Trials of Antioxidants

Trial	Study Population	Study Agents
Primary Prevention		
Continuation of Physician's Health Study	Physician's Health Study cohort	Factorial design of β-carotene, vitamin E, vitamin C, and multivitamins
Women's Health Study	40,000 U.S. women health professionals	Vitamin E
Heart Protection Study	20,000 higher-risk men and women	Combination of vitamin E, β-carotene, and vitamin C
Secondary Prevention		
Women's Antioxidant Cardiovascular Study (WACS)	8000 U.S. women health professionals with CVD	Factorial design of vitamin E, β-carotene, and vitamin C
Heart Outcomes Prevention Evaluation (HOPE)	9000 men and women following myocardial infarction	Vitamin E
Gruppo Italiano per lo Studio della Sopravvivenza nell'Infarto Miocardico (GISSI)	12,000 men and women following myocardial infarction	Vitamin E

CVD, cardiovascular disease.

Recent trials raise the possibility that some of the benefits from observational epidemiology may have been overestimated.[33] For β-carotene there appears to be no overall benefit in the primary prevention of cardiovascular disease among well-nourished people. However, whether there is a risk reduction among those with prior disease or even lower baseline levels of β-carotene remains unclear. For vitamin E there have been only two primary prevention trials, both of which had methodologic limitations. In both the ATBC Cancer Prevention Trial and the Chinese Cancer Prevention Trial, the dose of vitamin E was relatively low. Recent trial data are compatible with the possibility of a benefit of higher doses of vitamin E on reinfarction among those with coronary disease; however, this hypothesis requires confirmation in the current ongoing large-scale, randomized trials.

Based on the available evidence, antioxidants represent a possible but as yet unproven means to reduce the risks of cardiovascular disease. The ongoing randomized trials will provide valuable information on which rational clinical decision making for people and policy for the health of the general public can be reliably based. Although it remains unclear whether antioxidant supplementation will reduce the risks of cardiovascular disease, consumption of fruits and vegetables high in these micronutrients is an important part of a healthy diet.

REFERENCES

1. Steinberg D, Parthasarathy S, Carew T, et al. Beyond cholesterol—modifications of low-density lipoprotein that increase its atherogenicity. N Engl J Med 1989; 320(14):915–924.
2. Hessler JR, Morel DW, James LJ, Chisolm GM. Lipoprotein oxidation and lipoprotein-induced cytotoxicity. Arteriosclerosis 1983; 3(3):215–222.
3. Yagi K. Increased serum lipid peroxides initiate atherogenesis. Bioessays 1984; 1:58–60.
4. Quinn MT, Parthasarathy S, Steinberg D. Endothelial cell–derived chemotactic activity for mouse peritoneal macrophages and the effects of modified forms of low-density lipoprotein. Proc Natl Acad Sci USA 1985; 82:5949–5953.
5. Schuffner T, Taylor K, Bardic EA, et al. Arterial foam cells with distinctive immunomorphologic and histochemical features of macrophages. Am J Pathol 1980; 100:57–73.
6. Gerrity RG. The role of the monocyte in atherogenesis: I. Transition of blood-borne monocytes into foam cells in fatty lesions. Am J Pathol 1981; 103:181–190.
7. Fogelman AM, Schechter I, Hokom M, et al. Malondialdehyde alteration of low-density lipoproteins leads to cholesterol ester accumulation in human monocyte macrophages. Proc Natl Acad Sci USA 1980; 77:2214–2218.
8. Goldstein JL, Ho YK, Basu SK, Brown MS. Binding site on macrophages that mediates uptake and degradation of acetylated low-density lipoprotein, producing massive cholesterol deposition. Proc Natl Acad Sci USA 1979; 76:333–337.
9. Salonen JT, Yla-Herttuala S, Yamamoto R, et al. Autoantibody against oxidised LDL and progression of carotid atherosclerosis. Lancet 1992; 339:883–887.
10. Beckman JS, Beckman TW, Chen J, et al. Apparent hydroxyl radical production by peroxynitrite: Implications for endothelial injury from nitric oxide and superoxide. Proc Natl Acad Sci USA 1990; 87:1620–1624.
11. Marcus AJ, Silk ST, Safier LB, Ullman HL. Superoxide production and reducing activity in human platelets. J Clin Invest 1977; 59:149–158.
12. Saran M, Michael C, Bors W. Reaction of NO with O_2: Implications for the action of endothelium-derived relaxing factor (EDRF). Free Radic Res Commun 1990; 10:221–226.
13. Gaziano JM, Steinberg D. Natural antioxidants. *In* Manson JE, Ridker PM, Gaziano JM, Hennekens CH (eds). Prevention of Myocardial Infarction. New York, Oxford Press, 1996, pp 321–350.
14. Hennekens CH, Buring JE. Observational evidence. Ann NY Acad Sci 1993; 703:18–24.
15. Steinberg D, Workshop Participants. Antioxidants in the prevention of human atherosclerosis: Summary of the Proceedings of a National Heart, Lung, and Blood Institute Workshop, September 5–6, 1991, Bethesda, MD. Circulation 1992; 85(6):2337–2344.
16. Blot WJ, Li JY, Taylor PR, et al. Nutrition intervention trials in Linxian, China: Supplementation with specific vitamin/mineral combinations, cancer incidence, and disease-specific mortality in the general population. J Natl Cancer Inst 1993; 85:1483–1492.
17. Alpha-Tocopherol, Beta Carotene Cancer Prevention Study Group. The effect of vitamin E and beta carotene on the incidence of lung cancer and other cancers in male smokers. N Engl J Med 1994; 330:1029–1035.
18. Omenn GS, Goodman GE, Thornquist MD, et al. Effects of a combination of beta carotene and vitamin A on lung cancer and cardiovascular disease. N Engl J Med 1996; 334:1150–1155.
19. Hennekens CH, Buring JE, Manson JE, et al. Lack of effect of long-term supplementation with beta carotene on the incidence of malignant neoplasms and cardiovascular disease. N Engl J Med 1996; 334:1145–1149.
20. Rapola JM, Virtamo J, Haukka JK, et al. Effect of vitamin E and beta carotene on the incidence of angina pectoris: A randomized, double-blind, controlled trial. JAMA 1996; 275:693–698.
21. Stampfer MJ, Hennekens CH, Manson JE, et al. A prospective study of vitamin E consumption and risk of coronary disease in women. N Engl J Med 1993; 328:1444–1449.
22. Rimm EB, Stampfer MJ, Ascherio A, et al. Dietary intake and risk of coronary heart disease among men. N Engl J Med 1993; 328:1450–1456.
23. Greenberg ER, Baron JA, Karagas MR, et al. Mortality associated with low plasma concentration of beta carotene and the effect of oral supplementation. JAMA 1996; 275:660–703.
24. Livingston PD, Jones C. Treatment of intermittent claudication with vitamin E. Lancet 1958; 2:602–604.
25. Williams HTG, Fenna D, MacBeth RA. Alpha tocopherol in the treatment of intermittent claudication. Surg Gynecol Obstet 1971; 132:662–666.
26. Haeger K. Long-time treatment of intermittent claudication with vitamin E. Am J Clin Nutr 1974; 27:1179–1181.
27. Anderson TW, Reid W. A double-blind trial of vitamin E in the treatment of angina pectoris. Am Heart J 1974; 93:444–449.
28. Gillian RE, Mandell B, Warbasse JR. Quantitative evaluation of vitamin E in the treatment of angina pectoris. Am Heart J 1977; 93(4):444–449.
29. DeMaio SJ, King SB III, Lembo NJ, et al. Vitamin E supplementation, plasma lipids, and incidence of restenosis after percutaneous transluminal coronary angioplasty (PTCA). J Am Coll Nutr 1992; 11:131–138.
30. Gaziano JM, Manson JE, Ridker PM, et al. Beta carotene therapy for chronic stable angina. Circulation 1990; 82(4, Suppl 3):III–202.
31. Rapola JM, Virtamo J, Ripatti S, et al. Randomized trial of α-tocopherol and β-carotene supplements on incidence of major coronary events in men with previous myocardial infarction. Lancet 1997; 349:1715–1720.
32. Stephens NG, Parsons A, Schofield PM, et al. Randomized, controlled trial of vitamin E in patients with coronary disease: Cambridge Heart Antioxidant Study (CHAOS). Lancet 1996; 347: 781–786.
33. Hennekens CH, Buring JE, Peto R. Antioxidant vitamins—benefits not yet proven. N Engl J Med 1994; 330:1080–1081.

33 Dietary Factors

► Frank M. Sacks

Definitive trials using 3-hydroxy-3-methylglutaryl coenzyme A reductase inhibitors to lower blood low-density lipoprotein (LDL) cholesterol have now proven the LDL theory of coronary heart disease (CHD).[1–4] The causal relationship between LDL levels and CHD had been supported strongly by a consistent body of evidence from observational epidemiologic studies,[5–8] trials that used coronary angiography to assess change in atherosclerosis,[9] and early clinical trials that used treatments that had less effect on LDL cholesterol than the reductase inhibitors.[10] Lowering LDL cholesterol reduces coronary events in populations with or without clinical CHD and in populations with hypercholesterolemia[1–3, 9, 10] or average cholesterol levels.[4] The Cholesterol and Recurrent Events (CARE) trial showed that lowering an average LDL cholesterol (mean 140 mg/dL) with pravastatin reduced recurrent coronary events in patients with myocardial infarction. This result, applied to the general population, suggests that an average blood cholesterol level in Western societies is too high[11, 12] and is likely to cause coronary events. Since most adults could conceivably benefit from a lower cholesterol level, the importance of nonpharmacologic approaches is great. This chapter reviews the considerable body of evidence that dietary modification can prevent CHD.

National health organizations advocate dietary changes that decrease intake of saturated fat and cholesterol to prevent coronary heart disease.[13] A point of controversy concerns the nutrient that should replace the energy provided by saturated fat, that is, either carbohydrate or unsaturated oils.[14] Moreover, the *trans*-unsaturated fatty acids, produced during the industrial hydrogenation of vegetable oil to make shortenings and margarine, have recently been shown to have adverse effects on serum lipid levels and to be associated with CHD. The relationship between dietary fat and serum lipoprotein levels is central to understanding the link between diet and CHD and to evaluate different dietary approaches.

In addition to the dietary fats, evidence from epidemiologic studies and clinical trials suggests that dietary factors other than fats may protect against CHD. These include antioxidant vitamins (discussed in Chapter 32), folic acid, and vitamin B_6. The possible role of these nutrients in dietary therapy is discussed.

DIETARY FAT AND SERUM LIPOPROTEIN CONCENTRATIONS

Thirty years ago, experiments conducted on metabolic wards established that intake of saturated fatty acids having 12, 14, or 16 carbon atoms (lauric, myristic, and palmitic acids, respectively) raised serum total cholesterol levels.[15, 16] Myristic and palmitic acids are the most common saturated fatty acids in Western diets, whereas lauric acid is the major fatty acid in coconut and palm kernel oils. More recent studies confirmed that these saturated fatty acids raised LDL cholesterol levels, with descending order of potency, myristic, lauric, and palmitic.[17] Meta-analysis of controlled dietary trials demonstrated that the average effect in groups of persons of replacing 10% of energy from saturated fat by either carbohydrate or monounsaturated or polyunsaturated fat is a decrease in LDL of 13 mg/dL, 15 mg/dL, or 18 mg/dL, respectively.[17] Therefore, exchanging any of these nutrients for saturated fat lowers LDL cholesterol levels. Monounsaturated and particularly polyunsaturated fatty acids accentuate this effect compared with carbohydrate.

In contrast to their differential effects on LDL, all three major classes of fatty acids raise high-density lipoprotein (HDL) levels compared with carbohydrate, with saturated fat having the most and polyunsaturated fat the least effect.[17] HDL is well established as an independent protective factor for coronary disease.[18] In clinical trials of drug therapy, increases in HDL have been correlated with reductions in coronary events[19, 20] or with decreases in coronary stenosis.[21] The ratio of total cholesterol to HDL cholesterol concentrations is often used as a summary measure of blood lipid changes to estimate change in risk of

TABLE 33–1 • Examples of Two Dietary Approaches to Lower Blood Cholesterol Levels

	Low-Fat/High-Carbohydrate Diet (NCEP Step 2*)	High-Unsaturated-Fat Diet (Mediterranean)
Total fat	38% → 25%	38% → 38%
Saturated fat	20% → 6%	20% → 6%
Monounsaturated	11% → 12%	11% → 22%
Polyunsaturated	7% → 7%	7% → 10%
Carbohydrate	42% → 55%	42% → 42%
Cholesterol	400 mg → 100 mg	400 mg → 100 mg

* NCEP Step 2 recommends total fat ≤30%, saturated fat <7%, carbohydrate ≥55%, and cholesterol intake <200 mg/day.
NCEP, National Cholesterol Education Program.[13]

coronary heart disease.[22, 23] The ratio shows little change when saturated fat is replaced with carbohydrate since the percentage decreases in total cholesterol and HDL are about the same; however, the ratio is improved with monounsaturated or polyunsaturated fat, which lowers LDL and very-low-density lipoprotein (VLDL) more than HDL.[17]

Plasma triglycerides are an independent risk factor for coronary disease when measured in the fasting[24–27] or nonfasting states.[28] Carbohydrate raises fasting triglyceride levels when it replaces any type of fat.[17] A meal with mainly carbohydrate, compared with monounsaturated fat, raises postprandial triglyceride levels.[29–31]

Examples of changes in dietary intake with a high-carbohydrate/low-fat diet compared with a high-unsaturated-fat diet are shown in Table 33–1. In the first instance, a relatively high total fat intake, 38%, is reduced to 25% solely by decreasing saturated fat and increasing carbohydrate. This diet is consistent with the National Cholesterol Education Program Step 2 diet.[13] In the other instance, saturated fat is decreased by replacing it with primarily monounsaturated but also polyunsaturated fats, resulting in a diet similar to that eaten traditionally in Greece.[32] The dietary cholesterol intake is reduced similarly in both diets. Changes in intake of types of foods are shown in Table 33–2. The predicted percentage changes in blood lipids are calculated in a patient with mild combined hyperlipidemia who is at high risk for coronary events (Fig. 33–1). Both diets reduce LDL by similar amounts, 17% to 21%. However, the low-fat diet would reduce HDL by 18% compared with 6% with the high-unsaturated-fat diet. The total cholesterol to HDL ratio would increase by 5% on the low-fat diet compared with a decrease of 9% with the high-unsaturated-fat diet. Moreover, the low-fat diet would increase fasting triglycerides by 17% compared with 1% on the high-unsaturated-fat diet. Such decreases in HDL and increases in triglycerides with the low-fat diet raise questions about the eventual effects on risk of CHD.[14]

TABLE 33–2 • Changes in Foods to Achieve Nutritional Goals to Prevent Cardiovascular Disease

Increase	Decrease
Vegetables	Animal fats
Fruits	Hydrogenated vegetable oils (*trans*-fatty acids)
Whole grains	Sugar
Unsaturated oils	Refined (low-fiber) cereal grains
Fish	Red meat
Nuts	
Low-fat dairy foods	

The effects of *trans*-unsaturated fatty acids (*trans*-fatty acids) on lipoproteins and CHD need to be considered separately from the natural *cis*-unsaturated oils. Oils from plants have double bonds between carbon atoms that are exclusively in the *cis* orientation, and their effects have been discussed earlier. *Trans*-fatty acids are produced during industrial hydrogenation of vegetable oil in the manufacturing of vegetable shortening and margarine. The hydrogenation process uses high temperature, metallic catalysts, and hydrogen gas to reduce the double bonds between carbon atoms to single bonds; a byproduct of this process is the isomerization of *cis* to *trans* double bonds. *Trans*-fatty acids have a higher melting point than *cis*-isomers and contribute to solidity of these products. Hydrogenation does not occur during cooking with vegetable oil. *Trans*-fatty acids are also produced by bacteria in the gut of ruminant animals and are found in red meat and dairy fat. During the past 6 years, many careful dietary studies have shown that intake of *trans*-fatty acids has several harmful effects on plasma lipoprotein concentrations: LDL increases, HDL decreases, and lipoprotein(a), a potentially atherogenic lipoprotein, also increases.[33, 34] These adverse effects on plasma lipoproteins may explain why epidemiologic studies found an association between intake of *trans*-fatty acids and incidence of CHD.[35–37] Although a clinical endpoint trial has not, and probably never will be, conducted that alters *trans*-fatty acids as a single nutrient, the evidence for harmful effects is strong and should lead to avoidance of foods that contain hydrogenated oils. At this time, food labeling does not separately list the *trans*-fatty acids, but the term *partially hydrogenated* in the list of ingre-

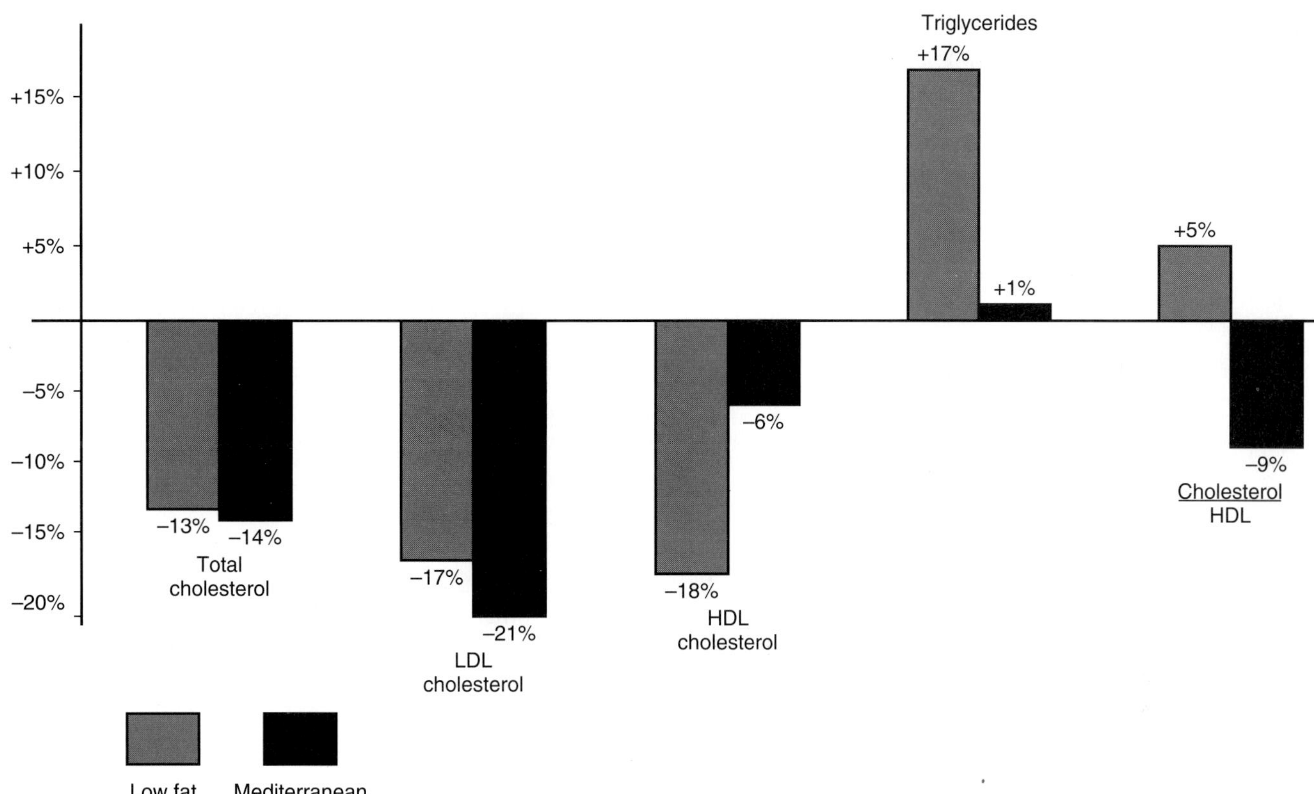

Figure 33–1 Expected effects of moderate dietary changes on blood lipids in a patient with mild combined hyperlipidemia. The pretreatment levels were as follows: total cholesterol 240 mg/dL, low-density lipoprotein (LDL) cholesterol 170 mg/dL, high-density lipoprotein (HDL) cholesterol 35 mg/dL, and triglycerides 175 mg/dL. The percentage changes in blood lipids were calculated for the changes in dietary fatty acids[17] and dietary cholesterol[15] shown in Table 33–1 for an example of a low-fat National Cholesterol Education Program (NCEP) Step 2 diet,[13] and a high-unsaturated-fat Mediterranean-type diet. Gray bars, low-fat diet; black bars, high unsaturated fat, Mediterranean-type diet.

dients indicates that *trans*-fatty acids are present. In the United States, they are ubiquitous in baked goods.

CONTROLLED TRIALS OF DIETARY THERAPY AND CORONARY EVENTS

Controlled dietary trials show a clear pattern of benefit in relation to CHD events. For this analysis, I have considered randomized dietary trials with at least 2 years of average follow-up,[38–43] since, in cholesterol-lowering therapy, 2 years appears to be the average duration before the treatment group begins to show a reduction in coronary events.[44] The Indian Heart Study,[45, 46] a controlled dietary trial with several unique aspects, is discussed separately. Multifactorial intervention programs are also considered separately because it is impossible to distinguish the effect of the diet from that of the other treatments. Two dietary approaches have been tested: one to lower total and saturated fat[38, 39] and the other to replace saturated with unsaturated fats, leaving total fat unchanged.[40–43] The high-unsaturated-fat diets were more successful than the low-fat diets in lowering serum cholesterol (mean 14% vs. 4%) and in lowering CHD (Table 33–3). Reduction in CHD in the high-unsaturated-fat diets averaged 21% and ranged from 14% to 43%, as opposed to −9% to +4% in the low-fat diet trials. Since, theoretically, the two types of diets should lower serum total cholesterol levels to a similar extent,[17] one must conclude that adherence to the low-fat diet was poorer than for the high-unsaturated-fat diets. To summarize, coronary events decreased significantly in all trials in which the diet lowered plasma total cholesterol by at least 10% (see Table 33–3). Overall, in these trials of hypercholesterolemic patients, the mean reductions in coronary events in the trials of unsaturated fat diets[40–43] averaged 21%, and compare favorably with that achieved with nicotinic acid[47] or cholestyramine,[19] but the magnitude of effect was less than that observed for pravastatin[1] or simvastatin.[2]

In the St. Thomas Atherosclerosis Regression Study (STARS), coronary arteriography was used to measure the luminal diameter or luminal obstruction of diseased coronary arteries, as the primary study endpoints, in a trial that compared dietary therapy with or without cholestyramine[48] (Table 33–4). The diet was designed to lower total and saturated fat and

TABLE 33–3 • Clinical Trials of Diet Therapy to Lower Blood Cholesterol Levels and Reduce Coronary Events

Trials†	N	Dietary Fat (% energy)	Duration (yr)	▲Cholesterol (%)	▲CHD (%)
Reduction in Total Fat					
MRC[38]	123	22	3	−5	+4
DART[39]	1015	"low fat"	2	−3.5	−9
Substitution of Unsaturated Fat for Saturated Fat					
Turpeinen[42]	676	34	6	−15*	−43*
Leren[43]	206	39	5	−14*	−25*
MRC soy oil[41]	194	46	4	−15*	−14
Dayton[40]	424	40	8	−13*	−23*

* $P < 0.05$.
† Trials with at least 2 years of average follow-up were included.
▲Cholesterol refers to the percentage change in serum cholesterol in the treatment group compared with the change in the control group. ▲CHD refers to the percentage difference in coronary event rates in the treatment group compared with the control group.

increase unsaturated oils and vegetables and fruits. LDL significantly decreased by 16%, but contrary to expectation,[17] HDL did not decrease, and triglycerides actually decreased rather than increased. Since the patients did not lose weight, it seems likely that saturated fat was replaced more by unsaturated oils than by carbohydrate; the specific dietary changes made by the patients were not reported. Relative to the control group, the dietary groups with or without cholestyramine both showed significant improvement in coronary stenosis, and there was little difference between the two treatments. One could speculate that the beneficial effects on coronary stenosis of the decrease in LDL caused by cholestyramine were counterbalanced by the increase in triglyceride levels relative to the diet only group. In this trial, the improvement in coronary stenosis with diet alone was greater than in other angiographic studies of diet or drug therapy.[49] Again, the evidence supports the conclusion that effective diet therapy produces considerable benefit to coronary disease.

The Lyon Diet Heart Study,[50] a secondary prevention trial, tested the effects of a "Mediterranean" diet compared with a standard low-fat diet (Table 33–5). The specific dietary changes were substitution of animal fat with polyunsaturated vegetable oil rich in α-linolenic acid (ALA) and replacement of meat, butter, and cream with fish, legumes, bread, fruits, and vegetables. Total fat intake did not change. Surprisingly, there were no changes in plasma lipid levels. Nonetheless, coronary events were reduced in the treatment group by 73%. Adherence to the diet was confirmed by increases in blood levels of oleic acid, the ω-3 fatty acids, ALA and eicosapentaenoic acid (EPA), and antioxidant vitamins. This trial suggests that aspects of the diet besides those that affect blood lipids can prevent coronary events. Which of these nutritional changes were responsible for the benefit cannot be determined.

FISH AND FISH OIL

A British trial tested the effects of three dietary therapies for 2 years in men with myocardial infarction: reduced fat, high-fiber cereal, or increased fatty fish.[39] In these men who usually did not eat much fatty fish, only two fish meals per week significantly reduced total mortality by 29% (Fig. 33–2) and coronary mortality by 33%. In contrast, neither the reduced-fat nor the increased-fiber diets showed any tendency to

TABLE 33–4 • Effectiveness of Diet Therapy on Coronary Stenosis in Men with Combined Hyperlipidemia: The St. Thomas Atherosclerosis Regression Study (STARS)[48]

	Control (%)	Diet (%)	Diet + Cholestyramine (%)
Change in Blood Lipids			
Total cholesterol	−2	−14*	−25*
LDL cholesterol	−3	−16*	−36*
HDL cholesterol	−1	0	−4
Triglycerides	+1	−20*	0
Coronary Atherosclerosis			
Change in stenosis†	+6	−1*	−2*

*$P < 0.05$ compared with control.
† For change in stenosis, a positive sign indicates worsening and a negative sign indicates improvement.
LDL, low-density lipoprotein; HDL, high-density lipoprotein.

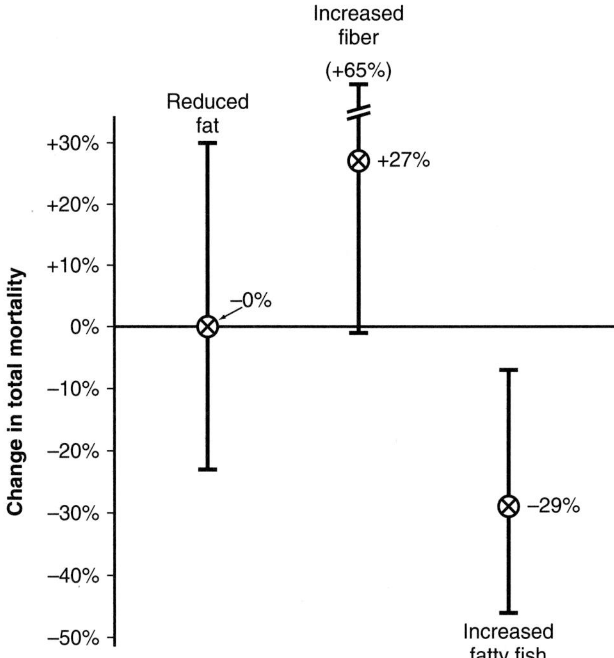

Figure 33–2 Three diet therapies after myocardial infarction from the Diet and Reinfarction Trial (DART).[39] Mean and 95% confidence intervals are shown. The study used a factorial design to randomize 2033 men, 2 months or sooner after myocardial infarction, to an active treatment group or control group. The resulting sample sizes for each treatment or control group were 1015 to 1018. The average duration of treatment was 2 years.

produce benefit. As with the Lyon Heart Study[50] (see Table 33–5), this trial suggests that ω-3 fatty acids could be beneficial against CHD.

The ω-3 fatty acids that are found in fish, EPA and docosahexaenoic acid (DHA) have several effects that could contribute to reducing clinical coronary events. In relatively high amounts, 3 to 12 g daily, as in 200 to 800 g of fatty fish, they lower the plasma triglyceride concentration,[51] accelerate the clearance of potentially atherogenic postprandial triglyceride-rich lipoproteins,[52] raise HDL_2 cholesterol concentration,[53] and lower blood pressure in patients with mild to moderate hypertension but not in patients with normal or high normal blood pressure.[53, 54] Recent evidence is consistent with an antiarrhythmic action of ω-3 fatty acids. In dogs who had sustained experimental myocardial infarction, intravenous infusion of ω-3 fatty acids raised the threshold for ischemia-induced ventricular fibrillation.[55] In a double-blind trial in patients who had ventricular premature complexes, fish oil supplementation using 16 mL of cod liver oil daily for 16 weeks reduced the daily incidence of such events.[56] In agreement with this hypothesis, a case-control study death found that dietary intake of ω-3 fatty acids was very low in persons who experienced sudden death.[57] Perhaps this antiarrhythmic action could have contributed to the reduction in coronary death in the Lyon Heart Study[50] and in the Diet and Reinfarction Trial (DART),[39] both of which increased intake of ω-3 fatty acids in patients who had acute myocardial infarction.

TABLE 33–5 • Mediterranean Dietary Approach to Prevent Death After Myocardial Infarction: The Lyon Heart Study[50]

Dietary Changes
Increased: fruits, vegetables, beans, bread, vegetable oil
Decreased: meats, butter, cream
Unchanged: total fat (31%)
Body Weight:
Decreased
Fatty Acid Changes
Increased: oleic, α-linolenic, ω-3 (EPA, DHA)
Decreased: linoleic, saturated
Unchanged: trans
Blood Levels
Increased: ascorbic acid, α-tocopherol, oleic acid, α-linolenic, EPA, DHA
Decreased: none
Unchanged: cholesterol, LDL, HDL, blood pressure, platelet aggregation
Coronary Events (*n*)
Control: 33/303
Experimental: 8/302
Change: −73% ($P = 0.001$)

EPA, eicosapentaenoic acid; DHA, docosahexaenoic acid; LDL, low-density lipoprotein; HDL, high-density lipoprotein.

DIET AND EXERCISE

Diet and vigorous exercise therapy for 1 year improved coronary stenosis in angiographic trials (Table 33–6). In one trial, adherence was enhanced by providing the patients with all of their food, and yoga and stress management training were integral components.[58] Adherence to the entire program was correlated with improvement in stenosis. In the other trial, improvement in exercise capacity was the most sig-

TABLE 33–6 • Dietary and Exercise Programs to Improve Coronary Atherosclerosis

Trial	Lifestyle Heart Study (Ornish[58])	Schuler[59]
Location	San Francisco, USA	Heidelberg, Germany
Intervention	Low-fat, strict vegetarian diet Exercise Stress management, yoga	Low-fat diet Exercise
Duration	1 yr	1 yr
*Blood Cholesterol**	−19	−10
Coronary Stenosis,†*	−5.6	−4

* Change in blood cholesterol level and coronary stenosis in treatment group compared with control group.
† For coronary stenosis, the change is expressed in percentage points of luminal narrowing. A negative sign indicates improvement.

nificant variable that predicted improved stenosis.[59] Comparing the various diet and drug trials, the diet trials with or without exercise had a greater benefit on coronary stenosis than could be expected from the reductions in LDL cholesterol.[49] Thus it seems likely that nonpharmacologic therapy has benefits that are independent of effects on LDL concentration. However, long-term adherence and clinical outcomes in these rigorous programs need to be studied.

EARLY BENEFITS FROM PROMPT INITIATION OF DIET THERAPY AFTER MYOCARDIAL INFARCTION (Table 33–7)

Several studies enrolled patients soon after myocardial infarction: 2 days,[45, 46] 2 weeks,[50, 60] and 6 weeks.[39] Diet therapy was used in three of the trials,[39, 45, 50] whereas diet, exercise, and smoking cessation were used in one.[60] All demonstrated reduction in coronary death at the end of the trials, which ranged from 1 to 3 years in average duration. However, the striking finding in these trials was the early benefit. The curves of the event rates of the treated groups began diverging from the control groups within 2 to 3 months of randomization[39, 45, 60] or before 6 months.[50]

The Indian Heart Study[45, 46] was unique in its population and intervention and in the demonstration of a significant reduction in coronary events after only 12 weeks of treatment. In this 1-year dietary trial in India,[45, 46] patients during hospitalization with acute myocardial infarction were taught to increase intake of vegetables, fruits, and whole grains and to decrease saturated fat and cholesterol. Unique to this trial, the patients were eating a low-fat, mainly vegetarian diet before treatment, and the total fat in both treatment groups was maintained at the customarily low level of 24% to 26%. Several coronary risk factors were significantly improved in the treatment compared with the control group. Serum cholesterol decreased by 8%, body weight decreased by 4 kg, blood pressure decreased by 8 mm Hg systolic and 6 mm Hg diastolic, and fasting glucose level was reduced. Coronary death was reduced by 41% and nonfatal myocardial infarction by 38% at the end of the trial. After 12 weeks, coronary events were reduced by 36% ($P < 0.01$).

The early benefit in these trials that started dietary therapy soon after myocardial infarction contrasts with a generally longer duration of latency, 2 years on average, in secondary prevention trials in which therapy is started later after myocardial infarction, or in most primary prevention trials.[44] This analysis suggests that timing of diet therapy after myocardial infarction is important to produce early benefit. There are no drug studies that have yet addressed the issue of when to initiate therapy, although prudence suggests also starting early.

DIETARY FACTORS THAT COULD BE PROTECTIVE AGAINST CHD

The diets that were used in CHD prevention trials usually made changes in many nutrients that could have been responsible for the reduction in CHD. Reduction in saturated fat and cholesterol lowers LDL cholesterol concentrations, and this has the most well-established relationship to coronary events. Increases in ω-3 fatty acids either from vegetable oils or fish oils favorably affect lipoproteins, blood pressure, and the threshold for ventricular arrhythmia. Intake of fruits and vegetables is often increased in diets to

TABLE 33–7 • Effect on Recurrent Coronary Events of Diet and Other Nonpharmacological Therapy Initiated Early After Myocardial Infarction

Trial	*N*	Therapy	When Started (post-MI)	Duration	Coronary Events: *Death* (N)	Coronary Events: *Nonfatal MI* (N)	Time to Earliest Discernible Benefit*
WHO Finland[60]	375	Diet Exercise No smoking	2 wk	3 yr	35 vs. 55**	34 vs. 21	≤3 mo
DART[39]	1015	Fatty fish	6 wk	2 yr	78 vs. 116**	49 vs. 33	<2 mo
Indian Heart Study[45,46]	406	Diet†	2 d	1 yr	21 vs. 38**	29 vs. 44**	12 wk§
Lyon Heart Study[50]	606	Mediterranean diet‡	2 wk	27 mo	3 vs. 6**	5 vs. 17**	<6 mo

* Earliest discernible benefit is defined as the point at which the event rate of the treatment group began to diverge from that of the control group, as estimated from Kaplan-Meier or survival curves.

† Increased fruits and vegetables, decreased saturated fat, cholesterol, and refined carbohydrate.

‡ See Table 33–5 for description of diet.

§ Significant reduction in coronary events by 12 weeks.

** $P < 0.05$.

MI, myocardial infarction.

prevent CHD, which increases antioxidant vitamins, folic acid, vitamin B_6, and fiber that are associated with a lower CHD event rate in epidemiologic studies. The dietary antioxidants, vitamin E, carotenoids, vitamin C, and selenium are discussed Chapter 32.

The plasma homocysteine concentration is a risk factor for CHD.[61, 62] Folic acid, vitamin B_6, and vitamin B_{12} are cofactors for enzymes that convert homocysteine to methionine, thereby lowering plasma concentrations. Elevated plasma homocysteine levels occur mainly in persons whose daily intake of folic acid is below 400 μg.[63] Primary sources of folic acid are vegetables and fruits. A standard multivitamin contains enough folic acid to normalize folic acid levels, as well as supplying the other cofactors, vitamins B_6 and B_{12}. The homocysteine hypothesis of atherosclerosis has not been examined in a controlled clinical trial by supplementing folic acid or the other cofactors. However, in view of the strength of the available evidence, it would appear reasonable to recommend daily use of a standard multivitamin in a program to prevent CHD.

Epidemiologic studies have found an inverse association between fiber intake and CHD.[64] Fruits, vegetables, and whole cereal grains are good sources of dietary fiber. Fiber is divided into two general categories: soluble and insoluble. Soluble fibers are like gels and gums and absorb water in the intestine. This may affect intestinal cholesterol and bile acid metabolism and result in lowered plasma LDL cholesterol.[65] However, the effect on LDL is small within practical ranges of intake[65–67] and cannot explain the inverse association between fiber and CHD in populations. Moreover, the protective association with CHD was found mainly with cereal fiber,[64] which is mostly insoluble and does not lower LDL concentrations. High intake of soluble fiber may reduce the glycemic index of foods to improve postprandial glucose and insulin levels,[68] although this effect does not appear to be present within the practical range of fiber intake.[69] Only one clinical trial exists that increased dietary fiber, and it showed no effect on recurrent coronary events in patients with recent myocardial infarction.[39] Therefore, the causal role for fiber is not well supported by clinical trials, and its inverse association with CHD in epidemiologic studies may be due to the fact that high-fiber intake occurs in persons with an entire constellation of healthy behaviors, dietary and other.[64, 70] Fiber should increase as a byproduct of adhering to diets that are recommended to prevent CHD. Eating foods that are high in fiber supplies other important nutrients such as antioxidants and folic acid that could be protective, as well as displacing foods that contain saturated fat and cholesterol.[67] The current state of knowledge supports overall changes in diet that are shown to prevent CHD rather than placing emphasis on fiber supplements.

MULTIFACTORIAL TRIALS

Multifactorial approaches to prevent cardiovascular disease have been difficult to interpret in view of conflicting results. Certain trials combined nonpharmacologic and pharmacologic therapy to treat hyperlipidemia,[71] others combined various nonpharmacologic interventions,[72] whereas still other trials combined diet and drug therapy to treat simultaneously both hyperlipidemia and hypertension.[73–75] Variable compliance to the nonpharmacologic intervention, and possible toxicity from drug therapies such as clofibrate[71] or high-dose diuretics[75] confound conclusions as to the benefits, if any, that can be expected. The Oslo Study Group[72] and the World Health Organization (WHO) Collaborative Program for primary prevention of cardiovascular disease[73, 74] both provide insight into such programs. The Oslo study intervened with diet to reduce serum cholesterol and body weight, and with smoking cessation. Each risk factor was significantly improved, and coronary events were reduced by 47%. The investigators estimated that lowered serum cholesterol was responsible for at least 75% of the benefit and smoking cessation for no more than 25%.[72] The WHO Collaborative Program was carried out with closely comparable methods for 5 to 6 years in 18,210 persons in Belgium[73] and 19,409 persons in the United Kingdom.[74] The intervention consisted of diet therapy and exercise to reduce blood cholesterol and body weight, smoking cessation, and hypertension control by diuretics with potassium supplementation. The Belgian program was successful in reducing significantly the coronary event rate by 25% and total mortality by 18% in the intervention compared with the control group, whereas in the United Kingdom, the coronary event rate was 6% higher (not significant) in the intervention group. The favorable result in Belgium compared to United Kingdom was attributed to better adherence as shown by greater improvements in risk factors. Finally, the perplexing Helsinki Businessmen Study of primary prevention[71] deserves comment. In this trial, 1222 men were randomized to a control group or to a multifactorial program of diet with or without clofibrate and/or probucol for hyperlipidemia, or diuretics and/or beta blockers for hypertension. The treated men were "frequently" given four or five agents.[76] The results were inconclusive after the 5-year planned duration of the randomized trial, but 10 years after the trial ended, coronary deaths were higher in the previously treated group. However, the patients who received only diet treatment did not have a higher death rate, and it may be considered that an adverse effect of the particular combination of drugs used could have been responsible. In conclusion, as regards multifactorial programs, good adherence to effective therapy for elevated blood cholesterol and/or blood pressure that does not have major side effects, as well as smoking cessation produces the desired benefits for coronary heart disease.

CONCLUSION USING EVIDENCE-BASED MEDICINE

Evidence-based medicine requires that guidelines for treatment be based on randomized clinical trials that show improvement in clinical event rates or in risk factors that are known to be in the causal pathway. Clinical trials demonstrate that diets that increase unsaturated fat and decrease saturated fat reduce coronary events without increasing other causes of morbidity or mortality. In contrast, the standard approach for diet therapy with the Step 1 and 2 diets has not shown efficacy either for improving the lipid profile or reducing coronary events either because of low adherence or adverse metabolic effects. Clinicians can recommend to patients or to dietitians who work with them cookbooks on Mediterranean-type diets to assist them in making diet changes. The use of unsaturated oils expands the range of cooking styles that are compatible with the dietary goals. Other dietary approaches that have reduced coronary events in single trials are increased intake of fatty fish,[39] increased fruits and vegetables,[45] and a Mediterranean diet.[50] Initiation of dietary therapy soon after myocardial infarction may produce early benefits. Multifactorial programs for hyperlipidemia and hypertension are more complicated to evaluate, but programs that demonstrably improve risk factors with diet therapy and use simple drug regimens that are known individually to reduce cardiovascular events and are not a cause of toxicity are likely to be effective.

REFERENCES

1. Shepherd J, Cobbe SM, Ford I, et al. Prevention of coronary heart disease with pravastatin in men with hypercholesterolemia. N Engl J Med 1995; 333:1301–1307.
2. Scandinavian Simvastatin Survival Study Group (4S). Randomized trial of cholesterol lowering in 4444 patients with coronary heart disease: The Scandinavian Simvastatin Survival Study (4S). Lancet 1994; 344:1383–1389.
3. Byington RP, Jukema JW, Salonen JT, et al. Reduction in cardiovascular events during pravastatin therapy: Pooled analysis of clinical events of the Pravastatin Atherosclerosis Intervention Program. Circulation 1995; 92:2419–2425.
4. Sacks FM, Pfeffer MA, Moye LA, et al. The effect of pravastatin on coronary events after myocardial infarction in patients with average cholesterol levels. N Engl J Med 1996; 335:1001–1009.
5. Martin MJ, Hulley SB, Browner WS, et al. Serum cholesterol, blood pressure, and mortality: Implications from a cohort of 361,662 men. Lancet 1986; 2:933–936.
6. Pekkanen J, Linn S, Heiss G, et al. Ten-year mortality from cardiovascular disease in relation to cholesterol level among men with and without preexisting cardiovascular disease. N Engl J Med 1990; 322:1700–1707.
7. Rose G, Reid DD, Hamilton PJ, et al. Myocardial ischemia, risk factors and death from coronary heart disease. Lancet 1977; 1:105–109.
8. Kannel WB. Range of serum cholesterol values in the population developing coronary artery disease. Am J Cardiol 1995; 76:69C–77C.
9. Rossouw JE. Lipid-lowering interventions in angiographic trials. Am J Cardiol 1995; 76:86C–92C.
10. Holme I. Cholesterol reduction and its impact on coronary artery disease and total mortality. Am J Cardiol 1995; 76:10C–17C.
11. Rubins HB, Robins SJ, Collins C, et al. Distribution of lipids in 8,500 men with coronary artery disease. Am J Cardiol 1995; 75:1196–1201.
12. Johnson CL, Rifkind BM, Sempos CT, et al. Declining serum total cholesterol levels among US adults: The National Health and Nutrition Examination Surverys. JAMA 1993; 269:3002–3008.
13. Expert Panel. Summary of the Second Report of the National Cholesterol Education Program (NCEP) Expert Panel on Detection, Evaluation, and Treatment of High Blood Cholesterol in Adults (Adult Treatment Panel II). JAMA 1993; 269:3015–3022.
14. Sacks FM, Willett WC. More on chewing the fat—the good fat and the good cholesterol. [Editorial]. N Engl J Med 1991; 325:1740–1742.
15. Keys A, Anderson JT, Grande F. Serum cholesterol response to changes in the diet. Metabolism 1965; 14:747–787.
16. Hegsted DM, McGandy RB, Myers ML, Stare FJ. Quantitative effects of dietary fat on serum cholesterol in man. Am J Clin Nutr 1965; 17:281–295.
17. Mensink RP, Katan MB. Effect of dietary fatty acids on serum lipids and lipoproteins: A meta-analysis of 27 trials. Arterioscl Thromb 1992; 12:911–919.
18. Gordon DJ, Rifkind BM. High-density lipoprotein—the clinical implications of recent studies. N Engl J Med 1989; 321:1311–1316.
19. Lipid Research Clinics Program. The Lipid Research Clinics Coronary Primary Prevention Trial Results: II. The relationship of reduction of incidence of coronary heart disease to cholesterol lowering. JAMA 1984; 251:365–374.
20. Manninen V, Elo O, Frick H, et al. Lipid alterations and decline in the incidence of coronary heart disease in the Helsinki Heart Study. JAMA 1988; 260:641–651.
21. Brown G, Albers JJ, Fisher LD, et al. Regression of coronary artery disease as a result of intensive lipid-lowering therapy in men with high levels of apolipoprotein B. N Engl J Med 1990; 323:1289–1298.
22. Kinosian B, Glick H, Garland G. Cholesterol and coronary heart disease: Predicting risks by levels and ratios. Ann Intern Med 1994; 121:641–647.
23. Stampfer MJ, Sacks FM, Salvini S, et al. A prospective study of lipids, apolipoproteins, and risks of myocardial infarction. N Engl J Med 1991; 325:373–381.
24. Manninen V, Tenkanen L, Koskinen P, et al. Joint effects of serum triglyceride and LDL cholesterol and HDL cholesterol concentrations on coronary heart disease risk in the Helsinki Heart Study. Circulation 1992; 85:37–45.
25. Austin M. Plasma triglyceride and coronary heart disease. Arterioscler Thromb 1991; 11:2–13.
26. Criqui MH, Heiss G, Cohn R, et al. Plasma triglyceride level and mortality from coronary heart disease. N Engl J Med 1993; 328:120–125.
27. Assmann G, Schulte H. Relation of HDL cholesterol and triglycerides to incidence of atherosclerotic coronary artery disease: The PROCAM experience. Am J Cardiol 1992; 70:733–737.
28. Stampfer MJ, Krauss RM, Ma J, et al. A prospective study of triglycerides, LDL particle diameter, and risk of myocardial infarction. JAMA 1996; 276:882–888.
29. Chen YD, Skowronski R, Coulston AM, et al. Effect of acute variations in dietary fat and carbohydrate intake on retinyl ester content of intestinally derived lipoproteins. J Clin Endocrinol Metab 1992; 74:28–32.
30. Lichtenstein AH, Ausman LM, Carrasco W, et al. Effects of canola, corn, and olive oils on fasting and postprandial plasma lipoproteins in humans as part of a National Cholesterol Education Program Step 2 diet. Arterioscler Thromb 1993; 13:1533–1542.

31. Grant KI, Marais MP, Dhansay MA. Sucrose in a lipid-rich meal amplifies the postprandial excursion of serum and lipoprotein triglyceride and cholesterol concentrations by decreasing triglyceride clearance. Am J Clin Nutr 1994; 59:853–860.
32. Tzonou A, Kalandidi A, Trichopoulou A, et al. Diet and coronary heart disease: A case-control study in Athens, Greece. Epidemiology 1993; 4:511–516.
33. Mensink RP, Zock PL, Katan MB, et al. Efect of dietary *cis* and *trans* fatty acids on serum lipoprotein(a) in humans. J Lipid Res 1992; 33:1493–1501.
34. Nestel P, Noakes M, Belling B, et al. Plasma lipoprotein and Lp(a) changes with substitution of elaidic acid for oleic acid in the diet. J Lipid Res 1992; 33:1029–1036.
35. Willett WC, Stampfer MJ, Colditz GA, et al. Intake of *trans* fatty acids and risk of coronary heart disease among women. Lancet 1993; 341:581–585.
36. Ascherio A, Hennekens CH, Buring JE, et al. *Trans* fatty acids and risk of myocardial infarction. Circulation 1994; 89:969–974.
37. Siguel EN, Lerman RH. *Trans* fatty acid patterns in patients with angiographically documented coronary artery disease. Am J Cardiol 1993; 71:916–920.
38. Research Committee. Low-fat diet in myocardial infarction. Lancet 1965; 2:501–504.
39. Burr ML, Fehily AM, Gilbert JF, et al. Effects of changes in fat, fish, and fibre intakes on death and myocardial infarction: Diet and Reinfarction Trial (DART). Lancet 1989; 2:757–761.
40. Dayton S, Pearce ML, Hashimoto S, et al. A controlled clinical trial of a diet high in unsaturated fat in preventing complications of atherosclerosis. Circulation 1969; 40(Suppl II):II1–II63.
41. Research Committee. Controlled trial of soya-bean oil in myocardial infarction. Lancet 1968; 2:693–700.
42. Turpeinen O, Karvonen MJ, Pekkarinen M, et al. Dietary prevention of coronary heart disease: The Finnish Mental Hospital Study. Int J Epidemiol 1979; 8:99–118.
43. Leren P. The Olso Diet-Heart Study: Eleven-year report. Circulation 1970; 42:935–942.
44. Law M, Wald NJ, Thompson NJ. By how much and how quickly does reduction in serum cholesterol concentration lower risk of ischaemic heart disease? BMJ 1994; 308:367–372.
45. Singh RB, Rostogi SS, Verma R, et al. Randomised, controlled trial of cardioprotective diet in patients with recent acute myocardial infarction: Results of one-year follow-up. BMJ 1992; 304:1015–1019.
46. Singh RB, Niaz MA, Ghosh S, et al. Effect on mortality and reinfarction of adding fruits and vegetables to a prudent diet in the Indian Experiment of Infarct Survival. J Am Coll Nutr 1993; 12:255–261.
47. The Coronary Drug Project Research Group. Clofibrate and niacin in coronary heart disease. JAMA 1975; 231:360–381.
48. Watts GF, Lewis B, Brunt JN, et al. Effects on coronary artery disease of lipid-lowering diet, or diet plus cholestyramine, in the St Thomas' Atherosclerosis Regression Study (STARS). Lancet 1992; 339:563–569.
49. Sacks FM, Gibson CM, Rosner B, et al, and the Harvard Atheroscleosis Reversibility Project Research Group. The influence of pretreatment low-density lipoprotein cholesterol concentrations on the effect of hypocholesterolemic therapy on coronary atherosclerosis in angiographic trials. Am J Cardiol 1995; 76:78C–85C.
50. De Lorgeril M, Renaud S, Mamelle N, et al. Mediterranean alpha-linolenic acid-rich diet in secondary prevention of coronary heart disease. Lancet 1994; 343:1454–1459.
51. Harris WS. Fish oils and plasma lipid and lipoprotein metabolism in humans: A critical review. J Lipid Res 1989; 30:785–807.
52. Weintraub MS, Zechner R, Brown A, et al. Dietary polyunsaturated fats of the omega-6 and omega-3 series reduce postprandial lipoprotein levels. J Clin Invest 1988; 82:1884–1894.
53. Sacks FM, Hebert P, Appel LJ, et al. The effect of fish oil on blood pressure and high-density lipoprotein cholesterol levels in phase 1 of the Trials of Hypertension Prevention. J Hypertension 1994; 12(Suppl 7):S23–S31.
54. Morris MC, Sacks F, Rosner B. Does fish oil lower blood pressure? A meta-analysis of controlled trials. Circulation 1993; 88:523–533.
55. Billman GE, Hallaq H, Leaf A. Prevention of ischemia-induced ventricular fibrillation by omega-3 fatty acids. Proc Natl Acad Sci USA 1994; 91:4427–4430.
56. Sellmayer A, Witzgall H, Lorenz RL, Weber PC. Effects of dietary fish oil on ventricular premature complexes. Am J Cardiol 1995; 76:974–976.
57. Siscovic DS, Raghunathan TE, King I, et al. Dietary intake and cell membrane levels of long-chain n-3 polyunsaturated fatty acids and the risk of primary cardiac arrest. JAMA 1995; 274:1363–1367.
58. Ornish D, Brown SE, Scherwitz LW, et al. Can lifestyle changes reverse coronary heart disease? The Lifestyle Heart Trial. Lancet 1990; 336:129–133.
59. Schuler G, Hambrecht R, Schlierf G, et al. Regular physical exercise and low-fat diet: Effects on progression of coronary artery disease. Circulation 1992; 86:1–11.
60. Kallio V, Hamalainen H, Hakkila J, Luurila OJ. Reduction in sudden deaths by a multifactorial intervention programme after acute myocardial infarction. Lancet 1979; 2:1091–1094.
61. Clarke R, Daly L, Robinson D, et al. Hyperhomocysteinemia: An independent risk factor for vascular disease. N Engl J Med 1991; 324:1149–1155.
62. Stampfer MJ, Malinow MR, Willett WC, et al. A prospective study of plasma homocysteine and risk of myocardial infarction. JAMA 1992; 268:877–881.
63. Selhub J, Jacques PF, Wilson PW, et al. Vitamin status and intake as primary determinants of homocystenemia in elderly populations. JAMA 1993; 270:2693–2698.
64. Rimm EB, Ascherio A, Giovannucci E, et al. Vegetable, fruit, and cereal fiber intake and risk of coronary heart disease among men. JAMA 1996; 275:447–451.
65. Jenkins DJ, Wolever TM, Rao AV, et al. Effect on blood lipids of very high intakes of fiber in diets low in saturated fat and cholesterol. N Engl J Med 1993; 329:21–26.
66. Ripsin CM, Keenan JM, Jacobs DR, et al. Oat products and lipid lowering: A meta-analysis. JAMA 1992; 267:3317–3325.
67. Swain JF, Rouse IL, Curley CB, et al. Comparison of the effects of oat bran and low-fiber wheat on serum lipoprotein levels and blood pressure. N Engl J Med 1990; 322:147–152.
68. Jenkins DJ, Leeds AR, Gassull MA, et al. Unabsorbable carbohydrate and diabetes: Decreased postprandial hyperglycemia. Lancet 1976; 2:172–174.
69. Hollenbeck CB, Coulston AM, Reaven GM. To what extent does increased dietary fiber improve glucose and lipid metabolism in patients with noninsulin-dependent diabetes mellitus (NIDDM)? Am J Clin Nutr 1986; 43:16–24.
70. Wynder EL, Stellman SD, Zang EA. High-fiber intake: Indicator of a healthy lifestyle [Editorial]. JAMA 1996; 275:486–487.
71. Strandberg TE, Salomaa VV, Naukkarinen VA, et al. Long-term mortality after 5-year multifactorial primary prevention of cardiovascular diseases in middle-aged men. JAMA 1991; 266:1225–1229.
72. Hjermann I, Velve Byre K, Holme I, Leren P. Effect on diet and smoking intervention on the incidence of coronary heart disease. Lancet 1981; 2:1303–1309.
73. Kornitzer M, DeBacker G, Dramaix M, et al. Belgian Heart Disease Prevention Project: Incidence and mortality results. Lancet 1983; 1:1066–1070.
74. Rose G, Tunstall-Pedoe HD, Heller RF. UK Heart Disease Prevention Project: Incidence and mortality results. Lancet 1983; 1:1062–1066.
75. The Multiple Risk Factor Intervention Trial Research Group. Mortality after 16 years for participants randomized to the Multiple Risk Factor Intervention Trial. Circulation 1996; 94:946–951.
76. Strandberg TE, Miettinen TA. Multifactorial primary prevention: Exploring the failures. J Myocard Ischemia 1994; 6:15–23.

34 Multiple Risk Factor Intervention Trials

▶ Dean Ornish
▶ Jacqueline A. Hart

Coronary artery disease (CAD) remains the leading cause of morbidity and mortality in the Western industrialized world. It was first discovered and diagnosed in the early nineteenth century; approximately 11 million people in the United States now have CAD. In 1995, 1.5 million Americans had myocardial infarctions (MIs), 500,000 had coronary bypass operations, and 600,000 had percutaneous transluminal coronary angioplasties, with an estimated cost of $56.3 billion.[1]

Increasing evidence supports the idea that much of this cost—both financial and in human suffering—may be greatly reduced by the implementation of comprehensive risk factor intervention strategies. These may include behavioral interventions for motivating patients to make and maintain comprehensive changes in lifestyle (e.g., very-low-fat, low-cholesterol diets, exercise, smoking cessation, stress management techniques, and psychosocial support) and drug therapy (e.g., lipid-lowering drugs and antihypertensive medications).

Although more research is always needed, we believe that, taken as a whole, the body of evidence is sufficient to make recommendations. This is especially true given that the risks of changing diet and lifestyle are quite low, whereas the potential benefits are often substantial. In short, the limiting factor is not a lack of scientific and clinical data; rather, it is a lack of education, infrastructure, and third-party reimbursement necessary to provide this information to the patients and health professionals who may benefit from it.

This chapter provides an overview of the literature and discusses what conclusions can be substantiated. Rather than providing an encyclopedic listing of all the multiple risk factor intervention trials that have been conducted, we focus on a few of the most important and representative studies and synthesize their key lessons and applications to patient care.

The emerging understanding of the pathophysiology of CAD is having a profound influence on the awareness of how comprehensive risk factor modification may help prevent and even reverse the progression of coronary heart disease. These mechanisms also provide a greater understanding of why intensive risk factor modification may cause rapid improvements in ventricular function and myocardial perfusion and reduction in cardiac events and angina more quickly than had once been believed possible.

This chapter focuses on nonpharmacologic approaches to risk factor modification, particularly studies that impact more than one risk factor simultaneously, because there is evidence that synergy often exists between various cardiac risk factors. We have not emphasized studies that relied primarily on a single pharmacologic intervention (e.g., lipid-lowering drugs and antihypertensive medications) since these are more fully described in other chapters. We have described studies that used these drugs if they also included one or more behavioral interventions that went beyond the conventional recommendations (e.g., a diet more restrictive than an American Heart Association (AHA) Step 1 or 2 diet).

To quote from the AHA's *Medical/Scientific Consensus Panel Statement on Preventing Heart Attack and Death in Patients with Coronary Disease*,[2]

> Compelling scientific evidence, including data from recent studies in patients with coronary artery disease, demonstrates that comprehensive risk factor interventions:
>
> - Extend overall survival
> - Improve quality of life
> - Decrease need for interventional procedures such as angioplasty and bypass grafting, and
> - Reduce the incidence of subsequent myocardial infarction
>
> Application of risk reduction tactics to the more than 11 million people with coronary disease—most of whom already receive medical care—will improve overall patient outcomes and should reduce the economic burden of heart disease. In selected patients with coronary artery disease, comprehensive risk intervention may provide

satisfactory initial management, allowing postponement of or even obviating revascularization procedures.

Clinical trial data that support these recommendations derive from studies of myocardial infarction survivors and other patients with diagnosed coronary disease. However, the rationale for this approach extends to patients with other documented atherosclerotic vascular disease—for example, transient ischemic attack, stroke, or aortic or peripheral vascular disease—because coronary artery disease is a leading cause of death and disability in these patient groups.

Although these risk reduction interventions significantly improve clinical outcomes, their application is inconsistent across medical care settings and patient groups. The American Heart Association urges that every effort be made throughout the spectrum of medical care to promote more comprehensive application of risk reduction in all eligible patients.

The present consensus summary is presented as a guide to help prevent further cardiac events and death in patients with coronary and other vascular disease. More intensive efforts in applying these risk reduction strategies to all patients at the time of first diagnosis will improve both quality of life and overall outcome for this group of patients and most likely will reduce healthcare costs.

Studies have demonstrated that only approximately one third of eligible patients continue risk factor interventions over the long term. However, data also show that this proportion can be significantly increased by a team approach in which healthcare professionals—including physicians, nurses, and dietitians—manage risk reduction therapy by using follow-up techniques that include office or clinic visits and telephone contact.

Attention to enhancing patient compliance is an integral part of any risk reduction program. In many healthcare settings, the team approach will be the preferred technique for optimizing risk reduction.

Multiple risk factor intervention trials are inherently messy. The scientific method and the randomized, controlled trial are easiest to implement in animal studies, where one has complete control over the environment, or with drug studies, where one can conduct double-blinded, placebo-controlled clinical trials. In a classic randomized, controlled trial, the investigators study one independent variable (e.g., a drug) and one dependent variable (e.g., the effect of that drug on a disease) while keeping constant other possible confounding variables.

When asking patients to make multiple changes in diet and lifestyle, however, the issues are much more complex. These include the following questions:

- How can patients be motivated to make and maintain intensive lifestyle changes?
- How does one control for the confounding effects of multiple interventions?
- Which social factors influence and may confound the interpretation of medical outcomes?
- Can one conduct a true randomized, controlled trial with behavioral interventions? By definition, double-blinded studies are usually impossible when one group of patients is asked to make diet and lifestyle changes since it is obvious to both patients and investigators which group is receiving the intervention.
- How can one assess the relative and potentially confounding contribution of each component of an intervention?
- How much change in behavior is required to achieve a significant change in a risk factor? How much change in a risk factor, in turn, is required to achieve a clinically significant effect? Which is more important—the relative reduction or absolute reduction in a risk factor?

The first section of this chapter outlines and classifies clinically accepted coronary risk factors and defines terms frequently used in this body of literature. The following sections are presented chronologically, starting with epidemiologic studies that began to recognize and identify coronary risk factors, followed by discussion of early intervention trials attempting to establish a cause-effect relationship between risk factors and CAD, description of community- or population-based studies that attempt to alter the disease process from a public health perspective, and review of some of the more recent regression studies designed to impact the presumed mechanism of the disease process. The last section summarizes the data, commenting on what conclusions can be drawn and what information may be clinically relevant and applicable. In that last section, we also discuss the role of possible future research.

EPIDEMIOLOGIC STUDIES AND THE DISCOVERY OF RISK FACTORS

Cardiovascular risk factors can be classified as either modifiable or nonmodifiable.

Modifiable Risk Factors Proven to Decrease Cardiovascular Risk

1. Cigarette smoking
2. Elevated low-density lipoprotein (LDL) cholesterol
3. Hypertension

Modifiable Risk Factors that May Decrease Cardiovascular Risk

1. Physical activity
2. Obesity
3. Psychological stress/hostility
4. Lack of social support
5. Lipoprotein(a)
6. Elevated levels of homocysteine
7. Low levels of antioxidants
8. Alcohol consumption

9. Estrogen replacement therapy
10. Plasma fibrinogen
11. Glucose intolerance/diabetes mellitus
12. Low high-density lipoprotein (HDL) levels
13. Elevated triglyceride level
14. Low educational level
15. Low socioeconomic status

Nonmodifiable Risk Factors

1. Age
2. Gender
3. Family history of CAD

These risk factors often confer not only an additive but also a multiplicative effect.[3] This synergy is particularly true of cigarette smoking and its relation to other risk factors.[4]

Although the concept of "risk factors" is now widely understood, this idea has been established only a relatively short time. Starting in the late 1940s and lasting well into the 1980s, several epidemiologic prospective studies found associations between certain factors and the development and progression of CAD.

The first and perhaps most important studies were the Seven Countries Study[5] and the Framingham Heart Study.[6] Later studies included the Albany study of male civil servants,[7] the Los Angeles study of male civil servants,[8] the Chicago Western Electric Study,[9] and a study of Minneapolis professional and businessmen.[10] The China Study[11] is an example of a more recent important epidemiologic investigation.

According to William Kannel, one of the principal investigators of the Framingham Heart Study,

> Epidemiology has become the basic science of preventive cardiology. . . . Clinicians now look to epidemiological research to provide definitive information about possible predisposing factors for cardiovascular disease and preventive measures that are justified. As a result, clinicians are less inclined to regard usual or average values as acceptable and are more inclined to regard optimal values as 'normal.' Cardiovascular events are coming to be regarded as a medical failure rather than the first indication of need for treatment.[12]

THE FRAMINGHAM HEART AND SEVEN COUNTRIES STUDIES

Cardiovascular disease epidemiology began in 1948 with the advent of the Seven Countries Study and the Framingham Heart Study. At that time, many believed that cardiovascular disease must have a single origin. Exercise was considered dangerous for most people who had cardiovascular disease, and the idea that dietary fat, high blood pressure, elevated blood cholesterol levels, and smoking were important causes of coronary heart disease was controversial.

As the importance of these risk factors became better documented, interest grew in studying what happens when these risk factors were modified. These studies became categorized as *primary prevention* (modification of diet and lifestyle in people without known risk factors), *secondary prevention* (risk factor modification in people with known risk factors), and *tertiary prevention* (risk factor modification in people with known disease). These terms can be confusing, because some authors refer to primary prevention as risk factor modification in people with known risk factors and secondary prevention as risk factor modification in people with known disease.

Although advances in conventional treatments were occurring rapidly (e.g., the advent of coronary artery bypass surgery and percutaneous transluminal coronary angioplasty and the development of new categories of medications), half of coronary heart disease deaths occur suddenly in people without prior diagnosis of heart disease and most strokes occur without prior transient ischemic attacks.[13] Therefore, the need for prevention—that is, intensive risk factor modification—became increasingly understood.

INTERVENTIONAL TRIALS

Randomized, Controlled Trials

THE MULTIPLE RISK FACTOR INTERVENTION TRIAL

Epidemiologic studies *observed* the evidence documenting the existence of risk factors. Based on these observations, a number of *interventional* studies were conducted to determine if some of these risk factors could be modified and, if so, the effects on primary, secondary, and tertiary prevention.

For example, The Multiple Risk Factor Intervention Trial (MRFIT) was a randomized, controlled clinical trial to test the effect of a multifactorial intervention program on mortality from coronary heart disease in 12,866 high-risk men aged 35 to 57 years.[14] Men were randomly assigned either to a special intervention (SI) program consisting of stepped-care treatment for hypertension, counseling for cigarette smoking, and dietary advice for lowering blood cholesterol levels, or to their usual sources of health care in the community (UC).

The primary outcome measure was death from CAD. Other outcome measures included death from other cerebrovascular diseases, all-cause mortality, nonfatal MI, change in lipid profiles with comparison between the SI and UC groups, change in resting electrocardiograms (ECGs), change in resting diastolic blood pressure, self-reported smoking histories with verification by serum thiocyanate levels, and change in exercise treadmill tests.

The specific risk factors for which they chose to intervene were hypertension, smoking, and elevated cholesterol. The modalities used in the SI group included

1. Weight reduction, sodium restriction, and a stepwise approach to blood pressure treatment using medication for hypertension (beginning with thiazide diuretics, then adding beta blockers, then other medications as needed).
2. Smoking cessation programs, including behavioral modification, aversive techniques, hypnosis in selected instances, and a 10-week group support session. This last approach, group support sessions, was the most successful modality for getting people to quit permanently. Of note, the investigators from MRFIT did not intervene with pipe or cigar smokers, only cigarette smokers.
3. Dietary counseling for hypercholesterolemia initially aimed to reduce saturated fat to no more than 10% of total calories and restrict cholesterol ingestion to 300 mg per day; in 1976, the study protocol was changed to no more than 8% of total calories from saturated fat and 250 mg or less of cholesterol per day. These differences approximate the AHA Steps 1 and 2 dietary guidelines (200 mg cholesterol per day), respectively.

The SI group was seen at least every 4 months by a variety of health care professionals on a multidisciplinary team. The UC group received treatment from their usual physician(s) and yearly checkups by health care providers of the MRFIT study. Outcome measures were examined annually for the duration of the study.[15]

Over an average follow-up period of 7 years, risk factor levels declined in both groups, but to a greater degree for the SI men. Mortality from coronary heart disease was 17.9 deaths per 1000 in the SI group and 19.3 per 1000 in the UC group, a statistically nonsignificant difference of 7.1% (90% confidence interval, −15% to 25%). Total mortality rates were 41.2 per 1000 (SI) and 40.4 per 1000 (UC).

The results of this primary analysis were disappointing for many people since the difference between groups was not statistically significant. In short, *patients in the SI group did not change risk factors as much as needed, whereas patients in the UC group changed risk factors more than expected compared with the general population.* Also, thiazide diuretics may have paradoxically increased the risk of sudden cardiac death by causing hypokalemia (low potassium levels) in SI men.

Despite some of the problems encountered in the MRFIT study, it was a landmark trial. It was the first intensive, comprehensive, long-term intervention looking at multiple risk factors simultaneously and using a multidisciplinary approach. In addition, given the size of this trial, the investigators did a remarkable job with recruitment and follow-up with less than a 10% total dropout rate over the 7-year time course. This study was an ambitious undertaking; only studies of this scope could begin to address questions about mortality. Finally, MRFIT illustrates that implementation of a comprehensive approach to lifestyle change can significantly impact on risk factor modification, which has been a prelude to subsequent research; the investigators of MRFIT had particular success in the area of smoking cessation.

THE OSLO STUDY

The Oslo Study, started in the early 1970s, was also designed to look at the causal relationship between coronary risk factor modification and coronary events in subjects without identified CAD, that is, a secondary prevention trial like MRFIT. In Oslo, Norway, 1232 male residents between 40 and 49 years of age with hypercholesterolemia (serum cholesterol levels between 290 and 380 mg/dL), systolic blood pressure less than 150 mm Hg, a coronary risk score in the upper quartile of risk (based on cholesterol levels, smoking, and blood pressure), and a normal ECG were randomly assigned to either intervention or control and followed for 5 years. The principal outcome measure was coronary events defined as nonfatal MI, fatal MI, or sudden death. The incidence of strokes was also followed.

The intervention group received an initial evaluation and educational training in a diet similar to a Step 1 diet as well as in smoking cessation, with follow-up every 6 months by a multidisciplinary team. The control group received follow-up examinations once per year by a physician.

At baseline, the two groups were similar with regard to cholesterol level, tobacco consumption, and blood pressure. Following 5 years of the intervention, total and LDL cholesterol levels were both 13% lower in the intervention group compared with the control group, and triglyceride levels were 20% lower while HDL levels remained unchanged in both groups. Tobacco consumption was decreased by 45% in the intervention group compared with control at the 5-year point. Degree of physical activity and level of blood pressure remained unchanged in both groups compared with baseline. Mean body weight was also significantly reduced in the intervention group compared with control.

In terms of cardiovascular events, unlike MRFIT, there was a significant reduction in fatal MI, nonfatal MI, sudden death, and cerebrovascular accidents in the intervention group compared with control. Although coronary mortality was 55% lower and total mortality was 33% lower in the intervention group, these differences did not reach statistical significance.[16]

In another segment of the Oslo Trial assessing treatment of hypertension in men with moderately elevated blood pressure (systolic between 150 and 179 mm Hg and/or diastolic between 90 and 110 mm Hg), 785 men between 40 and 59 years of age were randomly assigned to drug treatment or usual care without a placebo intervention. Like MRFIT, there was no difference in the treatment group compared with control in terms of cardiovascular events despite a statistically significant change in both diastolic and systolic blood pressure from baseline compared with the control group.[17] Antihypertensive drugs included hydrochlorothiazide, alpha methyldopa, and propranolol. As in the MRFIT study, these drugs may have had unanticipated side effects that outweighed the potential benefit of reducing blood pressure.

In conclusion, the Oslo Trial supports the impact of reducing two risk factors—cigarette smoking and hypercholesterolemia—on lowering the incidence of MIs, strokes, and cardiovascular deaths. Hypertension as a risk factor was separated in the Oslo Trial but was not in MRFIT. Even though the Oslo Trial investigators achieved significant reduction in blood pressure levels, there was no significant difference between groups with regard to major cardiovascular morbidity or mortality. Coronary heart disease, including sudden cardiac death, was *higher* in the treated group, although between-group differences were not statistically significant.

Community Intervention Trials

The first symposium defining and discussing the community trials epidemiologic approach was published in the *American Journal of Epidemiology* in 1978.[18] Several major community-based trials looking at prevention of CAD started around the time of that publication: the Minnesota Heart Health Program (MHHP), the Stanford Five-City Project (SFCP), the Pawtucket Heart Health Program (PHHP), and the North Karelia project in Finland.

From a population standpoint, most coronary events occur in the majority of people with moderately increased risk rather than the few with very high risk. The implication is that prevention efforts should, therefore, be concentrated on that larger population because there would be a greater theoretical benefit from a public health and a cost-efficacy standpoint.

However, many clinical trials show the greatest degree of clinical benefit—both in risk factor and coronary event reduction—in the highest-risk population. Also, potential unexpected adverse effects from drug treatments are more justifiable in patients who are at high risk or who have overt disease than in population-based strategies in which a large number of people have to be treated to save relatively few lives.

Some of the original community-based trials studying multiple risk factor modification for CAD took place in Europe and are known collectively as the *World Health Organization (WHO) European Collaborative Trial of Multifactorial Prevention of Coronary Heart Disease.* Another early trial in Europe known as the *North Karelia Project* took place in Finland. Each country involved in the WHO Collaborative was also evaluated individually. The countries involved included the United Kingdom, Belgium, Italy, Poland, and Spain. The locations functioned independently; however, the study design at each site was virtually identical, as were the methods of intervention for the purpose of pooling the data.

One variation between sites was how much time health care professionals spent with treatment subjects, which turned out to be a statistically significant factor. As one would expect, the more time spent with person or persons by health care providers, the more clinical improvement they achieved in terms of risk factor modification as well as morbidity and mortality reduction. This is discussed more completely as we review the results of the trial.

THE WHO MULTIFACTORIAL TRIAL

The WHO Multifactorial Trial was started in the United Kingdom in 1971; other countries joined the effort soon thereafter.[19] The two main questions were the following:

1. Can coronary risk factors be reduced using a population-based intervention?
2. If so, do changes in risk factors translate into decreased incidence of and mortality from coronary disease and from all causes?

Two factories in each country listed were paired—one received the intervention and the other acted as a control. Within study factories, all men 40 to 59 years of age were offered an initial screening examination followed by educational materials and/or individual counseling on risk factor modification in the areas of smoking cessation, low-fat, low-cholesterol diet, daily exercise, weight reduction, and treatment of hypertension. Eighty-six percent of those eligible agreed to participate. The authors of articles related to the WHO trial did not discuss any particular characteristics, demographic or otherwise, regarding those who agreed to participate and how they may have differed from those who did not. There is also no comment regarding whether those with already defined CAD were or were not excluded from the trial.[20]

The total decrease, with data from all centers combined, was 11.1% for the combined risk estimate and 19.4% in the high-risk subjects. The net overall reduction for coronary heart disease rates was 7.4%, for deaths was 3.9%, and for fatal coronary heart disease plus nonfatal MI was 3.9%. However, none of these differences was statistically significant for the whole group.[21]

Only the Belgian center showed statistically significant differences, even though the men at the Belgian intervention factory did not experience a much larger change in coronary risk factors compared with the Belgian control factory.[22] The one variable that distinguished the Belgian intervention site from the others was that the subjects received more attention from health care professionals. This suggests that the amount of time spent with subjects and not necessarily the amount of risk reduction was associated with decreased development of and death from cardiovascular disease. These benefits of close personal attention may simply be reflected in better adherence, but also the effects of social support on morbidity and mortality from cardiac and noncardiac events independent of changes in risk factors is well documented.[23, 24] These powerful social factors are often ignored as potentially confounding influences when the effects of multiple risk factor modification interventions are assessed.

The more health care personnel at a factory site and the more individual attention received, the better the subjects did clinically. The higher-risk subjects tended to receive more one-on-one counseling from the factory nurse, physician, and/or nutritionist (a reason they may have incurred more benefit). This particular variation in implementation of the intervention seemed to account for differences in the results of each of the countries.

THE NORTH KARELIA PROJECT

The power of social support was also seen clearly in the North Karelia Project, which, as mentioned earlier, was the first population-based cardiovascular disease prevention program. Even though the risk factor intervention achieved, as compared with the reference population, a sizeable reduction in smoking and a small reduction in blood pressure and serum cholesterol levels, the effect on coronary and cardiovascular mortality of the program remained equivocal. As seen in the other community trials and in the MRFIT study, the failure to show significant differences between the groups was owing to an insufficiently rigorous intervention and to secular trends in the comparison group.[25]

However, there was a significant association between the extent of social support (whether provided by the intervention or from other sources) and mortality from ischemic heart disease in the North Karelia Project. Those who were socially isolated had a 200% to 300% increased risk of death over 5 to 9 years when compared with those who had the greatest sense of social connection and community. These results were found even when there was extensive adjustment for traditional cardiovascular risk factors. Analyses using a variety of techniques provide no evidence that this association was owing to the impact of prevalent disease on the extent of social contacts. Furthermore, changes in social connections during one 9-year period were prospectively associated with increased risk of death from ischemic heart disease in a subsequent 9-year period. Finally, the level of social connections modified the association between diastolic blood pressure and risk of death from ischemic heart disease.[26]

THE MINNESOTA HEART HEALTH PROGRAM

The MHHP remains the largest community-based trial funded by the National Heart, Lung, and Blood Institute (NHLBI) to look at a community approach to primary prevention of CAD. The study design included 500,000 people from a total of six communities (three paired communities) in the upper Midwest. This was a community-wide intervention invoking multiple approaches to encourage changes in the population at large instead of in selected people in hopes that it would impact on the rate of overall development of CAD assessed by incidence of cardiac risk factors and occurrence of coronary events, including death. The intent would be to decrease the *population's* risk as opposed to an *individual's* risk and to measure the resulting impact on public health.

Following a few years of baseline data collection, the MHHP intervention was implemented between 1981 and 1984 and remained ongoing in the last treatment community until 1990. Each treatment community received five to six years of active intervention in the areas of hypertension prevention and control, dietary education and counseling for lowering cholesterol and blood pressure, smoking cessation, and encouragement of physical activity. All communities were assessed for lifestyle behaviors and risk factors for up to 7 years of follow-up and for morbidity and mortality for up to 13 years. The paired communities were matched on size, character, and distance from Minneapolis-St. Paul.

The sites within each matched pair were not randomly assigned to either intervention or comparison; however, the assignments were completed prior to collection of any data. Baseline and follow-up data were collected by two survey methods: *cross sectional* and *cohort*. The cross-sectional approach refers to independently conducted surveys of 300 to 500 randomly selected adults between 25 and 74 years of age conducted every 2 years in each of the six study communities. The cohort surveys were conducted on a group of randomly selected participants from the preintervention cross-sectional surveys who were recontacted for follow-up throughout the 6- to 7-year time course, that is, the same group followed longitudinally as opposed to the cross-sectional surveys, which were different individuals at any given survey point. Each approach is useful and provides somewhat different information. The cohort surveys allow for following behavioral trends and risk factor patterns in people over time; however, a potential bias stems from the involvement and contact with health care professionals conducting the surveys and measuring risk factors, a problem partly obviated by using data from independent samples via the cross-sectional surveys. In other words, the cross-sectional surveys theoretically examine the pure impact of the community-based learning programs on people without the influence of individualized attention.

Interventions were implemented on several different levels, including (1) individual exposure with structured programs geared to education and behavioral modification to reduce risk factors; (2) community organization with involvement of key respected community leaders, including physicians; and (3) mass media communication. Examples of approaches used included but were not limited to the following:

1. Adult education classes for weight control, exercise, and cholesterol lowering
2. Worksite weight control programs
3. Home correspondence course for weight loss and/or smoking cessation made available to those in the intervention communities by mass mailings
4. Incentive programs for weight loss and smoking cessation (including reimbursement of the cost of the program if smoking cessation was achieved or if the weight goal was obtained; "Quit and Win" contests)
5. School interventions for primary prevention in adolescents
6. Self-help materials and pamphlets available in the intervention communities and sent by direct mailings to peoples' homes
7. Telephone support (for those participating in programs)
8. Presence of education centers around town for screening blood pressure, weight, and cholesterol
9. Grocery store food labeling with education about "shopping smart for your heart"
10. Use of mass media, including newspapers, radio, and television

The results of this large, comprehensive, population-based study were not as positive or promising as anticipated. For most of the cardiac risk factors examined, the changes in the intervention groups were in a favorable direction relative to the comparison groups (namely, hypertension, smoking, weight, cholesterol, and physical activity); however, with a few rare exceptions, none of the changes was statistically significant. There was no significant difference in death rate from CAD when comparing the two groups, which is the only cardiac event data available.

As in the MRFIT study, (1) the experimental group was not asked to make changes large enough to cause substantial changes in risk factors, and (2) the control group began to make changes on their own, in part because of background secular trends—that is, a greater awareness in the general population of the importance of changing risk factors—and because the act of observing people in a study with surveys and questionnaires often influences their behavior. In addition, several influential events occurred during the particular time course of the trial, including public smoking restrictions, improved labeling of food products, and general increased availability of health information. More broadly, the existence of a trial such as MHHP influences and affects secular trends, presumably through advertising, media exposure, communication between participants and nonparticipants (including participating and nonparticipating health care providers), and migration of people from treatment community to nontreatment communities. It is difficult to control for these components, and their influence should not be underestimated.

There are other interesting lessons to learn from the MHHP study design and findings. The design is unusual and complicated in that communities are the units of analysis, while individuals within the communities are the units of observation and data collection. This lends to a bias for which it is difficult to control. The investigators learned that it would have been better to have a greater number of smaller communities, maximizing both the similarities within each community and the likelihood of identifying differences between communities.

Another problem in the study design was that the communities were not randomly selected for participation in the trial, nor were the communities within each pair randomly assigned to treatment versus comparison. Therefore, although the paired communities were matched based on the criteria discussed earlier in this section, there were baseline differences between the groups discovered from the initial surveys conducted; awareness of these differences by investigators may have influenced subsequent information gathered and comparisons made.

Finally, when tabulating results and differences between treatment and comparison groups, the investigators looked at all interventional programs together, despite the variety of treatment methods employed. Separate analysis of distinct approaches may have yielded more valuable information about which particular methods were most effective. In more recent publications, the MHHP investigators have begun to look at differences between the interventions to address this question of effectiveness. They state that the more intense types of behavioral change were the most effective in eliciting clinical improvement in the form of risk factor modification. However, recruitment to those particular interventional programs was more difficult than desired or expected. Therefore, as the trial proceeded, investigators focused their promotional efforts on the programs with greater "mass appeal," which were not always effective in altering cardiac risk factors or cardiac status.[18]

Understanding what is *effective* as opposed to what is *feasible* for lifestyle modification of risk factors is an extremely important concept. If a method is relatively easy to do but ineffective, it is misleading to tell people that it will help modify their risk for coronary disease. In addition, acknowledging and discussing what is effective makes that method more accessible over time by enhancing familiarity and, ultimately, changing belief patterns about what is feasible and desirable. By analogy, most physicians acknowledge to their patients the difficulty of quitting smoking, yet advise their patients to quit, not simply to cut back from three to two packs a day. It may be easier to cut back than to quit, but it may not be effective.

THE PAWTUCKET HEART HEALTH PROGRAM AND THE STANFORD FIVE-CITY PROJECT

The two other main studies in this category of community-based trials include the PHHP[27, 28] and the SFCP,[29, 30] both of which shared some similarities with MHHP and the WHO Collaborative but also had some differences. Like MHHP, the PHHP was funded by NHLBI. PHHP provided a more accurate prediction of secular trends than MHHP; therefore, the study was powered more appropriately. PHHP was designed in hopes of producing the following statistically significant results:

1. 6% reduction in mean total cholesterol
2. 6 mm Hg reduction in mean systolic blood pressure
3. 30% reduction in numbers of active smokers
4. 15% reduction in cardiovascular event rates

In comparison with the MHHP predictions, these values come closer to the actual values. SFCP had two treatment and three comparison cities (a total of 320,300 subjects), whereas PHHP had one of each (approximately 140,000 subjects).

Similar to MHHP, the groups in PHHP and SFCP were not randomly assigned. The investigators chose the cities based on two different criteria: (1) population between 40,000 and 100,000 from 1975 census data, and (2) stability of migration to try to ensure that the character of the population did not change tremendously over the study time course. That stability also facilitates follow-up in the cohort surveys and ensures greater accuracy of population-based statistics because the people who were being exposed to the interventions are the same people having their risk factors and cardiac event rate affected later. Unlike MHHP, baseline statistics from the two cities in PHHP were examined and considered before communities were chosen for the trial; therefore, they were demographically and clinically similar.

Selection criteria for the cities in the SFCP included location, size, and media market. The three control cities (Modesto, San Luis Obispo, and Santa Maria) were specifically chosen because, at the time, they were isolated from the treatment media market while the two treatment cities (Monterey and Salinas) shared a media market.

Although the five cities had been similar demographically according to 1970 census information, baseline surveys conducted at the start of the trial found significant differences between them: Monterey and San Luis Obispo had a higher mean level of education, and residents of San Luis Obispo had the younger mean age as well as a significantly higher percentage of men. To try to account for the demographic differences, the investigators not only looked at the results of the community at large but also broke them down into 24 smaller categories based on gender, age, and level of education. In addition to these demographic differences, there were clinical differences as well. The control groups were significantly more knowledgeable about coronary risk factors and had significantly lower baseline cholesterol, mean systolic and diastolic blood pressure, and lower basal metabolic index at baseline than the treatment group.

The intervention or implementation of community-based programs as well as the collection of data for PHHP and SFCP was similar to MHHP. As with MHHP, PHHP and SFCP conducted cohort and independent or cross-sectional surveys over time. The results of these two trials were more strongly positive than MHHP.

SFCP found significant changes in each of the following areas when comparing treatment groups with controls:

1. Improved knowledge of coronary disease risk factors—both treatment and comparison groups experienced improvement, but the treatment participants experienced significantly greater magnitude of change
2. Reduction in mean total cholesterol in the second and third surveys for the cohort groups—cholesterol values improved with each survey for the independent participants; however, that change was only statistically significant by the fourth measurement

3. Percentage of active smokers declined significantly in cohort participants but not among independent participants, reinforcing what was seen from the results of MHHP and the WHO Collaborative discussed earlier—the likelihood of smoking cessation seems to be enhanced by repeated contact by health care providers and reinforcement, direct and indirect, of behavior modification

Angiographic Trials

In the 1980s, a number of trials began to use angiography to measure changes in coronary atherosclerosis in relatively small groups of patients, rather than large community trials measuring risk factors and clinical events in large groups of people.[31–36] A few trials were able to look at morbidity and mortality; for the most part, though, these trials were not powered to examine clinical events. The major risk factor emphasized in all these trials was cholesterol, except the Lifestyle Heart Trial and the Stanford Coronary Risk Intervention Project (SCRIP), which examined multiple risk factors simultaneously.

Of these angiographic trials, only two used solely nonpharmacologic/nonsurgical treatments: The Heidelberg Trial and the Lifestyle Heart Trial. The SCRIP used a step-wise approach to treatment; therefore, there were some participants in the trial who did not receive medication. However, most subjects were on lipid-lowering medication by the end of the trial: 70.6% by the end of 1 year and 89.9% by the end of 4 years. In practical terms, therefore, SCRIP was a study of lipid-lowering drugs plus moderate lifestyle changes.

THE LIFESTYLE HEART TRIAL

The earliest studies to address the possibility of regression of coronary heart disease from lifestyle changes alone were a pilot study of the Lifestyle Heart Trial in 1977[37] and a randomized, controlled trial using noninvasive measures in 1980.[38] In the 1977 study, 10 patients with angiographically documented coronary heart disease were given an intensive lifestyle program for 1 month that included a low-fat vegetarian diet, moderate aerobic exercise, stress management training, smoking cessation, and group support.[39] Control group patients were not asked to make lifestyle changes, although they were free to do so. The diet contained approximately 10% of calories as fat (polyunsaturated/saturated [P/S] ratio >1), 15% to 20% protein, and 70% to 75% predominantly complex carbohydrates. Cholesterol intake was limited to 10 mg per day or less. The stress management techniques included stretching exercises, breathing techniques, meditation, progressive relaxation, and imagery. The purpose of each technique was to increase the patients' sense of relaxation, concentration, awareness, and well-being. Patients were asked to practice these stress management techniques for at least 1 hour per day. Participants were also asked to exercise a minimum of 3 hours per week and to spend a minimum of 30 minutes per session exercising within their prescribed target heart rates and/or perceived Borg exertion levels. Group support sessions were designed to increase social support and a sense of community by creating a safe environment for the expression of feelings and also to help patients adhere to the lifestyle change program. In 1980, the same intervention was studied in a randomized, controlled trial in which 48 patients were randomly assigned to an experimental group asked to make these lifestyle changes and a control group asked to follow usual-care guidelines.

In those two studies, experimental group patients showed more than a 90% average decrease in frequency of angina along with improvements in cardiac risk factors, functional status, myocardial perfusion as measured by exercise thallium scintigraphy, and left ventricular ejection fraction response as measured by exercise radionuclide ventriculography.

The Lifestyle Heart Trial[40] started in 1986 with 48 subjects randomized to either the intensive lifestyle intervention described earlier or to usual care. Approximately 50% of eligible subjects enrolled. Clinical entry criteria included age between 35 and 75 years; no coexisting life-threatening illness (other than CAD); lack of MI within 6 weeks of the start of the trial; not currently taking lipid-lowering medication; single-, double-, or triple-vessel coronary disease in nonrevascularized vessel(s); left ventricular ejection fraction greater than 25%; and lack of treatment with thrombolytics because these can affect the degree of coronary atherosclerosis. The original Lifestyle Heart Trial was a 1-year study; based on the results after 1 year, the NHLBI provided funding to extend the trial for 3 additional years.

Primary endpoint measurements included (1) quantitative coronary arteriography at baseline, 1 year, and 4 years to assess the extent of coronary atherosclerosis; (2) cardiac positron-emission tomography scans to measure myocardial perfusion[41]; and (3) lipoprotein and apolipoprotein profiles. Three-day diet diaries and other questionnaires were designed to measure adherence, and psychosocial questionnaires were administered to evaluate change in quality of life.

After 4 years, experimental patients were exercising an average of 3.6 hours per week, practicing stress management 5.7 hours per week, and consuming an average of 18.6 mg per day of cholesterol and 8.5% of total calories from fat. Control patients were exercising 2.9 hours per week, practicing stress management techniques 0.98 hours per week, and consuming an average of 138.7 mg per day of cholesterol and 25% of total calories from fat.

From baseline to 1 year, experimental group patients had a 91% reduction in reported frequency, a 42% reduction in duration, and a 53% reduction in severity of angina; at 4 years the corresponding figures were 72%, 71% and 40% reduction from baseline levels. In contrast, from baseline to 1 year, the control group had a 186% increase in reported frequency, a 138% increase in duration, and a 133% increase in severity of angina; at 4 years the corresponding figures were a 36% decrease in severity, a 69% decrease in duration, and a 0% change in severity from baseline levels. These decreases in the control group were in large part because three of the five patients who reported an increase in anginal episodes from baseline to 1 year underwent coronary angioplasty between years 1 and 4. Overall, 60% of control group patients underwent revascularization during the 4 years of the study versus only 21% of experimental group patients.

In the experimental group, 82% of the patients showed regression of coronary atherosclerosis after 1 year. The average percent diameter stenosis showed more improvement after 4 years than it did after 1 year (baseline, 38.9%; 1 year, 37.2%; 4 years, 35.9%), but in the control group the average stenosis continued to worsen (42.5%, 44.8%, and 54.3%, respectively; $P = 0.001$ between groups for changes from baseline to 4 years). These changes in percent diameter stenosis after 1 year and also after 4 years in the experimental group were strongly correlated with adherence to the lifestyle intervention. The number of cardiac events was less than half in the experimental group (1.53 events/patient) as in the control group (3.4 events/patient), including significantly lower rates of angioplasty, bypass surgery, and cardiac-related hospitalizations.[42]

THE HEIDELBERG TRIAL

The Heidelberg Trial[43] followed 113 subjects for 1 year who were randomized to either of the following: (1) a control group that received advice about the AHA Step 1 diet and moderate aerobic exercise; or (2) an intervention group that was asked to follow a lower-fat diet (20% fat, <200 mg per day of dietary cholesterol, P/S ratio >1) and a specific physical activity program involving 30 minutes of exercise daily at home plus two 60-minute group training sessions per week where they received ongoing advice and motivation for compliance.

Patients assigned to the intervention group stayed on a metabolic unit during the initial 3 weeks of the program, during which they were instructed in how to lower the fat content of their regular diet. Patients were asked to exercise daily at home on a bicycle ergometer for a minimum of 30 minutes close to their target heart rates, which were determined as 75% of the maximal heart rate during symptom-limited exercise. In addition, they were expected to participate in at least two group training sessions of 60 minutes each week.

During strict supervision on the metabolic unit, total cholesterol levels decreased 23% in the intervention group. In the following months after the group left the unit, there was a considerable erosion of dietary discipline; the average reduction in lipoproteins was only 10%. Cholesterol levels in the control group remained essentially unchanged.

Results of quantitative coronary arteriography were analyzed on both a per-patient and a per-lesion basis using both minimum diameter and percent diameter stenosis. According to minimal diameter reduction analyzed on a per-patient basis, progression was noted in 23%, no change in 45%, and regression in 32% of the patients in the experimental group. According to relative diameter reduction, progression was noted in 20%, no change in 50%, and regression in 30% of these patients. In the control group, according to minimal diameter reduction analyzed on a per-patient basis, the incidence of progression was noted in 48% of patients, no change in 35%, and regression in 17%. According to relative diameter reduction in the control group, coronary morphology deteriorated in 42%, no change was noted in 54%, and regression was noted in 4%. Both groups differed significantly from each other ($P < 0.001$). On a per-lesion basis, no significant change was noted either in relative diameter reduction (65 ± 24% vs. 64 ± 23%) or minimal diameter reduction (0.92 ± 0.72 mm vs. 0.91 ± 0.67 mm).

Exercise thallium scintigraphy performed in these patients showed statistically significant improvements in myocardial perfusion when compared with the control group. Of great interest is that this improvement occurred even though there was no significant improvement in coronary atherosclerosis as noted earlier, when all lesions were analyzed on a per-lesion basis. Indeed, the investigators found that a decrease in myocardial ischemia was not limited to patients with regression but also occurred in individual patients with no change or significant progression. Possible mechanisms of improvement in myocardial perfusion in the absence of regression of atherosclerosis might include exercise-induced stimulation of growth in collateral circulation and improvements in blood rheology.

THE STANFORD CORONARY RISK INTERVENTION PROJECT

The SCRIP[44] applied a step-wise approach combining intensive lifestyle change and medication. Quantitative coronary arteriography was the primary endpoint measure. From four institutions, 4771 patients were screened, of which 538 (11.3%) were eligible and 300 (56%) of those eligible agreed (259 men [86.3%] and 41 women [13.7%]) to be randomized to either usual care with their personal physician or to an individualized, multifactorial, risk-reduction program managed by the SCRIP staff and implemented in cooperation with the subject's personal physician. Recruitment took place between 1984 and 1987, and participants were followed for 4 years. Eligibility criteria included age less than 75 years, residence within a 5-hour drive of Stanford University, and lack of severe congestive heart failure, pulmonary disease, intermittent claudication, and noncardiac life-threatening illness.

The risk-reduction intervention included an initial risk stratification and goal-setting session with a SCRIP nurse. Follow-up for the intervention group was approximately every 2 to 3 months, whereas follow-up for the control group was determined by their usual physician. As part of the intake, the SCRIP staff would try to determine how likely it would be that a particular subject would meet the maximal clinical goal of an LDL cholesterol under 110 mg/dL within the first year without the use of medication. If the staff determined that a person was unlikely to meet the goal by lifestyle intervention (although it is not clear how that determination was made), then a lipid-lowering medication was prescribed. Cholesterol-lowering medication also was added during the trial if needed. By the end of the first year, 70.6% of the subjects in the SCRIP treatment arm were on medication, and 89.9% were on medication by the end of the fourth year; only 11% and 22.6% of the usual-care subjects were on lipid-lowering medication by the end of the first and fourth years, respectively.

The lifestyle interventions for this study included a moderately low-fat diet, physical activity, and counseling for smoking cessation. The recommended diet was less than 20% of calories from fat, less than 6% of calories from saturated fat, and less than 75 mg of cholesterol per day. The goal of the physical activity program for the risk-reduction group was to increase the individual subject's level from his or her baseline. Current and recent exsmokers were given stop-smoking and relapse-prevention programs, respectively, by staff psychologists. The risk-reduction subjects returned every 2 to 3 months, at which time lipids, body weight, and blood pressure all were measured and adherence to the individually prescribed lifestyle program was evaluated.

Data from 274 (91.3%) of the original 300 subjects randomized were completed at the end of the 4-year time course. There were significant baseline differences between the two groups: the intervention group had a higher percentage of women, a higher baseline HDL, lower average weight, significantly less daily cholesterol ingestion, and a better P/S fat ratio of intake. There were clinically significant improvements in percent body fat, weight, blood pressure (particularly systolic), LDL cholesterol, apolipoprotein B levels, triglycerides, HDL cholesterol, and exercise capacity based on metabolic equivalents (METS) in the treatment group compared with controls. Overall, these changes reduced the treatment arm's cardiac risk by 22% based on the calculated Framingham score. Although not statistically significant, risk factor profiles in the control group worsened in the areas of smoking, blood pressure, and weight, which may be of some clinical relevance despite the lack of statistical significance. There were no significant differences between the groups in the change in percentage of smokers during the trial nor in lipoprotein(a) levels; among the smokers in the treatment group, the number of cigarettes smoked per day decreased.

The primary endpoint for the SCRIP trial was minimum diameter as assessed by quantitative coronary arteriography. *Both groups had progression of disease* based on minimal diameter change, which was the factor by which the trial was powered. The risk-reduction group, though, had a 47% lower rate of progression per individual and a 58% lower rate of worsening in diseased vessel segments than the usual-care group. This difference was statistically significant. Women had the same rate of progression as men in the control group; however, women who received the treatment intervention had less progression than men in the same arm. A multivariate analysis showed that the three variables that best predicted potential rate of change in minimum diameter included exercise performance by treadmill (specifically METS), Framingham risk score (which is based on systolic blood pressure, total cholesterol, HDL, and smoking status), and dietary fat intake.

Although not designed for this purpose, SCRIP investigators reported the following clinical events:

5 cardiac related deaths (3 in usual care and 2 in risk reduction)
1 noncardiac-related death from cancer in the risk-reduction group
17 nonfatal MIs (11 in usual care, 6 in risk reduction; $P = 0.23$)

Most events (68%) for the risk-reduction group occurred in the first year compared with the usual-care group, which had only 20% of their coronary events occur in the first year of this 4-year trial.

Summary of Lessons Learned from Multiple Risk Factor Intervention Trials

1. Moderate changes in risk factors may not go far enough to cause statistically or clinically significant

reductions in morbidity and mortality. However, more intensive changes in risk factors with diet and lifestyle changes and/or drug therapy often cause improvements in morbidity and mortality that are clinically and statistically significant. This lesson was seen in a number of studies, including the MRFIT. Increasing evidence indicates that the Steps 1 and 2 diets used in MRFIT and still recommended by the AHA and the National Cholesterol Education Program do not go far enough to stop the progression of coronary atherosclerosis in most patients, whereas more intensive changes in diet may stop or reverse the progression of atherosclerosis.[45] When cholesterol levels in the 10-year follow-up of 361,662 men screened for the MRFIT program were correlated with coronary-related deaths, mortality decreased continuously and was directly related to cholesterol levels down to 140 mg/dL.[46]

2. Multiple risk factor intervention studies usually involve behavioral interventions. One can control access to new drugs but not to behavioral changes. Therefore, it is difficult to have a true nonintervention control group because many control group patients also may begin to make lifestyle changes. In many of the studies described in this chapter, "usual care" was dynamic and evolving. Patients in the control group were affected by secular trends and the general increase in awareness of the importance of addressing risk factors. Because of this, the actual mortality rate for the control groups was often lower than anticipated and the change in risk factor profile was often better. When the experimental group is asked to make only moderate changes in diet and lifestyle and the control group also begins to make similar changes on their own, then the likelihood of being able to demonstrate statistically significant between-group differences is greatly reduced. In the MRFIT study, for example, subjects enrolled and randomized in the trial were as aware of its goals as were the patients in the control group; indeed, control group patients often believed that they were in the intervention group when interviewed after the study was completed. Also, the level of health-related information available in the general public became much more widespread during the time frame of many of these studies, as was demonstrated in particular over the time course of the community-based trials. Later, population-based trials such as the PHHP and SFCP tried to better account for secular trends.[27, 30] Close personal attention frequently paid to control group patients increased the likelihood that they would also make changes.

3. It is easier to detect the benefits of risk factor modification in patients with documented disease than in those who have only risk factors. In the subgroup of men in the MRFIT study with a normal exercise ECG response, there was no significant SIUC difference in the CAD mortality rate (16.0 and 13.8 per 1000 for SI and UC men, respectively). In contrast, there was a 57% lower rate among men in the SI group with an abnormal baseline test result compared with men in the UC group (22.2 vs. 51.8 per 1000). The relative risks (SI/UC) in these two strata were significantly different ($P = 0.002$).[47] These findings suggest that men with elevated risk factors who have an abnormal exercise test response may benefit substantially from risk factor reduction. This finding was the opposite of what the authors hypothesized a priori, which was that the subgroup of men with a normal ECG response to a heart-rate–limited exercise test would experience particular benefit from intervention. Thus, those at the greatest risk or who have documented disease appear to benefit the most from intensive risk factor modification.

4. In angiographic trials, the percentage of subjects who achieved regression was greater for those participating in the nonpharmacologic trials compared with those in the pharmacologic trials (52% and 24.5%, respectively), despite the fact that the pharmacologic trials showed a greater change in LDL cholesterol. This suggests that absolute levels of cholesterol and degree of change in cholesterol may not be the only influences in terms of atherosclerotic plaque load and progression or regression of CAD.[48]

5. Pharmacologic interventions to reduce risk factors may have unanticipated side effects that may actually be detrimental. This was borne out primarily in earlier trials when effects of certain medications were not known. In the MRFIT study, for example, most of the subjects in the SI group were on thiazide diuretics for blood pressure control. The results of the MRFIT study revealed the unanticipated finding that thiazide diuretics can increase total cholesterol as well as triglycerides, which was not known at the time that the investigators designed the trial. Also, diuretics may cause hypokalemia which, in turn, may predispose to sudden cardiac death.

6. As noted earlier, those at the greatest risk or who have documented disease may benefit the most from intensive risk factor modification, and interventions to reduce risk factors may have unanticipated side effects that may be detrimental. Because of this, it is more difficult to demonstrate the benefit of using drugs for primary prevention in large groups of otherwise healthy people over long periods when the costs and potential risks of treatment may outweigh the hoped-for benefits.

7. Treatment of a single risk factor, such as hypertension, may not induce the expected reduction in occurrence of coronary events if other risk factors are not adequately treated.[49] Treatment of several risk factors simultaneously affords greater improvement in each compared with treatment of a single risk factor at a time. This synergy of risk factors works in

both directions: helping and harming. For example, in the MRFIT study, people with a diastolic blood pressure higher than 92 mm Hg and a cholesterol level higher than 245 mg/dL had a much higher coronary heart disease death rate per 10,000 if they were also smokers than if they were nonsmokers.[50] Conversely, treating all of these factors simultaneously affords greater improvement in risk than the additive benefit of treating each risk factor separately.

8. Related to Lesson 7, in our experience, we have observed a paradox that it is often easier to motivate patients to make substantial and multiple changes in diet and lifestyle all at once than to make small, gradual changes in only one risk factor. When patients make comprehensive lifestyle changes (e.g., stopping smoking, exercising, beginning a very low-fat, low-cholesterol diet, practicing stress management techniques, and seeking group support), most find that they feel much better, quickly, and this reframes the motivation for changing from simply risk factor modification to improving their quality of life. In addition, the behaviors have a unique way of reinforcing each other. For example, practicing stress reduction techniques tends to make dietary adherence easier for people.

9. Social factors, including social support, play an important role in adherence to comprehensive lifestyle changes and may have powerful effects on morbidity and mortality, independently of influences on known risk factors. An increasing number of studies have shown that those who feel socially isolated have three to five times the risk of premature death not only from coronary heart disease but also from all causes when compared with those who have a sense of connection and community.[51–53] In the community-based trials reviewed, those who participated in groups were more adherent to behavioral chenges. Unfortunately, though, groups were frequently eliminated despite their efficacy because of costs and/or intensity of labor.

10. Intensive risk factor modification can reduce cardiac events quite rapidly by stabilizing the endothelium, whether by comprehensive changes in diet and lifestyle or with lipid-lowering drugs, even before there is time for meaningful regression in coronary atherosclerosis. The most common cause of MI, sudden cardiac death, or unstable angina is rupture of an atherosclerotic plaque, often associated with localized coronary thrombosis and/or coronary artery spasm.[54–56] Research publications since 1990 have consistently shown the benefits of lipid-lowering therapy in reducing cardiac events. The benefits demonstrated in the more recent studies probably reflect more intensive and effective intervention both with lipid-lowering drugs and/or with diets lower in fat and cholesterol. The reduction in cardiac events by intensive risk factor modification contrasts with the fact that no studies have demonstrated that angioplasty reduces cardiac events when compared with conventional medical therapy, and bypass surgery has been shown to prevent cardiac events only in a relatively small subset of those undergoing revascularization.[57] There are more trials showing decreased coronary events by *intensive* multiple risk factor intervention than by elective angioplasty or bypass surgery in patients with stable coronary artery disease.[58] In addition, increasing evidence indicates that 30% to 40% obstructions may be more likely to rupture and cause a cardiac event than the 80% to 90% lesions, because the more severe lesions are generally more stable and well collateralized.[59] Intensive risk factor modification may help stabilize all lesions, including those of moderate size, whereas revascularization tends to be performed only on lesions that are more than 50% stenosed.

11. Similar to Lesson 10, improvements in myocardial perfusion and substantial reductions in angina may occur within weeks in response to comprehensive lifestyle changes and/or to lipid-lowering drugs.[60, 61] Mechanisms of rapid improvement are not fully understood but may include favorable changes in coronary vasomotor tone, decreased viscosity and improved collateral flow, and reductions in platelet aggregation.

In summary, risk factor intervention trials have made a major contribution to the understanding of the pathophysiology of coronary artery disease and of the best ways to intervene—as well as a greater understanding of approaches that are not as effective. Further studies are necessary to understand the most cost- and medically effective strategies for making intensive risk factor modification programs available to the large number of people who need and can benefit from them. This will of necessity include not only more rigorous, large-scale studies but also reimbursement from insurance companies, managed care organizations, and Medicare.

REFERENCES

1. American Heart Association. Heart and Stroke Facts: 1995 Statistical Supplement. Dallas, American Heart Association, 1995.
2. Smith C Jr, Blair N, Criqui H, et al. The Secondary Prevention Panel. AHA Medical/Scientific Statement: Consensus Panel Statement: Preventing Heart Attack and Death in Patients with Coronary Disease. Circulation 1995; 92:2–4.
3. Kannel WB. Contributions of the Framingham Study to the conquest of artery disease. Am J Cardiol 1988; 62:1109–1112.
4. Gordon T, Kannel WB, Castelli WP, et al. Lipoproteins, cardiovascular disease, and death: The Framingham Study. Arch Intern Med 1981; 141:1128–1132.
5. Verschuren WM, Jacobs DR, Bloemberg BP, et al. Serum total cholesterol and long-term coronary heart disease mortality in different cultures: Twenty-five-year follow-up of the Seven Countries Study. JAMA 1995; 274:131–136.
6. Kannel WB. Clinical misconceptions dispelled by epidemiological research. Circulation 1995; 92:3350–3360.

7. Doyle JT, Heslin SA, Hilleboe HE, et al. A prospective study of cardiovascular disease in Albany: Report of three years' experience: Ischemic heart disease. Am J Public Health 1957; 47:25–32.
8. Chapman JM, Goerke LS, Dixon W, et al. Measuring the risk of coronary heart disease in adult population groups: IV. Clinical status of a population group in Los Angeles under observation for two to three years. Am J Public Health 1957; 47:33–42.
9. Shekelle RB, Shryock AM, Paul O, et al. Diet, serum cholesterol, and death from coronary heart disease: The Western Electric Study. N Engl J Med 1981; 304:65–70.
10. Keys A, Taylor HL, Blackburn HB, et al. Coronary heart disease among Minnesota business and professional men followed 15 years. Circulation 1963; 28:381–395.
11. Campbell TC, Junshi C. Diet and chronic degenerative diseases: Perspectives from China. Am J Clin Nutr 1994; 59(5 Suppl): 1153S–1161S.
12. Kannel WB. Clinical misconceptions dispelled by epidemiological research. Circulation 1995; 92:3350–3360.
13. Kannel WB, Barry P, Dawber TR. Immediate mortality in coronary heart disease: The Framingham study. *In* Proceedings of the IV World Congress of Cardiology of the Mexican International Society of Cardiology 1963; IV-B:176–188.
14. Multiple Risk Factor Intervention Trial Research Group. Multiple Risk Factor Intervention Trial: Risk factor changes and mortality results (MRFIT). JAMA 1982; 248:1465–1477.
15. Grimm R. The Multiple Risk Factor Intervention Trial in the U.S.: A summary of results at four years in special intervention and usual care men. Prev Med 1983; 12:185–190.
16. Hjermann I. A randomized primary preventive trial in coronary heart disease: The Oslo study. Prev Med 1983; 12:181–184.
17. Wilhelmsen L. Risk factors for coronary heart disease in perspective: European intervention trials. Am J Med 1984; 76:37–40.
18. Murray D. Design and analysis of community trials: Lessons from the Minnesota Heart Health Program. Am J Epidemiol 1995; 142:569–575.
19. World Health Organization European Collaborative Group. European collaborative trial of multifactorial prevention of coronary heart disease: Final report on the 6-year results. Lancet 1986; 1:869–872.
20. World Health Organization European Collaborative Group. Multifactorial trial in the prevention of coronary heart disease: III. Incidence and mortality results. Eur Heart J 1983; 4:141–147.
21. Wilhelmsen L. Risk factors for coronary heart disease in perspective: European intervention trials. Am J Med 1984; 76:37–40.
22. Menotti A. The European Multifactorial Preventive Trial of Coronary Heart Disease: Four-year experience. Prev Med 1983; 12:175–180.
23. House JS, Landis KR, Umberson D. Social relationships and health. Science 1988; 241:540–545.
24. Ornish D. Love and Survival: The Scientific Basis for the Healing Power of Intimacy. New York, Harper Collins, 1998.
25. Salonen JT. Prevention of coronary heart disease in Finland—application of the population strategy. Ann Med 1991; 23:607–612.
26. Kaplan GA. Social contacts and ischaemic heart disease. Ann Clin Res 1988; 20:131–136.
27. Assaf AR, Banspach SW, Lasater TM, et al. The Pawtucket Heart Health Program: II. Evaluation strategies. RI Med J 1987; 70:541–546.
28. Carleton RA, Lasater TM. Primary prevention of coronary heart disease: A challenge for behavioral medicine. Circulation 1987; 76:I124–I1249.
29. Fortmann SP, Flora JA, Winkleby MA, et al. Community intervention trials: Reflections on the Stanford Five-City Project experience. Am J Epidemiol 1995; 142:576–586.
30. Farquhar JW, Fortmann SP, Flora JA, et al. Effects of community-wide education on cardiovascular disease risk factors: The Stanford Five-City Project. JAMA 1990; 264:359–365.
31. Blankenhorn DH, Nessim SA, Johnson RL, et al. Beneficial effects of combined colestipol-niacin therapy on coronary atherosclerosis and coronary venous bypass grafts. JAMA 1987; 257:3233–3240.
32. Brown GB, Albers JJ, Fisher LD, et al. Niacin or lovastatin combined with colestipol regresses coronary atherosclerosis and prevents clinical events in men with elevated apolipoprotein B. N Engl J Med 1990; 323:1289–1298.
33. Kane JP, Malloy MJ, Ports TA, et al. Regression of coronary atherosclerosis during treatment of familial hypercholesterolemia with combined drug regimens. JAMA 1990; 264:3007–3012.
34. Buchwald H, Vargo RL, Matts JP, et al. Effect of partial ileal bypass surgery on mortality and morbidity from coronary heart disease in patients with hypercholesterolemia. N Engl J Med 1990; 323:946–955.
35. Cashin-Hemphill L, Mack WJ, Pogoda JM, et al. Beneficial effects of colestipol-niacin on coronary atherosclerosis. JAMA 1990; 264:3013–3017.
36. Schuler G, Hambrecht R, Schlierf G, et al. Myocardial perfusion and regression of coronary artery disease in patients on a regimen of intensive physical exercise and low-fat diet. J Am Coll Cardiol 1992; 19:34–42.
37. Ornish DM, Gotto AM, Miller RR, et al. Effects of a vegetarian diet and selected yoga techniques in the treatment of coronary heart disease. Clin Res 1979; 27:720A.
38. Ornish DM, Scherwitz LW, Doody RS, et al. Effects of stress management training and dietary changes in treating ischemic heart disease. JAMA 1983; 249:54–59.
39. Ornish D. Dr. Dean Ornish's Program for Reversing Heart Disease. New York, Random House, 1990; Ballantine Books, 1992.
40. Ornish DM, Brown SE, Scherwitz LW, et al. Can lifestyle changes reverse coronary atherosclerosis? The Lifestyle Heart Trial. Lancet 1990; 336:129–133.
41. Gould KL, Ornish D, Kirkeeide R, et al. Improved stenosis geometry by quantitative coronary arteriography after vigorous risk factor modification. Am J Cardiol 1992; 69:845–853.
42. Ornish DM, Scherwitz LW, Brown SE, et al. Can intensive lifestyle changes reverse coronary heart disease? Four-year results of The Lifestyle Heart Trial. in press.
43. Schuler G, Hambrecht R, Schlierf G, et al. Regular physical exercise and low-fat diet effects on progression of coronary artery disease. Circulation 1992; 86:1–11.
44. Haskell WL, Alderman EL, Fair JM, et al. Effects of intensive multiple risk factor reduction on coronary atherosclerosis and clinical cardiac events in men and women with coronary artery disease: The Stanford Coronary Risk Intervention Project (SCRIP). Circulation 1994; 89:975–990.
45. Ornish D. Dietary treatment of hyperlipidemia. J Cardiovasc Risk 1994; 1:283–286.
46. National Cholesterol Education Program. Second Report of the Expert Panel on Detection, Evaluation, and Treatment of High Blood Cholesterol in Adults (Adult Treatment Panel II). Circulation 1994; 89:1329–1445.
47. Multiple Risk Factor Intervention Trial Research Group. Exercise electrocardiogram and coronary heart disease mortality in the Multiple Risk Factor Intervention Trial. Am J Cardiol 1985; 55:16–24.
48. Superko HR, Krauss, RM. Current perspectives: Coronary artery disease regression: Convincing evidence for the benefit of aggressive lipoprotein management. Circulation 1994; 90:1056–1069.
49. Borghi C, Ambrosioni E. Primary and secondary prevention of myocardial infarction. Clin Exp Hypertens 1996; 18:547–558.
50. Neaton JD, Wentworth D. Serum cholesterol, blood pressure, cigarette smoking, and death from coronary heart disease: Overall findings and differences by age for 316,099 white men. Arch Intern Med 1992; 152:56–64.
51. House JS, Landis KR, Umberson D. Social relationships and health. Science 1988; 241:540–545.
52. Berkman LF. The role of social relations in health promotion. Psychosom Med 1995; 57:245–254.
53. Ruberman W, Weinblatt E, Goldberg JD, Chaudhary BS. Psychosocial influences on mortality after myocardial infarction. N Engl J Med 1984; 311:552–559.
54. Fuster V, Badimon L, Badimon JJ, Chesebro JH. The pathogenesis of coronary artery disease and the acute coronary syndromes. N Engl J Med 1992; 326:242–318.
55. Brown BG, Zhao XQ, Sacco DE, Albers JJ. Lipid lowering

and plaque regression: New insights into prevention of plaque disruption and clinical events in coronary artery disease. Circulation 1993; 87:1781–1791.
56. van der Wal AC, Becker AE, van der Loos CM, Das PK. Site of intimal rupture or erosion of thrombosed coronary atherosclerotic plaques is characterized by an inflammatory process irrespective of the dominant plaque morphology. Circulation 1994; 89:36–44.
57. Yusuf S, Zucker D, Peduzzi P, et al. Effect of coronary artery bypass graft surgery on survival: Overview of 10-year results from randomised trials by the Coronary Artery Bypass Graft Surgery Trialists Collaboration. Lancet 1994; 344:563–570.
58. Gould K. Clinical cardiology frontiers: Reversal of coronary atherosclerosis: Clinical promise as the basis for noninvasive management of coronary artery disease. Circulation 1994; 90:1558–1571.
59. Fuster V, Badimon L, Badimon JJ, Chesebro JH. The pathogenesis of coronary artery disease and the acute coronary syndromes. N Engl J Med 1992; 326:242–318.
60. Ornish DM, Scherwitz LW, Doody RS, et al. Effects of stress management training and dietary changes in treating ischemic heart disease. JAMA 1983; 249:54–59.
61. Gould KL, Martucci JP, Goldberg DI, et al. Short-term cholesterol lowering decreases size and severity of perfusion abnormalities by positron emission tomography after dipyridamole in patients with coronary artery disease: A potential noninvasive marker of healing coronary endothelium. Circulation 1994; 89:1530–1538.

35 Prevention Strategies: From the Office to the Community

▶ Ira S. Ockene
▶ David Chiriboga

The clinical trials described in this book represent the best that medical science can offer: teams of well-trained people led by experienced investigators and focused on the project at hand. The results of these trials inform us as to those methodologies and interventions that have the potential to be truly useful. They leave us, however, with several important problems.

- In the realm of prevention, much of what needs to be done falls outside the purview of the traditional medical environment. What can be done to bring preventive interventions to the school, worksite, and community? Are there effective methodologies that will work at these levels?
- What is a population-based intervention? Is there a tension between interventions carried out at the level of the individual, in traditional physician-patient interactions, and interventions carried out at the population level? Or are these activities synergistic?
- How will these interventions work in the real world, as opposed to the world of the clinical trial? In the real world, health care providers may not be as well informed or trained as we would like them to be; therefore, they may not apply an intervention effectively or may fail to use it at all.

Thrombolysis has been the subject of numerous well-designed clinical trials, a number of which have been reviewed in this book. In an article reviewing some of the issues of concern in thrombolytic therapy, Hennekens and colleagues reviewed the advantages and disadvantages of the available thrombolytic agents. They pointed out that both thrombolytic therapy and aspirin clearly save lives in the setting of acute myocardial infarction. Yet

> Both therapies remain underutilized in the United States: as few as 40% of patients with myocardial infarction receive thrombolysis and 72% receive aspirin, . . . [with] comparable figures of as high as 68% and 84%, respectively, in the United Kingdom. Thus, the small differences in efficacy, safety, and ease of administration of different thrombolytic agents are far outweighed by the large benefits that would derive from wider utilization and earlier administration of any of the available agents.[1]

What we do in this chapter, therefore, is to place the issue of clinical trials in prevention into the largest possible perspective, beginning with a discussion of the concept of the "population-based" approach, then considering what can be done to improve the delivery of preventive interventions in the physician's office and practice, and, finally, evaluating the available evidence for intervention at the community level and beyond.

POPULATION APPROACH VERSUS THE HIGH-RISK APPROACH

"Population" and "high-risk," the two approaches to the prevention of coronary heart disease (CHD), are at times described as though they were mutually exclusive. This is not the case. Both are appropriate, although requiring differing levels of intensity. The high-risk approach is the usual modus operandi of physicians. Patients at high risk are looked for in physicians' offices or by screening programs and, when found, are treated to reduce their risk. In contrast, the population approach aims to lower the mean level of a risk factor in the entire population and thus shift the entire risk curve to the left (Fig. 35–1). Population interventions include antismoking campaigns, efforts to reduce the use of saturated fat in fast food restaurants, and national nutrition education campaigns.

Rose has pointed out that these two approaches relate to two different etiologic questions.[2] The individual-centered approach seeks the causes of cases and asks questions such as "Why does this person have an elevated cholesterol level?" The population-centered approach seeks the causes of incidence and asks the question "Why does this population of peo-

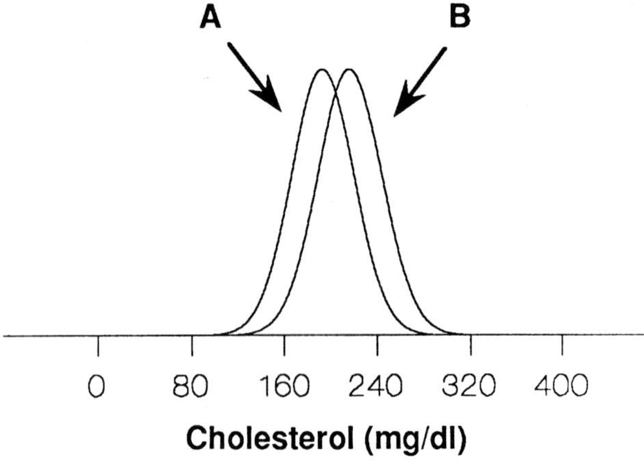

Figure 35–1 An example of the population-based approach to the prevention of coronary heart disease. The goal is to move the curve from B to A.

ple have a higher mean cholesterol level and many individuals with elevated levels, when in other populations elevated cholesterol levels are rare?" The relative advantages and disadvantages of these approaches are summarized in Tables 35–1 and 35–2.

The high-risk strategy uses an approach that is inherently appealing to physicians. Paying special attention to those at the high end of a risk distribution is a typical medical approach. The physician is treating a person who understands the need to be treated ("I have high cholesterol, and so I need to change my diet"), and this approach also applies resources to those people who will have the highest pay-off in terms of diminished risk. Likewise, any unfavorable consequences of the treatment will be seen as being part of a favorable risk-benefit ratio.

Nonetheless, this approach has a number of drawbacks. It is difficult to screen a population. Patients at highest risk are often least likely to be reached, and the level of compliance with recommended follow-up is often poor.[3] The younger, hyperlipidemic, smoking, physician-avoiding person is far less likely to appear at a screening site. The same logic applies to many other risk-altering situations: the population at highest risk is often least likely to voluntarily participate in risk-modifying behaviors.

TABLE 35–1 • The "High-Risk" Strategy

Advantages	Disadvantages
Intervention appropriate to the individual	Difficulties and cost of screening
Subject motivation	Does not deal with the root causes of disease
Physician motivation	Limited potential for both the individual and the population
Cost-effective use of resources	Imposes behavioral difficulties
Favorable risk-benefit ratio	Labels asymptomatic individuals as "sick"

TABLE 35–2 • The "Population Approach"

Advantages	Disadvantages
Radical—can alter the root causes of the disease	Small benefit to the individual (the "prevention paradox")
Larger potential for reducing disease incidence	Poor motivation of subject
Behaviorally appropriate	Poor motivation of physician
	Problematic risk-benefit ratio if intervention may not be entirely benign

There is an even more important disadvantage to the high-risk approach: treating only those most liable to be affected by a population-based condition such as a high-saturated fat diet does not affect the root cause of the problem, and the next generation will have the same burden of disease as the last. In addition, the prediction of risk for a given individual will always be poor for all but those at highest risk.[4] Most will always come from the middle of the risk distribution, because the great bulk of the population resides here.

The high-risk strategy may also require a person to change behavior in a fashion that is socially difficult. Eating in a different way than the rest of the family, exercising when your friends want to watch a football game—these are difficult changes to make.

The population-based strategy is quite different. Shifting the risk curve of a population can progressively lower the incidence of disease, and the decline in CHD mortality in the United States that has occurred over the last several decades is consistent with the risk factor change that has occurred over that period.[5] Furthermore, changes occurring in an entire population make it easier for an individual to change—it is easier to quit smoking when your workplace is smoke-free, and easier to follow a low-fat diet when such choices are widely available in the company or school cafeteria and in fast-food restaurants.

The population-based strategy does have an inherent downside, what Rose has called the *prevention paradox:* preventive measures that greatly benefit society as a whole may bring little benefit to each person who is individually at relatively low risk.[6] Because the gain for a given person is small, motivating that person to make lifestyle changes may be difficult. All that this means, however, is that the intensity of the intervention needs to be matched to the person's level of risk: individual, high-intensity, and relatively expensive approaches for those at high levels of risk, and population approaches such as those described in this chapter for the great bulk of the population at low or moderate risk. The combination of these approaches should be combined into an overall national strategy.

The importance of the population approach is made clear by simulations carried out by several investigators. Kottke and colleagues tested the effects of several intervention strategies on CHD mortality rates.[7, 8] Lowering serum cholesterol by 4%, smoking by 15%, and diastolic blood pressure by 3% for the entire population goals that are easily achievable and, in the case of cholesterol and smoking, already surpassed in the United States would be expected to reduce the incidence of nonfatal myocardial infarction by at least 13% and CHD deaths by at least 18%. On the other hand, lowering serum cholesterol by 34%, smoking by 20%, and diastolic blood pressure to 90 mm Hg in the subset of the population with all three risk factors in the highest quartile would only result in a 6% to 8% reduction in nonfatal myocardial infarction and a 2% to 9% reduction in deaths from CHD. Similarly, Goldman and colleagues[9] used Framingham Heart Study coefficients in a computer simulation (the Coronary Heart Disease Policy Model) to analyze the effect of a targeted program to reduce all cholesterol levels above 250 mg/dL to 250 mg/dL, as opposed to a population-wide program to reduce everyone's cholesterol level. Their model suggests that such a targeted program would reduce CHD incidence by 8% to 10% in men 35 to 54 years of age and by 1% to 4% in men 55 to 74 years of age. A similar reduction in CHD incidence could also be achieved by a 10 mg/dL population-wide reduction in serum cholesterol. Such a decline in cholesterol has already been seen in the United States and has been associated with an unprecedented decline in CHD mortality.

Thus, it is clear that efforts that target only high-risk segments of the overall population are inadequate to significantly reduce the population burden of disease. If we are to improve the cardiovascular health of the nation, we must develop population approaches that build on the high-risk approach offered by the individual practitioner.

THE HEALTH-CARE PROVIDER AND THE HEALTH-CARE SYSTEM

The medical profession has an important role to play in the reduction of cardiovascular risk. Some 76% of Americans visit a physician in any given year, with many of them (59% to 85%) reporting repeat visits within that year. Appropriate counseling of these patients regarding alteration of health risk behaviors could have a substantial public health impact.[10, 11] Yet our increasing knowledge of effective interventions for the prevention of cardiovascular disease (CVD) is often poorly translated into effective delivery of preventive care by the provider, and this is related to a number of barriers that exist to the delivery of effective preventive care.

- Traditionally, most physicians have been more interested in the delivery of therapeutic, rather than preventive care. They often express the belief that they are ineffective in health behavior interventions and often also state that patients do not want their physicians to intervene on risk factors (such as smoking) when they are seeing them for other problems.
- Physicians (and other health care providers) often believe that they have poor intervention skills. In reality, few have had training in behavioral counseling; yet the modification of behavior is the essence of patient-oriented preventive activities.
- Physicians have traditionally prided themselves on their autonomy. Following best-practice guidelines is foreign to them and is often derided as "cookbook" medicine.
- Physicians and other providers are increasingly pressured for time in today's cost-conscious environment. Thus they often have little time to fit preventive interventions into their practices, keeping in mind that lifestyle intervention is only one of their many responsibilities.
- There are few economic incentives for prevention-oriented activities. Taking the time to counsel patients effectively is rarely adequately reimbursed and does not yield the same financial rewards as do technologic interventions.
- Physicians' practices generally are also not set up to cue them to intervene and to facilitate integration of prevention activities with other more traditional medical needs.

Two general strategies have been shown to be effective in improving the delivery of preventive services to individual patients. These are (1) the training of individual providers in counseling methodologies in combination with office systems that facilitate the delivery of such counseling, and (2) the development of case-management systems that add onto the physician's activities a systematic risk-factor modification approach that is entirely separate from the usual office activities. Examples of both follow:

1. The Worcester-Area Trial for Counseling in Hyperlipidemia (WATCH) randomized 45 primary care health maintenance organization internists by site into three conditions: (I) usual care; (II) physician nutrition counseling training; and (III) physician nutrition counseling training plus a structured office practice environment for nutrition management.[12–14] The two physician intervention groups were provided with a 3-hour training program incorporating behavioral

principles for brief, patient-centered, interactive counseling. Group III was in addition provided with an office practice management system that included prompts, algorithms, and simple dietary assessment tools. Patient recruitment occurred over a 2-year period, and physician counseling skills were maintained over this period, despite the lack of any further training.[15] At 1 year of follow-up, significant improvement was seen in diet, weight, and blood lipid levels but was limited to patients in condition III. As compared with the control group, condition III patients had average reductions of 2.53 percentage points (an 8% decline) for energy intake from fat ($P = 0.03$); 1.33 percentage points for saturated fat (12% decline; $P = 0.01$); an average weight loss of 6.3 lb ($P = 0.0001$); and a 6.9 mg/dL decrease in low-density lipoprotein (LDL) cholesterol ($P = 0.05$). When patients placed on cholesterol-lowering medication were excluded, the LDL-cholesterol reduction increased to 9.3 mg/dL ($P = 0.009$), as more patients in the control condition were placed on lipid-lowering medication. Average time for the initial counseling intervention in condition III was 9.2 minutes. Patients of condition II physicians (trained but not supported) showed results no different from controls. The study demonstrated that brief physician nutrition counseling can produce beneficial changes in diet, weight, and blood lipids, but only if accompanied by an office support system that facilitates the intervention.

The lipid outcomes in a diet intervention study such as this may seem modest when compared with the results of recent studies involving pharmacologic intervention.[16, 17] The findings, however, must be placed in context. WATCH was a primary care study involving a low-cost, minimal-effort counseling intervention. To achieve a 12% reduction in calories from saturated fat and a 5.5% reduction in LDL-cholesterol levels in patients *not* placed on pharmacologic therapy, maintained 1 year out from the intervention, is clearly worthwhile. Such an LDL-cholesterol change, if maintained, should lead to an estimated 10% reduction in coronary event rates.[18]

In any analysis of the prevention literature, it is important to differentiate between primary and secondary intervention studies. In primary care the intervention needs to be of low intensity (and low cost), and the patient's motivation to change is much less than it is when a myocardial infarction or other clinical event has already occurred.

2. The Stanford Case Management System for Coronary Risk Factor Modification after Acute Myocardial Infarction[19] was a secondary prevention study designed to evaluate the efficacy of a physician-directed but nurse-managed case management system for coronary risk factor modification. Five hundred eighty-five patients with a recent myocardial infarction, all members of the Kaiser-Permanente medical system, were randomized to usual care or special intervention. Following an initial inhospital nurse intervention for smoking cessation, diet/drug intervention for hyperlipidemia, and exercise training, follow-up intervention (approximately 9 hours of nurse contact during the 1-year follow-up) was implemented primarily by telephone and mail.

The study had a number of interesting outcomes. The intervention group made significant dietary changes, achieving a better-than Step II American Heart Association (AHA) diet. Surprisingly, however, the usual-care group achieved almost the same level of dietary change. The special-care group had a significantly lower 1-year plasma LDL-cholesterol level (107 vs. 132 mg/dL special care vs. usual care, respectively), but this was primarily due to a much greater percentage of special-care patients being placed on pharmacologic lipid-lowering therapy (66% vs. 21% at 12 months, respectively). Smoking cessation rates were 70% for the special-care group and 53% for the usual-care group. Functional capacity at 1 year was also significantly higher in the special-care group.

There was no difference in the number of coronary events seen in the two groups over the 1 year of follow-up. However, it is known that lipid changes generally have a 1- to 2-year lag before clinical benefit is seen,[16, 17] and only 43.1% of the patients were smokers. The study clearly demonstrated that a relatively intensive case-management approach can result in significant and important changes in patients' risk factor profiles.

For risk-factor change on the level of the health care provider and the individual patient, then, we have learned that there is value to training practitioners in behavioral counseling methodology[12] and in setting up supportive office systems, as well as developing case-management systems that deliver a more intensive intervention that coordinates with the primary providers' efforts. It is also likely that dietitians can make an important contribution to patient behavior change, although this is not as well studied.[20, 21]

PREVENTION OF CARDIOVASCULAR DISEASE OUTSIDE THE TRADITIONAL HEALTH CARE ENVIRONMENT

Community Interventions

DESCRIPTION

The community approach is based on the premise that intervention at the level of the community organization can change the setting in which people live so as to support healthier lifestyles and thus lead to decreases in chronic disease morbidity and mortality.[22]

In the past few decades increasing attention has been paid to community organization as a means of accomplishing large-scale change for the prevention of chronic health problems.[23, 24] In general, community interventions for CVD attempt to reduce the prevalence of risk factors associated with the disease, such as high blood pressure, elevated serum cholesterol level, smoking, overweight, and sedentary lifestyle. Program components include community organization, needs assessment, prioritization and evaluation, and program maintenance. Activities include social marketing, direct behavior-change efforts (including skills training, health education, and contingency management), screening (including counseling and referral), and policy and environmental change. Such community intervention can be applied through a variety of channels: contacting community leaders and existing formal and informal community groups (such as social, religious, ethnic, and school programs; adult education programs; and self-help programs), using the existing mass media network, and supporting community organization efforts. The core of a successful program is the community organization process.[25] This involves identification and activation of key community leaders, stimulation of citizens and organizations to volunteer time and offer resources to CVD prevention, and the promotion of prevention as a community theme. Community health professionals play a vital role in providing program endorsement and stimulating the participation of other community leaders.

One of the earliest community trials for the reduction of cardiovascular risk was the Stanford Three-Community Study.[26] One community was monitored as a control site, one assigned to media intervention only, and the third to a combination of media and face-to-face intervention. In both treatment communities there was substantial and similar improvement in cardiovascular risk profiles by the end of the second year, although initially the level of improvement was greater in the community with face-to-face counseling. The study suggested that mass-media campaigns can be effective in modifying risk factors at the community level.

The North Karelia project carried out in Finland yielded comparable results.[27] After 10 years of followup, men in the intervention group demonstrated statistically significant differences in risk factors: a 1% decrease in mean diastolic blood pressure, a 3% decrease in mean systolic blood pressure, a 28% decrease in smoking prevalence, and a 3% decrease in serum cholesterol levels. This was associated with a 22% reduction in age-standardized CHD mortality in men and 43% in women. This study used community channels for cardiovascular risk factor modification, ranging from education and building of a strong social support system to point-of-purchase advertising and television campaigns.

The North Karelia Project has not only had an effect on reducing the mortality from CHD in all of Finland, but over a 20-year followup period (1972 to 1991), cancer mortality declined in North Karelia by 45.4% and in all of Finland by 32.7% ($P = 0.006$ for difference). The greater decline in North Karelia occurred particularly in the second decade of the follow-up and was related particularly to lung cancer. The results support the hypothesis that reduction in the population levels of cardiovascular risk factors leads to beneficial changes in cancer mortality rates, presumably via effects on smoking and diet, but such changes take a longer time to manifest than for CHD.[28]

After these initial efforts, a second generation of studies was funded by the National Heart, Lung, and Blood Institute to examine the effects of a community approach to change in cardiovascular risk factors, including the Pawtucket Heart Health Program, the Minnesota Heart Health Program, and the Stanford Five-City Project. All three studies used various community organization techniques to ensure participation by the community members.

The Stanford Five-City Project is typical of this group of studies.[29] Two treatment cities ($N = 122{,}800$) and two control cities ($N = 197{,}500$) were compared for changes in knowledge of risk factors, blood pressure, plasma cholesterol level, smoking rate, body weight, and resting pulse rate. Treatment cities received a 5-year, low-cost, comprehensive program using social learning theory, a communication-behavior change model, community organization principles, and social marketing methods that resulted in about 26 hours of exposure to multichannel and multifactor education. Surveys carried out at intervals varying from 30 to 64 months following the start of the study demonstrated significant reductions favoring the treatment communities: plasma cholesterol level (2%), blood pressure (4%), resting pulse rate (3%), and smoking rate (13%); a composite total mortality risk score fell 15% and a CHD risk score decreased 16%. Thus, such low-cost programs can have an impact on risk factors in broad population groups.

Some studies, however, have not been able to clearly demonstrate benefit. The Minnesota Heart Health Program found no overall effect on mean body mass index after 7 years of community intervention activities that included risk factor screening, mass-media education, adult education classes, worksite interventions, home correspondence programs, school-based programs, restaurant programs, and point-of-purchase education in supermarkets. However, a positive intervention effect was noted early in the intervention among those with elevated cholesterol levels or a history of obesity-related disease.[30] There was a marked secular trend for weight to increase in all study communities. The investigators note that explanations for a less-than-expected intervention effect include secular forces overwhelming intervention effects, an inadequately focused intervention effort, a population already highly aware of the issue at baseline, and inherent limitations in educational approaches for a difficult public health problem.

In the United States, state public health departments nationwide are implementing community-based CVD prevention programs,[25] with the development of a statewide CVD prevention plan being an important element of such efforts.[31] These programs must attend to factors such as affordability, acceptability, and adequacy of the intervention, given that efforts sponsored at the state level will rarely have the resources of federally funded demonstration projects.[32]

DISCUSSION

The overall results of these interventions suggests that there is great potential for community interventions.[22] Where differences between intervention and control groups have been less than expected, the following factors may be playing a role:

- In many community interventions, an initial favorable effect in groups that already have a given risk factor for CVD seems to abate with time, despite the increased level of awareness of the community as a whole. With few exceptions[33, 34] most studies have not looked at differences in subgroups within the community. It may be that for people at risk community interventions are useful to initiate change but that this "high risk" subgroup may ultimately need a more intensive intervention to maintain the desired behavior and to prevent a "rebound effect." On the other hand, the rest of the population (the majority) may slowly assimilate the information and work toward behavior modification.
- Another problem inherent to community-based intervention projects in this age of communication is that information can disseminate quickly and interfere with classic intervention/evaluation control designs through contamination. Therefore, alternative experimental designs for assessing the effectiveness of long-term intervention programs need to be considered. These should not rely solely on the use of reference populations but should balance the measurement of outcome with an assessment of the process of change in communities.[35]
- Populations of low socioeconomic status or of differing cultural backgrounds may require specific approaches that differ from those applicable to the general population. The New York State Healthy Heart Program studied a population of approximately 200,000 people, predominantly Hispanic and of low socioeconomic status, living in northern Manhattan in New York City.[33] Potential barriers to diffusion of the community-based disease prevention model in disadvantaged inner city communities were identified, including issues of scale and complexity, adaptation of the model to a "community" without geopolitical boundaries or infrastructure, linguistic and cultural diversity, competing problems, and sustainability of the program in a poor community. Strategies used to address obstacles to model adoption included legitimizing the program, building program infrastructure, setting realistic expectations, focusing on one risk factor at a time, defining target population segments, and emphasizing a small number of communication channels. The initial experience implementing this model in a disadvantaged urban setting supports the feasibility of this approach.

School Intervention

Most adult CVD is attributable to risk factor–related behaviors that are often established in early childhood.[36–39] By age 12 at least one modifiable risk factor for CHD exists in 36% to 60% of children in the United States.[40] There is also a general assumption that the psychosocial environment of childhood contributes to behaviors in adult life, including those related to CVD morbidity and mortality.[41] These behavioral risks—cigarette smoking, inappropriate dietary habits, and insufficient exercise—all are difficult to modify once established. In the United States more than 50 million children attend private and public schools, for an average of 5 to 8 hours a day, 5 days a week for 36 weeks a year, turning schools into a major window of opportunity for promoting health related behaviors among children.[42, 43]

For the most part, the model for school health services that has guided the development of school health programs in the United States includes three components: health instruction, a healthful school environment, and the provision of school health services. Health instruction includes teaching health-related knowledge, attitudes, and practices. The school environment relates to the actual physical setting, as well as to an awareness of its influence on the attitude and behavior of students. School health services include medical examinations, screening programs, communicable disease control, and correction of remediable problems. This model has been used to tailor CVD interventions as well as interventions in other acute and chronic diseases in the school setting.[36, 44]

Before 1980, the goal of most school health education programs was to transmit information with the hope that increased knowledge would lead students to adopt positive health behaviors.[36] However, there is substantial evidence that such an approach is ineffective. It is clear, for example, that most adults who smoke begin smoking while in their teens,[45] and rates of adolescent smoking have not declined as have those for other age groups. This has been particularly true for teenage girls, who now smoke more than their male counterparts.[46] Thus a modified approach has evolved that places less emphasis on knowledge acquisition and more on skills development, social influences, and behavioral competencies, with the goal of intervening before risk behaviors become established.[41] School-based smoking prevention programs incorporating these approaches have had generally positive results,[47, 48] the most successful being programs that are targeted to delay the onset of smoking, which is important in terms of reducing the likelihood of a person becoming a heavy smoker as an adult.[49] It is generally agreed that, at a minimum, a smoking prevention program in the school setting should offer information about the short-term physiologic effects of tobacco and the social influences that lead to smoking, training in refusal skills, and facts on the social consequences of smoking.[46]

The school environment also must support smoking prevention, and a nonsmoking policy for both staff and students should be the norm.[50] A California study demonstrated that in schools with the most restrictive smoking policies and a strong emphasis on prevention, fewer students used tobacco.[51] Recognizing the importance of school smoking policies, the National Cancer Institute recommended establishment of restrictive smoking policies by schools as one of the essential elements of school-based tobacco use prevention programs.[46]

The social-influences approach is frequently described as the most effective model for prevention of adolescent smoking, and it is, in fact, the only program with demonstrated results.[52] With up to 5 years of follow-up, these programs have consistently demonstrated the ability to delay the onset of smoking.[53] However, there is evidence suggesting that the benefits in early adolescence may disappear entirely by the time a student graduates from high school.[54]

Dietary recommendations are a major component of national chronic disease prevention strategies, particularly for CVD and cancer. National recommendations include reducing total- and saturated-fat consumption, increasing the consumption of fruits, vegetables, and whole-grain products, and reducing alcohol, sugar, and salt intake. Although these recommendations are for adults, they seem to be appropriate as well for children older than 2 years of age.[55] The Bogalusa Heart Study has shown that the total-fat, saturated-fat, and sodium consumption of 10 year-old children exceeds recommended levels and that the food preferences of children and adolescents are like those of their community and culture.[56] Parents have a powerful influence on their children's eating behavior, an influence that is probably even greater than it is in the case of cigarette smoking.[57] Although parents usually select most of their children's food, these selections take into account the needs and expressed demands of children.[58] These demands are often shaped by the advertising of foods on television.[41]

An analysis of school lunches carried out as part of a CVD prevention program demonstrated that total fat accounted for 38.8% of the total calories children consumed at lunch, nearly a third above the recommendations of the National School Lunch Program.[55] These results were consistent with the findings of other school-based heart disease prevention programs[56] and showed little change even after the U.S. Department of Agriculture published guidelines in 1983 for reducing the fat, sugar, and sodium content of school lunches.[55] Because 60% of public school students participate in school lunch programs and consume 25% to 33% of their total daily calories at school, cafeteria and school lunch interventions are a common component of comprehensive school-based nutrition programs.[42]

The value of nutritional interventions in the schools has been shown in a number of studies. Ellison and colleagues[59] tested the influence of an environmental nutrition program aimed at changing the food buying and preparation practices of school food service workers. Although there was no student education component, the diet of the students in the intervention group contained 15% to 20% less sodium and 20% less saturated fat than that of a control group. A multifactorial approach as used in the Heart Smart cardiovascular school health project (a school lunch program providing cardiovascular healthful food choices, a physical education program promoting personal fitness and aerobic conditioning, and cardiovascular risk factor screening) has also been shown to be of value.[60] Screening participants showed greater improvement in health knowledge than did nonparticipants. School lunch choices were successfully altered, and children whose lunch choices were cardiovascular healthful demonstrated the greatest cholesterol reduction. Improvements in run/walk performance were related in predicted directions to the overall cardiovascular risk profile.

A supportive and reinforcing school environment increases the likelihood that the students will develop health-promoting skills and attitudes.[50] The student activities should be based on sound behavioral and learning theory and, whenever possible, be those that have already been shown to be effective in achieving positive outcomes.[61] However, although schools can be instrumental in promoting the health of school-aged children, they cannot be expected to do the job alone. A supportive and reinforcing family and home setting is particularly important in encouraging children to establish healthy behaviors.[62, 63] Reviewing the literature on the role of families in influencing health-related behaviors, Perry and colleagues concluded that children can also influence their parents' health behavior, that parents are often difficult to recruit to traditional health education classes, and that more flexible learning methods are needed that can be used at home.[64] Schools can also provide an effective channel for rural health promotion efforts, where community intervention programs face the challenge of disseminating health information to widely scattered populations.[65]

One problem of particular concern is the relative lack of attention directed at high-risk, hard-to-reach youth. With a few notable exceptions,[66, 67] most CVD prevention programs have been targeted at nonminority, middle-class populations. Health professionals and schools must be continually alert to providing appropriate programming for high-risk, difficult-to-reach groups, particularly while they can still be reached in the formal school system.

In adults there is substantial evidence that lack of physical activity is related to obesity, hypertension, high blood lipid levels, and early death from CHD.[68] National physical fitness surveys indicate that only a minority of adults engage in regular physical activity at a level likely to maintain cardiac and respiratory fitness.[69] Physical inactivity in adulthood often has its roots in childhood.[70, 71] Most observers have concluded that the current generation of children is not as fit as the previous one, today's youth having more body fat than children in the 1960s.[55] The goal of school-based physical education programs should be, at least partially, to create favorable attitudes, experiences, and skills to increase the likelihood that children will continue being physically active as adults.[72] At least 80% of 10- to 18-year olds are enrolled in physical education programs at school, but these programs often do not focus on health-related fitness that is likely to lead to greater activity by adults.[73] Data from the Class of 1989 Study (part of the Minnesota Heart Health Program), however, suggest that multiple intervention components such as behavioral education in schools and complementary community-wide strategies can produce lasting improvement in adolescent physical activity.[74]

Some programs have targeted multiple cardiovascular risk factors among elementary school students,[75–77] high school students,[78] and minority populations.[67] Most notable among these is a National Heart, Lung, and Blood Institute–funded cooperative project: The Child and Adolescent Trial for Cardiovascular Health (CATCH).[41] This study's overall goal is to determine the effect of school-based intervention on promoting healthy behavior and reducing CVD risk factors among elementary school students. It uses programs promoting exercise, a healthful diet, and fitness. Interventions focus on school curricula and environment and on fostering parental involvement.

The relationship of home and school-based programs has been examined in several studies. In the San Diego Family Health Project, Mexican-American and Anglo-American families with children in the fifth or sixth grade were randomized to either a control condition or to a year-long education program designed to change dietary and exercise habits using classes held in local schools.[66] After 1 year, positive changes had occurred in the intervention families' dietary practices, but their cardiovascular fitness levels had not changed significantly. The authors concluded that involving families in health education programs using school-based resources is effective and that this is a promising area for future research.

In another study, the benefits of school-based programs were compared with those aimed directly at the home environment.[63] Conducted in Minnesota and North Dakota, the study compared the results of a 5-week school-based program for third graders with that of a 5-week program of written information sent to the homes of third graders; both programs required parental involvement. Eighty-six percent of eligible parents participated in the home-based program, and 71% completed the five-week course. Students in the home-based program had greater reductions in dietary fat and saturated fat than did those in the school-based program. The study showed that a large number of parents are willing to participate in home-based programs and that this type of parental participation can initiate changes in the eating patterns of young children as well as the parents.

One of the limitations of school-based programs is that they do not influence the high-risk adolescents who drop out of school. These adolescents are not only untouched by school-based interventions, but their risk behaviors often exceed those of their peers who are still in school. This is true of smoking and may also be the case for other cardiovascular risks.[54, 79] Other barriers to CVD prevention programs in the schools include overcrowded curricula, overburdened teachers, the desire for broad and locally controlled programs, inadequate funding, and lack of teacher training.[46]

Worksite Intervention

The worksite provides a vehicle for helping people reduce risk through changes in the work organization and environment. CHD risks may be reduced by eliminating or reducing exposures to hazardous substances such as cigarette smoke or by altering work conditions that are associated with increased disease incidence, such as the stressful work combination of high demand and low control.[80–82]

Seventy percent of adults between 18 and 65 years of age are employed.[83] Even a small intervention effect in this large segment of the population has the potential to change health behaviors so as to result in substantial changes in CHD event rates.[6, 84] This target population includes many people with low income and educational levels who may not be reached through other intervention channels. Interventions addressing multiple risk-related behaviors, such as smoking, diet, and exercise, can be offered in worksites repeatedly over time, thus increasing the likelihood of motivating change in persons who are at various points of readiness for such change.[85, 86] Because much of our lives are spent working, the potential for the worksite to be an effective force for risk factor modification is considerable. Increasingly, businesses themselves are taking an active role in this process, as they perceive prevention as a way of holding down health care costs related to absenteeism, insurance claims, and disability.[87, 88]

The number of health promotion programs in the worksite has increased in recent years, with most of the programs aimed at individual behavior change.[89] Results of the first National Survey of Worksite Health Promotion Activities found that 65.5% of responding worksites had one or more types of health promotion activities.[90] Worksite preventive health programs typically include, in decreasing order of frequency, smoking cessation, health risk assessment, back care regimens, stress management, exercise and fitness programs, accident prevention, nutrition education, high blood pressure treatment, and weight control. The frequency of these activities is directly related to the size of the worksite and varies by industry type.[89]

Typical of the type of studies carried out in the workplace is IBM's "A Plan for Life" program, which evaluated changes in blood pressure; serum total, high-density lipoprotein, and non–high-density lipoprotein cholesterol; body mass index; and cigarette smoking over a 1- to 5-year period among nonrandomized program participants and nonparticipants initially found to be at risk. After adjustment for age, sex, time to follow-up, and baseline values, the proportion of participants no longer at high risk was significantly greater than the corresponding proportion of nonparticipants, with meaningful changes occuring in blood pressure, total and non–high-density lipoprotein cholesterol, and smoking cessation.[91]

Few systematic studies have provided evidence that health promotion is a cost-effective means of decreasing health care costs, although the evidence for tangible benefits is beginning to accumulate.[87, 92–96] A landmark study conducted at the DuPont Company compared 41 intervention sites and 19 control sites, with a total of more than 40,000 hourly employees.[92] Over a 2-year period, blue-collar employees at intervention sites experienced a significant decline in disability days (14%), as compared with a smaller decline in the control sites (5.8%). Savings due to lower disability costs at intervention sites provided a return of $2.05 for every dollar invested in the program by the end of the second year. There is also evidence suggesting that a comprehensive health promotion program may have other benefits for employers, including improved attitudes of employees toward the company, reductions in corporate health benefits costs, and decreased utilization of inpatient services.[97, 98] For some employers, the major motivation for sponsoring health promotion efforts may be the potential savings resulting from healthier employee lifestyles; in such cases, accurate estimates of cost savings can improve the program's chances of adoption.[99] Other employers may be primarily interested in programs as a means to improve employee morale or the company's public image and may be especially responsive to employee requests when offering programs.[100]

In a randomized, controlled worksite nutrition intervention program that focused on promoting eating patterns low in fat and high in fiber (The Treatwell Study), 16 worksites from Massachusetts and Rhode Island were randomly assigned to either an intervention or a control condition.[101] The intervention included direct education and environmental programming tailored to each worksite; control worksites received no intervention. A cohort of workers randomly sampled from each site was surveyed both prior to and following the intervention. Dietary patterns were assessed using a semiquantitative food frequency questionnaire. Adjusting for worksite, the decrease in mean dietary fat intake was 1.1% of total calories more in intervention sites than in control sites ($P < 0.005$). There was no difference in dietary fiber intake between intervention and control sites. Thus a worksite nutrition intervention program can effectively influence the dietary habits of workers.

POLITICAL ISSUES

Smoking and diet have been increasingly a source of concern on the national level, with regulatory agencies and Congress progressively more involved in suggesting or enacting rules and regulations that respond to public concern. The Surgeon General's office has taken the lead in marshalling the evidence against smoking, much of which has been used in the legislative process whereby smoking in this country has been progressively curtailed.[47, 102] Such approaches have included increased taxation on cigarettes, the banning of smoking in public places, and the support of media campaigns against smoking by public agencies such as the National Cancer Institute.

The U.S. food supply is regulated by a series of laws administered by the Department of Health and Human Services and the Department of Agriculture. The Food and Drug Administration's (FDA) requirements concerning the provision of basic, standard-format nutrition information ("nutrition labeling") on food products have changed dramatically over the past 50 years. The new FDA regulations that become effective in 1994 require standardized nutrition labeling on most food products carried in interstate commerce.[103] Under the new FDA regulations, it is illegal to use any health claim or nutrient content claim in food labeling unless the claim has been approved in advance by the FDA.

In response to the new law, on January 6, 1993, the FDA promulgated regulations that described general requirements for health claims on foods in conventional food forms and specific requirements for seven authorized health claim topics. Three authorized claims are related to heart disease: dietary saturated fat and cholesterol and CHD; fruits, vegetables and grain products that contain fiber, particularly soluble fiber, and risk of CHD; and the relationship of sodium intake to hypertension. Approval for health claims is based on the totality of publicly available scientific evidence and significant agreement among experts qualified by scientific training and experience to evaluate the relationship. On January 4, 1994, the FDA finalized similar requirements for health claims on dietary supplements.[104]

In the dietary area, three proposals to reduce the availability of atherogenic foods are

1. Use of warning labels on atherogenic foods
2. Prohibition of advertising for such high-risk foods
3. Imposition of an excise tax on the same foods[105]

Food labeling is an especially important and interesting interface between policy and preventive medicine. Dietary choices are complex, and in contrast to cigarette smoking the consumer needs a great deal of information to make intelligent choices. The awareness of the nutritional content of foods influences people's choices.[106–109] A study performed at the University of Utah to estimate the effects of changing nutrition information format assessed consumer preferences for 12 label alternatives used to provide nutrition information on Campbell's Soup cans. Consumers clearly preferred the nutrition label that displayed all nutrient values using a bar graph format, offered the most information load, and expressed nutrient values using both absolute numbers and percentages. Consumers also preferred nutrition information arranged in an order that grouped nutrients that should be consumed in adequate amounts on the top, calories in the middle, and nutrients that should be consumed in lesser amounts on the bottom of the label.[110] Another study concluded that consumer choices may be overly influenced by industry-directed claims placed on the front of a product package.[111]

The use of labels seems to be an effective way to spread knowledge. However, many studies also show that the general public is currently overloaded with nutritional information and that many basic concepts regarding healthful dietary choices are not clear.[112] There are also problems in the implementation of labeling guidelines. A New York City study carried out to determine the accuracy of caloric labeling demonstrated that all locally prepared foods had more actual than labeled kilocalories, with the mean local dish underestimating caloric content by 85.4%.[113] Regionally distributed foods also had significantly more kilocalories than reported on the label, but the average discrepancy was considerably smaller (25.22%). On the other hand, the labeling of nationally advertised foods was quite accurate, with only a 2.2% underestimate of caloric content. These findings suggest that labels on foods produced by small enterprises without extensive resources to carry out or commission appropriate testing may be inadequate sources for caloric monitoring.

CONCLUSIONS

To be truly effective, a strategy for the prevention of CVD must incorporate intervention at many levels. The physician and other health care workers remain central to this strategy, but their care needs to incorporate newer methodologies that enhance the delivery of preventive services. Beyond this, to reduce the national burden of CVD, it is necessary to intervene at the level of the school, worksite, and community and also to influence the political process so as to facilitate the prevention of disease. Only by expanding our horizons in this manner will we shift the entire population risk profile in a favorable direction, so that the next generation will see a much-lessened incidence of CVD.

REFERENCES

1. Hennekens CH, O'Donnell CJ, Ridker PM, et al. Current issues concerning thrombolytic therapy for acute myocardial infarction. J Am Coll Cardiol 1995; 25[suppl]:18S–22S.
2. Rose G. Sick individuals and sick populations. Int J Epidemiol 1985; 14:32–38.
3. Fischer PM, Guinan KH, Burke JJ, et al. Impact of a public

cholesterol screening program. Arch Intern Med 1990; 150:2567–2572.
4. Kannel WB, Garcia MJ, McNamara PM, et al. Serum lipid precursors of coronary heart disease. Hum Pathol 1971; 2:129–151.
5. Goldman L, Cook EF. The decline in ischemic heart disease mortality rates. Ann Intern Med 1984; 101:825–836.
6. Rose G. Strategy of prevention: Lessons from cardiovascular disease. BMJ 1981; 282:1847–1851.
7. Kottke TE, Puska P, Salonen JT, et al. Projected effects of high-risk versus population-based prevention strategies in coronary heart disease. Am J Epidemiol 1985; 121:697–704.
8. Kottke TE, Gatewood LC, Wu SC, et al. Preventing heart disease: Is treating the high risk sufficient? J Clin Epidemiol 1988; 41:1083–1093.
9. Goldman L, Weinstein MC, Williams LW. Relative impact of targeted versus population-wide cholesterol interventions on the incidence of coronary heart disease: Projections of the Coronary Heart Disease Policy Model. Circulation 1989; 80:254–260.
10. Ockene JK. Physician-delivered interventions for smoking cessation: Strategies for increasing effectiveness. Prev Med 1987; 16:723–737.
11. Ockene IS, Ockene JK. Barriers to lifestyle change, and the need to develop an integrated approach to prevention. Cardiol Clin North Am 1996; 14:159–169.
12. Ockene JK, Ockene IS, Quirk ME, et al. Physician training for patient-centered nutrition counseling in a lipid intervention trial. Prev Med 1995; 24:563–570.
13. Ockene IS, Hebert J, Ockene JK, et al. Effect of physician-delivered nutrition counseling training and a structured office environment on diet and serum lipid measurements. Circulation 1996; 94(Suppl):I–177.
14. Ockene IS, Hebert JR, Ockene JK, et al. Effect of physician-delivered nutrition counseling training and a structured office practice on diet and serum lipid measurements in a hyperlipidemic population: The Worcester-Area Trial for Counseling in Hyperlipidemia (WATCH). 1996. submitted.
15. Ockene IS, Hebert JR, Ockene JK, et al. Effectiveness of physician training and a structured office practice setting on physician-delivered nutrition counseling: The Worcester-Area Trial for Counseling in Hyperlipidemia (WATCH). Am J Prev Med 1996; 12:252–258.
16. Pedersen TR, Kjekshus J, Berg K, et al. Randomised trial of cholesterol lowering in 4444 patients with coronary heart disease: The Scandinavian Simvastatin Survival Study (4S). Lancet 1994; 344:1383–1389.
17. Shepherd J. The West of Scotland Coronary Prevention Study: A trial of cholesterol reduction in Scottish men. Am J Cardiol 1995; 76:C113–C117.
18. The Lipid Research Clinics Program. The Lipid Research Clinics Coronary Primary Prevention Trial results: II. The relationship of reduction in incidence of coronary heart disease to cholesterol lowering. JAMA 1984; 251:365–374.
19. Debusk RF, Miller NH, Superko HR, et al. A case-management system for coronary risk factor modification after acute myocardial infarction. Ann Intern Med 1994; 120:721–729.
20. Hebert JR, Ockene IS, Ockene JK, et al. Reductions in dietary fat, relative weight, and total serum cholesterol from a nutritionist-based, patient-centered intervention: The Worcester Area Trial for Counseling in Hyperlipidemia. submitted.
21. Shaffer J, Wexler LF. Reducing low-density lipoprotein cholesterol levels in an ambulatory care system: Results of a multidisciplinary collaborative practice lipid clinic compared with traditional physician-based care. Arch Intern Med 1995; 155:2330–2335.
22. Thompson B, Pertschuk M. Community Intervention and Advocacy. *In* Ockene IS, Ockene JK (eds). Prevention of Coronary Heart Disease. Boston, Little, Brown, 1992.
23. Blackburn H. Research and demonstration projects in community cardiovascular disease prevention. J Public Health Pol 1983; 4:398–421.
24. Farquhar J. The community-based model of life style intervention trials. Am J Epidemiol 1978; 108:103–111.
25. Mittelmark MB, Hunt MK, Heath GW, et al. Realistic outcomes: Lessons from community-based research and demonstration programs for the prevention of cardiovascular diseases [Review]. J Public Health Pol 1993; 14:437–462.
26. Farquhar JW, Wood PD, Breitrose H, et al. Community education for cardiovascular health. Lancet 1977; 1:1192–1195.
27. Puska P, Nissinen A, Tuomilehto J, et al. The community-based strategy to prevent coronary heart disease: Conclusions from the ten years of the North Karelia Project. Annu Rev Public Health 1985; 6:147–193.
28. Puska P, Korhonen HJ, Torppa J, et al. Does community-wide prevention of cardiovascular diseases influence cancer mortality? Eur J Cancer Prev 1993; 2:457–460.
29. Farquhar JW, Fortmann SP, Flora JA, et al. Effects of communitywide education on cardiovascular disease risk factors: The Stanford Five-City Project. JAMA 1990; 264:359–365.
30. Jeffery RW, Gray CW, French SA, et al. Evaluation of weight reduction in a community intervention for cardiovascular disease risk: Changes in body mass index in the Minnesota Heart Health Program. Int J Obes Metab Disord 1995; 19:30–39.
31. Schwartz R, Smith C, Speers MA, et al. Capacity building and resource needs of state health agencies to implement community-based cardiovascular disease programs. J Public Health Pol 1993; 14:480–494.
32. Elder JP, Schmid TL, Dower P, et al. Community heart health programs: Components, rationale, and strategies for effective interventions. J Public Health Pol 1993; 14:463–479.
33. Shea S, Basch CE, Lantigua R, et al. The Washington Heights–Inwood Healthy Heart Program: A third-generation community-based cardiovascular disease prevention program in a disadvantaged urban setting. Prev Med 1992; 21:203–217.
34. Jousilahti P, Tuomilehto J, Korhonen HJ, et al. Trends in cardiovascular disease risk factor clustering in eastern Finland: Results of 15-year follow-up of the North Karelia Project. Prev Med 1994; 23:6–14.
35. Nutbeam D, Smith C, Murphy S, et al. Maintaining evaluation designs in long-term community-based health promotion programmes: Heartbeat Wales case study. J Epidemiol Comm Health 1993; 47:127–133.
36. Eriksen MP. School intervention. *In* Ockene IS, Ockene JK (eds). Prevention of Coronary Heart Disease. Boston, Little, Brown, 1992.
37. Hunter SM, Bao WH, Berenson GS. Understanding the development of behavior risk factors for cardiovascular disease in youth: The Bogalusa Heart Study. Am J Med Sci 1995; 310:S114–S118.
38. Gidding SS, Bao WH, Srinivasan SR, et al. Effects of secular trends in obesity on coronary risk factors in children: The Bogalusa Heart Study. J Pediatr 1995; 127:868–874.
39. Berenson GS. Prevention of heart disease beginning in childhood through comprehensive school health: The Heart Smart Program. Prev Med 1993; 22:507–512.
40. Williams C, Carter B, Wynder E. Prevalence of selected cardiovascular and cancer risk factors in a pediatric population: The Know Your Body Project. Prev Med 1981; 10:235–250.
41. Perry CL, Stone EJ, Parcel GS, et al. School-based cardiovascular health promotion: The Child and Adolescent Trial for Cardiovascular Health (CATCH). J School Health 1990; 60:406–413.
42. Frank GC. Primary prevention in the school arena: A dietary approach. Health Values 1983; 7:14–21.
43. Iverson DC, Kolbe LJ. Evolution of the national disease prevention and health promotion strategy: Establishing a role for the schools. J School Health 1983; 54:33–38.
44. Stone E. ACCESS: Keystones for school health promotion. J School Health 1990; 60:298–300.
45. Escobedo LG, Anda RF, Smith PF, et al. Sociodemographic characteristics of cigarette smoking initiation in the United States. JAMA 1990; 264:1550–1555.
46. Glynn TJ. Essential elements of school-based smoking prevention programs. J School Health 1989; 59:181–188.
47. U.S. Department of Health and Human Services. Reducing the Health Consequences of Smoking: 25 Years of Progress. A Report of the Surgeon General. DHHS Publication No (CDC) 89–8411. Atlanta, Centers for Disease Control, 1989.
48. Rundall TG, Bruvold WH. A meta-analysis of school-based smoking and alcohol use prevention programs. Health Educ Q 1988; 15:317–334.

49. Best JA, Thomson SJ, Santi SM, et al. Preventing cigarette smoking among children. Annu Rev Public Health 1988; 9:161–201.
50. Stevens NH, Davis LG. Exemplary school health education: A new change from HOT districts. Health Educ Q 1988; 15:63–70.
51. Pentz MA, Brannon BR, Charlin VL, et al. The power of policy: The relationship of smoking policy to adolescent smoking. Am J Publ Health 1989; 79:857–862.
52. Pentz MA, Dwyer JH, MacKinnon DP, et al. A multicomponent community trial for primary prevention of adolescent drug abuse: Effects on drug use prevalence. JAMA 1989; 261:3259.
53. Perry CL, Klepp KI, Sillers C. Community-wide strategies for cardiovascular health: The Minnesota Heart Health Program youth program. Health Educ Res 1989; 4:87–101.
54. Flay BR, Koepke D, Thomson SJ, et al. Six-year follow-up of the first Waterloo School Smoking Prevention Trial. Am J Public Health 1989; 79:1371–1376.
55. Parcel GS, Simons-Morton BG, O'Hara NM, et al. School promotion of healthful diet and exercise behavior: An integration of organizational change and social learning theory interventions. J School Health 1987; 57:150–156.
56. Frank GC, Berenson GS, Webber LS. Dietary studies and the relationship of diet to cardiovascular risk factor variables in 10-year old children: The Bogalusa Heart Study. Am J Clin Nutr 1978; 31:228–240.
57. Crockett SJ, Mullis R, Perry CL, et al. Parent education in youth-directed nutrition interventions. Prev Med 1989; 17:475–491.
58. Wadden TA, Brownell KD. The development and modification of dietary practices in individuals, groups and large populations. *In* Matarazzo JD, Weiss SM, Herd JA, Miller NE (eds): Behavioral Health: A Handbook of Health Enhancement and Disease Prevention. New York, John Wiley, 1984.
59. Ellison RC, Goldberg RJ, Witschi JC, et al. Use of fat-modified food products to change dietary fat intake of young people. Am J Public Health 1990; 80:1374–1376.
60. Arbeit ML, Johnson CC, Mott DS, et al. The Heart Smart Cardiovascular School Health Promotion: Behavior correlates of risk factor change. Prev Med 1992; 21:18–32.
61. Parcel GS, Simons-Morton BG, Kolbe LJ. Health promotion: Integrating organizational change and student learning strategies. Health Educ Q 1988; 15:435–450.
62. Cohen RY, Felix MRJ, Brownell KD. The role of parents and older peers in school-based cardiovascular prevention programs: Implications for program development. Health Educ Q 1990; 16:245–253.
63. Perry CL, Luepker RV, Murray DM, et al. Parent involvement with children's health promotion: A one-year follow-up of the Minnesota Home Team. Health Educ Q 1989; 16:171–180.
64. Perry CL, Crockett SJ, Pirie P. Influencing parental health behavior: Implications of community assessments. Health Educ 1987; 18:68–77.
65. Barthold J, Pearson J, Ellsworth A, et al. A cardiovascular health education program for rural schools. J School Health 1993; 63:298–301.
66. Nader PR, Sallis JF, Patterson TL, et al. A family approach to cardiovascular risk reduction: Results from the San Diego Family Health Project. Health Educ Q 1989; 16:229–244.
67. Bush PJ, Zuckerman AE, Taggart VS, et al. Cardiovascular risk factor prevention in black school children: The "Know Your Body" evaluation project. Health Educ Q 1989; 16:215–227.
68. Blair SN, Horton E, Leon AS, et al. Physical activity, nutrition, and chronic disease. Med Sci Sports Exerc 1996; 28:335–349.
69. Crespo CJ, Keteyian SJ, Heath GW, et al. Leisure-time physical activity among US adults: Results from the Third National Health and Nutrition Examination Survey. Arch Intern Med 1996; 156:93–98.
70. Riopel DA, Boerth RC, Coates TJ, et al. Coronary risk factor modification in children: Exercise. Circulation 1986; 74:1189A–1191A.
71. Iverson DC, Fielding JE, Crow RS, et al. The promotion of physical activity in the United States populations: The status of programs in medical, worksite, community, and school settings. Public Health Rep 1985; 100:212–214.
72. Simons-Morton BG, Parcel GS, O'Hara NM, et al. Health-related physical fitness in childhood: Status and recommendations. Annu Rev Public Health 1988; 9:403–425.
73. Ross JG, Pate RR. The National Children and Youth Fitness Study: II. A summary of findings. J Phys Educ Recreat Dance 1987; 58:51–56.
74. Kelder SH, Perry CL, Klepp KI. Community-wide youth exercise promotion: Long-term outcomes of the Minnesota Heart Health Program and the Class of 1989 Study. J School Health 1993; 63:218–223.
75. Walter HJ. Primary prevention of chronic disease among children: The school-based "Know Your Body" intervention trials. Health Educ Q 1989; 16:201–214.
76. Simons-Morton BG, Parcel GS, O'Hara NM. Implementing organizational changes to promote healthful diet and physical activity at school. Health Educ Q 1988; 15:115–130.
77. Butcher AH, Frank GC, Harsha DW, et al. Heart Smart: A school health program meeting the 1990 objectives for the nation. Health Educ Q 1988; 15:17–34.
78. Killen JD, TN Robinson, Telch MJ, et al. The Stanford Adolescent Heart Health Program. Health Educ Q 1989; 16:263–283.
79. Pirie PL, Murray DM, Luepker RV. Smoking prevalence in a cohort of adolescents, including absentees, dropouts, and transfers. Am J Public Health 1988; 78:176–178.
80. Theriault GP. Cardiovascular disorders. *In* Levy BS, Wegman DH (eds). Occupational Health: Recognizing and Preventing Work-Related Disease, 2nd ed. Boston, Little, Brown, 1988.
81. Karasek RA, Theorell T, Alfredsson L, et al. Job psychological factors and coronary heart disease. Adv Cardiol 1982; 29:62–67.
82. Karasek RA, Theorell T, Alfredsson L, et al. Job characteristics in relation to the prevalence of myocardial infarction in the U.S. Health Examination Survey (HES) and the Health and Nutrition Examination Survey (HANES). Am J Public Health 1988; 78:910–918.
83. U.S. Bureau of the Census. Statistical Abstract of the United States. Washington, DC, U.S. Government Printing Office, 1986.
84. Terborg JR. The organization as a context for health promotion. *In* Oskamp S (ed). Social Psychology and Health: The Clargmont Symposium on Applied Social Psychology. Newbury Park, CA, Sage, 1988.
85. Terborg JR. Health promotion at the worksite: A research challenge for personnel and human resources management. Res Personnel Hum Resources Manage 1986; 4:225–267.
86. Heaney CA, Inglish P. Are employees who are at risk for cardiovascular disease joining worksite fitness centers? J Occup Envir Med 1995; 37:718–724.
87. Warner KE, Wickizer TM, Wolfe RA, et al. Economic implications of workplace health promotion programs: Review of the literature. J Occup Med 1988; 30:106–112.
88. Sloan RP, Gruman JC, Allegrante JP. Investing in Employee Health: A Guide to Effective Health Promotion in the Workplace. San Francisco, Josey-Bass, 1987.
89. Sorensen G, Himmelstein J. Worksite intervention. *In* Ockene IS, Ockene JK (eds). Prevention of Coronary Heart Disease. Boston, Little, Brown, 1992.
90. Fielding JE, Piserchia PV. Frequency of worksite health promotion activities. Am J Public Health 1989; 79:16–20.
91. Goetzel R, Sepulveda M, Knight K, et al. Association of IBM's "A Plan for Life" health promotion program with changes in employees' health risk status. J Occup Med 1994; 36:1005–1009.
92. Bertera RL. The effects of workplace health promotion on absenteeism and employment costs in a large industrial population. Am J Public Health 1990; 80:1101–1105.
93. Jones RD, Bly JL, Richardson JE. A study of a worksite health promotion program and absenteeism. J Occup Med 1990; 32:95–99.
94. Reed RW, Mulvaney D, Bellingham R, et al. Health Promotion Service: Evaluation Study. Indianapolis, Blue Cross–Blue Shield of Indiana, 1985.
95. Baun WP, Bernack EJ, Tsai SPA. A preliminary investigation:

Effect of a corporate fitness program on absenteeism and health care cost. J Occup Med 1986; 28:18–22.
96. Blair SN, Piserchia PV, Wilbur CS, et al. A public health intervention model for work-site health promotion. JAMA 1986; 225:921–926.
97. Holzbach RL, Piserchia PV, McFadden DW, et al. Effect of a comprehensive health promotion program on employee attitudes. J Occup Med 1990; 32:973–970.
98. Bly JL, Jones RC, Richardson JE. Impact of worksite health promotion on health care costs and utilization: Evaluation of Johnson and Johnson's Live for Life Program. JAMA 1986; 256:3235–3240.
99. Sorensen G, Glasgow R, Corbett K. Involving worksites and other organizations. *In* Bracht N (ed). Organizing for Community Health Promotion: A Guide. Newbury Park, CA, Sage, 1990.
100. Brownell KD. Weight control at the workplace: The power of social and behavioral factors. *In* MF Cataldo, Coates TJ (eds). Health Promotion in Industry: A Behavioral Medicine Perspective. New York, John Wiley, 1986, pp 143–161.
101. Sorensen G, Morris DM, Hunt MK, et al. Work-site nutrition intervention and employees' dietary habits: The Treatwell program. Am J Public Health 1992; 82:877–880.
102. U.S. Department of Health and Human Services. The Health Consequences of Smoking: Cardiovascular Disease. A Report of the Surgeon General. DHHS Publication No. (PHS) 84–50204. Bethesda, MD, U.S. Department of Health and Human Services, Public Health Service, Office on Smoking and Health, 1983.
103. McNamara SH. The brave new world of FDA nutrition regulation—some thoughts about current trends and long-term effects. Crit Rev Food Sci Nutr 1994; 34:215–221.
104. Yetley EA, Park YK. Diet and heart disease: health claims. J Nutr 1995; 125(Suppl):679S–685S.
105. Bodenheimer T. A public health approach to cholesterol: Confronting the "TV-auto-supermarket society." West J Med 1991; 154:344–348.
106. Shide DJ, Rolls BJ. Information about the fat content of preloads influences energy intake in healthy women. J Am Diet Assoc 1995; 95:993–998.
107. Daillant-Spinnler B, Issanchou S. Influence of label and location of testing on acceptability of cream cheese varying in fat content. Appetite 1995; 24:101–105.
108. Aaron JI, Mela DJ, Evans RE. The influences of attitudes, beliefs, and label information on perceptions of reduced-fat spread. Appetite 1994; 22:25–37.
109. Tuorila H, Cardello AV, Lesher LL. Antecedents and consequences of expectations related to fat-free and regular-fat foods. Appetite 1994; 23:247–263.
110. Geiger CJ, Wyse BW, Parent CR, et al. Nutrition labels in bar graph format deemed most useful for consumer purchase decisions using adaptive conjoint analysis. J Am Diet Assoc 1991; 91:800–807.
111. Hrovat KB, Harris KZ, Leach AD, et al. The new food label, type of fat, and consumer choice: A pilot study. Arch Fam Med 1994; 3:690–695.
112. Goldberg JP. Nutrition and health communication: The message and the media over half a century. Nutr Rev 1992; 50:71–77.
113. Allison DB, Heshka S, Sepulveda D, et al. Counting calories—caveat emptor. JAMA 1993; 270:1454–1456.

Index

Note: Page numbers in *italics* refer to illustrations; page numbers followed by t refer to tables.

A

Abciximab (ReoPro), 167–168
in myocardial infarction, 180, 181
in percutaneous coronary intervention, 170–175, *172–173, 175,* 177, 178t, 180–181
as c7E3, 194
vs. small molecule platelet inhibitors, 180–181
ACE inhibitors, contraindications to, 302
for hypertension, 351, 353t, 356
in diabetes, 351, 356–357
in congestive heart failure, 298–303
after MI, 100, 101, 102, 103, 302, 303
contraindications to, 302
exercise capacity and, 299, 300, *300*
for hypertension, 351
hemodynamic improvement and, 98, 298–299, *299,* 300, 302
left ventricular dysfunction and, 301
overview analysis of, 301–302, 302t
survival and, 300–302, *301,* 302t
symptomatic improvement and, 298, 299, 300, 302
with digoxin, 305
with diuretics, 298
in diabetes, for hypertension, 351, 356–357
in MI, 103
in myocardial infarction, 95–103
and additivity with other therapies, 95, 100
animal studies of, 96
ejection fraction and, 102
hemodynamic effects of, 98
in elderly patients, 103
long-term trials of, 98–100, 99t, *99,* 102, 302, *303–304*
meta-analysis of, 102–103
neuroendocrine effects of, 96–97
nitrates with, 134–135, 136, *136–137,* 138, 141, 142
short-term acute trials of, 99, *100,* 100–103, 101t, 302–303
summary of results with, 103
ventricular remodeling and, 96, 97t, 97–98, 103
with aspirin, 102
with congestive heart failure, 102
left ventricular dysfunction and, after MI, 97t, 97–98, 99–100, 102–103, 302–303, *303–304*
in heart failure, 301
neutral endopeptidase inhibitor with, 311
nitrate tolerance and, 132, 141
original synthesis of, 95
pharmacologic actions of, 95–96
Acebutolol, after MI, 85–86
for mild hypertension, 383t, 386
in heart failure, 307t
Acenocoumarol, after MI, 251, 252
in atrial fibrillation, 261
N-Acetylcysteine (NAC), for nitrate tolerance, 132, *132*
with nitroglycerin, in acute MI, 141
in unstable angina, 140–141
ACT (activated clotting time), during angioplasty, 154, 187, 190
Acute coronary syndromes. See also *Myocardial infarction (MI); Non–Q wave MI; Unstable angina.*
classification of, 55, 145
platelet activation in, 245
Adenosine, in supraventricular tachyarrhythmias, 232–233, *233*
stress testing with, 280
Adenosine triphosphate, in supraventricular tachyarrhythmias, 233
Adrenaline. See *Epinephrine.*
Adrenergic activation, in heart failure, *87,* 87–88
Adrenergic α_1-antagonist. See also *Doxazosin.*
for hypertension, 351, 353t, 356
Adrenergic α_2-agonist, in atrial fibrillation, 241
Aerobic capacity, bed rest and, 278–279, 279t
prognostic significance of, 280, 280t
African Americans, hypertension in, 341, 356, 386
Age. See also *Elderly patients.*
blood pressure reduction and, 347, 349t
cholesterol reduction and, 333–334, 334t
Aggrastat. See *Tirofiban (Aggrastat).*
Aldosterone. See *Renin-angiotensin-aldosterone system.*
Alteplase. See *t-PA (tissue-type plasminogen activator, alteplase).*
American Heart Association dietary guidelines, 321, 435, 443
AMI. See *Myocardial infarction (MI), acute.*
Amiloride, for hypertension, 78t, 79, 114t, 353t
Amiodarone, after MI, 222–226, *225,* 227
vs. metoprolol, 224
in atrial fibrillation, after cardiac surgery, 240
chronic, 239
for acute termination, 235, 235t, 236
in congestive heart failure, 226–227, 310
pharmacologic actions of, 222, 226–227
Amlodipine, 106
atherogenesis and, 110
for hypertension, 114t, 353t
Amlodipine *(Continued)*
mild, 383t, 386
in heart failure, 113, 309–310
Analysis by treatment received, 11
Analytic epidemiology, 4t, 4–7
Aneurysm, aortic, smoking and, 362
myocardial, 96
Aneurysmal subarachnoid hemorrhage, nimodipine in, 115
Angina pectoris. See also *Coronary artery disease (CAD); Myocardial ischemia.*
angioplasty in, complications and, 156
direct antithrombins during, 157–158, *158,* 159, *160,* 162–163
vs. bypass surgery, 267, 268t, 268–277, *271, 274–275,* 276t, 277t
vs. medical therapy, 267–268, 268t, 269–270
aspirin in, 245–246, 249, 392, 393, 394
calcium channel blockers in, 106, 112–113, 351
estrogen and, 407, 408
exercise programs in, 204, 205, 389
exercise-induced, 280, 280t
lifestyle intervention in, 204–205, 315, 318, 388, 440, 441, 444
lipid-lowering drug(s) in, lovastatin as, 205
simvastatin as, 205, 207
nitrates in, tolerance with, 141
vs. angioplasty, 267–268, 268t
postinfarction, angioplasty in, 156
bivalirudin during, 159, *160,* 162–163
tirofiban in, 177–179
Prinzmetal's, magnesium in, 120
psychosocial intervention in, 319
smoking and, 362
unstable. See *Unstable angina.*
variant, 109. See also *Coronary artery spasm.*
vitamin E and, 419
Angiogenesis, estrogen and, 407
Angioplasty, percutaneous transluminal coronary, after thrombolysis, 186t, 186–187, 191–193
antiplatelet therapy after, 249, 392
aspirin during, 153–154
complication(s) of, 152, 155–156, *156,* 170
abrupt closure as, 156, 159–160, 187, 193
arterial injury as, 152–153, 154–155, 170
hemorrhagic, 160
coronary blood flow after, 193–194, *194*
direct antithrombin(s) during, 151–163
advantages of, 154–155, 160, *161–162,* 161–163

Angioplasty *(Continued)*
bivalirudin as, 157–158, *158,* 159–160, *160,* 162–163
hirudin as, 154–155, 156–157, *157,* 159, 160, 162
limitations of, 158–160
rationale for, 151–156
with GPIIb/IIIa antagonists, 160–161
failure of, stenting for, 191
for left anterior descending CAD, 267, 268, 269–270
GPIIb/IIIa antagonist(s) during, abciximab as, 170–175, *172–173, 175,* 177, 178t, 180–181
eptifibatide as, 169, 170, 175–176, 177, 178t, 180
tirofiban as, 168, 170, 176–177, 178t, 180
with direct antithrombins, 160–161
heparin during, 151–152, 153–154, 155, 156–157, *157–158,* 160, 162–163
high-risk, 153, 155–156, *156*
in acute MI, after failed thrombolysis, 191–193
nonrandomized studies of, 187–188, 188t
vs. thrombolysis, *72,* 72–73, 188–190, 189t
with thrombolysis, 186t, 186–187
in chronic angina, vs. bypass surgery, 267, 268t, 268–277, *271, 274–275,* 276t, 277t
vs. medical therapy, 267–268, 268t, 269–270
rehabilitation after, 279
repeat, 152, 156, 170, 254
rescue, after failed thrombolysis, 191–193
restenosis after, 152, 170
angioplasty for, 152, 156, 170
bypass surgery and, 152, 269
hirudin and, 155, 157
smoking and, 369
stents and, 267
vitamin E and, 419
vitronectin receptors and, 167
smoking cessation after, 369
vs. multiple risk factor intervention, 444
Angiotensin II. See *Renin-angiotensin-aldosterone system.*
Angiotensin II receptor antagonists, 310–311
Angiotensin-converting enzyme inhibitors. See *ACE inhibitors.*
Animal research, 3–4
Anistreplase (Eminase), aspirin or anticoagulation after, 253
Anorexiant medications, 381t, 381–382
Antiarrhythmic agent(s). See also *Arrhythmias.*
after MI, amiodarone as, 222–226, *225,* 227
CAST trial of, 34, 35t, 39, 40, 217–220, *218–219*
vs. beta blockers, 86
future trials of, 228
meta-analysis of, for 51 trials, 219–220
patient selection for, 217, 218
sotalol as, 220–222, *221–222,* 227
vs. implantable defibrillators, 217, 227–228
beta blockers as, 76, 86
fatty acids as, 427
in atrial fibrillation, after cardiac surgery, *239,* 239–240
Antiarrhythmic agent(s) *(Continued)*
chronic, for heart rate control, 240–242
for suppression, 234, *238,* 238–239
paroxysmal, for prevention, 236–238
for termination, 232, 234–236, 235t
in heart failure, amiodarone as, 310
in supraventricular tachycardias, 231–242
for acute termination, 232–233, *233*
of atrial fibrillation, 234–236, 235t
for heart rate control, acute, 232
chronic, in atrial fibrillation, 240–242
for long-term suppression, 233–234
of atrial fibrillation, 234, *238,* 238–239
for prevention, after surgery, *239,* 239–240
of atrial fibrillation, 236–238
limitations of trials with, 231t, 231–232
magnesium as, 120
magnesium as, 119–120
Anticoagulant therapy. See also *Antiplatelet agent(s); Antithrombins, direct; Heparin; Warfarin.*
after MI, recommendations for, 254–255
secondary prevention trials of, 251–252
vs. aspirin, 252–253
with aspirin, 253–254
in atrial fibrillation. See *Atrial fibrillation, stroke prevention in.*
pathophysiologic basis of, 245, 246
Antihypertensive drug trials, 342–357. See also *Hypertension.*
CHD and stroke reduction in, 343, 345t, 345–346, *345–347,* 357
by age, 347, 349t
by drug type, 347, *351,* 351–352, 352t, 353t
by gender, 347
by level of BP, 342, 346–347, 348t
by trial duration, 347, 350t
unpublished trials and, 352, 352t, 354t–355t, 356–357
vs. observational studies, 5
in African Americans, 356
of ACE inhibitors, 351, 353t, 356
in diabetes, 351, 356–357
of beta blockers, 77, 78t, 79, 344t, 352, 353t
in diabetes, 357
vs. diuretics, 79–81, 343, 347, 351, *351,* 353t
chlorthalidone in, 81, 383t, 386
meta-analysis of, 81, 82t
of calcium channel blockers, 106, 114, 114t, 351, 352, 353t, 356–357
optimal blood pressure goals in, 356–357
participant characteristics in, 343, 344t
summary of, 357
Antioxidant, carvedilol as, 86, 91
estrogen as, 403–404
Antioxidant vitamins, 415–421
basic research on, 415t, 415–416
need for more evidence about, 420–421
observational studies of, 6, 416
randomized trials of, 6–7, 416–417
in primary prevention, 417t, 417–418, 420, 420t
in secondary prevention, 208, 417t, 419–420, 420t
Antiplatelet agent(s). See also *Aspirin; Glycoprotein IIb/IIIa antagonists; Platelets.*
after MI, pathophysiologic basis for, 245–246
Antiplatelet agent(s) *(Continued)*
recommendations for, 254–255
secondary prevention trials of, 245–247
duration of treatment and, 250
meta-analyses of, 44, 247–250, *248–249*
vs. anticoagulants, 252–253
with anticoagulants, 253–254
beta blockers as, 82
magnesium as, 120
new, 254
nitrates as, 131
Antithrombin III, 56, 145, 146, *146*
in menopause, 404, 405
Antithrombins, direct, 145–146
cost of, 163
critique of, *161–162,* 161–163
during angioplasty, 151–163
advantages of, 160, *161–162,* 161–163
bivalirudin as, 157–158, *158,* 159–160, *160,* 162–163
hirudin as, 154–155, 156–157, *157,* 159, 160, 162
limitations of, 158–160
rationale for, 151–156
with GPIIb/IIIa antagonists, 160–161
mechanism of action of, 146, *146,* 161–162, *161–162*
Phase II trials of, 146–149, *147, 149*
Phase III trials of, 149–151, 150t, *151–153,* 154t, 155t, 162
thrombin rebound with, 158–159
vs. thrombolysis, 145
with thrombolysis, 146–148, *147*
Antithrombotic therapy. See *Anticoagulant therapy; Antiplatelet agent(s).*
Anturane (sulfinpyrazone), after MI, 247, 248, *249*
Aortic regurgitation, nifedipine in, 113–114
apo C-III, atherosclerosis regression and, 201
Apoptosis, calcium channel blockers and, 116
in heart failure, 87, *87,* 91
APSAC (anisoylated plasminogen-streptokinase activator complex), 60t, 69, 72
Argatroban, 146
in MI, 148, 162
Arginine vasopressin, in heart failure, 96
Arm exercises, 283–284, *283–284*
Arrhythmias. See also *Antiarrhythmic agent(s); Supraventricular tachycardias; Ventricular arrhythmias; Ventricular fibrillation; Ventricular tachycardia.*
after myocardial infarction, 217
behavioral factors and, 318
reperfusion, 125
estrogen and, 407
smoking and, 361, 369
Aspirin, adverse effects of, 250, 252, 254, 393, 393t
after MI, 392
cost effectiveness of, 291, 291t
dosage of, 250, 254
recommendation for, 250–251
trials of, 246–251, *248–249*
underutilization of, 62, 251
vs. anticoagulants, 252–253
with ACE inhibitors, 102
with anticoagulants, 253–254
with dipyridamole, 246–247, 248
after stent placement, 254

Aspirin *(Continued)*
controlled-release, 250, 254
during angioplasty, 153–154
for primary prevention, 393t, 393–397, 394t, 395t, 396t
recommendations for, 396–397
with warfarin, 254, 255, 396
in acute MI, 55, *58,* 58–59, 59t, 60t, 61–62, 392–393
in atrial fibrillation, 257–263, 258t, 259t
in stable angina, 245–246
in unstable CAD, 55–57, 61–62
platelet function and, 56, 392
with fibrinolytic therapy, 59, 245
with fibrinolytic therapy, *58,* 58–59, 60t, 61, 245
Asthma, beta blockers in, 77, 86
AT_1 receptor antagonists, 310–311
Atenolol, for arrhythmia prevention, after surgery, 240
for hypertension, 77, 78t, 79, 343, 353t
in type II diabetes, 357
vs. diuretics, 80, 343, 353t, 383t, 386
in acute MI, 83, *83,* 84t
in stable angina, vs. nifedipine, 112
Atherectomy, directional coronary, abciximab in, 173, 174, 177
eptifibatide in, 169
laser, 174
transluminal extraction catheter, 174
Atherogenic diet, 200
Atherosclerosis. See also *Coronary artery disease (CAD); Thrombus formation.*
ACE inhibitors and, 298
antioxidant vitamins and, 415, 416, 420
arteriography of, quantitative, 110, *111*
beta blockers and, 77, 79, 80, 82
cholesterol reduction and, 327, 423, 443
clopidogrel and, 254
estrogen and, 403, 406, 407
homocysteine and, 43, 429
pathologic processes in, 208–212
plaque composition in, 209–210, 212
plaque disruption in, 145, 199–200, 209, 210–213, *211,* 444
acute MI and, 58, 245
angioplasty causing, 153
aspirin and, 392
beta blockers and, 82, 86
exercise-related, 288
healing of, 200
lesion size and, 444
smoking-related, 362
thrombus formation and, 166, 210, 211, *211,* 213
plaque histology in, 200, *200,* 210
progression of, 199, 315
aspirin and, 245, 394
calcium channel blockers and, 110t, 110–112, *111,* 112t
risk reduction program and, 388
rabbit model of, 110
regression of, 315
antihypertensive treatment and, 346
definitions of, 200
diet vs. cholestyramine and, 425–426, 426t
exercise and, 287–288, *289*
in arteriographic trials, 200–202, 202t, 203t, *204–205,* 205, 212, 443
in multiple risk factor trials, 292, 440–442
lifestyle modification and, 318, 387, 387t, 427t, 427–428
mechanisms of, 200, 213
plaque stabilization and, 199–200, 212, 213, 292, 444
Atherosclerosis *(Continued)*
smoking and, 361, 362, 370
thrombin receptor and, 245
vasomotor impairment in, 131, 209, 406
Atrial fibrillation, after cardiac surgery, *239,* 239–240
anticoagulant therapy in, 255
antiplatelet therapy in, 249, 250, 392
chronic, suppression of, 234, *238,* 238–239
heart rate control in, 232, 240–242
limitations of antiarrhythmic trials in, 231, 231t
paroxysmal, acute termination of, 232, 234–236, 235t
prevention of, 236–238
stroke prevention in, 257–265
clinical practice and, *264,* 264–265
cost effectiveness of, 264
future research in, 264–265
need for, 257
optimal INR level for, *263,* 263–264
primary prevention trials of, 257–263, 258t, 259t, 261t
risk factors and, 260–261, 265
secondary prevention trial of, 259t, 261
thrombus formation and, 257
Atrial natriuretic factor, in MI, 96
Atrial tachycardia, automatic, 232
multifocal, magnesium and, 120
Atrioventricular block, beta blockers and, 86
Atrioventricular nodal reentrant tachycardia, 231, 232, 233–234
Atrioventricular reentrant tachycardia, 231, 232, 233–234
Autoantibodies, atherogenesis and, 415

B

Basic research, 3–4
vs. randomized trials, 6, 7
BBB (bundle branch block), fibrinolytic therapy in, 65, 66, *67,* 67–68, 73
Benazepril, for nitrate tolerance, 141
Bendrofluazide, for hypertension, 353t
vs. beta blockers, 77, 78t, 80
with atenolol, 77
Bepridil, in stable angina, 112
Beta blockers, 76–91. See also specific agent.
after cardiac surgery, for arrhythmia prevention, *239,* 239–240
after MI, 77, 81, 84t, 84–87, *85–86*
cost effectiveness of, 291, 291t
recommendations for, 86–87
vs. amiodarone, 223, 224
cardioselectivity of, 76, 76t, 77, 91
contraindications to, 86
amiodarone and, 223
for hypertension, 77, 78t, 79, 344t, 352, 353t
in diabetes, 357
vs. diuretics, 79–81, 343, 347, 351, *351,* 353t
chlorthalidone as, 81, 383t, 386
meta-analysis of, 81, 82t
in acute MI, 77, 81–84, *83,* 84t
recommendations for, 86
in atrial fibrillation, 240–242
in chronic angina, vs. angioplasty, 267–268, 268t
in congestive heart failure, 77, 87–91, 306–309, 307t
exercise capacity and, 307t, 307–308
Beta blockers *(Continued)*
future research needed with, 91
hemodynamic effects of, *90,* 91, 307
large trials of, 88–90, 89t, *89,* 308, *308*
mechanisms of benefit with, *87,* 87–88, 88t, *90,* 91
meta-analyses of, 90–91, 309, *309*
ongoing trials of, 90t, 91
third-generation, *90,* 91
in multiple risk factor trials, 429, 435
in supraventricular tachycardias, 232, 233, 240–242
pharmacology of, 76t, 76–77
d,l-sotalol as, 220, 222
Beta-adrenergic receptors, regulation of, 87–88
Beta-carotene, 415, 416
in cancer prevention trials, 417t, 417–418, 419
in cardiovascular trials, 7, 419, 420, 420t, 421
Bezafibrate, 202t
Bias(es). See also *Confounding variables.*
deviations from protocol and, 11–12
in assessing moderate effects, 25t, 25–26, 28–29
in control group selection, 10
in meta-analyses, 28–29, 49–50
in observational studies, 28
in outcome assessment, 10–11
in reviews of research, 43
in risk estimation, cholesterol and, 327
in subgroup analyses, 26, 29
in treatment selection, 10
interim trial results and, 38
publication bias as, 29, 49–50
unbiasedness and, 9, 9t
Biofeedback, 317
Bisoprolol, in heart failure, 88–89, 89t, 90t, 307t, 308
Bivalirudin (Hirulog), 146
during angioplasty, 157–158, *158,* 159–160, *160,* 162–163
phase II trials of, 148, 149
Blacks, hypertension in, 341, 356, 386
Blood pressure. See also *Hypertension.*
increase in, smoking and, 361
reduction of, by ACE inhibitors, 98
by atherosclerosis regression, 201
by beta blockers, 76, 77
by magnesium, 120
by resistance exercise training, 285
Breast cancer, hormone replacement therapy and, 408, 408t, 409, *409*
Bronchodilation, β_2-mediated, 76–77
Bruce treadmill protocol, 279–280
Bucindolol, in heart failure, 88, 90t, *90,* 307t
Bundle branch block (BBB), fibrinolytic therapy in, 65, 66, *67,* 67–68, 73
Bypass, cardiopulmonary, calcium channel blockers during, 114, 115
magnesium during, 122–123
Bypass graft. See *Coronary artery bypass graft (CABG).*

C

CABG. See *Coronary artery bypass graft (CABG).*
CAD. See *Coronary artery disease (CAD).*
Calcium, in heart failure, 87, 88, 306
in platelet activation, 126, 127
in reperfusion, 125
magnesium and, 119, 120
Calcium channel blockers, 106–116. See also specific agent.

Calcium channel blockers *(Continued)*
adverse effects of, 115–116, 351
atherosclerosis and, 110t, 110–112, *111*, 112t
cerebrovascular trials of, 114–115
chemical structures of, 106, *106–107*
controversy about, 115–116
estrogen as, 407
for hypertension, 81, 106, 114, 114t, 351, 352, 353t, 356
in type II diabetes, 356–357
in atrial fibrillation, 240, 241, 242
in elderly patients, adverse effects of, 115–116
in heart failure, 108, 113–114, 241, 309–310
in myocardial infarction, 106–108, 109t
in stable angina, 106, 112–113, 351
vs. angioplasty, 267–268, 268t
in supraventricular tachycardias, 233–234
atrial fibrillation as, 240, 241, 242
in unstable angina, 108–110, 109t
vs. nitroglycerin, 140
pharmacologic actions of, 106
Cancer, antioxidant vitamins and, 415, 417t, 417–418
cholesterol reduction and, 331–332, 332t
of breast, hormone replacement therapy and, 408, 408t, 409, *409*
Candoxatril, 311
Captopril, for hypertension, cost effectiveness of, 291, 291t
in type II diabetes, 357
for nitrate tolerance, 141
in congestive heart failure, 299–300, *300*
vs. digoxin, 300, 304
with digoxin, 304–305
in MI, animal studies of, 96
clinical studies of, 96–98, 97t
left ventricular dysfunction and, 302, *303–304*
long-term trials of, 99t, *99*, 99–100
short-term trials of, *100*, 101t, 101–102
vs. magnesium, 122
original synthesis of, 95
Carbohydrate, dietary, 423, 424
Carbon monoxide, smoking and, 361, 362
Cardiac. See also *Heart* entries.
Cardiac arrest, after MI, 217
cerebrovascular injury in, calcium channel blockers and, 115
physical exertion and, 288, 289
smoking and, 361, 368, 369
Cardiac catheterization, 185, 186, 193
Cardiac output, beta blockers and, 76
captopril and, 98
estrogen and, 406
in congestive heart failure, 297
Cardiac psychology, 315
Cardiac rehabilitation. See also *Exercise training.*
multifactorial, 278, 286, 287, 291–292, 320, 388–389
Cardiac rupture, beta blockers and, 82, 83
Cardiac transplantation, diltiazem after, 111
exercise therapy and, 291
Cardiogenic shock, angioplasty in, 72–73
captopril and, 101, 102
fibrinolytic therapy in, 68
magnesium and, 122
Cardiomyopathy. See also *Congestive heart failure.*
amiodarone in, 310
amlodipine in, 310
Cardiomyopathy *(Continued)*
beta blockers in, 88–90, 89t, *89*, 307, 308
in dilated cardiomyopathy, 88, 89t, 306, 307, 308
dilated, beta blockers in, 88, 89t, 306, 307, 308
diltiazem in, 113
enalapril in, 301
Cardiopulmonary bypass, calcium channel blockers during, 114, 115
magnesium during, 122–123
Carotene. See *Beta-carotene.*
Carotid atherosclerosis, isradipine vs. hydrochlorothiazide in, 111–112
Carvedilol, in heart failure, exercise capacity and, 88, 307t, 307–308
hemodynamic effects of, *90*, 91
left ventricular function and, 86–87, 308, *308*
mortality reduction and, *89*, 89–91, 90t, 308, 309, *309*
pharmacologic actions of, 86, 88
Case management, for risk factor modification, 449, 450
Case-control studies, 4–6
CAST (Cardiac Arrhythmia Suppression Trial), beta blockers and, 86
termination of, 34, 35t, 39, 40, 218–220
Cause-effect relationship, 4
observational studies and, 5–6
randomized clinical trials and, 6, 7
c7E3 Fab. See *Abciximab (ReoPro).*
Cerebrovascular disease. See also *Stroke.*
calcium channel blockers in, 114–115
CHD (coronary heart disease). See *Coronary artery disease (CAD).*
Children, cardiovascular risk factors in, 452–454
Chlorthalidone, for hypertension, 353t
vs. beta blockers, 81, 383t, 386
Cholesterol. See also *HDL cholesterol; LDL cholesterol; Lipid-lowering therapy.*
dietary, 200, 423, 424
in atherosclerotic plaque, 201, 210, 212
platelet aggregability and, 209
total serum, dietary fats and, 423
exercise training and, 287t
mortality rates and, 443, 449
smoking and, 362
vasodilatory dysfunction and, 209
Cholestyramine, after bypass graft, 201
cost effectiveness of, 336, 337
primary prevention trials of, 328, 328t, 332, 332t
secondary prevention trials of, 202t
vs. diet, 425–426, 426t
Claudication, vitamin E and, 419
Clinical trials. See also *Randomized clinical trials.*
administrative structure for, 31, *32*
early termination of, 31, 32–36, 33t, 35t, 39, 40
monitoring of. See *Data and Safety Monitoring Board (DSMB).*
phases of, 31–32
Clofibrate, primary prevention trials of, 328, 328t, 331, 429
secondary prevention trial of, 11, 33, 207
Clonidine, in atrial fibrillation, 241
Clopidogrel, vs. aspirin, 254
Cluster randomization, 18, 22
Cochrane Collaboration, 44
Cohort studies, 4–6
randomized clinical trials as, 6
Colestipol, cost effectiveness of, 291, 291t
primary prevention trial of, 328, 328t
Colestipol *(Continued)*
secondary prevention trials of, 202t, *212*
Collagen, coronary artery, 200, 201, 210, 211
estrogen and, 407
Community intervention trials, 436–440, 450–452
Concealed bypass tract, verapamil in, 233–234
Conditional power, 33
Confidence intervals, 12, 13
Confounding variables. See also *Bias(es).*
in meta-analysis, 48
in observational studies, 5–6, 7, 28
in randomized trials, 6–7, 10, 28
Congestive heart failure, 296–311. See also *Cardiomyopathy; Left ventricular dysfunction.*
ACE inhibitors in. See *ACE inhibitors, in congestive heart failure.*
after MI, fibrinolytic therapy in, 68
magnesium and, 121, 122
propranolol and, 85
ventricular dilation and, 96
aims of treatment for, 296–297, 297t
amiodarone in, 226–227
angiotensin II receptor antagonists in, 310–311
assessment of, in clinical trials, 297t, 297–298
atrial fibrillation in, stroke and, 261, 262
beta blocker(s) in. See *Beta blockers, in congestive heart failure.*
calcium channel blocker(s) in, 108, 113–114, 309–310
diltiazem as, 241, 309
definitions of, 297
digoxin in, 300, 303–306, *305*
diuretics in, 298
early trials in, 296
economic costs of, 296
evidence-based medicine and, 297
exercise capacity in, beta blockers and, 307t, 307–308
exercise training with, 278, 290–291, 291t, 389
in antihypertensive drug trials, 81, 82t
inotropic alternative agents in, 306
management of, principles of, 296–297
mechanisms of improvement in, 297–298, 298t
mortality in, ACE inhibitors and, 300–302, *301*
beta blockers and, 308–309, *309*
outcomes assessment and, 297, 298, 298t
rates of, 296
neurohormonal mechanisms in, *87*, 87–88, 88t, 96
calcium channel blockers and, 113
survival and, 298
neutral endopeptidase inhibitor in, 311
new treatments for, 310–311
nitrate tolerance in, 132
prevalence of, 296
Control group, 10
Coronary artery(ies). See also *Atherosclerosis.*
endothelial dysfunction in, 209
antioxidant vitamins and, 415, 520
smoking and, 362
remodeling of, 200, 209
thrombosis of, 245. See also *Thrombus formation.*
Coronary artery bypass graft (CABG), after stenting, 191, 191t, 254

Coronary artery bypass graft (CABG) *(Continued)*
antiplatelet therapy after, 249
arrhythmias after, *239*, 239–240
magnesium and, 123
emergency, 189
after angioplasty, 152, 156, 170, 188, 188t
in chronic angina, after angioplasty, 276, 277t
vs. angioplasty, 267, 268–277, *271, 274, 275*
for isolated LAD disease, 268, 269–270
recommendations for, 276–277
summary of trials with, 274–276, 276t
lifestyle intervention after, 318, 320
lipid-lowering therapy after, 201, 267
magnesium with, 123
new techniques for, 267
psychological depression after, 316
rehabilitation after, 279
repeat, 292
smoking cessation after, 369
vs. multiple risk factor intervention, 444
Coronary artery disease (CAD). See also *Atherosclerosis; Myocardial ischemia.*
left anterior descending (LAD), angioplasty in, 267, 268, 269–270
bypass graft in, 269–270
medical therapy in, 269–270
risk status in, 278, *279*
exercise testing and, 280, 280t
treatment goals in, 199–200
Coronary artery spasm, 199
calcium channel blockers for, 108, 109, 138
plaque disruption and, 444
smoking and, 362
unstable angina and, 109
Coronary atherectomy, directional, abciximab in, 173, 174, 177
eptifibatide in, 169
laser, 174
transluminal extraction catheter, 174
Coronary blood flow. See also *Myocardial perfusion.*
beta blockers and, 82
lifestyle modification and, 318
PTCA or thrombolysis and, 193–194, *194*
Coronary steal, nitrates causing, 132, 133
Coronary syndromes, acute. See also *Myocardial infarction (MI); Non-Q wave MI; Unstable angina.*
classification of, 55, 145
platelet activation in, 245
Coronary thrombosis, 245. See also *Thrombus formation.*
Costs. See *Economic costs.*
C-reactive protein, 246
Cyclo-oxygenase, aspirin and, 56, 57, 392
sulfinpyrazone and, 247

D

Dalteparin, with aspirin, for unstable CAD, 57
Data analysis, intention-to-treat analysis in, 11–12
Data and Safety Monitoring Board (DSMB), 31–41
communication by, 40
constitution of, 36–37
data input to, 32
data reports to, 38–39
Data and Safety Monitoring Board (DSMB) *(Continued)*
design modifications by, 32
documentation of, 40
early termination and, 32–36
communication of, 40
considerations for, 32–33, 33t
data reporting and, 39
external information and, 39
for treatment benefit, 33–34, 34t
for treatment harm, 34–35, 35t
with Physicians' Health Study, 35t, 35–36
external information for, 39–40
meetings of, 37–38
rationale for, 31–32
statistical analysis center and, 37
Databases, research using, 10
Defibrillators, implantable, 217, 227–228
Denial, psychological, 320, 321
Depression, after bypass graft, 316
beta blockers and, 77
prognosis and, 315, 316
psychosocial intervention and, 319, 320
Descriptive epidemiology, 4, 4t
Desulfohirudin, with t-PA, 147
Dexfenfluramine, 381t, 382
Diabetes, ACE inhibitors in, 103, 351, 356–357
angioplasty vs. bypass surgery in, 274, 276
antihypertensive trials in, 351, 352, 356–357
antiplatelet therapy in, 250
atrial fibrillation in, stroke and, 261
beta blockers in, 77
after MI, 85
in acute MI, 83
lipid-lowering therapy in, guidelines for, 337, 337t
in secondary prevention trials, 207, 208
vasodilatory dysfunction and, 209
weight loss and exercise programs in, 375, 384, 387
Diastolic dysfunction, primary, 297, 302
Dietary modification, 423–430. See also *Antioxidant vitamins; Lipid-lowering therapy; Multiple risk factor intervention; Weight loss.*
AHA guidelines for, 321, 435, 443
controlled trials of, 425–426, 426t, 427t
with exercise, 427t, 427–428
with fish and fish oil, 426–427, *427*, 428, 430
food groups and, 424t
high-carbohydrate vs. high-unsaturated fat in, 424, 424t
in multifactorial trials, 429–430
low-fat vs. high-unsaturated fat in, 425, 426t
nutrient factors in, 428–429
recommendations for, 430
school-based programs of, 453
serum lipoproteins and, 423–424, *425*
worksite program of, 455
Digoxin, after cardiac surgery, *239*, 239–240
in atrial fibrillation, acute, 235, 235t, 236
chronic, 240–241, 242
in heart failure, 300, 303–306, *305*
in supraventricular arrhythmias, 234
atrial fibrillation as, acute, 235, 235t, 236
chronic, 240–241, 242
Dihydropyridines, 106, *106–107*, 110, 112. See also specific agent.
Diltiazem, 106, *106*
adverse effects of, 115–116
atherosclerosis and, 110, 111, 112t
for hypertension, 114, 353t
in atrial fibrillation, 241
in heart failure, 241, 309
in myocardial infarction, 107–108, 109t
in stable angina, 112
in supraventricular arrhythmias, 233, 234, 241
in unstable angina, 109t, 110
vs. nitroglycerin, 140
Dipyridamole, stress testing with, 280
with aspirin, reinfarction and, 246–247, 248, *249*
Directional coronary atherectomy, 169, 173, 174, 177
Disopyramide, for atrial fibrillation, chronic, 238
postoperative, 239–240
Diuretics, in antihypertensive trials, 343, 344t, 346, 352, 353t, 356, 357, 429
vs. beta blocker(s), 79–81, 343, 347, 351, *351*, 353t
atenolol as, 383t, 386
meta-analysis of, 81, 82t
in congestive heart failure, 298
in multiple risk factor trials, 435, 436
adverse effects of, 443
nitrate tolerance and, 132
Dobutamine, in heart failure, 306
stress testing with, 280
Double blind trials, 10–11
Doxazosin, for hypertension, 353t, 383t, 386
DSMB. See *Data and Safety Monitoring Board (DSMB).*

E

Echocardiography, exercise, 280
Economic costs, cost effectiveness of interventions and, 291t, 291–292
for cholesterol reduction, 334–337, 335t
of clinical trials, 9
factorial designs and, 14
of health care, worksite prevention and, 455
of heart failure, 296
EDRF (endothelium-derived relaxing factor). See *Nitric oxide.*
Efegatran, 146
in MI, 148, 162
Effect size, meta-analysis and, 44
Effectiveness trials, 20–21
Efficacy trials, 20–21
Efficiency, relative, 9
Elastin, coronary artery, 200, 201
Elderly patients, blood pressure reduction in, 347, 349t
calcium channel blockers in, 115–116
cholesterol reduction in, 333–334, 334t
exercise training in, 290
smoking cessation in, 366–367
Electrocardiography (ECG), in exercise testing, 280, 280t
Eminase (anistreplase), aspirin or anticoagulation after, 253
Enalapril, for hypertension, 353t, 383t, 386
in acute MI, 35, 97, *100*, 100–101, 101t
in heart failure, *299*, 300–301, *301*
left ventricular dysfunction and, 302
Encainide, after MI, 34, 35t, 39, *218*, 218–220
Endothelin-1, estrogen and, 406
Endothelium-derived relaxing factor (EDRF). See *Nitric oxide.*

Enoxaparin, in unstable CAD, 57, 162
Enoximone, in heart failure, 306
Epidemiologic studies. See also *Clinical trials; Observational studies.*
cause-effect relationships and, 4, 5–6, 7
design strategies for, 4, 4t
vs. basic research, 3, 4
Epinephrine, in MI, 96
in myocardial infarction, ACE inhibitors and, 97
smoking and, 361
Eptifibatide (Integrelin), 168–169
in canine model, 161
in coronary atherectomy, 169
in MI, 179, 180, 181
in non–Q wave MI, 177
in percutaneous coronary intervention, 169, 170, 175–176, 178t, 180
in unstable angina, 177, 180
Esmolol, in supraventricular arrhythmias, 232
Estrogen, hemodynamic and vascular effects of, 209, 405–407
Estrogen receptors, vasoreactivity and, 406
Estrogen therapy, in men, with prior MI, 207
in women. See *Hormone replacement therapy (HRT).*
Ethical issues. See also *Clinical trials, early termination of.*
data monitoring and, 31
randomization and, 27
Ethyl biscoumacetate, after MI, 252
Exercise, angina induced by, 280, 280t
cardiovascular disease risk and, 292, 375
clinical trials of, for cardiac rehabilitation, 285–287, 286t, *286,* 287t, 288t, 291–292, 388–389
in cardiovascular disease, 387t, 387–388
in healthy people, 376, 377t, 378–381
in people with risk factors, 382, 383t, 384–385
limitations of, 375–376
in angina, 204, 205, 389
in atrial fibrillation, 240–241
in CAD, vasoconstriction caused by, 209
in heart failure, 87, 88
in hypertension prevention trials, 385–387
in lifestyle modification programs, 318, 320, 322, 427t, 427–428
in myocardial ischemia, 317, 318
multiple short periods of, 379
school-based programs of, 454
Exercise testing, early postinfarction, 279–280
prognostic variables in, 280, 280t
symptom-limited, 279
Exercise training, 278–292
assessment for, 279–280
cardiac transplantation and, 291
clinical trials of, 285–287, 286t, *286,* 287t, 288t, 291–292, 388–389
cost effectiveness of, 291t, 291–292
eligibility for, 278, *279*
in congestive heart failure, 278, 290–291, 291t, 389
in elderly patients, 290
in women, 290, 290t
inpatient and early convalescent, 278–279, 279t
meta-analyses of, 286, 287, 287t, *288*
pathophysiologic outcomes in, 287–288, *289*
physiologic alterations in, 288–289, *289*
Exercise training *(Continued)*
program for, 280–285
arm exercises in, 283–284, *283–284*
duration in, 282–283, 283t
frequency in, 281, *283*
intensity in, 281–282, 282t
prescription form for, 281, *282*
resistance training in, 284–285, 285t
session format in, 280–281, *281*
safety of, 288–290, 289t, *289,* 290t
underutilization of, 278

F

Factor VII, menopause and, 404, 405
smoking and, 362
warfarin and, 246
Factor Xa, heparin and, 56
Factorial designs, 14–15, 15t
False-positive results, 33
Family of patient, adjustment by, 320, 321
Fats, dietary, 423–425, 424t, *425*
omega-3 fatty acids as, 426–427, *427,* 428
Felodipine, 106, *107*
for hypertension, 114t, 353t
in heart failure, 309
Fenfluramine, 381, 381t, 382
Fiber, dietary, 426–427, *427,* 429
Fibrin, in thrombus formation, 126, 166
Fibrinogen, elevated, CAD and, 209, 404
smoking and, 362
hormone replacement therapy and, 400, 404–405
platelet binding of, 126, 166
Fibrinolytic capacity, impaired, 209
aspirin and, 246
menopause and, 405
smoking and, 362
Fibrinolytic (thrombolytic) therapy, 65–73. See also *r-PA (recombinant plasminogen activator, reteplase); Streptokinase (SK); t-PA (tissue-type plasminogen activator, alteplase).*
angioplasty after, 186t, 186–187
aspirin vs. anticoagulant after, 253
aspirin with, *58,* 58–59, 60t, 61, 245
beta blockers with, 83–84, 84t
comparison of regimens for, with APSAC, 69, 72
with r-PA, 69, 71, 72
with streptokinase vs. t-PA, 68–69, 70t, *71,* 71–72
coronary blood flow after, 193–194, *194*
direct antithrombins with, 146–148, *147*
early hazard of, 65, 66, 66t, 67, 68
failed, rescue angioplasty and, 191–193
GPIIb/IIIa antagonists with, 167, 179–180, 181
heparin with, 59, 60t, 61, 62
historical background of, 185
in elderly patients, 68, *68,* 69, 73
in very-high-risk patients, 68
in women, underuse of, 73
magnesium with, 121, 124, 126–128
new agents for, 194
platelet aggregation in, 59, 126–127
recommendations for, 73
reinfarction risk with, 59
smoking and, 369–371
underutilization of, 73, 447
vs. angioplasty, *72,* 72–73, 188–190, 189t
vs. no fibrinolytic therapy, 65–68, *66–68*
Fibrinopeptide A, during angioplasty, 153
Fish oil, 426–427, *427,* 428, 430
Fixed-effects model, 45, 46, 47, 48
Flecainide, after MI, 34, 35t, 39, *218,* 218–220
in supraventricular arrhythmia(s), 233, 234
atrial fibrillation as, acute, 235t, 235–236
chronic, 238–239
for prevention, 236–237
Flosequinan, in heart failure, 34–35, 306
Fluvastatin, 202t
Foam cells, 210, 211, 212, 213, 415
Folic acid, 423, 429
Follow-up, in clinical trials, 13
Food labeling, 456
Fosinopril, for hypertension, 353t
Free radicals, atherogenesis and, 415, 416
magnesium and, 120, 126
reperfusion injury and, 126

G

Gemfibrozil, 328, 328t, 332, 332t
Glyceryl trinitrate, in acute MI, 134–135
Glycoprotein IIb/IIIa antagonists, 167–170. See also specific agent.
comparative efficacies of, 180–181
hemorrhage risk with, 167
in coronary atherectomy, 169
in myocardial infarction, 167, 179–180, 181
in non–Q wave MI, 177
in percutaneous coronary intervention, 168, 169, 170–177, *172–173, 175,* 178t, 180–181
in thrombolytic therapy, 167, 179–180, 181
in unstable angina, 177–179, 180, 181
thienopyridines as, 254
vitronectin receptors and, 167, 168, 181
with hirudin, in canine model, 160–161
Glycoprotein IIb/IIIa receptors, 153, 166–167
magnesium and, 126, 127
nitrates and, 131
Golden hour, for fibrinolytic therapy, 67, 71
Greenberg Report, 31, *32*
Group psychotherapy, 315, 318, 319, 322
Group randomization, 18, 22
Group sequential procedure, 33
Guanethidine, for hypertension, 77
Guanylate cyclase, nitrates and, 131, *132,* 140

H

HDL cholesterol, arterial benefit and, 201, 202
beta blockers and, 77
coronary disease risk and, 423–424
dietary changes and, 423, 424, *425,* 426, 426t, 427
exercise and, in cardiac rehabilitation, 283, 287t
in healthy people, 376, 377t, 378–381
hormone replacement therapy and, 399–404, 400t, 401t, *401, 403*
obesity and, 375
pravastatin monotherapy and, 207
smoking and, 362
vasodilatory dysfunction and, 209
Health-care costs, worksite prevention and, 455
Health-care system, prevention and, 449–450
Heart. See also *Cardiac* entries.

Heart *(Continued)*
failure of. See *Congestive heart failure.*
Heart rate, beta blockers and, 76, 81, 86
control of, in supraventricular arrhythmias, 232
atrial fibrillation as, 240–242
in heart failure, 87, *87*
smoking and, 361
Heparin, after stent placement, 254
after thrombolysis, 253
disadvantages of, 145
during angioplasty, complications and, 156, *156*, 159
disadvantages of, 151–152, 153–155
thrombin generation and, 153, 159
vs. direct antithrombins, 156–158, *157–158*, 160–161
in acute MI, 58, 59, 59t, 60t, 61, 62
assessment of trials with, 55
vs. direct antithrombins, *147*, 147–148
in fibrinolytic therapy, 59, 60t, 61, 62
in unstable CAD, 55, 56–57, 62
low-molecular-weight preparations of, 56
mechanism of action of, 146, *146*, 161–162, *161–162*
nitroglycerin interaction with, 140
thrombocytopenia caused by, 145, 160, 163
vs. direct antithrombins, during angioplasty, 156–158, *157–158*, 160–161
in ST-segment MI, *147*, 147–148
in unstable angina/non–Q wave MI, 148, 149, *149*
phase III trials of, 149–151, 150t, *151–153*, 154t, 155t
thrombin generation and, 159, 161
High-density-lipoprotein cholesterol. See *HDL cholesterol.*
High-risk strategy, for prevention, 447–449, 448t
Hirudin, 146
during angioplasty, 156–157, *157*, 159, 160, 162
balloon injury and, 154–155
mechanism of action of, 146, *146*, 161–162, *161–162*
phase II trials of, 146–149, *147*, *149*
phase III trials of, 149–151, 150t, *151–153*, 154t, 155t, 162
thrombin generation and, 159, 161
with GPIIb/IIIa antagonist, 161
Hirulog. See *Bivalirudin (Hirulog).*
Historical controls, 10
HMG-CoA (hydroxymethylglutaryl–coenzyme A) reductase inhibitors, 201, 328, 423. See also *Statins.*
Homocysteine, atherosclerosis and, 43
coronary heart disease and, 429
estrogen and, 407
Hormone replacement therapy (HRT), 399–410
CHD and, epidemiology of, 407t, 407–409, 408t, *409*
HDL/LDL effects of, 399–404, 400t, 401t, *401*, *403*
hemodynamic and vascular effects of, 209, 405–407
hemostatic effects of, 404–405
limitations of existing data on, 399
ongoing trials of, 409
Hydralazine, in heart failure, 301
Hydrochlorothiazide, for hypertension, 343, 353t
vs. beta blockers, 80, 81
with beta blockers, 78t, 79
Hydrochlorothiazide *(Continued)*
in carotid atherosclerosis, 111–112
Hydrogenated vegetable oils, 424–425
Hypercholesterolemia. See also *Cholesterol.*
platelet aggregability in, 209
vasodilatory dysfunction in, 209
Hypertension. See also *Antihypertensive drug trials; Blood pressure.*
as risk factor, for cardiovascular disease, 341–342
for renal disease, 342
atherosclerosis and, 209
criteria for, 341
diastolic dysfunction and, 297
dietary modification and, 427, 429
in atrial fibrillation, stroke and, 261, 262
in multiple risk factor intervention trials, 434, 435, 436
malignant, 342
obesity and, 375
prevalence of, 341
primary prevention of, 342
recommended first-line agents for, 77, 81
smoking and, 362
stage classification of, 342
systolic vs. diastolic, 341
weight loss trial in, 385–387
Hypomagnesemia, during cardiopulmonary bypass, 122–123
Hypotension, ACE inhibitors causing, 98, 103
captopril as, 101, 102
enalapril as, 100–101
lisinopril as, 101
beta blockers and, 86
exertional, 280, 280t
magnesium and, 122
nitrates causing, 132, 133, 135

I

Ibopamine, in heart failure, 305
Ilial bypass, for cholesterol lowering, 202t, 207
Indapamide, for hypertension, 353t
Indication bias, 28
Infarct expansion, 96
Inogatran, 146
in unstable angina/non–Q wave MI, 149, 162
Inotropic agents, alternative, 306
Insulin resistance, coronary artery disease and, 292
hormone replacement therapy and, 407
Integrelin. See *Eptifibatide (Integrelin).*
Integrin receptors, 166–167
Intention-to-treat analysis, 11–12, 25
Intervention studies. See *Randomized clinical trials.*
Intrinsic sympathomimetic activity (ISA), 76, 76t, 77, 85–86
Ischemia. See *Myocardial ischemia.*
Ischemic injury. See also *Reperfusion injury.*
calcium channel blockers and, 114
estrogen and, 407
Ischemic syndromes, acute. See also *Myocardial infarction (MI); Non–Q wave MI; Unstable angina.*
classification of, 55, 145
platelet activation in, 245
Isosorbide dinitrate (ISDN), 131
in heart failure, vs. enalapril, 301
mechanism of action of, *132*
tolerance with, 132
Isosorbide mononitrate, in acute MI, 133, 135
Isosorbide mononitrate *(Continued)*
vs. magnesium, 122
Isradipine, 106
for hypertension, 351, 353t
in carotid atherosclerosis, 111–112, 112t

K

Kininase, 95

L

Labetalol, in atrial fibrillation, 240
in heart failure, 307t
Lacidipine, for hypertension, 353t
LAD (left anterior descending) coronary artery disease, angioplasty in, 267, 268, 269–270
bypass graft in, 269–270
medical therapy in, 269–270
Lamifiban, 169–170
in MI, with thrombolytic therapy, 179, 180, 181
in non–Q wave MI, 179
in unstable angina, 170, 179, 180
Laser atherectomy, 174
LDL (low-density lipoprotein). See also *Lipoprotein(a).*
atherogenicity of, 201
in vessel wall, 209–210, 211
oxidation of, atherogenesis and, 415, 416
estrogen and, 406
LDL cholesterol, arterial benefit and, 201, 202
coronary disease risk and, 327, 423
dietary changes and, 423, 424, *425*, 426, 426t
fiber as, 429
exercise training and, 287t
hormone replacement therapy and, 399–404, 400t, 401t, *401*, *403*
lifestyle intervention and, 318
smoking and, 362
statin(s) and, 330
lovastatin as, 329
pravastatin as, 207–208
treatment goal for, 337t, 337–338
vasodilatory dysfunction and, 209
Left anterior descending (LAD) coronary artery disease, angioplasty in, 267, 268, 269–270
bypass graft in, 269–270
medical therapy in, 269–270
Left ventricular dysfunction. See also *Congestive heart failure.*
ACE inhibitors and, after MI, 97t, 97–98, 99–100, 102–103, 302–303, *303–304*
in heart failure, 301
asymptomatic, 297
after MI, 298, 302, *303*
in heart failure, 301
progression of, 87
beta blocker(s) and, 307, 307t
carvedilol as, 308, *308*
calcium channel blockers and, 108
in aortic regurgitation, 114
digoxin and, 304
exercise testing and, 280
in heart failure, 297, 298, 298t, 301
mechanisms of, 87, 96
Left ventricular hypertrophy, diuretics and, 80
vs. congestive heart failure, 297
Lidoflazine, in cardiac arrest, 115
in myocardial infarction, 107
in stable angina, 112

Lifestyle intervention, 315–316, 316t. See also *Multiple risk factor intervention.*
clinical trials of, 316–320, 317t
enrollment in, timing of, 321
patient choices in, 321–322
psychological issues in, 315–316, 320–321
Linsidomine, in acute MI, 136
Lipid profiles, exercise training and, 285, 286, 287t
in women, 290
Lipid-lowering therapy. See also *Dietary modification.*
for primary prevention, 327–338
coronary heart disease and, 327–329, 328t, 338, 423
cost effectiveness of, 334–337, 335t
guidelines for, 337t, 337–338
in elderly, 333–334, 334t
in women, 334t, 334–336
nonvascular mortality and, 330–332, 332t, 338
stroke and, 329–330, 338
total mortality and, 332–333, 338
for secondary prevention, 199–213
after revascularization, 201, 267
age and, 334t
arteriographic trials of, 201–202, *204–205,* 205, 212, *212,* 440–442
descriptions of, 202t
outcomes of, 203t
pending, 208
clinical endpoint trials of, 205, 206t, 207–208
cost effectiveness of, 335t, 335–337
in angina, 204–205
in women, 202, 207, 208, 334t
lifestyle intervention as, 318
mechanisms of benefit in, 199–201, 208–213
Lipoprotein. See *HDL cholesterol; LDL (low-density lipoprotein); LDL cholesterol; VLDL (very-low-density lipoprotein).*
Lipoprotein(a), CAD and, 201, 209–210
hormone replacement therapy and, 400, 402–403, 404t
trans-fatty acids and, 424
Lisinopril, in acute MI, GISSI-3 trial of, 97t, 98, *100,* 101, 101t, 134–135
in antihypertensive drug trials, 353t
Losartan, for hypertension, 353t
in heart failure, 310–311
Lovastatin, after bypass graft, 201
cost effectiveness of, 291, 291t, 336, 337
in angina, 205, 209
primary prevention trial of, 328t, 329, 335t
secondary prevention trials of, 202t, 208, *212,* 335t
Lp(a), CAD and, 201, 209–210
hormone replacement therapy and, 400, 402–403, 404t
trans-fatty acids and, 424
Luindione, after MI, 252
Lung disease, beta blockers in, 77
passive smoking and, 363

M

Macrophages, foam cells as, 210, 211, 212, 213
Magnesium, cardiovascular pharmacology of, 119–120
during cardiopulmonary bypass, 122–123
in acute MI, 119–128
conflicting evidence with, 119, 123–124
Magnesium *(Continued)*
current status of, 128
hypothesis-testing trials of, 119, 121–122, *122*
platelet function and, 120, *126–127,* 126–128
reperfusion injury and, 124–126, 125t, 127, 128
time dependency of, 124–126, 127, *127*
unpowered trials of, 119, 120–121, *121,* 122
in thrombolytic therapy, 121, 124, 126–128
platelet function and, 120, *126–127,* 126–128
Mediterranean diet, 424t, 426, 428t, 430
MET (metabolic equivalent), 278
Meta-analysis, 43–50
as hypothesis-generating technique, 120
benefits of, 44
biases in, 28–29, 49–50
clinical application of, 50
heterogeneity in, 45, 48, 50
historical background of, 44
information resources on, 43, 44
methodologic guidelines for, 43, 47–48
models used in, 45–47
of observational studies, 44, 47
of ongoing trials, 39–40
publication bias and, 49–50
quality of studies in, 48–49
subgroup analysis and, 26, 29, 44, 47–48
Metabolic equivalent (MET), 278
Methionine, for nitrate tolerance, 132
Methodology of trials. See *Bias(es); Clinical trials; Meta-analysis; Randomized clinical trials.*
Methyldopa, for hypertension, 77
Metoprolol, after MI, 85, 86
vs. amiodarone, 224
for hypertension, 79, 353t
vs. diuretics, 80, 81
in acute MI, 82–83, 84t
in heart failure, 88, 90t, 91, 307t
hemodynamic effects of, acute, *90*
in dilated cardiomyopathy, 88, 89t, 306, 308
mortality reduction and, 309
in stable angina, vs. verapamil, 112
with thrombolytic therapy, 83–84, 84t
MI. See *Myocardial infarction (MI).*
Milrinone, in heart failure, 34, 304, 306
Mitral stenosis, stroke prevention in, 257
MK-383. See *Tirofiban (Aggrastat).*
Moduretic, for hypertension, 353t
Molsidomine, in acute MI, 136, *137*
Monoclonal antibodies. See *Abciximab (ReoPro).*
Monounsaturated fatty acids, 423, 424
Moricizine, after MI, 218, 219, *219,* 220
Multiple risk factor intervention, 432–444. See also *Lifestyle intervention.*
angiographic trials of, 440–442
community trials of, 436–440
complexity of, 433
in children and adolescents, 454
modifiable risk factors and, 433–434
randomized controlled trials of, 429–430, 434–436
rationale for, 432–433
summary of trial results in, 442–444
Myocardial contractility, beta blockers and, 88
calcium channel blockers and, 106
Myocardial infarction (MI), ACE inhibitors in. See *ACE inhibitors, in myocardial infarction.*
Myocardial infarction (MI) *(Continued)*
acute, ACE inhibitors in, 99, *100,* 100–103, 101t, 302–303
after angioplasty, 156, 170, 174–175
angioplasty in, 186t, 186–190, 188t, 189t
after failed thrombolysis, 191–193
anticoagulants in, 251
antiplatelet trials in, overview of, *248*
aspirin in, 55, *58,* 58–59, 59t, 60t, 61–62, 392–393
beta blockers in, 81–84, *83*
direct antithrombins in, with thrombolysis, 146–148, *147*
exercise after, 278–280, 279t, 280t
exertion-related, 288–289, 289t
fibrinolytic therapy in. See *Fibrinolytic (thrombolytic) therapy.*
GPIIb/IIIa antagonists in, with thrombolysis, 167, 179–180, 181
heparin in, 58, 59, 59t, 60t, 61, 62
assessment of trials with, 55
vs. direct antithrombins, *147,* 147–148
Lp(a) in, 209
magnesium in. See *Magnesium, in acute MI.*
nitrates in, 131, 133–138, *134, 137,* 141–142
pathophysiology of, 245
plaque disruption and, 57–58, 210, *211,* 245, 315
platelet activation in, 245
psychological triggers of, 316
smoking and, 361
stenting in, 191, 191t
anticoagulant therapy after, 251–252
recommendations for, 254–255
vs. aspirin, 252–253
with aspirin, 253–254
antioxidant vitamins and, 419
arrhythmias after. See *Antiarrhythmic agent(s), after MI.*
aspirin after, 392
cost effectiveness of, 291, 291t
dosage of, 250, 254
recommendation for, 250–251
trials of, 246–251, *248–249*
underutilization of, 62, 251
vs. anticoagulants, 252–253
with ACE inhibitors, 102
with anticoagulants, 253–254
with dipyridamole, 246–247, 248
calcium channel blockers in, 106–108, 109t
case management after, 450
C-reactive protein and, 246
dietary modification after, 426–427, *427,* 428, 428t
exercise after. See *Exercise training.*
implantable defibrillators after, 227–228
lifestyle modification after, 318, 319, 320
neurohormones and, 96–97
non-Q wave. See *Non-Q wave MI.*
recurrent, ACE inhibitors and, 100, 102, 302
antiplatelet agents and, 245, 246–251, *248–249,* 392
beta blockers and, 84, 85, 86
calcium channel blockers and, 107–108
exercise training and, 389
fibrinolytic therapy causing, 59
lifestyle modification and, 318, 319
prevention of, 245
risk factors for, 217, 280
vitamin E and, 421

Myocardial infarction (MI) *(Continued)*
  risk of, hormone replacement therapy and, 407
    lipid-lowering therapy and, 211, *212*
    with calcium channel blockers, 351
  smoking and, 362, 363
    cessation and, 366, 368–370, 370t
    prognosis and, 369–370, 370t
  ventricular remodeling after, 96
    ACE inhibitors and, 96, 97t, 97–98, 103
    carvedilol and, 86–87
    nitrates and, 133, 134
Myocardial ischemia, 199. See also *Acute coronary syndromes; Angina pectoris; Coronary artery disease (CAD).*
  beta blockers and, 82
  exercise testing and, 280
  exercise training and, 287–288
  hormone replacement therapy and, 407
  lipid-lowering therapy and, 204–205
  magnesium and, 120, 124–126, 125t, 127, 128
  nitrates and, 132, 133, 139
  platelet activation in, 245
  psychosocial intervention and, 318–319
  silent, 319
  smoking and, 361, 362
Myocardial perfusion. See also *Coronary blood flow.*
  imaging of, 205
  multiple risk factor intervention and, 440, 441, 444
  nitrates and, 131–132, 133
  smoking and, 362
Myocyte dysfunction, 87, *87*
  beta blockers and, 88

N

NAC (*N*-acetylcysteine), for nitrate tolerance, 132, *132*
  with nitroglycerin, in acute MI, 141
    in unstable angina, 140–141
Nadolol, in atrial fibrillation, 240
Naughton treadmill protocol, 279–280
Nebivolol, in heart failure, 307, 307t
Neuroendocrine system, in heart failure, *87*, 87–88, 88t, 96
    calcium channel blockers and, 113
    survival and, 298
  in myocardial infarction, 96
    ACE inhibitors and, 96–97
Neutral endopeptidase inhibitor, 311
Nevibolol, in heart failure, 88
Niacin (nicotinic acid), in secondary prevention trials, 202t, 207, 208, *212*
  vs. dietary modification, 425
Nicardipine, 106, *107*
  atherosclerosis and, 110–111, 112t
  for hypertension, 353t
  in stable angina, 112
Nicotine, cardiovascular disease and, 361, 362
Nicotinic acid. See *Niacin (nicotinic acid).*
Nicoumalone, after MI, 252
Nifedipine, 106, *106–107*
  adverse effects of, 115–116
  atherosclerosis and, 110, 112, 112t
  for hypertension, 114, 114t, 351, 353t
  in heart failure, 113–114, 309
  in myocardial infarction, 107, 109t
  in stable angina, 112, 113
  in unstable angina, 109t, 109–110
Nimodipine, 106, *107*
  cerebrovascular trials of, 114–115
Nisoldipine, 106, *107*
Nisoldipine *(Continued)*
  for hypertension, 353t
  in heart failure, 309
  in stable angina, 112–113
Nitrates, 131–143
  antiplatelet activity of, 131
  hemodynamic effects of, 131–132
  historical background of, 131
  in acute MI, 133–138
    ACE inhibitors with, 134–135, 136, *136–137*, 138, 141, 142
    adverse effects of, 133
    large trials of, 134–136, *136–137*, 138
    N-acetylcysteine with, 141
    rationale for, 131, 133
    recommendations for, 138, 141–142
    smaller trials of, 133–134, *134*, 136, *136–137*, 138
  in chronic angina, tolerance with, 141
    vs. angioplasty, 267–268, 268t
  in unstable angina, 131, 138–141
    heparin interaction with, 140
    N-acetylcysteine with, 140–141
    nitroglycerin vs. nitroprusside as, 140
    observational studies of, 138–139, 139t
    recommendations for, 142
    vs. calcium channel blockers, 140
  mechanisms of action of, 131–132, *132*
  tolerance with, 132, *132*, 141
  withdrawal of, rebound ischemia in, 139
Nitrendipine, 106, *107*
  for hypertension, 114, 353t, 356
Nitric oxide, estrogen and, 406, 407
  in hypercholesterolemia, 209
  nitrates and, 131, 132, *132*
  smoking and, 362
  vasodilation and, 131–132, *132*, 209, 406
Nitroglycerin (NTG), hemodynamic effects of, 131–132
  in acute MI, 133–135, *134*
  in unstable angina, heparin interaction with, 140
    observational studies of, 138–139, 139t
    vs. calcium channel blockers, 140
    vs. nitroprusside, 140
    with *N*-acetylcysteine, 140–141
  mechanism of action of, 131, *132*
  tolerance with, 132, 141
  with rt-PA, 133
Nitroprusside, disadvantages of, 132
  in acute MI, 133, *134*
  in unstable angina, 140
Noncompliance, intention-to-treat analysis and, 11, 25
  reduction of, 14
  statistical power and, 13–14
Non–Q wave MI. See also *Unstable coronary artery disease.*
  antiarrhythmic drugs after, 220, 221
  diagnostic features of, 55
  diltiazem in, 107
  direct antithrombins in, 148–149, *149*
  exercise-induced ST depression in, 280, 280t
  lamifiban in, 179
  pathophysiology of, 55, 145
  tirofiban in, 177–178
Nonrandomized study designs, 25, 28
Norepinephrine, beta blockers and, 76
  in heart failure, 87, 88
  in myocardial infarction, 96
    ACE inhibitors and, 96, 97
  smoking and, 361
NTG. See *Nitroglycerin (NTG).*
Nutrition. See *Antioxidant vitamins; Dietary modification.*
Nutrition counseling, 449–450
Nutrition labeling, 456

O

Obesity, 375. See also *Weight loss.*
Observational studies, 4–7
  biases in, 28
  meta-analysis of, 44, 47
Odds ratios, 47
Open artery hypothesis, 185, 192
Oral contraceptives, smoking and, 363
Outcomes research, 28
Overview analysis. See *Meta-analysis.*
Oxford database in perinatal medicine, 44, 49
Oxprenolol, for hypertension, 80

P

Palmaz-Schatz coronary artery stent, 254
Passive smoking, 363
PCI (percutaneous coronary intervention). See *Angioplasty, percutaneous transluminal coronary; Atherectomy; Stenting, intracoronary.*
PDGF (platelet-derived growth factor), smoking and, 362
Pentaerythritol tetranitrate, in acute MI, 133
Percutaneous transluminal coronary angioplasty. See *Angioplasty, percutaneous transluminal coronary.*
Perindopril, for hypertension, 353t
Peripheral vascular disease, antiplatelet therapy in, 249, 392
  C-reactive protein and, 246
  smoking and, 361–362
Persantine. See *Dipyridamole.*
Phase I trials, 31, 32
Phase II trials, 31, 32
Phase III trials, 31–32. See also *Data and Safety Monitoring Board (DSMB).*
Phase IV trials, 32
Phenindione, after MI, 252
Phenprocoumon, after MI, 251, 252
    with aspirin, 247
  after stent placement, 254
  in atrial fibrillation, 261
Phentermine, 381, 381t
Phosphodiesterase inhibitors, 306
Physical activity, 375. See also *Exercise.*
Physicians' Health Study, early termination of, 35t, 35–36, 40
Pimobendan, in heart failure, 306
Pindolol, for hypertension, 79, 343
  in atrial fibrillation, chronic, 240–241
Pirmenol, in atrial fibrillation, acute, 235, 235t
Plaque. See *Atherosclerosis.*
Plasminogen activator inhibitor–1, in menopause, 404, 405
  myocardial infarction risk and, 246
  nitroglycerin and, 133
  thrombogenesis and, 209
Plasminogen activators. See *r-PA (recombinant plasminogen activator, reteplase); t-PA (tissue-type plasminogen activator, alteplase); Urokinase-type plasminogen activator.*
Platelet-derived growth factor (PDGF), smoking and, 362
Platelets. See also *Antiplatelet agent(s); Thrombocytopenia.*
  activation of, 126, 153
    by exercise, 288–289

Platelets *(Continued)*
during angioplasty, 153
GPIIb/IIIa receptor and, 153, 166
in acute MI, 245
smoking and, 362
adhesion of, 166, 167
hormone replacement therapy and, 405
in thrombus formation, 126, 145, 166–167
hypercholesterolemia and, 209
inhibition of, by *N*-acetylcysteine, 140
by aspirin, 56, 392
by estrogens, 405
by magnesium, 120, *126–127,* 126–128
by nitrates, 131
Policy Advisory Board, 31, *32*
Polyunsaturated fatty acids, 423, 424, 426
Population-based intervention, 447–449, 448t, *448*
Potassium channel blockers, for supraventricular arrhythmias, 220–222, *221–222*
in heart failure, 310
Potsdam Consultation, 43, 47
Power of trials. See *Statistical power.*
Practolol, after MI, 369
Prasozin, in heart failure, 301
Pravastatin, primary prevention trial of, 328t, 328–329
secondary prevention trials of, 207–208, 423
in elderly, 333, 334t
vs. dietary modification, 425
Precision, in clinical trials, 9, 9t, 12
Preintervention-to-postintervention design, 18
Premature ventricular contractions (PVCs), exercise-induced, 280
Prevention paradox, 448, 448t
Prevention strategy(ies), 447–456
community intervention as, 436–440, 450–452
health-care delivery and, 449–450
politics of, 455–456
population-based vs. high-risk, 447–449, 448t, *448*
real-world use of, 447
school intervention as, 438, 452–454
worksite intervention as, 438, 454–455
Prevention trials, 17–22
analysis of results in, 21–22
design of, 17–19
duration of, 20–21
eligibility criteria for, 20
management of, 21
noncompliance in, 14
of efficacy vs. effectiveness, 20–21
outcomes measured in, 19
recruitment for, 19–20
settings of, 19–20
types of, 17
Primary prevention, definitions of, 17, 434
Primordial prevention, definition of, 17
Prinzmetal's angina, magnesium in, 120
Proarrhythmia, drug-induced, 220, 222
Probucol, 429
Procainamide, in atrial fibrillation, after cardiac surgery, 239
for acute termination, 235, 235t
Progestins, in postmenopausal hormone replacement, 399, 400, 401–402, 405, 408
vasoreactivity and, 406
Propafenone, after cardiac surgery, for arrhythmia prevention, 240
in atrial fibrillation, chronic, 238
for acute termination, 235t, 235–236
for prevention, 237–238

Propafenone *(Continued)*
in supraventricular arrhythmia(s), for acute termination, 233
of atrial fibrillation, 235t, 235–236
for long-term suppression, 234
of atrial fibrillation, 238
for prevention, of atrial fibrillation, 237–238
Propranolol, after cardiac surgery, for arrhythmia prevention, 239
after MI, BHAT trial of, 84t, 84–85, *85*
early termination of, 33–34, 34t, 39, 40
for hypertension, 80, 436
in atrial fibrillation, chronic, 241
in heart failure, after MI, 85
hemodynamic effects of, *90*
in supraventricular arrhythmia(s), atrial fibrillation as, 241
for heart rate control, 232
for long-term suppression, 234
in unstable angina, 109t, 110
vs. carvedilol, in animal studies, 86
Prostacyclin, aspirin and, 250, 254
estrogens and, 405
Prostatic hypertrophy, α_1-receptor blockers with, 351
Providers, health care, prevention and, 447, 449–450
Psychological adjustment to CHD, 320–322
Psychosocial factors, 315–322. See *Lifestyle intervention.*
Psychotherapy, group, 315, 318, 319, 322
individual, 319
PTCA. See *Angioplasty, percutaneous transluminal coronary.*
Publication bias, 29, 49–50
Pulmonary artery wedge pressure, captopril and, 98
Pulmonary congestion, in heart failure, 297
diuretics and, 298
Pulmonary embolism, hormone replacement therapy and, 408
PVCs (premature ventricular contractions), exercise-induced, 280

Q

Quasi-experimental design, 18
Quinapril, for hypertension, 353t
Quinidine, in atrial fibrillation, after cardiac surgery, 240
chronic, 238
paroxysmal, for acute termination, 235t, 236
for prevention, 236–237, 238

R

Radiofrequency ablation, for supraventricular tachycardias, 231–232, 234, 242
Raloxifene, 409
Ramipril, after acute MI, *99*, 99t, 100
in heart failure, 302, *304*
for hypertension, 353t
Random errors, in meta-analyses, 29
moderate treatment effects and, 25t, 26–27, 28–29
sample size and, 9
Random-effects model, 45, 46, 47, 48
Randomization, biases and, 25
by groups, 18, 22
need for, 9–11
uncertainty principle and, 27–28
Randomized clinical trials, 6–7. See also *Bias(es); Clinical trials; Meta-analysis.*
aim of, 9

Randomized clinical trials *(Continued)*
costs of, 9, 14
methodology of, 9–15
factorial designs in, 14–15, 15t
follow-up duration in, 13
intention-to-treat analysis in, 11–12, 25
noncompliance in, 11, 13–14
randomization in, 9–11, 18, 22, 25, 27–28
sample size in, *12,* 12–13
three principles in, 9, 9t
of moderate treatment effects, 24–29
biases in, 25t, 25–26, 28–29
random errors in, 25t, 26–27, 28–29
successful examples of, 29
vs. outcomes research, 28
simplicity as virtue in, 27
vs. observational studies, 6–7
Reentrant supraventricular tachycardia, magnesium and, 120
Reentry, infarct, 217
Regression dilution bias, 327
Rehabilitation. See also *Exercise training.*
multifactorial, 278, 286, 287, 291–292, 320, 388–389
Reinfarction. See *Myocardial infarction (MI), recurrent.*
Relative efficiency, 9
Relative risk, 5–6
Relaxation techniques, 204, 317, 317t, 318, 319, 320
Renal disease, hypertension and, 352, 356
in diabetes, ACE inhibitors in, 298
Renin-angiotensin-aldosterone system, 95
ACE inhibitors and, 95–96, 97
angiotensin II receptor antagonists and, 310–311
beta blockers and, 76
in heart failure, 87, *87*
diuretics and, 298
in myocardial infarction, 96, 97
ReoPro. See *Abciximab (ReoPro).*
Reperfusion, measures of, 193–194, *194*
spontaneous, 124
Reperfusion injury, components of, 124–125
estrogen and, 407
magnesium and, 120, 123, 124–126, 125t, 127, 128
oxidative damage in, 415
Rescue angioplasty, 191–193
Research synthesis, 43–44, 47–48. See also *Meta-analysis.*
Reserpine, for hypertension, 343
Restenosis. See *Angioplasty, percutaneous transluminal coronary, restenosis after.*
Reteplase. See *r-PA (recombinant plasminogen activator, reteplase).*
Retinol, in primary prevention trial, 418
Revascularization. See *Angioplasty; Coronary artery bypass graft (CABG); Fibrinolytic (thrombolytic) therapy; Stenting.*
Rheumatic heart disease, stroke prevention in, 257
Risk differences, 45, 46, 47
Risk factors, cardiovascular, 433–434
synergy of, 443–444
Risk ratios, 47
Ro 44–9883. See *Lamifiban.*
r-PA (recombinant plasminogen activator, reteplase), stroke risk with, 69
vs. angioplasty, 189, 190
vs. streptokinase or t-PA, 71, 72
with abciximab, 180
with angioplasty, 186, 187, 193
with nitroglycerin, 133

S

Safety, of clinical trials. See *Data and Safety Monitoring Board (DSMB).*
Salvage angioplasty, 191–193
Sample size, moderate treatment effects and, 26–27
  random error and, 9
  statistical power and, *12,* 12–13, 14
  with group randomization, 18
Saturated fat, 423, 430
School interventions, 438, 452–454
Secondary prevention, definitions of, 17, 434
Second-hand smoke, 363
Selection bias, 49
Selenium, in primary prevention trial, 417
Sensitivity analyses, 48
Serotonin, in thrombus formation, 166, 167
Simvastatin, cost effectiveness of, 207, 291, 291t, 335t, 336–337
  secondary prevention trials of, 202t, 205, 207, 208
    cost effectiveness and, 207, 335t, 336–337
    in elderly, 333, 334t
    nonvascular deaths in, 331
  vs. dietary modification, 425
SK. See *Streptokinase (SK).*
Smoker's paradox, 370
Smoking, 361–371
  as political issue, 455–456
  cardiovascular disease risk and, 362–363, 364t–365t
    observational studies of, 5–6, 362
    other risk factors and, 434
  mortality rates and, 361
  passive, 363
  pathophysiologic effects of, 361–362
  prevalence of, 361
Smoking cessation, cardiovascular disease risk and, 363, 364t–365t, 365
  cost effectiveness of, 291, 291t
  exercise training and, 286
  in multifactorial trials, 363, 367, 368t, 429, 430, 434, 435, 436, 438
  methods for, 435
  primary prevention of CVD and, 363, 365–367, 366t, 368t, 369t
  school-based programs for, 453
  secondary prevention of CVD and, 367–371, 370t
Social support, in risk factor intervention, 444
Sodium restriction, 435
Sotalol, after MI, 220–222, *221–222,* 227
  atrial fibrillation and, after cardiac surgery, 239–240
    chronic, 238, 239, 241
    paroxysmal, 235t, 236, 237
  in heart failure, 310
  in stable angina, aspirin with, 246
  in supraventricular arrhythmias, for acute termination, 233
ST segment depression, exercise-induced, 280, 280t
  fibrinolytic therapy and, 66
ST segment elevation, 145
  exercise-induced, 280, 280t
  fibrinolytic therapy and, 65, 66, *67,* 67–68, 73, 145
Statins. See also *Fluvastatin; Lovastatin; Pravastatin; Simvastatin.*
  cost effectiveness of, 335t, 336
  trials of, 328t, 328–329, 334t
    in elderly patients, 333–334, 334t
    in women, 334, 335t
    nonvascular deaths in, 331, 332
Statins *(Continued)*
    stroke risk in, 330, 330t
    total mortality in, 333
Statistical power, definition of, 12
  duration of follow-up and, 13
  in meta-analysis, 44
  rule of thumb for, 13
  sample size and, *12,* 12–13, 14
Steal, coronary, nitrates causing, 132, 133
Stenting, intracoronary, 185, 191, 191t
    abciximab with, 171, 174, 177, 178t
    abrupt vessel closure and, 159–160, 187
    antithrombotic therapy after, 254
    conditional, 191
    restenosis and, 267, 276
Stochastic curtailment, 33
Streptokinase (SK), age and, *68*
  in heart failure, 68
  platelet aggregation and, 126–127
  statistical analysis of, 12, 13, 45–47, 46t, 48
  stroke risk with, 69, 189
  vs. angioplasty, 190
  vs. rTPA, 189
  vs. t-PA, 68–69, 70t, *71,* 71–72
  with angioplasty, 187
  with aspirin and heparin, *58,* 60t, 61
  with captopril, 98
  with direct antithrombins, 147, 148, 162
  with GPIIb/IIIa antagonists, 179
  with nitroglycerin and NAC, 141
Stress management, 317–318, 319, 320, 427, 440
Stress testing, early postinfarction, 280
Stroke. See also *TIA (transient ischemic attack).*
  anticoagulant therapy and, 251, 252, 254
  antihypertensive drug trials and, 343, 345t, 345–346, *346–347,* 357
    age and, 347, 349t
    by drug type, 347, *351,* 351–352, 352t, 353t
    gender and, 347
    level of BP and, 342, 346–347, 348t
    trial duration and, 347, 350t
    unpublished, 352, 352t, 354t–355t, 356–357
    with beta blockers, 77, 79, 80, 81, 82t
  antioxidant vitamins and, 416, 417, 417t, 418, 419
  aspirin and, for primary prevention, 393, 394, 394t, 395, 396
    for secondary prevention, 247–248, *248,* 249–250, 253, 392, 393
  aspirin causing, 250, 254
  atrial fibrillation and. See *Atrial fibrillation, stroke prevention in.*
  calcium channel blockers in, 114–115
  cholesterol reduction and, 329–330, 330t
  C-reactive protein and, 246
  fibrinolytic therapy and, 68, 69, 70t, *71,* 71–72, 73
    with rTPA vs. PTCA, 190
    with rTPA vs. streptokinase, 189
  hormone replacement therapy and, 408
  smoking and, 361, 362, 363
  unstable CAD and, 55
Stromalysin, in plaque disruption, 212
Stunning, myocardial reperfusion and, 125, 126
Subadditive effects, 15
Subarachnoid hemorrhage, calcium channel blockers in, 114, 115
  oral contraceptives and, 363
  smoking and, 363
Subgroup analysis, 26, 29, 44, 47–48
Sulfinpyrazone (Anturane), after MI, 247, 248, *249*
Superoxide ion, vasodilatory dysfunction and, 209
Supraventricular tachycardias. See also *Antiarrhythmic agents, in supraventricular tachycardias; Atrial fibrillation.*
  radiofrequency ablation for, 231–232, 234, 242
Surrogate dilution bias, 327

T

TABP (type A behavior pattern), 315, 316, 317t, 318–319
Tamoxifen, prevention trials with, 19
Teprotide, 95, 98
Tertiary prevention, definition of, 434
Thiazide, for hypertension, 353t
Thienopyridines, 254
Thrombin, generation of, abciximab and, 167
    during angioplasty, 153
    plaque disruption and, 166
  heparin and, 56, 159, 161
  inhibition of, 146, *146,* 161–162, *162*
    balloon injury and, 154–155
  platelet activation by, 153, 245
Thrombin hypothesis, 146
Thrombin inhibitors. See *Antithrombins, direct; Heparin.*
Thrombin paradox, 148
Thrombin rebound, 158–159
Thrombocytopenia, heparin causing, 145, 160, 163
  tirofiban causing, 168
β-Thromboglobulin, 245
Thrombolytic therapy. See *Fibrinolytic (thrombolytic) therapy.*
Thrombosis, coronary, MI and, 245
  deep venous, bivalirudin for, 160
    hormone replacement therapy and, 408
Thromboxane A_2, aspirin and, 56, 250, 392
  hormone replacement therapy and, 405
  in thrombus formation, 145, 166
  magnesium and, 127
Thromboxane B_2, aspirin and, *126*
  estrogen and, 405
  in acute MI, 245
Thrombus formation, 145, 166
  aspirin and, 392
  during angioplasty, 152–153, 156
  exercise-related, 288–289
  GPIIb/IIIa receptor and, 166, 167
  hyperlipidemia and, 209
  in atrial fibrillation, embolism and, 257
  magnesium and, 120, 127, *127*
  oxidative damage and, 415
  plaque disruption and, 166, 210, 211, *211,* 213
  platelets in, 126, 145, 166–167, 209
  smoking and, 362
Thyroxine, secondary prevention trial of, 207
TIA (transient ischemic attack), antiplatelet agents after, 247, 248, *248,* 249, 250, 392, 393
Tiapamil, in MI, 107
Ticlopidine, secondary prevention trials of, 250, 254
TIMI flow grades, 193–194, *194*
Timolol, after MI, 84, 84t, 85, 86
    smoking cessation and, 369
Tioclomarol, after MI, 252
Tirofiban (Aggrastat), 168
  in non–Q wave MI, 177–178
  in percutaneous coronary intervention, 168, 170, 176–177, 178t, 180

Tirofiban (Aggrastat) *(Continued)*
in unstable angina, 177–179, 180, 181
Tissue-type plasminogen activator. See *t-PA (tissue-type plasminogen activator, alteplase).*
α-Tocopherol. See *Vitamin E.*
Torsades de pointes, *d,l*-sotalol and, 220, 221, 222
magnesium and, 119–120
t-PA (tissue-type plasminogen activator, alteplase). See also *r-PA (recombinant plasminogen activator, reteplase).*
endogenous, 209, 246, 405
platelet aggregation and, 126–127
stroke risk with, 69, *71,* 71–72
vs. streptokinase, 68–69, 70t, *71,* 71–72
with aspirin and heparin, 60t, 61, 62, 245
with direct antithrombins, 147, *147,* 148
with GPIIb/IIIa antagonists, 179–180
with metoprolol, 83–84, 84t
Trandolapril, after acute MI, *99,* 99t, 100, 302
trans-fatty acids, 424–425
Transient ischemic attack (TIA), antiplatelet agents after, 247, 248, *248,* 249, 250, 392, 393
Transluminal extraction catheter atherectomy, 174
Transplantation. See *Cardiac transplantation.*
Trauma deaths, cholesterol reduction and, 332, 332t
Treadmill tests, early postinfarction, 279–280, 280t
Treatment protocols, deviations from, 11–12
Trichlormethiazide, for hypertension, 353t
Triglycerides, beta blockers and, 77
coronary disease risk and, 424
dietary changes and, 424, 426, 427
exercise and, in cardiac rehabilitation, 287t
in healthy people, 376, 377t, 378
hormone replacement therapy and, 400, 400t, 402
smoking and, 362
Type A behavior pattern (TABP), 315, 316, 317t, 318–319

U

Unbiasedness, 9, 9t
Uncertainty principle, 27–28
Unit randomization, 18, 22
Unsaturated fats, 423, 424t, 424–425, 426, 426t, 430
Unstable angina. See also *Angina pectoris; Unstable coronary artery disease.*
angiographic progression in, 315
angioplasty in, abciximab with, 170, 171–173, 174, 181
complications of, 156, *156,* 157, 159
hirudin with, 156–157, *157,* 162–163
Hirulog (bivalirudin) with, 159
tirofiban with, 176
vs. bypass graft, 268–269, 271
antiplatelet therapy in, 62, 247, 248, 249, 392
with anticoagulation, 253
bypass graft in, magnesium with, 123
vs. angioplasty, 268–269, 271
calcium channel blockers in, 108–110, 109t
diagnostic features of, 55
direct antithrombins in, 148–149, *149,* 156
Unstable angina *(Continued)*
with angioplasty, 156–157, *156–157,* 159, 162–163
endothelial dysfunction in, 209
GPIIb/IIIa antagonists in, 177–179, 180, 181
lifestyle changes and, 315
lipid-lowering therapy and, *212*
nitrates in, 131, 138–141, 139t, 142
pathogenesis of, 55, 109, 145, 210, 211, *211*
smoking and, 361
Unstable coronary artery disease. See also *Non–Q wave MI; Unstable angina.*
aspirin in, 55, 56–57
definition of, 55
diagnostic features of, 55
fibrinolytic therapy in, 66–67
heparin in, 55, 56–57
lysis of thrombi in, 200
pathogenesis of, 55
Urokinase-type plasminogen activator, 209

V

Valve replacement, antiplatelet therapy in, 249
with anticoagulation, 253, 254
calcium channel blockers in, 114, 115
Variant angina, 109. See also *Coronary artery spasm.*
Vasoconstriction, adrenergic activation and, 87, *87*
angiotensin II causing, 95, 96
beta blockers causing, 76
exercise causing, in CAD, 209
in atherosclerosis, 406
smoking causing, 362
thromboxanes causing, 245
Vasodilation, ACE inhibitors causing, 98, 298
calcium channel blockers causing, 106
carvedilol causing, 86, 91
dysfunction of, in atherosclerosis, 209
smoking and, 362
estrogen and, 406–407
nitric oxide and, 131–132, *132,* 209
Vegetarian diet, 204, 318, 322, 387, 387t, 428, 440
Ventricular arrhythmias, after bypass, magnesium and, 123
exercise-induced, 280, 288, 289, *289*
fatal, after MI, 217
beta blockers and, 86
torsades de pointes as, *d,l*-sotalol and, 220, 221, 222
magnesium and, 119–120
Ventricular dysfunction. See *Left ventricular dysfunction.*
Ventricular fibrillation, after MI, 217
beta blockers and, 82
carvedilol as, 86
exercise-related, 288, 289
fatty acids and, 427
reperfusion causing, 125
Ventricular remodeling, after MI, 96
ACE inhibitors and, 96, 97t, 97–98, 103
carvedilol and, 86–87
nitrates and, 133, 134
in heart failure, 87, *87*
beta blockers and, 88
Ventricular tachycardia, after MI, 217
magnesium and, 120
reperfusion causing, 125
Verapamil, 106, *106*
Verapamil *(Continued)*
adverse effects of, 115–116
after cardiac surgery, 239, *239*
atherosclerosis and, 110
for hypertension, 114, 114t, 353t
in atrial fibrillation, acute, 235, 235t
chronic, 238, *238,* 241
in heart failure, 309
in MI, 106–107, 108, 109t
in stable angina, 112
in supraventricular arrhythmias, atrial fibrillation as, acute, 235, 235t
chronic, 238, *238,* 241
for acute termination, 232–233
for long-term suppression, 233–234
Vesnarinone, in heart failure, 306
Vital exhaustion, 315, 316
Vitamin B_6, 423, 429
Vitamin B_{12}, 429
Vitamin C, 415, 416
Vitamin E, 415, 416, 420
Vitamins, antioxidant. See *Antioxidant vitamins.*
Vitronectin receptor, 167
abciximab and, 181
tirofiban and, 168
VLDL (very-low-density lipoprotein), dietary fats and, 424
hormone replacement and, 402

W

Warfarin, after MI, 252, 255
with aspirin, 253–254
after thrombolysis, 253
chronic, after hirudin, 162
factor VII and, 246
for primary prevention, with aspirin, 254, 255, 396
in atrial fibrillation, 257–265, 258t, 259t, 261t, *263–264*
Weight loss, clinical trials of, in healthy people, 376, 377t, 378–381
in people with CVD, 387t, 387–388
in people with risk factors, 382, 383t, 384–385
limitations of, 375–376
to prevent hypertension, 385–387
with anorexiant medications, 381t, 381–382
with multiple risk factors, 435
dietary composition and, 375
Wolff-Parkinson-White syndrome. See *Atrioventricular reentrant tachycardia.*
Women, aspirin in, for primary prevention, 396
atherosclerotic plaques in, 210
exercise training in, 290, 290t
lipid-lowering therapy in, 202, 207, 208, 334–336, 335t
psychosocial intervention in, 315, 319
Worksite interventions, 438, 454–455

X

Xamoterol, in heart failure, 304, 306

Y

Yoga, 318, 427

Z

Zofenopril, after MI, 97, 97t, 98, 102
in acute MI, 303

ISBN 0-7216-6867-4